Basic
Medical
Biochemistry

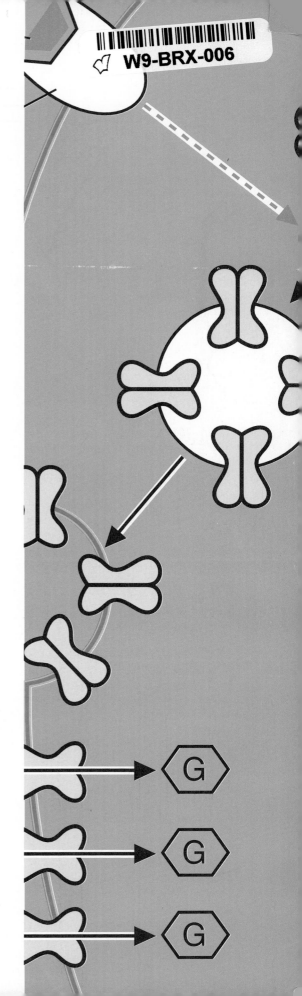

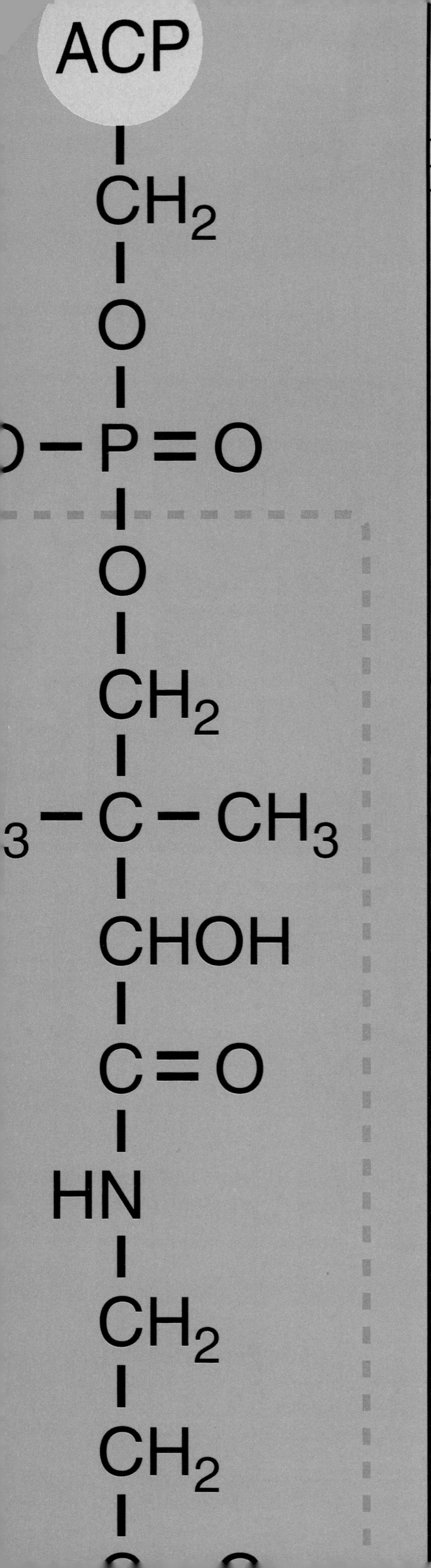

ACP

CH₂

O

O—P=O

O

CH₂

C—CH₃

CHOH

C=O

HN

CH₂

CH₂

Dawn B. Marks, Ph.D.

Professor of Biochemistry
Department of Biochemistry
Temple University School of Medicine
Philadelphia, Pennsylvania

Allan D. Marks, M.D.

Associate Professor of Internal Medicine
Department of Internal Medicine
Temple University School of Medicine
Philadelphia, Pennsylvania

Colleen M. Smith, Ph.D.

Associate Professor of Biochemistry
Department of Biochemistry
Temple University School of Medicine
Philadelphia, Pennsylvania

Basic
Medical
Biochemistry

A CLINICAL APPROACH

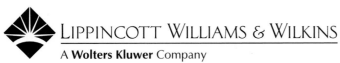

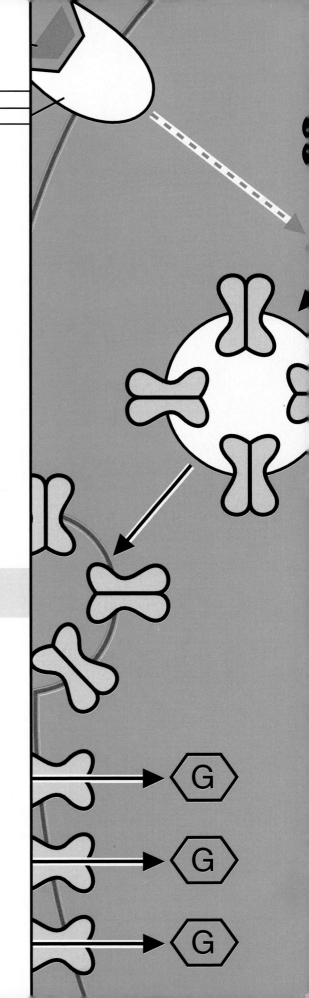

LIPPINCOTT WILLIAMS & WILKINS
A **Wolters Kluwer** Company

Philadelphia · Baltimore · New York · London
Buenos Aires · Hong Kong · Sydney · Tokyo

LW&W

Editor: Jane Velker
Development Editor: Kathleen Scogna
Production Coordinator: Anne Stewart Seitz
Copy Editor: Janet M. Krejci
Designer: Karen S. Klindedinst
Illustrations: Chansky, Inc.
Illustration Planner: Lorraine Wrzosek
Cover Designer: Dan Pfisterer
Composition: Donna M. Smith and Mario Fernández
Printer: R.R. Donnelley & Sons

Copyright © 1996
Lippincott Williams & Wilkins
351 West Camden Street
Baltimore, Maryland 21201-2436 USA

530 Walnut Street
Philadelphia, Pennsylvania 19106-3621 USA

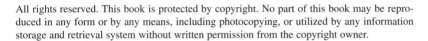

Accurate indications, adverse reactions and dosage schedules for drugs are provided in this book, but it is possible that they may change. The reader is urged to review the package information data of the manufacturers of the medications mentioned.

Printed in the United States of America

Library of Congress Cataloging-in-Publication Data

Marks, Dawn B.
  Basic medical biochemistry: a clinical approach/Dawn B. Marks, Allan D. Marks,
Colleen M. Smith
    p. cm.
  Includes indexes.
  ISBN 0-683-05595-X
  1. Biochemistry. 2. Clinical biochemistry. I. Marks, Allan D.
II. Smith, Colleen M. III. Title
  [DNLM: 1. Biochemistry. QU 4 M346b 1996]
QP514.2.M27 1996
574.19'2—dc20
DNLM/DLC
for Library of Congress   95-33624
                                                                          CIP

The publishers have made every effort to trace the copyright holders for borrowed material. If they have inadvertently overlooked any, they will be pleased to make the necessary arrangements at the first opportunity.

To purchase additional copies of this book, call our customer service department at **(800) 638-3030** or fax orders to **(301) 824-7390.** For other book services, including chapter reprints and large quantity sales, ask for the Special Sales Department. International customers should call **(301) 714-2324**.

Visit Lippincott Williams & Wilkins on the Internet: http://www.lww.com. Lippincott Williams & Wilkins customer service representatives are available from 8:30 am to 6:00 pm, EST.

02 03
7 8 9 10

Preface

This book is intended to cover human biochemistry in a reasonably comprehensive fashion, but without excessive detail. The aim of the book is to help students learn to use biochemistry in the process of clinical problem solving. The basic text follows a somewhat traditional format to provide students with a comprehensive, coherent base of information. Other components of the book are designed to encourage students to use this information within a clinical context.

A major unifying concept of the book is fuel metabolism. What happens when we eat, when we fast, or when we fast for long periods of time? How does the body get the energy and precursors it needs to keep functioning, to survive? The regulation of metabolic pathways by intracellular and hormonal mechanisms is emphasized because an understanding of metabolic regulation is essential if students are to grasp the implications of biochemistry for pathological conditions.

The clinical material is presented in the form of "real patients," who are composites of the patients seen by one of the authors (A.D. Marks) in his many years of practicing internal medicine. The patients in the book have names intended to serve as mnemonics that help students remember the case histories. As the chapters evolve, the patients appear and reappear as their problems are examined in the light of the biochemical concepts covered in the text. Many of the patients are seen repeatedly throughout the book with exacerbations or new facets of their original problem or with totally unrelated problems that require medical attention. The patients are not just dry initials, but people with personalities and quirks that must be considered in their treatment. Some patients comply with their treatment plan, and some do not. Some are cured, some get progressively worse in spite of appropriate treatment, and, as in real life, some die.

HOW TO USE THIS BOOK

Icons identify the various components of the book: the patients who are presented at the start of each chapter; the clinical notes, biochemical notes, questions, and answers that appear in the margins; and the clinical and biochemical comments that are found at the end of each chapter.

Each chapter starts with an abstract that summarizes the information so that students can recognize the key words and concepts they are expected to learn. The next component of each chapter is a "Waiting Room," containing patients with complaints and a description of the events that lead them to seek medical help.

 indicates a female patient

 indicates a male patient

 indicates a patient who is a baby or a young child

As each chapter unfolds, icons appear in the margin, identifying information related to the material presented in that portion of the text.

 indicates a clinical note, usually related to the patients who appear in the waiting room for that chapter. These notes explain the signs or symptoms of a patient or give some other clinical information relevant to the text.

 indicates a book note, which elaborates on some aspect of the basic biochemistry presented in the text. These notes provide tidbits, pearls, or just reemphasize a major point of the text.

"Questions" and "Answers" also appear in the margin and should help to keep students thinking as they read the text.

 indicates a question, numbered so that the appropriate answer can be identified.

 indicates the answer to the question of the same number. It is usually located at some distance from the question (further down the page or on a subsequent page) so it is difficult for the student to simply read the question and the answer without pausing to think in between.

Each chapter ends with "Clinical Comments" and "Biochemical Comments."

 indicates clinical comments that give additional clinical information, often describing the treatment plan and the outcome.

 indicates biochemical comments that add biochemical information not covered in the text or that explore some facet of biochemistry in more detail or from a more philosophical angle.

"Suggested Readings" are listed at the end of the chapter, for students who would like to pursue a particular topic in more depth. The references suggested are generally recent review articles at the level most suitable for beginning medical students. Due to space limitations, we were unable to appropriately credit the original investigators or to list more advanced review articles.

Finally, "Problems" are presented, usually of a clinical nature, that ask the student to apply the biochemistry covered in the chapter to problems more complex than those that appear as questions in the margin. Generally, "Answers" are given for each problem.

Acknowledgments

We would like to thank the many students, patients, and colleagues who inspired the design of the manuscript. We would also like to thank the staff at Williams & Wilkins (particularly Tim Satterfield, Nancy Evans, Anne Stewart Seitz, and Janet Krejci) and the reviewers who patiently aided us with the strenuous task of turning our ideas into the pages of a textbook. We are especially grateful to Matthew Chansky, the artist who, with amazing speed, turned our scribbles into crisp illustrations.

Dawn B. Marks
Allan D. Marks
Colleen M. Smith

Contents

Fuel Metabolism

In order to survive, we require fuel to provide the energy that drives the chemical reactions of our bodies. These reactions enable us to carry out such diverse functions as seeing, moving, thinking, and reproducing. Without fuel, life ends. The source of our fuel is obvious: our food provides us with energy. But what happens when we are not eating—between meals, and while we sleep? What is the source of our energy during these periods? And what happens when we fast for an extended period—when we cannot afford the local supermarket prices, or when we are sick? How long can the hunger-striker in the morning headlines expect to survive, or the 1,400-lb person who gets stuck in the bathroom doorframe and vows not to eat until he can fit into normal spaces? Are the skeletal fashion models who parade through our magazine and TV ads in metabolic danger?

We will deal with these questions by describing the fuels in our diet, the compounds produced by their digestion, and the basic patterns of fuel metabolism in the tissues of our bodies. We will describe how these patterns change when we eat, when we fast for a short time, and when we starve for prolonged periods. Patients with medical problems that involve an inability to deal normally with fuels will be introduced. These patients will appear repeatedly throughout the book, and they will be joined by others as we delve deeper into the subject of biochemistry.

1   Metabolic Fuels and Dietary Components

We obtain our fuel mainly from the carbohydrates, fats, and proteins in our diet. As we eat, our foodstuffs are digested and absorbed. The products of digestion circulate in the blood, enter various tissues, and are eventually taken up by cells and oxidized to produce energy. To completely convert our foodstuffs to carbon dioxide (CO_2) and water (H_2O), molecular oxygen (O_2) is required. We breathe in order to obtain this oxygen and to eliminate the CO_2 that is produced by the oxidation of our foodstuffs.

Any dietary fuel that exceeds the body's immediate energy needs is stored, mainly as triacylglycerol (fat) in adipose tissue, as glycogen (a carbohydrate) in muscle and liver, and, to some extent, as protein in muscle. When we are fasting, between meals and overnight while we sleep, fuel is drawn from these stores and is oxidized to provide energy.

We require enough energy each day to drive the basic functions of our bodies and to support our physical activity. If we do not consume enough food each day to supply that much energy, the body's fuel stores supply the remainder, and we lose weight. Conversely, if we consume more food than required for the energy we expend, our body's fuel stores enlarge, and we gain weight.

In addition to providing energy, the diet provides precursors from which the body's components are derived. Among these are the essential fatty acids and amino acids, which the body needs but cannot synthesize. The diet also supplies vitamins, minerals, and water. Water is the solvent of life.

Ronald Templeton is a 25-year-old medical student who was very athletic during high school and college. However, since he started medical school, he has been gaining weight, and he has decided to consult a physician at the student health service before the problem gets worse.

Thomas Appleman is a 56-year-old accountant who has been morbidly obese for a number of years. His major recreational activities are watching TV, while drinking Scotch and soda, and doing some occasional gardening. At a company picnic, he became very "winded" while playing baseball and decided it was time for a general physical examination. At the examination, he was found to weigh 264 lb at 5 feet 10 inches tall. His blood pressure was slightly elevated, 155 mm Hg systolic (normal = 140 mm Hg or less) and 95 mm Hg diastolic (normal = 90 mm Hg or less).

Priscilla Twigg is a 23-year-old buyer for a woman's clothing store. Despite the fact that she is 5 feet 7 inches tall and currently weighs 99 lb, she is convinced that she is overweight. Two months ago, she started a daily exercise program that consists of 1 hour of jogging every morning and 1 hour of walking every evening. She also decided to consult a physician about a weight reduction diet.

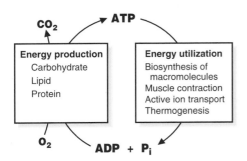

Fig. 1.1. The ATP-ADP cycle.

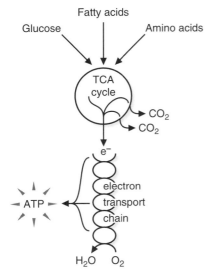

Fig. 1.2. Generation of ATP from fuels during respiration. Dietary carbohydrates are converted mainly to glucose, dietary lipids to fatty acids, and dietary protein to amino acids. The TCA cycle is described in Chapter 19, and the electron transport chain is discussed in Chapter 20. e^- = electrons.

"Calorie" meaning kilocalorie was originally spelled with a capital C (to indicate "large" calories), but the capitalization was dropped as the term became popular.

Nutritional "calories" = kilocalories.

Teresa Livermore is a 49-year-old homemaker who was in good health until her husband died suddenly a year ago. Since that time she has experienced an increasing degree of fatigue and has lost interest in many of the activities she previously enjoyed. Shortly after her husband's death, her only child married and moved far from home. Since then, Mrs. Livermore has had little appetite for food. When a neighbor found Mrs. Livermore sleeping in her clothes, unkempt, and somewhat confused, she called an ambulance. Mrs. Livermore was admitted to the hospital psychiatry unit with a diagnosis of mental depression associated with dehydration and malnutrition.

DIETARY FUELS

The major fuels we obtain from our diet are carbohydrates, proteins, and lipids. When these fuels are oxidized to CO_2 and H_2O in our cells, energy is released by the transfer of electrons to O_2. The energy from this oxidation process generates heat and adenosine triphosphate (ATP). Carbon dioxide travels in the blood to the lungs where it is expired, and water is excreted in urine, sweat, and other secretions. Although the heat that is generated by fuel oxidation is used to maintain body temperature, the main purpose of fuel oxidation is to generate ATP. ATP provides the energy that drives most of the energy-consuming processes in the cell, including biochemical reactions, muscle contraction, and active transport across membranes. As these processes utilize energy, ATP is converted back to ADP and inorganic phosphate (P_i). The generation and utilization of ATP is referred to as the ATP-ADP cycle (Fig. 1.1).

The oxidation of fuels to generate ATP is called respiration (Fig. 1.2). The pathways for oxidizing these dietary components have many features in common. Most of the oxidation of fuels occurs in a series of reactions termed the tricarboxylic acid (TCA) cycle (see Chapter 19). Electrons are transferred to O_2 by a series of proteins in the electron transport chain (see Chapter 20). The energy of electron transfer is used to convert ADP and P_i to ATP by a process known as oxidative phosphorylation.

In discussions of metabolism and nutrition, energy is often expressed in units of calories. "Calorie" in this context really means "kilocalorie" and we will abbreviate it "kcal." Energy is also expressed in joules. One kilocalorie equals 4.18 kilojoules (kJ). Physicians tend to use units of calories, in part because that is what their patients use and understand.

Carbohydrates

The major carbohydrates in the human diet are starch, sucrose, lactose, fructose, glucose, and indigestible fiber, such as cellulose. The polysaccharide starch is the storage form of carbohydrates in plants. Sucrose (table sugar) and lactose (milk sugar) are disaccharides, and fructose and glucose are monosaccharides. Digestion converts the larger carbohydrates to monosaccharides, which can be absorbed into the bloodstream. Glucose, a monosaccharide, is the predominant sugar in human blood (Fig. 1.3).

Oxidation of carbohydrates to CO_2 and H_2O in the body produces approximately 4 kcal/g (Table 1.1). In other words, every gram of carbohydrate we eat yields approximately 4 kcal of energy. Note that carbohydrate molecules contain a significant amount of oxygen (see Fig. 1.3).

Table 1.1. Caloric Content of Dietary Components

	kcal/g
Carbohydrate	4
Protein	4
Fat	9
Alcohol	7

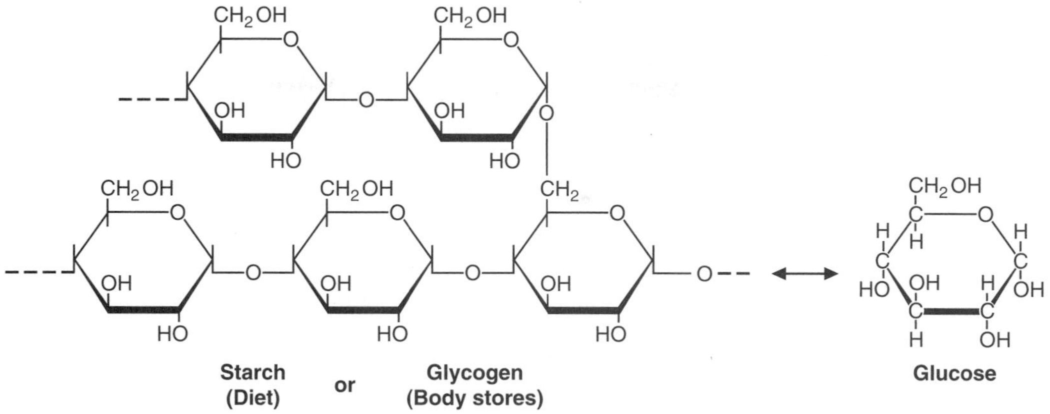

Fig. 1.3. General structure of the major carbohydrates. Glucose is a monosaccharide. Two monosaccharides may be linked together to form a disaccharide. Polysaccharides, such as starch or glycogen, are composed of many monosaccharides linked together.

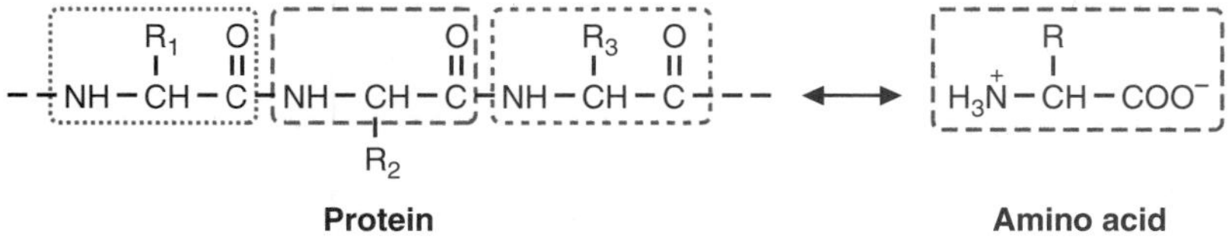

Fig. 1.4. General structure of proteins and amino acids. R = side chain. Different amino acids have different side chains. For instance, R_1 might be $-CH_3$; R_2, $-\bigcirc$; R_3, $-CH_2-COO^-$.

Proteins

Proteins are composed of amino acids that are joined to form linear chains (Fig. 1.4). In addition to carbon, hydrogen, and oxygen, proteins contain about 16% nitrogen by weight. The digestive process breaks down proteins to their constituent amino acids, which enter the bloodstream. The complete oxidation of proteins to CO_2 and H_2O in the body produces approximately 4 kcal/g.

Lipids

The lipids in our diet consist mainly of triacylglycerols (also called triglycerides). A triacylglycerol molecule contains 3 fatty acids esterified to one glycerol moiety (Fig. 1.5).

Fats contain much less oxygen than is contained in carbohydrates or proteins. Therefore, fats are more reduced and yield more energy when oxidized. The complete oxidation of triacylglycerols to CO_2 and H_2O in the body produces approximately 9 kcal/g, more than twice the energy produced by an equivalent amount of carbohydrate or protein.

Alcohol

Many people used to believe that alcohol (ethanol, in the context of the diet) has no caloric content (Fig. 1.6). In fact, alcohol is oxidized to CO_2 and H_2O in the body and yields about 7 kcal/g, that is, more than carbohydrate but less than fat.

BODY FUEL STORES

Although some of us may try, it is virtually impossible to eat constantly. Therefore, it is fortunate that we carry supplies of fuel within our bodies (Fig. 1.7). These fuel

Q 1.1: An analysis of **Priscilla Twigg's** diet indicated that she ate 100 g of carbohydrate, 20 g of protein, and 15 g of fat each day. How many calories did she consume per day?

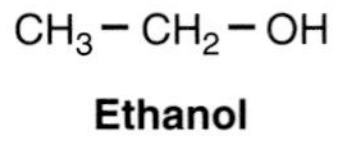

$$CH_3 - CH_2 - OH$$

Ethanol

Fig. 1.6. Structure of ethanol.

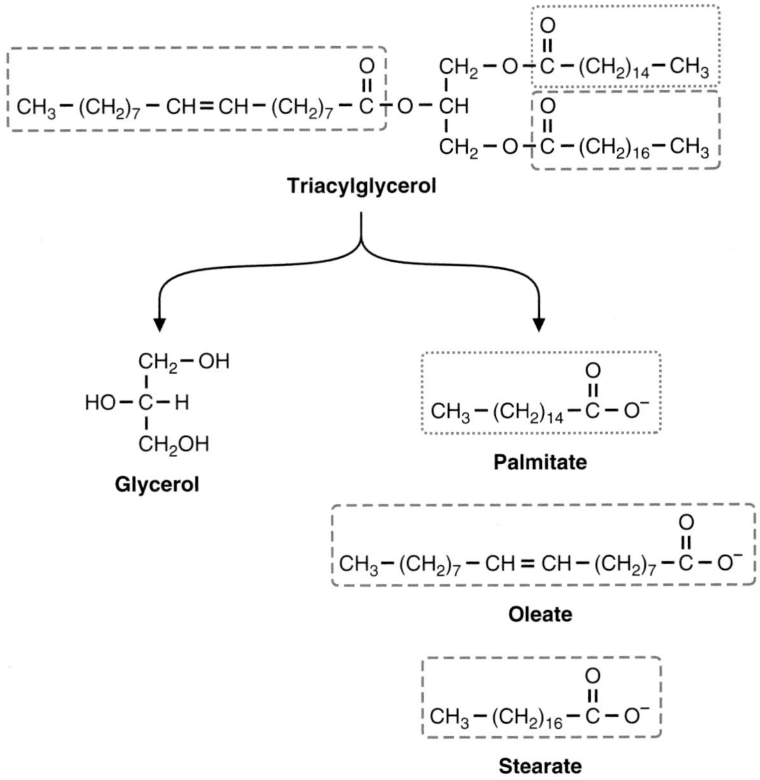

Triacylglycerol

Glycerol

Palmitate

Oleate

Stearate

Fig. 1.5. Structure of a triacylglycerol. Palmitate and stearate are saturated fatty acids, i.e., they have no double bonds. Oleate is monounsaturated (one double bond). Polyunsaturated fatty acids have more than one double bond.

Q 1.2: An analysis of **Thomas Appleman's** diet indicated that he ate 585 g of carbohydrate, 150 g of protein, and 95 g of fat each day. In addition, he drank 45 g of alcohol. How many calories did he consume per day?

stores are light in weight, large in quantity, and readily converted into oxidizable substances.

Most of us are familiar with fat, our major fuel store, which is located in adipose tissue. Although fat is distributed throughout our bodies, it tends to increase in quantity in our hips and thighs and in our abdomens as we advance into middle age. In addition to these familiar fat stores, we also have important although much smaller stores of carbohydrate in the form of glycogen located mainly in our liver and muscles. Glycogen consists of glucose residues joined together to form a large, branched polysaccharide. Body protein, particularly the protein of our large muscle masses, also serves to some extent as a fuel store and we draw on it for energy when we fast.

It is not surprising that our body fuel stores consist of the same kinds of compounds that dominate our diet, because the plants and animals we eat also store fuels in the form of starch or glycogen, triacylglycerols, and proteins.

Triacylglycerols

Our major fuel store is adipose triacylglycerol (triglyceride). The average 70-kg man has about 15 kg of stored triacylglycerol, which accounts for about 85% of his total stored calories (see Fig. 1.7).

Two characteristics make adipose triacylglycerol a very efficient fuel store: the fact that triacylglycerol contains more calories per gram than carbohydrate or protein (9 kcal/g versus 4 kcal/g) and the fact that adipose tissue does not contain much water. Muscle tissue contains about 80% water; adipose tissue contains about 15%. That means that the 70-kg man, who has 15 kg of stored triacylglycerol, has only about 18 kg of adipose tissue. What would happen if this man stored the same amount of energy as protein in muscle? The stored fuel itself would amount to about 34 kg of protein. In addition, there would be 4 times that weight in tissue water. Thus, the man would end up carrying a total of about 170 kg of extra muscle tissue, and he would weigh more than 3 times what he now weighs.

Glycogen

Our stores of glycogen in liver and muscle are relatively small in quantity but are nevertheless important. Liver glycogen is used to maintain blood glucose levels between meals. Thus, the size of this glycogen store fluctuates during the day: an average 70-kg man might have 200 g or more of liver glycogen after a meal but only 80 g after an overnight fast. Muscle glycogen supplies energy for muscle contraction during exercise. At rest, the 70-kg man has about 150 g of muscle glycogen.

Protein

Protein serves many important roles in the body, and it is, therefore, not solely a fuel store like fat and glycogen. Muscle protein is essential for body movement. Other proteins serve as enzymes (catalysts of biochemical reactions) or as structural components of the body. Only a limited amount of body protein can be degraded, about 6 kg in the average 70-kg man, before our body functions are compromised.

DAILY ENERGY EXPENDITURE

If we want to stay in energy balance, neither gaining nor losing weight, we must, on average, consume an amount of food that meets our daily energy expenditure. The daily energy expenditure includes the energy to support our basal metabolism and our physical activities plus the energy required to process the food we eat (diet-induced thermogenesis).

Basal Metabolic Rate (BMR)

The basal metabolic rate is a measure of the energy required to maintain life: the functioning of the lungs and kidneys, the pumping of the heart, the maintenance of ionic gradients across membranes, the reactions of biochemical pathways, and so forth. The BMR is usually determined from a measurement of the rate at which oxygen is consumed or heat is produced by a resting person who has recently awakened

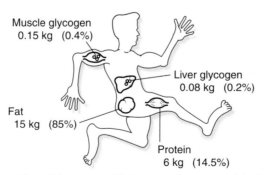

Fig. 1.7. Fuel composition of the average 70-kg man after an overnight fast (in kilograms and as percentage of total calories).

In biochemistry and nutrition, the standard reference is often the 70-kg (154 lb) man. This standard probably was chosen because in the early part of the 20th century, when many nutritional studies were performed, young healthy medical and graduate students (who were mostly men) volunteered to serve as subjects for these experiments.

Adipose tissue contains:
• fat stores (9 kcal/g)
• only 15% water

Protein:
• has essential roles other than providing fuel
• can be oxidized for energy in only limited amounts
• is 20% of muscle tissue (80% is water)

Daily energy expenditure = Energy expended at rest + physical activity + diet-induced thermogenesis

1.1:
Miss Twigg consumed

100 × 4 = 400 kcal as carbohydrate
 20 × 4 = 80 kcal as protein
 15 × 9 = 135 kcal as fat
for a total of 615 kcal/day.

1.2:
Mr. Appleman consumed

585 × 4 = 2,340 kcal as carbohydrate
150 × 4 =   600 kcal as protein
 95 × 9 =   855 kcal as fat
 45 × 7 =   315 kcal as alcohol
for a total of 4,110 kcal/day.

Q 1.3: What is **Mr. Appleman's** BMR? (Use the method for a rough estimate.)

in the morning after fasting for at least 12 hours. In practice, therefore, the BMR is really the resting metabolic rate (RMR).

BMR is usually expressed in kilocalories required per day. Obviously, the amount of energy required for basal functions in a large person will be greater than the amount required in a small person, a fact that restaurants and even hospitals often do not recognize when offering portions of food to their patrons.

Although an individual's BMR depends mainly on body weight, many other factors affect it (Table 1.2). The BMR is lower for women than for men of the same weight because women usually have more adipose tissue. Adipose tissue is much less metabolically active than is lean tissue. Body temperature also affects the BMR. Women who have passed on the saying "feed a fever; starve a cold" may have made some valid scientific observations, because the BMR increases by 12% with each degree centigrade increase in body temperature. The ambient temperature affects the BMR, which increases slightly in colder climates. Excessive secretion of thyroid hormone (hyperthyroidism) causes the BMR to increase, while diminished secretion (hypothyroidism) causes it to decrease. The BMR increases during pregnancy and lactation. Growing children have a higher BMR per kilogram body weight than adults, because a greater portion of their bodies is composed of brain, muscle, and other more metabolically active tissues. Whether the BMR decreases to a constant level by age 20 or continues to decline with age is somewhat controversial. Certainly, the BMR decreases in aging individuals whose metabolically active tissue is shrinking and body fat is increasing.

There are large variations in BMR from one adult to another. Nevertheless, it is clear that BMR depends on body weight. A rough estimate of the BMR may be obtained by assuming it is 24 kcal/day/kg body weight and multiplying by the body weight. An easy way to remember this is 1 kcal/kg/hour. Other methods are also used by clinicians for calculating the BMR (Table 1.3). Such calculations are, of course, only estimates because of the wide variation among individuals.

Q 1.4: What is **Miss Twigg's** BMR? (Use the method for a rough estimate.)

Physical Activity

In addition to the BMR, the energy required for physical activity contributes to the daily energy expenditure. The difference in physical activity between a student and a

Table 1.2. Factors That Affect BMR/kg Body Weight

Gender (males higher than females)
Body temperature (increased with fever)
Environmental temperature (increased in cold climates)
Thyroid status (increased in hyperthyroidism)
Pregnancy and lactation (increased)
Age (increased in childhood)

Table 1.3. Methods for Calculating BMR[a]

Rough Estimate: BMR = 24 × weight in kg
Owen Equations[b]:
$$BMR_{WOMEN} = 795 + (7.18 \times \text{weight in kg})$$
$$BMR_{MEN} = 879 + (10.2 \times \text{weight in kg})$$
Harris and Benedict Equations:
$$BMR_{WOMEN} = 655 + (9.6 \times W) + (1.8 \times H) - (4.7 \times A)$$
$$BMR_{MEN} = 66 + (13.7 \times W) + (5 \times H) - (6.8 \times A)$$
   where W is weight in kg, H is height in cm, and A is age in years.

[a]Units of BMR are kcal/kg/day.

[b]Owen uses the term RMR rather than BMR because the RMR (resting metabolic rate) is what is actually measured.

lumberjack is enormous, and a student who is relatively sedentary during the week may be much more active during the weekend. Table 1.4 gives factors for calculating the approximate energy expenditures associated with typical activities.

A rough estimate of the energy required per day for physical activity can be made by using the following approximate values:

- 30% of the BMR for a very sedentary person (such as a medical student who does little but study)
- 60–70% of the BMR for a person who engages in about 2 hours of moderate exercise a day (see Table 1.4)
- 100% or more of the BMR for a person who does several hours of heavy exercise a day.

Diet-Induced Thermogenesis

In addition to the BMR, our daily energy expenditure includes a component related to the intake of food known as diet-induced thermogenesis (DIT). DIT was formerly called the specific dynamic action (SDA) or the thermic effect of food. Following the ingestion of food, our metabolic rate increases because energy is required to digest, absorb, distribute, and store nutrients.

The energy required to process the types and quantities of food in the typical American diet is probably equal to about 10% of the kilocalories ingested. This amount is about equivalent to the caloric content of carbohydrate, fat, and protein lost by rounding off these values to 4, 9, and 4, respectively. Therefore, DIT is often ignored and calculations are based simply on the BMR and the energy required for physical activity.

Calculations of Daily Energy Expenditure

The total daily energy expenditure is usually calculated as the sum of the BMR (in kilocalories/day) plus the energy required for the amount of time spent in each of the various types of physical activity (see Table 1.4).

An approximate value for the daily energy expenditure can be determined from the BMR and the appropriate percentage of the BMR required for physical activity (given above). For example, a very sedentary medical student would have a daily energy expenditure equal to the BMR plus 30% of the BMR (or 1.3 × BMR). A mod-

 Based on the activities listed in Table 1.4, the average U.S. citizen is rather sedentary. Sedentary habits correlate strongly with risk for cardiovascular disease, so it is not surprising that cardiovascular disease is the major cause of death in this country.

Table 1.4. Typical Activities with Corresponding Activity Factors

Activity Category	Activity Factor/ Unit Time[a] (in hrs)
Resting: sleeping, reclining	1.0
Very light: seated and standing activities: driving, laboratory work, typing, sewing, ironing, cooking, playing cards, playing a musical instrument	1.5
Light: walking on a level surface at 2.5–3 mph, garage work, electrical trades, carpentry, restaurant trades, house cleaning, golf, sailing, table tennis	2.5
Moderate: walking 3.5–4 mph, weeding and hoeing, carrying loads, cycling, skiing, tennis, dancing	5.0
Heavy: walking uphill with a load, tree felling, heavy manual digging, mountain climbing, basketball, football, soccer	7.0

Reprinted with permission from Recommended Dietary Allowances, 10th edition. © 1989 by the National Academy of Sciences. Courtesy of the National Academy Press, Washington, DC.

[a]The activity factor is multiplied by the BMR/24 (or BMR expressed as kcal/hr) times the number of hours spent performing the activity. Summing these values for all the activities engaged in for 24 hours gives the total energy expenditure for the day. This sum includes the BMR.

A 1.3: Mr. **Appleman** weighs 264 lb or 120 kg (264 lb divided by 2.2 lb/kg). His BMR = 24 kcal/kg/day × 120 = 2,880 kcal/day.

A 1.4: **Miss Twigg** weighs 99 lb or 45 kg (99/2.2 lb/kg). Her BMR = (24 kcal/kg/day) × (45 kg) = 1,080 kcal/day.

1.5: What is a reasonable estimate for **Mr. Appleman's** daily energy expenditure?

 1.6: What is a reasonable estimate for **Miss Twigg's** daily energy expenditure?

 1.7: Are **Mr. Appleman** and **Miss Twigg** gaining or losing weight?

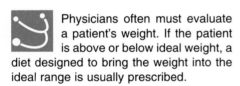 Physicians often must evaluate a patient's weight. If the patient is above or below ideal weight, a diet designed to bring the weight into the ideal range is usually prescribed.

erately active person's daily energy expenditure would be about 1.6 or 1.7 times the BMR, and an active person's daily expenditure could be 2 or more times the BMR.

Maintenance of Body Weight

To maintain our body weight, we must stay in caloric balance. We are in caloric balance if the kilocalories in the food we eat equal our daily energy expenditure. Ideally, we should strive to maintain a weight consistent with good health. From this perspective, what is a person's ideal or desirable weight? Life insurance companies have concluded that it is the weight at which a person is most likely to live for the longest time. They periodically publish tables of average weights for healthy people, based on sex, height, and body frame size (Table 1.5). Overweight people are frequently defined as more than 20% above their ideal weight. The body mass index (BMI), calculated as weight/height^2 (kg/m^2), is another measure often used to determine whether a person's weight is in the desirable range. Individuals with BMI values below 20 or above 25 are considered to be underweight or overweight, respectively.

Weight Gain and Loss

If we eat less food than we require for our daily energy expenditure, our body fuel stores supply the additional calories, and we lose weight. On the other hand, if we eat more food than we require for our energy needs, the excess fuel is stored (mainly in our adipose tissue), and we gain weight (Fig. 1.8).

When we draw upon our adipose tissue to meet our energy needs, we lose approximately 1 lb whenever we expend 3,500 calories more than we consume (see Problems at end of Chapter 3).

In other words, if we eat 1,000 calories less than we expend per day, we will lose about 2 lb/week. Since the average food intake is only about 2,000–3,000 calories/day, eating one third to one half the normal amount will cause a person to lose weight rather slowly. Fad diets that promise a loss of weight much more rapid than this have no scientific merit. In fact, the rapid initial weight loss the fad dieter

Table 1.5. 1983 Metropolitan Height and Weight Tables

Men[a]				Women[b]			
Height feet inches	Small Frame	Medium Frame	Large Frame	Height feet inches	Small Frame	Medium Frame	Large Frame
5 2	128–134	131–141	138–150	4 10	102–111	109–121	118–131
5 3	130–136	133–143	140–153	4 11	103–113	111–123	120–134
5 4	132–138	135–145	142–156	5 0	104–115	113–126	122–137
5 5	134–140	137–148	144–160	5 1	106–118	115–129	125–140
5 6	136–142	139–151	146–164	5 2	108–121	118–132	128–143
5 7	138–145	142–154	149–168	5 3	111–124	131–135	131–147
5 8	140–148	145–157	152–172	5 4	114–127	124–138	134–151
5 9	142–151	148–160	155–176	5 5	117–130	127–141	137–155
5 10	144–154	151–163	158–180	5 6	120–133	130–144	140–159
5 11	146–157	154–166	161–184	5 7	123–136	133–147	143–163
6 0	149–160	157–170	164–188	5 8	126–139	136–150	146–167
6 1	152–164	160–174	168–192	5 9	129–142	139–153	149–170
6 2	155–168	164–178	172–197	5 10	132–145	142–156	152–173
6 3	158–172	167–182	176–202	5 11	135–148	145–159	155–176
6 4	162–176	171–187	181–207	6 0	138–151	148–162	158–179

Courtesy of Metropolitan Life Insurance Company, *Statistical Bulletin.*

[a]Weights at ages 25–59 based on lowest mortality. Weight in pounds according to frame in indoor clothing weighing 5 lb, shoes with 1-inch heels.

[b]Weights at ages 25–59 based on lowest mortality. Weight in pounds according to frame in indoor clothing weighing 3 lb, shoes with 1-inch heels.

typically experiences is due largely to loss of body water. This loss of water occurs in part because muscle tissue protein and liver glycogen are degraded rapidly to supply energy during the early phase of the diet. When muscle tissue (which is about 80% water) and glycogen (about 70% water) is broken down, this water is excreted from the body.

DIETARY REQUIREMENTS

In addition to supplying us with fuel and with general-purpose building blocks for biosynthesis, our diet also provides us with specific nutrients that we need to remain healthy. Among these are the essential fatty acids and the essential amino acids, the small number of fatty acids and amino acids that the body cannot synthesize from other molecules and which it must therefore obtain from the diet. We also need a regular supply of vitamins and minerals.

The Recommended Dietary Allowances (RDA) (Table 1.6) are the amounts of various nutrients that should be ingested each day. They vary with age and gender and are higher during pregnancy and lactation. These values are reviewed regularly by the National Research Council and updated at least every 10 years. They represent the quantities of nutrients required to keep the general population in good health and are considerably higher than the minimum amounts required to prevent deficiency symptoms.

Carbohydrates

No specific carbohydrates have been identified as dietary requirements. Carbohydrates can be synthesized from amino acids. However, the less carbohydrate we eat, the more fat and protein we must oxidize to obtain the energy we require.

Essential Fatty Acids

Fatty acids of the linoleic and α-linolenic series are required or "essential" in our diet because we cannot synthesize fatty acids with these particular arrangements of double bonds. The essential fatty acids are the precursors of the eicosanoids (a set of hormone-like molecules that are secreted by cells in small quantities and have numerous important effects on neighboring cells) and are also precursors of compounds that decrease the permeability of the skin to water. The essential fatty acids are converted in the body to larger polyunsaturated fatty acids, such as arachidonic acid, which enter the biosynthetic pathway for the production of the eicosanoids and other related compounds.

Protein

The RDA for protein is about 0.8 g of high quality protein per kilogram of ideal body weight, or about 60 g/day for men and 50 g/day for women. "High quality" protein contains all the essential amino acids in adequate amounts. Proteins of animal origin (milk, egg, and meat proteins) are high quality. The proteins in plant foods are generally of lower quality, which means they are low in one or more of the essential amino acids. Vegetarians may obtain adequate amounts of the essential amino acids by eating mixtures of vegetables that complement each other in terms of their amino acid composition.

ESSENTIAL AMINO ACIDS

Amino acids are used in the body as precursors for the synthesis of proteins and other nitrogen-containing compounds. The nine amino acids that are essential for an adult

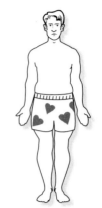

Consumption > Expenditure

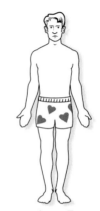

Consumption = Expenditure

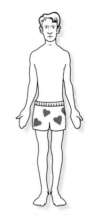

Consumption < Expenditure

Fig. 1.8. Food consumption, energy expenditure, and body weight.

A 1.5: **Mr. Appleman's** BMR is 2,880 kcal/day. He is sedentary, so he only requires approximately 30% more calories for his physical activity. Therefore, his daily expenditure is approximately 2,880 + (0.3 × 2,880) or 1.3 × 2,880 or 3,744 kcal/day.

Table 1.6. Food and Nutrition Board, National Academy of Sciences—National Research Council Recommended Dietary Allowances,[a] Revised 1989
Designed for the maintenance of good nutrition of practically all healthy people in the United States

Category	Age (yrs) or Condition	Weight[b] (kg)	(lb)	Height[b] (cm)	(in)	Protein (g)	Fat-Soluble Vitamins Vita-min A (µg RE)[c]	Vita-min D (µg)[d]	Vita-min E (mg α-TE)[e]	Vita-min K (µg)	Water-Soluble Vitamins Vita-min C (mg)	Thia-min (mg)	Ribo-flavin (mg)	Niacin (mg NE)[f]	Vita-min B6 (mg)	Fo-late (µg)	Vitamin B12 (µg)	Minerals Cal-cium (mg)	Phos-phorus (mg)	Mag-nesium (mg)	Iron (mg)	Zinc (mg)	Iodine (µg)	Sele-nium (µg)
Infants	0.0–0.5	6	13	60	24	13	375	7.5	3	5	30	0.3	0.4	5	0.3	25	0.3	400	300	40	6	5	40	10
	0.5–1.0	9	20	71	28	14	375	10	4	10	35	0.4	0.5	6	0.6	35	0.5	600	500	60	10	5	50	15
Children	1–3	13	29	90	35	16	400	10	6	15	40	0.7	0.8	9	1.0	50	0.7	800	800	80	10	10	70	20
	4–6	20	44	112	44	24	500	10	7	20	45	0.9	1.1	12	1.1	75	1.0	800	800	120	10	10	90	20
	7–10	28	62	132	52	28	700	10	7	30	45	1.0	1.2	13	1.4	100	1.4	800	800	170	10	10	120	30
Males	11–14	45	99	157	62	45	1,000	10	10	45	50	1.3	1.5	17	1.7	150	2.0	1,200	1,200	270	12	15	150	40
	15–18	66	145	176	69	59	1,000	10	10	65	60	1.5	1.8	20	2.0	200	2.0	1,200	1,200	400	12	15	150	50
	19–24	72	160	177	70	58	1,000	10	10	70	60	1.5	1.7	19	2.0	200	2.0	1,200	1,200	350	10	15	150	70
	25–50	79	174	176	70	63	1,000	5	10	80	60	1.5	1.7	19	2.0	200	2.0	800	800	350	10	15	150	70
	51+	77	170	173	68	63	1,000	5	10	80	60	1.2	1.4	15	2.0	200	2.0	800	800	350	10	15	150	70
Females	11–14	46	101	157	62	46	800	10	8	45	50	1.1	1.3	15	1.4	150	2.0	1,200	1,200	280	15	12	150	45
	15–18	55	120	163	64	44	800	10	8	55	60	1.1	1.3	15	1.5	180	2.0	1,200	1,200	300	15	12	150	50
	19–24	58	128	164	65	46	800	10	8	60	60	1.1	1.3	15	1.6	180	2.0	1,200	1,200	280	15	12	150	55
	25–50	63	138	163	64	50	800	5	8	65	60	1.1	1.3	15	1.6	180	2.0	800	800	280	15	12	150	55
	51+	65	143	160	63	50	800	5	8	65	60	1.0	1.2	13	1.6	180	2.0	800	800	280	10	12	150	55
Pregnant						60	800	10	10	65	70	1.5	1.6	17	2.2	400	2.2	1,200	1,200	300	30	15	175	65
Lactating	1st 6 mos.					65	1,300	10	12	65	95	1.6	1.8	20	2.1	280	2.6	1,200	1,200	355	15	19	200	75
	2nd 6 mos.					62	1,200	10	11	65	90	1.6	1.7	20	2.1	260	2.6	1,200	1,200	340	15	16	200	75

Reprinted with permission from Recommended Dietary Allowances, 10th edition. © 1989 by the National Academy of Sciences. Courtesy of the National Academy Press, Washington, DC.

[a]The allowances, expressed as average daily intakes over time, are intended to provide for individual variations among most normal persons as they live in the United States under usual environmental stresses. Diets should be based on a variety of common foods in order to provide other nutrients for which human requirements have been less well defined. See text for detailed discussion of allowances and of nutrients not tabulated.

[b]Weights and heights of Reference Adults are actual medians for the U.S. population of the designated age, as reported by NHANES II. The median weights and heights of those under 19 years of age were taken from Hamill et al. (1979) see pages 16–17). The use of these figures does not imply that the height-to-weight ratios are ideal.

[c]Retinol equivalents. 1 retinol equivalent = 1 µg retinol or 6 µg β-carotene. See text for calculation of vitamin A activity of diets as retinol equivalents.

[d]As cholecalciferol. 10 µg cholecalciferol = 400 IU of vitamin D.

[e]α-Tocopherol equivalents. 1 mg d-α-tocopherol = 1 α-TE. See text for variation in allowances and calculation of vitamin E activity of the diet as α-tocopherol equivalents.

[f]One NE (niacin equivalent) is equal to 1 mg of niacin or 60 mg of dietary tryptophan.

human—that is, the ones that cannot be synthesized in the body and must therefore be obtained in the diet—are lysine, isoleucine, leucine, threonine, valine, tryptophan, phenylalanine, methionine, and histidine (Table 1.7).

The adult requirement for histidine is small. In fact, adults can survive for extended periods of time with no serious consequences if histidine is not consumed. This amino acid is present in only small quantities in proteins, and the adult has substantial supplies, which can be reutilized.

Children and pregnant women have additional amino acid requirements because they are manufacturing proteins to support growth. They need more dietary histidine and they require dietary arginine. The body can synthesize arginine, but not at the rate needed for growth.

NITROGEN BALANCE

The proteins in the body undergo constant turnover, that is, they are constantly being degraded to amino acids and resynthesized. When a protein is degraded, its amino acids are released into the pool of free amino acids in the body. The amino acids from dietary proteins also enter this pool. Free amino acids can have one of two fates: either they are synthesized into proteins and other essential nitrogen-containing compounds, or they are oxidized as fuel to yield energy. When amino acids are oxidized, their nitrogen atoms are excreted in the urine principally in the form of urea. The urine also contains smaller amounts of other nitrogenous excretory products (uric acid, creatinine, and NH_4^+) derived from the degradation of amino acids and compounds synthesized from amino acids (Table 1.8).

Nitrogen balance is the difference between the amount of nitrogen taken into the body each day (mainly in the form of dietary protein) and the amount of nitrogen-containing compounds lost in urine, sweat, feces, and cells that slough off (Table 1.9). Most of the amino acid nitrogen is excreted in urine. Healthy adults are in zero nitrogen balance, that is, the amount of nitrogen obtained from the diet is equal to the amount that is lost.

If more nitrogen is lost than is obtained from the diet, the person is said to be in negative nitrogen balance. Conversely, if more nitrogen is ingested than is excreted, the person is said to be in positive nitrogen balance.

A negative nitrogen balance develops in two circumstances: if a person is eating too little protein, or if a person is eating protein that has too little of one or more of the essential amino acids. The reason the lack of an essential amino acid causes a negative nitrogen balance is that the body needs a complete complement of the 20 common amino acids to synthesize its proteins. An essential amino acid that is in short supply will limit the total amount of protein made. If a negative nitrogen balance persists for too long, bodily function will be impaired because of the net loss of critical proteins. When a person is producing new tissue, positive nitrogen balance occurs (for example, during childhood, adolescence, and pregnancy).

Vitamins and Minerals

Vitamins and minerals are required in the human diet. The RDA are given in Table 1.6.

VITAMINS

The vitamins are a diverse group of complex organic molecules that are required in very small quantities in the diet. Although we cannot synthesize most vitamins, some vitamins or their functional derivatives are produced in the body but in quantities that

Table 1.7. Essential Amino Acids for an Adult[a]

Lysine
Isoleucine
Leucine

Threonine
Valine

Tryptophan

Phenylalanine[b]
Methionine[c]

Histidine[d]

Additional Amounts Required for Growth

Histidine
Arginine

[a]Medical students sometimes use silly mnemonics to remember such lists. Here is one: LIL TV To PM (HA). (Little TV tonight (PM). HA.)

[b]Larger amounts of phenylalanine are required if the diet is low in tyrosine. (Tyrosine is synthesized in the body from phenylalanine.)

[c]Larger amounts of methionine are required if the diet is low in cysteine. (The sulfur of methionine is used in the synthesis of cysteine.)

[d]Histidine is not required in large quantities for the adult.

Table 1.8. Major Nitrogenous Excretory Products

Urea
Creatinine
Uric acid
NH_4^+

A 1.6: **Miss Twigg's** BMR is 1,080 kcal/day. She performs 2 hours of moderate exercise per day (jogging and walking), so she requires approximately 65% more calories for her physical activity. Therefore, her daily expenditure is approximately 1,080 + (0.65 × 1,080) or 1.65 × 1,080 or 1,782 kcal/day.

A 1.7: **Mr. Appleman** expends 3,744 kcal/day and consumes 4,110. Therefore, he consumes 366 more kcal than he expends each day, so he is gaining weight.

Miss Twigg expends 1,782 kcal/day while she consumes only 615. Therefore, she expends 1,167 more kcal/day than she consumes, so she is losing weight.

Protein contains approximately 16% nitrogen.

Table 1.9. Nitrogen Balance

Positive nitrogen balance Growth	Dietary Nitrogen > Excretory Nitrogen
Nitrogen balance Normal adult	Dietary Nitrogen = Excretory Nitrogen
Negative nitrogen balance Dietary deficiency of total protein or of one or more essential amino acids	Dietary Nitrogen < Excretory Nitrogen

are not sufficient to meet our needs. Most vitamins are converted to cofactors, compounds that are required by enzymes for the catalysis of biochemical reactions.

The vitamins are often divided into two classes, the fat-soluble vitamins and the water-soluble vitamins. This classification has little relationship to their function. The sources of the vitamins and the signs and symptoms of deficiencies are listed in Table 1.10. Excessive intake of vitamins as well as dietary deficiencies may cause deleterious effects. Megadoses of some of the fat-soluble vitamins are particularly troublesome, causing problems ranging from desquamation of the skin to birth defects. We will consider the roles played by the individual vitamins in metabolism as we progress through the subsequent chapters of this text.

MINERALS

The minerals that are required in the diet may be divided into two groups, those that are required in relatively large quantities and those that are required in only trace amounts (Table 1.11; see also Table 1.6).

Calcium and phosphorus serve as structural components of bones and teeth. Calcium (Ca^{2+}) plays many other roles in the body; for example, it is involved in hormone action and blood clotting. Phosphorus is required for the formation of ATP and of phosphorylated intermediates in metabolism. Magnesium activates many enzymes and also forms a complex with ATP.

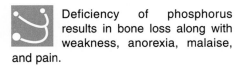
A dietary deficiency of calcium can lead to osteoporosis, a disease in which bones are insufficiently mineralized and consequently are fragile and easily fractured. Osteoporosis is a particularly common problem among elderly women.

Sulfur is ingested principally in the amino acids cysteine and methionine. It is found in connective tissue, particularly in cartilage and skin. It has important functions in metabolism, which we will describe when we consider the action of coenzyme A, a compound used to activate carboxylic acids. Sulfur is excreted in the urine as sulfate.

Sodium (Na^+), potassium (K^+), and chloride (Cl^-) are the major electrolytes (ions) in the body. They establish ion gradients across membranes, maintain water balance, and neutralize positive and negative charges on proteins and other molecules.

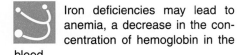
Deficiency of phosphorus results in bone loss along with weakness, anorexia, malaise, and pain.

Minerals required in very small quantities in the diet (see Table 1.11) are known as the trace minerals. Iron is a particularly important trace element because it functions as a component of hemoglobin (the oxygen-carrying protein in the blood) and is part of many enzymes.

Problems associated with dietary excesses or deficiencies of vitamins and minerals will be described in subsequent chapters in conjunction with their normal metabolic functions.

Water

Water constitutes one half to four fifths of the weight of the human body. The intake of water required per day depends on the balance between the amount produced by body metabolism and the amount lost in the urine and stool as well as through the skin and in expired air.

Iron deficiencies may lead to anemia, a decrease in the concentration of hemoglobin in the blood.

The Prudent Diet

Many studies have shown an association between diet and certain diseases. As a result, dietary recommendations were proposed initially to reduce the risk of heart attacks and strokes. Subsequently, studies indicated that similar dietary recommendations might lower the incidence of cancer. These recommendations were merged into guidelines sometimes called "the prudent diet."

CARBOHYDRATES

- Five or more servings of vegetables and fruits should be eaten each day, particularly green and yellow vegetables and citrus fruits.
- Six servings of starches and other complex carbohydrates should be eaten each day, in the form of breads, cereals, and legumes. In addition to energy, foods of this type supply vitamins, minerals, and fiber. Fiber, the indigestible part of plant food, has various beneficial effects, including relief of constipation.
- The consumption of refined sugar should be reduced below the American norm. Refined sugar has no nutritional value other than its caloric content, and it promotes tooth decay.

FATS

- Fat should account for no more than 30% of total dietary calories.
- Saturated fatty acids should account for 10% or less of total dietary calories.
- Polyunsaturated fatty acids should account for about 10% of total dietary calories (about one third of the total fat intake).
- Cholesterol intake should be less than 300 mg/day.

PROTEINS

- Protein intake for adults should be about 0.8 g/kg ideal body weight per day.

ALCOHOL

- No more (and probably less) than 1 oz (approximately 15 g) of ethanol should be consumed per day. This amount is contained in about two small glasses of wine. Pregnant women should drink no alcohol.

VITAMINS AND MINERALS

- No more than 3 g of table salt should be eaten per day, and individuals prone to salt-sensitive hypertension should eat less than 3 g/day.
- Low fat or nonfat dairy products and dark-green leafy vegetables should be consumed to ensure adequate calcium intake.
- Dietary supplementation in excess of the RDA (for example, megavitamin regimens) should be avoided.
- Fluoride should be present in the diet, at least during the years of tooth formation, as a protection against dental caries.

CLINICAL COMMENTS. **Ronald Templeton** sought help in reducing his weight to his previous level of 154 lb. Because he was a medical student, he felt he should approach his weight loss as scientifically as possible. His height was 68 inches, his body weight was 187 lb without clothes, and he had a moderate-sized

1.8: In the hospital, it was learned that **Mrs. Livermore** had lost 39 lb in the 8 months since her last visit to her family physician. On admission, her hemoglobin (the iron-containing compound in the blood which carries O_2 from the lungs to the tissues) was 10.7 g/dL (reference range = 12–15.5), her serum iron was 42 µg/dL (reference range = 60–120), and other hematological indices were also abnormal. Her serum folic acid level was 0.9 ng/mL (reference range = 2–11), her vitamin B_{12} level was 98 pg/mL (reference range = 200–1,200), and her serum albumin was 2.2 g/dL (reference range = 3.5–5.0).

What caused these abnormal values and what consequences would result from them? (Consult the Clinical Comments at the end of this chapter for the answers.)

Cholesterol is obtained from the diet and synthesized in most cells of the body. It is a component of cell membranes and the precursor of steroid hormones and of the bile salts used for fat absorption. High concentrations of cholesterol in the blood, particularly the cholesterol in lipoprotein particles called low density lipoproteins (LDL) contribute to the formation of atherosclerotic plaques. These plaques (fatty deposits on arterial walls) are associated with heart attacks and strokes. A high content of saturated fat in the diet tends to increase circulatory levels of LDL cholesterol and contributes to the development of atherosclerosis.

The high intake of sodium and chloride (in table salt) of the average American diet appears to be related to the development of hypertension (high blood pressure) in individuals who are genetically predisposed to this disorder.

Table 1.10. Sources of Vitamins and Manifestations of Deficiency

Fat–Soluble Vitamins	Sources	Manifestations of Deficiency
Vitamin A	Liver Fish liver oil Whole and fortified milk Eggs Carrots Dark-green leafy vegetables	Night blindness Xerophthalmia
Vitamin D	Exposure of skin to sunlight Fortified milk	Inadequate bone mineralization Rickets in children
Vitamin E	Vegetable oils Margarine Wheat germ Nuts Green leafy vegetables	Reproductive failure Muscular dystrophy Neurological abnormalities
Vitamin K	Bacterial flora of intestine Green leafy vegetables	Defective coagulation of blood
Water–Soluble Vitamins	**Sources**	**Manifestations of Deficiency**
Vitamin C	Citrus fruits Potatoes Green & red peppers Broccoli Tomatoes Spinach Strawberries	Scurvy
Thiamin	Unrefined cereal grains Brewer's yeast Liver Pork Legumes Seeds Nuts	Beriberi
Riboflavin	Meats Poultry Fish Dairy products	Oral-buccal cavity lesions
Niacin	Meat Lime-treated or fortified cereals[a] Tryptophan in protein[b]	Pellagra
Vitamin B_6 (pyridoxine)	Chicken Fish Liver Pork Eggs Unmilled rice Soy beans Oats Whole-wheat products Peanuts Walnuts	Convulsions Dermatitis Anemia
Folate	Liver Yeast Leafy vegetables Legumes	Impaired cell division and growth
Vitamin B_{12}	Animal products[c]	Megaloblastic anemia Neurological symptoms
Biotin	Liver Egg yolk Soy flour Cereals Yeast	Anorexia Nausea Vomiting Glossitis Alopecia Dry, scaly dermatitis
Pantothenic acid	Wide distribution in foods especially animal tissues, whole grain cereals, legumes	Listlessness Fatigue "Burning feet" syndrome

Summarized from Recommended Dietary Allowances. National Research Council. Washington, DC: National Academy Press, 1989.

[a]Most of the niacin in cereal grains has low bioavailability.

[b]The dietary requirement for niacin may be met in part by biosyntheses from the amino acid tryptophan.

[c]Produced by bacteria in animal products. Not present in plants.

Table 1.11. Major Minerals and Trace Elements Required in the Human Diet

Major Minerals	Sources	Manifestations of Deficiency
Calcium	Dairy products Broccoli Kale Collards Sardine & salmon bones (soft)	Inadequate bone mineralization in children Bone loss in adults
Phosphorus	Most foods	Hypophosphatemic rickets (children) Bone loss Weakness Anorexia Malaise Pain
Magnesium	Seeds Nuts Legumes Unmilled grains Chlorophyll of green vegetables	Nausea Muscle weakness Irritability Mental derangement
Sulfur	Protein (Cys, Met)	
Na^+	Many foods, particularly table salt	Lethargy, weakness, seizures, etc.
K^+	Nuts, whole grains, meats, fruits	Muscle cramps Weakness Polyuria Cardiac arrhythmias
Cl^-	Many foods, particularly table salt	

Trace Elements	Sources	Manifestations of Deficiency
Iron	Meat Eggs Vegetables Fortified cereals	Low iron stores Deficient red blood cell formation Iron deficiency anemia
Zinc	Meat Liver Eggs Seafood, especially oysters	Loss of appetite Growth retardation Hypogonadism Dwarfism
Iodine	Seafood Foods grown on coastal land Iodized table salt	Cretinism Goiter
Selenium	Seafood Liver	Muscle weakness Cardiomyopathy
Copper	Liver Seafood Nuts Seeds	Anemia Neutropenia Bone demineralization
Manganese	Whole grains & cereals Tea	Poor reproductive performance Growth retardation Congenital malformations Abnormal bone and cartilage formation Impaired glucose tolerance
Fluoride	Tea Marine fish bones Fluoridated water	Dental caries
Chromium	Brewer's yeast Calf's liver American cheese Wheat germ	Impaired glucose tolerance
Molybdenum	Milk Beans Breads Cereals	Amino acid intolerance Irritability Decreased urinary excretion of uric acid and sulfate

Summarized from Recommended Dietary Allowances. National Research Council. Washington, DC: National Academy Press, 1989.

skeletal frame. According to the Metropolitan height and weight table (see Table 1.5), the highest ideal weight for a male with these measurements is 157 lb.

A Lange calipers was used to measure his skinfold (fatfold) thickness in the triceps area. Obesity by this physical anthropometric technique is defined as a fatfold thickness greater than the 85th percentile for young adults; that is 18.6 mm for males and 25.1 mm for females. Ron's skinfold thickness was 18.2 mm, just under the threshold for obesity. With this information and assurances from the physician that he was otherwise in good health, Ron embarked on a weight loss program (see Problem 4, below).

Thomas Appleman weighed 264 lb and was 70 inches tall with a heavy skeletal frame. According to the Metropolitan height and weight tables, a male of these proportions should weigh no more than 180 lb. His weight exceeded this level by 84 lb (47% above maximal ideal weight).

Mr. Appleman's physician cautioned him that exogenous obesity (caused by overeating) represents a risk factor for atherosclerotic vascular disease, particularly when the distribution of fat is primarily "central" or in the abdominal region (android obesity—apple shape in contrast to pear shape). In addition, obesity may lead to other cardiovascular risk factors such as hypertension, hyperlipidemia (high blood lipid levels), and glucose intolerance. Although Mr. Appleman has not yet developed glucose intolerance, he already has a mild elevation in both systolic and diastolic blood pressure. Furthermore, his total serum cholesterol level was 296 mg/dL, well above the desired normal value, which is currently considered to be 200 mg/dL.

Mr. Appleman was referred to the hospital's weight reduction center where a team of physicians, dieticians, and psychologists will assist him in reaching his ideal weight range.

Because of her history and physical examination, **Priscilla Twigg** was diagnosed as having early anorexia nervosa, a behavioral disorder that involves both emotional and nutritional disturbances. Miss Twigg was referred to a psychiatrist with special interest in anorexia nervosa, and a program of psychotherapy and behavior modification was initiated.

Teresa Livermore weighed 94 lb and was 63 inches tall (without shoes) with a medium frame. Her range of ideal weight was 124–138 lb. Her triceps skinfold measured 16.5 mm (12th percentile).

Mrs. Livermore's malnourished state was reflected in her admission laboratory profile. The results of hematological studies were consistent with an iron deficiency anemia complicated by low levels of folic acid and vitamin B_{12}, two vitamins which can affect the development of normal red blood cells. Her low serum albumin level was caused by an insufficient protein intake and a shortage of essential amino acids, which result in a reduced ability to synthesize body proteins. Because of decreased intake, her serum cholesterol level was 127 mg/dL, a value in the lowest quintile for women of her age. The psychiatrist requested a consultation with a hospital dietician to evaluate the extent of Mrs. Livermore's marasmus (malnutrition caused by a deficiency of both protein and total calories) as well as her vitamin and mineral deficiencies.

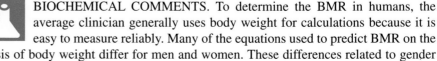 BIOCHEMICAL COMMENTS. To determine the BMR in humans, the average clinician generally uses body weight for calculations because it is easy to measure reliably. Many of the equations used to predict BMR on the basis of body weight differ for men and women. These differences related to gender can be eliminated if the BMR is calculated on the basis of the fat-free mass (FFM), which is equal to the total body mass minus the mass of the person's adipose tissue.

With FFM, the BMR is calculated using the equation BMR = 186 + FFM $\times$ 23.6 kcal/kg/day. This formula is applicable to both sexes and is similar to the one for obtaining a rough estimate of the BMR, i.e., 24 kcal/kg/day (see Table 1.3). However, determining FFM is relatively cumbersome—it requires weighing the patient under-water and measuring the residual lung volume.

Suggested Readings

For the recommended dietary allowances and the prudent diet see: Recommended Dietary Allowances. National Research Council. Washington, DC: National Academy Press, 1989.

For calculation of the BMR see: Owen OE, Tappy L, Mozzoli MA, Smalley KJ. Acute starvation. In: Cohen RD, Lewis B, Alberti KGMM, Denman AM (eds): The metabolic and molecular basis of acquired disease. London: Bailliere Tindall, 1990:550.

To determine the content of the food in the diet: Nutritive Value of American Foods in Common Units. Agriculture Handbook No. 456, Washington, DC: U.S. Department of Agriculture. (Can be obtained from the U.S. Government Printing Office, 100 N. 7th St., Philadelphia, PA.)

Laveille GA, Zabik MA, Morgan KJ. Nutrients in foods. Cambridge, MA: Academic Guild, 1983. This book provides nutrient values for pre-prepared and packaged foods as well as basic foods.

PROBLEMS

1. Calculate your own BMR. Determine your daily energy expenditure, considering the amount of time you spend in each type of activity (see Table 1.4). Compare this value to one obtained by multiplying your BMR by the appropriate factor.

2. Keep track of your food intake for at least 3 or 4 days. Compare your caloric intake with your daily energy expenditure. Are you in caloric balance, or are you gaining or losing weight? (See Suggested Readings for sources of data on the nutritive content of foods.)

3. Is your vitamin, mineral, and protein intake adequate?

4. **Ronald Templeton** was an ideal 70-kg man when he entered medical school. He weighed 154 lb. What was his BMR at that time? As a sedentary medical student, what was his approximate daily energy expenditure?

5. **Ron** realized that he was not as active during medical school as he was as a college athlete, but he continued to eat the same amount of food each day and, in addition, each night when he finished studying he drank a glass of beer and ate some pretzels. As a consequence, he gained 33 lb by the time of the last final exam of his second year. What was his BMR and daily energy expenditure at this time?

6. **Ron** wanted to lose the 33 lb that he had gained, so that he would be at his ideal weight by the autumn of his third year of medical school. He decided to undertake a weight reduction program during the 12 weeks of his summer clinical clerkships. He planned to reduce his caloric intake to the level for a person at his ideal weight (154 lb) with a light pattern of activity. How much weight would he lose in the 12 weeks of the summer only by restricting his diet? If he decided to play tennis for a few hours each evening after he finished working in the hospital, how many hours of tennis would he have to play each day to lose the additional weight?

ANSWERS

1, 2, and 3. The answers to these questions will vary for each individual student.

4. At 154 lb, Ron's BMR was 1,680 kcal/day (154 lb/2.2 lb/kg = 70 kg × 24 kcal/kg/day = 1,680 kcal/day). As a sedentary medical student, his daily energy expenditure was approximately 1.3 × 1,680 kcal/day or 2,184 kcal/day (BMR + 30% BMR).

5. Ron gained 33 lb, so he now weighed 154 + 33 or 187 lb, which is 187/2.2 or 85 kg. At this time, his BMR was 85 kg × 24 kcal/kg or 2,040 kcal/day. As a sedentary medical student, his daily energy expenditure was 1.3 × 2,040 or 2,652 kcal/day.

6. The BMR for a 70-kg man is 1,680 kcal/day. If he spent a number of hours each day walking in the hospital during his summer rotations, his activity level could be considered to be light (see Table 1.4), and his daily energy expenditure would be 1,680 × 1.6 (BMR + 60% BMR) or 2,688 kcal/day. Ron's actual BMR at 187 lb (85 kg) was 2,040 kcal/day, and during his summer hospital rotation, his daily expenditure was 2,040 × 1.6 or 3,264 kcal/day.

Ron had gained 33 lb, the equivalent of 115,500 kcal of adipose tissue. (One pound of adipose tissue is equivalent to about 3,500 kcal.) Therefore, in the 12-week period, he had to consume 115,500 kcal less than he expended. He decreased his caloric intake to that for a 70-kg man engaged in light activity (2,688 kcal/day), but at 187 lb he was actually expending 3,264 kcal/day, so he was in caloric deficit to the extent of 576 kcal/day. In the 12-week period (12 × 7 = 84 days), therefore, he ate 576 kcal/day × 84 days or 48,384 kcal less than he expended. His weight loss due to the decreased caloric intake was 48,384/3,500 or 13.8 lb. (A 3,500-kcal deficit results in the loss of approximately 1 lb of adipose tissue.)

Of the 33 lb he had gained, Ron still needed to lose 19.2 lb (the equivalent of 67,200 kcal of adipose tissue). For a 187-pound (85 kg) person, tennis requires about 425 kcal/hour (calculated from Table 1.4). For 1 hour, Ron's BMR is 2,040 kcal/24 hour = 85 kcal. Tennis increases the BMR 5-fold, so 1 hour of tennis is equivalent to 85 kcal × 5 or 425 kcal). Therefore, he would have to play tennis for 67,200/425 or 158 hours during the 12-week period or 158/12 = 13.2 hours/week. In other words, Ron had to play tennis for about 1.9 hours/day for 12 weeks. These calculations, of course, are estimates. As Ron lost weight, his BMR decreased and his total energy expenditure, therefore, also decreased, and he lost weight at a slower rate. However, if he continued to consume the appropriate number of calories for a 154-lb man, he would eventually equilibrate at that weight.

After 12 weeks of daily tennis and dieting, Ron began his September clerkship much closer to his ideal weight and in much better physical condition.

2 The Fed or Absorptive State

During a meal, we ingest carbohydrates, lipids, and proteins, which are subsequently digested and absorbed. Some of this material is used in ATP-generating pathways to meet the immediate energy needs of the body. Fuel that is consumed in excess of the body's energy needs is transported to the fuel depots, where it is stored. During the period from the start of absorption until absorption is completed, we are in the fed, or absorptive, state.

Dietary carbohydrates are digested to monosaccharides, which are absorbed into the bloodstream. The major monosaccharide in the blood is glucose. After a meal, glucose is oxidized by various tissues for energy and stored as glycogen, mainly in liver and muscle. The liver also converts glucose to triacylglycerols, which are packaged as very low density lipoproteins (VLDL) and released into the blood. The fatty acids of the VLDL are used to some extent to meet the energy needs of cells, but mainly they are stored as triacylglycerols in adipose tissue.

Dietary proteins are digested to amino acids, which are absorbed into the blood. The amino acids may either be oxidized for energy or used by tissues for biosynthesis. Most of the amino acids used for biosynthesis are converted to proteins; the remainder is used to make various important nitrogen-containing compounds such as neurotransmitters, hormones, heme, and the purine and pyrimidine bases of DNA and RNA.

Triacylglycerols are the major fats in the diet. They are digested to fatty acids and 2-monoacylglycerols, which are resynthesized into triacylglycerols in intestinal epithelial cells, packaged in chylomicrons, and secreted by way of the lymph into the blood. The fatty acids of the chylomicrons may be oxidized for energy in various tissues, but mainly they are stored as triacylglycerols in adipose cells.

 Fuel metabolism is often discussed as though the body consisted only of brain, skeletal and cardiac muscle, liver, adipose tissue, red blood cells, kidney, and intestinal epithelial cells ("the gut"). These are the dominant tissues in terms of overall fuel economy, and they are the tissues we will describe most often. Of course, all tissues use fuels.

 In the liver and most other tissues, the major way in which glucose, fats, and other fuels are oxidized to CO_2 to obtain energy requires their conversion to a 2-carbon activated acetyl group, acetyl CoA. CoA is a cofactor (coenzyme A) derived from the vitamin pantothenate, which makes the acetyl group more reactive.

The 2-carbon acetyl group ($CH_3-\overset{\overset{O}{\|}}{C}-$) is a central intermediate in most of the pathways of ATP generation from fuel oxidation.

Thomas Appleman returned to his doctor for a second visit. His initial efforts to lose weight had failed dismally. In fact, he now weighed 270 lb, an increase of 6 lb since his first visit 2 months ago. He reported that the recent death of his 45-year-old brother from a heart attack had made him realize that he must pay more attention to his health. Because Mr. Appleman's brother had a history of hypercholesterolemia and because Mr. Appleman's serum total cholesterol had been significantly elevated (296 mg/dL) at his first visit, his blood lipid profile was determined and a number of other blood tests were ordered. (The blood lipid profile is a test that measures the content of the various triacylglycerol- and cholesterol-containing particles in the blood.) His blood pressure was 162 mm Hg systolic and 98 mm Hg diastolic or 162/98 mm Hg (normal = 140/90 mm Hg or less).

 Enzymes are proteins that catalyze biochemical reactions, i.e., that increase the speed at which reactions occur. Their names usually end in "ase."

DIGESTION AND ABSORPTION

After a meal is consumed, the dietary components are digested by a series of enzymes in the mouth, stomach, and small intestine. The products of digestion eventually enter the bloodstream. Figure 2.1 illustrates the main features of metabolism during the fed state.

Carbohydrates

Digestive enzymes convert complex sugars to single sugar units for absorption. Sugars are saccharides, and the prefixes "mono" (one), "di" (two), "tri" (three), "oligo" (some), and "poly" (many) refer to the number of sugars linked together.

Starch, a polymer of glucose, is the major carbohydrate of the diet. It is digested by salivary α-amylase, and then by an α-amylase produced by the pancreas, which acts in the small intestine. The di-, tri-, and oligosaccharides that are produced by these α-amylases are cleaved to glucose by the action of digestive enzymes located on the surface of the brush border of the intestinal epithelial cells. The disaccharides of the diet are also cleaved to their component monosaccharides by enzymes on this brush border. Sucrase converts sucrose (table sugar) to glucose and fructose, and lactase converts lactose (milk sugar) to glucose and galactose. The monosaccharides produced by digestion, along with any free glucose and fructose that are consumed in the diet, are absorbed by the intestinal epithelial cells and released into the hepatic portal vein.

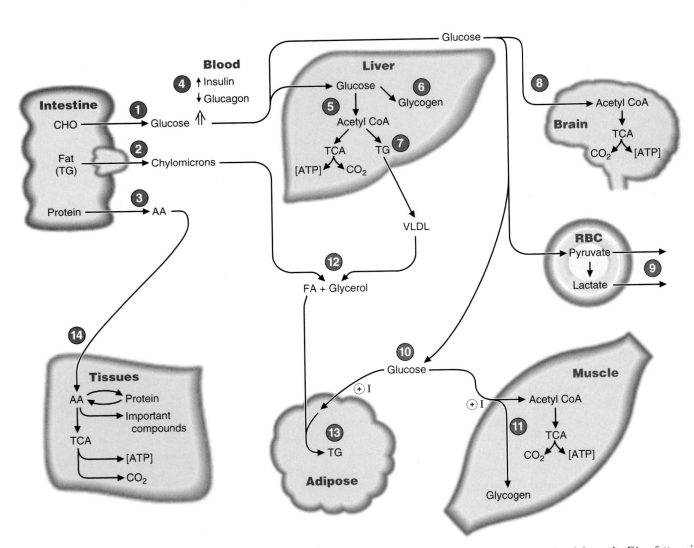

Fig. 2.1. The fed state. The circled numbers indicate the approximate order in which the processes occur. TG = triacylglycerols; FA = fatty acid; AA = amino acid; RBC = red blood cell; VLDL = very low density lipoprotein; I = insulin; ⊕ = stimulated by.

Proteins

Dietary proteins are cleaved by a series of enzymes working in concert to convert proteins to amino acids for absorption in the intestine. Pepsin acts in the stomach, and the proteolytic enzymes produced by the pancreas (trypsin, chymotrypsin, elastase, and the carboxypeptidases) act in the lumen of the small intestine. Aminopeptidases and di- and tripeptidases associated with the intestinal epithelial cells complete the conversion of dietary proteins to amino acids, which pass through these cells into the hepatic portal vein.

Proteins are amino acids linked through peptide bonds. Dipeptides have 2 amino acids, tripeptides have 3 amino acids, and so on. Digestive enzymes cleave the peptide bonds between the amino acids.

Fats

The digestion of fats is more complex than that of carbohydrates or proteins because they are not very soluble in water. The triacylglycerols of the diet are emulsified in the intestine by bile salts, which are synthesized in the liver and stored in the gall-bladder. Pancreatic lipase converts the triacylglycerols in the lumen of the intestine to fatty acids and 2-monoacylglycerols (glycerol with a fatty acid esterified at carbon 2). These products interact with bile salts to form tiny microdroplets called micelles, and they are absorbed from these micelles into the intestinal epithelial cells. In these cells, the fatty acids and 2-monoacylglycerols are resynthesized into triacylglycerols, which are packaged with proteins, phospholipids, cholesterol, and other compounds into the lipoprotein complexes known as chylomicrons, which are secreted into the lymph and ultimately enter the bloodstream.

Even in the blood, fats must be transported bound to protein or in lipoprotein complexes because they are not very water soluble.

CHANGES IN HORMONE LEVELS FOLLOWING A MEAL

After a typical high carbohydrate meal, the pancreas is stimulated to release insulin, and glucagon release is inhibited. The subsequent changes in circulating hormone levels cause changes in the body's metabolic patterns, involving a number of different tissues.

FATE OF GLUCOSE AFTER A MEAL

Conversion to Glycogen and Triacylglycerols in the Liver

Because glucose leaves the intestine via the hepatic portal vein, the first tissue it passes through is the liver. The liver extracts a portion of this glucose from the bloodstream. Some of the glucose that enters liver cells is oxidized in ATP-generating pathways to meet the immediate energy needs of these cells, and the remainder is converted to glycogen and triacylglycerols. In the liver, insulin promotes the uptake of glucose, its use as a fuel, and its storage as glycogen and triacylglycerols (Fig. 2.2).

Liver glycogen stores reach a maximum of about 200–300 g after a high carbohydrate meal, whereas the body's fat stores are relatively limitless. As the glycogen stores begin to fill, the liver also begins converting some of the glucose it receives to triacylglycerols. Both the glycerol and the fatty acid moieties of the triacylglycerols are synthesized from glucose. Triacylglycerol is not stored in the liver, however, but instead is packaged along with proteins, phospholipids, and cholesterol in the lipoprotein complexes known as very low density lipoproteins (VLDL), which are secreted into the bloodstream. Some of the fatty acids from the VLDL are taken up by tissues for their immediate energy needs, but most are stored in adipose tissue as triacylglycerol.

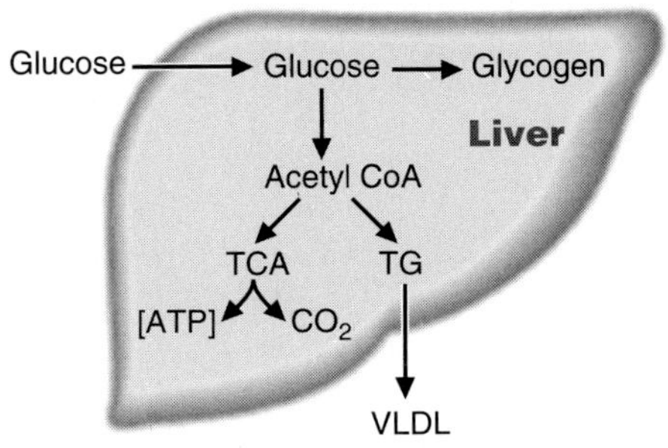

Endocrine hormones are compounds in the blood carrying messages to the different tissues concerning the overall physiological state of the body. They integrate the metabolic pathways of the tissues. Insulin, a hormone which is secreted from the pancreas in response to a high carbohydrate meal, carries the message that dietary glucose is available. The release of another hormone, glucagon, from the pancreas is suppressed by glucose. Glucagon carries the message that glucose must be generated from endogenous fuel stores.

Fig. 2.2. Fate of dietary glucose in the liver. TG = triacylglycerol.

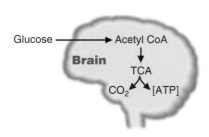

Fig. 2.3. Oxidation of glucose by the brain.

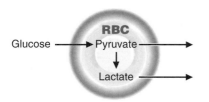

Fig. 2.4. Oxidation of glucose in red blood cells.

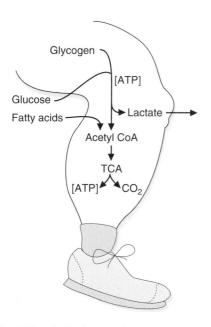

Fig. 2.5. Oxidation of fuels in exercising skeletal muscle. Exercising muscle uses more energy than resting muscle, and, therefore fuel utilization is increased to supply more ATP.

GLUCOSE METABOLISM IN OTHER TISSUES

The glucose from the intestine that is not metabolized by the liver travels in the blood to peripheral tissues, where it may be oxidized for energy. Glucose is the one fuel that can be utilized by all tissues. Many tissues store small amounts of glucose as glycogen. Muscle has relatively large glycogen stores.

Insulin greatly stimulates the transport of glucose into the two tissues that have the largest mass in the body, muscle and adipose tissue. It has much smaller effects on the transport of glucose into other tissues.

Brain and Other Nervous Tissue

The brain and other nervous tissues are very dependent on glucose for their energy needs. They oxidize glucose to CO_2 and H_2O, generating ATP (Fig. 2.3). Except under conditions of starvation, glucose is their only major fuel. If our blood glucose drops much below normal levels, we become dizzy and light-headed. If blood glucose continues to drop, we become comatose and ultimately die. Under normal, non-starving conditions, the brain and the rest of the nervous system require about 150 g of glucose each day.

Red Blood Cells

Red blood cells can use only glucose as fuel because they lack mitochondria. Other fuels, including fatty acids, are oxidized in mitochondria, the site of most of the body's fuel oxidation and ATP-generating reactions. Glucose, in contrast, undergoes glycolysis, its initial phase of catabolism, in the cytoplasm. Red blood cells obtain their energy by this process. Glycolysis involves the conversion of glucose to pyruvate. In red blood cells, pyruvate is either released directly into the blood or converted to lactate and then released (Fig. 2.4). In cells with mitochondria, the pyruvate produced by glycolysis can be converted to the 2-carbon acetyl unit of acetyl CoA and oxidized fully to CO_2 and H_2O.

Without glucose, red blood cells could not survive. Red blood cells carry O_2 from the lungs to the tissues. Without red blood cells, most of the tissues of the body would suffer from a lack of energy because they require O_2 in order to completely convert their fuels to CO_2 and H_2O.

Muscle

An exercising skeletal muscle can use glucose from the blood or from its own glycogen stores, converting it to lactate via glycolysis or to CO_2 and H_2O. Exercising muscle also uses other fuels from the blood, such as fatty acids (Fig. 2.5). After a meal, glucose is used by muscle to replenish the glycogen stores that were depleted during exercise. Glucose is transported into muscle cells and converted to glycogen by processes that are stimulated by insulin.

Adipose Tissue

Insulin stimulates the transport of glucose into adipose cells as well as into muscle cells. Adipocytes oxidize glucose for energy, and they also use glucose as the source of the glycerol moiety of the triacylglycerols they store.

FATE OF LIPOPROTEINS IN THE FED STATE

Two types of lipoproteins, chylomicrons and VLDL, are produced in the fed state. The major function of these lipoproteins is to transport triacylglycerols in the blood.

The triacylglycerols of chylomicrons are formed in intestinal epithelial cells from the products of digestion of dietary triacylglycerols. The triacylglycerols of VLDL are synthesized in the liver, mainly from dietary glucose.

When these lipoproteins pass through blood vessels in adipose tissue, their triacylglycerols are degraded to fatty acids and glycerol. The fatty acids enter the adipose cells and combine with a glycerol moiety that is produced from blood glucose. The resulting triacylglycerols are stored as large fat droplets in the adipose cells. The remnants of the chylomicrons are cleared from the blood by the liver. The remnants of the VLDL may be cleared by the liver, or they may form low density lipoproteins (LDL).

Most of us have not even begun to reach the limits of our capacity to store triacylglycerols in adipose tissue. The ability of humans to store fat appears to be limited only by the amount of tissue we can carry without overloading the heart.

FATE OF AMINO ACIDS IN THE FED STATE

The amino acids derived from dietary proteins leave the intestine through the bloodstream and are taken up by various tissues, where they are either used as substrates for biosynthesis or oxidized to yield energy. Most of the amino acids that are used in biosynthesis go into the construction of proteins. Proteins undergo turnover; they are constantly being synthesized and degraded. The amino acids released by protein breakdown enter the same pool of free amino acids as the amino acids from the diet. These pools supply the precursors for protein synthesis.

Cells also use amino acids to synthesize a wide variety of important nitrogen-containing compounds, including ATP, some hormones, neurotransmitters, the skin pigment melanin, and the heme component of hemoglobin.

Some tissues, such as the gut, can oxidize certain amino acids to obtain energy.

SUMMARY OF THE FED (ABSORPTIVE) STATE

After a meal, the fuels that we eat are oxidized to meet our immediate energy needs. Any excess fuel is stored, mainly as triacylglycerol in adipose tissue but also as glycogen in muscle and liver. Amino acids from dietary proteins are converted to body proteins, particularly in muscle.

 CLINICAL COMMENTS. **Mr. Appleman** was advised that his obesity represents a risk factor for future heart attacks and strokes. He was told that his body has to maintain a larger volume of circulating blood to service his extra fat tissue. This expanded blood volume not only contributes to his elevated blood pressure (itself a risk factor for vascular disease) but also puts an increased workload on his heart. This increased load will cause his heart muscle to thicken and eventually to fail.

Mr. Appleman's increasing adipose mass has also contributed to his development of NIDDM. The mechanism behind this breakdown in glucose tolerance is, at least in part, a resistance by his triacylglycerol-rich adipose cells to the action of insulin.

In addition to NIDDM, Mr. Appleman has a hyperlipidemia (high blood lipid level—elevated cholesterol and triacylglycerol), another risk factor for cardiovascular disease. A genetic basis for Mr. Appleman's disorder is inferred from a positive family history of hypercholesterolemia and premature coronary artery disease in a brother.

At this point, the first therapeutic steps should be nonpharmacologic. Mr. Appleman's obesity should be treated with caloric restriction and a carefully moni-

 2.1: The laboratory studies ordered at the time of his second office visit indicate that **Mr. Appleman** has developed glucose intolerance (an inability to utilize glucose in a normal manner). This results in hyperglycemia, elevations of blood glucose above normal values. At the time of this visit, his 2-hour postprandial blood glucose level was found to be 205 mg/dL. (Postprandial refers to the glucose level measured 2 hours after a meal, when glucose should have been taken up by tissues and blood glucose returned to the fasting level, approximately 80–100 mg/dL.) When he returned to the hospital laboratory to have his blood glucose determined after an overnight fast, it was found to be 162 mg/dL. Because both of these blood glucose measurements were significantly above normal, a diagnosis of non-insulin-dependent diabetes mellitus (NIDDM) was made. In this disease, muscle, adipose tissue, and liver are relatively resistant to the action of insulin in promoting glucose uptake into cells and conversion to glycogen.

If Mr. Appleman eats a high carbohydrate meal, what consequences would you predict?

A 2.1: Because **Mr. Appleman** has NIDDM, the uptake of glucose into his adipose tissue and muscle is not stimulated by insulin to the normal extent after a high carbohydrate meal. Particularly because he is so overweight, his adipose and muscle tissue contribute a considerable amount to the mass of his body. The larger than normal amounts of these tissues help to explain the slower than normal decrease in his blood glucose after a high carbohydrate meal.

Mr. Appleman's total cholesterol level is now 315 mg/dL, slightly higher than his previous level of 296. (The currently recommended level for total serum cholesterol is 200 mg/dL or less.) His triacylglycerol level is 250 mg/dL (normal is between 60 and 160 mg/dL). These lipid levels clearly indicate that Mr. Appleman is at risk for the future development of atherosclerosis and its consequences, such as heart attacks and strokes.

The liver makes triacylglycerols from a caloric excess of both carbohydrate and protein. The fatty acids of these triacylglycerols, together with the fatty acids of chylomicrons (derived from dietary fat), are deposited in adipose tissue. Thus, **Thomas Appleman's** increased adipose tissue is coming from his intake of all fuels in excess of his caloric need.

tored program of exercise. A reduction of dietary fat and sodium would be advised in an effort to correct his hyperlipidemia and his hypertension, respectively.

 BIOCHEMICAL COMMENTS. Fat stores are distributed in the body in two different patterns, android and gynecoid. After puberty, men tend to store fat in and on their abdomens (an android pattern), while women tend to store fat around their breasts, hips, and thighs (a gynecoid pattern). The typical male tends to have more of an apple shape than the typical female, who is more pear-shaped. However, these two classifications overlap to a considerable extent. When waist and hip circumference was measured at the umbilicus and iliac crest, respectively, in standing individuals, the average waist-to-hip ratio for men was 0.93 (with a range of 0.75–1.10) and the average for women was 0.83 (with a range of 0.70–1.00).

Body fat stores correlate well with the body mass index (BMI) which is the weight/height^2. Values within the normal or desirable range of 20–25 kg/m^2 are associated with longer life spans than values that are lower or higher. Individuals with large fat stores have BMI values that are above the normal range, and these individuals are considered to be obese. A higher incidence of atherosclerosis, diabetes, and other diseases is associated with obesity, particularly the android type.

Suggested Reading

Garrow JS. In: Cohen RD, Lewis B, Alberti KGMM, Denman AM (eds). Obesity. In: The metabolic and molecular basis of acquired disease. London: Bailliere Tindall, 1990:583–601.

PROBLEMS

1. If a patient has high levels of chylomicrons in the blood, what dietary therapy might be helpful in lowering the chylomicron levels?

2. If a patient has high levels of VLDL in the blood, what dietary therapy might be helpful in lowering the VLDL levels?

ANSWERS

1. Because chylomicrons are produced from dietary triacylglycerols, a diet low in fat should help to lower the chylomicron levels.

2. Because the triacylglycerols of VLDL are produced mainly from dietary carbohydrate, a diet low in carbohydrate should help to lower the VLDL levels.

3 Fasting

Within about 1 hour after a meal, blood glucose levels begin to fall. Consequently, insulin levels decline and glucagon levels rise (Fig. 3.1). These changes in hormone levels trigger the release of fuels from the body stores. Liver glycogen is degraded by the process of glycogenolysis, supplying glucose to the blood. Adipose triacylglycerols are mobilized by the process of lipolysis, releasing fatty acids and glycerol into the blood. These fatty acids serve as the major fuel that is oxidized during fasting, which occurs between the time that blood glucose levels return to the fasting range after one meal and the time that blood glucose levels begin to rise after the start of the next meal.

Glucose is oxidized by tissues such as the brain and red blood cells, and fatty acids are oxidized by tissues such as muscle and liver. While muscle converts fatty acids completely to CO_2 and H_2O, the liver only partially oxidizes most of the fatty acids it takes up, producing small molecules called ketone bodies, which are released into the blood. This partial oxidation of fatty acids by the liver is completed by tissues such as muscle and kidney, in which the ketone bodies are completely oxidized to CO_2 and H_2O.

As fasting progresses, the liver produces glucose not only by glycogenolysis (the release of glucose from glycogen), but also by a second process known as gluconeogenesis (the synthesis of glucose from noncarbohydrate compounds (see Fig. 3.1)). The major sources of carbon for gluconeogenesis are lactate, glycerol, and amino acids. When the carbons of the amino acids are converted to glucose by the liver, their nitrogen is converted to urea.

When we fast for 2 or more days, muscle continues to burn fatty acids but decreases its use of ketone bodies. As a result, the concentration of ketone bodies rises in the blood to a level where the brain begins to oxidize them for energy. The brain then needs less glucose, so the liver decreases its rate of gluconeogenesis. Consequently, muscle protein, which supplies amino acids for gluconeogenesis, is spared, and its vital functions are preserved as long as possible.

Because of these changes in the fuel utilization patterns of various tissues, humans can survive for extended periods of time without ingesting food.

 Pathways named with the suffix "lysis" are ones in which complex molecules are broken down or "lysed" into smaller units. For instance, in glycogenolysis, glycogen is lysed into glucose subunits; in glycolysis, glucose is lysed into 2 pyruvate molecules; in lipolysis, triacylglycerols are lysed into fatty acids and glycerol; in proteolysis, proteins are lysed into their constituent amino acids.

 Gluconeogenesis means formation (genesis) of new (neo) glucose, and by definition, converts new (noncarbohydrate) precursors to glucose.

During the first week of her hospital stay, **Teresa Livermore** continued to eat very modest portions of her meals and refused all nutritional supplements. She lost an additional 2 lb after admission. To continue assessing the degree of Mrs. Livermore's undernutrition, several tests were ordered, including measurements of fasting blood glucose and serum albumin. In addition, the serum ketone body concentration and the quantity of ketone bodies in a 24-hour urine specimen were measured.

Priscilla Twigg saw her gynecologist because she had not had a menstrual period for 5 months. In addition, she complained of becoming easily fatigued. The physician recognized that her body weight of 85 lb was now less than 65% of her ideal weight. Immediate hospitalization was recommended. The admission diagnosis was severe malnutrition secondary to anorexia nervosa. Clinical findings included decreased body core temperature, blood pressure, and pulse (adaptive responses to malnutrition). To assess the degree of malnutrition, measurements of blood glucose and ketone body levels were ordered and a spot urine check for ketone bodies was made.

Q 3.1: If the blood glucose level continued to decrease during fasting, the function of which tissues would be most affected?

BLOOD GLUCOSE AND THE ROLE OF THE LIVER DURING FASTING

Blood glucose levels peak about an hour after eating and then decrease as tissues oxidize glucose or convert it to storage forms of fuel. By 2 hours after a meal, the level returns to the fasting range (between 80 and 100 mg/dL). This decrease in blood glucose causes the pancreas to decrease its secretion of insulin, and the serum insulin level falls. The liver responds to this hormonal signal by starting to degrade its glycogen stores and release glucose into the bloodstream.

If we eat another meal within a few hours, we return to the fed state. However, if we continue to fast for a 12-hour period, we enter the basal state (also known as the postabsorptive state). A person is generally considered to be in the basal state after an overnight fast, when no food has been eaten since dinner the previous evening. By this time, the serum insulin level is low and glucagon is rising. Figure 3.1 illustrates the main features of the basal state.

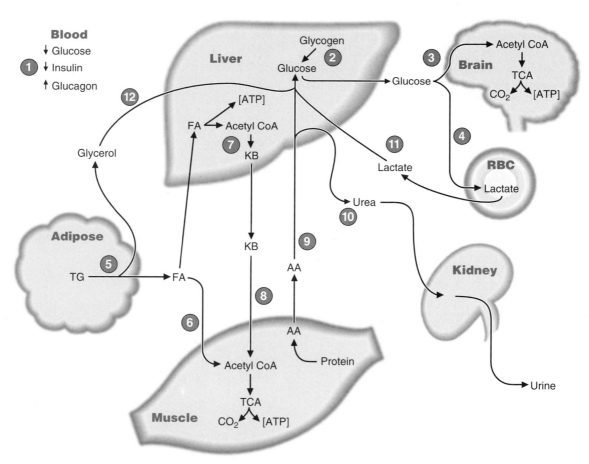

Fig. 3.1. Basal state. This state occurs after an overnight (12 hour) fast. The circled numbers serve as a guide indicating the approximate order in which the processes begin to occur. KB = ketone bodies. Other abbreviations are defined in Figure 2.1.

The liver maintains blood glucose levels during fasting, and its role is thus critical. Glucose is the major fuel for tissues such as the brain and nervous tissue, and the sole fuel for red blood cells. Because these tissues depend on glucose for energy, it is imperative that blood glucose not decrease too rapidly or fall too low.

Initially, liver glycogen stores are degraded to supply glucose to the blood, but these stores are limited. Although liver glycogen levels may increase to 200–300 g after a meal, only about 80 g remain after an overnight fast. Fortunately, the liver has another mechanism for producing blood glucose. This process, known as gluconeogenesis, uses carbon sources which include lactate, glycerol, and amino acids. After a number of hours of fasting, gluconeogenesis begins to add to the glucose produced by glycogenolysis in the liver.

Lactate is a product of glycolysis in red blood cells and exercising muscle, glycerol is obtained from lipolysis of adipose triacylglycerols, and amino acids are generated by the breakdown of muscle protein. These compounds travel in the blood to the liver where they are converted to glucose by gluconeogenesis. Because the nitrogen of the amino acids can form ammonia, which is toxic to the body, the liver converts this nitrogen to urea, which is a very soluble, nontoxic compound that can be readily excreted by the kidneys (Fig. 3.2).

As fasting progresses, gluconeogenesis becomes increasingly more important as a source of blood glucose. After about 30 hours of fasting, liver glycogen stores are depleted and gluconeogenesis is the only source of blood glucose.

It is important to realize that most fatty acids cannot provide carbon for gluconeogenesis. Thus, of the vast store of food energy in adipose tissue triacylglycerols, only a minor fraction, represented mainly by the glycerol moieties, can be used to produce blood glucose.

ROLE OF ADIPOSE TISSUE DURING FASTING

Adipose triacylglycerols are the major source of energy during fasting. They provide glycerol for gluconeogenesis but, more importantly, they supply fatty acids, which are quantitatively the major fuel for the human body. Fatty acids are not only oxidized directly by various tissues of the body, they are also converted in the liver to compounds known as ketone bodies which are subsequently oxidized by other tissues.

As blood insulin levels decrease and blood glucagon levels rise, adipose triacylglycerols are mobilized by a process known as lipolysis. They are converted to fatty acids and glycerol which enter the bloodstream.

Fatty acids serve as a fuel for tissues such as muscle and kidney, where they are oxidized to acetyl CoA, and subsequently to CO_2 and H_2O, producing energy in the form of ATP. Muscle uses ATP for contraction, and the kidney uses it for urinary resorptive and secretory processes.

Most of the fatty acids that enter the liver are converted to ketone bodies rather than being completely oxidized. The process of conversion of fatty acids to acetyl CoA produces a considerable amount of energy (ATP) which drives the reactions of the liver under these conditions. The acetyl CoA is converted to the ketone bodies acetoacetate and β-hydroxybutyrate, which are released into the blood (Fig. 3.3). These ketone bodies may be further oxidized by tissues such as muscle and kidney. In these tissues, acetoacetate and β-hydroxybutyrate are converted to acetyl CoA and then to CO_2 and H_2O with the production of energy.

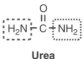

After the first week of hospitalization, **Mrs. Livermore's** blood glucose level was 72 mg/dL (normal = 80–100), and her serum albumin was 2.3 g/dL (normal = 3.5–5.0).

$$H_2N - \overset{\overset{\displaystyle O}{\|}}{C} - NH_2$$

Urea

Fig. 3.2. Urea. This nitrogen-containing excretion product of amino acid catabolism has two amino groups for every carbon and thus is an efficient means of disposing of excess nitrogen.

A 3.1: If blood glucose continued to decrease during fasting, the brain would suffer. The brain is very dependent on glucose for energy. Insufficient energy production would lead to coma, and ultimately death. Many other tissues are also totally or partially dependent on glucose for energy.

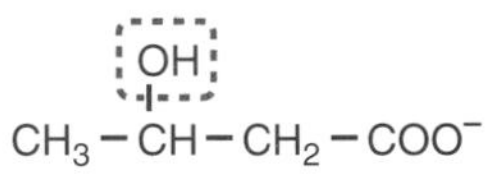

$$CH_3 - \overset{\overset{\displaystyle OH}{|}}{CH} - CH_2 - COO^-$$

β–Hydroxybutyrate

$$CH_3 - \overset{\overset{\displaystyle O}{\|}}{C} - CH_2 - COO^-$$

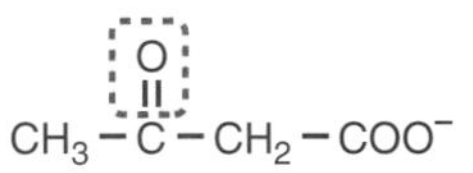

Acetoacetate

Fig. 3.3. β-Hydroxybutyrate and acetoacetate. These compounds are ketone bodies. A third compound, acetone

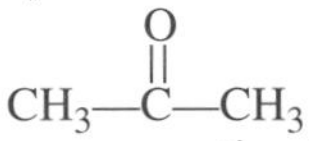

$$CH_3 - \overset{\overset{\displaystyle O}{\|}}{C} - CH_3$$

produced by nonenzymatic decarboxylation of acetoacetate, is also considered one of the ketone bodies. However, acetone does not provide a significant source of energy for the body.

On the seventh day of her hospitalization, **Mrs. Livermore's** serum ketone body level was 110 µM. (In a well-nourished, normal subject, after a 12-hour fast, the blood ketone body level would be about 70 µM.) No ketone bodies were detectable in her urine.

SUMMARY OF THE METABOLIC CHANGES DURING A BRIEF FAST

In the initial stages of fasting, stored fuels are used for energy (see Fig. 3.1). The liver plays a key role by maintaining blood glucose levels, first by glycogenolysis and subsequently by gluconeogenesis. Lactate, glycerol, and amino acids serve as carbon sources for gluconeogenesis. Amino acids are supplied by muscle. Their nitrogen is converted in the liver to urea, which is excreted by the kidneys.

Fatty acids, which are released from adipose tissue by the process of lipolysis, serve as the body's major fuel during fasting. Most tissues can oxidize fatty acids. However, the liver oxidizes most of its fatty acids only partially, converting them to ketone bodies, which are released and used by other tissues.

Overall, during the initial stages of fasting, blood glucose levels are maintained in the range of 80–100 mg/dL, and the levels of fatty acids and ketone bodies increase. Muscle uses fatty acids, ketone bodies, and (when exercising and while supplies last) glucose from muscle glycogen. Many other tissues use a mixture of fatty acids and ketone bodies. Red blood cells, the brain, and other nervous tissue use mainly glucose.

METABOLIC CHANGES DURING PROLONGED FASTING

If the pattern of fuel utilization that occurs during a brief fast were to persist for an extended period, the body's protein would be quite rapidly consumed to the point

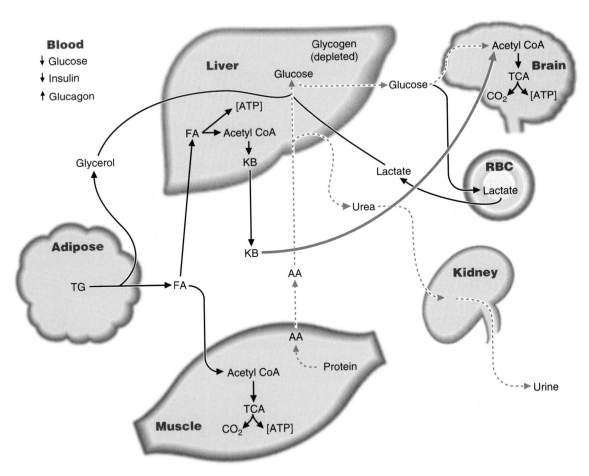

Fig. 3.4. Starved state. Abbreviations are defined in Figures 2.1 and 3.1. Dashed lines indicate processes that have decreased and the heavy solid line indicates a process that has increased relative to the fasting state.

where critical functions would be compromised. Fortunately, metabolic changes occur during prolonged fasting that conserve (spare) muscle protein. Figure 3.4 shows the main features of metabolism during prolonged fasting (starvation).

After 4 or 5 days of fasting, when the body enters the starved state, muscle decreases its use of ketone bodies and depends mainly on fatty acids for its fuel. The liver, however, continues to convert fatty acids to ketone bodies. The result is that the concentration of ketone bodies rises in the blood (Fig. 3.5). The brain begins to take up these ketone bodies from the blood and to oxidize them for energy. Therefore, the brain needs less glucose than it did after an overnight fast (Table 3.1).

Glucose is still required, however, as an energy source for red blood cells, and the brain continues to use a limited amount of glucose, which it oxidizes for energy and utilizes as a source of carbon for the synthesis of neurotransmitters. Overall, however, glucose is "spared" (conserved). Less glucose is used by the body, and therefore, the liver needs to produce less glucose during prolonged fasting than during shorter periods of fasting.

Because the stores of glycogen in the liver are depleted by about 30 hours of fasting, gluconeogenesis is the only process by which the liver can supply glucose to the blood if fasting continues. Amino acids, produced by the breakdown of muscle protein, continue to serve as a major source of carbon for gluconeogenesis. However, as a result of the decreased rate of gluconeogenesis during prolonged fasting, muscle protein is "spared," that is, not as much muscle protein is degraded to supply amino acids for gluconeogenesis.

During the conversion of amino acid carbon to glucose by the process of gluconeogenesis, the nitrogen of the amino acids is converted to urea. Consequently, because of decreased production of glucose, the production of urea also decreases during prolonged fasting compared to its production early in a fast (Fig. 3.6).

ROLE OF ADIPOSE TISSUE DURING PROLONGED FASTING

During prolonged fasting, adipose tissue continues to break down its triacylglycerol stores, providing fatty acids and glycerol to the blood. These fatty acids serve as the major source of fuel for the body. The glycerol is converted to glucose, while the fatty acids are oxidized to CO_2 and H_2O by tissues such as muscle. In the liver, they are converted to ketone bodies which are oxidized by tissues, including the brain.

The amount of adipose tissue in our bodies is a major determinant of the length of time we can fast, because adipose tissue supplies the body with its major source of fuel. Glucose, however, is still used to some extent, even during prolonged fasting. Although we degrade muscle protein to supply amino acids for gluconeogenesis at a slower rate during starvation than during the early period of a fast, we still continue losing protein as long as we are fasting.

Eventually, we develop problems, e.g., we run out of fuel (mainly adipose tissue), protein becomes so depleted that the heart, the kidney, and other vital tissues stop functioning, or we develop an infection and do not have adequate reserves to mount an immune response. Ultimately, we die of starvation.

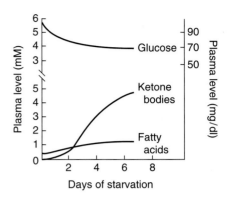

Fig. 3.5. Changes in the concentration of fuels in the blood during prolonged fasting.

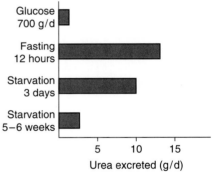

Fig. 3.6. Changes in urea excretion during prolonged fasting. The decrease in urea excretion as fasting progresses reflects the decreased breakdown of muscle protein. Because the brain meets some of its energy needs by oxidizing ketone bodies after 3–5 days of fasting, gluconeogenesis decreases, sparing muscle protein and also protein in kidney and other tissues.

Priscilla Twigg's admission laboratory studies revealed a blood glucose level of 65 mg/dL (normal fasting blood glucose = 80–100). Her serum ketone body concentration was 4,200 μM (normal = about 70). The Ketostix urine test was moderately positive, indicating that ketone bodies were present in the urine.

Table 3.1. Metabolic Changes during Prolonged Fasting

Muscle	↓	utilization of ketone bodies
Brain	↑	utilization of ketone bodies
Liver	↓	gluconeogenesis
Muscle	↓	protein degradation
Liver	↓	production of urea

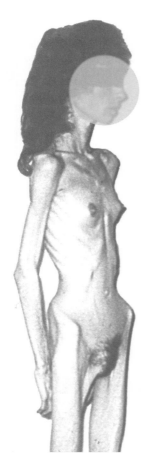

Fig. 3.7. Photograph of a patient with anorexia nervosa. From a MedCom slide, 1970.

 CLINICAL COMMENTS. As a result of her severely suppressed appetite for food, **Mrs. Livermore** has developed a degree of protein-calorie undernutrition. When prolonged, this type of undernutrition can cause changes in the villi of the small intestine that reduce its absorptive capacity for what little food is ingested.

Despite her insufficient intake of dietary carbohydrates, Mrs. Livermore's blood glucose level is 72 mg/dL, close to the lower limit (80 mg/dL) of the normal range for a well-nourished, healthy person after a 12-hour fast. This is the finding you would expect: it reflects the liver's capacity to maintain adequate levels of blood glucose by means of gluconeogenesis, even during prolonged and moderately severe caloric restriction.

The albumin level in the blood is subnormal (2.3 g/dL vs. normal of 3.5–5.0) because dietary protein intake is low and because of the intestine's diminished capacity to absorb dietary amino acids. Consequently, fewer amino acids are available to the liver cells for the synthesis of albumin, and the serum albumin concentration falls.

At this stage, ketone bodies were only moderately elevated in the blood (110 μM vs. normal of 70 μM) and did not appear in the urine.

Treatment consists of continued attempts, mainly through psychological counseling, to convince Mrs. Livermore that she needs to resume her normal eating pattern.

Priscilla Twigg has anorexia nervosa, a chronic disabling disease in which poorly understood psychological and biological factors lead to disturbances in the patient's body image. These patients typically insist they are overweight in spite of a sometimes grotesque "skeletal" appearance (Fig. 3.7).

Amenorrhea (lack of menses) usually develops when a woman's body fat content falls to about 22% of her total body weight. The immediate cause of amenorrhea is a reduced production of the gonadotropic hormones, luteinizing hormone and follicle-stimulating hormone, by the anterior pituitary; the connection between this hormonal change and body fat content is not yet understood.

Ms. Twigg is suffering from the consequences of severe caloric restriction. Fatty acids, released from adipose tissue by lipolysis, are being converted to ketone bodies in the liver, and the level of ketone bodies in the blood is extremely elevated (4,200 μM vs. normal of 70 μM). The fact that her kidneys are excreting ketone bodies is reflected in the moderately positive urine test for ketone bodies noted on admission.

As would be expected, Ms. Twigg's blood glucose is only slightly below the normal fasting range (65 mg/dL vs. normal of 80) despite her severe, near starvation diet. This reflects her body's ability to maintain an adequate level of blood glucose by means of gluconeogenesis.

The general therapeutic plan, outlined in Chapter 1, of nutritional restitution and identification and treatment of those emotional factors which led to the patient's anorectic behavior was continued.

 BIOCHEMICAL COMMENTS. Complex interactions occur among the various tissues of the body. Not all tissues use the same fuels, and the pattern of fuel utilization changes with changes in fuel availability as the body shifts from one physiological state to another (Table 3.2).

Tissues interact chemically by passing compounds through the bloodstream. For example, during fasting, the liver oxidizes fatty acids and produces ketone bodies. It also produces glucose from amino acids derived from muscle protein. The nitrogen of the amino acids is converted to urea. The ketone bodies, glucose, and urea are released from the liver into the blood. Glucose and ketone bodies are taken up by various tissues and oxidized. The urea is excreted by the kidney via the urine.

Table 3.2. Metabolic Capacities of Various Tissues

Process	Liver	Adipose Tissue	Kidney Cortex	Muscle	Brain	RBC
TCA cycle (acetyl CoA→ CO_2 + H_2O)	+++	+++	+++	+++	+++	–
β-Oxidation of fatty acids	+++	–	+++	+++	–	–
Ketone body formation	+++		+	–	–	–
Ketone body utilization	–	+	++	+++	– (fed) +++ (prolonged starvation)	–
Lipogenesis (glucose → fatty acids)	+++	+	–	–	–	–
Gluconeogenesis (lactate → glucose)	+++	–	+	–	–	–
Glycogen metabolism (synthesis and degradation)	+++	+	+	+++	(+)	–
Lactate production (glucose → lactate)	+	+	+	+++ exercise	(+)	+++

When a patient develops a metabolic problem, it is difficult to examine cells to determine the cause. In order to obtain tissue for metabolic studies, biopsies must be performed. These procedures can be difficult, dangerous, or even impossible, depending on the tissue. Cost is an additional problem.

However, both blood and urine can readily be obtained from patients, and measurements of substances in the blood and urine can help in diagnosing a patient's problem. Concentrations of substances that are higher or lower than normal indicate which tissues are malfunctioning. For example, if blood urea nitrogen (BUN) levels are low, a problem centered in the liver might be suspected because urea is produced in the liver. On the other hand, high blood levels of urea would suggest that the kidney is not excreting this compound normally. If high levels of ketone bodies are found in the blood or urine, the patient's metabolic pattern is that of the starved state. If the high levels of ketone bodies are coupled with elevated levels of blood glucose, the problem is most likely a deficiency of insulin, that is, the patient probably has insulin-dependent diabetes mellitus.

These relatively easy and inexpensive tests on blood and urine can be used to determine which tissues need to be studied more extensively to diagnose and treat the patient's problem. A solid understanding of fuel metabolism helps in the interpretation of these simple tests.

Suggested Reading

Owen OE, Tappy L, Mozzoli MA, Smalley KJ. Acute starvation. In: Cohen RD, Lewis B, Alberti KGMM, Denman AM (eds). The metabolic and molecular basis of acquired disease. London: Bailliere Tindall, 1990:550–601.

PROBLEMS

1. A person is eating a diet that contains enough protein and enough carbohydrate to meet the needs of glucose-requiring tissues, but that provides fewer calories than the person expends. Whenever this person expends 3,500 kcal more energy than is obtained in the diet, 1 lb of adipose tissue will be lost.

   A. Show with calculations that 3,500 kcal of fat are stored in 1 lb of adipose tissue.

   B. How much of each pound that is lost under these conditions will be water?

2. If a person is not eating an adequate amount of carbohydrate to meet the needs of tissues such as the brain and red blood cells, then muscle protein will be degraded, providing amino acids which will be converted to glucose by gluconeogenesis.

   A. Calculate the number of kilocalories released as amino acids when 1 lb of muscle tissue is lost.

   B. How much of each pound of muscle tissue that is lost under these conditions is water?

3. Suppose that an average 70-kg man went on a hunger strike. He developed no other problems, but died only because he ran out of stored fuel. Calculate the approximate length of time he survived during this prolonged fast.

ANSWERS

1A. When adipose tissue is lost because its triacylglycerol (fat) store is used to supply energy to the body,

$$3{,}500 \text{ kcal} \times \frac{1 \text{ g fat}}{9 \text{ kcal}} \times \frac{100 \text{ g adipose tissue}}{85 \text{ g fat}} \times \frac{2.2 \text{ lb}}{1{,}000 \text{ g}}$$
$$= 1 \text{ lb of adipose tissue.}$$

1B. Adipose tissue contains about 85% fat and 15% water. Therefore, whenever 1 lb of adipose tissue is lost, 0.15 lb of water is lost.

2A. Whenever 1 lb of muscle tissue is degraded to provide amino acids for gluconeogenesis,

$$1 \text{ lb muscle tissue} \times \frac{1{,}000 \text{ g}}{2.2 \text{ lb}} \times \frac{20 \text{ g protein}}{100 \text{ g muscle}} \times \frac{4 \text{ kcal}}{1 \text{ g protein}}$$
$$= 364 \text{ kcal.}$$

2B. In contrast to adipose tissue which contains about 15% water, muscle tissue contains about 80% water. Therefore, 0.8 lb of water is lost whenever 1 lb of muscle tissue is lost. Loss of muscle tissue, therefore, is mainly loss of water. Very few kilocalories are obtained, in contrast to adipose tissue. One pound of muscle has about 360 calories and is 80% water. One pound of adipose tissue has about 3,500 calories and is 15% water.

3. The average 70-kg man has about 15 kg (that is, 15,000 g) of fat or, at 9 kcal/g, 135,000 kcal stored in adipose tissue as triacylglycerol (see Chapter 1, Fig. 1.7).

   At 70 kg, his basal metabolic rate would be about 24 kcal/kg/day × 70 kg or 1,680 kcal/day. While fasting, he would most likely be rather sedentary. With an activity factor of 1.3, his total caloric expenditure would be about 2,184 kcal/day (1.3 × 1,680). If we consider only his fat stores, the average 70-kg man has enough fuel to last for about 62 days (135,000 kcal stored / 2,184 kcal expended/day = 62 days). The 6 kg of protein (about one third to one half of the body's total protein) that can be used as fuel (most of it oxidized as glucose produced from amino acids by gluconeogenesis) would provide the equivalent of 11 additional days of fuel (6,000 g × 4 kcal/g = 24,000 kcal ÷ 2,184 kcal/day = about 11 days). (Of course, the fat and protein will be used concurrently, not on separate days.)

   Glycogen stores are extremely small (80 g in liver and 150 g in muscle) and would not add appreciably to his lifespan.

   Overall, the average 70-kg man has enough fuel to last a maximum of 73 days, if he dies only because he has run out of fuel and not because he develops an infection or some other problem.

Chemical and Biological Foundations of Biochemistry

The discipline of biochemistry developed as chemists began to study the molecules of cells and as biologists began to study the molecular basis of their observations of living organisms. Therefore, a student who intends to learn biochemistry must have an adequate understanding of cell biology and of chemistry, particularly the chemistry of carbohydrates, lipids, proteins, and nucleic acids. This section is designed to cover this fundamental information. It is not meant to be comprehensive, but to focus on the concepts that are most relevant to biochemistry as it applies to medicine.

The relationship of metabolic acids to blood pH is described in Chapter 4. Chapter 5 focuses on the terminology of the common organic compounds in the body. In Chapter 6, the structures of the major classes of biochemical compounds are described with emphasis on carbohydrates and lipids (which serve not only as fuels, but also as structural components of cells and tissues) and on nucleotides (which provide energy for biochemical reactions and serve as the building blocks for the synthesis of nucleic acids).

Because a knowledge of protein structure is so critical for understanding the physiological functions of the body, Chapters 7 and 8 are devoted to amino acid and protein structure. Amino acids serve as a major source of fuel and as the precursors for the synthesis of our body proteins. The functions of proteins are myriad. They transport compounds through the bloodstream and across membranes. They are the components that allow muscles to contract, thus permitting movement. In the form of antibodies and other components of the immune system, they protect us from infection by foreign organisms. They also prevent blood loss by producing the cascade of events that lead to clot formation.

An important function of proteins is to serve as enzymes, the catalysts that increase the speed of biochemical reactions. Without these protein catalysts, reactions would occur so slowly that life would not be possible. The subject of enzymes is treated in Chapter 9.

Proteins and all the other compounds of the body are organized into organs and tissues, which are composed of cells. Therefore, this section ends in Chapter 10 with a brief description of the structural components of cells and their organization into membranes and subcellular organelles.

4 Acids, Bases, and Buffers

Many compounds in the body contain chemical groups that can act as acids or bases, releasing or accepting protons. Therefore, they may carry a charge at physiological pH. These compounds range from small molecules such as ATP to large polymers such as the protein hemoglobin. Because the charges on these molecules are due to acidic and basic groups and these charges are very important in determining structure and function, the subject of acids and bases needs to be considered among the chemical foundations of biochemistry.

Most biochemical reactions occur in aqueous solutions. Water dissociates to a slight extent to form H^+ and OH^-. The concentration of hydrogen ions, $[H^+]$, determines the acidity of the solution, which is usually expressed in terms of pH. The pH of a solution is the negative log of its hydrogen ion concentration (Fig. 4.1).

An acid is a substance that can release hydrogen ions (protons), whereas a base is a substance that can accept hydrogen ions. In solution, almost all the molecules of a strong acid dissociate, but only a small number of the total molecules of a weak acid dissociate. A weak acid has a characteristic dissociation constant, K_a.

The negative log of the dissociation constant K_a is defined as the pK_a. The relationship between pH, pK_a, and the concentrations of a weak acid and its conjugate base is described by the Henderson-Hasselbalch equation (Fig. 4.2).

A buffer is a mixture of an undissociated acid and its conjugate base that causes a solution to resist changes in pH when either H^+ or OH^- are added. A buffer has its greatest buffering capacity in the pH range near its pK_a.

Because acids are produced in the course of normal metabolism, the body must have buffers that can maintain the pH in a range compatible with life.

$$pH = -\log [H^+]$$

Fig. 4.1. Definition of pH.

$$pH = pK_a + \log \frac{[A^-]}{[HA]}$$

Fig. 4.2. Henderson-Hasselbalch equation. pK_a, analogous to pH, is the negative log of the dissociation constant, K_a. [HA] = concentration of the undissociated acid; $[H^+]$ = concentration of the hydrogen ions; and $[A^-]$ = concentration of the conjugate base.

Dianne Beatty is a 26-year-old woman who was diagnosed with diabetes mellitus at the age of 12. She depends on daily injections of insulin to prevent severe elevations of glucose and ketone bodies in her blood. When she could not be aroused from an afternoon nap, her roommate called an ambulance, and Di Beatty was brought to the emergency room of the hospital in a coma. Her roommate reported that Di was nauseated and had been vomiting for 24 hours and complained of feeling drowsy. Di is clinically dehydrated and her blood pressure is low. Her respirations are deep and rapid, and her pulse rate is rapid. Her breath has the odor of acetone.

Blood samples are drawn for measurement of her arterial blood pH, arterial partial pressure of carbon dioxide (P_aCO_2), serum glucose, and serum bicarbonate (HCO_3^-). In addition, serum and urine are tested for the presence of ketone bodies and Di is treated with intravenous normal saline and insulin.

Dennis Livermore, age 3, was brought to the emergency department by his grandmother Teresa Livermore. While Dennis was visiting his grandmother, he had climbed up on a chair and taken from the kitchen counter a half-full 500-tablet bottle of 325 mg aspirin (acetylsalicylic acid) tablets. When his grand-

Di Beatty has a ketoacidosis. Because she has insulin-dependent diabetes mellitus, her pancreas is unable to produce an adequate amount of insulin and, therefore, she needs to inject insulin on a regular basis. If she neglects to take her insulin, she remains in a condition similar to a fasting state even though she ingests food (see Chapters 2 and 3). Her liver continues to produce the ketone bodies acetoacetic acid and β-hydroxybutyric acid, and she develops a type of metabolic acidosis called a ketoacidosis. In a patient with an acidosis, the hydrogen ion concentration of the blood increases and the blood pH decreases below the normal range. The lab report indicates that Ms. Beatty's blood pH is 7.08 (reference range = 7.37–7.43) and that ketone bodies are present in both blood and urine.

37

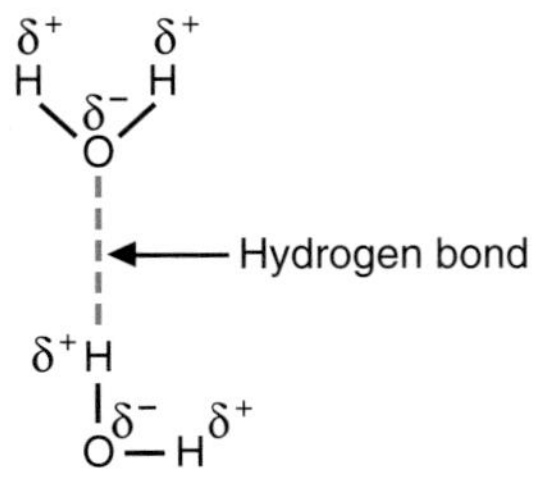

Fig. 4.3. Hydrogen bond between water molecules.

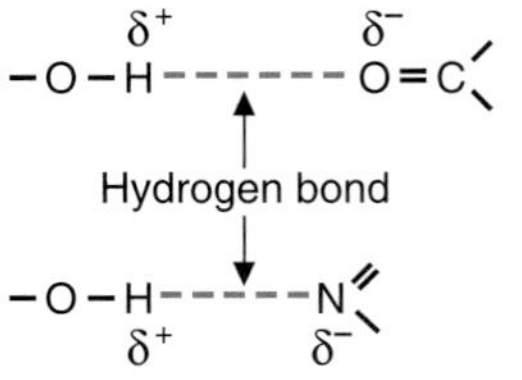

Fig. 4.4. Examples of types of hydrogen bonds.

$$H_2O \rightleftharpoons H^+ + OH^-$$

Fig. 4.5. Dissociation of water.

$$K = \frac{[H^+] \, [OH^-]}{[H_2O]}$$

Fig. 4.6. Dissociation constant of water.

$$K_w = [H^+] \, [OH^-] = 1 \times 10^{-14}$$

Fig. 4.7. Ion product of water.

$$pH = -\log [H^+]$$

Fig. 4.8. Relationship of pH and $[H^+]$.

$$CO_2 + H_2O \longrightarrow H_2CO_3$$

Carbon dioxide   **Water**   **Carbonic acid**

Fig. 4.9. Conversion of carbon dioxide to carbonic acid.

mother discovered him with a mouthful of aspirins, which she removed, she could not tell how many tablets he had already ingested. When they arrived at the emergency room, the child appeared bright and alert, but his grandmother was hyperventilating.

WATER

Water is the solvent of life. About two thirds of our body weight is water. With the exception of reactions that occur in lipid membranes, the reactions of the body occur in an aqueous medium. Because water molecules are polar, they can interact with each other. Each of the 2 hydrogen atoms in a water molecule shares its electrons with the unshared electrons of the oxygen atom. Because the oxygen atom has a greater attraction for the shared electrons than the hydrogen atoms (i.e., is more electronegative), the oxygen has a partial negative charge (δ^-) and the hydrogens each have a partial positive charge (δ^+). These partial charges cause one water molecule to be attracted to another by means of weak interactions known as hydrogen bonds (Fig. 4.3). A large number of such bonds form between the molecules of liquid water. Each molecule may form hydrogen bonds with as many as 4 neighboring molecules. Water may also form hydrogen bonds with other electronegative atoms (generally oxygen or nitrogen) (Fig. 4.4). Therefore, it is a solvent in which polar molecules can readily dissolve.

Water molecules can dissociate to a slight extent, producing hydrogen ions, H^+, and hydroxide ions, OH^- (Fig. 4.5). Hydrogen ions are also called protons. Although hydrogen ions (H^+) react with water to form hydronium ions (H_3O^+) and species that are more extensively hydrated, for the sake of simplicity they are usually represented as H^+.

At equilibrium, the product of the concentrations of the dissociated ions divided by the concentration of the undissociated water is a constant, K (Fig. 4.6). Because the extent of dissociation is very small, the concentration of pure water, $[H_2O]$, remains essentially at 55.5 M and is incorporated into another constant designated as the ion product of water, K_w (Fig. 4.7). This product does not change. If H^+ is added to an aqueous solution, $[OH^-]$ decreases proportionately. Conversely, if OH^- is added, $[H^+]$ decreases. $K_w = 1 \times 10^{-14}$.

The hydrogen ion concentration of pure water is 0.0000001 M. In order to avoid dealing with such small numbers, chemists developed the term pH. The pH of a solution is the negative log of the hydrogen ion concentration (Fig. 4.8). H^+ for pure water is 1×10^{-7}; therefore, the pH is 7.

ACIDS AND BASES

Acids are compounds that donate protons to a solution, and bases are compounds that accept protons. The body produces a number of acids during normal metabolism (Table 4.1). Carbon dioxide, which is produced during the oxidation of fuels, reacts with water to form carbonic acid (Fig. 4.9).

Table 4.1. Acids Produced by the Body

Carbonic acid
Sulfuric acid
Phosphoric acid
Lactic acid
Citric acid
Ammonium ions
Ketone bodies:
Acetoacetic acid
β-Hydroxybutyric acid

Acids undergo dissociation (Fig. 4.10). Strong acids, such as sulfuric acid, dissociate completely. Weak acids, such as acetic acid, dissociate only to a limited extent.

$$HA \leftrightharpoons H^+ + A^-$$

(where HA and A$^-$ are an acid-base conjugate pair). HA, the undissociated acid, can release a proton, and A$^-$, the conjugate base, can accept a proton.

At the pH in the blood, most organic acids are completely dissociated. The name of the conjugate base ends in "ate" (see Fig. 4.10).

The value of the dissociation constant (K_a) for a weak acid indicates the tendency of the acid (HA) to lose its proton and form its conjugate base (A$^-$) (Fig. 4.11). Stronger acids have a greater tendency to dissociate and, therefore, have higher dissociation constants than do weaker acids.

Henderson and Hasselbalch rearranged the formula for the dissociation constant of a weak acid (see Fig. 4.11), expressing the terms in logarithmic form. The result is an equation that bears their names (Fig. 4.12).

BUFFERS

A buffer consists of a weak acid and its conjugate base that cause a solution to resist changes in pH when an acid or a base is added (Fig. 4.13). A buffer has this property because it is able to compensate partially for an influx or removal of hydrogen ions. If hydrogen ions are added (via an acid), they combine with the weak base. If hydrogen ions are removed (by combining with a base that is added to the solution), the weak acid dissociates, replacing them. In either case, the pH of the solution is returned toward its original level.

Two factors determine the effectiveness of a buffer: its pK_a relative to the pH of the solution and its concentration. A buffer works best within 1 pH unit of its pK_a. Because pH is on a logarithmic scale, this translates into saying that a buffer works best when the concentration ratio of the undissociated acid to its conjugate base is between 1/10 and 10/1 (i.e., between 1 pH unit below and 1 unit above the pK_a). A buffer is also more effective the more concentrated it is, simply because a more concentrated solution contains more buffer molecules. A 1 M solution of a given buffer has 1 million times more buffering molecules than a 1 μM solution.

Body fluids must be protected against changes in pH because most enzymes are very pH sensitive. Moreover, the protective mechanisms must be constantly active, because metabolism involves the production of acids and bases (especially acids). In the long run, excess acid or base is eliminated via the kidneys and the lungs. In the short run, the body is protected against pH changes by buffering systems. Two main buffers occur in the blood: the bicarbonate buffer and a buffer involving the oxygen-carrying protein hemoglobin. These mechanisms normally act to maintain blood pH between 7.37 and 7.43.

Fig. 4.10. Dissociation of acids. The acids in the body are produced by metabolism or they are ingested. Sulfuric acid is a strong acid that dissociates completely. It is produced in the body during degradation of the amino acid cysteine. Acetic acid (a weak acid) is produced by metabolism or ingested in the form of vinegar and other food. Acetylsalicylic acid (another weak acid) is not produced in the body, but may be ingested in the form of aspirin.

$$K_a = \frac{[H^+]\,[A^-]}{[HA]}$$

Fig. 4.11. Dissociation constant (K_a) for a weak acid. HA = the undissociated acid; A$^-$ = the conjugate base.

$$pH = pK_a + \log \frac{[A^-]}{[HA]}$$

Fig. 4.12. Henderson-Hasselbalch equation. pK_a, analogous to pH, is the negative log of the dissociation constant, K_a. Note that when the concentrations of HA and A$^-$ are equal, pH = pK_a.

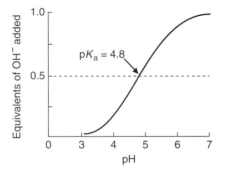

Fig. 4.13. Titration of acetic acid.

Dennis Livermore has ingested an unknown number of acetylsalicylic acid (aspirin) tablets. Acetylsalicylic acid is rapidly converted to salicylic acid in the body. Excessive ingestion of aspirin can produce a complex metabolic acidosis, caused in part by salicylic acid itself and in part by the accumulation of other organic acids in the blood.

Although adults would find it difficult to swallow a large number of aspirin tablets, children sometimes ingest lethal quantities. It was appropriate for Mrs. Livermore to bring her grandson to the emergency room.

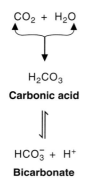

$$CO_2 + H_2O$$

$$H_2CO_3$$
Carbonic acid

$$HCO_3^- + H^+$$
Bicarbonate

Fig. 4.14. Conversion of carbon dioxide to bicarbonate.

The partial pressure of CO_2 (P_aCO_2) in **Di Beatty's** blood was 30 mm Hg (reference range = 38–42), and her serum bicarbonate level was 13 mEq/L (reference range = 24–28). Elevated levels of ketone bodies had produced a ketoacidosis, and Di Beatty was breathing deeply and frequently (Kussmaul breathing) to compensate. As a result, her P_aCO_2 and $[HCO_3^-]$ were low.

Both **Di Beatty** and **Mrs. Livermore** were hyperventilating when they arrived at the emergency room, Di in response to her primary metabolic acidosis and Mrs. Livermore because of anxiety. Hyperventilation raised blood pH in both cases; in Di's case it partially countered the acidosis, and in Mrs Livermore's case it produced a respiratory alkalosis (abnormally high pH).

The bicarbonate buffer depends on the fact that the carbon dioxide produced by fuel oxidation reacts reversibly with water to produce a weak acid, carbonic acid, which undergoes partial dissociation to produce the conjugate base, bicarbonate (Fig. 4.14).

The reaction of carbon dioxide with water to produce carbonic acid is catalyzed by the enzyme carbonic anhydrase, which is located in red blood cells and other cell types. The acid-base pair H_2CO_3/HCO_3^- acts as a buffer. Moreover, the total amount of carbonic acid in the blood can be reduced by breathing more deeply and thus eliminating more CO_2 via the lungs. This strategy allows the body to counter an influx of acid (a metabolic acidosis) by reducing its total concentration of acid via a compensatory respiratory mechanism (a compensatory respiratory alkalosis). Conversely, if the pH of the blood rises (if a metabolic alkalosis occurs), breathing becomes more shallow, CO_2 is retained, and the blood pH decreases (a compensatory respiratory acidosis occurs).

Hemoglobin acts as a buffer because it carries the basic amino acid histidine in a number of exposed positions. These histidine residues can combine reversibly with hydrogen ions, producing protonated and unprotonated forms of hemoglobin. This effect is more complicated than indicated here; it will be described in detail in Chapter 8.

These buffers in the blood act in conjunction with mechanisms in the kidneys for excreting protons as well as with mechanisms in the lungs for exhaling CO_2 to maintain the pH within the normal range (Fig. 4.15).

CLINICAL COMMENTS. Di Beatty has insulin-dependent diabetes mellitus (IDDM). Unless she injects insulin daily under her skin, her blood insulin levels fall too low. One result is that free fatty acids leave her fat cells and are converted by the liver to ketone bodies. As these acids accumulate in the blood, a metabolic acidosis known as diabetic ketoacidosis (DKA) develops. Until insulin is administered to reverse this trend, several compensatory mechanisms oper-

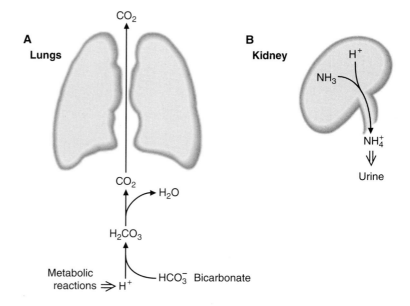

Fig. 4.15. Action of the lungs and the kidneys in decreasing $[H^+]$ in the body. **A.** Reactions in the lungs. **B.** Reactions in the kidneys.

ate to minimize the extent of the acidosis. One of these mechanisms is a central stimulation of the respiratory center induced by the acidosis, which leads to deeper and more frequent respirations (Kussmaul respiration). CO_2 is expired more rapidly than normal, and the blood pH rises. The results of the laboratory studies performed on Di Beatty in the emergency room were consistent with a moderately severe DKA. Her arterial blood pH and serum bicarbonate were low, and ketone bodies were present in her blood and urine. In addition, her serum glucose level was 648 mg/dL (reference range = 80–100 fasting and no higher than 140 after a meal).

Treatment was initiated with intravenous saline solutions to replace fluids lost as a result of the osmotic diuresis which occurs when large amounts of glucose are excreted in the urine with appropriate amounts of water and as water of respiration during hyperventilation.

A loading dose of regular insulin was given as an intravenous bolus followed by additional insulin each hour as needed. The patient's metabolic response to these and other measures was monitored closely.

Dennis Livermore remained alert in the emergency room. While awaiting the report of his initial serum salicylate level, his stomach was lavaged and several white tablets were found in the stomach aspirate. He was examined repeatedly and showed none of the early signs or symptoms of salicylate toxicity, such as respiratory stimulation, upper abdominal distress, nausea, or headache.

His serum salicylate level was reported as 92 µg/mL (usual level in an adult on a therapeutic dosage of 4–5 g/day is 120–350 µg/mL, and a level of 800 µg/mL is considered potentially lethal). He was admitted for overnight observation and continued to do well. A serum salicylate level the following morning was 24 µg/mL. He was discharged later that day.

When **Teresa Livermore** brought her grandson to the emergency room, she complained of light-headedness and "pins and needles" in her hands and around her lips in response to her anxiety concerning her grandson's aspirin ingestion. After being reassured that Dennis would be fine, she was asked to breath slowly into a small paper bag placed around her nose and mouth to allow her to re-inhale the CO_2 being exhaled through hyperventilation. Within 20 minutes, her symptoms disappeared.

🔬 BIOCHEMICAL COMMENTS. The concentrations of compounds in the blood are expressed in various ways. A 1 molar (M) solution contains 1 mole of solute per liter (L) of solution. A mole is 1 g molecular weight (the molecular weight in grams). Therefore, a 1 M solution of glucose (molecular weight = 180) contains 180 g/L. The normal fasting blood glucose is about 0.005 M, which is 5 mM. One mole equals 1,000 millimoles (mmol).

Because 1 g contains 1,000 mg, a 5 mM glucose solution contains 180 mg × 5 mmol or 900 mg/L. Physicians usually express blood glucose concentrations as milligrams per deciliter (mg/dL). A deciliter (dL) is 100 mL. Values for fasting blood glucose according to this system will be 90 mg/dL. An older system which is still in use would call this value 90 mg%. The % stands for "in a volume of 100 mL."

To review the relationships among the prefixes used for various units (such as weight, volume, and length) in the metric system, see Table 4.2. Micro, milli, deci, and kilo are the prefixes most commonly used. As methods for measuring small amounts of substances, such as hormones, are developed, nano and pico are being used more frequently.

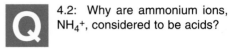

Q 4.1: When the pH of a solution equals the pK_a, what is the concentration of the conjugate base relative to the concentration of the undissociated acid?

Q 4.2: Why are ammonium ions, NH_4^+, considered to be acids?

A 4.1: When the pH equals the pK_a, according to the Henderson-Hasselbalch equation,

$$pH - pK_a = 0 = \log \frac{[A^-]}{[HA]}$$

The log of 1 equals 0, so when log $[A^-]/[HA] = 0$, $[A^-]/[HA] = 1$, and the concentration of the conjugate base is equal to the concentration of the undissociated acid. These are the conditions under which the buffer is most effective at resisting changes caused by the addition of acid or base.

A 4.2: Ammonium ions can dissociate a proton, forming ammonia.

$$pK_a = 9.25$$

NH₄⁺ ⇌ $NH_3 + H^+$
Ammonium ion   Ammonia

Ammonium ions are acids, while ammonia (NH_3) is a base because it can accept a proton to form the acid, NH_4^+. Note that the pK_a for this dissociation is 9.25. Therefore, the acid form (NH_4^+) predominates at physiological pH.

Table 4.2. Frequently Used Prefixes in the Metric System

Prefix	Symbol	Value Relative to the Unprefixed Unit
femto	f	10^{-15}
pico	p	10^{-12}
nano	n	10^{-9}
micro	μ	10^{-6}
milli	m	10^{-3}
centi	c	10^{-2}
deci	d	10^{-1}
unit		10^{0}
kilo	k	10^{3}

Suggested Reading

For more information on aspirin and its therapeutic and side effects, see: Gilman AG, Rall T, Nies A, Taylor P (eds). Goodman and Gilman's the pharmacological basis of therapeutics. New York: Pergamon Press, 1990:638–654.

PROBLEMS

1. Derive the Henderson-Hasselbalch equation from the equation for the dissociation of a weak acid.

2. Di Beatty was infused with normal saline (0.9% NaCl). What was the concentration of the NaCl in g/dL? In g/L? In mg/mL?

ANSWERS

1. The dissociation constant for a weak acid is:

$$K_a = \frac{[H^+][A^-]}{[HA]} = [H^+] \frac{[A^-]}{[HA]}$$

Take the log of each of the terms of this equation.

$$\log K_a = \log[H^+] + \log \frac{[A^-]}{[HA]}$$

Rearrange as follows (remember to change signs):

$$-\log[H^+] = -\log K_a + \log \frac{[A^-]}{[HA]}$$

Substitute pH for $-\log[H^+]$ and pK_a for $-\log K_a$.

$$pH = pK_a + \log \frac{[A^-]}{[HA]}$$

2. The saline solution of 0.9% NaCl was 0.9 g/dL. Since 10 dL = 1 L, this is 9 g/L. Since 1 g = 1,000 mg, and 1 L = 1,000 mL, the saline solution was also 9 mg/mL.

5 Relationship of Organic Chemistry to Biochemistry

The underlying principle of biochemistry is that every aspect of life involves chemical reactions between biological molecules. These reactions obey the laws of physics and chemistry. In addition to carbon (C), the organic molecules of the body also contain hydrogen (H), oxygen (O), nitrogen (N), sulfur (S), and phosphorus (P). These atoms are joined together by covalent bonds. The properties of these atoms dictate the types of reactions that can occur.

In addition to covalent bonds, weaker interactions may allow one portion of a molecule to associate with another portion of the same molecule or these interactions may cause one molecule to associate with other molecules.

The functional groups of molecules affect their solubility and reactivity. Compounds containing charged or polar groups dissolve more readily in water than do compounds containing uncharged or nonpolar groups. Functional groups of opposite polarity tend to react with each other. The compounds of the body undergo a number of different types of reactions that are catalyzed by enzymes.

 Dianne Beatty was hospitalized in diabetic ketoacidosis. After 10 hours of rehydration with intravenous saline solutions and hourly infusions of insulin, her ketoacidosis is improved, and she has regained consciousness. Her blood glucose level has fallen from 648 to 282 mg/dL (fasting reference range = 80–100) and her arterial blood pH has risen from 7.08 to 7.29 (reference range = 7.37–7.43). Her serum bicarbonate (HCO_3^-) level, which was 13 mEq/L on admission to the emergency room, has increased to 20 mEq/L (reference range = 24–28).

BIOLOGICAL COMPOUNDS

The molecules of the body consist mainly of the elements carbon, hydrogen, oxygen, nitrogen, sulfur, and phosphorus which are joined together by covalent bonds. The key element is carbon, which has a tetrahedral structure and can form covalent bonds with other carbon atoms and also with atoms of hydrogen, oxygen, nitrogen, and sulfur. Phosphorus is usually linked to carbon by an oxygen atom. Single and double bonds join the atoms of these elements in various combinations to form a large number of compounds of different degrees of complexity (Fig. 5.1).

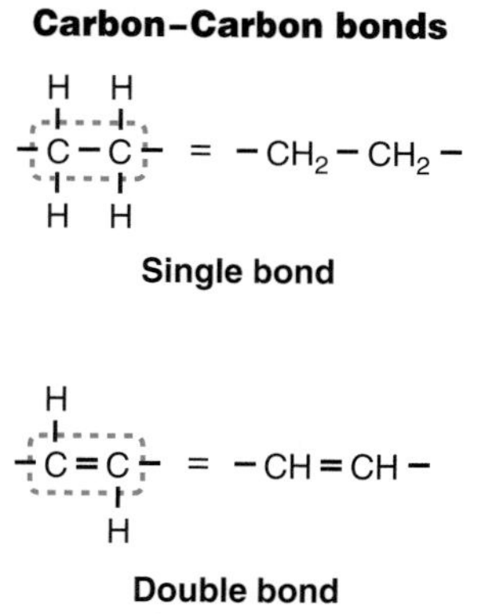

FUNCTIONAL GROUPS

Figure 5.2 shows the major functional groups found in the molecules of the body. These groups are responsible for many of the properties of biomolecules, including their solubility and reactivity. They include hydroxyl groups (sometimes called alcohols), aldehydes, ketones, carboxylic acids, ethers, acid anhydrides, sulfhydryl groups, amines, carbonyl groups, esters, thioesters, phosphoesters, and amides.

Functional groups are often part of the common name of a compound. For

Carbon–Carbon bonds

$$-\overset{\overset{\displaystyle H}{|}}{C}-\overset{\overset{\displaystyle H}{|}}{C}- \;=\; -CH_2-CH_2-$$

Single bond

$$-\overset{\overset{\displaystyle H}{|}}{C}=\overset{\overset{\displaystyle H}{|}}{C}- \;=\; -CH=CH-$$

Double bond

Fig. 5.1. Examples of single and double bonds.

Di Beatty has a metabolic acidosis resulting from an increased hepatic production of ketone bodies. Although her condition has improved with treatment, screening tests using the nitroprusside reaction for the presence of ketones in her blood and urine are still positive.

43

5.1: The ketone bodies synthesized in the liver are acetoacetic acid and β-hydroxybutyric acid. At physiological pH, these compounds form their conjugate bases, acetoacetate and β-hydroxybutyrate.

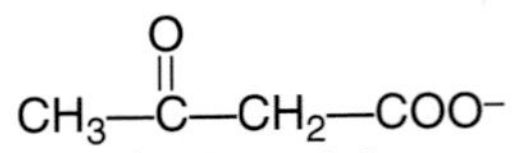

$$CH_3—\overset{\overset{\text{O}}{\|}}{C}—CH_2—COO^-$$
Acetoacetate

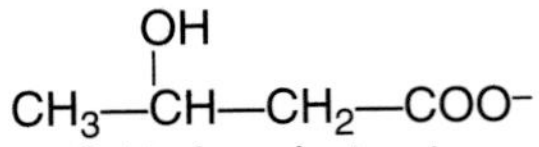

$$CH_3—\overset{\overset{\text{OH}}{|}}{CH}—CH_2—COO^-$$
β-Hydroxybutyrate

A third ketone body, acetone, is formed by the nonenzymatic decarboxylation of acetoacetate.

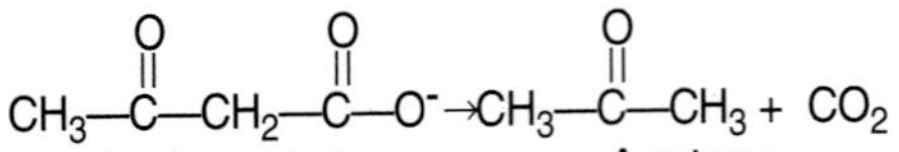

$$CH_3—\overset{\overset{\text{O}}{\|}}{C}—CH_2—\overset{\overset{\text{O}}{\|}}{C}—O^- \rightarrow CH_3—\overset{\overset{\text{O}}{\|}}{C}—CH_3 + CO_2$$
Acetoacetate   Acetone

Ketotic patients, like **Di Beatty**, produce acetone, which has a characteristic smell. Their breath is sometimes described as having a "sweet mousy" odor.

What functional groups do the ketone bodies contain?

A **5.1:** Acetoacetate contains a ketone group and a carboxyl group; β-hydroxybutyrate contains a hydroxyl group and a carboxyl group; and acetone contains a ketone group. Because β-hydroxybutyrate does not contain a ketone group, the general term for these compounds, ketone bodies, is really a misnomer.

Q **5.2:** Which of these compounds is glycerol, and which is glyceraldehyde?

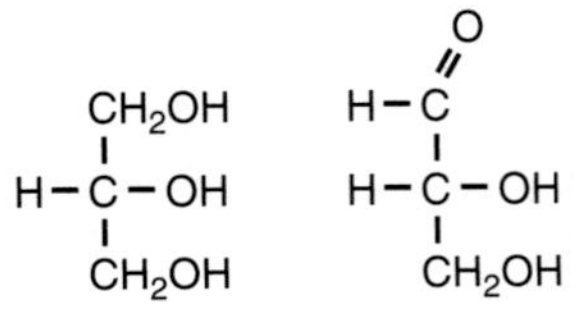

$$\begin{array}{cc} CH_2OH & H-\overset{\overset{\text{O}}{\|}}{C} \\ H-\overset{|}{\underset{|}{C}}-OH & H-\overset{|}{\underset{|}{C}}-OH \\ CH_2OH & CH_2OH \\ \mathbf{A} & \mathbf{B} \end{array}$$

Carbon–Oxygen groups

$-CH_2\!-\!\boxed{OH}$
Alcohol

$\boxed{\overset{\overset{\text{O}}{\|}}{C}-H}$
Aldehyde

$-CH_2\!-\!\boxed{\overset{\overset{\text{O}}{\|}}{C}}\!-\!CH_2-$
Ketone

$\boxed{\overset{\overset{\text{O}}{\|}}{C}-OH}$
Carboxylic acid

$\boxed{\overset{|}{\underset{|}{C}}-O-\overset{|}{\underset{|}{C}}}$
Ether

$\boxed{\overset{\overset{\text{O}}{\|}}{C}-O-\overset{\overset{\text{O}}{\|}}{C}}$
Acid anhydride

Carbon–Sulfur groups

$-\overset{|}{\underset{|}{C}}-\boxed{SH}$
Sulfhydryl group

$-\overset{|}{\underset{|}{C}}-\boxed{S-S}-\overset{|}{\underset{|}{C}}-$
A disulfide

Carbon–Nitrogen groups

$-CH_2-CH_2\!-\!\boxed{NH_2}$
Amino group

$-CH_2\!-\!\boxed{\overset{\overset{CH_3}{|}}{\underset{\underset{CH_3}{|}}{N^+}}-CH_3}$
Quaternary amine

Esters and Amides

$\boxed{\overset{\overset{\text{O}}{\|}}{C}-O-CH_2}-$
Ester

$\boxed{\overset{\overset{\text{O}}{\|}}{C}-S-CH_2}-$
Thioester

$HO\!-\!\boxed{\overset{\overset{\text{O}}{\|}}{\underset{\underset{OH}{|}}{P}}-O-\overset{|}{C}}$
Phosphoester

$\boxed{\overset{\overset{\text{O}}{\|}}{C}-NH}-$
Amide

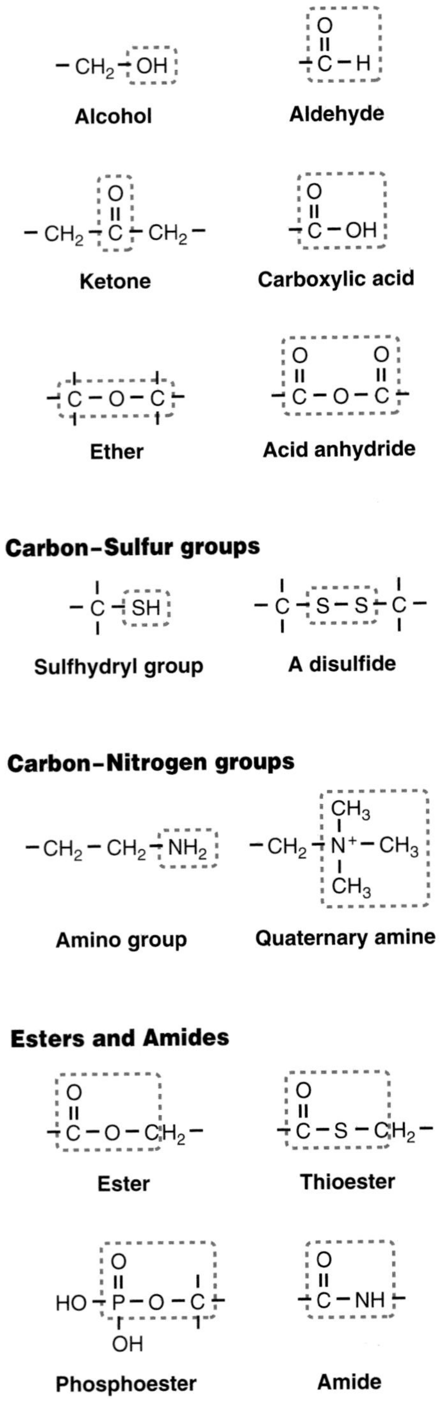

Fig. 5.2. Types of chemical groups commonly found in biochemical compounds.

instance, a ketone might have a name which ends in "one," like acetone, and a compound that contains a hydroxyl (alcohol) group (OH) might end in "ol." The presence of a carbonyl (acyl) group (the C=O in an ester or amide linkage) is also usually incorporated into the name. For example, the fat stores of the body are tri**acyl**glycer**ol**s. Three **acyl** groups are esterified to glycer**ol** (a compound that contains alcohol groups). Sugars, for the most part, end in "ose," as in gluc**ose**. Enzymes usually end in "ase."

Groups That Carry a Charge

Acidic groups contain a proton that can dissociate, leaving the remainder of the molecule with a negative charge (see Chapter 4). The major acidic compounds in the body contain carboxyl groups, phosphate groups, or sulfate groups (Fig. 5.3).

Compounds containing nitrogen are usually basic and may acquire a positive charge. Nitrogen has 5 electrons in its valence shell. If only 3 of these electrons form covalent bonds with other atoms, the nitrogen has no charge. If the remaining 2 electrons form a bond (e.g., with a proton or a carbon atom), the nitrogen carries a positive charge (Fig. 5.4).

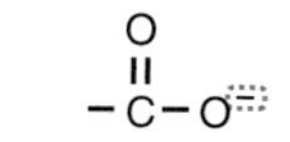

Carboxyl group

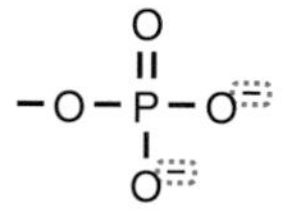

Phosphate group

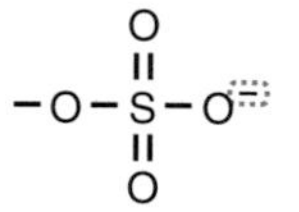

Sulfate group

Fig. 5.3. Examples of negatively charged groups.

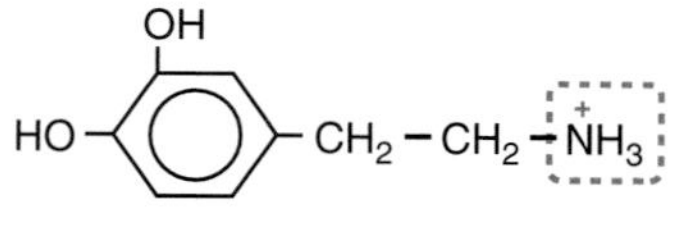

Dopamine (a primary amine)

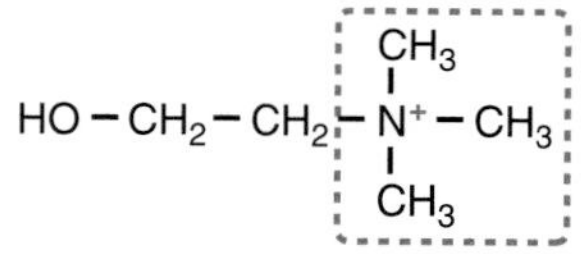

Choline (a quaternary amine)

Fig. 5.4. Examples of positively charged groups.

Polarity of Bonds and Partial Charges

Covalent bonds result from the sharing of electrons between 2 atoms to complete their electron shells. In carbon-carbon bonds and carbon-hydrogen bonds, the electrons are shared almost equally between the carbon atoms, or between the carbon and hydrogen atoms. The bond is, thus, nonpolar. Polar bonds occur when the electron cloud is more dense around 1 atom, the atom with the greater electronegativity. Oxygen is more electronegative than carbon, and in a carbon-oxygen bond (—C=O) the electron cloud is centered on the oxygen atom. Therefore, the oxygen atom has a partial negative charge, indicated by the symbol δ^-, and the carbon atom has a partial positive charge, indicated by the symbol δ^+. Nitrogen and sulfur are also more electronegative than carbon or hydrogen (Fig. 5.5).

Fig. 5.5. Partial charges on carbon-oxygen, carbon-nitrogen, and carbon-sulfur bonds.

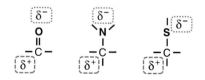

Solubility

Water is a very polar molecule. It participates in biochemical reactions both as a reactant and as a catalyst. As described in Chapter 4, the oxygen atom of a water molecule is far more electronegative than are the hydrogen atoms. Therefore, the oxygen has a partial negative charge, and each hydrogen has a partial positive charge. Water has a lattice-like structure in which the oxygen of a water molecule attracts the hydrogens of other water molecules.

In order for molecules to be soluble in water, they must contain charged or polar bonds which can associate with the partial positive and negative charges of water. Water diminishes the interactions between negative and positive charges of other molecules (i.e., electrostatic or ionic interactions). Thus, salt (NaCl) is able to dissociate into separate Na^+ and Cl^- ions and dissolve in an aqueous environment. Organic compounds that contain hydrophilic (water-loving) groups also tend to dissolve in water. Hydroxyl groups on glucose, for instance, are polar and make glucose almost infinitely soluble in water. The water molecules interacting with a polar or ionic compound form a hydration shell around the compound.

Compounds or regions of compounds that are nonpolar cannot be attracted to the partial positive and negative charges on water molecules and are, therefore, water insoluble. These nonpolar regions of compounds are termed hydrophobic (water-fearing). They tend to cluster together in an aqueous environment because they cannot form energetically favorable interactions with water.

A 5.2: "B" contains an aldehyde group, and is glyceraldehyde. "A" is glycerol. It contains three alcohol groups.

Amphipathic molecules contain both polar and nonpolar regions. For example, phospholipids are composed of a hydrophobic (nonpolar) "tail" region, usually derived from long chain fatty acids, and a hydrophilic (polar) "head" region which contains a phosphate group with a negative charge and, in some instances, a group with a positive charge. This difference in the regions at the two ends of phospholipid molecules causes them to concentrate at interfaces between aqueous and nonaqueous phases within the cell. Their role as the primary constituents of cellular membranes will be considered in more detail in Chapter 10.

Reactivity

The consequence of bond polarity is that atoms which carry a partial (or full) negative charge will be attracted to atoms which carry a partial (or full) positive charge, and vice versa. These partial or full charges dictate the course of biochemical reactions—which follow the same principles of electrophilic and nucleophilic attack characteristic of organic reactions in general.

For example, the oxidation of fatty acids begins by their conversion to thioesters of coenzyme A (CoASH). Because this process is energy-requiring, it occurs in two steps. In the first step, the acid reacts with adenosine triphosphate (ATP) to form an adenosine monophosphate (AMP) derivative. In the second step, the sulfur atom of CoASH, which has a partial negative charge, attacks the carboxyl carbon, which has a partial positive charge (Fig. 5.6).

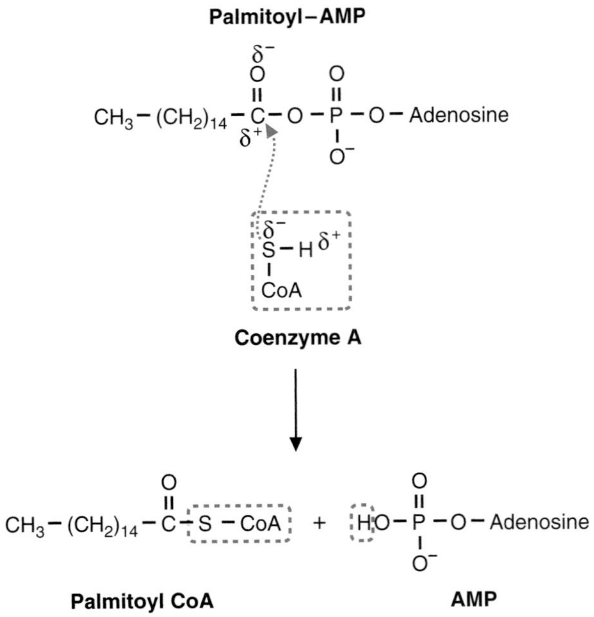

The steps of biochemical reactions follow the same general mechanisms as ordinary chemical reactions. However, because of enzymes, nature's protein catalysts, they can occur faster.

Fig. 5.6. Formation of a fatty acyl CoA.

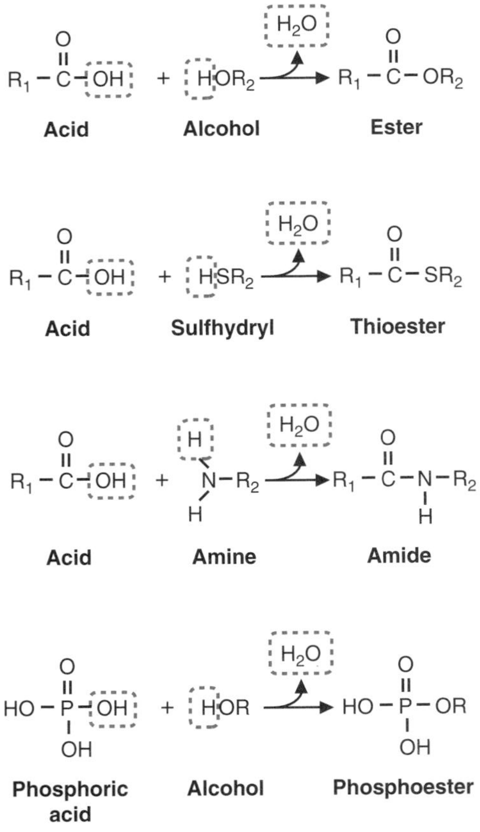

Fig. 5.7. Formation of esters, thioesters, amides, and phosphoesters.

The partial positive charge on the carboxyl carbon accounts for many of the reactions of carboxylic acids. An ester is formed when a carboxylic acid and an alcohol react, splitting out water. Similarly, a thioester is formed when an acid and a sulfhydryl group react. An amide is formed when an acid reacts with an amine. Similar reactions result in the formation of a phosphoester from phosphoric acid and an alcohol, and by the reaction of two acids to produce anhydrides (Figs. 5.7 and 5.8).

EXAMPLES OF TYPES OF REACTIONS

Five types of reactions occur frequently in metabolism: group transfer, cleavage, condensation, rearrangement, and oxidation-reduction reactions.

Group Transfer Reactions

One type of group transfer reaction that occurs is phosphorylation, that is, a phosphate group is transferred from one compound to another. The source of the phosphate group is often ATP, which transfers one of its phosphate groups to a hydroxyl group on the other compound, thus forming a phosphoester (see Fig. 5.7). After glucose enters a cell, for example, it is phosphorylated by ATP (Fig. 5.9).

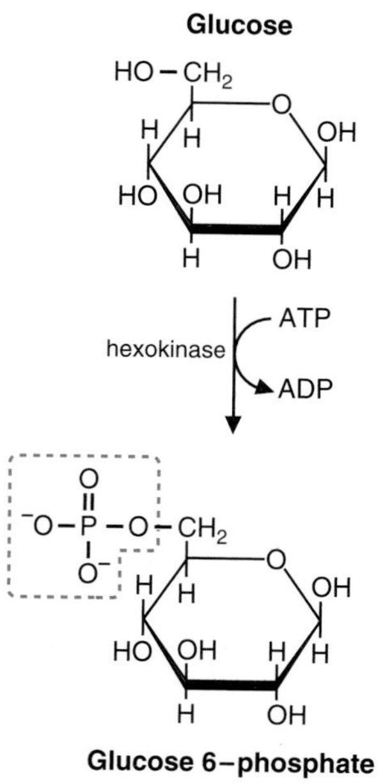

Cleavage Reactions

Bonds in compounds are often cleaved by the addition of water. Specifically, as shown in Figure 5.10, the components of a water molecule are added to the 2 atoms involved in the bond, which is thereby broken. This reaction is the reverse of the reaction in Figure 5.9, except that phosphate is released in the form of inorganic phosphate (HPO_3^{2-}; abbreviated P_i) instead of being used directly to reconstitute ATP from ADP.

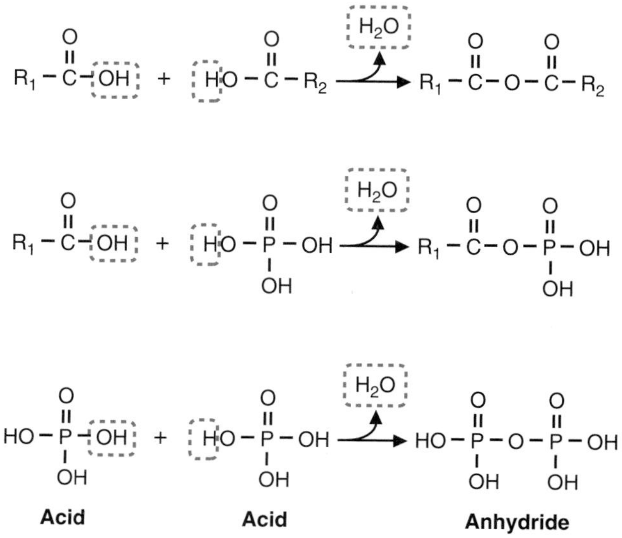

Fig. 5.9. A group transfer reaction: the phosphorylation of glucose.

Fig. 5.8. Formation of anhydrides.

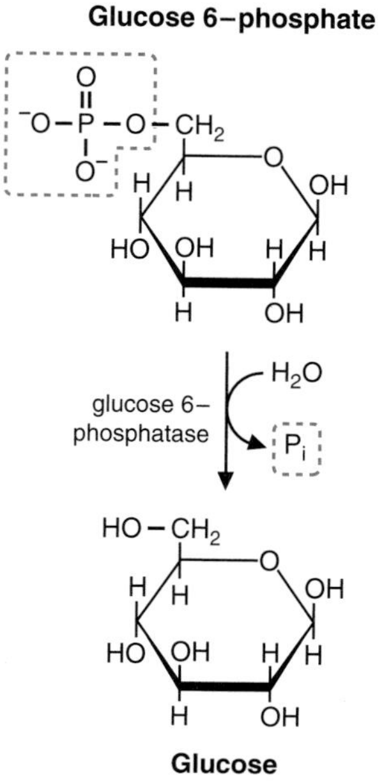

Fig. 5.10. A cleavage reaction: the hydrolysis of glucose 6-phosphate. P_i = inorganic phosphate.

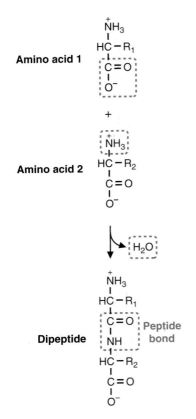

Condensation Reactions

Compounds usually condense by eliminating water. For example, 2 amino acids condense to form a peptide bond (a type of amide). In the body, this condensation occurs by a very complex mechanism. A simple overview is shown in Figure 5.11. The details of the process are described in Chapter 14.

Rearrangement Reactions

The bond structure in a compound can rearrange to produce a different compound. For example, aldehydes may rearrange to form ketones (Fig. 5.12).

Oxidation-Reduction Reactions

The carbon atoms in organic molecules have different oxidation states, depending on whether they are involved in single or double bonds, or whether they are part of an alcohol, aldehyde, ketone, or carboxylic acid group. The oxidation of a molecule involves the loss of electrons.

The most common way of oxidizing organic molecules in the body is through a reaction in which electrons are transferred from a compound to an electron acceptor (Fig. 5.13). The electrons may be transferred as hydrogen with its electrons (the hydrogen atom, H•) or the hydride ion (a hydrogen atom with 2 electrons, H:). The compound losing electrons is oxidized, and the electron acceptor, which is usually an electron-accepting coenzyme, is reduced in this process (Fig. 5.13). Thus the carbons in a double bond have a higher oxidation state than do the carbons in a single bond, and the carbon atom in an aldehyde group has a higher oxidation state than does the carbon in an alcohol group.

Another way animals oxidize compounds is through the direct addition of oxygen or a hydroxyl group, using oxygen atoms obtained from O_2. In these reactions, O_2 is the electron acceptor and is reduced to H_2O or H_2O_2.

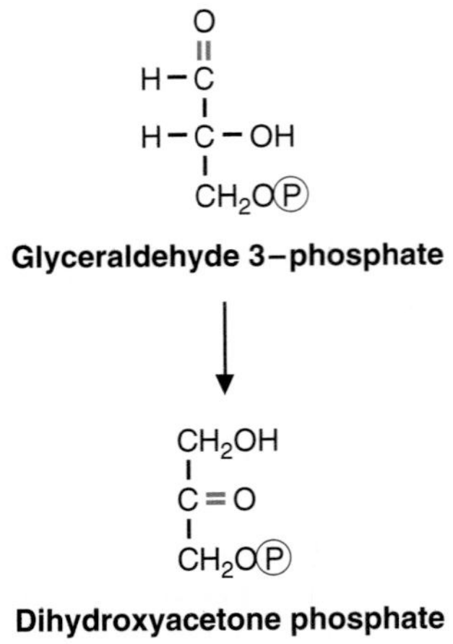

Fig. 5.11. A condensation reaction: the formation of a peptide bond.

Fig. 5.12. A rearrangement reaction: the conversion of glyceraldehyde 3-phosphate to dihydroxyacetone phosphate. circled P = phosphate group.

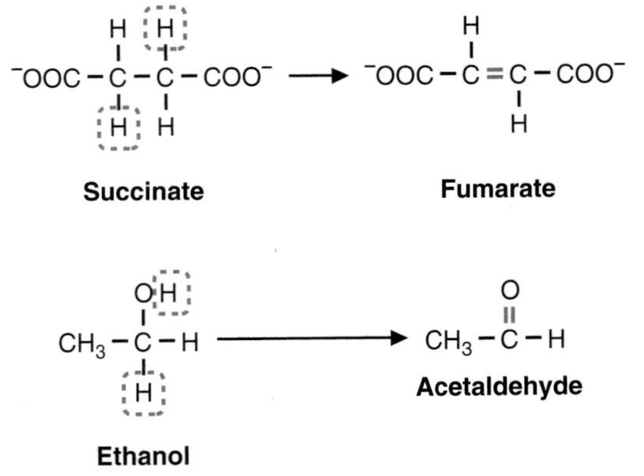

Fig. 5.13. Oxidation-reduction reactions: the oxidation of succinate to fumarate and of ethanol to acetaldehyde. In each case, hydrogens and electrons are transferred to an electron acceptor, and the compound is oxidized. Ethanol is an alcohol.

NOMENCLATURE

Use of Trivial Names

In biochemistry, the common or trivial names of compounds are used rather than the systematic nomenclature favored by organic chemists. Sometimes such names reflect the source from which the compound was first isolated.

Identification of Carbon Atoms

Biochemists use two systems for the identification of the carbons in a chain. In the first system, the carbons in a compound are numbered, starting with the carbon in the most oxidized group. In the second system, the carbons are given Greek letters, starting with the carbon **next** to the most oxidized group. Hence, the compound in Figure 5.14 is known as 3-hydroxybutyrate or β-hydroxybutyrate.

 In biochemistry, you will encounter compounds with names such as acetate, glutamate, palmitate, pyruvate, lecithin, pantothenic acid, arachidonic acid, and taurocholic acid. Applying systematic names to these compounds, many of which are very complex, would make them far more difficult to remember than the trivial names, which eventually give them a personality.

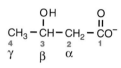

Fig. 5.14. Two systems for identifying the carbon atoms in a compound. This compound may be called 3-hydroxybutyrate or β-hydroxybutyrate.

 CLINICAL COMMENTS. The severity of clinical signs and symptoms in patients, such as **Di Beatty**, with diabetic ketoacidosis (DKA) is directly correlated with the concentration of ketone bodies in the blood. Direct quantitative methods for measuring acetoacetate and β-hydroxybutyrate are not routinely available. As a result, clinicians usually rely on semiquantitative reagent strips (Ketostix) or tablets (Acetest) to estimate the level of acetoacetate in the blood and the urine. The nitroprusside on the strips and in the tablets reacts with acetoacetate and to a lesser degree with acetone (both of which have ketone groups) but does not react with β-hydroxybutyrate (which does not have a ketone group). Since β-hydroxybutyrate is the predominant ketone body present in the blood of a patient in DKA and since its concentration may decline at a disproportionately rapid rate compared to the concentrations of acetoacetate and acetone following appropriate therapy, tests employing the nitroprusside reaction to monitor the success of therapy in such patients may be misleading.

 BIOCHEMICAL COMMENTS. Many students "memorize" biochemistry, which is an overwhelming task. Biochemistry is much easier to learn (and remember) if it is viewed as a series of predictable chemical reactions. During evolution, cells did not devise a totally new set of chemical reactions whenever they developed a new function. Instead, they adapted existing reactions, applying them to new sets of compounds. (A less anthropomorphic but more precise explanation for this phenomenon involves the transfer of certain domains (or regions) of previously existing enzymes to newly developed enzymes during evolution by recombinational events at the level of the gene.) Successful students usually recognize these patterns of reactions and look for their repetition.

 5.3: Which of the following compounds is more reduced and which is more oxidized?

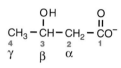

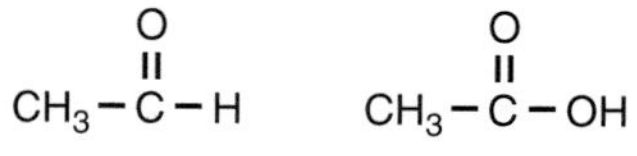

A   B

Suggested Readings

This chapter is a review of certain aspects of organic chemistry related to biochemistry. Therefore, if you need more extensive explanations, try thumbing through your old, well-worn organic chemistry textbook from your undergraduate course.

PROBLEMS

1. What do you think the "β" means in the pathway of β-oxidation of fatty acids?

 5.4: In patients in diabetic ketoacidosis, such as **Di Beatty**, the liver produces the ketone bodies acetoacetate and β-hydroxybutyrate which appear in elevated levels in the blood. What type of reaction is involved in the conversion of β-hydroxybutyrate to acetoacetate?

A 5.3: "B" is acetic acid, and it is more oxidized than acetalde-hyde ("A"). The carboxyl carbon contains more oxygen, relative to hydrogen, than does the aldehyde carbon. To count electrons for the purpose of determining an oxidation state, the electrons in carbon-oxygen bonds are not counted with the carbon, but with the oxygen. Thus the carboxyl carbon has fewer electrons (compared to the aldehyde carbon) and has lost electrons to oxygen.

A 5.4: Acetoacetate is enzymatically reduced to form β-hydroxy-butyrate. The electrons are transferred from the electron donor, NADH + H$^+$ to acetoacetate.

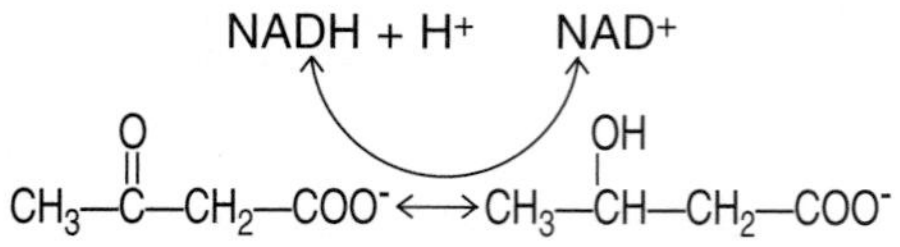

NADH + H$^+$ NAD$^+$

CH$_3$–C–CH$_2$–COO$^-$ ⟷ CH$_3$–CH–CH$_2$–COO$^-$

Acetoacetate   β-Hydroxybutyrate

This reaction is reversible, and β-hydroxybutyrate may be oxidized to form acetoacetate.

2. Compound A and compound B shown below are both vitamins. Which is water-soluble and which is water-insoluble?

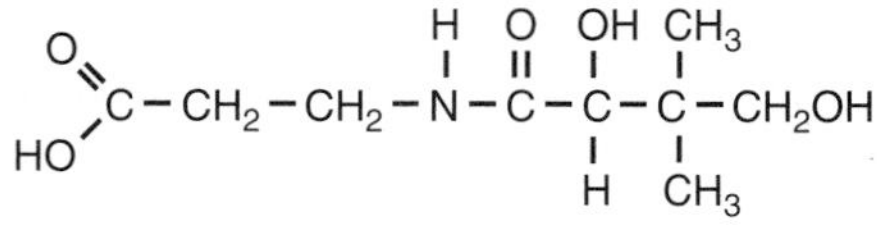

Compound A

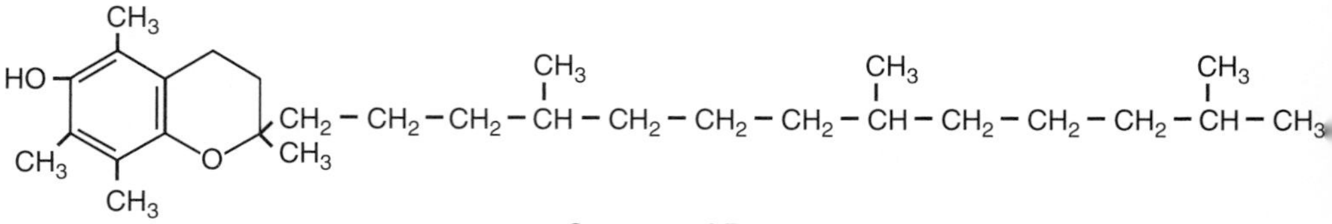

Compound B

ANSWERS

1. The reactions in β-oxidation involve the β-carbon of the fatty acyl group.

CH$_3$—(CH$_2$)$_{14}$—CH$_2$—CH$_2$—C~SCoA

2. Compound A is pantothenic acid, a water-soluble vitamin. At physiological pH, the carboxylic acid dissociates into an H$^+$ and a negatively charged carboxylate ion (pantothenate). The carboxylate group, the alcohol groups, the amide N, and the carbonyl group are polar and can hydrogen bond with H$_2$O.

Compound B is the fat-soluble vitamin E. The long nonpolar side chain and the nonpolar ring structure prevent it from associating with water and dissolving.

6 Structures of the Major Compounds of the Body

The body contains compounds of great structural diversity, ranging from relatively simple molecules such as sugars and amino acids to enormously complex polymers such as proteins and nucleic acids. The structures of these compounds are intimately related to their physiological functions.

In this chapter, we will describe the structures of the major carbohydrates, lipids, and nucleotides. The structures of amino acids, proteins, and the nucleic acids will be mentioned briefly and covered in more detail in subsequent chapters. Because the structures of the vitamins are so complex and diverse, they will be described in the sections related to their role in metabolism.

Carbohydrates, commonly known as sugars, are divided into four different classes according to their size: monosaccharides, disaccharides, oligosaccharides, and polysaccharides. Monosaccharides, such as glucose, galactose, and fructose, are the smallest sugars. They may be joined together by glycosidic bonds to form the other classes of carbohydrates. Disaccharides, such as sucrose, maltose, and lactose, each consist of 2 monosaccharides joined by a glycosidic bond. Oligosaccharides, such as the carbohydrate components of glycoproteins and glycolipids, contain from 3 to about 12 monosaccharide units. Polysaccharides, such as starch and glycogen, contain tens to thousands of monosaccharide units.

Although the major function of carbohydrates is to serve as a source of fuel for the body, they also serve as precursors for the synthesis of lipids, amino acids, glycolipids, glycoproteins, and proteoglycans.

The structures of lipids are very heterogeneous. Their common feature is their hydrophobicity; they are not very soluble in water. Lipids serve as the major source of fuel for the body, and they also function as components of membranes and as precursors for the synthesis of compounds such as bile salts and eicosanoids. The major lipids of the human body are the fatty acids, which are often found esterified to glycerol, forming compounds such as triacylglycerols (triglycerides) or phosphoacylglycerols (phosphoglycerides). In the sphingolipids, serine, rather than glycerol, is the precursor of the backbone to which fatty acids are attached. Polyunsaturated fatty acids are the precursors of the eicosanoids (the prostaglandins, thromboxanes, and leukotrienes).

Cholesterol, the major steroid in the body, is the precursor of other compounds that contain the steroid nucleus, such as the bile salts and the steroid hormones. In animals, isoprene units, used in the synthesis of cholesterol, are also precursors for the synthesis of dolichol and ubiquinone (coenzyme Q).

Amino acids are the monomeric units of proteins. Each amino acid contains a carboxyl group, an amino group, and a side chain, all attached to the α-carbon. Amino acids are joined by peptide bonds to form the linear chains of proteins. Proteins have many roles in the body. They serve, for example, as enzymes, hormones, cell surface receptors, antibodies, and contractile elements.

A nucleoside is composed of a nitrogenous base and a sugar. The addition of phosphate produces a nucleotide. One, two, or three phosphate groups may be linked to the sugar to form nucleoside mono-, di-, and triphosphates, respectively. Nucleotides, particularly ATP, serve to transfer energy from one compound to another. They also are the monomeric units of the nucleic acids.

A solution frequently used for intravenous infusions is a 5% solution (5 g/100 mL) of D-glucose. It is sometimes called dextrose, an old name for glucose.

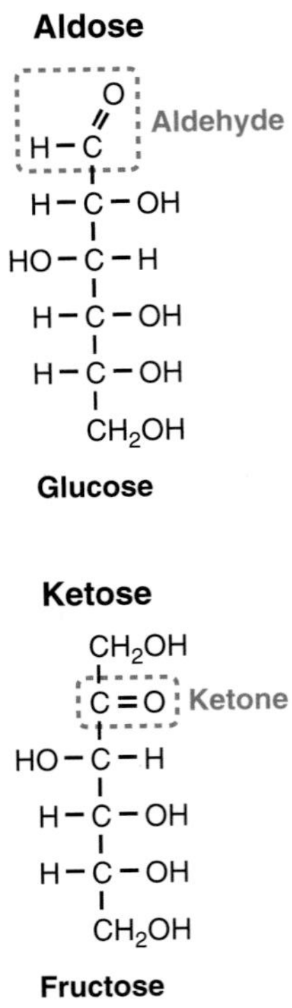

Aldose

H – C (=O) Aldehyde
H – C – OH
HO – C – H
H – C – OH
H – C – OH
CH₂OH

Glucose

Ketose

CH₂OH
C = O Ketone
HO – C – H
H – C – OH
H – C – OH
CH₂OH

Fructose

Fig. 6.1. An aldose and a ketose. Aldoses contain an aldehyde group and ketoses contain a ketone group.

Di Beatty recovered from her bout of diabetic ketoacidosis and was discharged from the hospital. She has returned for a follow-up visit as an outpatient. She reports that she has been compliant with her recommended American Diabetes Association diet and that she faithfully gives herself insulin by subcutaneous injection twice daily. Her serum glucose levels are monitored in the hospital laboratory approximately every 2 weeks, and she self-monitors her blood glucose levels every other day.

Yves Topaigne is a 47-year-old man who came to the physician's office complaining of a severe throbbing pain in the right great toe that began 8 hours earlier. The toe has suffered no trauma but appears red and swollen. It is warmer than the surrounding tissue and is exquisitely tender to even light pressure. Mr. Topaigne is unable to voluntarily flex or extend the joints of the digit and passive motion of the joints causes great pain.

CARBOHYDRATES

Monosaccharides

A monosaccharide, the smallest sugar unit, may be represented as a straight chain of carbon atoms, one of which forms a carbonyl group via a double bond with oxygen. The other carbons of a monosaccharide usually contain hydroxyl groups. If the carbonyl group is an aldehyde, the sugar is called an aldose. A sugar with a ketone group is called a ketose (Fig. 6.1). In the most common monosaccharides, the number of carbons ranges from 3 (called trioses) to 7 (called heptoses). Those with 4, 5, and 6 carbons are called tetroses, pentoses, and hexoses, respectively (Fig. 6.2).

D- and L-Sugars

A carbon atom that contains four different chemical groups forms an asymmetric (or chiral) center (Fig. 6.3). The triose glyceraldehyde has one asymmetric carbon. Therefore, there are two different optically active isomers (or enantiomers), D-glyceraldehyde and L-glyceraldehyde (Fig. 6.4).

Other monosaccharides are designated D or L, depending on the configuration of the asymmetric carbon farthest from the carbonyl group (the aldehyde or ketone group). Those with the same configuration as D-glyceraldehyde belong to the D series and those similar to L-glyceraldehyde belong to the L series (Fig. 6.5). Because most

To monitor her own blood glucose levels, **Di Beatty** pricks her finger with a lancet to obtain a drop of blood. The blood is placed on a reagent strip which, through a color change, gives a close estimate of her blood glucose concentration.

The suffix "-emia" (from the Greek "haima" meaning blood) is used to indicate that a compound is present in the blood. The prefix "hyper-" indicates that the concentration of the compound is high, and "hypo-" indicates that it is low. Thus, hyperglycemia means that the blood glucose level is high and hypoglycemia means that it is low.

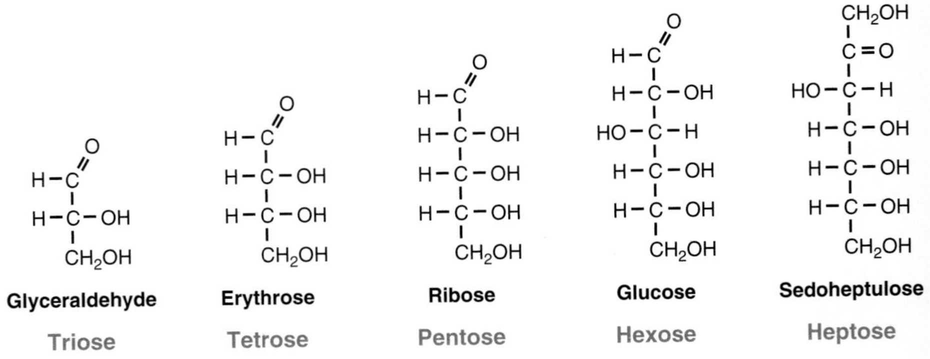

H – C (=O)
H – C – OH
CH₂OH

Glyceraldehyde

Triose

H – C (=O)
H – C – OH
H – C – OH
CH₂OH

Erythrose

Tetrose

H – C (=O)
H – C – OH
H – C – OH
H – C – OH
CH₂OH

Ribose

Pentose

H – C (=O)
H – C – OH
HO – C – H
H – C – OH
H – C – OH
CH₂OH

Glucose

Hexose

CH₂OH
C = O
HO – C – H
H – C – OH
H – C – OH
H – C – OH
CH₂OH

Sedoheptulose

Heptose

Fig. 6.2. Examples of monosaccharides.

of the sugars in living organisms belong to the D series, sugars are assumed to be D-isomers unless L is specifically indicated. Thus, "glucose" refers to D-glucose, the major sugar in human blood.

STEREOISOMERS, ENANTIOMERS, AND EPIMERS

Stereoisomers have the same chemical formula but differ in the position of the hydroxyl group on one or more of their asymmetric carbons (Fig. 6.6). A sugar with n asymmetric centers has 2^n stereoisomers unless it has a plane of symmetry.

Enantiomers are stereoisomers that are mirror images of each other. D-Glyceraldehyde and L-glyceraldehyde are enantiomers (see Fig. 6.4), as are D-glucose and L-glucose. No matter how the D and L forms of a sugar are rotated, their atoms cannot be superimposed.

Epimers are stereoisomers that differ in the position of the hydroxyl group at only one of their asymmetric carbons. D-Glucose and D-galactose are epimers, differing only at position 4 (Fig. 6.7).

RING STRUCTURES

Although monosaccharides are often represented as straight chains, they exist in solution mainly as ring structures in which the carbonyl (aldehyde or ketone) group has reacted with a hydroxyl group in the same molecule, forming a ring. Hexoses, such as the aldohexose, glucose, and the ketohexose, fructose, form either six-membered rings (called pyranoses) or five-membered rings (called furanoses) (Fig. 6.8). The

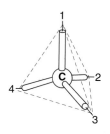

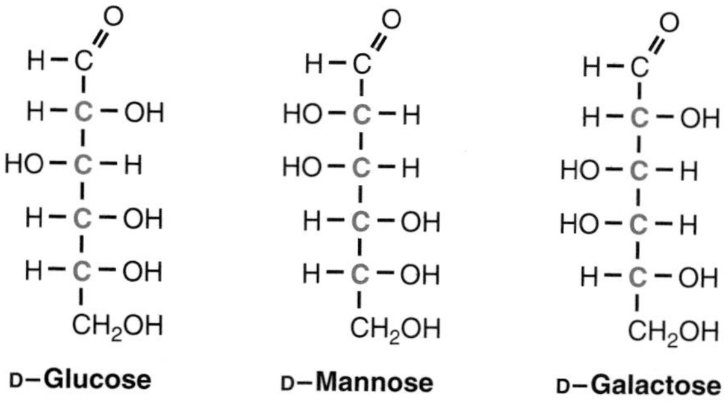

Fig. 6.3. An asymmetric carbon atom. The carbon atom (C) contains four different substituent groups (1, 2, 3, 4). The four single bonds formed by the carbon atom with its substituents have a tetrahedral arrangement.

D–Glyceraldehyde   L–Glyceraldehyde

Fig. 6.4. The simplest D- and L-sugars.

D–Glucose   D–Mannose   D–Galactose

Fig. 6.6. Examples of stereoisomers. These compounds have the same chemical formula ($C_6H_{12}O_6$) but differ in the positions of the hydroxyl groups on their asymmetric carbons (in blue).

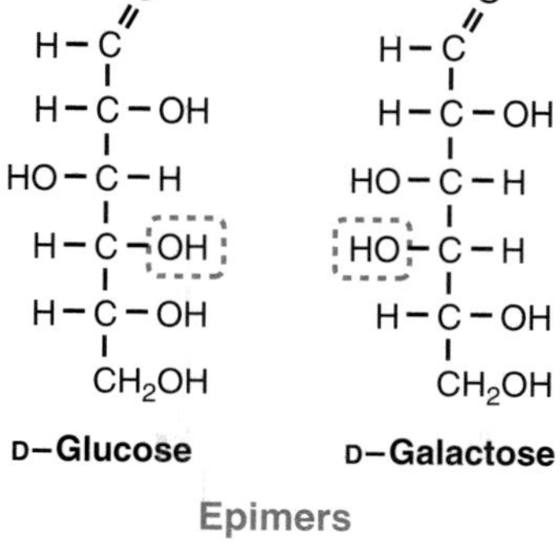

D–Glucose   D–Galactose

Epimers

Fig. 6.7. Epimers. These sugars differ only in the position of the hydroxyl group on one asymmetric carbon.

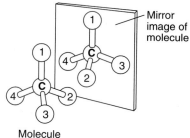

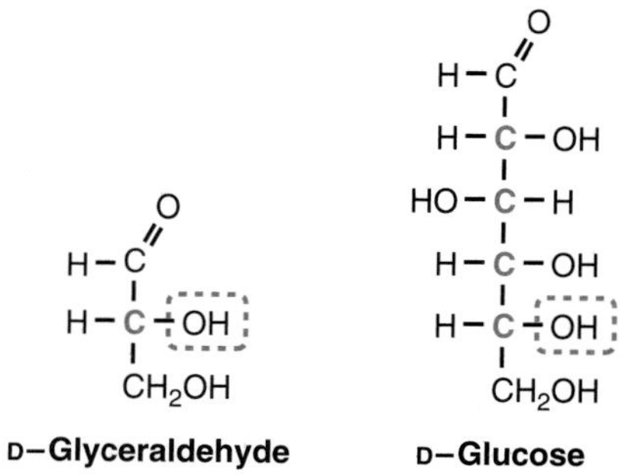

D–Glyceraldehyde   D–Glucose

Fig. 6.5. D-Glyceraldehyde and D-glucose. These sugars have the same configuration at the asymmetric carbon atom farthest from the carbonyl group. They both belong to the D series. Asymmetric carbons are shown in blue.

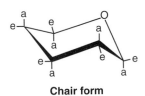

Chair form

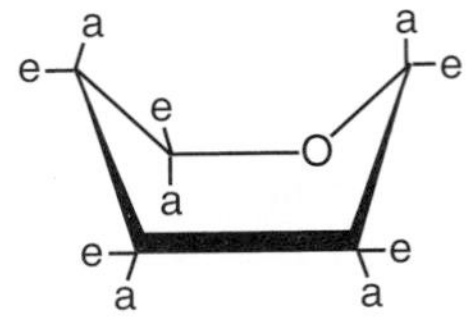

Boat form

Fig. 6.9. Chair and boat forms of pyranose rings. Axial substituents (a) are essentially perpendicular to the plane of the ring while equatorial substituents (e) are parallel.

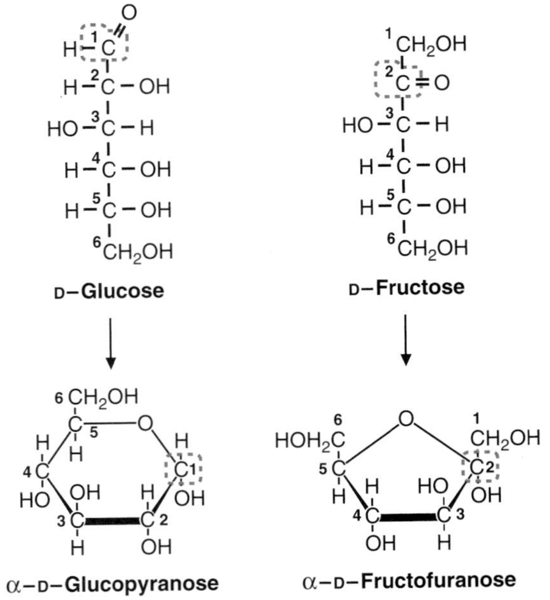

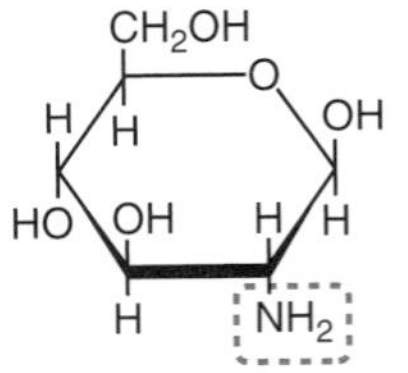

β−D−**Glucosamine**

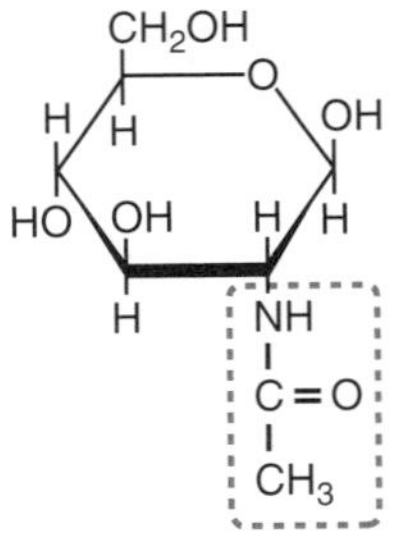

N−Acetyl−β−D−**glucosamine**

Fig. 6.11. An amino and an *N*-acetylated sugar.

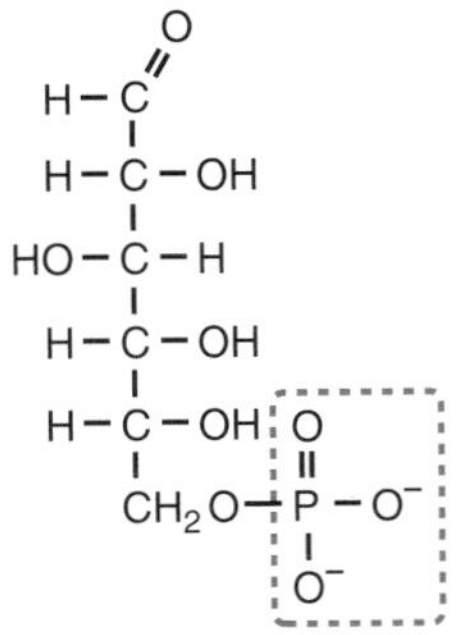

D−**Glucose**

D−**Fructose**

α−D−**Glucopyranose**

α−D−**Fructofuranose**

Fig. 6.8. Pyranose and furanose rings formed from glucose and fructose. The anomeric carbons are highlighted.

aldehyde or ketone carbon forms a hemiacetal or hemiketal, respectively, generating a new asymmetric center. The carbon atom of the original aldehyde or ketone group, which is now bound to oxygen within the ring, is known as the anomeric carbon. The sugars can be depicted more accurately as chair or boat forms (Fig. 6.9). In solution, the chair form predominates.

Sugars may exist either in α or in β configurations (Fig. 6.10). If the sugar is depicted with the ring in the plane of the paper, the hydroxyl group covalently attached to the anomeric carbon is in the α position if it is below the plane of the ring. In the β position, this hydroxyl group is above the plane.

In solution, the sugar ring can open and close. When it is open, the straight chain aldehyde or ketone is formed. When the ring recloses, the hydroxyl group on the anomeric carbon may be either in the α or the β position. The process by which the α and β forms equilibrate in solution is called mutarotation (see Fig. 6.10).

Mutarotation of free monosaccharides is enzymatically catalyzed in the cell and occurs rapidly. However, when the anomeric carbon joins the sugar to another compound, the bond is fixed in the α or the β configuration. Enzymes differentiate between these configurations and are specific for only one.

Glucose 6−phosphate

Fig. 6.12. A phosphorylated sugar.

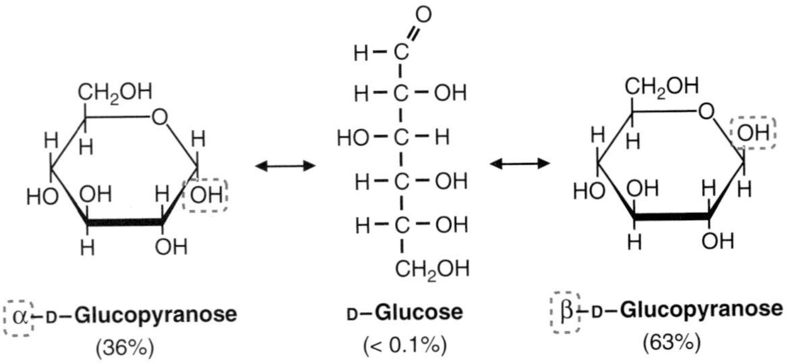

α−D−**Glucopyranose**
(36%)

D−**Glucose**
(< 0.1%)

β−D−**Glucopyranose**
(63%)

Fig. 6.10. Mutarotation of glucose in solution, with percentages of each form at equilibrium.

AMINO SUGARS

Sugars may contain amino groups (Fig. 6.11). Glucosamine and galactosamine are examples of amino sugars. The amino groups are often acetylated.

PHOSPHORYLATED SUGARS

Within cells, monosaccharides usually contain phosphate groups (Fig. 6.12). The addition of phosphate groups prevents sugars from crossing membranes. As a consequence of phosphorylation, sugars are "trapped" within the cell. When glucose enters cells, it is phosphorylated at position 6, forming glucose 6-phosphate.

Phosphate groups may join sugars to nucleosides. For example, glucose 1-phosphate may react with UTP to form UDP-glucose (Fig. 6.13).

SULFATED SUGARS

Some sugars contain sulfate groups, particularly the sugars of the glycosaminoglycans, such as chondroitin sulfate and heparin, which are major components of connective tissue (Fig. 6.14).

OXIDATION AND REDUCTION OF CARBOHYDRATES

In the body, the aldehyde group of a sugar or carbon 6 of a hexose is sometimes oxidized to a carboxylic acid. For example, glucose may be oxidized at carbon 1 to form gluconic acid or at carbon 6 to form glucuronic acid (Fig. 6.15).

Sugars that can be oxidized at carbon 1 are known as reducing sugars. As they are oxidized, they cause another compound to be reduced (see Biochemical Comments).

If the aldehyde group of a sugar (which contains the anomeric carbon) is reduced, the sugar becomes a polyalcohol (polyol). For example, glucose may be reduced to the corresponding polyol sorbitol, and galactose to galactitol (Fig. 6.16).

GLYCOSIDES

When the hydroxyl group on the anomeric carbon of a monosaccharide reacts with an —OH or an —NH group of another compound, glycosides are formed. The bonds joining the monosaccharides are called glycosidic or glycosyl bonds. The linkage may be either α or β, depending on the position of the atom attached to the anomer-

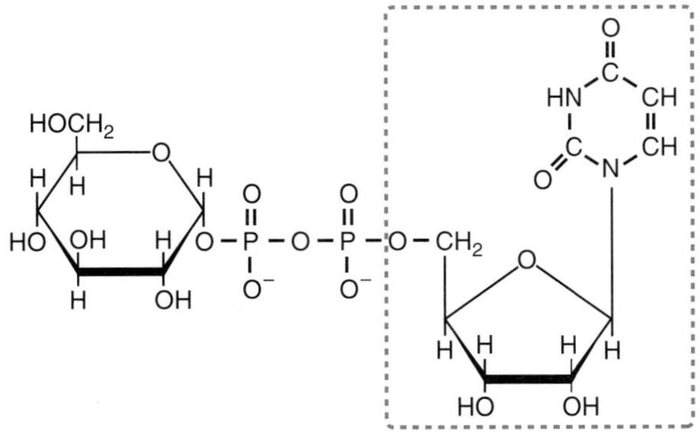

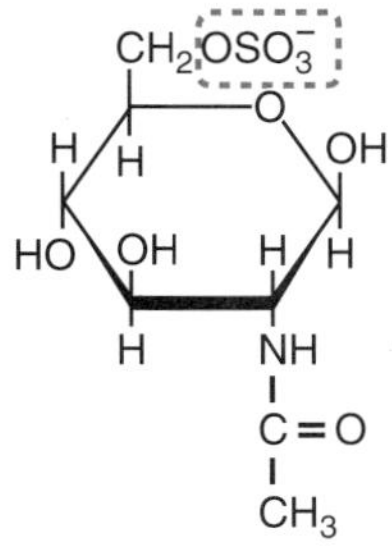

N–Acetylglucosamine 6–sulfate

Fig. 6.14. A sulfated sugar.

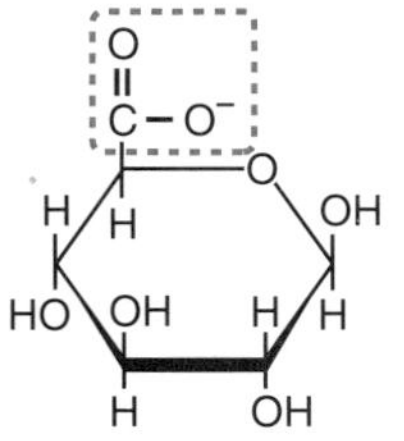

β–D–Glucuronate

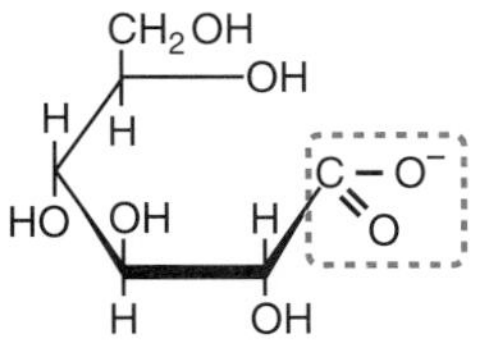

D–Gluconate

Fig. 6.15. Glucuronic and gluconic acids. Dissociation of the carboxyl group produces the salt forms glucuronate and gluconate.

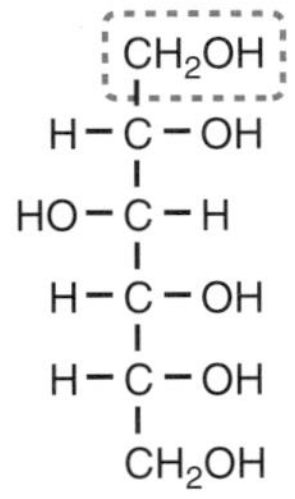

D–Sorbitol 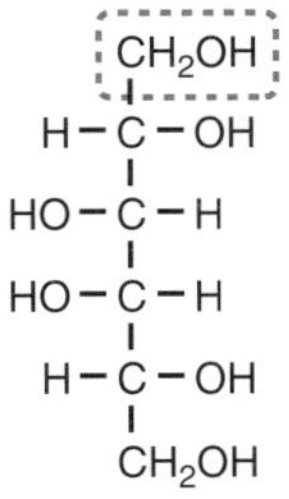   **D–Galactitol**

Fig. 6.16. Polyols.

**Uridine diphosphate glucose
(UDP-glucose)**

Fig. 6.13. Uridine diphosphate glucose (UDP-glucose). The nucleoside uridine is highlighted.

 6.1: How do sorbitol and galactitol differ?

6.2: Is the glycosidic bond of ATP in the α or the β configuration?

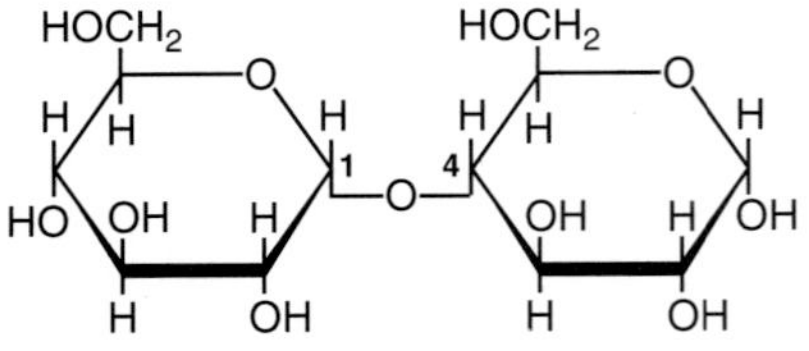

Maltose
(Glucose–α(1→4)–glucose)

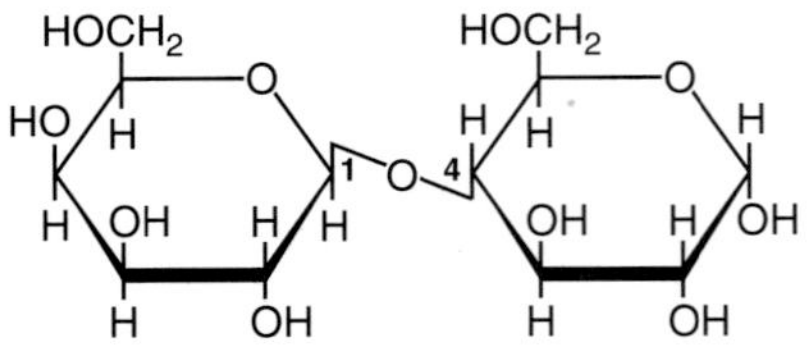

Lactose
(Galactose–β(1→4)–glucose)

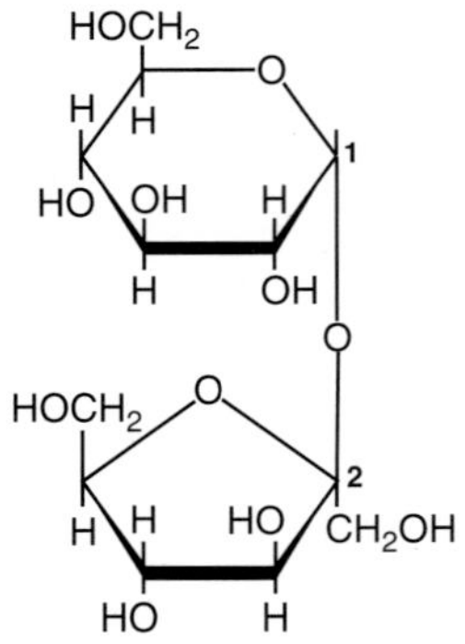

Sucrose
(Glucose–α(1→2)–fructose)

Fig. 6.18. The most common disaccharides. Maltose is produced during the digestion of starch. Lactose is milk sugar, and sucrose is table sugar.

6.1: Like their aldehyde forms glucose and galactose, sorbitol and galactitol differ only in the position of the hydroxyl group on carbon 4.

6.2: ATP has a β-glycosidic bond.

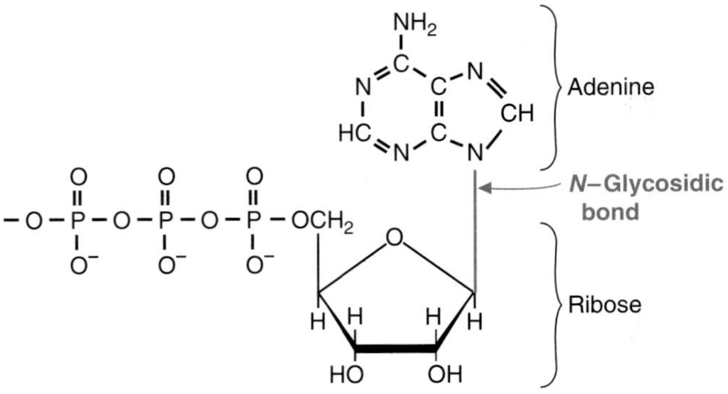

Fig. 6.17. The *N*-glycosidic bond of adenosine triphosphate (ATP).

ic carbon of the sugar. Monosaccharides may be joined together by *O*-glycosidic bonds to form disaccharides, oligosaccharides, and polysaccharides.

N-Glycosidic bonds are found in nucleotides. For example, in the adenosine moiety of ATP, the nitrogenous base adenine is linked to the sugar ribose via an *N*-glycosidic bond (Fig. 6.17). Because nucleotides are the monomeric units of nucleic acid polymers, *N*-glycosidic bonds join the sugars to the bases in DNA and RNA.

Disaccharides

A disaccharide contains two monosaccharides joined by an *O*-glycosidic bond. The most common disaccharides are maltose, lactose, and sucrose (Fig. 6.18). Maltose consists of 2 glucose units linked α(1→4). In lactose, a galactose and a glucose are linked β(1→4). In sucrose, glucose and fructose are joined α(1→2) through their anomeric carbons.

Oligosaccharides

Oligosaccharides are carbohydrates that contain from 3 to about 12 monosaccharides. They are found in the carbohydrate components of glycoproteins and glycolipids, and among the digestive products of starch. Proteins that are secreted from cells, such as the immunoglobulins and the blood clotting proteins, usually contain oligosaccharide chains and, therefore, are glycoproteins. The carbohydrate groups of the glycoproteins and glycolipids embedded in the cell membrane are located on the extracellular surface.

Polysaccharides

Polysaccharides contain tens to thousands of monosaccharides joined by glycosidic bonds. They exist as linear chains or as branched structures.

STARCH

Starch, the storage form of carbohydrates in plants, contains amylose and amylopectin. Amylose is composed of long, unbranched chains of glucose units linked α(1→4). Amylopectin is composed of α(1→4) linked chains of glucose units that are joined together at branch points via α(1→6) linkages (Fig. 6.19). Amylopectin is similar to glycogen except that it has fewer branches.

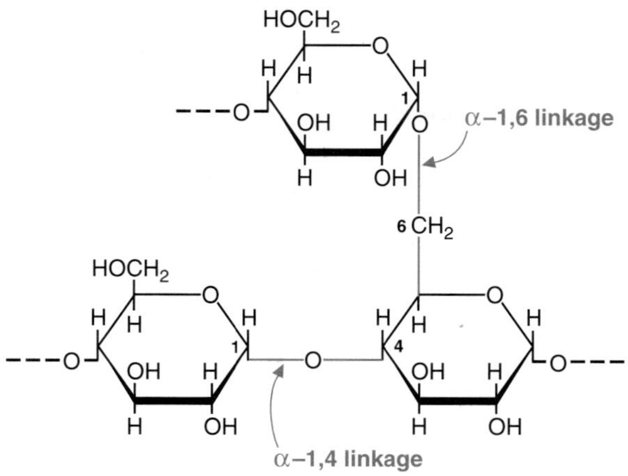

HOCH$_2$

α–1,6 linkage

$_6$CH$_2$

HOCH$_2$

α–1,4 linkage

Fig. 6.19. α-1,4 and α-1,6 linkages between glucose residues in starch and glycogen.

GLYCOGEN

Glycogen, the storage form of carbohydrates in animals, is a large, branched poly-saccharide composed of glucose residues (Fig. 6.20). In overall structure, each glyco-gen molecule resembles a tree. The linkage between the glucose units is $\alpha(1\rightarrow4)$ except at branch points where the linkage is $\alpha(1\rightarrow6)$. Branches are more frequent in the interior of the molecule, occurring about every 4 glucose residues. At the periph-ery, branching is less frequent so that, in each molecule, branches occur an average of every 8–10 residues.

A glycogen molecule contains only one glucose residue that does not have its anomeric carbon attached to another glucose residue. The portion of the molecule containing this glucose residue is known as the reducing end. The glucose residue at the reducing end is linked to a protein known as glycogenin. All the other glucose residues of glycogen contain anomeric carbons that are involved in forming glyco-sidic bonds with other glucose residues. The ends of the chains that contain glucose residues in glycosidic linkage are known as the nonreducing ends.

Q 6.3: How many nonreducing ends does a glycogen molecule have?

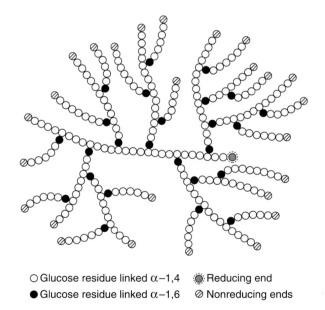

○ Glucose residue linked α–1,4   ◉ Reducing end
● Glucose residue linked α–1,6   ⊘ Nonreducing ends

Fig. 6.20. Structure of glycogen.

A 6.3: A glycogen molecule con-tains only one reducing end but many nonreducing ends, one on every branch. The reactions of glycogen synthesis and degradation occur at the nonreducing ends of the branches. (See Biochemical Comments for an explana-tion of the term "reducing sugar.")

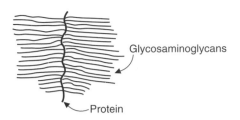

Fig. 6.21. "Bottle brush" structure of a proteoglycan.

Margarine, the major source of most *trans* fatty acids found in humans, is produced by the chemical hydrogenation of vegetable oils, which have a high content of polyunsaturated fatty acids.

PROTEOGLYCANS

Proteoglycans are composed of long, unbranched polysaccharide chains (glycosaminoglycans), radiating from a core protein and forming a structure that resembles a bottle brush (Fig. 6.21). Proteoglycans are found in the extracellular matrix, the synovial fluid of joints, the vitreous humor of the eye, secretions of mucus-producing cells, and in cartilage.

LIPIDS

Fatty Acids

Fatty acids are straight aliphatic chains with a methyl group at one end (the ω-carbon) and a carboxyl group at the other end (Fig. 6.22). Most fatty acids in the human have an even number of carbon atoms, usually between 16 and 20. They may be saturated or unsaturated (Fig. 6.23).

Monounsaturated fatty acids contain one double bond, and polyunsaturated fatty acids contain two or more double bonds (Fig. 6.24). The position of a double bond is indicated by the number of the first carbon involved in the bond. For example, oleic acid, which contains 18 carbon atoms and a double bond between positions 9 and 10, may be indicated as $18:1,\Delta^9$. The number 18 indicates the number of carbon atoms, 1 (one) indicates the number of double bonds, and the Δ and superscript indicate the position of the double bond (Table 6.1). Sometimes the Δ is omitted, and oleic acid is indicated as 18:1(9). Fatty acids may also be classified by the distance of the first double bond from the ω-carbon. Oleic acid is, thus, an ω9 fatty acid. Arachidonic acid, which has 20 carbon atoms and four double bonds, may be described as $\omega6,20:4,\Delta^{5,8,11,14}$.

The double bonds in most naturally occurring fatty acids are in the *cis* configuration (Fig. 6.25). The designation *cis* means that the acyl chains are on the same side of the double bond. *Trans* means that the acyl chains are on opposite sides of the double bond.

The melting point of a fatty acid increases with chain length and decreases with the degree of unsaturation. Consequently, the fatty acid composition of membrane phospholipids determines the fluidity of membranes at body temperature.

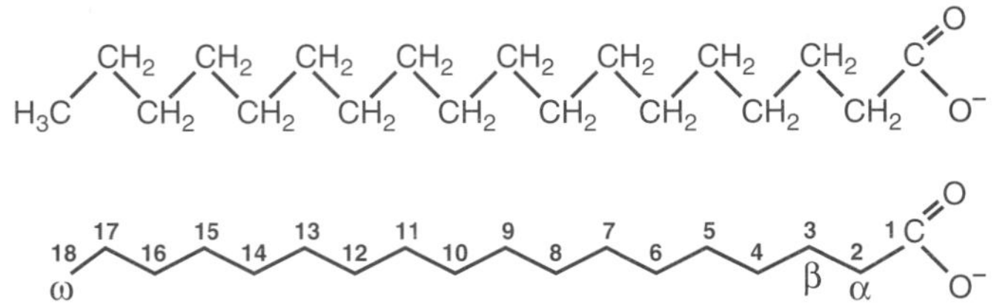

Stearic acid
18:0

Fig. 6.22. A saturated fatty acid. In the molecule at the top, all the atoms are shown. Another way of depicting the same structure is shown below. The carbons are numbered starting with the carboxyl group, or they are given Greek letters starting with the carbon next to the carboxyl group. The methyl (or ω) carbon at the end of the chain is always called the ω-carbon regardless of the chain length. 18:0 refers to the number of carbon atoms (18) and the number of double bonds (0).

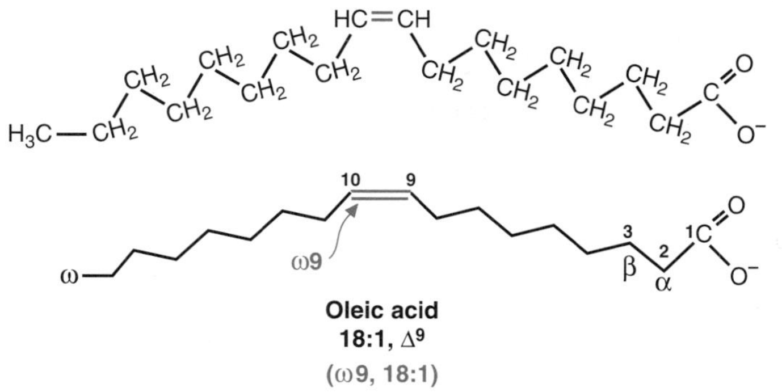

Oleic acid
18:1, Δ⁹
(ω9, 18:1)

Fig. 6.23. An unsaturated fatty acid. Two methods for depicting the same molecule are shown. 18:1,Δ⁹ means that oleic acid has 18 carbons and one double bond (Δ⁹). The double bond is at position 9 (between carbons 9 and 10). It is also at the ninth carbon from the ω-end (ω9).

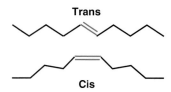

Fig. 6.25. *Cis* and *trans* double bonds in fatty acid chains. Note that the *cis* double bond causes the chain to bend.

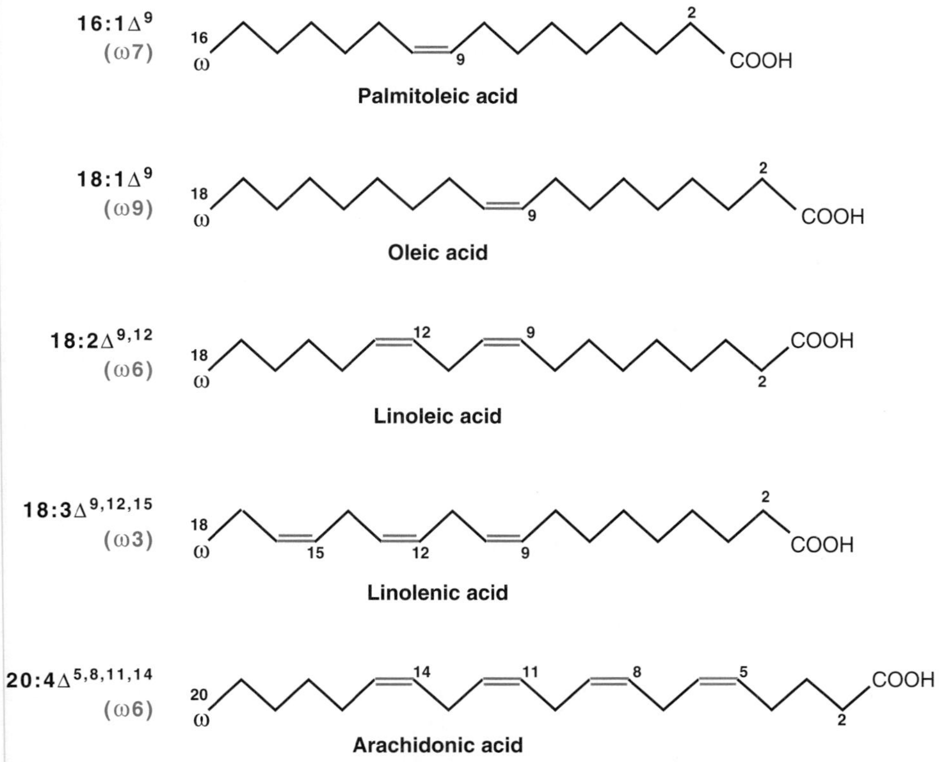

16:1Δ⁹
(ω7)
Palmitoleic acid

18:1Δ⁹
(ω9)
Oleic acid

18:2Δ⁹,¹²
(ω6)
Linoleic acid

18:3Δ⁹,¹²,¹⁵
(ω3)
Linolenic acid

20:4Δ⁵,⁸,¹¹,¹⁴
(ω6)
Arachidonic acid

Fig. 6.24. Some common unsaturated fatty acids. Note that the double bonds are *cis* and spaced at 3-carbon intervals.

Table 6.1. Names and Composition of Some Common Carboxylic Acids

Composition	Name	
1	Formic	Produced in body as acid or as CoA derivative
2:0	Acetic	
3:0	Propionic	
4:0	Butyric	In food, particularly milk products such as butter
5:0	Valeric	
6:0	Caproic	
8:0	Caprylic	
10:0	Capric	
12:0	Lauric	In food of plant origin
14:0	Myristic	
16:0	Palmitic	Product of fatty acid synthesis
$16:1\Delta^9$	Palmitoleic	Produced from palmitic acid
18:0	Stearic	
$18:1\Delta^9$	Oleic	
$18:2\Delta^{9,12}$	Linoleic	Essential fatty acids; obtained from plant oils
$18:3\Delta^{9,12,15}$	Linolenic	
$20:4\Delta^{5,8,11,14}$	Arachidonic	Produced from linoleic acid; precursor of eicosanoids

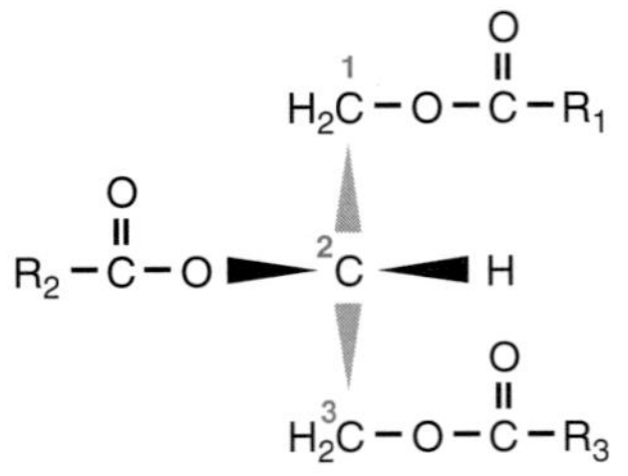

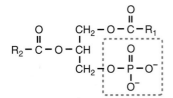

Triacyl–*sn*–glycerol

Fig. 6.26. A triacylglycerol. Note that carbons 1 and 3 of the glycerol moiety are not identical.

Acylglycerols

Fatty acids react with alcohol (hydroxyl) groups to form esters (Fig. 6.26). The three hydroxyl groups of glycerol can react with fatty acids to form monoacylglycerols, diacylglycerols, and triacylglycerols, which contain 1, 2, or 3 fatty acids esterified to glycerol, respectively. A triacylglycerol rarely contains the same fatty acid at all three positions. Therefore, they are "mixed" triacylglycerols.

In the three-dimensional configuration of glycerol, carbons 1 and 3 are not identical (see Fig. 6.26). Enzymes are usually specific for carbon 1 or for carbon 3.

Phosphoacylglycerols

Phosphoacylglycerols contain fatty acids esterified to positions 1 and 2 of glycerol and a phosphoryl group at position 3. If only a phosphate group is attached to position 3, the compound is known as a phosphatidic acid (Fig. 6.27). Phosphatidic acids are intermediates in the synthesis of triacylglycerols and phosphoacylglycerols.

Compounds derived from phosphatidic acid that contain substituents on the phosphate group include the most common phosphoacylglycerols: phosphatidylcholine (lecithin), phosphatidylethanolamine, and phosphatidylserine (Fig. 6.28). These compounds are major components of cellular membranes. The removal of a fatty acid from these compounds produces a lysophosphoacylglycerol, e.g., lysolecithin (Fig. 6.29).

Phosphatidylinositol bisphosphate is another important membrane component (Fig. 6.30). It is cleaved in response to extracellular signals to form diacylglycerol and inositol trisphosphate, which serve as intracellular signals known as second messengers (see Section VIII).

Sphingolipids

Sphingolipids are derivatives of ceramide, which is synthesized from serine, palmitic acid, and an additional fatty acid (Fig. 6.31). A sphingolipid does not contain a glycerol moiety. Phosphorylcholine is esterified to ceramide in sphingomyelin, and sugars are attached to ceramide in cerebrosides and gangliosides. Sphingolipids are major components of myelin and of the membranes of brain and other nervous tissue.

Phosphatidic acid

Fig. 6.27. Phosphatidic acid.

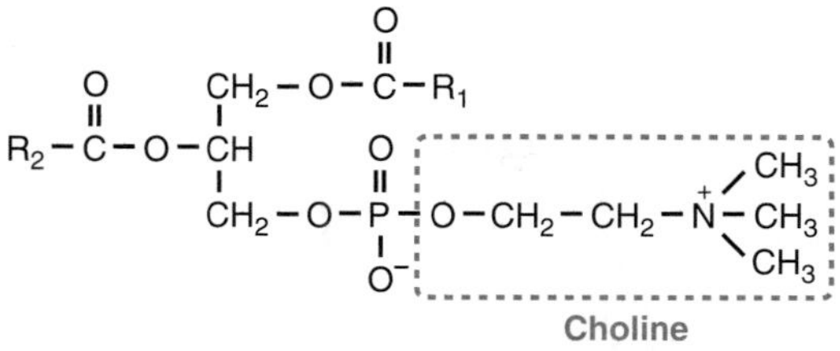

Phosphatidylcholine

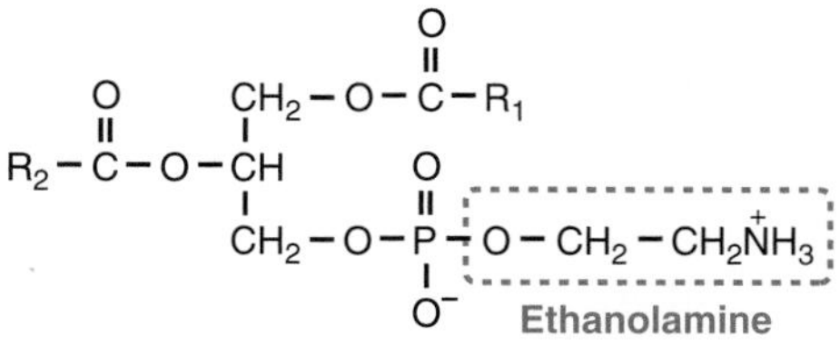

Phosphatidylethanolamine

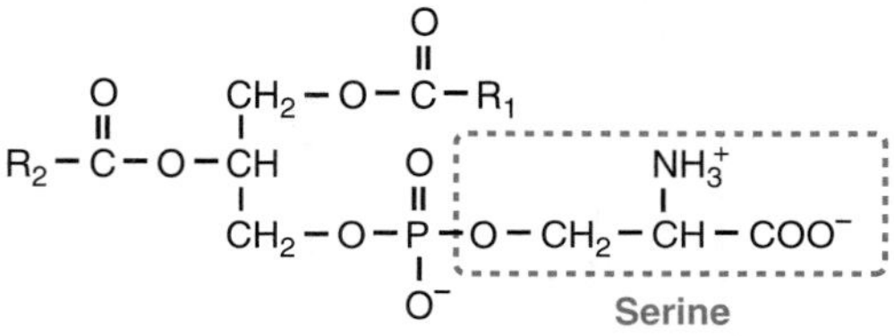

Phosphatidylserine

Fig. 6.28. The major phosphoacylglycerols.

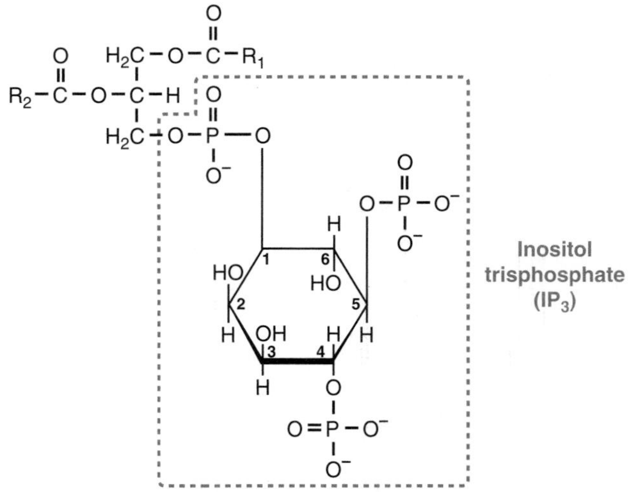

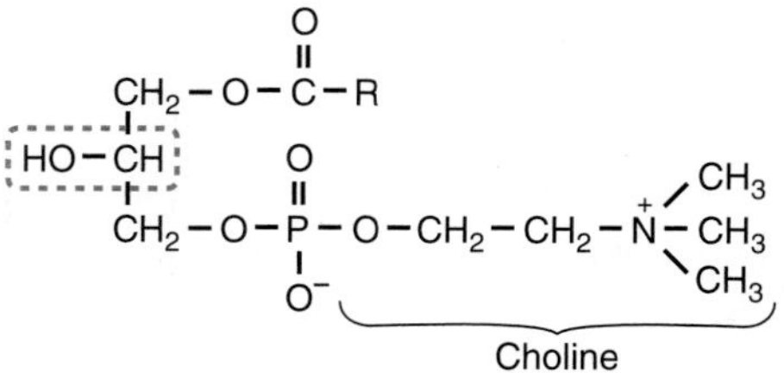

Lysolecithin

Fig. 6.29. Lysolecithin. This compound is produced by removal of a fatty acid from position 2 of the glycerol moiety of phosphatidylcholine (lecithin).

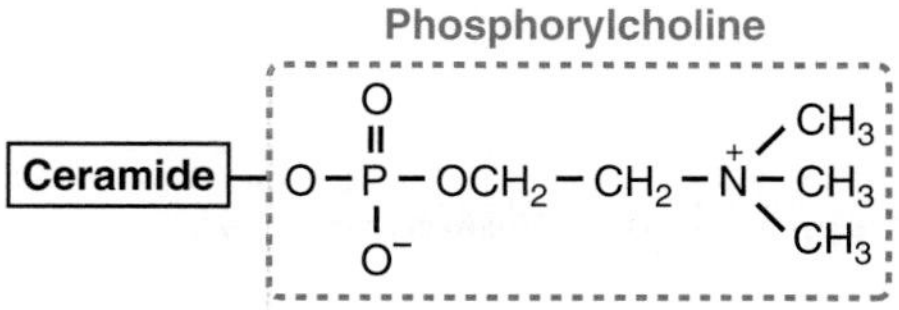

Sphingomyelin

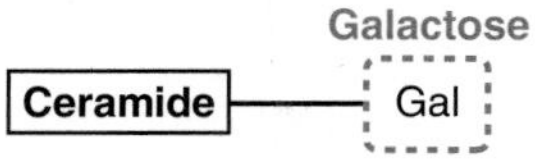

Galactocerebroside

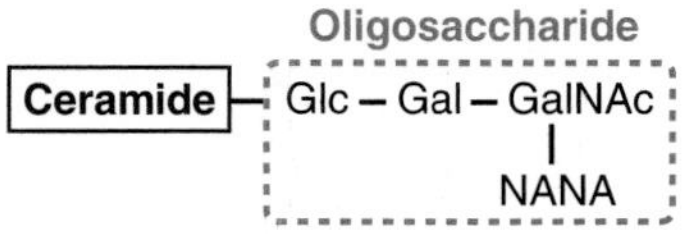

Ganglioside

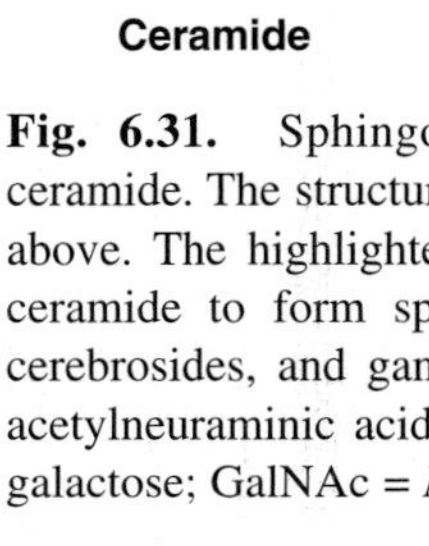

Ceramide

Fig. 6.31. Sphingolipids, derivatives of ceramide. The structure of ceramide is shown above. The highlighted groups are added to ceramide to form sphingomyelins, galactocerebrosides, and gangliosides. NANA = N-acetylneuraminic acid; Glc = glucose; Gal = galactose; GalNAc = N-acetylgalactosamine.

Phosphatidylinositol 4,5–bisphosphate (PIP$_2$)

Fig. 6.30. Phosphatidylinositol bisphosphate (PIP$_2$). PIP$_2$, a membrane phospholipid, is cleaved to form inositol trisphosphate (in blue) and diacylglycerol, which serve as second messengers.

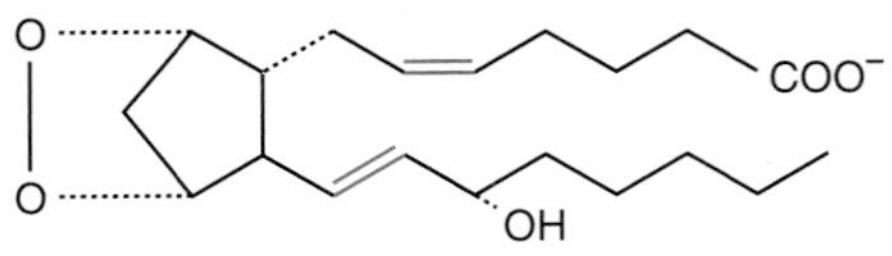

A prostaglandin (PGH$_2$)

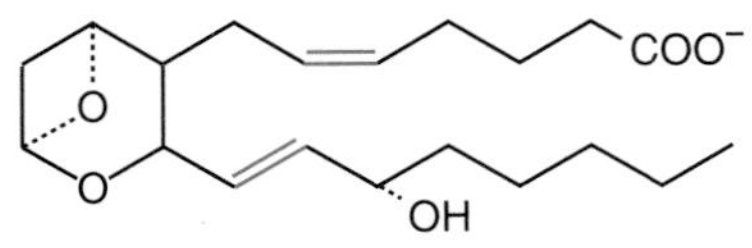

A thromboxane (TXA$_2$)

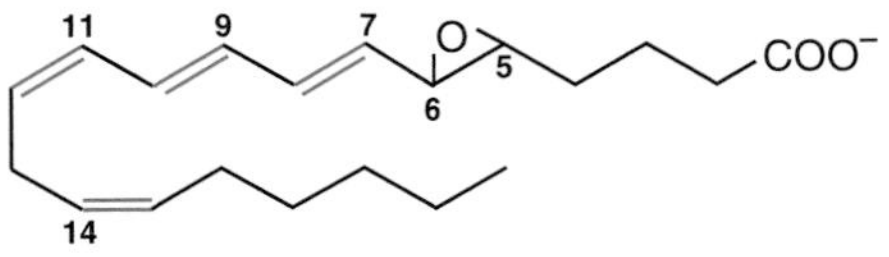

A leukotriene (LTA$_4$)

Fig. 6.32. Some eicosanoids.

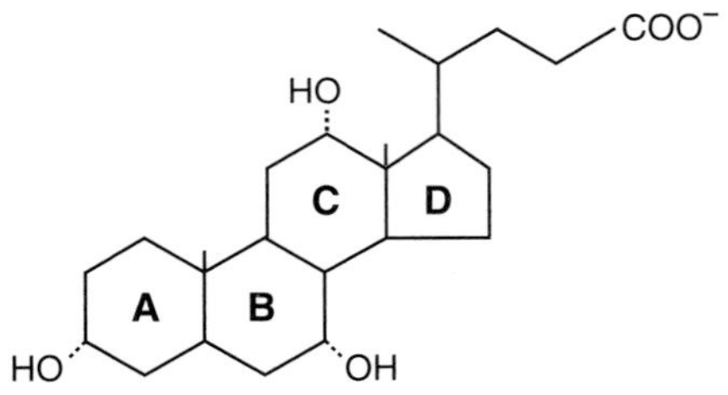

Cholic acid

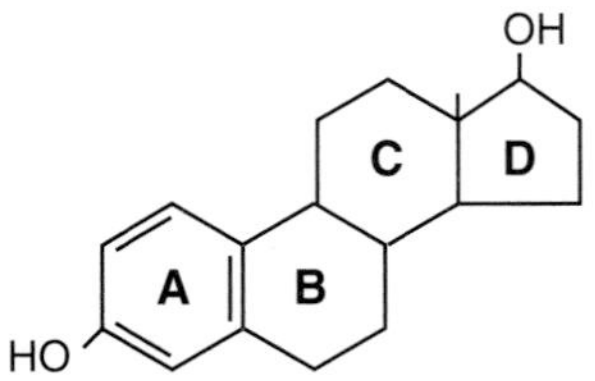

17β–Estradiol

Fig. 6.34. A bile salt (cholic acid) and a steroid hormone (17β-estradiol).

Q 6.4: Which portion of the bile salt cholic acid (see Fig. 6.34) is hydrophobic and which is hydrophilic?

Eicosanoids

The eicosanoids are a group of hormone-like compounds, produced by many cells in the body. They are synthesized from polyunsaturated fatty acids containing 20 carbon atoms (eicosanoic acids) with 3, 4, or 5 double bonds. The prostaglandins, thromboxanes, and leukotrienes belong to this group of compounds (Fig. 6.32).

Steroids

The steroids are a group of compounds that contain a structure with four rings known as the steroid nucleus. Cholesterol, which is synthesized in animals but not in plants, is the parent compound from which other steroids are produced in humans (Fig. 6.33). It is converted to bile salts, the adrenocortical steroids, and the sex hormones (Fig. 6.34).

The 3-hydroxyl group of cholesterol allows it to react with fatty acids, forming cholesterol esters. These esters are even less soluble than cholesterol and, therefore, are the form in which cholesterol is stored as droplets in cells. Cholesterol esters also are found in the blood lipoproteins.

The bile salts serve as good examples of the amphipathic nature of many lipids. Amphipathic compounds contain both hydrophobic and hydrophilic regions. Therefore, they are often found at the interface between lipids and water, their hydrophobic regions interacting with the lipid and their hydrophilic regions interacting with the water. Bile salts are good detergents, serving to emulsify the lipids in the digestive tract.

PROTEINS

Amino acids are the building blocks from which proteins are constructed. They also are oxidized for fuel and serve as precursors for the synthesis of other nitrogen-containing compounds, such as neurotransmitters, heme, and the purine and pyrimidine bases. The α-carbon of an amino acid contains a carboxyl group, an amino group, and a side chain (Fig. 6.35). Amino acids differ in the structure of their side chains (Fig. 6.36).

Proteins are synthesized from amino acids that are joined together by peptide bonds to form linear chains (Fig. 6.37). These chains fold in various ways to form the three-dimensional structure of a protein. The structures of amino acids and proteins are described in more detail in Chapters 7 and 8.

NUCLEOTIDES

A nucleotide is composed of a nitrogenous base, a sugar, and phosphate (Fig. 6.38). Two types of nitrogenous bases occur: the purines and the pyrimidines. The sugar, generally ribose or deoxyribose, is joined to the base by an N-glycosidic bond.

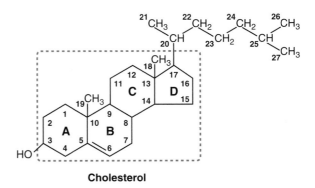

Cholesterol

Fig. 6.33. Cholesterol. The steroid nucleus is shown in blue.

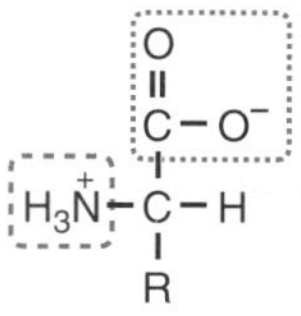

Fig. 6.35. General structure of an amino acid. The side chain (R) differs from one amino acid to another.

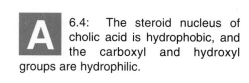

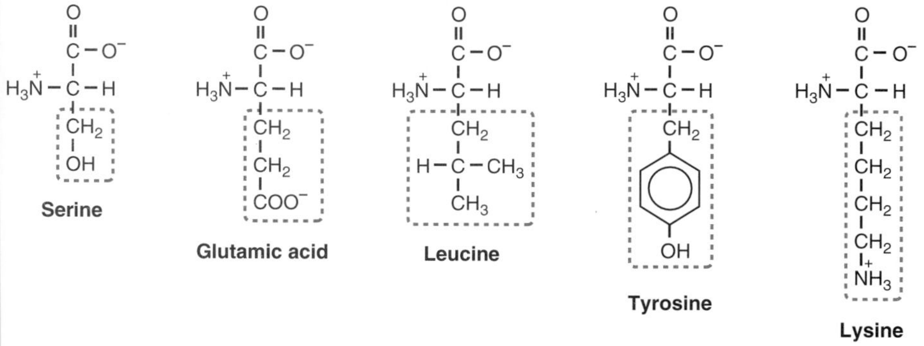

A 6.4: The steroid nucleus of cholic acid is hydrophobic, and the carboxyl and hydroxyl groups are hydrophilic.

Serine

Glutamic acid

Leucine

Tyrosine

Lysine

Fig. 6.36. Examples of amino acids.

Q 6.5: Which nitrogenous bases are similar to uric acid?

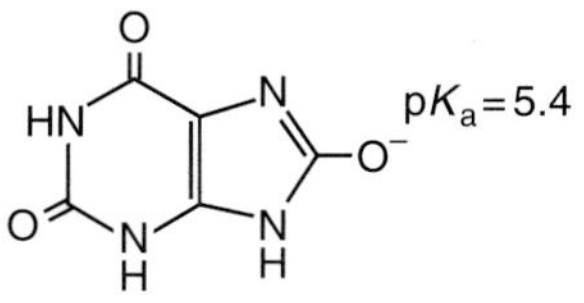

$pK_a = 5.4$

Uric acid

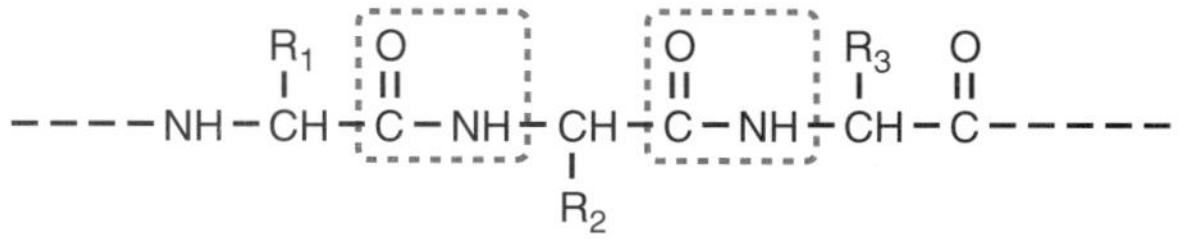

Fig. 6.37. A protein chain. The side chains of the amino acids are represented by R_1, R_2, and R_3. Peptide bonds are shown in blue.

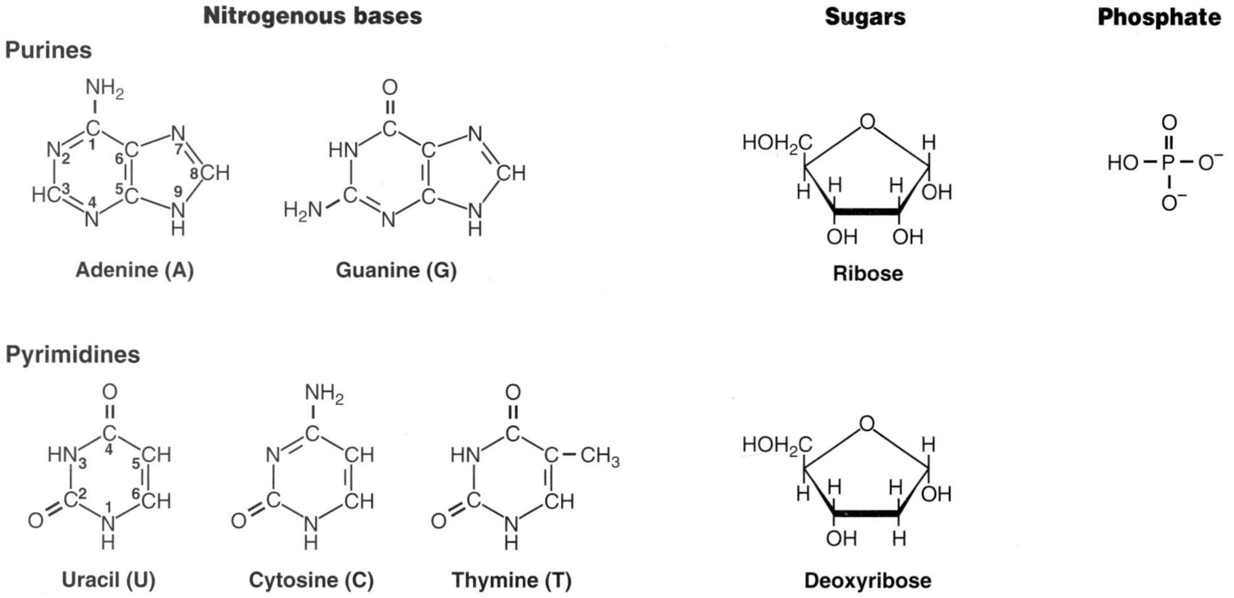

Nitrogenous bases

Purines

Adenine (A)

Guanine (G)

Sugars

Ribose

Phosphate

Pyrimidines

Uracil (U)

Cytosine (C)

Thymine (T)

Deoxyribose

Fig. 6.38. Components of nucleotides.

A 6.5: Uric acid contains two rings and is similar to the purines adenine and guanine. In fact, uric acid is a degradation product of these purine bases and is excreted in the urine. Uric acid is not very soluble in water. It tends to precipitate in joints, causing the severe pain of gout, the condition that plagues **Yves Topaigne.**

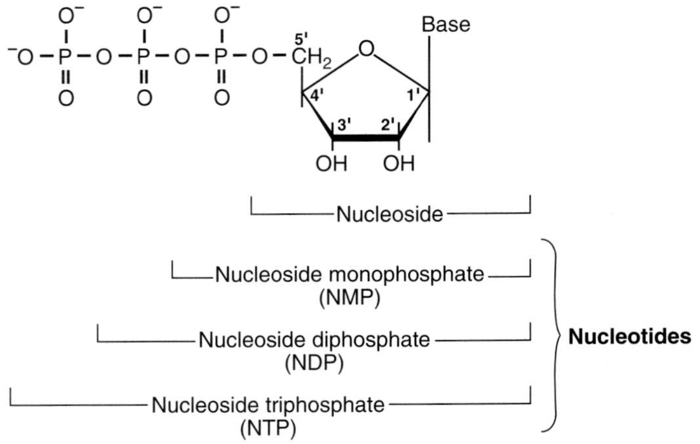

Fig. 6.39. Structures of nucleosides and nucleotides. For specific nucleotides, the letter N in the general abbreviation (NMP, NDP, or NTP) is replaced by the first letter of the name of the base (see Fig. 6.38).

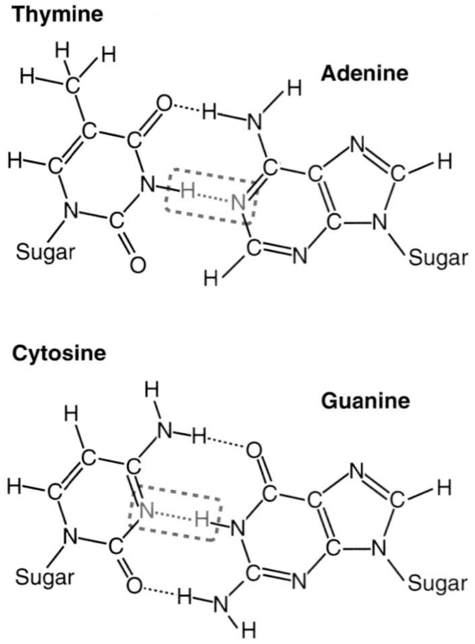

Thymine

Adenine

Cytosine

Guanine

Fig. 6.40. Base pairs of DNA. The hydrogen bonds formed by the nitrogen atoms in the rings are shown in blue.

A nucleoside consists only of a base and a sugar. Phosphate groups may be attached to nucleosides to produce nucleotides (Fig. 6.39). An ester bond joins the first phosphate group to the sugar, usually at the 5′-carbon, producing a nucleoside monophosphate. A second phosphate may form an anhydride bond with the first phosphate, producing a nucleoside diphosphate. The addition of a third phosphate group also occurs by means of an anhydride bond, producing a nucleoside triphosphate.

Nucleotides serve to transfer energy from one compound to another in the body. The major nucleotide involved in energy transfers within the body is adenosine triphosphate (ATP). However, in certain reactions, other nucleoside triphosphates may play this role.

Nucleotides serve as the monomeric units of the nucleic acids, DNA and RNA. Base pairing, which involves hydrogen bonds, is essential for the function of the nucleic acids. The purine and pyrimidine bases would not be able to form base pairs if they contained only carbon and oxygen. These bases have special properties because of the presence of nitrogen atoms, which each contain two unshared electrons. These electrons allow nitrogen to participate in hydrogen bonding while still covalently bound in a ring (Fig. 6.40).

CLINICAL COMMENTS. Diabetic patients, like **Di Beatty,** can self-monitor blood glucose levels at home, markedly reducing the time and expense of the many blood glucose determinations required over their lifetimes. Blood obtained from a pricked finger is placed on the pad of a plastic strip. The strip contains a reagent consisting of an enzyme (usually glucose oxidase) that converts the glucose in the blood to a substance that reacts with a dye, producing a color. The intensity of the color is directly related to the concentration of glucose in the patient's blood.

Like many patients with insulin-dependent diabetes mellitus (IDDM, type I diabetes mellitus), Di's blood glucose levels vary considerably in spite of her improved compliance with diet, exercise, insulin administration, and frequent follow-up with her physician.

Diabetes is derived from a Greek word meaning "to pass through" and "melos" meaning sugar. Diabetes mellitus, therefore, means excretion of sweet urine.

Yves Topaigne has acute gouty arthritis (podagra) involving his right great toe. Needle aspiration of the joint space yielded fluid which under polarized light microscopy was seen to contain crystals of monosodium urate phagocytosed by white blood cells. The presence of the relatively insoluble urate crystals within the joint space activates an inflammatory cascade leading to the classic components of joint inflammation (pain, redness, warmth, swelling, and limitation of joint motion).

BIOCHEMICAL COMMENTS. Over the years, methods of testing for the presence of sugars in urine and blood have been developed. Initially, blood could not readily be obtained, so urine was used. The urine of individuals with a condition subsequently called diabetes mellitus was found to have a sweet taste. Therefore, a "taste test" became the method for identifying individuals with diabetes mellitus who were excreting glucose in their urine. When chemists developed other tests for sugars, the tasting method was abandoned, and when sterile methods for obtaining blood from patients were developed, blood as well as urine could be analyzed.

The reducing sugar test is a colorimetric test that is based on the principle that an oxidation is always accompanied by a reduction (Fig. 6.41). When the anomeric carbon of a sugar is oxidized, another compound is reduced. If the compound that is reduced develops a color, the intensity of the color can be used to determine the amount of the sugar that was oxidized. The sugar that is oxidized is called a "reducing" sugar because it reduces another compound.

A major problem with the reducing sugar test is that it is not specific for glucose. Other sugars, such as fructose and galactose, also react. Fructose is a reducing sugar because the reducing sugar test is performed in an alkaline solution in which fructose, through an intermediate enediol, forms both glucose and mannose (Fig. 6.42). Under

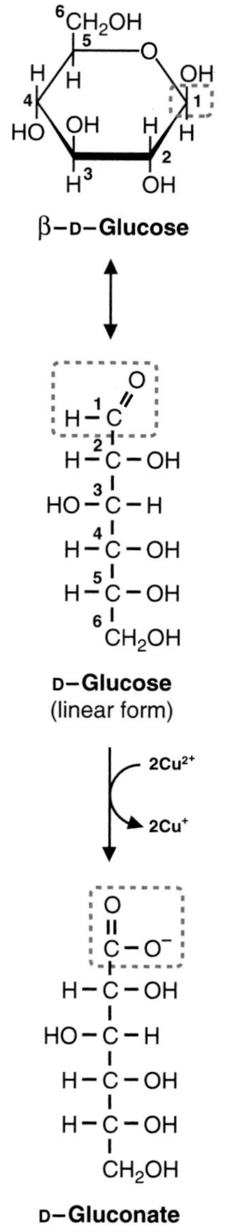

Fig. 6.41. The reducing sugar test. Carbon 1 of glucose undergoes oxidation, and copper is reduced, producing a blue color.

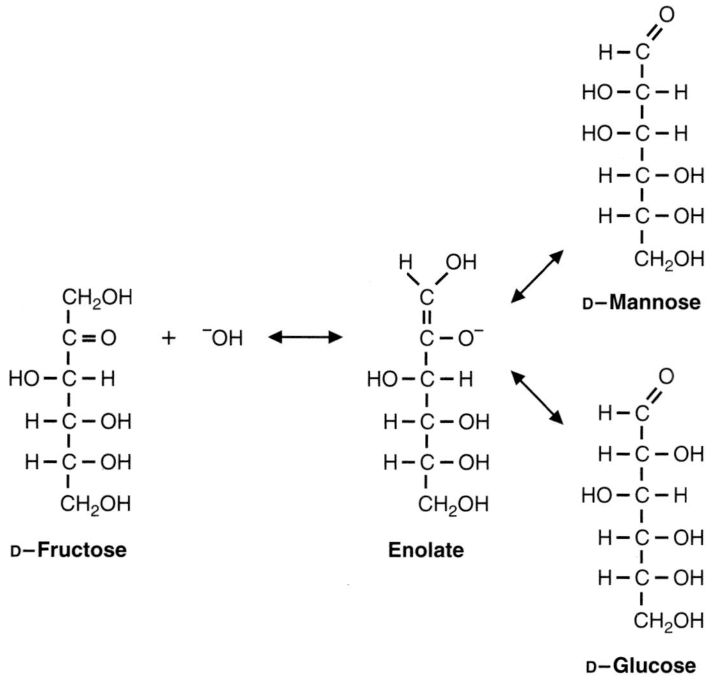

Fig. 6.42. Conversion of fructose to glucose and mannose in alkaline solution.

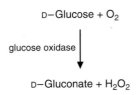

Fig. 6.43. Glucose oxidase reaction. Hydrogen peroxide (H_2O_2) reacts with a dye in the solution, producing a color.

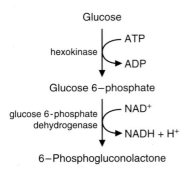

Fig. 6.44. Hexokinase/glucose 6-phosphate dehydrogenase coupled reaction. The amount of glucose in the solution is determined by measuring the amount of NAD^+ reduced to NADH.

normal fasting conditions, glucose is the predominant sugar in the blood, and fructose and galactose are present in negligible amounts. Therefore, the reducing sugar test can be used to determine blood glucose with reasonable accuracy. In fact, automated machinery was developed for performing this test.

Eventually, the automated machinery in clinical laboratories was adapted to perform tests using enzymes specific for glucose. The first enzymatic test employed glucose oxidase, a microbial enzyme (Fig. 6.43). Currently, hexokinase is being used. The hexokinase reaction is coupled to another reaction using a form of glucose 6-phosphate dehydrogenase that has NAD^+ rather than $NADP^+$ as a cofactor. The change in absorbance at 340 nm is measured to determine the amount of NAD^+ that is reduced to NADH, which, in turn, serves as a measure of the amount of glucose in the original solution (Fig. 6.44).

Suggested Readings

For additional information on the structures of biochemical compounds, see undergraduate biochemistry textbooks, such as the one by L. Stryer.

PROBLEM

Although enzymes specific for glucose currently are used for determining glucose levels in blood and urine, pediatricians still use the reducing sugar test, particularly for the urine of neonates (newborns). What is the rationale for using the reducing sugar test for newborn infants?

ANSWER

Certain genetic defects prevent galactose or fructose from being metabolized. If an individual with such a defect consumes a sugar that cannot be metabolized, the concentration of the sugar rises in the blood, and it may be excreted in the urine. A strip of paper coated with the components required for the reducing sugar test can be dipped into the individual's urine, and a color will be produced if a reducing sugar is present. Further tests can then be performed to identify the sugar.

Galactosemia (high levels of galactose in the blood) occurs when galactose cannot be phosphorylated or converted to UDP-galactose at a normal rate in cells. After birth, when infants with a defect in galactose metabolism receive lactose (the major source of dietary galactose) in their feedings, blood levels of galactose will be elevated, and the sugar may appear in the urine.

Fructosemia (high levels of fructose in the blood) and fructosuria (high levels of fructose in the urine) occur when fructose cannot be phosphorylated at a normal rate. This condition has no serious consequences and is known as benign fructosuria. In infants with fructose intolerance, fructose can be phosphorylated to fructose 1-phosphate, but the phosphorylated compound cannot be cleaved at a normal rate. This condition, which also results in fructosemia and fructosuria, may have devastating consequences. When an infant with a problem in fructose metabolism receives fructose in its diet, fructose levels rise in the blood and urine.

7 Amino Acids Found in Proteins

Amino acids are the monomeric units from which proteins are assembled, and they are the primary products of protein degradation. Twenty common amino acids are used during the synthesis of proteins, which occurs on ribosomes. The α-carbon of amino acids contains a carboxylic acid group, an amino group, and a side chain arranged in an L configuration. Some amino acids are chemically modified after incorporation into proteins.

The side chains of the amino acids are chemically diverse. Their chemical properties determine the specific characteristics of the proteins within which the amino acids reside. At physiological pH, in addition to the positive charge on the amino group and the negative charge on the carboxyl group, some amino acids also carry a charge on their side chain. Other side chains are polar, but some are nonpolar (hydrophobic). Some of the hydrophobic side chains are aromatic, containing rings with conjugated double bonds. Two amino acids have side chains that contain sulfur, two contain amide groups, and one is cyclic (its amino group is incorporated into a ring).

Michael Sichel is a 17-year-old male who presented to the hospital emergency room with severe pain in his lower back, abdomen, and legs which began after a 2-day history of nausea and vomiting caused by gastroenteritis. He was diagnosed as having sickle cell disease at age 3 years and has been admitted to the hospital on numerous occasions for similar vasoocclusive "sickle cell" crises.

The patient's hemoglobin level in the peripheral venous blood on admission was 7.8 g% (reference range = 12–16). (Hemoglobin is the protein in red blood cells which reversibly binds to oxygen.) The hematocrit or packed cell volume (the percentage of the total volume of blood made up by red blood cells) was 23.4% (reference range = 41–53). His serum total bilirubin level (a pigment derived from hemoglobin degradation) was 2.3 mg/dL (reference range = 0.2–1.0).

An x-ray of his abdomen showed radiopaque stones in his gallbladder. These stones are the result of the chronic excretion of excessive amounts of bilirubin from the liver into the bile leading to bilirubinate crystal deposition in the gallbladder lumen.

Cal Kulis is an 18-year-old male who was brought to the hospital by his mother because of the sudden onset of severe pain in the left flank radiating around his left side toward his pubic area. His urine was noted to be reddish-brown in color, and his urinalysis revealed the presence of many red blood cells. When his urine was acidified with acetic acid, clusters of flat hexagonal transparent crystals were noted. An x-ray of his abdomen showed radiopaque calculi (stones) in both kidneys. There was no family history of kidney stone disease.

Fig. 7.1. Structure of an amino acid. The α-carbon contains four substituents; an amino group, a carboxyl group, a hydrogen atom, and a side chain (R). Both the amino and carboxyl groups carry a charge at physiological pH.

Fig. 7.2. Dissociation of the α-carboxyl and α-amino groups of amino acids. At physiological pH (~7), a form in which both the α-carboxyl and α-amino groups are charged predominates. Some amino acids also have ionizable groups on their side chains.

D-Amino acids rarely occur in living organisms. Those of medical importance are found in bacterial cell walls and in some antibiotics produced by bacteria.

In aqueous solutions, nonpolar amino acids are frequently found in the interior of globular proteins, where their hydrophobic side chains form clusters that exclude water. In the proteins of membranes, nonpolar amino acids are on the surface, where they interact with the hydrophobic portions of the membrane lipid.

STRUCTURES OF THE AMINO ACIDS

As the name implies, an amino acid contains both an amino and a carboxylic acid group (Fig. 7.1). In all amino acids used for protein synthesis, these groups are attached to the α-carbon atom (carbon 2). At physiological pH, the amino group carries a proton and is positively charged, while the carboxyl group has dissociated a proton and is negatively charged. Although the values vary for the different amino acids, the pK_a for the α-carboxyl group is about 2 and the pK_a for the α-amino group is about 9–10 (Fig. 7.2).

In addition to the amino and carboxyl groups, each amino acid contains a side chain, called an R group, which is also attached to the α-carbon (see Fig. 7.1). The side chains differ for each of the 20 common amino acids which are used in the synthesis of proteins. For 19 of these amino acids, the α-carbon has four different substituents, the amino group, the carboxyl group, the side chain, and a hydrogen atom. Thus, the α-carbon is asymmetric, and amino acids may exist in either the D or the L configuration. The D and L forms cannot be superimposed because they are mirror images of each other (Fig. 7.3).

All of the amino acids found in body proteins, except glycine, are of the L configuration. The α-carbon of glycine is not asymmetric because it contains two groups which are identical: the two hydrogen atoms, one of which serves as the side chain.

The functions of the individual amino acids and their roles in protein structure are related mainly to the chemical properties of their side chains (Fig. 7.4). Therefore, the amino acids are usually divided into groups based on the relative polarity of these chains, which indicates their tendency to react. Overall, the side chains range through a spectrum from very nonpolar to very polar. Some amino acids have very hydrophobic (nonpolar) side chains. Others are more hydrophilic, bearing polar but uncharged R groups. The most hydrophilic amino acids have side chains with either a negative or a positive charge at physiological pH. Three-letter and sometimes one-letter abbreviations represent the amino acids (Table 7.1). The one-letter abbreviations are generally used to give the amino acid sequences of long protein chains.

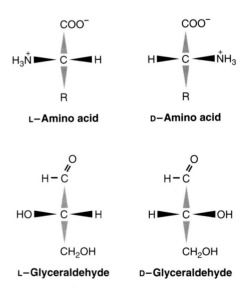

Fig. 7.3. L- and D-amino acids. The L forms are the only ones found naturally in humans. Bonds coming out of the paper (black arrows); those going in (shaded arrows). The α-amino groups and H-atom come toward the reader, while the α-carboxyl and side chains go away. The L and D forms are mirror images. They cannot be superimposed by rotating the molecule. The reference for the L and D forms are the stereoisomers of glyceraldehyde (see Fig. 6.4).

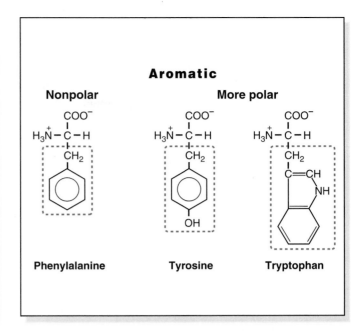

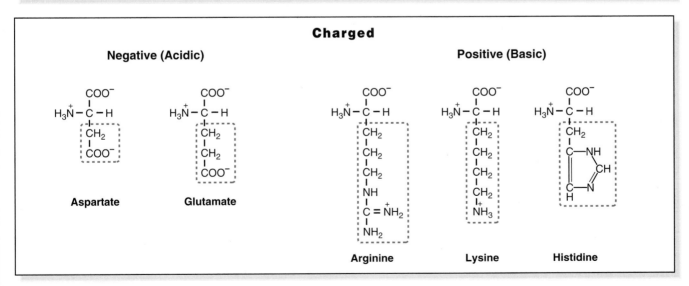

Fig. 7.4. The side chains of the amino acids. The side chains are highlighted. The amino acids are grouped by the polarity of their side chains. These groupings are not absolute, however. Tyrosine and tryptophan, listed with the nonpolar amino acids, are relatively polar because of their phenolic and indole rings, respectively.

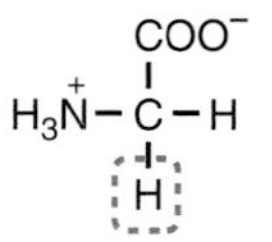

Glycine

Fig. 7.5. Glycine, the simplest amino acid. The α-carbon is not asymmetric because the R group (highlighted) is a hydrogen atom. Therefore, glycine is neither D nor L.

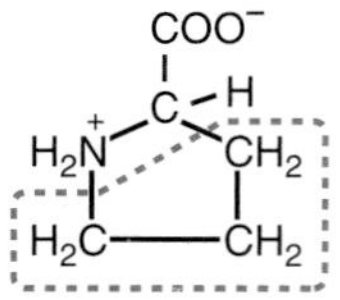

Proline

Fig. 7.6. Proline, a cyclic amino acid. The α-amino nitrogen is incorporated into a ring, which has a rigid structure.

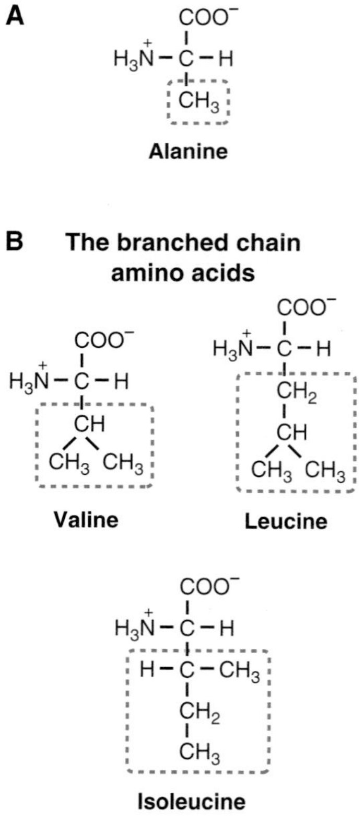

A

Alanine

B   The branched chain amino acids

Valine   **Leucine**

Isoleucine

Fig. 7.7. Amino acids with aliphatic side chains. **A.** Alanine. **B.** Branched chain amino acids (valine, leucine, and isoleucine). The side chains of these amino acids are hydrophobic.

Table 7.1. Abbreviations for the Amino Acids

Name	Abbreviations[a]	
	Three-Letter	One-Letter
Alanine	Ala	A
Arginine	Arg	R
Asparagine	Asn	N
Aspartate	Asp	D
Cysteine	Cys	C
Glutamate	Glu	E
Glutamine	Gln	Q
Glycine	Gly	G
Histidine	His	H
Isoleucine	Ile	I
Leucine	Leu	L
Lysine	Lys	K
Methionine	Met	M
Phenylalanine	Phe	F
Proline	Pro	P
Serine	Ser	S
Threonine	Thr	T
Tryptophan	Trp	W
Tyrosine	Tyr	Y
Valine	Val	V

[a]Three-letter abbreviations are generally used. One-letter abbreviations are used mainly to list the amino acid sequences of long protein chains.

Amino Acids with Nonpolar, Aliphatic Side Chains

GLYCINE AND PROLINE

Glycine has a hydrogen atom for a side chain, so it is the simplest amino acid and the least interactive (Fig. 7.5). Because the hydrogen atom is small, it produces minimal steric hindrance (i.e., it does not significantly impinge on the space occupied by other atoms or chemical groups). Therefore, glycine allows the greatest structural flexibility when it is present in a protein. The amino acid proline, on the other hand, allows little flexibility in protein structure (Fig. 7.6). Its nitrogen atom is covalently attached to its side chain, forming a rigid ring.

ALANINE AND THE BRANCHED CHAIN AMINO ACIDS

Alanine and the branched chain amino acids (valine, leucine, and isoleucine) have bulky, nonpolar, aliphatic side chains. Alanine contains a methyl group. Valine, leucine, and isoleucine have branched chains that are very hydrophobic (Fig. 7.7).

Amino Acids with Aromatic Side Chains

The aromatic amino acids are structurally related to alanine (Fig. 7.8). In each case,

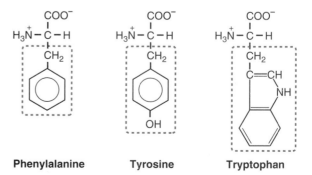

Phenylalanine   **Tyrosine**   **Tryptophan**

Fig. 7.8. The aromatic amino acids.

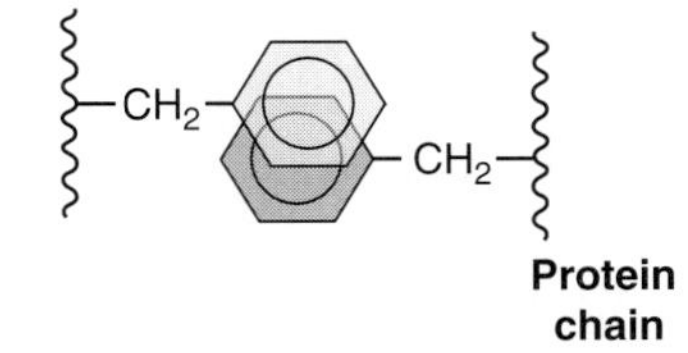

Fig. 7.9. Stacking of aromatic groups to form strong hydrophobic interactions.

an aromatic ring is attached to carbon 3 (the β-carbon), which is in the methyl group of alanine.

Phenylalanine contains a phenyl group, which is very hydrophobic. The rings can stack on each other (Fig. 7.9). Although tyrosine and tryptophan are also hydrophobic, they are more polar than phenylalanine because tyrosine contains a phenolic group, which is a weak acid (pK_a ~ 10), and tryptophan contains a nitrogen in its indole group.

Amino Acids with Polar, Uncharged Side Chains

A group of amino acids are polar, but uncharged. These amino acids are hydrophilic ("water-loving") and, in aqueous solutions, are frequently found on the surface of globular proteins where they interact with water. The side chains of serine and threonine contain polar hydroxyl groups. Asparagine and glutamine are amides of the amino acids aspartate and glutamate. They are polar because of the carbonyl and nitrogen atoms in their amide groups. Cysteine and methionine are relatively polar because they each contain a sulfur atom (Fig. 7.10). However, they are more hydrophobic than the other amino acids in this class.

The hydroxyl groups of serine and threonine and the amide groups of asparagine and glutamine allow these amino acids to form hydrogen bonds with each other, with water, or with other polar compounds that bind to proteins (Fig. 7.11). Although tyrosine is hydrophobic, its hydroxyl group allows it to form hydrogen bonds.

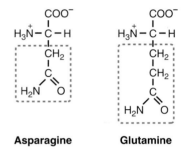

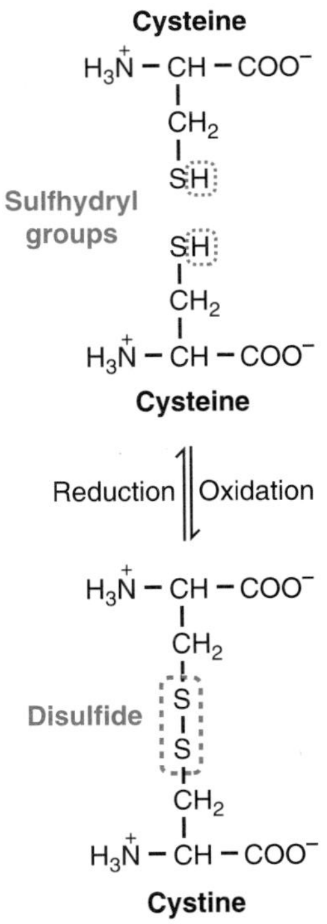

A. Hydroxy

Serine   Threonine

B. Amide

Asparagine   Glutamine

C. Sulfur–containing

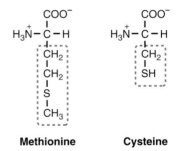

Methionine   Cysteine

Fig. 7.10. Hydroxy-, amide-, and sulfur-containing amino acids. Asparagine and glutamine are formed from aspartate and glutamate. Serine, threonine, asparagine, and glutamine can form hydrogen bonds. Cysteine can form covalent disulfide bonds.

Cysteine

Sulfhydryl groups

Cysteine

Reduction ⇅ Oxidation

Disulfide

Cystine

Fig. 7.12. A disulfide bond. Covalent disulfide bonds may be formed between 2 molecules of cysteine or between 2 cysteine residues in a protein. The disulfide compound is called cystine. The hydrogens (with their electrons) of the sulfhydryl groups of cysteine are lost during oxidation.

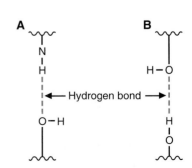

Fig. 7.11. Hydrogen bonds involving nitrogen or oxygen.

Cal Kulis passed a renal stone shortly after admission with immediate relief of flank pain. Stone analysis revealed its major component to be cystine. Normally, amino acids are filtered by the renal glomerular capillaries into the tubular urine, but are almost entirely reabsorbed from this fluid back into the blood via the proximal tubular cells of the kidney. Mr. Kulis' urine, however, contained significant amounts of the amino acids cystine (the result of the oxidation of 2 cysteines to form a disulfide), arginine, and lysine, a finding consistent with a diagnosis of the genetic disorder known as cystinuria. In this disorder, cystine, which is less soluble than cysteine, precipitates in the urine, forming renal stones.

Because of its sulfhydryl group, cysteine may interact with other sulfhydryl groups to form disulfides. For example, 2 molecules of cysteine may be oxidized to form cystine, which is composed of 2 cysteine molecules linked by a disulfide bond (Fig. 7.12). Disulfide formation may also occur between 2 cysteine residues in a protein.

Amino Acids with Charged Side Chains

At physiological pH, 5 amino acids carry charges on their side chains (Fig. 7.13). Two other amino acids are uncharged, but become negatively charged in a higher pH range. Positively or negatively charged groups can participate in electrostatic interactions with groups of opposite charge on other amino acids or on other compounds (Fig. 7.14).

ASPARTATE AND GLUTAMATE, THE NEGATIVELY CHARGED AMINO ACIDS

Aspartic and glutamic acids contain carboxylic acids in their side chains and, therefore, are called the acidic amino acids. At physiological pH, the protons are dissociated, and the side chains carry a negative charge (Fig. 7.15). The negatively charged forms of these amino acids are called aspartate and glutamate.

The pK_a for the acidic groups in the side chains of these amino acids is about 4 (Table 7.2). When the pH equals the pK_a, the protonated (uncharged) species are equal in number to the negatively charged species, that is, the number of molecules with zero charge on the side chain is equal to the number with a negative charge (see

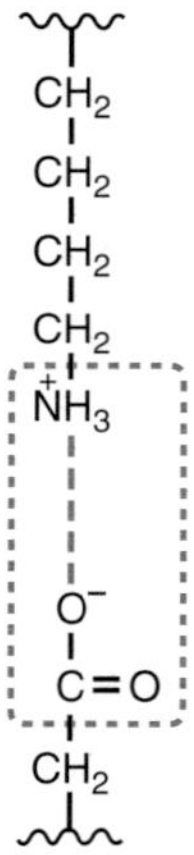

Fig. 7.14. Electrostatic interaction between the positively charged side chain of lysine and the negatively charged side chain of aspartate.

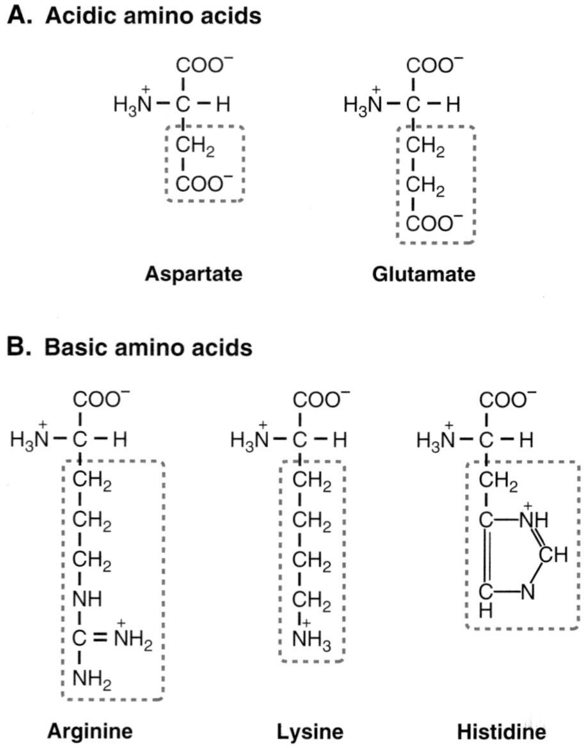

7.1: **Michael Sichel** has sickle cell anemia, in which a point mutation causes the sixth amino acid in the β-globin chain of hemoglobin to change from glutamate to valine. What differences would you expect to find in the chemical properties of sickle cell hemoglobin compared to normal hemoglobin based on this change in amino acid composition?

Fig. 7.13. The acidic and basic amino acids. These amino acids have side chains that carry a charge at physiological pH. The side chains of the acidic amino acids have a carboxyl group that is negatively charged, while the side chains of the basic amino acids have a nitrogen-containing group that is positively charged.

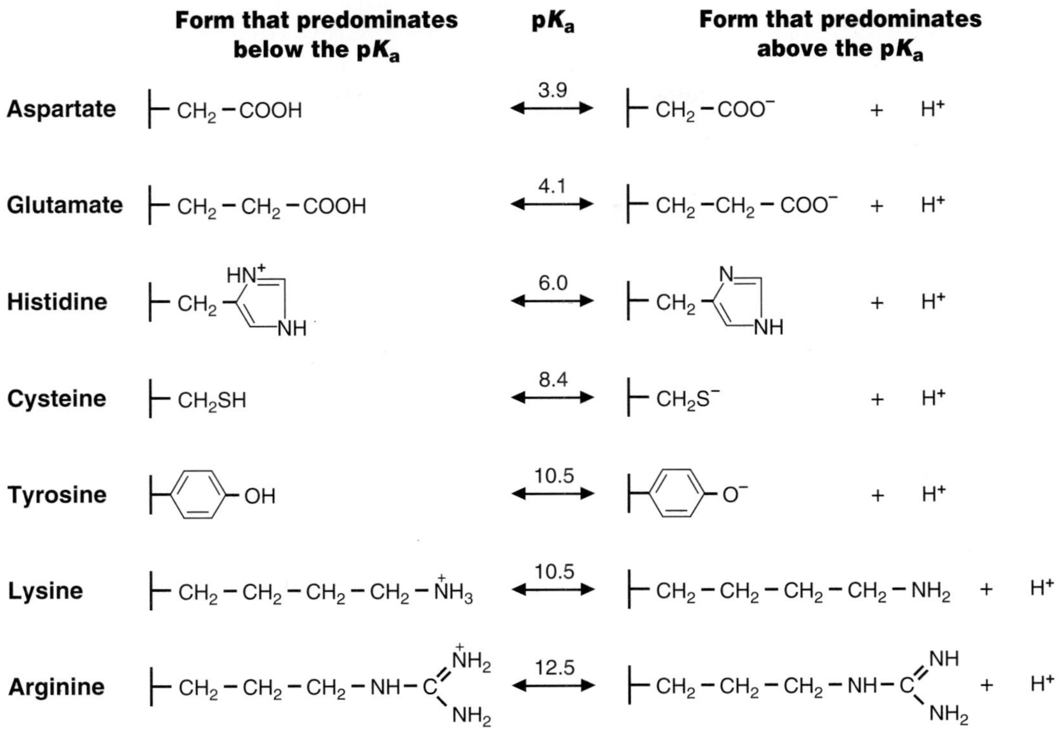

	Form that predominates below the pK_a	pK_a	Form that predominates above the pK_a

Aspartate $-CH_2-COOH$ 3.9 $-CH_2-COO^-$ + H^+

Glutamate $-CH_2-CH_2-COOH$ 4.1 $-CH_2-CH_2-COO^-$ + H^+

Histidine $-CH_2-$(imidazole HN^+)   6.0 $-CH_2-$(imidazole N)   + H^+

Cysteine $-CH_2SH$ 8.4 $-CH_2S^-$ + H^+

Tyrosine   (ring)$-OH$ 10.5   (ring)$-O^-$ + H^+

Lysine $-CH_2-CH_2-CH_2-CH_2-\overset{+}{N}H_3$ 10.5 $-CH_2-CH_2-CH_2-CH_2-NH_2$ + H^+

Arginine $-CH_2-CH_2-CH_2-NH-C\overset{\overset{+}{N}H_2}{\underset{NH_2}{}}$ 12.5 $-CH_2-CH_2-CH_2-NH-C\overset{NH}{\underset{NH_2}{}}$ + H^+

Fig. 7.15. Dissociation of the side chains of the amino acids. As the pH increases, the charge on the side chain goes from 0 to + or from + to 0. The pK_a is the pH at which half the molecules of an amino acid in solution have side chains that are charged. Half are uncharged.

Table 7.2. Properties of the Common Amino Acids

Amino Acid	pK_{a1}* (Carboxyl)	pK_{a2} (Amino)	pK_{aR} (R Group)	Hydropathy Index**
Nonpolar aliphatic				
Glycine	2.4	9.8		−0.4
Proline	2.0	11.0		−1.6
Alanine	2.3	9.7		1.8
Leucine	2.4	9.6		3.8
Valine	2.3	9.6		4.2
Isoleucine	2.4	9.7		4.5
Aromatic				
Phenylalanine	1.8	9.1		2.8
Tyrosine	2.2	9.1	10.5	−1.3
Tryptophan	2.4	9.4		−0.9
Polar uncharged				
Cysteine	2.0	10.3	8.4	2.5
Methionine	2.3	9.2		1.9
Threonine	2.1	9.6	13.6	−0.7
Serine	2.2	9.2	13.6	−0.8
Aspargine	2.0	8.8		−3.5
Glutamine	2.2	9.1		−3.5
Charged — negative				
Aspartate	1.9	9.6	3.9	−3.5
Glutamate	2.2	9.7	4.1	−3.5
Charged — positive				
Histidine	1.8	9.3	6.0	−3.2
Lysine	2.2	9.0	10.5	−3.9
Arginine	2.2	9.0	12.5	−4.5
Average	2.2	9.5		

*When these amino acids reside in proteins, the pK_a for the side chains may vary to some extent from the value for the free amino acid depending on the local environment of the amino acid in the three-dimensional structure of the protein.

**The hydropathy index is a measure of the hydrophobicity of the amino acid (the higher the number, the more hydrophobic). Values based on Kyte J, Doolittle RF. J Mol Biol 1982;157:105–132.

A 7.1: In normal hemoglobin, a glutamate is in position 6 of the β-chain of hemoglobin. This amino acid carries a negative charge on its side chain at physiological pH and, thus, can engage in electrostatic interactions. The mutation that causes sickle cell anemia results in the substitution of this glutamate by a valine. Valine is a hydrophobic amino acid and, therefore, tends to interact with other hydrophobic compounds. (The structure of hemoglobin will be described in more detail in Chapter 8.)

Chapter 4, the Henderson-Hasselbalch equation). Below pH 4, the number of molecules that carry a proton and, thus, have no charge is greater than the number of negatively charged molecules. Above pH 4, the molecules that predominate have lost a proton and, therefore, are negatively charged.

ARGININE, LYSINE, AND HISTIDINE, THE POSITIVELY CHARGED AMINO ACIDS

Because the side chains of arginine, lysine, and histidine contain nitrogen, they may be protonated and positively charged (see Fig. 7.15 and Table 7.2). For each of these amino acids, the protonated, positively charged form predominates below the pK_a and the dissociated, uncharged form above the pK_a. Arginine has a guanidinium group on its side chain ($pK_a \sim 12.5$), and lysine contains an amino group on the ε (epsilon) carbon ($pK_a \sim 10.5$). Therefore, these amino acids are positively charged at physiological pH (~ 7.4). Histidine has an imidazole ring ($pK_a \sim 6$). In proteins, the pK_a of the imidazole group is between 6 and 7. Therefore, it titrates in the physiological pH range, and small changes in the pH or in the local environment can alter the charge. This property allows histidine to play an important role in protein function.

CYSTEINE AND TYROSINE

The side chains of cysteine ($pK_a \sim 8.4$) and tyrosine ($pK_a \sim 10.5$) are predominately protonated below their pK_a and have no charge (see Fig. 7.15 and Table 7.2). Above the pK_a, the protons dissociate, and the side chains carry a negative charge. In proteins, therefore, these amino acids are usually uncharged at physiological pH.

TITRATION OF AMINO ACIDS

When amino acids that do not have ionizable side chains are titrated, two pK_a values are observed, the first corresponding to the α-carboxyl group and the second to the α-amino group (Fig. 7.16).

At low pH, both groups carry protons. The amino group has a positive charge, and the carboxyl group has zero charge. As the pH is increased by the addition of alkali (OH^-), the proton dissociates from the carboxyl group, and its charge changes from zero to negative with a pK_a between 2 and 3. The amino group titrates at a much higher pH (between 9 and 10), and the charge on this group changes from positive to zero as the pH rises. Thus, amino acids that carry charges only on their α-carboxyl and α-amino groups have an overall positive charge at low pH, both a positive and a negative charge (overall or net charge of zero) at physiological pH (about 7.4), and a negative charge at a higher pH.

In addition to the pK_a values corresponding to their α-carboxyl and α-amino groups, amino acids with ionizable side chains have a third pK_a (Fig. 7.17). This third pK_a corresponds to the pH range in which the proton on the side chain dissociates.

The pH at which the net charge on the molecules in solution is zero is called the isoelectric point (pI). At this pH the molecules (called zwitterions) will not migrate in an electric field because the number of negative charges on each molecule is equal to the number of positive charges.

CLINICAL COMMENTS. After 3 days of parenteral narcotics for the pain of his vasoocclusive crisis, in addition to hydration, nasal inhalation of oxygen, and hydroxyurea therapy, **Michael Sichel's** acute symptoms gradually subsided. Had his severe pain persisted, partial exchange blood transfusions would

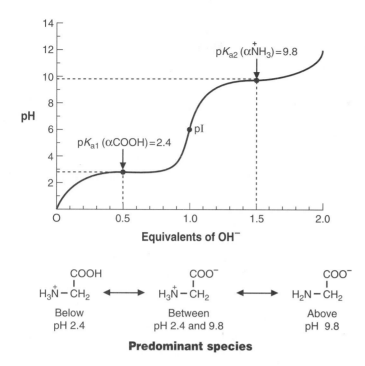

Fig. 7.16. Titration curve of glycine. The ionic species that predominates in each region is shown below the graph. pI is the isoelectric point (at which there is no net charge on the molecule).

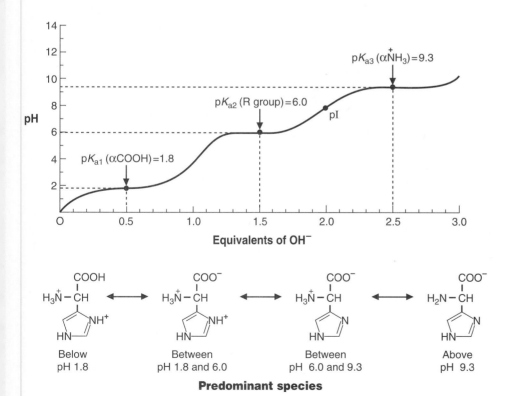

Fig. 7.17. Titration curve of histidine. The ionic species that predominates in each region is shown below the graph. pI is the isoelectric point (at which there is no net charge on the molecule).

have been considered since no other effective therapy is currently available. Because patients with sickle cell anemia periodically experience sickle cell crises, Michael's physician urged him to seek medical help whenever symptoms reappeared.

Mr. Kulis has cystinuria, a relatively rare disorder, with a prevalence that ranges between 1 in 2,500 to 1 in 15,000, depending on the population studied. It is a genetically determined disease with a complex recessive mode of inheritance resulting from allelic mutations. These mutations lead to a reduction in the activity of renal tubular cell transport proteins which normally carry cystine from the tubular lumen into the renal tubular cells. The transport of the basic amino acids, lysine, arginine, and ornithine (an amino acid found in the urea cycle but not in proteins) is also often compromised, and they appear in the urine.

Because cystine is produced by oxidation of cysteine, conservative treatment of cystinuria includes reducing the amount of cysteine within the body and, hence, the amount of cystine eventually filtered by the kidneys. Reduction of cysteine levels is accomplished by restricting dietary methionine, a precursor for cysteine formation.

To increase the amount of cystine that remains in solution, the volume of fluid ingested daily is increased. Crystallization of cystine is further prevented by chronically alkalinizing the urine. Finally, drugs may be administered to enhance the conversion of urinary cystine to more soluble compounds.

If these conservative measures fail to prevent continued cystine stone formation, existing stones may be removed by a surgical technique that involves sonic fracture. The fragmented stones may then pass spontaneously or may be more easily extracted surgically because of their smaller size.

 BIOCHEMICAL COMMENTS. The 20 common amino acids (described in this chapter) that are used for the synthesis of proteins are not the only amino acids that are found in the body. Modified amino acids are present in protein chains, and "free" amino acids (i.e., not part of protein chains) are intermediates in various pathways.

Modification of amino acids occurs after they are incorporated into proteins. For example, proline can be oxidized to hydroxyproline in collagen. The activity of many enzymes is regulated by phosphorylation of serine, threonine, and tyrosine residues. Galactose, glucose, mannose or other sugars or oligosaccharides are attached to serine, threonine, or asparagine in glycoproteins. Tyrosine is converted to the thyroid hormones triiodothyronine (T_3) and thyroxine (T_4) in the protein thyroglobulin. These types of modifications are discussed in more detail in the following chapter.

Free amino acids are intermediates in certain pathways. For example, ornithine and citrulline are intermediates of the urea cycle (see Section VII). Dihydroxyphenylalanine (dopa) is an intermediate on the pathway from tyrosine to the catecholamines dopamine, norepinephrine, and epinephrine that serve as neurotransmitters and hormones.

PROBLEM

Calculate the isoelectric point (pI) for glycine and for histidine.

ANSWER

The numerical value of the pI is the average of the two pK_a values between which the amino acid has no net charge.

For glycine (see Fig. 7.16), which does not have an ionizable side chain, the pI will be the average between the pK_a for the α-carboxyl group and the pK_a for the α-amino group

$$pI = \frac{pK_{a1} + pK_{a2}}{2}$$

or (2.4 + 9.8) / 2 which equals 6.1. At this pH, the negative charge on the carboxyl group is balanced by the positive charge on the amino group.

For histidine (see Fig. 7.17), which has an ionizable side chain, the α-carboxyl group will have no charge, while the imidazole ring and the α-amino group will each carry a positive charge at low pH. As the pH rises, the carboxyl group loses its proton and becomes negatively charged. After the imidazole group is titrated and loses its positive charge, the molecule will contain one negative charge (on the carboxyl group) and one positive charge (on the amino group). Thus, the pI will be between the second and third pK_a values, that is,

$$pI = \frac{pK_{a2} + pK_{a3}}{2}$$

or (6.0 + 9.3) / 2 which equals 7.7.

8 Protein Structure

Four different levels of structure are found in proteins (Fig. 8.1). The primary structure of a protein is the linear sequence of amino acids in the polypeptide chain. Secondary structure (which includes α-helices and β-sheets) consists of local regions of polypeptide chains that have a regular conformation which is stabilized by hydrogen bonds. The total three-dimensional conformation of an entire polypeptide chain is its tertiary structure, which includes α-helices, β-sheets, and regions that are globular (or spherical). Some proteins exhibit quaternary structure; the three-dimensional conformation of a multisubunit protein composed of a number of polypeptide chains (or subunits) joined by noncovalent interactions.

Proteins within the cell are in their "native" state. Heat, acid, and other agents cause the proteins to be denatured, that is, to unwind and lose their native three-dimensional conformation.

In their native state within the cell, many proteins bind other substances, ranging from ions to complex molecules such as coenzymes. These ligands are necessary for the function of the proteins.

A multitude of different proteins can be formed from only 20 common amino acids, because these amino acids can be linked together in an enormous number of different combinations. Differences in the sequence of amino acids along the protein chains result in different three-dimensional structures and, therefore, different functions.

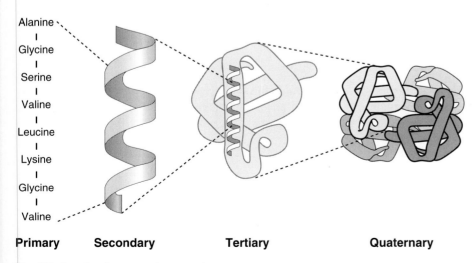

Alanine
|
Glycine
|
Serine
|
Valine
|
Leucine
|
Lysine
|
Glycine
|
Valine

Primary　　**Secondary**　　　**Tertiary**　　　　**Quaternary**

Fig. 8.1. Levels of structure in a protein.

Michael Sichel was readmitted to the hospital with symptoms indicating that he was experiencing another sickle cell crisis. His parents were concerned that their youngest daughter might also have sickle cell disease.

Amy Lloyd is a 62-year-old woman who complains of increasing muscle weakness and fatigue over the last 5 months. Two weeks ago, Mrs. Lloyd noted sudden severe pain in the area of her second lumbar vertebra which has improved slightly. Her family notes that the patient experienced periods of confusion which are gradually becoming more frequent and more severe.

Initial laboratory studies showed an anemia with a hemoglobin of 10.2 g% (reference range = 12–16), mild renal failure with a serum creatinine of 1.9 mg/dL (reference range [females] = 0.5–1.1), an elevated total calcium of 11.8 mg/dL (reference range = 8.4–10.2), and normal serum albumin and phosphorus levels. A urinalysis revealed the presence of a moderate proteinuria and numerous white blood cells and bacteria in the urinary sediment.

William Hartman is a 54-year-old male who is 68 inches tall and weighs 198 lb. He has a history of high blood pressure and elevated serum cholesterol levels. Following a heated argument with a neighbor, Mr. Hartman experienced a "tight pressure-like band of pain" across his chest, associated with shortness of breath, sweating, and a sense of light-headedness.

After 7 hours of intermittent chest pain, he went to the hospital emergency room, where his electrocardiogram showed changes consistent with an acute infarction of the anterior wall of his heart. He was admitted to the cardiac care unit. Blood was sent to the laboratory for tests, including the total creatine phosphokinase (CK) level as well as the MB ("muscle-brain") fraction of CK in the blood.

Ann Sulin is a 39-year-old woman who was in good health until 6 months ago when she noted the gradual onset of increased thirst, frequency of urination, and fatigue. She lost 4 lb over a 5-week period in spite of a good appetite and normal activity. Her physician's initial suspicion of diabetes mellitus was confirmed when her 2-hour postprandial (after a meal) blood glucose was found to be elevated at 242 mg/dL. In spite of compliance with an appropriate diabetic diet, and maximal doses of the antidiabetic sulfonylurea agent glipizide, her 2-hour postprandial blood glucose levels remained unacceptably elevated. Therefore, her physician initiated therapy with Iletin II NPH beef insulin.

PEPTIDE BONDS

Amino acids join together by amide linkages (peptide bonds) to form linear chains called polypeptides. In a peptide bond, the α-carboxyl group of one amino acid is covalently attached to the α-amino group of the next amino acid (Fig. 8.2). The amino

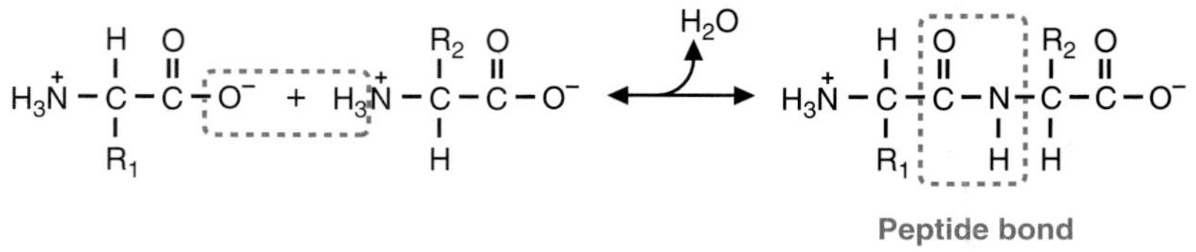

Fig. 8.2. A peptide bond between two amino acids.

acids within the protein chain are called amino acid residues. The amino acid residue at one end of the chain has a free amino group, and the one at the other end of the chain has a free carboxyl group.

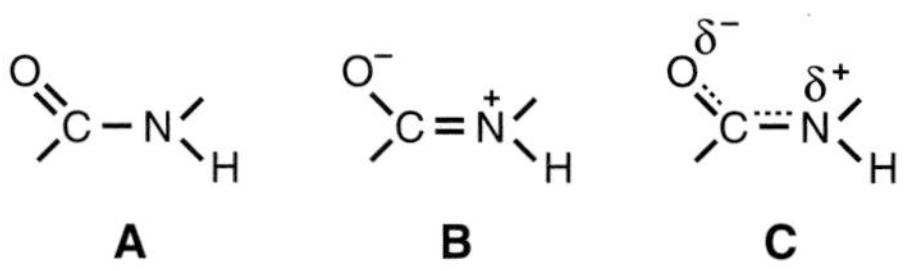

Nomenclature for Amino Acid Sequences

By convention, the amino acid sequence of a protein is written from the amino- or N-terminus on the left to the carboxyl- or C-terminus on the right. The ending of the name of each amino acid in a peptide chain is changed to "yl" except the one at the C-terminal end. Three-letter abbreviations for the amino acids are also used, and for very long sequences the amino acid residues are represented by single letters (Fig. 8.3 and Table 7.1).

Properties of Peptide Bonds

Peptide bonds are very stable, and chemical hydrolysis requires extreme conditions. In the body, peptide bonds are cleaved by proteolytic enzymes called proteases or peptidases.

Because the peptide bond is a hybrid of two resonance states, it has a partial double-bond character (Fig. 8.4). Therefore, the structure is planar, and free rotation does not occur around the carbon-nitrogen bond (Fig. 8.5). Furthermore, the oxygen of the carbonyl group has a partial negative charge, and the nitrogen has a partial positive charge.

In a polypeptide, the α-carbons of adjacent amino acids are usually in a *trans* configuration, that is, they are on opposite sides of the peptide bond (Fig. 8.6). Therefore, the side chains of the adjacent amino acids are also *trans*, and steric interference is minimized.

In contrast to the rigid peptide bond, free rotation can occur around the bonds between the nitrogen of a peptide bond and the adjacent α-carbon, as well as between this α-carbon and its carbonyl carbon, which is involved in the next peptide bond in the chain (see Fig. 8.5). A proline residue causes limited flexibility because its nitrogen is incorporated into the pyrrolidine ring.

Despite the rigidity of its peptide bonds, the flexibility around the bonds of the other atoms of a protein would allow an enormous number of possible conformations for each molecule. However, each molecule of a protein actually folds into its most stable conformation, assuming a shape that is identical to the shape of the other molecules of the same protein. This shape is known as the native conformation.

LEVELS OF PROTEIN STRUCTURE

The sequence of amino acid residues in a protein and the types of interactions that occur between these residues, particularly between their side chains or between the atoms of their peptide bonds, determine the native conformation of the protein.

Fig. 8.4. Resonance forms of peptide bonds. The actual bond is a hybrid (**C**) between (**A**) and (**B**). The carbonyl oxygen has a partial negative charge, and the nitrogen has a partial positive charge.

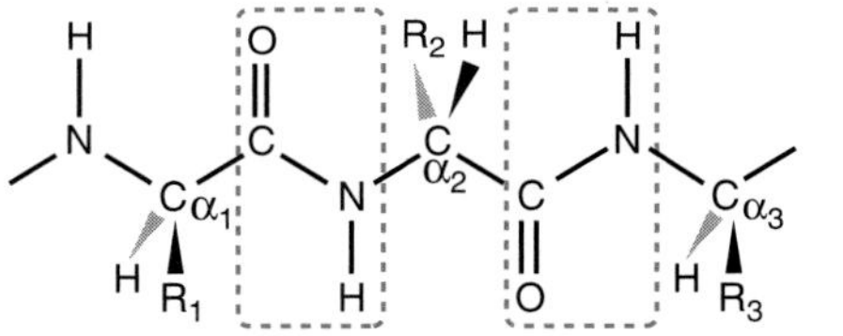

Fig. 8.5. Planar nature of peptide bonds. Because of the partial double bond character of the peptide bond, free rotation does not occur around the C—N bond. Therefore, these atoms and the O and H atoms attached to them all lie in the same plane. Two planar peptide groups are shown connected by carbon α_2. The planar peptide groups can pivot around their shared α-carbon.

N-terminal ➡ Alanylglycylserylglutamylphenylalanine ⬅ C-terminal

Ala – Gly – Ser – Glu – Phe   3 letter abbreviation

A   G   S   E   F   1 letter abbreviation

Fig. 8.3. Nomenclature and abbreviations for a polypeptide chain.

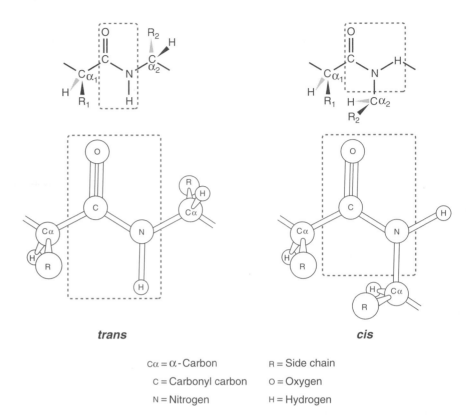

Cα = α - Carbon	R = Side chain
C = Carbonyl carbon	O = Oxygen
N = Nitrogen	H = Hydrogen

Fig. 8.6. *Trans* and *cis* configurations around peptide bonds. The *trans* configuration is favored because, in the *cis* configuration, the bulky side chains on adjacent α-carbons can interfere with each other.

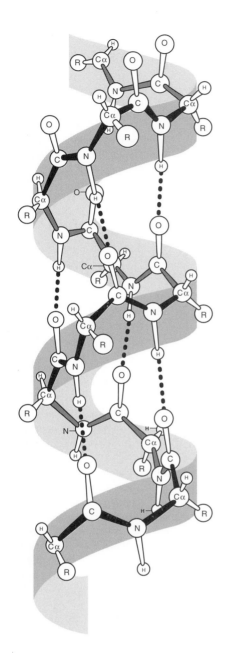

Fig. 8.7. α-Helix. Each oxygen of a carbonyl group of a peptide bond forms a hydrogen bond with the hydrogen atom attached to a nitrogen in a peptide bond 4 amino acids further along the chain.

Primary Structure

The primary structure of a protein is simply the linear sequence of amino acids that are linked together by peptide bonds. Branching of the chains does not occur.

Secondary Structure

Regions within polypeptide chains can form regular, recurring, localized structures that result from hydrogen bonding between atoms of the peptide bonds. These regions, known as secondary structures, include the α-helix and the β-sheet.

α-HELIX

In an α-helix, hydrogen bonds are formed between each carbonyl oxygen atom of a peptide bond and the hydrogen attached to the amide nitrogen atom of a peptide bond 4 amino acid residues further along the polypeptide chain (Fig. 8.7). Thus, a regular coiled structure exists in which each peptide bond is connected by hydrogen bonds to the peptide bond 4 amino acid residues ahead of it and 4 amino acid residues behind it in the primary sequence.

The side chains of the amino acid residues of an α-helix extend outward from the central axis (Fig. 8.8). Bulky side chains or side chains with charges that repel each other can prevent α-helix formation. Proline residues interrupt α-helical structures in proteins because they exert geometric constraints due to their ring structure and because, in peptide linkage, the nitrogen does not contain the hydrogen atom required to form a hydrogen bond.

β-SHEETS

In contrast to α-helical coils, β-sheets are formed by hydrogen bonding between linear regions of polypeptide chains as depicted in Figure 8.9. These hydrogen bonds occur between the carbonyl oxygen of one peptide bond and the nitrogen of another. The hydrogen bonds can form between two separate polypeptide chains or between two regions of a single chain that folds back on itself. This folding frequently involves a 4 amino acid structure known as a β-turn (Fig. 8.10). The chains or portions of chains that interact with each other may either be parallel or antiparallel.

SUPERSECONDARY STRUCTURES

Certain combinations of secondary structures occur in a number of proteins, forming supersecondary structures (Fig. 8.11). These include the helix-turn-helix, the β-α-β unit, the leucine zipper, and the zinc finger. Distinct structural units within the tertiary structure of a protein (known as domains) consist of various combinations of α and β structures and the more random sequences of the loops that join them together.

Tertiary Structure

The overall three-dimensional conformation of a protein is its tertiary structure. The shape of a globular protein involves interactions between amino acid residues that may be located at considerable distances from each other in the primary sequence of the polypeptide chain and includes α-helices and β-sheets. Noncovalent interactions

 Amy Lloyd's clinical presentation and initial laboratory studies suggested that she had a disorder involving white blood cells. Additional tests revealed the presence of Bence Jones protein in the urine. Bence Jones proteins consist of chains or fragments of the chains of immunoglobulins (antibodies) that have extensive β structure.

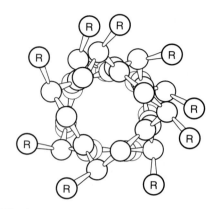

Fig. 8.8. A view down the axis of an α-helix. The side chains (R) jut out from the helix. If they sterically interfere with each other or there is charge repulsion, a stable helix cannot form. Adapted from Biochmistry, 4th ed. Copyright © 1975, 1981, 1988, 1995 by Lubert Stryer. Used with permission of W.H. Freeman and Company.

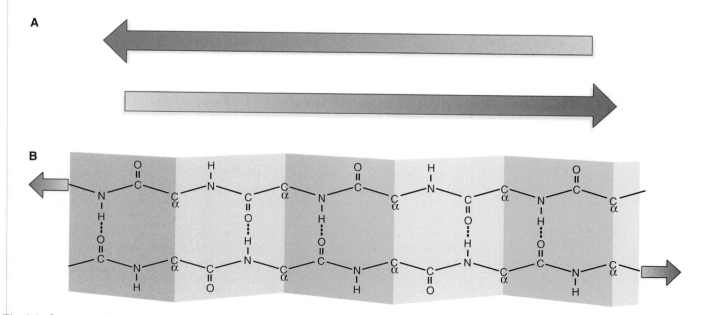

Fig. 8.9. β-Sheet. In this case, the chains are oriented in opposite directions (antiparallel), depicted by arrows (**A**). The α-carbons shown in **B** contain the side chains (R groups). Chains may also be oriented in the same direction. Two polypeptide chains may interact to form a β-sheet, or one chain may fold back on itself.

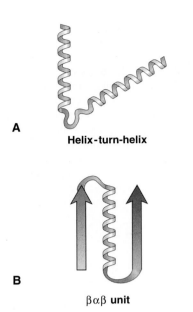

A

Helix-turn-helix

B

βαβ unit

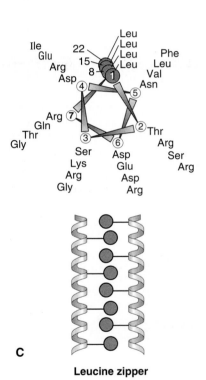

C

Leucine zipper

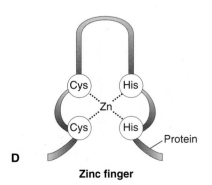

D

Zinc finger

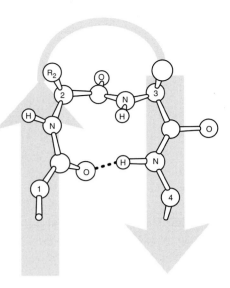

Fig. 8.10. β-Turn. A polypeptide chain that folds back on itself to form an antiparallel β-sheet usually contains a β-turn with 4 amino acid residues. The example shown above is a Type I β-turn. β-Turns are also called hairpin loops. Longer loops may connect parallel β-sheets.

Fig. 8.11. Supersecondary structures. **A** and **B.** Combinations of α-helices and β-sheets joined by loops or turns. **C.** The leucine zipper is a variation of the α-helix in which leucine residues are present at intervals such that they can interdigitate with similar leucine residues in another α-helix, forming a zipper. The upper diagram is a view down the axis of one helix, and the lower diagram is a side view of two helices with their leucine residues "zippered." **D.** In the zinc finger, Zn^{2+} is bound to 2 cysteine and to 2 histidine (or additional cysteine) residues. The helix-turn-helix, leucine zipper, and zinc finger motifs are frequently found in DNA binding proteins. **C** Reprinted with permission from Landschultz WH, et al. Science 1988;240:1759, 1763. Copyright 1988, American Association for the Advancement of Science.

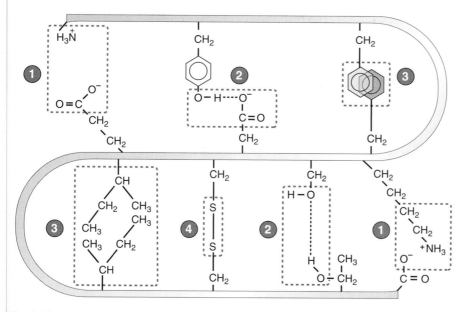

Fig. 8.12. Interactions between the side chains of amino acid residues in proteins. **1** = electrostatic interactions; **2** = hydrogen bonds; **3** = hydrophobic interactions; **4** = disulfide bonds.

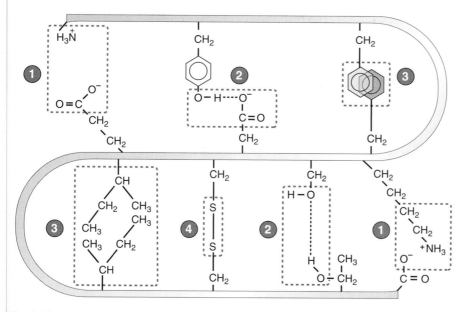

Fig. 8.13. Space-filled model of a protein. From Bennett WS, Steitz TA. J Mol Biol 1980;140:219.

between the side chains of amino acid residues are important in stabilizing the tertiary structure and include hydrophobic and electrostatic interactions as well as hydrogen bonds (Fig. 8.12). In addition, covalent linkages may occur involving disulfide bond formation between cysteine residues. Proteins tend to fold so that the atoms are packed closely together (Fig. 8.13). Therefore, van der Waals forces between the atoms play an important role in stabilizing the structure of proteins.

Hydrophobic interactions are particularly important in the structure of proteins. Hydrophobic amino acids tend to associate in the interior of a globular protein where they are not in contact with water, while hydrophilic amino acids are usually located on the surface of the protein where they interact with the surrounding water.

Certain types of conformational domains, which are composed of an assortment of α and β structures, occur repeatedly in proteins and include barrels, bundles, and saddles (Fig. 8.14). Large globular proteins consist of a number of different domains, each of which may contain a variety of these different structural motifs.

Regions of irregular structure can also occur within a protein. These regions are sometimes called random coils. However, they are not truly random in that they do not vary from one molecule of a protein to another.

Quaternary Structure

Quaternary structure is the three-dimensional structure of a protein composed of multiple subunits (Fig. 8.15). These subunits are held together by the same types of noncovalent interactions involved in tertiary structure, that is, hydrophobic and electrostatic interactions and hydrogen bonds. In hemoglobin, the subunits are similar. All four contain heme and bind oxygen. The pyruvate dehydrogenase complex, however, has several different types of subunits. This complex contains a large number of proteins including enzymes that catalyze the overall reaction, regenerate the cofactors, and regulate the activity.

A myocardial infarction (heart attack) is caused by a blockage in a coronary artery that prevents the flow of blood to an area of heart muscle. Thus, heart cells in this region suffer from a lack of oxygen and blood borne fuel. Because the cells cannot generate ATP, the membranes become damaged, and enzymes leak from the cells into the blood.

CK is one of these enzymes. It has quaternary structure because it is composed of two subunits, which may be either of the muscle (M) or the brain (B) type. The MB form, containing one M and one B subunit, is found primarily in cardiac muscle. After a heart attack, blood levels of CK rise, and the MB fraction constitutes more than 5% of the total.

On admission to the hospital, **William Hartman's** total CK was 182 units/L (reference range = 38–174). His MB fraction was 6.8% (reference range 5% or less of the total CK). Although these values are only slightly elevated, they are typical of the phase immediately following a myocardial infarction.

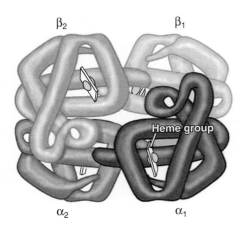

β_2 β_1

Heme group

α_2 α_1

Fig. 8.15. A multisubunit protein. The four chains of hemoglobin are illustrated. From Geoffrey Zubay, Biochemistry, 3rd ed. © 1993 Wm. C. Brown Communications, Inc. Reprinted by permission of Times Mirror Higher Education Group, Inc., Dubuque, Iowa. All rights reserved.

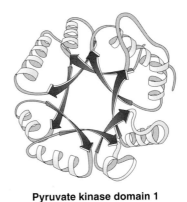

Pyruvate kinase domain 1

A. β-Barrel

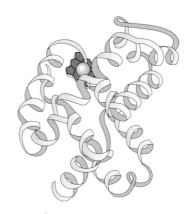

β-chain of hemoglobin

B. Bundle

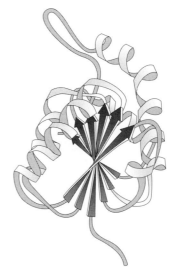

Lactate dehydrogenase domain 1

C. Saddle

Fig. 8.14. Common structural domains in proteins. Modified from Richardson JS. Adv Protein Chem 1981;34:167.

Charges on Proteins

Charges on proteins are mainly due to the side chains of the amino acid residues. Only the N-terminal amino and C-terminal carboxyl groups contribute to the charge because all the other α-amino and α-carboxyl groups are involved in peptide bonds. The pK_a values for these ionizable groups in proteins may differ to some extent from those for the free amino acids (those not joined by peptide bonds) (see Table 7.2). In proteins, the pK_a values are affected by other amino acid residues in adjacent regions of the molecule.

Because of their charge, proteins can migrate in an electrical field. This property of proteins is used to separate and identify proteins (Fig. 8.16).

Protein Folding

The primary structure of a protein determines its three-dimensional conformation. The amino acid sequence of a protein, that is the type of side chain each residue contains, dictates the way in which the chain will fold to form its native structure. If a protein in its native conformation is heated, subjected to extremes of pH, or treated with chemicals such as urea, it will denature, forming a random coil (Fig. 8.17). When certain proteins, such as ribonuclease, are denatured, and then returned to

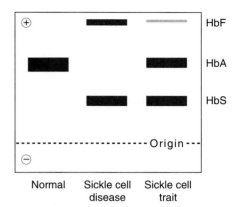

Fig. 8.16. Use of paper electrophoresis to distinguish hemoglobin S (HbS) from hemoglobin A (HbA). Samples of protein solutions are applied to filter paper in the region labeled "Origin." The paper is placed in a buffered solution and an electrical field is applied. Positively charged proteins migrate toward the cathode (⊖) and negatively charged proteins migrate toward the anode (⊕). This figure shows red blood cell lysates subjected to electrophoresis at pH 8.6 for 1 hour. HbA = normal hemoglobin; HbS = sickle cell hemoglobin; HbF = fetal hemoglobin.

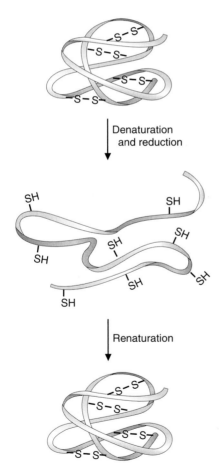

Fig. 8.17. Denaturation and renaturation. Denaturation by heat causes the molecule to unfold; however, disulfide bonds stay intact. An agent such as mercaptoethanol reduces the disulfide bonds. Under the appropriate conditions, the molecule may renature, that is, return to its native conformation. Renaturation may occur even if the disulfide bonds have been reduced.

On three hemoglobin electrophoretic patterns obtained with **Michael Sichel's** blood during earlier hospital admissions, his adult hemoglobin (HbA) level was consistently not detectable (reference range > 95% of total hemoglobin). His sickle hemoglobin (HbS) made up 85–95% of total hemoglobin (reference range = 0%). His fetal hemoglobin (HbF) made up 10% of total hemoglobin (reference range < 5%). See Figure 8.16 for an example of electrophoresis of human hemoglobins.

To determine if Michael's 4-year-old sister, **Amanda Sichel**, carried the gene for sickle hemoglobin, a hemoglobin electrophoresis of her blood was performed. The composition of her hemoglobin was: HbA 55%, HbS 44%, and HbF 1%. These values are consistent with a diagnosis of sickle cell trait. Such individuals are heterozygous for the gene coding for the structurally abnormal sickle hemoglobin. They have one normal gene that produces HbA and one mutant gene that produces HbS. They have normal total hemoglobin levels and experience vasoocclusive symptoms only under conditions of severe hypoxia.

Q 8.1: Four minor components of adult hemoglobin (HbA) result from posttranslational, nonenzymatic glycosylation (HbA$_{1a1}$, HbA$_{1a2}$, HbA$_{1b1}$, and HbA$_{1c}$). HbA$_{1c}$ makes up about 6% of the total hemoglobin in normal adults. Glycosylation of hemoglobin occurs continuously in red blood cells. It does not affect the ability of the cells to carry oxygen.

Red blood cells, which are derived from reticulocytes, have a lifespan of about 120 days. They are phagocytosed, and their hemoglobin is degraded. Therefore, the extent of glycosylation of hemoglobin is a direct reflection of the average serum glucose concentration to which the cell is exposed over its 120-day lifespan, and determination of the percentage of total hemoglobin that is present in the HbA$_{1c}$ fraction is a reasonable indicator of the extent to which the blood glucose level has been elevated on average over the preceding weeks or months.

When **Ann Sulin** was seen by her doctor after taking beef insulin for 2 months, her serum glucose measured 2 hours after finishing breakfast was in the normal range but her serum HbA$_{1c}$ level was elevated. What conclusions can you draw from this information?

physiological conditions, they will spontaneously refold into their native conformation, regaining their original function. However, they do not refold by a random search mechanism. Certain elements of the structure fold initially and these structures then help orchestrate the subsequent folding of other elements in the protein.

It is unlikely that proteins fold spontaneously as they are synthesized in the cell. A class of proteins known as chaperones appear to bind to proteins as they are being synthesized, ensuring that the completed proteins assume their appropriate conformation. After the protein has folded, cysteine residues that are in close contact in the tertiary structure can react to form disulfide bonds.

Ligand Binding to Proteins

Many proteins bind other substances known as ligands in order to perform their functions. These substances range from ions to complex coenzymes, and they fit into special pockets and crevices of proteins. Some ligands are loosely associated with their protein. Larger ligands that are tightly bound, such as the heme of hemoglobin, are known as prosthetic groups. The proteins that bind the ligand are called apoproteins. The proteins with their attached ligands are called holoproteins.

POSTTRANSLATIONAL MODIFICATIONS

After synthesis of a protein has been completed, certain amino acid residues may be chemically modified. Because protein synthesis occurs by a process known as translation, these changes are called posttranslational modifications. A common modification is phosphorylation which can occur on serine, threonine, or tyrosine residues (Fig. 8.18). Phosphorylation is frequently used by the cell to alter the activity of enzymes. Fatty acids, ADP-ribose, and methyl, acetyl, and carbohydrate groups may also be added to proteins posttranslationally by specific enzymes.

Many proteins, particularly those secreted by the cell or bound to the cell surface, are modified by the addition of carbohydrates. The addition of sugar moieties, by a process known as glycosylation, occurs on serine, threonine, or asparagine residues of a protein.

Addition of glucose moieties to proteins also occurs spontaneously (without the aid of enzymes), in proportion to the blood glucose concentration. The aldehyde group of glucose forms a Schiff base with the N-terminal amino group of the protein (or with another amino group), and a spontaneous, irreversible Amadori rearrangement produces a ketone derivative (Fig. 8.19).

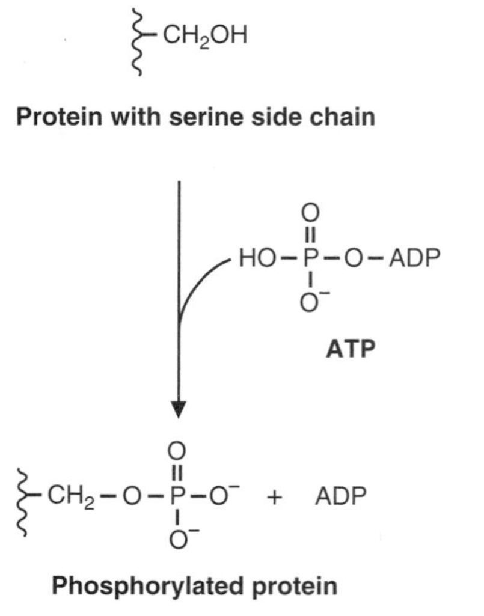

Fig. 8.18. Phosphorylation of proteins. In this example, ATP provides the phosphate group that forms an ester with the side chain of a serine residue in a protein.

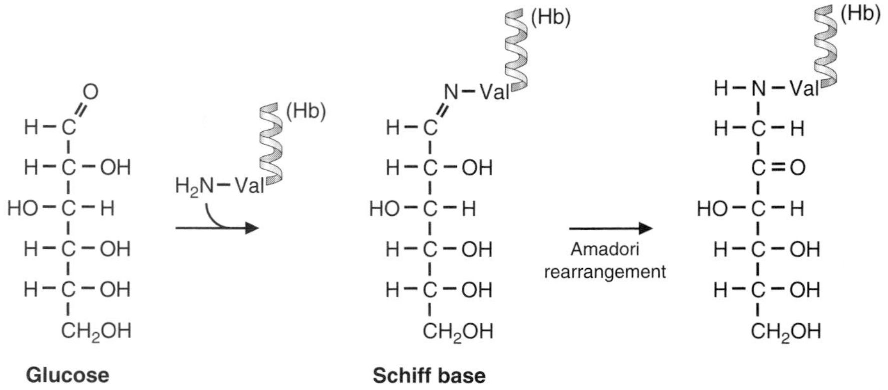

Fig. 8.19. Glycosylation of proteins. In this example, glucose becomes covalently attached by a nonenzymatic reaction to the N-terminal amino group of the β-chain of hemoglobin.

RELATIONSHIP BETWEEN PROTEIN STRUCTURE AND FUNCTION

The structure of a protein determines the function that it serves in the body. Some examples of proteins with different functions are (*a*) hemoglobin, which transports oxygen in the blood, (*b*) the antibodies, which react with antigens to combat infection, (*c*) collagen, which provides tensile strength for many structures of the body, (*d*) insulin, which acts as a hormone by binding to receptors on the cell membrane, transmitting signals to the interior of the cell, and (*e*) hexokinase, which is an enzyme that catalyzes the phosphorylation of glucose, converting it into a form that can be metabolized by the cell to generate energy.

Descriptions of each of these proteins will be used to illustrate the diversity of protein structure and its correlation with function.

Hemoglobin

STRUCTURE OF HEMOGLOBIN

Myoglobin and hemoglobin, the major oxygen-binding proteins of the body, were the first proteins for which the structures were determined in detail. X-ray crystallography showed that each of the four subunits of hemoglobin has a three-dimensional structure that is very similar to the single polypeptide chain of myoglobin (Fig. 8.20).

Myoglobin stores oxygen in muscle cells so that it is available for the oxidation of fuels that produce energy for muscle contraction. Heme serves as its prosthetic group. The single polypeptide chain contains 153 amino acids, arranged in eight α-helical regions, with most of the polar residues on the surface and the nonpolar residues in the interior of the molecule. Heme, which consists of a hydrophobic porphyrin ring that complexes with iron, binds in a hydrophobic pocket of the protein that contains 2 histidine residues. One of these histidine residues complexes with the heme iron.

Hemoglobin, which transports oxygen from the lungs to the tissues so it is available for fuel oxidation, contains four subunits: two α- and two β-chains. Even though the amino acid sequences differ, the three-dimensional structures of the α- and β-chains of hemoglobin are similar to each other and to the single polypeptide chain of myoglobin. The α- chains of hemoglobin have 141 amino acid residues, while the β-chains have 146.

Many hemoglobin molecules have been studied and over 300 instances have been found in which one amino acid has been substituted for another. Most of the substitutions are conservative, that is, they have little effect on the overall shape and function of the molecule. However, some substitutions have serious consequences, such as the substitution of a valine residue for glutamate that results in sickle cell anemia.

TRANSPORT OF OXYGEN BY HEMOGLOBIN

When the amount of oxygen bound to the protein is plotted against the partial pressure of oxygen (pO_2), a hyperbolic curve is obtained for myoglobin whereas that for hemoglobin is sigmoidal (Fig. 8.21). These curves show that when the pO_2 is high, both myoglobin and hemoglobin are saturated with oxygen. At lower levels of pO_2, however, myoglobin contains more oxygen than hemoglobin. Hemoglobin, therefore, serves as an effective transporter of oxygen, binding it in the lungs where the pO_2 is high and releasing it in the tissues where the pO_2 is low. Myoglobin, on the other hand, is still very saturated with oxygen at the pO_2 of tissues. Thus, in resting muscle cells, myoglobin binds oxygen released in the blood by hemoglobin. As muscles exercise and the oxygen tension declines, myoglobin releases oxygen.

This difference in function between myoglobin and hemoglobin stems from their

Heme is responsible for the color of red blood cells, which contain hemoglobin, and skeletal and heart muscle, which contain myoglobin.

Michael Sichel continues to experience severe low back and lower extremity pain 6 hours after admission. The diffuse pains of sickle cell crises are believed to result from occlusion of small vessels in a variety of tissues causing ischemic or anoxic damage to cells. Vasoocclusion occurs because the valine, which is on the surface of the abnormal β-globin chain of HbS, forms a hydrophobic protrusion which fits into a hydrophobic pocket present on other HbS molecules. These hydrophobic pockets are present only when hemoglobin is in its deoxygenated state, and HbS molecules polymerize in the capillaries where the partial pressure of oxygen (pO_2) is low. This polymerization causes the red blood cells to change from a biconcave disc to a sickle-like shape. These sickled cells lose their deformability and cannot readily pass through the capillary lumen. They pile up or aggregate, occluding the capillaries and preventing blood flow to the distal tissues. The subsequent hypoxia causes cellular damage and even death. The sickled cells are sequestered and destroyed mainly by phagocytic cells, particularly those in the spleen. An anemia results as the number of circulating red blood cells decreases, and bilirubin levels rise in the blood as hemoglobin is degraded.

A 8.1: Based on her postprandial blood glucose and HbA$_{1c}$ levels, **Ann Sulin's** physician concluded that, although her blood glucose was currently normal, her average serum glucose level over the last 6 weeks or longer had been above the normal range despite her compliance with her prescribed diet and therapy with beef insulin.

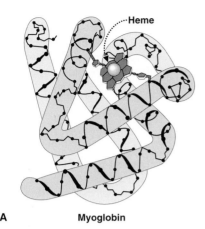

A   **Myoglobin**

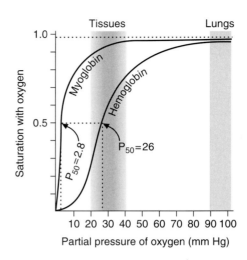

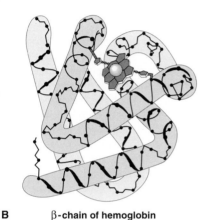

B   **β-chain of hemoglobin**

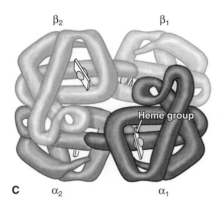

C α_2 α_1

Fig. 8.20. Structures of myoglobin (**A**), the β-chain of hemoglobin (**B**), and the four subunits of hemoglobin (**C**). Myoglobin consists of a single chain which is similar to the α- and β-chains of hemoglobin. **A** and **B** From *Enzyme Structure and Mechanism* by Fersht. Copyright © 1977 by WH Freeman and Company. Used with permission. **C** From Geoffrey Zubay, Biochemistry, 3rd ed. Copyright © 1993 Wm. C. Brown Communications, Inc. Reprinted by permission of Times Mirror Higher Education Group, Inc., Dubuque, Iowa. All rights reserved.

Fig. 8.21. Oxygen saturation curves for myoglobin and hemoglobin. Note that the curve for myoglobin is hyperbolic, while that for hemoglobin is sigmoidal. P_{50} is the partial pressure of O_2 (pO_2) when the protein is half-saturated with O_2. P_{50} for myoglobin is 2.8, and that for hemoglobin is 26.

difference in structure. Oxygen molecules bind independently of each other to the single polypeptide chain of myoglobin. On the other hand, the four subunits of hemoglobin act cooperatively in the binding of oxygen. Hemoglobin can exist in either an inactive "taut" or "tense" (T) state or an active "relaxed" (R) state (Fig. 8.22). When it is in the T state, it resists the binding of oxygen. In the R state, the binding of oxygen is facilitated. The binding of the first oxygen to a subunit of deoxygenated hemoglobin (which is in the T state) requires considerable energy to break electrostatic (salt) links between the subunits. However, when a subunit binds oxygen, conformational changes occur that permit other subunits to bind oxygen more readily. This phenomenon, known as positive cooperativity, is responsible for the sigmoidal oxygen saturation curve of hemoglobin (see Fig. 8.21).

When the amount of oxygen in the blood (pO_2) is low, pO_2 must increase considerably to permit the initial oxygen to bind to hemoglobin. However, once some oxygen is bound, only small increases in pO_2 cause large increases in the percent saturation of hemoglobin with oxygen. The result is a sigmoidal oxygen saturation curve.

AGENTS THAT AFFECT OXYGEN BINDING (FIG. 8.23)

2,3-Bisphosphoglycerate

2,3-Bisphosphoglycerate (2,3-BPG) is formed in red blood cells from the glycolytic intermediate 1,3-bisphosphoglycerate. 2,3-BPG binds to hemoglobin in the central cavity formed by the four subunits, increasing the energy required for the conformational changes that facilitate the binding of oxygen. Thus, 2,3-BPG lowers the affinity of hemoglobin for oxygen. Therefore, oxygen is less readily bound (i.e., more readily released in tissues) when hemoglobin contains 2,3-BPG.

During development, changes occur in the composition of hemoglobin. Fetal hemoglobin (HbF) consists of two α-globin chains and two γ-globin chains. In the first few weeks after birth, HbF is replaced by adult hemoglobin (HbA = $\alpha_2\beta_2$). The difference in amino acid composition between the β-chains of HbA and γ-chains of HbF results in structural changes that cause HbF to have a lower affinity for 2,3-BPG than adult hemoglobin (HbA) and, thus, a greater affinity for oxygen. Therefore, the oxygen released from the mother's hemoglobin (HbA) is readily bound by HbF in the fetus. Thus, the

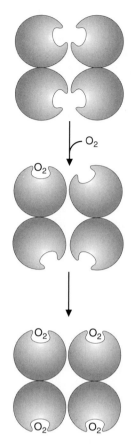

Fig. 8.22. Cooperative binding of O$_2$ to hemoglobin. Initially, the four subunits are in the T (taut or tense) state, in which they resist the binding of O$_2$. As O$_2$ binds, the subunits change their conformation, increasing the likelihood of additional O$_2$ binding. This example of positive cooperativity results in a sigmoidal O$_2$ saturation curve. As O$_2$ binds, the conformation of hemoglobin changes from the T to the R (relaxed) state.

transfer of oxygen from the mother to the fetus is facilitated by the structural difference between the hemoglobin molecule of the mother and that of the fetus.

Proton Binding

The binding of protons by hemoglobin lowers its affinity for oxygen (Fig. 8.24), contributing to a phenomenon known as the Bohr effect (Fig. 8.25). The pH of the blood decreases as it enters the tissues (and the proton concentration rises) because the CO$_2$ produced by metabolism is converted to carbonic acid by the reaction catalyzed by carbonic anhydrase in red blood cells. Dissociation of carbonic acid produces protons which react with several amino acid residues in hemoglobin, causing conformational changes that promote the release of oxygen.

In the lungs, this process is reversed. Oxygen binds to hemoglobin, causing a release of protons which combine with bicarbonate to form carbonic acid. This decrease of protons causes the pH of the blood to rise. Carbonic anhydrase cleaves the carbonic acid to H$_2$O and CO$_2$, and the CO$_2$ is exhaled. Thus, in tissues where the pH of the blood is low because of the CO$_2$ produced by metabolism, oxygen is released from hemoglobin. In the lungs where the pH of the blood is higher because CO$_2$ is being exhaled, oxygen binds to hemoglobin.

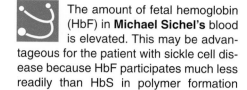

The amount of fetal hemoglobin (HbF) in **Michael Sichel's** blood is elevated. This may be advantageous for the patient with sickle cell disease because HbF participates much less readily than HbS in polymer formation within the red blood cell.

Normally, about 1% of hemoglobin in adult blood is HbF. It is found in a class of red blood cells known as F cells. In patients who are homozygous for HbS, the population of F cells increases in the bone marrow. Red cells with higher levels of HbF are more likely to survive than those with HbS. Therefore, in these individuals, a much larger than normal fraction of total hemoglobin is HbF.

Certain cytotoxic agents actually increase the production of hemoglobin F in patients with sickle cell disease. Hydroxyurea, although relatively toxic, is currently being used for this purpose with limited success.

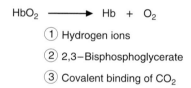

① Hydrogen ions
② 2,3–Bisphosphoglycerate
③ Covalent binding of CO$_2$

Fig. 8.23. Agents that affect O$_2$ binding by hemoglobin. Binding of hydrogen ions, 2,3-bisphosphoglycerate, and CO$_2$ to hemoglobin decrease its affinity for O$_2$.

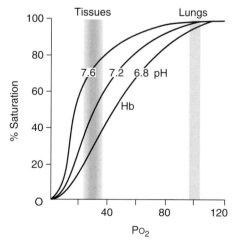

Fig. 8.24. Effect of pH on oxygen saturation curves. As the pH decreases, the affinity of hemoglobin for O$_2$ decreases, producing the Bohr effect.

A

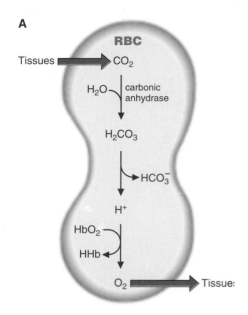

B

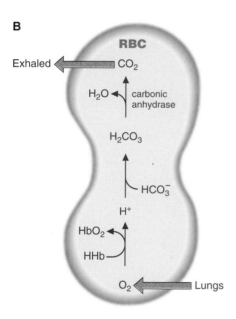

Fig. 8.25. Effect of H^+ on oxygen binding by hemoglobin (Hb). **A.** In the tissues, CO_2 is released. In the red blood cell, this CO_2 forms carbonic acid, which releases protons. The protons bind to Hb, causing it to release O_2 to the tissues. **B.** In the lungs, the reactions are reversed. O_2 binds to protonated Hb, causing the release of protons. They bind to bicarbonate (HCO_3^-), forming carbonic acid which is cleaved to H_2O and CO_2, which is exhaled.

Carbon Dioxide

Although most of the CO_2 produced by metabolism in the tissues is carried to the lungs as bicarbonate, some of the CO_2 is covalently bound to hemoglobin (Fig. 8.26). In the tissues, CO_2 forms carbamate adducts with the N-terminal amino groups of deoxyhemoglobin. In the lungs where the pO_2 is high, oxygen binds to hemoglobin and this bound CO_2 is released.

Immunoglobulins

The immunoglobulins (or antibodies) are one line of defense against invasion of the body by foreign organisms. They function by binding to antigens on the invading organisms, initiating the process by which these organisms are inactivated or destroyed. (An antigen is a molecule that elicits the production of antibodies that are capable of binding to that specific antigen.) Antibodies mark foreign invaders for destruction by phagocytic cells.

There are five major classes of immunoglobulins in the body. They are listed in Table 8.1. These proteins are similar in structure and are composed of multiple domains. Each antibody molecule contains four polypeptide chains: two identical small chains known as the light (L) chains and two identical large chains known as the heavy (H) chains. Disulfide bonds join an L chain to an H chain, and the two H chains (each bonded to an L chain) are joined by disulfide bonds (Fig. 8.27).

The most abundant immunoglobulins in human blood belong to the IgG class. These proteins, also known as γ-globulins, have approximately 220 amino acids in their light chains and 440 in their heavy chains. Carbohydrates are attached to the heavy chains. Both the light and heavy chains consist of variable (V) and constant (C) regions. The variable regions of the L and H chains interact, producing two regions at the ends of the molecule which each can bind one antigen molecule. Thus, 2 antigen molecules can be bound by each immunoglobulin molecule.

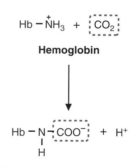

Fig. 8.26. Binding of CO_2 to hemoglobin. CO_2 forms carbamates with the N-terminal amino groups of hemoglobin chains. About 15% of the CO_2 in blood is carried to the lungs bound to hemoglobin. The reaction releases protons, which contribute to the Bohr effect.

Table 8.1. Types of Immunoglobulins

	Heavy (H) Chain Class	Normal Serum Concentration (mg/dL)
IgG	γ	1,000
IgA	α	200
IgM	μ	120
IgD	δ	3
IgE	ε	0.05

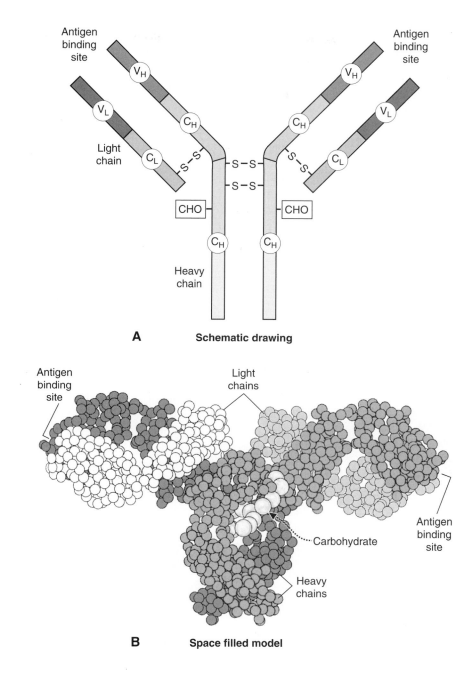

Fig. 8.27. Structure of immunoglobulins. **A.** Each antibody molecule contains two light (L) and two heavy (H) chains joined by disulfide bonds. Each chain contains a variable (V) and a constant (C) region. The variable regions are specific for the antigen that is bound, while the constant regions are the same for all antibody molecules of a given class. Carbohydrate (CHO) is bound as indicated within the constant region of the heavy chains (C_H). **B.** In the space filled model, the light chains are light in color and the heavy chains are two different shades of gray. Modified from Silverton EW, et al. Proc Natl Acad Sci USA 1977;11:5142.

Amy Lloyd's serum protein electrophoresis revealed the presence of a sharp peak or homogeneous "spike" in the γ-globulin zone known as an M-component. On immunoelectrophoresis of her serum, this immunoglobulin M-component was found to be derived from a single clone of antibody-producing cells (monoclonal, i.e., having a single type of H chain and a single type of L chain).

When the concentration of the immunoglobulins secreted by this clone of proliferating cells exceeds the renal threshold, Bence Jones proteins appear in the urine. The proteins may also infiltrate tissues producing protein aggregates known as amyloid deposits.

Gelatin and glue are both products made from animal collagen. Gelatin is not a very nutritious food because of its limited amino acid composition.

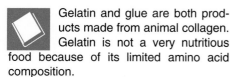

V_L domain

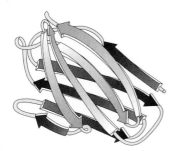

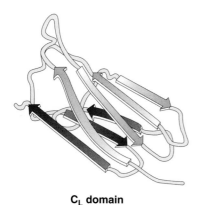

C_L domain

Fig. 8.29. Immunoglobulin fold. Layers of antiparallel β-sheets are stacked in these domains. **Top** modified from Richardson JS. Adv Protein Chem 1981;34:167; **bottom** reprinted in part with permission from Edmundson AB, et al. Biochemistry 1975;14:3954. © 1975 American Chemical Society.

The L chain contains one domain in the variable region and one in the constant region, while the H chain contains four domains, one in the variable region and three in the constant region (Fig. 8.28). These domains have a similar structure known as the immunoglobulin fold, which consists of a number of β-sheets that form a β-barrel (Fig. 8.29). This type of domain has been observed not only in immunoglobulins, but also in other proteins, many of which are involved in cell recognition.

Collagen

Collagen is a fibrous protein that is the major component of connective tissue and the most abundant protein in mammals. It is found in bone, tendons, skin, blood vessels, and the cornea of the eye. Collagen contains about 33% glycine and 21% proline and hydroxyproline, an amino acid produced by posttranslational modification of proline residues.

Tropocollagen, the precursor of collagen, is a triple helix composed of three polypeptide chains that are twisted around each other, forming a rope-like structure which has great tensile strength (Fig. 8.30). The individual polypeptide chains each contain about 1,000 amino acid residues. When three of these polypeptide chains wrap around each other, they form the supercoil which is tropocollagen.

The three polypeptide chains of the triple helix are linked by hydrogen bonds. Each turn of the triple helix contains 3 amino acid residues, so that every third amino acid is in close contact with the other two strands in the center of the structure. Only glycine, which lacks a side chain, could fit in this position, and indeed, every third amino acid residue of tropocollagen is glycine. Proline residues frequently follow the glycine residues in the sequence, which can be depicted as Gly-X-Y, where X is frequently proline and Y is any other amino acid found in collagen.

Tropocollagen is an example of a protein that undergoes extensive posttranslational modifications. Hydroxylation reactions produce hydroxyproline residues from proline residues and hydroxylysine from lysine residues. These reactions occur after the protein has been synthesized (Fig. 8.31) and require vitamin C (ascorbic acid). Hydroxyproline residues are involved in hydrogen bond formation that helps to sta-

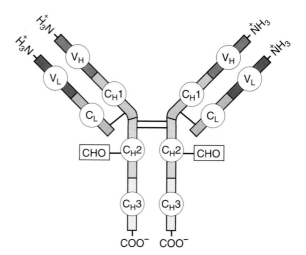

Fig. 8.28. Domains of immunoglobulins. The light chain has two domains (V_L and C_L). The heavy chain has one variable domain (V_H) and three constant domains (C_H1, C_H2, and C_H3). Carbohydrate (CHO) is attached to C_H2. These domains contain layers of β-sheets (see Fig. 8.29). The domains are circled.

bilize the triple helix, whereas hydroxylysine residues are the sites of attachment of carbohydrate moieties.

The side chains of lysine residues may also be oxidized to form the aldehyde allysine. These aldehyde residues produce covalent cross-links between tropocollagen molecules (Fig. 8.32). An allysine residue on 1 tropocollagen molecule reacts with the amino group of a lysine residue on another molecule, forming a covalent Schiff base which is converted to more stable covalent cross-links. Aldol condensation may also occur between 2 allysine residues, which form a structure known as lysinonorleucine.

Insulin

Insulin, one of the major hormones that regulate the metabolism of nutrients (see Chapter 24), is a small protein that contains 51 amino acids. It is composed of two polypeptide chains, the A chain which contains 21 amino acids and the B chain which contains 30 amino acids (Fig. 8.33). The chains are joined together by two disulfide bonds. In addition, the A chain contains an intrachain disulfide bond.

The primary structure of insulin has been studied in a number of animal species. Except for positions 8, 9, and 10 of the A chain and position 30 of the B chain, the sequences are homologous, and the changes at the variable positions are generally conservative.

Although much effort has been expended in many different research laboratories, the details of the mechanism of action of insulin are still a mystery. The synthesis of insulin and its metabolic effects are described in Chapter 24 and in Sections V, VI, and VII (carbohydrate, lipid, and nitrogen metabolism, respectively).

Hexokinase

Hexokinase is an extremely important enzyme in metabolism. It catalyzes the phosphorylation of glucose to form glucose 6-phosphate. The hexokinase molecule con-

 Severe vitamin C deficiencies result in scurvy, which affects tissues that are rich in collagen. Because proline and lysine residues are not hydroxylated, hydrogen bonding within triple helices and cross-linking between triple helices cannot occur. Therefore, collagen molecules are unstable. Scurvy is characterized by bleeding gums, loose teeth, skin lesions, and weakened blood vessel walls.

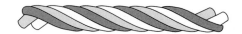

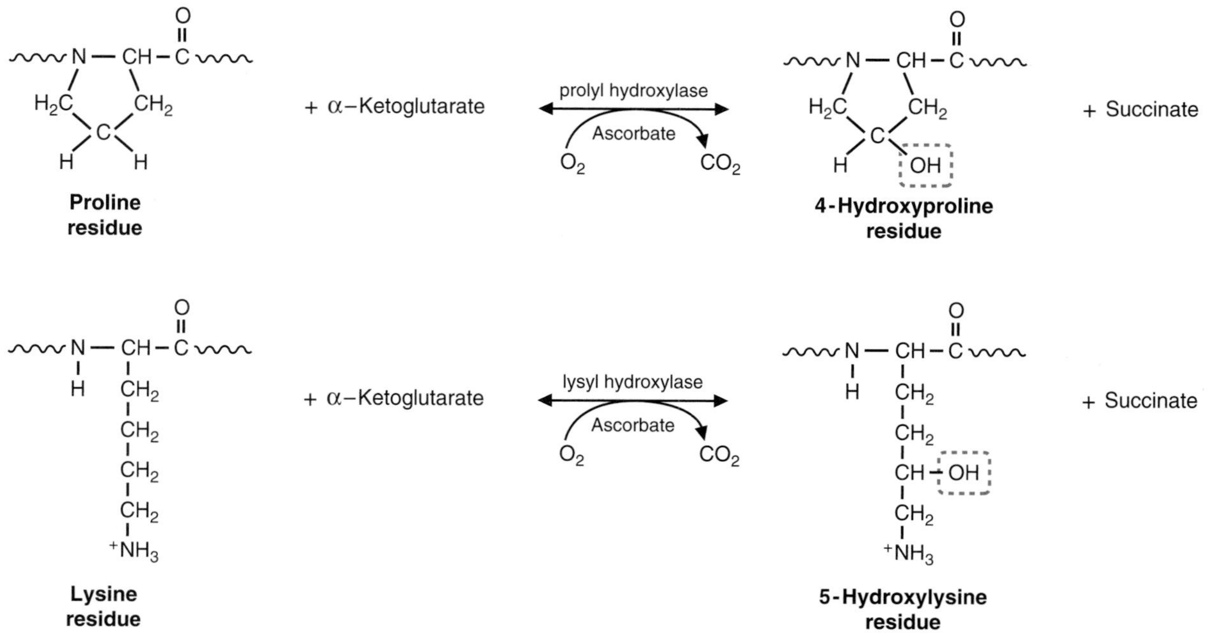

Fig. 8.30. Triple helix of collagen.

Fig. 8.31. Hydroxylation of proline and lysine residues in collagen. Proline and lysine residues within the collagen chain are hydroxylated by reactions that require ascorbate (vitamin C).

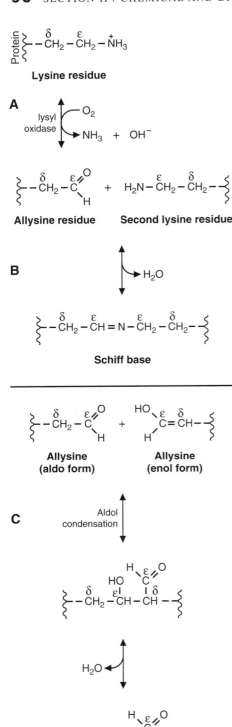

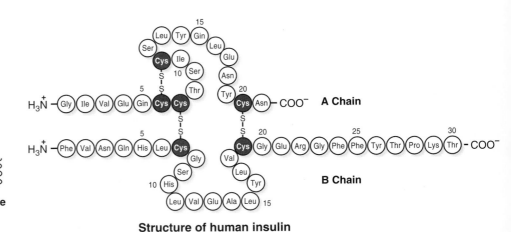

Structure of human insulin

Fig. 8.33. Primary structure of human insulin. Porcine insulin differs in only one position from human insulin; alanine replaces threonine as the C-terminal amino acid in the B chain. In addition to this replacement, bovine insulin also differs from human insulin in the A chain in that alanine replaces threonine at position 8 and valine replaces isoleucine at position 10.

tains two domains that are connected by a hinge region. Two different conformations of the molecule have been observed, an "open" and a "closed" structure. When glucose binds, the conformation of the enzyme changes from open to closed (Fig. 8.34). In this closed state, the enzyme is catalytically active.

The change in the conformation of hexokinase that is produced by the binding of glucose shows that protein structures are not static: they have enough structural flexibility to allow conformational changes which alter the functional activity of the protein.

 CLINICAL COMMENTS. After a few days of treatment, **Michael Sichel's** crisis was resolved. In the future, should Michael suffer a cerebrovascular accident as a consequence of vascular occlusion or have recurrent life-threatening episodes, a course of long term maintenance blood transfusions to prevent repeated sickle crises may be indicated. Iron chelation would have to accompany such a program to prevent or delay the development of iron overload.

Although a few individuals with this disease have survived into the sixth decade, mean survival is probably into the fourth decade. Death usually results from renal failure and/or cardiopulmonary disease.

Amy Lloyd has multiple myeloma, a plasma cell disorder. Multiple myeloma belongs to a group of related neoplastic diseases characterized by the proliferation of a single clone of immunoglobulin-secreting plasma cells. Normally, immunoglobulin molecules are produced by numerous clones of plasma cells.

The symptoms and signs of multiple myeloma are related to (a) the growth of the abnormal cell clone and (b) products secreted by the tumor cells. The proliferating myeloma cells in the bone marrow may replace the red cell precursors, leading to anemia. Myeloma cells may produce several peptides with osteolytic (bone resorbing) action, leading to focal skeletal destruction described as "Swiss cheese-like lesions" on skeletal x-rays. Pathologic fractures associated with bone pain and hypercalcemia (high serum calcium levels) secondary to extensive bone lysis may occur. Hypercalcemia, in turn, is associated with muscle weakness and myalgias, lethargy, and eventually confusion. Chronic hypercalcemia may damage renal tubular cells.

Fig. 8.32. Formation of cross-links in collagen. **A.** Lysine residues are oxidized to allysine (an aldehyde). Allysine may react with a lysine residue to form a Schiff base (**B**), or 2 allysine residues may undergo an aldol condensation (**C**).

Renal failure may occur as a result of the tubular injury associated with significant Bence Jones proteinuria.

Because patients with myeloma usually have severely suppressed levels of normal immunoglobulins, they are highly susceptible to infections and often present with pneumonia and other types of systemic infections.

Treatment involves (*a*) systemic chemotherapy to suppress the proliferative cell clone and (*b*) supportive care for the complications of the disorder (e.g., the consequences of hypercalcemia, sepsis, anemia, renal failure, and bone pain).

William Hartman continued to be monitored in the cardiac care unit. His initial CK levels were elevated, and the MB fraction was high (>5% of the total). Within 2 hours of the onset of an acute myocardial infarction, the MB form of CK begins leaking from those heart cells which were injured by the ischemic process. These rising serum levels of the MB fraction (and, therefore, of the total CK) reach their peak 12–36 hours later, and usually return to normal within 3–5 days from the onset of the infarction.

Ann Sulin has non-insulin-dependent diabetes mellitus (NIDDM), also called Type II, or adult-onset diabetes mellitus. Such patients sometimes require insulin injections to control their blood glucose levels. In contrast, patients with insulin-dependent diabetes mellitus (IDDM), also called Type I, or juvenile-onset diabetes mellitus, always require insulin injections. The IDDM patients are unable to synthesize adequate amounts of insulin to maintain normal blood glucose levels.

There are 12–15 million diabetic patients in the United States, the great majority of whom have NIDDM. Of IDDM and NIDDM patients who are taking insulin injections, the incidence of both local allergic and systemic reactions has fallen markedly because synthetic insulin preparations, which are structurally identical to human insulin, are now commercially available.

BIOCHEMICAL COMMENTS. This chapter was not intended to turn medical students into experts on protein structure, but rather to describe the general principles that will aid students in understanding protein function relevant to medicine. For those students interested in learning more about protein structure, textbooks that emphasize structures are available (see Suggested Readings).

Suggested Readings

Lehninger A, Nelson D, Cox M. Principles of biochemistry. New York: Worth, 1993.

Stryer L. Biochemistry. New York: W.H. Freeman, 1995.

PROBLEMS

1. Michael Sichel's hemoglobin (HbS) differs from normal adult hemoglobin (HbA) only in the amino acid sequence of the N-terminal region of the β-globin chain.

Determine the charge on HbA and HbS in this region of the β-chain at physiological pH from the sequences given below.

HbA   Val-His-Leu-Thr-Pro-Glu-Glu-Lys-Ser-Ala-Val-Thr – – – – – –

HbS   Val-His-Leu-Thr-Pro-Val-Glu-Lys-Ser-Ala-Val-Thr – – – – – –

Which of these proteins will migrate further toward the anode in an electrical field?

Ten weeks after initiating daily beef insulin injections, **Ann Sulin** noted redness and localized swelling at the injection site, generalized pruritus (itching), mild bronchospasm (wheezing), and a generalized rash. These symptoms worsened with continued injections.

Her physician recognized that Mrs. Sulin was experiencing an allergic reaction to the beef insulin which was both local (usually due to a contaminant in the insulin administered) and systemic (usually due to the insulin molecule itself). The beef insulin was immediately discontinued and therapy initiated with a small dose of Humulin insulin (a synthetic insulin produced by recombinant DNA technology and having a structure identical to that of human insulin).

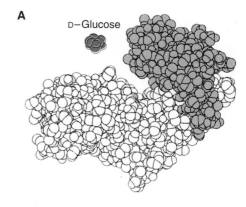

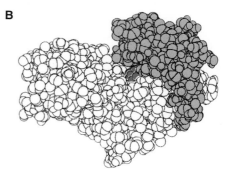

Fig. 8.34. Conformational change induced by the binding of glucose to hexokinase. Free enzyme (**A**). With glucose bound (**B**). From Bennett WS, Steitz TA. J Mol Biol 1980; 140:219.

ANSWERS

1. At pH 7.4, the N-terminal valine has a positive charge on its free amino group. Charges are also present on some of the side chains. Histidine has a partial positive charge ($pK_a \sim 6.0$), the glutamates have negative charges, and lysine has a positive charge.

Sickle cell hemoglobin (HbS) contains one less negative charge than does normal hemoglobin (HbA) because a hydrophobic valine residue has been substituted for a negatively charged glutamate. Therefore, **Michael Sichel's** sickle cell hemoglobin would not migrate as far toward the anode (the positive electrode) in an electrical field as normal hemoglobin (see Fig. 8.16).

9 Enzymes

Enzymes are proteins that act as catalysts, compounds that increase the rate of chemical reactions (Fig. 9.1). Enzyme catalysts bind the reactants, called substrates, convert them to products, and release the products. Although enzymes may be modified during this sequence, they return to their original form at the end of the reaction. In addition to increasing the speed of reactions, enzymes provide a means for regulating the rate of reactions in the metabolic pathways of the body. This chapter is divided into two parts: the first part explains the properties of enzymes as catalysts, and the second part presents the mechanisms of enzyme regulation.

Enzymes as catalysts. An enzyme binds the substrates of the reaction and converts them to products. The substrates are bound to specific substrate binding sites on the enzyme through interactions with the amino acid residues of the enzyme. The spatial geometry required for all the interactions between the substrate and the enzyme makes each enzyme selective for its substrates, and ensures that only specific products are formed.

The substrate binding sites overlap in the active catalytic site of the enzyme, the region of the enzyme where the reaction occurs. Within the active site, functional groups of other amino acid residues of the enzyme, compounds called coenzymes, and tightly bound metals participate in the reaction. The functional groups in the active site of the enzyme activate the substrates and decrease the energy needed to form the high energy intermediate stage of the reaction known as the transition state. Some of the catalytic strategies employed by enzymes, such as general acid-base catalysis, formation of covalent intermediates, and stabilization of the transition state, are illustrated by chymotrypsin.

The effectiveness of many drugs and toxins depends on their ability to inhibit an enzyme. The strongest inhibitors form covalent bonds with a reactive group in the enzyme active site, or are analogues of an intermediate stage of the reaction, such as the transition state.

Regulation of enzymes. The rate of an enzyme can be influenced by the concentrations of substrates, products, activators, and inhibitors. For many enzymes, the relationship between the velocity of the reaction and substrate concentration is described by the Michaelis-Menten equation. Products and other reversible physiological inhibitors may compete with a substrate for binding in the active site, thereby slowing the rate of the reaction.

Physiological regulation of metabolic pathways depends on the ability to alter flux through a pathway by activating enzymes which catalyze the slowest steps in the pathway. These enzymes often have allosteric activators or inhibitors, compounds that bind at sites other than the active catalytic site and regulate the enzyme through conformational changes in the enzyme.

Enzyme activity may also be regulated by phosphorylation or by modulator proteins. Some enzymes are synthesized as inactive precursors, called zymogens, and activated by proteolytic cleavage (e.g., the blood clotting proteins).

Enzymes that have different amino acid sequences but catalyze exactly the same reaction are known as isoenzymes. Tissue-specific isoenzymes often have properties consistent with different roles in different tissues (e.g., glucokinase and hexokinase).

After one year in the absence of enzyme

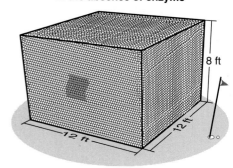

After one second with one molecule of enzyme

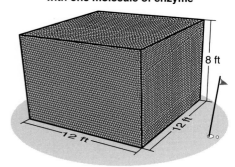

Fig. 9.1. Catalytic power of enzymes. Many enzymes increase the rate of a chemical reaction by a factor of 10^{11} or higher. To appreciate an increase in reaction rate by this order of magnitude, consider a room-sized box of golf balls which "reacts" by releasing energy and turning blue. The 12 ft × 12 ft × 8 ft box contains 380,000 golf balls. If the rate of the reaction in the absence of enzyme were 100 golf balls per year, in the presence of 1 molecule of enzyme the entire box of golf balls would turn blue in 1 second.

Sloe Klotter, a 6-month-old male infant, was brought to his pediatrician's office with a painful, expanding mass in his right upper thigh which was first noted just hours after he fell down three uncarpeted steps in his home. The child appeared to be in severe distress.

An x-ray revealed no fractures, but a soft tissue swelling, consistent with a hematoma (bleeding into the tissues). Sloe's mother related that soon after he began to crawl, his knees occasionally became swollen and seemed painful.

The pediatrician suspected a disorder of coagulation. A screening coagulation profile suggested a possible deficiency of Factor VIII, a protein involved in the formation of blood clots. Sloe's plasma Factor VIII level was found to be only 6% of the average level found in normal subjects. A diagnosis of hemophilia A was made.

Al Martini, a 44-year-old male who has been an alcoholic for the past 5 years, has a markedly diminished appetite for food. One weekend he became unusually irritable and confused after drinking two fifths of scotch and eating very little. His landlady convinced him to visit his doctor. Physical examination revealed a heart rate of 104 beats per minute. His blood pressure was slightly low, and he was in early congestive heart failure. He was poorly oriented to time, place, and person.

Several weeks after his acute gout attack subsided, **Yves Topaigne** was started on allopurinol in an oral dose of 150 mg twice a day.

While playing in his grandmother's basement, **Dennis Livermore** drank an unknown amount of the insecticide malathion, sometimes used for killing fruit flies. Malathion is similar in structure to the insecticide parathion, but not nearly as toxic. Nausea, coma, convulsions, respiratory failure, and death have resulted from the use of parathion by farmers who have gotten it on their skin. These compounds, like the nerve gas sarin, are organophosphorus compounds (Fig. 9.2). Fortunately, Dennis told his grandmother what he had done. She retrieved the bottle and rushed Dennis to the emergency room of the local hospital. On the way, Dennis vomited repeatedly and complained of abdominal cramps. As they arrived at the hospital, Dennis began salivating, sweating heavily, and tearing. He had an uncontrollable defecation.

In the emergency room, physicians passed a nasogastric tube for stomach lavage, started intravenous fluids, and recorded vital signs. Dennis' pulse rate was 48 beats per minute (slow) and his blood pressure was 78/48 mm Hg (low). The physicians noted involuntary twitching of the muscles in his extremities.

William Hartman's cardiovascular status stabilized 35 hours after his admission to the hospital cardiac care unit with severe chest pain, and his original electrocardiographic abnormalities improved. He remained in the hospital for observation and testing for a number of days.

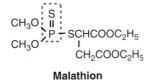

Malathion

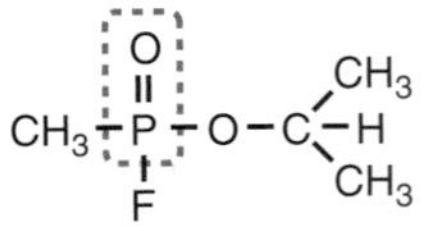

Sarin

Fig. 9.2. Organophosphorus compounds.

ENZYMES AS CATALYSTS

Enzymes, in general, provide speed, specificity, and regulatory control to reactions in the body. Enzymes are proteins that act as catalysts, compounds that increase the rate of chemical reactions. An enzyme binds the substrates and brings them together at the right orientation to react. The enzyme then participates in the making and breaking of bonds required for product formation, releases the products, and returns to its original state once the reaction is completed. The catalytic power of an enzyme, the rate of the catalyzed reaction divided by the rate of the uncatalyzed reaction, is usually in the range of 10^6 to 10^{14}. Each enzyme usually catalyzes a specific biochemical reaction. It reacts with just one set of substrates, and converts them to just one set of products. Enzymes also provide the body with a means of controlling the rate of reactions. Hormones and other regulatory factors change the rates of key steps in metabolic pathways by affecting the activity of enzymes. The speed, specificity, and regulatory control of enzymatic reactions are a result of the unique sequence of specific amino acids which form the enzyme and bind and activate substrate molecules.

GENERAL PROPERTIES OF ENZYMES

CLASSIFICATION AND NOMENCLATURE OF ENZYMES

Enzymes have been systematically classified by the International Commission on Enzymes into six major groups, according to the type of reaction catalyzed (Table 9.1). The major groups are further subdivided so that each enzyme has an individual Enzyme Commission number and a formal name that ends in "ase." In addition, most enzymes have common or trivial names, which are shorter and usually reflect the activity of the enzyme in a less standardized way. For example in the common name "glucokinase," "kinase" refers to the transfer of a phosphate from ATP to glucose, the compound in the prefix of the name (Fig. 9.3). The formal Enzyme Commission name for this enzyme is ATP:D-glucose 6-phosphotransferase, and its enzyme commission number is EC 2.7.1.2. Although a name ending in "ase" always denotes an enzyme, not all common names for enzymes end in "ase." Chymotrypsin is a common name for a peptidyl hydrolase, or protease (Fig. 9.4).

ACTIVE SITE OF THE ENZYME

To catalyze a chemical reaction, the enzyme binds the substrates and forms an enzyme-substrate complex (Fig. 9.5). The reaction occurs in a relatively small dynamic region of the enzyme, the active, or catalytic site. The proximity and orientation of substrate molecules in the active site contribute to the catalytic power of the enzyme. The active site may also contain cofactors, which are metal or nonprotein organic compounds that participate in the reaction. Interactions between the substrate and functional reactive groups on amino acid residues or cofactors of the enzyme promote the electronic rearrangements necessary for the reaction. For instance, an amino acid side chain might abstract a proton from the substrate, or form a covalent intermediate with the substrate. The active site is in a cleft, crevice, or cavity in the enzyme. This spatial arrangement permits the exclusion of water and allows func-

 Enzymes do not invent new reactions. They just make a reaction occur faster. Without the catalytic power of enzymes, reactions such as those involved in nerve conduction, heart contraction, and digestion of food would occur too slowly for life to exist.

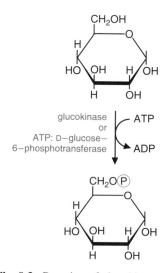

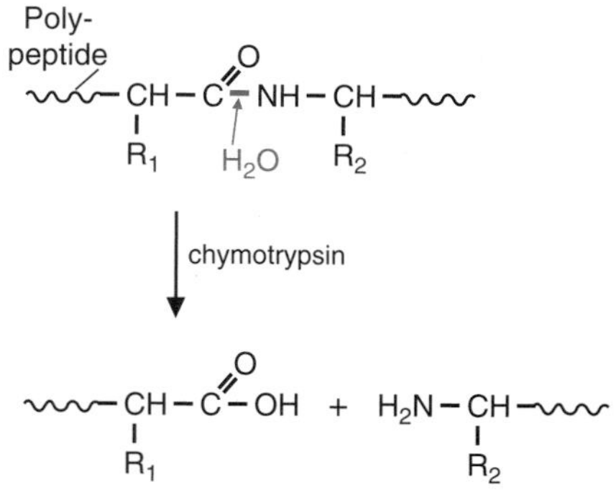

Fig. 9.3. Reaction of glucokinase.

Poly-peptide

chymotrypsin

Fig. 9.4. Chymotrypsin hydrolyses certain peptide bonds in proteins. Chymotrypsin is synthesized by the pancreas and secreted into the digestive tract, where it acts with other hydrolases to break food proteins into individual amino acids. The prefix "chyme" refers to the digestive juice which passes from the stomach into the intestine.

Table 9.1. Classification of Enzymes by the Type of Reaction Catalyzed

EC[a]	Class of Enzyme	Type of Reaction
1	Oxidoreductases	Transfer of electrons (as an e−, hydrogen atoms, or hydride ion) from one compound to an acceptor
2	Transferases	Transfer of a functional group, such as an acyl, amino, methyl, or phosphate group
3	Hydrolases	Cleavage of a C–O, C–N, or C–S bond by the addition of H_2O across the bond
4	Lyases	Addition of groups to double bonds or formation of double bonds
5	Isomerases	Transfer of groups within molecules to yield isomeric forms
6	Ligases	Formation of C–C, C–S, C–O, and C–N bonds coupled to cleavage of a high energy bond, such as ATP

[a]The Enzyme Commission (EC) number of the general class appears first, followed by a period and the number of the subclass.

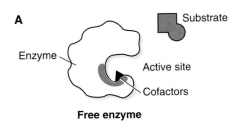

Free enzyme

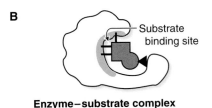

Enzyme–substrate complex

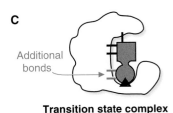

Transition state complex

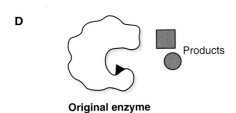

Original enzyme

Fig. 9.5. Reaction in the enzyme active site. **A.** The enzyme contains an active site, shown in dark blue, with a region or domain where the substrate binds. The active site may also contain cofactors, nonprotein components that assist in catalysis. **B.** The substrate forms bonds with amino acid residues in the substrate binding domain, shown in light blue. Substrate binding induces a conformational change in the active site. **C.** Functional groups of amino acid residues and cofactors in the active site participate in the reaction. During the course of the reaction, the enzyme forms a strained transition state complex which is stabilized by additional bonds with the enzyme, shown in blue. **D.** As the products of the reaction dissociate, the enzyme returns to its original conformation.

tional groups to approach the reacting substrates from three dimensions.

The activated substrates and enzyme form a transition state complex, an unstable high energy complex with a strained electronic configuration intermediate between substrate and product (see Fig. 9.5C). Functional groups within the active site stabilize the transition state complex and decrease the energy required for its formation. The transition state complex decomposes to products, which dissociate from the enzyme. The free enzyme then binds another set of substrates and repeats the process.

ENZYME SPECIFICITY

The specificity of the enzymatic reaction results from the three-dimensional arrangement of specific amino acid residues in the enzyme that form the binding sites for the substrates and activate the substrates during the course of the reaction. The "lock-and-key" and "induced-fit" models for substrate binding describe different aspects of the binding interaction between the enzyme and substrate.

Lock-and-Key Model for Substrate Binding

The substrate binding site contains amino acid residues arranged in a complementary three-dimensional surface which bind the substrate through multiple hydrophobic interactions, electrostatic interactions, and hydrogen bonds (Figs. 9.6 and 9.7). These amino acid residues can come from very different parts of the linear amino acid sequence of the enzyme, as seen in glucokinase (see Fig. 9.7). Steric hindrance and charge-repulsion in the substrate binding site may prevent the binding of even closely related compounds. In the lock-and-key model, the complementarity between the substrate and its binding site is compared to that of a key fitting into a rigid lock.

"Induced Fit" Model for Substrate Binding

As the substrate binds, almost all enzymes undergo a conformational change, an "induced fit," which repositions the side chains of the amino acids in the active site and increases the number of binding interactions (see Fig. 9.5). The induced fit model for substrate binding recognizes that the substrate binding site is not a rigid "lock," but a dynamic surface created by the flexible overall three-dimensional structure of the enzyme.

The function of the conformational change induced by substrate binding is usually to rearrange amino acid residues in the active site in ways that promote the reaction. For instance, the induced fit after glucose binding to glucokinase or hexokinase involves changes in the conformation of the whole enzyme which result in the exclusion of water from the active site (see Fig. 8.34). The induced fit after substrate binding to chymotrypsin moves a serine in the active site to a position where it can be activated and participate in the reaction (see Fig. 9.7). The induced fit might cause a conformational change which improves the binding site of a cosubstrate, or cause a conformational change in an adjacent subunit of the enzyme (e.g., hemoglobin, see Chapter 8). The multiple interactions between the substrate and the enzyme in the enzyme binding site, therefore, serve both for substrate recognition and for rearranging the active site for the next stage of the reaction.

Catalytic Power

Different enzymes achieve their catalytic power by employing the same types of catalytic strategies, or general mechanisms, for increasing the reaction rate (Table 9.2). One of these catalytic strategies, proximity and orientation, is an intrinsic fea-

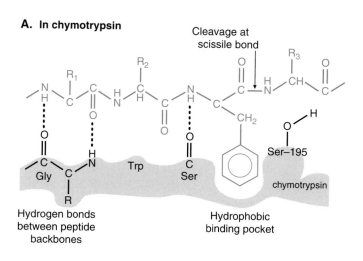

A. In chymotrypsin

Cleavage at
scissile bond

Ser–195

chymotrypsin

Trp

Gly

Ser

Hydrogen bonds
between peptide
backbones

Hydrophobic
binding pocket

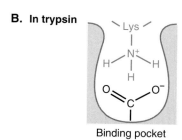

B. In trypsin

Lys

Binding pocket

Fig. 9.6. Binding sites of chymotrypsin and trypsin. The substrate protein is blue and the enzyme amino acid residues are named in the shaded area. **A.** Chymotrypsin hydrolyzes the peptide bond on the carbonyl side of a phenylalanine, tyrosine, or tryptophan in denatured proteins. The bond which is cleaved is called the scissile bond. The hydrophobic amino acid residues fit into a binding pocket in the active site referred to as the substrate recognition site. The denatured substrate protein is held more rigidly in place by hydrogen bonds with the chymotrypsin peptide backbone. Binding of the substrate induces a change in the conformation of chymotrypsin which moves serine-195 into a position where it can be activated to form a covalent intermediate. **B.** In trypsin, the substrate recognition binding pocket contains an aspartate, which binds arginine or lysine of the substrate protein. The remainder of the active site is very similar to that of chymotrypsin.

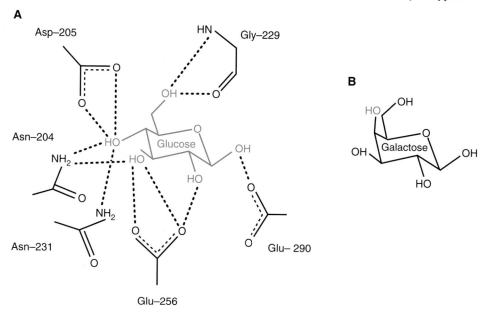

A

Asp–205

HN Gly–229

Asn–204

NH₂

Glucose

Asn–231

NH₂

Glu–256

Glu–290

B

Galactose

Fig. 9.7. Glucose binding site in glucokinase. **A.** Glucose, shown in blue, is held in its binding site by multiple hydrogen bonds between each hydroxyl group and polar amino acids from different regions of the enzyme amino acid sequence. (The position of the amino acid residue in the linear sequence is given by its number.) The multiple interactions enable glucose to induce large conformational changes in the enzyme. **B.** Enzyme specificity is illustrated by the comparison of galactose and glucose. Galactose differs from glucose only in the position of the –OH group shown in blue. However, it is not phosphorylated by the enzyme. Cells therefore require a separate galactokinase for the metabolism of galactose. **A** modified from Pilkis SJ, et al. J Biol Chem 1994;269:21927.

Q 9.1: General acid-base catalysis usually involves several amino acids working cooperatively in the active site to abstract a proton from the substrate in the first stage of the reaction (base catalysis), and donate it at a later stage of the reaction (acid catalysis). Why is histidine the amino acid most often involved?

The pancreatic digestive enzymes trypsin and chymotrypsin are part of an enzyme family that utilizes serine to hydrolyze peptide bonds; these enzymes are called serine proteases. Chymotrypsin and trypsin have similar amino acid sequences and three-dimensional structure, nearly identical active sites, and are presumably derived from a common ancestral serine protease through divergent evolution. However, differences in the amino acid residues that form the binding pocket give these enzymes different specificities (see Fig. 9.6).

Nucleophiles carry full or partial negative charges or have electron donating groups, such as the two unbonded electrons on N. Nucleophiles can form a covalent bond with atoms carrying full and partial positive charges, and thus nucleophilic catalysis is a specific type of covalent catalysis. Electrophiles carry full or partial positive charges and are attracted to atoms with full or partial negative charges. Electrophilic catalysis refers to the stabilization of a negative charge in an intermediate of the reaction by a metal or a positively charged group on the enzyme. The stabilization of developing positive charges in the substrates by a nucleophile on the enzyme or the stabilization of developing negative charges in the substrates by an electrophile on the enzyme are sometimes referred to as electrostatic catalysis.

ture of substrate binding and part of the catalytic mechanism of all enzymes. All enzymes also stabilize the transition state by electrostatic interactions. The catalytic mechanism of chymotrypsin provides an explanation of many of these catalytic strategies. Chymotrypsin employs proximity and orientation, transition state stabilization, acid-base catalysis, covalent catalysis, and nucleophilic catalysis to increase reaction rate.

CATALYTIC MECHANISM OF CHYMOTRYPSIN

Chymotrypsin hydrolyzes specific peptide bonds of denatured proteins (see Figs. 9.4 and 9.6). In the absence of enzyme, the negatively charged hydroxyl group of water attacks the positively charged carbonyl carbon (Fig. 9.8). An unstable oxyanion tetrahedral transition state complex is formed in which the oxygen atom carries a full negative charge. According to transition state theory, the overall rate of the reaction is determined by the number of molecules which can acquire the activation energy necessary to form the transition state complex (Fig. 9.9). The rate of the chemical reaction in the absence of chymotrypsin is slow because there are very few OH⁻ molecules in H₂O at neutral pH, and even fewer which have enough energy when they collide to form the transition state complex.

Functional Groups in the Chymotrypsin Active Site

The rate of the reaction in the presence of chymotrypsin is faster because functional groups in the enzyme active site activate the attacking hydroxyl group and stabilize the oxyanion transition state complex. The reaction takes place in two stages: (a) cleavage of the peptide bond in the denatured substrate protein and formation of a covalent acyl-enzyme intermediate (Fig. 9.10, steps 1–5), and (b) hydrolysis of the acyl-enzyme intermediate to release the remaining portion of the substrate protein (Fig. 9.10, steps 6–9).

In the first stage of the reaction, the peptide bond of the denatured protein substrate is cleaved as an active site serine attacks the carbonyl carbon of the scissile bond. The —OH of serine is not a particularly good nucleophilic attacking group. However, an active site histidine acts as a general base catalyst and abstracts a proton from the serine-OH; the histidine is activated by the negative charge of a nearby aspartate. The aspartate-histidine-serine combination, referred to as the catalytic triad, is an example of cooperative interactions between amino acid residues in the active site. The strong nucleophilic attacking group created by this charge-relay system has the same general effect on reaction rate as increasing the concentration of hydroxyl ions available for collision in the uncatalyzed reaction.

At two different times in the reaction sequence, an oxyanion tetrahedral transition state complex is formed which is stabilized by hydrogen bonds with –NH groups in the peptide backbone. Enzymes were originally viewed as distorting the bonds or bond angles of the reacting substrates to form the transition state complex. However, many transition state complexes, like the oxyanion tetrahedral complex, are better described as exhibiting "electronic strain," an electrostatic surface which would be highly improbable if it were not stabilized by bonds with functional groups on the

Table 9.2. Some General Strategies of Enzymatic Catalysis

Proximity and orientation
Transition state stabilization
Acid-base catalysis
Nucleophilic catalysis
Electrophilic catalysis
Covalent catalysis

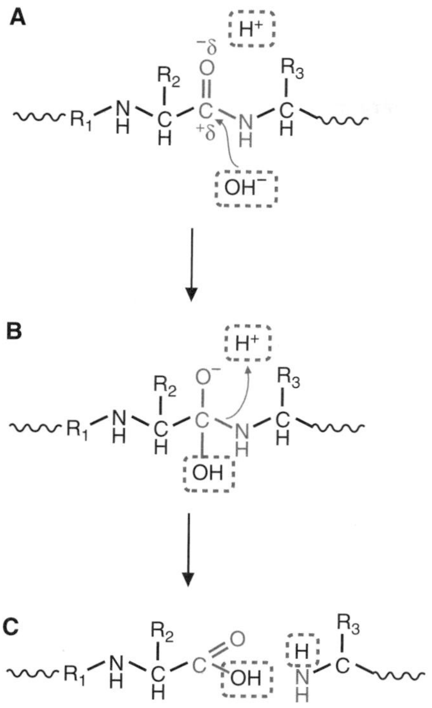

A

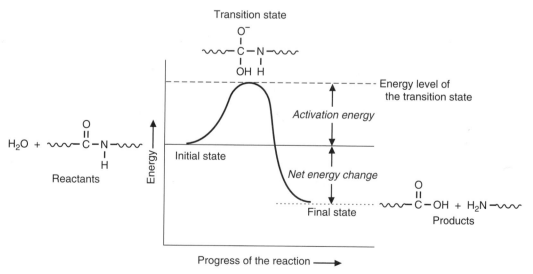

Fig. 9.8. Proteolysis in the absence of chymotrypsin. The scissile bond is shown in blue. **A.** The carbonyl carbon, which carries a partial positive charge, is attacked by a hydroxyl group from water. **B.** An unstable tetrahedral oxyanion intermediate is formed, which is the transition state complex. **C.** As the electrons return to the carbonyl carbon, the remaining proton from water adds to the leaving group to form an amine.

A 9.1: An imidazole nitrogen of histidine has a pK_a of 6.3, which means that it is 50% protonated at this pH. The aspartate residue of the enzyme increases this pK_a, so that histidine can both donate and accept a proton during different stages of the reaction.

Fig. 9.9. Energy diagram showing the energy levels of the substrates as they progress toward products in the absence of enzyme. The substrates must pass through the high energy transition state during the reaction.

Although there is a favorable loss of energy during the reaction, the rate of the reaction is slowed by the energy barrier to forming the transition state. The energy barrier is referred to as the activation energy.

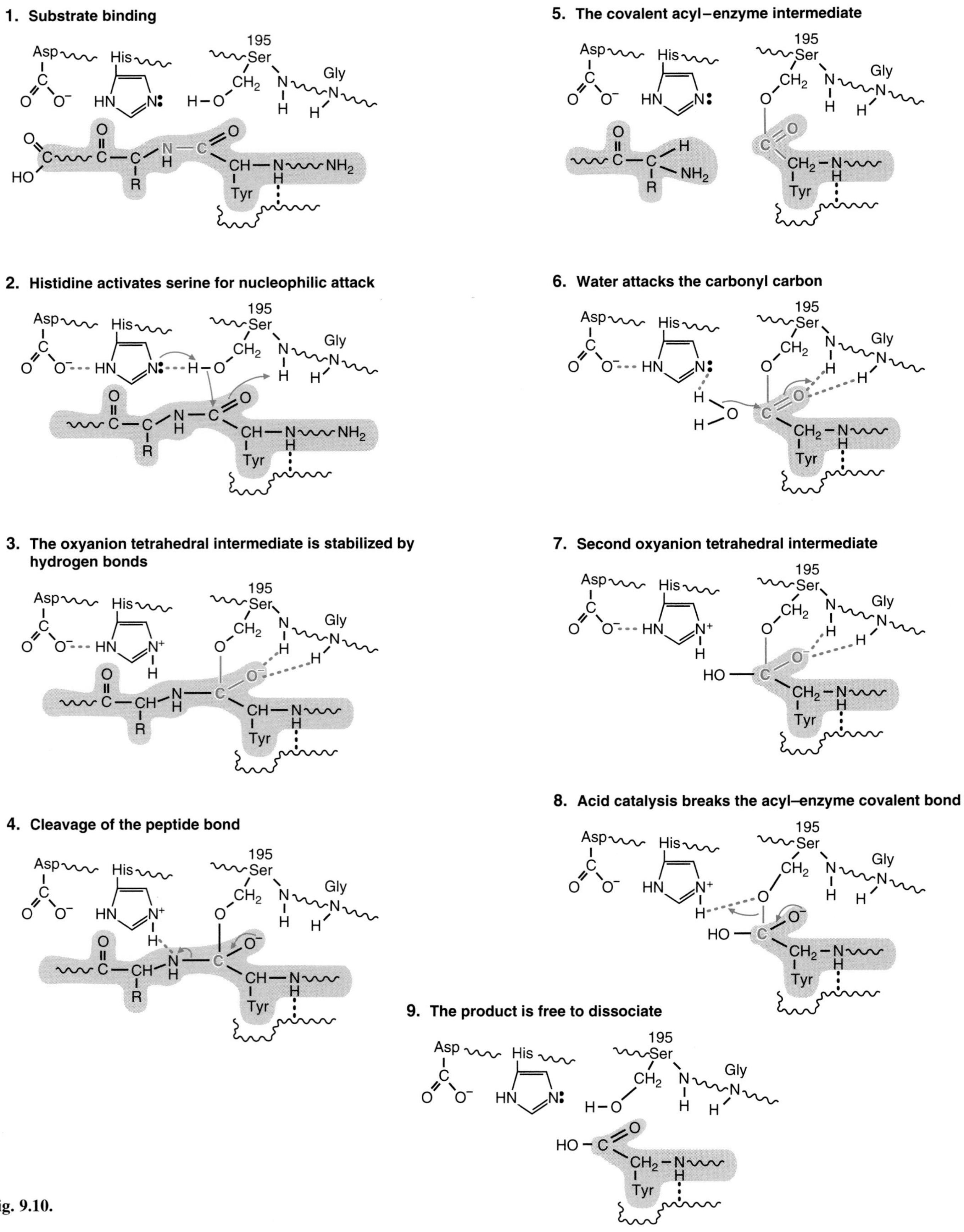
1. Substrate binding
2. Histidine activates serine for nucleophilic attack
3. The oxyanion tetrahedral intermediate is stabilized by hydrogen bonds
4. Cleavage of the peptide bond
5. The covalent acyl–enzyme intermediate
6. Water attacks the carbonyl carbon
7. Second oxyanion tetrahedral intermediate
8. Acid catalysis breaks the acyl–enzyme covalent bond
9. The product is free to dissociate

Fig. 9.10.

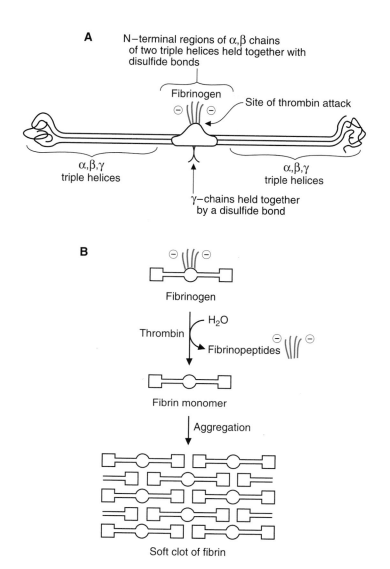

A. N-terminal regions of α,β chains
of two triple helices held together with
disulfide bonds

Fibrinogen

Site of thrombin attack

α,β,γ
triple helices

α,β,γ
triple helices

γ-chains held together
by a disulfide bond

B.

Fibrinogen

Thrombin — H_2O

Fibrinopeptides

Fibrin monomer

Aggregation

Soft clot of fibrin

Fig. 9.11. Cleavage of fibrinogen results in clot formation. **A.** Fibrinogen, the precursor protein of fibrin, is formed from two triple helices joined together at their N-terminal ends. The α,β-peptides are held together by disulfide bonds, and the γ-peptides are joined to each other by disulfide bonds. The terminal α,β-peptide regions, shown in blue, contain negatively charged glutamate and aspartate residues that repel each other and prevent aggregation. **B.** Thrombin, a serine protease, cleaves the terminal portions of fibrinogen containing negative charges. The fibrin monomers can then aggregate and form a "soft" clot. The soft clot is subsequently cross-linked by another enzyme.

Serine proteases in blood coagulation. The utilization of an active site serine to cleave a peptide bond is common to a variety of enzymes referred to as serine proteases. Serine proteases are essential for activating the formation of a blood clot from fibrin (Fig. 9.11). Fibrin and many of the other proteins involved in blood coagulation are present in the blood as inactive precursors or zymogens which must be activated by proteolytic cleavage. Thrombin, the serine protease which converts fibrinogen to fibrin, has the same aspartate-histidine-serine catalytic triad found in chymotrypsin and trypsin.

Thrombin is activated by proteolytic cleavage of its precursor protein, prothrombin. The sequence of proteolytic cleavages leading to thrombin activation requires Factor VIII, the blood-clotting protein deficient in **Sloe Klotter.**

Fig. 9.10. Catalytic mechanism of chymotrypsin. The substrate (a denatured protein) is in the shaded area. **1.** As the substrate protein binds to the active site, serine-195 and histidine-57 are moved closer together and at the right orientation for the nitrogen electrons on histidine to attract the hydrogen of serine. Without this change of conformation on substrate binding, the catalytic triad cannot form. **2.** Histidine serves as a general base catalyst as it abstracts a proton from the serine, increasing the nucleophilicity of the serine-oxygen, which attacks the carbonyl carbon. **3.** The electrons of the carbonyl group form the oxyanion tetrahedral intermediate. The oxyanion is stabilized by the N-H groups of serine-195 and glycine-193 in the chymotrypsin peptide backbone. **4.** The amide nitrogen in the peptide bond is stabilized by interaction with the histidine proton. Here the histidine acts as an general acid catalyst. As the electrons of the carbon-nitrogen peptide bond withdraw into the nitrogen, the electrons of the carboxyanion return to the carbonyl carbon, resulting in cleavage of the peptide bond. **5.** The cleavage of the peptide bond results in formation of the covalent acyl-enzyme intermediate, and the amide half of the cleaved protein dissociates. **6.** The nucleophilic attack by H_2O on the carbonyl carbon is activated by histidine, whose nitrogen electrons attract a proton from water. **7.** A tetrahedral oxyanion intermediate, the transition state complex, is formed. It is again stabilized by hydrogen bonds with the peptide backbone bonds of glycine and serine. **8.** As the histidine proton is donated to the electrons of the bond between the serine oxygen and the substrate carbonyl group, the electrons from the oxyanion return to the carbon, and the acyl-enzyme bond is broken. **9.** The enzyme, as it releases substrate, returns to its original state.

Transition state analogues. Because the transition state complex binds more tightly to the enzyme than does the substrate, compounds that resemble its electronic and three-dimensional surface are more potent inhibitors than are substrate analogues. Some bacteria and molds produce transition state analogues, sometimes called tight binding inhibitors, as self-defense mechanisms. For instance penicillin, which is produced by a mold to inhibit bacterial cell growth, contains a strained bond analogous to the transition state of a reaction required for bacterial cell wall synthesis (Fig. 9.13).

Abzymes. An abzyme is an antibody with the catalytic activity of an enzyme. Abzymes are made as antibodies against analogues of the transition state complex. They have an arrangement of amino acid side chains similar to the active site of the enzyme in the transition state and can, therefore, act as artificial enzymes. It is hoped that abzymes will find a therapeutic use in the correction of enzyme deficiencies.

enzyme. Stabilization of the transition state complex lowers its energy level and increases the number of molecules which reach this energy level.

The dissociating products of an enzyme-catalyzed reaction are often "destabilized" by some charge repulsion in the active site. In the case of chymotrypsin, the amino group formed after peptide bond cleavage is destabilized or "uncomfortable" in the presence of the active site histidine.

Energy Diagram in the Presence of Chymotrypsin

A major part of the catalytic power of enzymes arises from their ability to decrease the activation energy required for formation of the transition state complex (Fig. 9.12). Enzymes do not affect the energy levels of the substrate or product.

Energy for formation of the transition state complex is provided by the intrinsic energy of substrate binding, the energy arising from formation of bonds between the substrate and enzyme as the reaction progresses to products. At the initial stage of the reaction, energy is needed to restrict the freedom of translational and rotational movement of the separate enzyme and substrate molecules and separate the substrate and enzyme active site residues from water. This energy is provided by the formation of the initial multiple weak bonds between the substrate and enzyme. However, as the reaction progresses, these bonds are replaced by ever tighter bonds that stabilize the transition state complex. Semi-stable covalent intermediates of the reaction have lower energy levels than do the transition state complexes, and are present in the reaction diagram as dips in the energy curve. The final transition state complex,

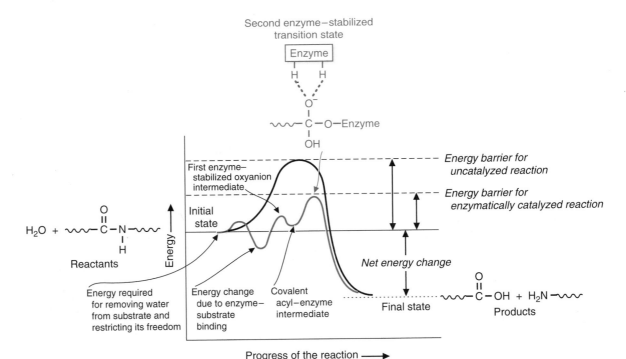

Fig. 9.12. A postulated energy diagram for the reaction catalyzed by chymotrypsin is shown for the presence of enzyme (blue) and the absence of enzyme (black). The energy barrier to the transition state is lowered by the formation of additional bonds between the substrate and enzyme in the transition state complex. The energy is provided by substrate binding to the enzyme. The enzyme does not, however, change the energy levels of the substrate or product.

which has the highest energy level in the reaction and is therefore the most unstable state, can collapse back to substrates or decompose to form products.

COMMON STRATEGIES IN ENZYME CATALYSIS

The catalytic strategies employed by chymotrypsin are common to many enzymes, but different enzymes may utilize different functional groups of amino acids or cofactors in the enzyme active site. Most polar amino acid side chains are nucleophilic and participate in reactions by stabilizing a developing positive charge. In some enzymes, serine and cysteine stabilize a positive charge through formation of a covalent intermediate (Table 9.3). In other enzymes, nucleophilic groups in the enzyme active site may polarize a hydrogen bond in the substrate, or stabilize the transition state complex. For instance, in alcohol dehydrogenase, described below, the active site serine oxygen polarizes the –OH group of the substrate. The opposite situation in which an amino acid residue stabilizes a developing negative charge requires an electrophile in the active site. NH groups in the peptide backbone, and the positively charged amino group of lysine and guanidinium group of arginine, can act as electrophiles.

Cofactors in Catalysis

Enzymes increase their repertoire of functional groups by binding cofactors, nonprotein compounds that participate in the catalytic process. Cofactors include metal ions (e.g., Fe^{2+}, Mg^{2+}, or Zn^{2+}), organic coenzymes (e.g., thiamine pyrophosphate and nicotinamide adenine dinucleotide), and metallocoenzymes (e.g., Fe^{2+}-heme). Coenzymes are complex organic structures which can be classified as activation-transfer coenzymes or oxidation-reduction coenzymes. A cofactor which is covalently bound to the enzyme is usually called a prosthetic group. An enzyme containing all its cofactors is called a holoenzyme. The protein portion, without the cofactors, is referred to as the apoenzyme or apoprotein.

ACTIVATION-TRANSFER COENZYMES

The activation-transfer coenzymes usually participate in catalysis by forming a covalent bond with a portion of the substrate; the tightly held substrate moiety is then activated for transfer, addition of water, or some other reaction. Each coenzyme has unique structural features which make it specific for the types of reactions in which it participates. For example, thiamine pyrophosphate cleaves the bond next to a keto group by forming a covalent bond with the carbonyl carbon (Fig. 9.14). Coenzyme A (CoASH) and biotin also have nucleophilic groups which participate in the formation

 Many similar enzymes, such as the serine proteases, are related by divergent evolution. Kinases that have similar ATP binding domains may also arise through divergent evolution. Convergent evolution, in contrast, results in enzymes carrying out similar reactions with similar catalytic strategies, but using different functional groups. Convergent evolution may occur because there are only so many ways certain types of reactions can occur.

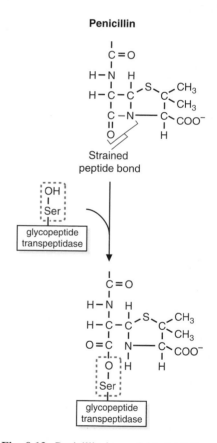

Fig. 9.13. Penicillin is a suicide inhibitor of bacterial glycopeptide transpeptidase. The bacterial transpeptidase is a serine protease which normally cleaves a peptide bond in the bacterial cell and reforms a peptide cross-link. The strained bond in the β-lactam ring of penicillin resembles the transition state of the normal reaction. As the enzyme attempts to cleave the β-lactam ring, penicillin becomes covalently and irreversibly attached to the active site serine.

Table 9.3. Some Functional Groups in the Active Site

Function of Amino Acid	Enzyme Example
Covalent intermediates	
cysteine–**SH**	Glyceraldehyde 3–phosphate dehydrogenase
serine–**OH**	Acetylcholinesterase
lysine–**NH₂**	Aldolase
histidine–**NH**	Phosphoglucomutase
Acid-base catalysis	
histidine–**NH**	Chymotrypsin
aspartate–**COOH**	Pepsin
Stabilization of anion	
peptide backbone–**NH**	Chymotrypsin
arginine–**NH**	Carboxypeptidase A
serine–**OH**	Alcohol dehydrogenase
Stabilization of cation	
aspartate–**COOH**	Lysozyme

Q 9.2: Although coenzymes seem autonomous in their catalytic structure, they have almost no catalytic power when not bound to the enzyme. Why?

Many alcoholics like **Al Martini** develop thiamine deficiency because alcohol inhibits the transport of thiamine through the intestinal mucosal cells. In the body, thiamine is converted to thiamine pyrophosphate (TPP). TPP acts as a coenzyme in the decarboxylation of α-keto acids such as pyruvate and α-ketoglutarate (see Fig. 9.14) and in the utilization of pentose phosphates in the pentose phosphate pathway. As a result of thiamine deficiency, the oxidation of α-keto acids is impaired. Dysfunction occurs in the central and peripheral nervous system, the cardiovascular system, and other organs.

Recently, a new class of organic catalysts has been discovered which is comprised of RNA and not protein. The catalytic RNAs, termed ribozymes, cleave RNA phosphodiester bonds at specific sites within their own RNA sequence (cis cleavage reactions) or in other RNA molecules (trans cleavage reactions). In self-cleavage reactions, unlike enzymatic reactions, the ribozyme is not acting like a true catalyst because it is modified during the course of the reaction. Ribozymes use many of the same catalytic strategies as enzymes; they specifically bind their substrates, and the –OH groups can even form covalent intermediates.

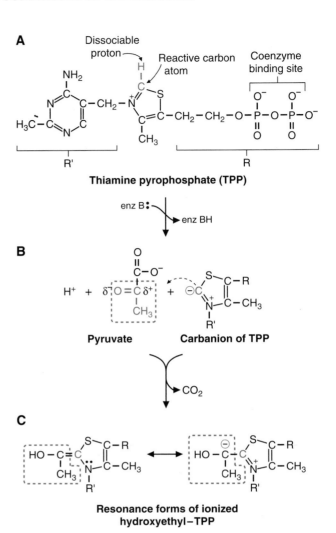

Fig. 9.14. The functional group of thiamine pyrophosphate (shown in blue) participates in formation of a covalent intermediate. **A.** A base on the enzyme (B:) abstracts a proton from thiamine, creating a carbanion (general acid-base catalysis). **B.** The carbanion is a strong nucleophile, and attacks the positively charged keto group on the substrate. **C.** A covalent intermediate is formed, which is stabilized by resonance forms. The uncharged intermediate is the stabilized transition state complex.

of a covalent intermediate of the reaction (Fig. 9.15). Pyridoxal phosphate also forms a covalent bond, but its positively charged ring nitrogen is a strong electron-withdrawing center. Therefore, it participates in electrophilic catalysis and forms a covalent complex with the amino groups of amino acids (Fig. 9.16).

Most coenzymes, like functional amino acids of the enzyme, are regenerated during the course of the reaction. However, CoASH and a few of the oxidation-reduction coenzymes are transformed during the reaction into products which dissociate from the enzyme at the end of the reaction (e.g., CoASH is converted to an acyl CoA derivative, and NAD+ is reduced to NADH). These dissociating coenzymes are nonetheless classified as coenzymes rather than substrates because they are synthesized from vitamins and are regenerated by other reactions.

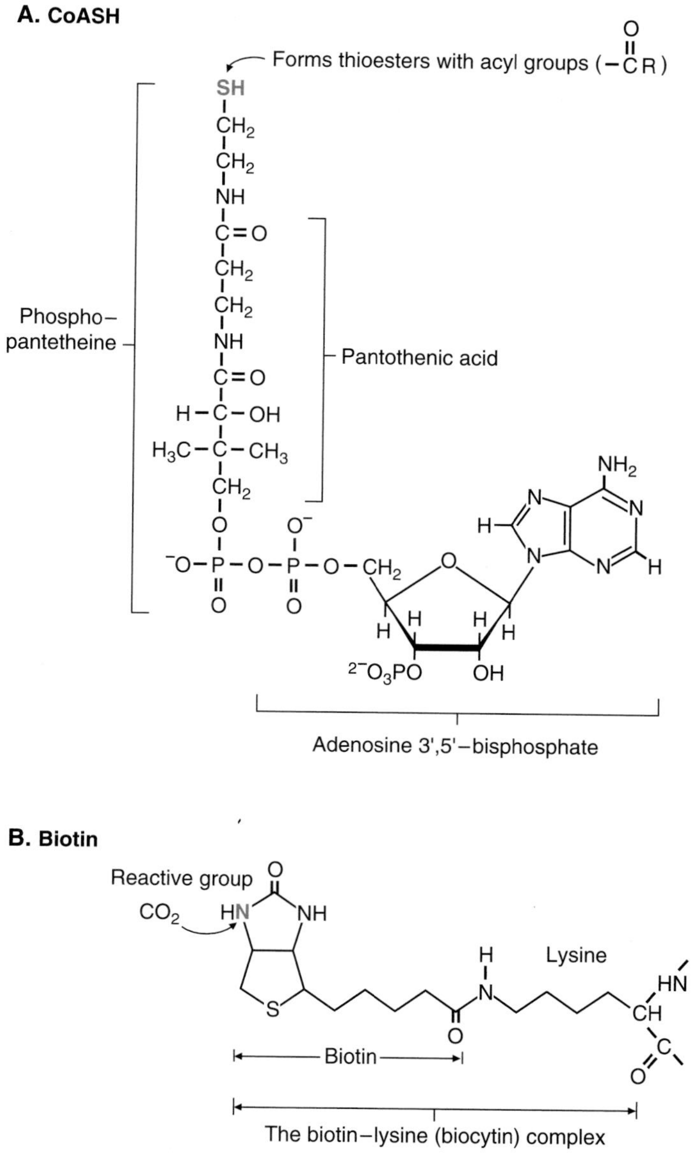

A. CoASH

B. Biotin

Fig. 9.15. CoA and biotin are activation-transfer coenzymes. **A.** Coenzyme A (CoA or CoASH) and phosphopantetheine are synthesized from the vitamin pantothenate (pantothenic acid). The active sulfhydryl group, shown in blue, is where acyl (e.g., acetyl, succinyl, or fatty acyl) groups bind to form thioesters. **B.** Biotin activates and transfers CO_2 to compounds in carboxylation reactions. The reactive N is shown in blue. The covalent attachment to a lysine residue of a carboxylase enzyme gives it a long flexible arm.

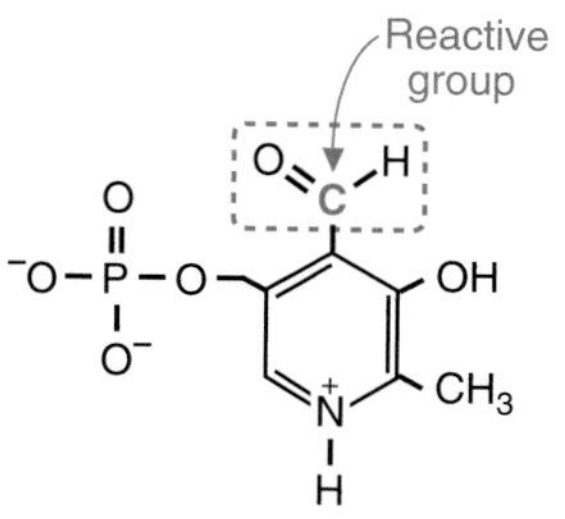

Pyridoxal phosphate (PLP)

Fig. 9.16. Reactive sites of pyridoxal phosphate. Pyridoxal phosphate contains a reactive aldehyde which forms a covalent intermediate with amino groups of amino acids (a Schiff base). The positively charged pyridine ring is a strong electron-withdrawing group which pulls electrons into it from the bonds around the amino acid α-carbon (electrophilic catalysis).

OXIDATION-REDUCTION COENZYMES

A large number of coenzymes are involved in oxidation-reduction reactions in which electrons are transferred from one compound to another. Some coenzymes, like NAD^+ and FAD, transfer electrons together with hydrogen and have unique roles in the generation of ATP from the oxidation of fuels. Other oxidation-reduction coenzymes work with metals to transfer single electrons to oxygen. Vitamins E and C are oxidation-reduction coenzymes which can act as antioxidants and protect against

A 9.2: The enzyme provides proximity, orientation, and other functional groups for the reaction and for stabilization of the transition state. For example, a basic amino acid residue in enzymes removes a proton from thiamine to activate it (see Fig. 9.14).

In humans, about 90% of ingested ethanol is oxidized to acetaldehyde in the liver by alcohol dehydrogenase. The acetaldehyde is responsible for liver injury associated with chronic alcoholism in patients such as **Al Martini.**

oxygen free radical injury. The different functions of oxidation-reduction coenzymes in metabolic pathways are explained in Chapters 18–21.

NAD$^+$-dependent dehydrogenases illustrate the principle that enzymes can use different functional groups in the active site to catalyze similar reactions. NAD$^+$-dependent dehydrogenases usually have similar three-dimensional binding domains for NAD$^+$, but very little sequence homology (i.e., sequences comprised of identical or similar amino acids) in the active site. They all catalyze the transfer of a hydride ion (H:$^-$) from a carbon on the substrate to NAD$^+$ in oxidation reactions such as the oxidation of alcohols to ketones or aldehydes to acids (Fig. 9.17). The positively charged pyridine ring nitrogen of NAD$^+$ activates the carbon opposite it to accept the hydride ion. If the reaction is oxidation of an alcohol to a ketone, the alcohol proton is released into water at the end of the reaction. Although a common feature of the reaction mechanism is polarization of the dissociating alcohol hydrogen, different types of dehydrogenases use different functional groups for this purpose; lactate dehydrogenase uses histidine, but liver alcohol dehydrogenase uses zinc and serine (Fig. 9.18).

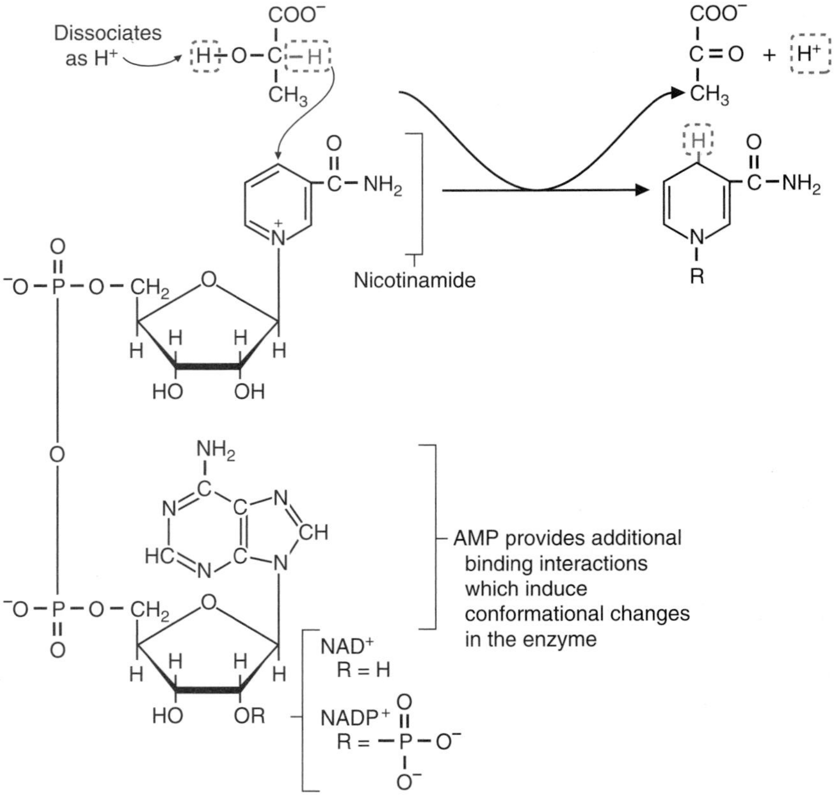

Fig. 9.17. NAD$^+$ accepts a hydride ion, shown in blue. NAD$^+$-dependent dehydrogenases catalyze the transfer of a hydride ion (H:$^-$) from a carbon to NAD$^+$ in oxidation reactions such as the oxidation of alcohols to ketones or aldehydes to acids. The positively charged pyridine ring nitrogen of NAD$^+$ increases the electrophilicity of the carbon opposite it in the ring. This carbon then accepts the negatively charged hydride ion. The alcoholic proton is released into water. NADP functions by the same mechanism, but is usually involved in pathways of reductive synthesis.

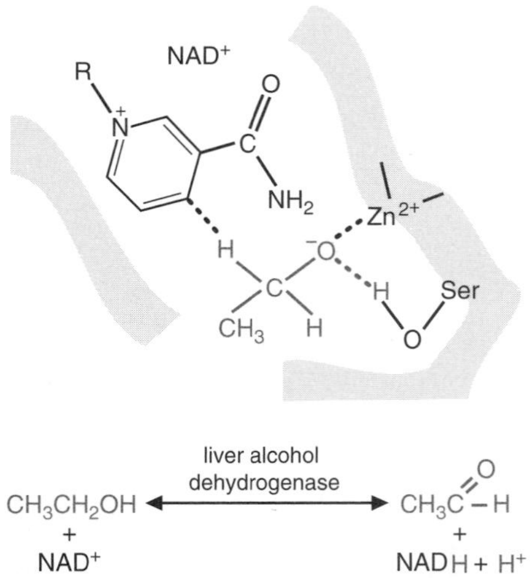

Fig. 9.18. Liver alcohol dehydrogenase catalyzes the oxidation of ethanol (shown in blue) to acetaldehyde. The active site of liver alcohol dehydrogenase contains an enzyme-bound zinc and a serine, which stabilize the partial negative charge on the oxygen.

COENZYME SYNTHESIS

Most of the coenzymes are synthesized from vitamins. The symptoms of vitamin deficiencies reflect the loss of specific enzyme activities dependent on the coenzyme form of the vitamin.

The biosynthetic pathways for coenzyme biosynthesis from vitamins add functional groups which participate in the reaction or increase the binding of the coenzyme to the enzyme. Hydrophobic regions or phosphate groups in the coenzymes can tightly bind the coenzyme to the enzyme while leaving the functional group free for the reaction. Thus many coenzymes, like thiamine, CoA, NAD^+, and pyridoxal phosphate have phosphate or an adenosine phosphate group attached to the reactive portion of the coenzyme (see Figs. 9.14–9.16).

METAL IONS IN CATALYSIS

Metal ions contribute to the catalytic process by acting as electrophiles (electron-attracting groups). They assist in the binding of the substrate, accept and donate electrons, and withdraw electrons to alter the distribution of partial charges in the substrate molecule.

The ability of certain metals to bind multiple ligands in their coordination sphere enables them to participate in binding substrates and coenzymes to enzymes and polarizing reactive groups in the active site. Zinc in alcohol dehydrogenase, for instance, contributes to the polarization of the alcohol group (see Fig. 9.18). Mg^{2+} plays a role in the binding of the negatively charged phosphate groups of ATP, and the nitrogen groups of heme chelate and hold Fe^{2+} in place.

Metal ions provide a range of energy levels for the transfer of single electrons, and are able to chelate ligands which can stabilize this transfer. For example, xanthine oxidase, which is discussed under mechanism-based inhibitors, donates electrons to xanthine while it is bound to a molybdenum-sulfide complex in the enzyme active site. The cytochromes of the electron transport chain bind Fe in structures similar to those of hemoglobin, except that the Fe^{3+} accepts and donates electrons. There are also metal-heme complexes which are able to interact directly with oxygen.

Mechanism-Based Inhibitors

Inhibitors are compounds that decrease the rate of an enzymatic reaction. Mechanism-based inhibitors mimic or participate in an intermediate step of the catalytic reaction. The term includes transition state analogues and compounds that can react irreversibly with functional groups in the active site.

IRREVERSIBLE INHIBITORS

Irreversible inhibitors form covalent or extremely tight bonds with functional groups in the active site. These functional groups are activated by their interactions with other amino acid residues of the enzyme, and are far more susceptible to forming irreversible covalent bonds with drugs and toxins than amino acid side chains in the remainder of the enzyme.

An irreversible inhibitor can be relatively nonspecific for the enzyme it inhibits. For instance, diisopropylphosphofluoridate is the organophosphorus compound that served as a prototype for the development of sarin, a nerve gas, and other organophosphorus toxins. It forms a covalent intermediate in the active site of all those enzymes that utilize serine for hydrolytic cleavage (Fig. 9.19). The covalent bond that is formed dissociates so slowly that the inhibition is essentially irreversible and activity can only be recovered as new enzyme is synthesized.

Vitamin deficiencies can result from drugs and toxins that inhibit vitamin transport proteins, enzymes in the biosynthetic pathway, or coenzyme binding proteins. A compound that causes a vitamin deficiency is sometimes called an antivitamin. Ethanol is an antivitamin which decreases the cellular content of almost every coenzyme. For example, ethanol inhibits the absorption of thiamine, and acetaldehyde produced from ethanol oxidation displaces pyridoxal phosphate from its protein binding sites, thereby accelerating its degradation.

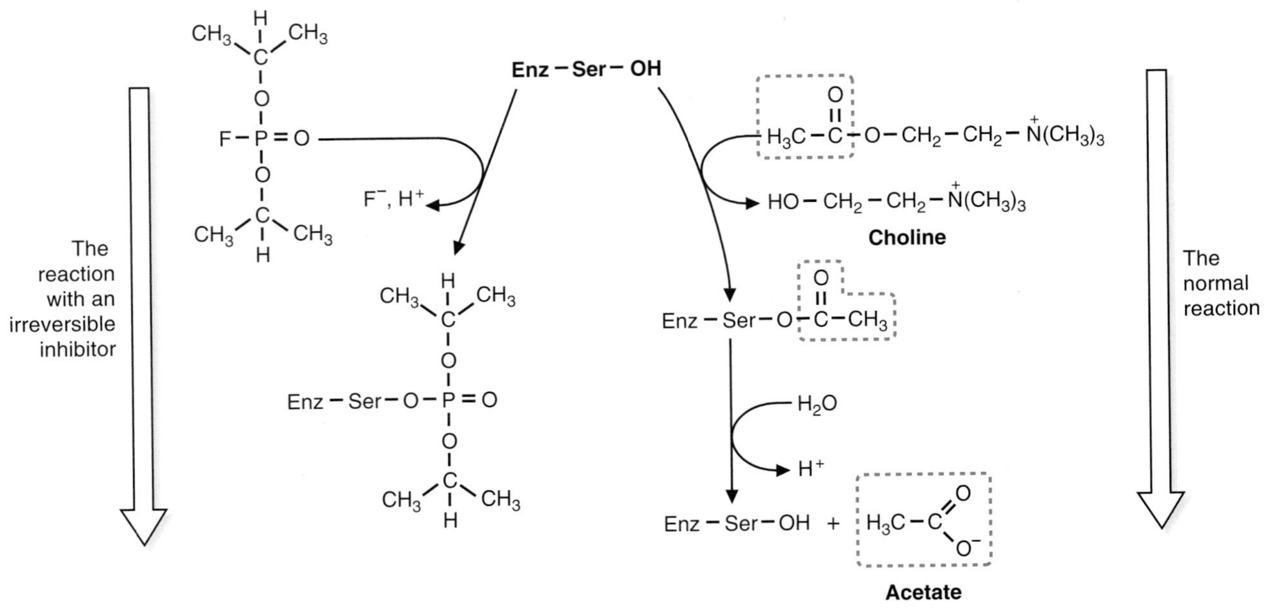

Fig. 9.19. Acetylcholinesterase normally catalyzes the hydrolytic inactivation of the neurotransmitter acetylcholine. The active site serine forms a covalent intermediate with the substrate during the course of the reaction. Diisopropyl phosphofluoridate, the ancestor of current organophosphorus nerve gases and pesticides, also forms a covalent complex with the active site serine, resulting in acetylcholine accumulation. Recovery of acetylcholinesterase activity depends on synthesis of new enzyme.

To avoid toxic reactions with enzymes, therapeutic drugs are designed to be much more specific and resemble the substrate or an intermediate stage of the reaction. For example, aspirin (acetylsalicylic acid) exerts its pharmacological effect by the covalent acetylation of an active site serine in the enzyme prostaglandin endoperoxide synthase. Aspirin resembles a portion of the prostaglandin which is a physiological substrate for the enzyme. However, therapeutic drugs may also cause side effects from the covalent inhibition of an enzyme other than the target enzyme.

SUICIDE INHIBITORS

Active site inhibitors that undergo partial reaction and form irreversible inhibitors in the active site are termed "suicide inhibitors." Penicillin, for example, is converted to a compound which cannot dissociate from the glycopeptidyl transpeptidase of bacterial cell wall synthesis (see Fig. 9.13). Allopurinol, a drug that is used to treat gout, owes its effectiveness to suicide inhibition of xanthine oxidase (Fig. 9.20).

TRANSITION STATE ANALOGUES AND COMPOUNDS THAT RESEMBLE INTERMEDIATE STAGES OF THE REACTION

Transition state analogues are extremely potent and specific inhibitors of enzymes because they bind so much more tightly to the enzyme than do substrates or products. Drugs cannot be designed which precisely mimic the transition state because of its highly unstable structure. However, substrates undergo progressive changes in their overall electrostatic structure during the formation of a transition state complex, and effective drugs often resemble an intermediate stage of the reaction more closely than they resemble the substrate. Medical literature often refers to such compounds as substrate analogues, even though they bind more tightly than substrates.

Organophosphorus compounds, such as the nerve gas sarin and the insecticides parathion and malathion, are irreversible inhibitors of enzymes containing reactive serines. Although many enzymes are inhibited by these compounds, the symptoms experienced by **Dennis Livermore** resulted from inhibition of the active site serine in the enzyme acetylcholinesterase. Acetylcholinesterase cleaves the neurotransmitter acetylcholine to acetate and choline in the postsynaptic terminal, thereby terminating the transmission of the neural signal (see Fig. 9.19). Inhibition of acetylcholinesterase results in accumulation of acetylcholine, causing the wide variety of Dennis Livermore's clinical symptoms.

A

GMP ⟶ Guanine

AMP ⟶ Hypoxanthine

Xanthine ⟶ Urate

xanthine oxidase

Inhibited by allopurinol

B

Hypoxanthine

Mo = S
xanthine
oxidase

H_2O
$+ H^+$ $3H^+, 2e^-$

Xanthine

H_2O
$+ H^+$ $3H^+, 2e^-$

Xanthine–enzyme
complex

⟶ Urate

enz

Mo^{VI}

Mo^{IV}

C

Allopurinol

xanthine
oxidase

Alloxanthine
(oxypurinol)

Fig. 9.20. Allopurinol is a suicide inhibitor of xanthine oxidase. **A.** Xanthine oxidase catalyzes the oxidation of hypoxanthine to xanthine, and xanthine to uric acid (urate) in the pathway for degradation of purines. Electrons and oxygen are donated from water. **B.** The oxidation is carried out by a molybdenum-oxo-sulfide coordination complex in the active site which complexes with the group being oxidized. **C.** Xanthine oxidase is able to carry out the first oxidation step and convert allopurinol to alloxanthine (oxypurinol). As a result, the enzyme has committed suicide, because the oxypurinol remains bound in the molybdenum coordination sphere during the next step of the reaction.

Optimal pH and Temperature

If the activity of most enzymes is plotted as a function of the pH of the reaction, an increase of reaction rate is usually observed as the pH goes from a very acidic level to the physiological range, and a decrease of reaction rate as the pH goes from the physiological range to a very basic range (Fig. 9.21). The shape of this curve in the acid region reflects the ionization of specific functional groups in the active site (or in the substrate) by the increase of pH, and the more general formation of hydrogen bonds important for the overall conformation of the enzyme. The loss of activity on the basic side usually reflects the inappropriate ionization of amino acid residues in the enzyme.

Most human enzymes also have an optimal temperature around 37°C. An increase of temperature from 0°C to 37°C increases the rate of the reaction by increasing the vibrational energy of the substrates. The maximum activity for most human enzymes occurs near 37°C because denaturation (loss of secondary and tertiary structure) occurs at higher temperatures.

REGULATION OF ENZYMES

The rate of metabolic pathways in cells is regulated to correspond to changing conditions, such as an increased need for ATP in skeletal muscles during exercise or an

Yves Topaigne is being treated with allopurinol for gout, which is caused by an accumulation of uric acid. Allopurinol is a suicide inhibitor of the enzyme xanthine oxidase, which is involved in the degradation of purine nucleotides to uric acid (urate) (Fig. 9.20). Xanthine oxidase catalyzes the hydroxylation of hypoxanthine to xanthine and the further hydroxylation of xanthine to uric acid in oxidation-reduction reactions. The enzyme contains a molybdenum-sulfide (Mo-S) complex which binds the substrates and transfers the electrons required for these hydroxylation reactions. Allopurinol, a structural analogue of hypoxanthine, is oxidized by xanthine oxidase to oxypurinol, an analogue of xanthine. Once oxypurinol is formed it remains bound to the Mo-S complex, and the reduced Mo-S complex cannot be regenerated. As a consequence, less uric acid is formed.

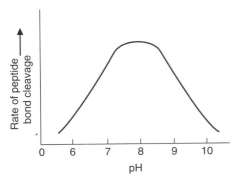

Fig. 9.21. pH profile of an enzyme. The rate of the reaction increases as the pH increases from 6 to 7.4. The exact shape of the curve depends on the protonation state of active site amino acid residues or on the hydrogen and ionic bonding required for maintenance of three-dimensional structure. In the enzyme shown in the figure, the increase of reaction rate corresponds to deprotonation of the active site histidine. At a pH above 8.5, deprotonation of an amino-terminal $-NH_3^+$ alters the conformation at the active site and the activity decreases. Other enzymes might have a lower pH maximum, a broader peak, or retain their activity in the basic side of the curve.

The parietal cells of the stomach secrete HCl into the lumen of the stomach, causing the pH of the contents to decrease to less than 1. This strongly acid environment is capable of irreversibly denaturing most proteins by protonating amino acids, thereby preventing the hydrogen bond formation necessary ·for tertiary structure. Many of the peptide bonds in proteins would not be accessible to digestive proteases unless they were denatured. Pepsin, a digestive protease present in the stomach, is exceptional because its pH optimum is about 1.6 and it is active in the acidic environment of the stomach.

As denatured dietary proteins pass into the intestinal lumen, the pH is raised by secretion of bicarbonate from the exocrine pancreas. At the higher pH, chymotrypsin and other proteases from the pancreas can act on the irreversibly denatured proteins.

increased availability of glucose for glycogen synthesis after a high carbohydrate meal. Changes in the flux of pathways occur because at least one enzyme in that pathway, the regulatory enzyme, has been activated or inhibited. Regulatory enzymes usually catalyze the rate-limiting or slowest steps in pathways. Thus changes in their activity can influence flux through the entire pathway.

Mechanisms of Enzyme Regulation

The rate of regulatory enzymes in the cell can be increased or decreased by changes in the concentration of substrate or product, by compounds or enzymes that alter the availability of functional groups in the active site, or by changes in the amount of enzyme present (Table 9.4). The regulatory mechanism employed depends on the function of the metabolic pathway in which the enzyme resides and the purpose of the regulation. For example, the pathways of energy production must be regulated by a mechanism which can respond rapidly to requirements for more ATP, but storage pathways can be regulated by a mechanism which responds more slowly to changing conditions.

VELOCITY AND SUBSTRATE CONCENTRATION

The velocity of all enzymes is dependent on the concentration of substrate. This dependence can regulate metabolic pathways if the supply of substrate to the rate-limiting enzyme varies with the need for the pathway. Storage pathways and toxic waste disposal pathways are partially regulated in this way. The equations of enzyme kinetics provide a quantitative way of describing enzymes with respect to their dependence on the concentration of substrate.

Michaelis-Menten Equation

The Michaelis-Menten equation relates the initial velocity of an enzyme-catalyzed reaction, v_i, to the concentration of substrate, S, and two parameters, K_m and V_{max} (Fig. 9.22). V_{max} is the velocity of the reaction extrapolated to infinite substrate concentration and K_m is the substrate concentration at which the initial velocity equals one-half V_{max}.

In the Michaelis-Menten model of enzyme kinetics, the rate of the reaction is proportionate to the concentration of enzyme-substrate complexes. The model applies to the simplest reaction, the conversion of a single substrate to a single product (Fig. 9.23). The enzyme and substrate form an enzyme-substrate complex (ES) with the rate constant k_1. The complex dissociates with the rate constant k_2, or is converted to product with the rate constant k_3. v_i, the rate of the reaction before a significant amount of substrate has been converted to product, is equal to k_3 times the concentration of ES. The higher the substrate concentration, the higher the ES concentration, and the higher the reaction rate. However, as the fraction of total enzyme present as ES increases, progressively larger increases of S are required to increase the concentration of ES by the same amount. At a hypothetical infinitely high substrate concen-

Table 9.4. Mechanisms of Enzyme Regulation

- Substrate concentration
- Reversible inhibition by products or other compounds
- Allosteric activation or inhibition
- Covalent modification
- Modulator protein binding
- Proteolytic cleavage
- Amount of enzyme present

tration, all of the enzyme molecules contain bound substrate. The Michaelis-Menten equation is therefore a rectangular hyperbola, and v_i approaches the maximal velocity V_{max} at infinite substrate concentration (see Fig. 9.22). The hyperbolic approach to a finite maximum limit in rate is referred to as saturation kinetics, and is a characteristic property of rate processes which depend on the binding of a compound to a protein.

The K_m of the enzyme for a substrate is defined as the concentration of substrate at which v_i equals one-half V_{max}. The K_m is generally equal to $(k_2 + k_3)/k_1$ or a more complex combination of rate constants in which the rate of dissociation appears in the numerator and the rate of binding in the denominator. If an enzyme mutated in a way that decreased its affinity for the substrate, the K_m of the enzyme for that substrate would increase. In general, the higher the K_m, the higher the substrate concentration required to reach one-half V_{max}.

The velocity of an enzyme is most sensitive to changes in the concentration of substrate at substrate concentrations below the K_m for the substrate. At substrate concentrations less than 1/10th of the K_m, a doubling of substrate concentration nearly doubles the velocity of the reaction; at substrate concentrations 10 times the K_m, doubling the substrate concentration has little effect on the velocity (see Fig. 9.23).

The constant k_{cat} is related to V_{max}. k_{cat} is the turnover number of the enzyme, the rate of product formation per active site of the enzyme determined under saturating substrate conditions. For the simple enzyme shown in Figure 9.23, k_{cat} is k_3. k_{cat} is equivalent to the V_{max} of the pure enzyme (expressed in units such as $M^{-1}\ min^{-1}$) divided by the concentration of active enzyme subunits present during the measurement of V_{max}. It has the units of reciprocal time, such as min^{-1}.

Hexokinase Isozymes Have Different K_m Values for Glucose

Hexokinase exists as a number of different tissue-specific isoenzymes (isozymes), proteins with different amino acid sequences which catalyze the same reaction. Tissues frequently contain characteristic isozymes which differ in their properties in ways that reflect differences in tissue function. A comparison between hexokinase I, the isozyme found in the erythrocyte and glucokinase (hexokinase IV) found in the liver illustrates the significance of the K_m of an enzyme for its substrate.

The isozymes of hexokinase found in skeletal muscles, brain, and most other tissues are similar to hexokinase I; they have kinetics which follow the Michaelis-Menten curve and have K_m values for glucose in the range of 0.02–0.13 mM. Glucokinase, the hexokinase isozyme present in liver and a few other cell types, does not follow the rectangular hyperbola of Michaelis-Menten kinetics. Instead, the curve for glucokinase is sigmoidal, or S-shaped (Fig. 9.24). The concentration of substrate required to reach half V_{max}, or half-saturation, is generally termed $S_{0.5}$, or $K_{0.5}$, rather than K_m. From the curve, the $S_{0.5}$ for glucokinase can be determined to be about 6 mM. The reported K_m determined by computer fit to a portion of the curve is about 5 mM. Occasionally, for simplification purposes, the K_m and the $S_{0.5}$ are used interchangeably in the medical literature.

Lineweaver-Burk Transformation

The K_m and V_{max} for an enzyme can be visually determined from a plot of 1/v versus 1/S, called a Lineweaver-Burk or a double reciprocal plot. The reciprocal of both sides of the Michaelis-Menten equation generates an equation which has the form of a straight line, y = mx + b (Fig. 9.25). K_m and V_{max} can be determined from intercepts on the abscissa and ordinate, respectively.

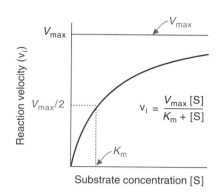

Fig. 9.22. A graph of the Michaelis-Menten equation. V_{max} (shown in blue) is the initial velocity extrapolated to infinite [S]. K_m (shown in blue) is concentration of S at which $v_i = V_{max}/2$.

For the reaction

$$E + S \underset{k_2}{\overset{k_1}{\rightleftharpoons}} ES \xrightarrow{k_3} P$$

The initial velocity is proportionate to [ES]

$$v_i = k_3\ [ES] = \frac{k_3\ [E_T]\ [S]}{K_m + [S]} = \frac{V_{max}\ [S]}{K_m + [S]}$$

Where $V_{max} = k_3\ [E_T]$ *and*

$$K_m = \frac{k_2}{k_1} \quad or \quad K_m = \frac{k_2 + k_3}{k_1}$$

Fig. 9.23. The Michaelis-Menten equation relates the initial velocity (v_i) of the reaction to the concentration of enzyme substrate complexes (ES). This equation is derived for a reaction in which a single substrate (S) is converted to a single product (P). The enzyme (E) and (S) associate to form an enzyme-substrate complex (ES) with the rate constant of k_1. The complex dissociates with the rate constant of k_2, or is converted to product with the rate constant k_3. Under the conditions in which the concentration of substrate is much higher than the concentration of enzyme, the amount of substrate converted to product is negligible, and the rate of conversion of ES to an enzyme-product complex is very fast, the initial velocity of the reaction is equal to $k_3 \times$ [ES]. The concentration of ES is a fraction of ET, the total amount of enzyme present as ES and E. If one assumes that $k_3 >>$ than k_1 or k_2, $K_m = k_2/k_1$. On the other hand, if one assumes only that [ES] does not change with time (steady-state conditions), $K_m = (k_2 + k_3)/k_1$. Note that k_2 is in the numerator and k_1 is in the denominator in both conditions. V_{max} is defined as equal to $k_3 E_T$.

Q 9.3: The K_m of human erythrocyte hexokinase for glucose is 0.04 mM. At the concentration of ATP found in tissues, all of the hexokinase molecules will contain an ATP in their ATP binding sites. Assume that the product concentration is zero, and that the Michaelis-Menten equation applies to these conditions. What is the velocity of hexokinase relative to V_{max} (v_i/V_{max}), when the intracellular [glucose] is at the fasting concentration of 5 mM? What fraction of enzyme molecules are present as ES complexes?

Q 9.4: Which enzyme, hexokinase I or glucokinase, would have the largest increase of velocity as the intracellular glucose concentration increases from 5 mM (the fasting level) to 10 mM (the level after a high carbohydrate meal)?

V_{max} is a rate constant times the total amount of enzyme present. In current literature, V_{max} can also be used to refer to the activity of an enzyme in a gram of tissue measured under conditions of saturating substrate concentration. In this case, an increase of V_{max} (micromoles/min/g tissue) can refer to either an increase in the amount of enzyme present or an increase of its catalytic power, k_{cat}.

The hexokinase isozymes, like many other groups of isozymes, apparently arose through gene duplication. Glucokinase, the low affinity hexokinase found in liver, is a single polypeptide chain with a molecular weight of 55 kD. The hexokinases found in erythrocytes, skeletal muscles, and most other tissues are 110 kD, and are essentially 2 mutated glucokinase molecules synthesized as one polypeptide chain. However, only one active site in hexokinase is functional.

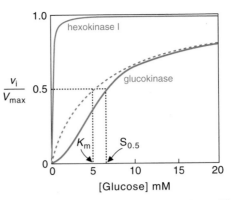

Fig. 9.24. A comparison between hexokinase I and glucokinase. The initial velocity as a fraction of V_{max} is graphed as a function of glucose concentration. The plot for glucokinase (solid blue line) is sigmoidal, possibly because the rate of an intermediate step in the reaction or of a conformational change is so slow that the enzyme does not follow Michaelis-Menten kinetics. The dashed blue line has been derived from the Michaelis-Menten equation fitted to the data for concentrations of glucose above 5 mM. At $v_i/V_{max} = 0.5$, the K_m is 5 mM, and the $S_{0.5}$ is 6.7 mM.

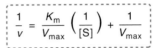

$$\frac{1}{v} = \frac{K_m}{V_{max}}\left(\frac{1}{[S]}\right) + \frac{1}{V_{max}}$$

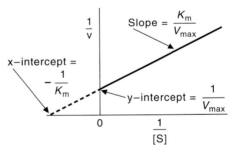

Fig. 9.25. The Lineweaver-Burk transformation (shown in blue) for the Michaelis-Menten equation converts it to a straight line of the form y = mx + b. When [S] is infinite, 1/[S] = 0, and the line crosses the ordinate (y-axis) at $1/v = 1/V_{max}$. The slope of the line is K_m/V_{max}. Where the line intersects the abscissa (x-axis), $1/[S] = -1/K_m$.

Multisubstrate Reactions

Most enzymes, like hexokinase, have more than one substrate, and the substrate binding sites overlap in the active site. For some enzymes, there is an ordered sequence of substrate binding, and the binding of the first substrate changes the conformation of the enzyme in a way that permits the second substrate to bind.

When an enzyme has more than one substrate, the sequence of substrate binding and product release affect the rate equation. As a consequence, the apparent value of K_m ($K_{m,app}$) may depend on the concentration of cosubstrate (Fig. 9.26). However, as with hexokinase, the dependence of velocity on concentration of one substrate at a constant concentration of cosubstrate, such as ATP, will often generate a simple Michaelis-Menten curve.

REVERSIBLE INHIBITION AT THE ACTIVE SITE

An inhibitor of an enzyme is a compound that decreases the velocity of the reaction by binding to the enzyme. Reversible inhibitors are compounds which are not covalently bound to the enzyme and can dissociate from the enzyme at a significant rate. All products, for instance, are reversible inhibitors of the enzymes which produce them. However, in many cases, the inhibition does not occur at physiological concentrations of product.

Competitive Inhibition

Reversible inhibitors that bind at the active site of enzymes can be competitive, noncompetitive, or uncompetitive with respect to a substrate of the reaction (Fig. 9.27). A competitive inhibitor "competes" with a substrate for binding at its substrate binding site, and binds to exactly the same forms of the enzyme as does the substrate. It is usually a close structural analogue of the substrate with which it competes. Increases of substrate concentration can overcome competitive inhibition—when the substrate concentration is increased to a high enough level, the substrate binding sites are occupied by substrate and no inhibitor molecules can bind. Competitive inhibitors therefore increase the K_m of the enzyme, but not the V_{max} (Fig. 9.28).

Noncompetitive Inhibition

In contrast, noncompetitive inhibition with respect to a substrate occurs when the inhibitor does not compete with that substrate for the same binding site on the enzyme. The inhibitor can bind to the enzyme in either the presence or absence of that substrate, and raising the substrate concentration will not prevent the inhibitor from binding. The inhibitor, in effect, lowers the concentration of the active enzyme. A noncompetitive inhibitor will always change the V_{max} of the enzyme, and may change the $K_{m,app}$ by binding with different affinities to different forms of the enzyme (Fig. 9.28).

Uncompetitive Inhibition

An inhibitor can also be uncompetitive with respect to a substrate of a multisubstrate reaction. An uncompetitive inhibitor binds only to the enzyme-substrate complex. Uncompetitive inhibition frequently occurs with enzymes which have an ordered sequence of substrate binding. The first substrate to bind induces a conformational change which "opens" the second binding site for either the cosubstrate or the inhibitor. Uncompetitive inhibitors decrease both K_m and V_{max}.

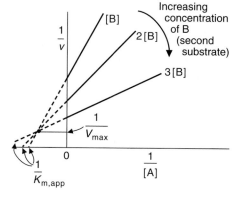

Fig. 9.26. A Lineweaver-Burk plot for a two-substrate reaction in which A and B are converted to products. In the graph, $1/[A]$ is plotted against $1/v$ for three different concentrations of the cosubstrate, [B], 2[B], and 3[B]. As the concentration of B is increased, the intersection on the abscissa, equal to $1/K_{m,app}$ is increased. The $K_{m,app}$ is the K_m at whatever concentration of cosubstrate, inhibitor, or other factor is present.

A 9.3: To calculate v_i/V_{max}, divide both sides of the Michaelis-Menten equation by V_{max}, and substitute the values for S and K_m into the equation. The result is

$$\frac{v_i}{V_{max}} = \frac{[S]}{K_m + [S]} = \frac{5}{0.04 + 5} = 0.992$$

Because v_i is proportionate to the concentration of ES, and at V_{max} all of the enzyme is present as ES and can form product, the fraction of total enzyme present as ES = v_i/V_{max} = 0.992.

A 9.4: From the Michaelis-Menten equation, the rate of hexokinase at 5 mM glucose is 99.2% of V_{max}, and the rate at 10 mM glucose is 99.6% of V_{max}, a 0.4% increase. From the graph, the rate of glucokinase increases from 40% of V_{max} at 5 mM to 70% of V_{max} at 10 mM glucose. On the basis of this comparison, only the rate of glucokinase can increase to a significant extent after a high carbohydrate meal. The properties of glucokinase permit excess glucose to be taken up by the liver, phosphorylated, and stored as glycogen after a high carbohydrate meal.

Product inhibition can contribute to the regulatory control of a pathway. For example, the rate of hexokinase I in red blood cells is regulated by the concentration of its product, glucose 6-phosphate. The phosphate group of glucose 6-phosphate makes it a competitive inhibitor with respect to ATP, and a noncompetitive inhibitor with respect to glucose. Thus the inhibition by glucose 6-phosphate cannot be totally reversed by increased levels of blood glucose.

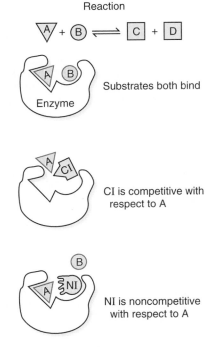

Reaction

Substrates both bind

CI is competitive with respect to A

NI is noncompetitive with respect to A

Fig. 9.27. Competitive or noncompetitive inhibition with respect to a given substrate. A and B are substrates for the reaction. The enzyme has separate binding sites for each substrate, which overlap in the active site. The competitive inhibitor (CI) competes for the binding site of A, the substrate it most closely resembles. NI is a noncompetitive inhibitor with respect to the substrate A, and A can still bind to its binding site in the presence of NI. However, NI is competitive with respect to B because it binds to the B binding site. In contrast, an inhibitor that is uncompetitive with respect to A might resemble NI, but it could only bind to the B site after A is bound.

ALLOSTERIC ENZYMES AND FEEDBACK REGULATION

Allosteric inhibitors have a much stronger effect on enzyme velocity than competitive, noncompetitive, and uncompetitive inhibitors, and need not resemble a substrate of the reaction. Allosteric enzymes can also have activators, compounds which increase the rate of the enzyme. These features of allosteric enzymes are essential for the regulation of certain types of metabolic pathways.

Allosteric Enzymes

Allosteric enzymes bind activators and inhibitors at sites separate from the active site (allosteric sites). Allosteric effectors (allosteric activators and inhibitors) change or stabilize the conformation of the enzyme in a way which influences the active (catalytic) site (Fig. 9.29). This conformational change in the position of amino acid side chains in the active (catalytic) site may affect substrate binding and/or the V_{max} of the reaction.

Allosteric enzymes contain multiple subunits and exhibit positive cooperativity; the binding of substrate to the active site on one subunit facilitates the binding of substrate to one or more of the remaining subunits (see Hemoglobin, Chapter 8). Allosteric activators change the enzyme to the active state, or stabilize the active state of the enzyme, thereby facilitating substrate binding in their own and other subunits. As a consequence, the characteristic sigmoidal v_i versus [S] curve of the allosteric enzyme becomes more like a rectangular hyperbola and $S_{0.5}$ is decreased. Allosteric inhibitors bind to allosteric enzymes at their own separate allosteric sites, or at the substrate or activator site, and stabilize the inactive form of the enzyme. Allosteric inhibitors increase the amount of activator or substrate required to saturate or stabilize the active form of the enzyme. Consequently, they increase $S_{0.5}$ and/or decrease V_{max}.

Feedback Inhibition and Allosteric Enzymes

Feedback regulation refers to a situation in which the endproduct of a pathway controls its own rate of synthesis (Fig. 9.30). This type of regulation, like other types of regulation, usually takes place at the first committed step of a pathway, or at an early step in the pathway. It also occurs at metabolic branchpoints.

In feedback inhibition, the endproduct of a pathway inhibits, or a related metabolite activates, a regulatory enzyme in the pathway. Feedback regulation often makes use of the properties of allosteric enzymes because the allosteric inhibitor or activator need not resemble a substrate or bind in the active site. Furthermore, small changes in the concentration of activator or inhibitor can have a very strong effect on the velocity of the enzyme. Activators become involved in feedback inhibition when their concentration in the cell is inversely related to the concentration of endproduct, i.e., the activator concentration increases when the concentration of the endproduct of the pathway is low.

Allosteric activation and inhibition are not the only mechanisms involved in feedback regulation. The endproduct of a pathway may also control its own synthesis by inducing or repressing the gene for the transcription of the rate-limiting enzyme in the pathway. This type of regulation is much slower to respond to changing conditions than allosteric regulation.

PHOSPHORYLATION

Many hormones exert their influence over enzymes by regulating the activity of a protein kinase. Protein kinases usually transfer a phosphate from ATP to the hydroxyl group of a specific serine or tyrosine residue on the target protein (Fig. 9.31). The

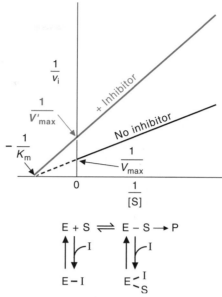

A. Competitive inhibition

$\frac{1}{v_i}$

+ Inhibitor

No inhibitor

$-\frac{1}{K_m}$

$\frac{1}{V_{max}}$

$-\frac{1}{K'_m}$

0

$\frac{1}{[S]}$

$E + S \rightleftharpoons E-S \rightarrow P$

$E - I$

B. Pure noncompetitive inhibition

$\frac{1}{v_i}$

$\frac{1}{V'_{max}}$

+ Inhibitor

No inhibitor

$-\frac{1}{K_m}$

$\frac{1}{V_{max}}$

0

$\frac{1}{[S]}$

$E + S \rightleftharpoons E-S \rightarrow P$

$E - I$

Fig. 9.28. Lineweaver-Burk plots of competitive and pure non-competitive inhibition. **A.** $1/v_i$ versus $1/[S]$ in the presence of a competitive inhibitor. The competitive inhibitor alters the intersection on the abscissa. The new intersection is $1/K_{m,app}$ (also called $1/K'_m$). A competitive inhibitor does not affect V_{max}. **B.** $1/v_i$ versus $1/[S]$ in the presence of a pure noncompetitive inhibitor. The non-competitive inhibitor alters the intersection on the ordinate, $1/V_{max,app}$ or $1/V'_{max}$, but does not affect $1/K_m$. A pure noncompetitive inhibitor binds to E and ES with the same affinity. If the inhibitor has different affinities for E and ES, the lines will intersect above or below the abscissa, and the noncompetitive inhibitor will change both the K'_m and the V'_m.

kinase is therefore classified as either a serine protein kinase or a tyrosine protein kinase. Phosphate is a bulky, negatively charged residue which interacts with other nearby amino acid residues of the protein to create a conformational change at the active catalytic site. This conformational change can make the enzyme more active or less active.

Glycogen phosphorylase, which catalyzes the degradation of glycogen to glucose 1-phosphate, is an example of an enzyme regulated by phosphorylation (Fig. 9.31). The activity of glycogen phosphorylase kinase, the enzyme which transfers a phosphate from ATP to glycogen phosphorylase, is influenced by the blood levels of insulin, glucagon, and other hormones. Enzyme phosphorylation is the major mechanism employed by hormones to control the rate of metabolic pathways.

MODULATOR PROTEINS

Modulator proteins are proteins which regulate the activity of another protein by conformational changes or steric hindrance created upon binding or dissociation. They can either activate or inhibit the enzyme to which they bind. Ca^{2+}-calmodulin, for example, is a modulator protein which binds to a number of proteins as a dissociable subunit and changes their activity (Fig. 9.32).

One of the enzymes activated by Ca^{2+}-calmodulin is glycogen phosphorylase kinase, the same enzyme that is regulated by hormonally activated phosphorylation (see Fig. 9.31). When calmodulin is activated by the Ca^{2+} released from the sarcoplasmic reticulum during muscle contraction, Ca^{2+}-calmodulin binds to muscle glycogen phosphorylase kinase and activates it. As a result, muscle glycogen is degraded to glucose 1-phosphate during exercise to provide the muscle with fuel.

Isocitrate dehydrogenase is an allosteric regulatory enzyme in the TCA cycle, a pathway that obtains energy from fuel oxidation for the generation of ATP from ADP. ATP can be considered the endproduct of the pathway. As ATP concentration begins to increase in cells, the concentration of ADP begins to decrease. ADP is an allosteric activator of isocitrate dehydrogenase, and even a small decrease in its concentration decreases the activity of the enzyme. Thus, feedback regulation of the TCA cycle has been carried out by an allosteric activator.

A model of an allosteric enzyme

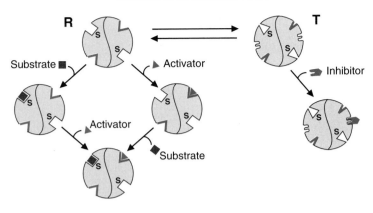

Most of the proteins involved in blood clotting, such as fibrinogen and prothrombin, are zymogens. Their activity is controlled through cleavage by enzymes attached to the site of injury (see Fig. 9.11).

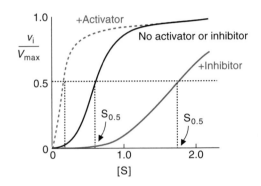

Serine controls its own rate of synthesis from glucose by induction/repression of transcription of the gene for 3-phosphoglycerate dehydrogenase, a regulatory enzyme in the pathway.

Fig. 9.29. Model of an allosteric enzyme. This enzyme has two identical subunits, each containing three binding sites: one for the substrate (s), one for the allosteric activator (blue triangle), and one for the allosteric inhibitor (two-pronged figure). The enzyme has two conformations, a relaxed active conformation (R) and an inactive conformation (T). Binding of the substrate at its binding site stabilizes the active conformation so that the second substrate binds more readily, resulting in a sigmoidal response of v_i/V_{max} to the substrate concentration. The activator binds only to its activator site when the enzyme is in the R configuration. The inhibitor binding site is open only when the enzyme is in the T state. As a consequence of these restrictions, the graph of v_i/V_{max} becomes hyperbolic in the presence of activator, and more sigmoidal with a higher $S_{0.5}$ in the presence of inhibitor.

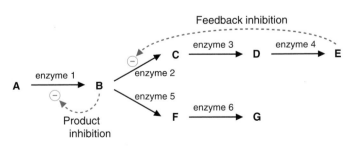

Fig. 9.30. A common pattern for feedback inhibition of metabolic pathways. The letters represent compounds formed from different enzymes in the reaction pathway. Compound B is at a metabolic branchpoint; it can go down one pathway to E, or down an alternate pathway to G. The endproduct of the pathway, E, might control its own synthesis by allosterically inhibiting enzyme 2, the first committed step of the pathway. As a result of the feedback inhibition, B accumulates. As a consequence, more B enters the pathway for conversion to G, which could be a storage, or disposal pathway. In this hypothetical pathway, B is a product inhibitor of enzyme 1, competitive with respect to A.

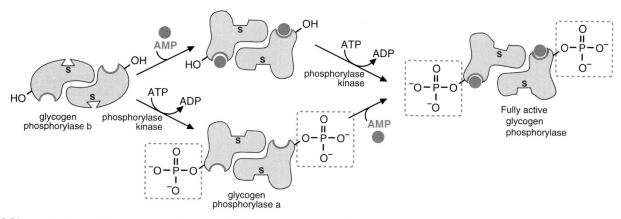

Fig. 9.31. Activation of glycogen phosphorylase by phosphorylation and AMP. Muscle glycogen phosphorylase is a dimer composed of two identical subunits. It can be activated either by its allosteric activator AMP, or by phosphorylation at specific serine residues. Glycogen phosphorylase kinase can transfer a phosphate from ATP to one serine residue in each subunit. Either phosphorylation or binding of AMP at its allosteric site causes a conformational change in the active site which converts the enzyme to a nearly fully active form. The first event at one subunit facilitates the subsequent events which convert the enzyme to the fully active form.

PRECURSOR CLEAVAGE

A number of proteolytic enzymes found in the blood or in the digestive tract are present as precursor proteins, called zymogens, which must be cleaved to be activated. Their synthesis in a precursor form prevents them from catalyzing reactions in the cells where they are synthesized. For example, chymotrypsin is secreted by the pancreas as chymotrypsinogen. It is activated in the digestive tract by the proteolytic enzyme trypsin, which cleaves off a small peptide from the N-terminal region. The cleavage changes the conformation of the enzyme and creates the binding cleft for the substrate. Precursor protein names have the prefix "pro," like prothrombin, or the suffix "ogen," like chymotrypsinogen.

AMOUNT OF ENZYME PRESENT

Tissues continuously adjust the rate of protein synthesis to vary the amount of different enzymes present. The expression for V_{max} in the Michaelis-Menten equation incorporates the concept that the rate of a reaction is proportional to the amount of enzyme present. The mechanisms by which the rate of protein synthesis is varied, such as induction/repression of gene transcription or stabilization of messenger RNA, are covered in the next section of the book.

Isoenzymes

Isoenzymes (isozymes) catalyze the same reaction, but have different amino acid sequences and different properties. The differences in properties between isoenzymes is usually a reflection of different roles for the isozymes in different tissues, different stages of development, or different intracellular compartments. (For example, the pattern of distribution of the hexokinase and glucokinase isozymes reflects the need of the red blood cell and certain other tissues to be independent of variability in blood glucose concentration.) There is also a fetal isozyme for some enzymes which matches the metabolic needs of cells which have not fully differentiated. The isozyme which appears in cancerous cells is often similar or identical to the fetal isozyme. If a reaction occurs in both the cytosol and mitochondrial compartments of the cells, it is usually catalyzed by different isozymes.

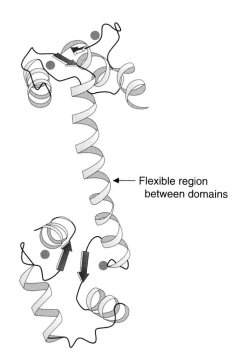

Fig. 9.32. Calcium-calmodulin has four binding sites for calcium (shown in blue). The ability of calcium to form a multiligand coordination sphere with a number of groups on the protein enables calcium to create large conformational changes in calmodulin and other calcium-binding proteins. There is a flexible region connecting the two domains which allows the protein to fold around and bind other proteins when calcium is present. From *Biochemistry* 4/E by Stryer. Copyright © 1995 by Lubert Stryer. Used with permission of W.H. Freeman and Company.

Creatine kinase isozymes in blood

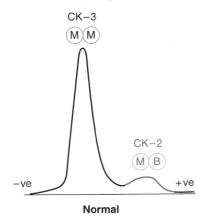

Normal

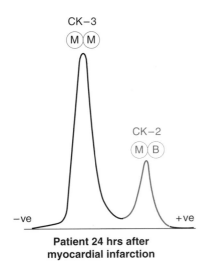

Patient 24 hrs after myocardial infarction

Fig. 9.33. Electrophoretic separation of serum creatine kinase isozymes from a normal healthy adult and from a patient who had a myocardial infarction 24 hours previously. Creatine kinase catalyzes the reversible transfer of a phosphate from ATP to creatine to form phosphocreatine and ADP. The reaction is an important part of energy metabolism in heart, muscle, and brain. Creatine kinase (CK) is composed of two subunits, M or B. Three different pairs of subunits can exist: BB (or CK-1, found in brain), MB (or CK-2, found only in heart), and MM (or CK-3, found in skeletal and heart muscle). These three isoenzymes are found in the cytosol or associated with myofibrillar structures and are released into the blood following damage to a tissue. Isoenzymes in the blood can be separated by electrophoresis, so that the amount of each isozyme can be determined. The appearance of CK-2 in the blood is diagnostic of a myocardial infarction because the heart is the only tissue containing significant amounts of CK-2. –ve = cathode; +ve = anode.

The existence of tissue-specific isozymes has provided a clinically useful diagnostic tool for the location of sites of tissue injury (Fig. 9.33). For example, cytosolic creatine phosphokinase isozymes (CK) consist of 2 subunits which may be either of the brain (B) or muscle (M) type. The brain isozyme is a dimer of 2 B subunits (BB), and the skeletal muscle has principally the isozyme formed of 2 M subunits (MM). Cardiac tissue contains the MM isozyme and is the only tissue which has the mixed MB isozyme. The appearance of the MB isozyme in the blood is characteristic of damage to heart tissue from a myocardial infarction.

CLINICAL COMMENTS. **Sloe Klotter** has hemophilia A, the most frequently encountered serious disorder of blood coagulation, occurring in 1 in every 10,000 males. In the majority of patients, the disease is genetically determined with an X-linked pattern of inheritance.

The most common manifestations of hemophilia A are those caused by bleeding into soft tissues such as muscle or into body spaces such as the peritoneal cavity or the lumen of the gastrointestinal tract. When bleeding occurs repeatedly into joints (hemarthrosis), the joint may eventually become deformed and immobile.

In the past, bleeding episodes have been managed primarily by administration of Factor VIII, sometimes referred to as the antihemophilia cofactor. These preparations, derived from multiple human donors, carry the risk of donor blood contamination with a variety of viruses such as hepatitis and HIV. Recombinant Factor VIII, free of this contamination risk, is commercially available. However, its widespread use may be limited by its considerable expense.

Al Martini was admitted to the hospital after intravenous thiamine was initiated at a dose of 100 mg/day (Recommended Dietary Allowance or RDA is approximately 0.5 mg/1,000 kcal ingested). His congestive heart failure was believed to be the result, in part, of the cardiomyopathy (heart muscle dysfunction) of acute thiamine deficiency known as beriberi heart disease. This nutritional cardiac disorder and the peripheral nerve dysfunction usually respond to thiamine replacement.

Within 2 days of starting allopurinol therapy, **Yves Topaigne's** serum uric acid level began to fall. Several weeks later, the level in the blood was normal. He remained free of further attacks of acute gouty arthritis and had no symptoms to suggest the formation of uric acid renal calculi.

Lethal doses of oral malathion are estimated at 1 g/kg of body weight for humans. **Dennis Livermore** survived his intoxication because he had ingested a small amount of the chemical, because he vomited shortly after the agent was ingested, and because the emergency room physicians were able to antagonize the action of the excessive amounts of acetylcholine which were accumulating in cholinergic receptors throughout his body. Intravenous atropine, an anticholinergic (antimuscarinic) agent, was the main drug used for this purpose.

After several days of intravenous therapy, the signs and symptoms of acetylcholine excess abated and therapy was slowly withdrawn. Dennis made an uneventful recovery.

William Hartman remained in the hospital following his heart attack until his CK enzyme levels had returned to normal and he had been free of chest pain for 7 days. He was discharged on a low fat diet and was asked to participate in the hospital's outpatient exercise program for patients recovering from a recent heart attack. He was scheduled for regular examinations by his physician.

BIOCHEMICAL COMMENTS. **Proteins of Blood Coagulation.** Damage to a blood vessel triggers three sequences of events to correct the injury and prevent loss of blood: vasoconstriction to diminish blood flow, clumping of platelets at the site of injury, and aggregation of the protein fibrin into an insoluble network, or clot, at the ruptured site. Hemostasis, maintaining a constant blood volume, requires rapid activation of blood coagulation, localization of the clot to the ruptured site on the blood vessel, and rapid termination of the process once the clot is formed. The proteins involved in the activation of blood coagulation, such as Factor VIII and thrombin, fall into three categories; proteases, protein cofactors, and regulatory proteins.

BLOOD COAGULATION CASCADE

Blood coagulation involves a sequence or cascade of reactions in which zymogens are converted to active proteases and cofactors through cleavage of one or more of their peptide bonds (Fig. 9.34). For example, Factor XIa, which is a serine protease, activates Factor IX, which is also a serine protease, by cleaving it to Factor IXa. Rapid activation and an enormous acceleration of the rate of clot formation occur because, at each stage of the cascade, 1 enzyme molecule forms many active enzyme molecules that catalyze the next step in the cascade. The cascade terminates in the cleavage of prothrombin to thrombin, which converts fibrinogen to fibrin and Factor XIII to XIIIa. The fibrin aggregates to form the "soft clot," which is then cross-linked by Factor XIIIa. Factor XIIIa is a transglutaminase which produces peptide bonds between the glutamyl portion of a glutamine on one fibrin monomer and a lysine residue on another. This meshwork of fibrin fibers traps the aggregated platelets and other cells, forming the thrombus or blood clot that plugs the leak in the vascular bed.

ROLE OF VITAMIN K IN BLOOD COAGULATION

Vitamin K is required for normal blood coagulation. It serves as an oxidation-reduction cofactor for the enzyme that forms γ-carboxyglutamate residues in a number of the blood coagulation proteins (Fig. 9.36). Vitamin K epoxide formed during the reaction is converted back to reduced vitamin K in a two-enzyme step catalyzed by epoxide reductase. Therapeutic drugs in the dicumarol family, such as warfarin, are analogues of vitamin K that inhibit blood clotting by blocking γ-carboxylation of the coagulation proteins (Fig. 9.37).

FIBRINOLYSIS

Once the damaged region of the vascular bed is repaired, the clot is no longer needed and is dissolved by plasmin, a serine protease which is able to cleave fibrin in the blood clot (Fig. 9.38). Plasmin is formed from its inactive precursor, plasminogen, by tissue plasminogen activator (TPA). TPA binds to both plasminogen and fibrin, so that plasmin is liberated directly on the clot.

A review of **Bill Hartman's** serum total CK and MB subunit (CK-2) concentrations showed the following:

Admission:

| CK | 182 units/L (reference range = 38–174) |
| CK-2 fraction | 6.8% (reference range < 5% of total CK) |

12 hours after admission:

| CK | 228 units/L |
| CK-2 fraction | 8% |

24 hours after admission:

| CK | 286 units/L |
| CK-2 fraction | 10.8% |

Both values returned to normal within 4 days of the patient's admission to the hospital.

Suggested Readings

Dressler D, Potter H. Discovering enzymes. Scientific American Library. New York: W.H. Freeman, 1991.

Fersht A. Enzyme structure and mechanism, 2nd ed. New York: W.H. Freeman, 1985.

Lerner RA. Catalytic antibodies: the concept and the promise. Hosp Pract 1993;(Jul 15):53.

Pilkis SJ, Weber IT, Harrison RW, Bell GI. Glucokinase: structural analysis of a protein involved in susceptibility to diabetes. J Biol Chem 1994;269:21925–21928.

In several of the key steps in the blood coagulation cascade, the protease is bound in a complex attached to the surface of platelets which have aggregated at the site of injury. Factors VII, IX, X, and prothrombin contain a domain in which 1 or more glutamate residues are carboxylated to γ-carboxyglutamate. Ca^{2+} forms a coordination complex with the negatively charged platelet membrane phospholipids and the γ-carboxylates of the blood coagulation factors. Protein cofactors such as tissue factor, Factor VIII, and Factor V are partially embedded in the membrane, and serve as "nests" for assembling enzyme-cofactor complexes on the platelet surface. For example, Factor VIIIa in the membrane forms a complex with Factor IXa, which is attached to the membrane by chelation of Ca^+ (Fig. 9.35).

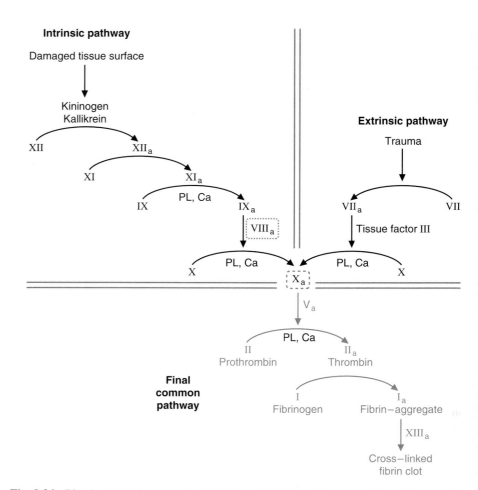

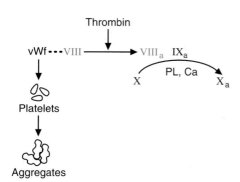

Fig. 9.35. Factor VIII, shown in blue, is a protein cofactor, or modulator protein, and not an enzyme. In the blood it circulates bound to von Willebrand factor (vWf). As thrombin cleaves and activates Factor VIII, vWf dissociates and binds to the ruptured endothelial surface where it activates platelet aggregation. Factor VIII$_a$ forms a complex with Factor IX$_a$ and Ca^{2+}-phospholipid (PL,Ca), which localizes the site of clot formation to the injured vessel. Hemophilia A, or classical hemophilia, is a deficiency of Factor VIII.

Fig. 9.34. Blood coagulation cascade. Activation of clot formation occurs through a cascade of proenzymes which sequentially activate each other through proteolytic cleavage. Activation of clot formation occurs through two separate pathways, termed the intrinsic and extrinsic pathways. The intrinsic pathway is activated when plasma proteins react with the exposed subendothelium of the damaged blood vessel. Platelets and the protein called von Willebrand factor bind to the exposed subendothelium, and the platelets, in turn, bind fibrinogen. The extrinsic pathway is activated by tissue factor (TF or Factor III) which is a membrane-bound protein exposed on the surface of cells following trauma. Trauma also activates conversion of Factor VII to VIIa, and tissue factor and Factor VIIa form a complex which cleaves Factor X to Factor Xa. The intrinsic and extrinsic pathways converge at the proteolytic activation of Factor X to Xa. Factors XII, XI, IX, VII, X, and thrombin are serine proteases. Finally thrombin cleaves fibrinogen to fibrin, and the initial "soft" clot is formed. Factor XIII$_a$ is a transglutaminidase. Factors VIII and V are cofactors which form complexes with the endothelial surface and Factors IXa and Xa, respectively. The reactions designated by "PL, Ca" are occurring via cofactors bound to phospholipids (PL) on the cell surface in a Ca^{2+} coordination complex.

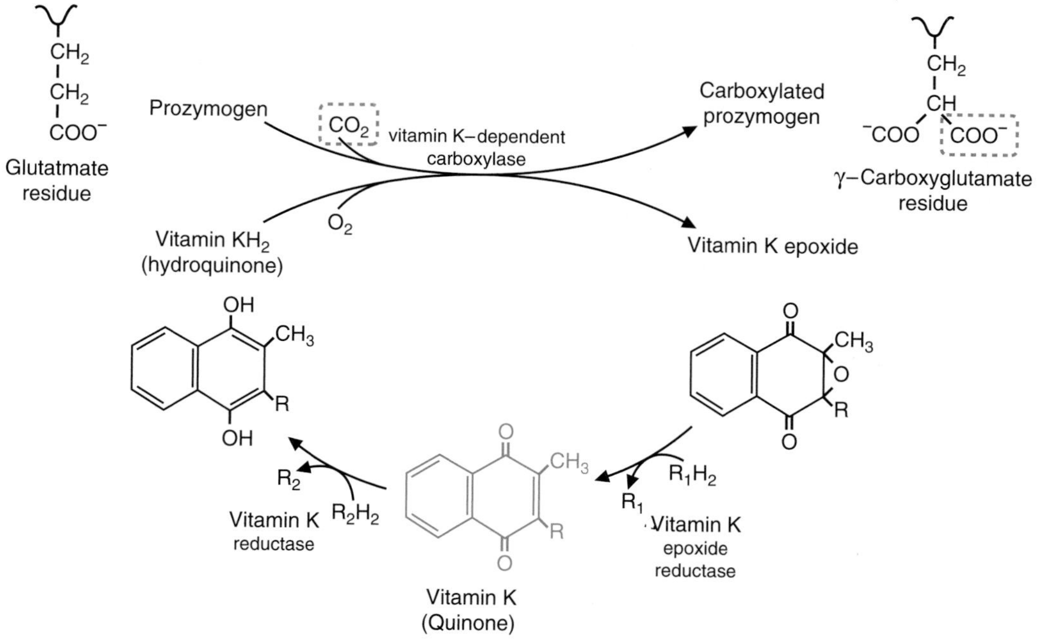

Fig. 9.36. Vitamin K-dependent formation of ;gg-carboxyglutamate residues. Prothrombin (II), Factor VII, Factor IX, and Factor X are bound to their phospholipid activation sites on cell membranes by Ca^{2+}. To bind calcium, 10 or more glutamic acid residues at the amino-terminal end of the clotting factors are converted by γ-carboxyglutamate amino acid residues that have a high affinity for calcium. The vitamin K-dependent carboxylase, which adds the extra carboxyl group, uses a reduced form of vitamin K (KH<->2<P>) as the electron donor and converts vitamin K to an epoxide. Vitamin K is reduced back to its active form by two enzymes, vitamin K epoxide reductase and vitamin K reductase.

Schramm VL, Horenstein BA, Kline PC. Transition state analysis and inhibitor design for enzymatic reactions. J Biol Chem 1994;269:18259–18262.

Symons RH. Small catalytic RNAs. Annu Rev Biochem 1992;61:641–671.

PROBLEMS

1. The effect of a number of single missense mutations on the kinetic properties of pancreatic B-cell glucokinase has been determined. A few of these are summarized in Table 9.5. The first three shown in the table are in glucokinases synthesized by site-directed mutagenesis for the purpose of examining the role of functional amino acids in the active site. Mutations 4–6 (and a large number of other mutations) have been found in individuals with maturity-onset diabetes of the young (MODY). Questions 1a–1c refer to Figure 9.23 and the mutations described in Table 9.5.

1a. Why would a change in Asn-204 to a glutamine increase the K_m more than a change to a serine?

1b. Changing a Glu-256 to an Ala (site-directed mutagenesis) or a Lys (natural mutation) affect both the K_m and the V_{max} of the enzyme in different ways. Which mutation decreases the activity of glucokinase most at a glucose concentration of 6 mM? (The Michaelis-Menten equation provides an approximate fit to the data for glucose concentrations above 5 mM, and can be used in the calculation).

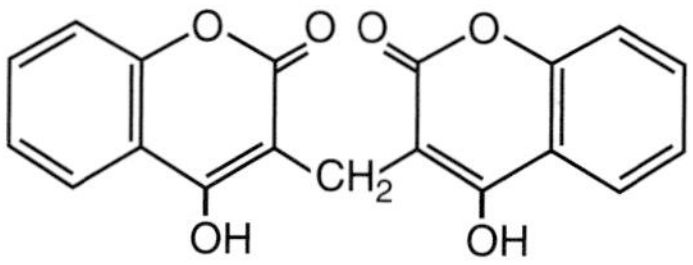

Dicumarol

Fig. 9.37. Dicumarol is a vitamin K analogue which inhibits vitamin K epoxide reductase and vitamin K reductase and thus blocks the conversion of vitamin K epoxide and vitamin K to the reduced coenzyme form. Drugs modeled after dicumarol, such as warfarin, are able to inhibit blood coagulation and are thus administered to patients to prevent clotting.

Deficiencies of vitamin K can result in uncontrolled bleeding (hemorrhage). Adult dietary deficiencies are uncommon because bacteria in the gut produce about half the requirement for vitamin K. Newborn infants, however, have a sterile digestive tract and very little in the way of vitamin K stores. They are usually given a vitamin K injection shortly after birth.

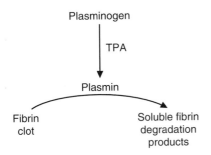

Plasminogen

TPA

Plasmin

Fibrin clot → Soluble fibrin degradation products

Fig. 9.38. Plasmin, the enzyme responsible for clot dissolution, is formed by the cleavage of plasminogen by the enzyme tissue plasminogen activator (TPA). TPA cleaves plasminogen to plasmin and remains tightly bound to the plasmin. TPA also has a high affinity for fibrin, and thus binds the plasmin to the fibrin clot. While plasmin is bound to the clot it is protected from protease inhibitors. Once the clot is dissolved, plasmin is inactivated by two other proteins, α_2-antiplasmin and α_2-macroglobulin. In vivo, stress, hypoxia, and a large number of low molecular weight organic compounds promote synthesis and release of TPA from tissues into the blood.

Patients with maturity onset diabetes of the young (MODY) have a rare genetic form of diabetes mellitus in which the amount of insulin being secreted from the pancreas is too low, resulting in hyperglycemia. The disease is caused by mutations in the gene for pancreatic glucokinase, a close isozyme of liver glucokinase. Glucokinase is part of the mechanism which controls the release of insulin from the pancreas. A decreased activity of glucokinase results in lower insulin secretion for a given blood glucose level.

Table 9.5. Mutations in Glucokinase[a]

Enzyme	K_m (mM)	V_{max} (units/mg)
Native B-cell glucokinase	6	93
Site-directed mutations:		
1) Asn-204→Ser	8	38
2) Asn-204→Gln	57	6
3) Glu-256→Ala	456	2
Mutations associated with decreased insulin release:		
4) Glu 256→Lys	92	0.2
5) Leu 309→Pro	2.2	0.9
6) Ser 131→Pro	110	46

Data from Pilkis SJ, Weber IT, Harrison RW, Bell GL. Glucokinase: structural analysis of a protein involved in susceptibility to diabetes. J Biol Chem 1994;269:21925–21928.

[a]The values of K_m and V_{max} were obtained by fitting the velocity versus substrate concentration curve measured in the presence of 5 mM ATP to a Michaelis-Menten equation.

1c. The Leu-309→Pro mutation is in a surface helix far from the active site. Yet it decreases the K_m of the enzyme and decreases the V_{max}. Can you postulate a mechanism for this?

2. How low would the blood glucose concentration have to fall to decrease the rate of glucose phosphorylation in the erythrocyte to 90% of V_{max}? (Assume that the Michaelis-Menten equation is applicable.)

ANSWERS

1a. Asn-204 is hydrogen-bonded to two —OH groups of the glucose molecule. Serine, which has a —CH_2OH side chain compared to a —CH_2—$CONH_2$ for asparagine, may still be able to make the same hydrogen bonds. The glutamine side chain ($CH_2CH_2CONH_2$) is longer than asparagine, and thus decreases the fit of glucose into the glucose binding site through steric hindrance. These changes will decrease the rate of glucose binding and increase its rate of dissociation, thereby increasing the K_m.

1b. To calculate v_i for each mutant enzyme, substitute the values for S = 6 mM, and V_{max} and K_m from the table into the Michaelis-Menten equation. v_i for the Glu-256→Ala mutant is 0.0259 unit/mg; v_i for the Glu-256→Lys mutant is 0.0122. The Glu-256→Lys mutation is the worst.

1c. Catalysis by glucokinase requires large conformational changes to close the active site to exclude water. The change of a leucine to a proline can affect the conformation of the enzyme in a way which makes the enzyme a tighter binding site for glucose, but makes it more difficult for the conformational changes to promote the stabilization of the transition state. This mutation illustrates the principle that a tighter binding of the substrate can increase the energy barrier between the enzyme-substrate complex and the transition state complex.

2. The substrate concentration at 90% of V_{max} can be obtained by substituting $v_i/V_{max} = 0.90$ and $K_m = 0.04$ mM into the Michaelis-Menten equation, and solving for [S]. The answer is [S] = 0.36 mM. Hexokinase catalyzes the first step of glycolysis, the only pathway in the erythrocyte which generates ATP. This calculation shows us that the blood glucose level would have to fall to less than 10% of its fasting level to significantly decrease the rate of ATP generation in the erythrocyte.

10 Relationship between Cell Biology and Biochemistry

Living organisms, ranging in complexity from bacteria to humans, are composed of cells. The architecture of a cell is intimately involved in regulating the flow of compounds through the sequences of reactions that constitute the pathways of biochemistry. A major architectural feature is the cell membrane that separates the contents of the cell from the surrounding environment and serves as a selective barrier, permitting only certain compounds to enter the cell and only certain compounds to leave.

Cells are divided into two major groups, the prokaryotes and the eukaryotes, based on the types of membranes they contain and the complexity of their genetic material. This chapter will concentrate on animal cells (a type of eukaryotic cell). However, we will briefly describe bacteria (as examples of prokaryotic cells) and the viruses that infect bacterial and animal cells.

Bacterial cells, including those that infect humans, are surrounded by a cell membrane and an exterior cell wall. Although the genetic material, DNA, is concentrated in a region of the bacterial cell, it is not separated from the cytoplasm by a membrane. In fact, bacteria do not contain organelles (membrane-bound subcellular structures) such as those found in eukaryotic cells.

Eukaryotes are much more complex than prokaryotes. Eukaryotic cells contain internal membrane systems which segregate various materials into organelles that have discrete functions. These organelles include nuclei (which contain the genetic material), mitochondria, the endoplasmic reticulum (both rough and smooth), the Golgi complex, lysosomes, and peroxisomes. The membranes of these internal organelles, like the cell membrane, determine which substances may enter or exit from the region they enclose.

Viruses are not really living cells, but rather collections of genetic material surrounded by a protein or a membrane coat. Whereas cells can replicate their DNA and divide to produce daughter cells, viruses cannot reproduce independently of other organisms. They exist only because they can parasitize living cells, using the biochemical machinery of prokaryotes or eukaryotes to generate their viral progeny. Viruses that grow in human cells can produce infections that range in severity from the common cold to AIDS.

Di Beatty returned for another follow-up visit with her physician. She reports that the glucose levels she measured on capillary blood by finger stick have ranged between 105 and 135 mg/dL after an overnight fast and 2 hours after a meal (postprandial). Her 2-hour postprandial blood glucose level, determined that morning by the hospital laboratory, was 145 mg/dL.

Before **Yves Topaigne** was treated with allopurinol, his physician administered acetyltrimethylcolchicinic acid (colchicine) for the acute attack of gout that affected his big toe. After taking a total of 3.6 mg of colchicine by mouth in divided doses over 6 hours, Mr. Topaigne reported that the throbbing pain in the toe had abated significantly. The redness and swelling also seemed to have lessened slightly.

Ron Templeton has embarked on an exercise program in an effort to continue losing weight and improve his level of physical conditioning. While jogging, he sprained his ankle and came to the sports medicine center for treatment. Although his exercise endurance has improved somewhat, he continues to tire relatively easily with jogging, noting shortness of breath within 5 minutes of starting his run. He is slightly discouraged and asks for additional advice regarding his training program. He also asks what cellular processes will take place as healing of his sprained ligament occurs.

CELL MEMBRANE

All cells are enclosed by a cell membrane, and eukaryotic cells also contain intracellular membranes surrounding subcellular organelles. As shown in Figure 10.1, membranes are composed of a lipid bilayer with embedded proteins. The bilayer is formed primarily by phospholipids, which are arranged with their hydrophilic heads facing the aqueous medium on either side of the membrane and their fatty acyl tails forming a hydrophobic membrane core (Fig. 10.2). Most of the membrane phospholipids are phosphoacylglycerols. In addition to phospholipids, the cell membrane may contain smaller quantities of sphingolipids, particularly in nerve cells of animals. Cholesterol is also present, but only in animal cells. The cell membrane in animal cells is also called the plasma membrane.

The proteins that span the cell membrane, from one side to the other, are called integral membrane proteins. The proteins embedded in only one side of the mem-

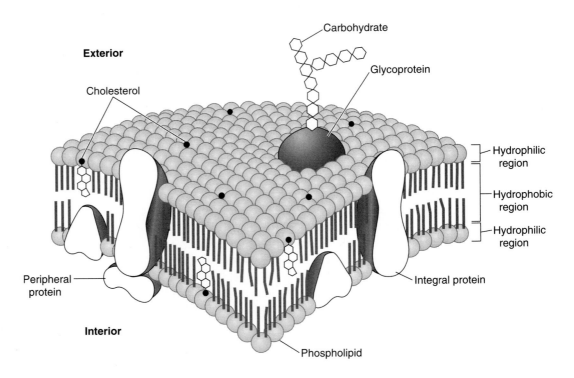

Fig. 10.1. Basic structure of an animal cell membrane.

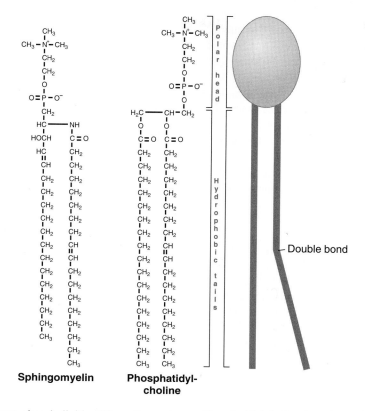

Sphingomyelin   **Phosphatidyl-choline**

Fig. 10.2. Some phospholipids of the cell membrane. Phosphatidylcholine is a phosphoacyl-glycerol, and sphingomyelin is a sphingolipid. Double bonds cause fatty acyl chains to bend.

brane are called peripheral proteins. Some of the proteins and lipids also bear short chains of carbohydrates on the exterior side of the membrane. Because the membrane consists of a mosaic of proteins and lipids, and because these components are free to drift about in the plane of the membrane, the membrane has been referred to as a fluid mosaic. (Some proteins are anchored to structural elements inside the cell and therefore are prevented from drifting.)

Membrane proteins serve various functions. Some are enzymes; some are transport proteins that conduct substances into or out of the cell; some are structural proteins that influence the cell's shape or movement; and some are involved in detecting signal molecules on the outside of the cell and transmitting the signal to the interior of the cell.

PROKARYOTES

Prokaryotes are cells that live and reproduce independently. The two major groups of prokaryotes are the bacteria and the cyanobacteria (blue-green algae). We will consider only the bacteria because members of this class are capable of growing within the human body, producing infections that range from gastrointestinal upsets to pneumonia.

As the term prokaryote (*pro*, before; *karyon*, nucleus) indicates, bacterial cells do not contain a nucleus. In fact, they do not contain any distinct subcellular organelles.

Bacterial cells have a membrane surrounding the cytoplasm (Fig. 10.3). External to this membrane is a cell wall which is composed of long chains of polysaccharides forming a protective shield on the surface of the cell. The genetic material (DNA) is concentrated in the central region of the cell, which is known as a nucleoid rather than a nucleus because it is not separated from the rest of the cellular contents by a membrane.

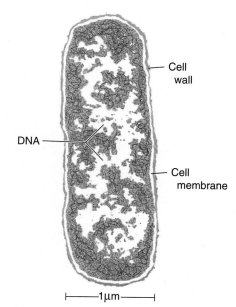

Fig. 10.3. Structure of a bacterial cell (*Escherichia coli*). E coli is a gram-negative rod. External to the cell membrane, it has a cell wall that is composed of periplasm, a thin layer of peptidoglycan (long chains of polysaccharides with peptide cross-bridges), and an outer membrane.

Bacterial cells usually contain a large circular chromosome. In contrast to eukaryotic cells, the DNA of this chromosome is not complexed with histones. Proteins are produced from the information in this DNA by processes similar to those in eukaryotic cells (see Section III).

Bacterial cells obtain nutrients from the medium on which they grow. They have pathways for obtaining energy from these fuels that are similar to those in eukaryotes. Bacteria, such as *Escherichia coli*, contain enzymes of the tricarboxylic acid (TCA) cycle and the components of the electron transport chain, which are located in the cell membrane.

Because the focus of this book is human biochemistry, we will describe the metabolism of prokaryotes only peripherally and will concentrate mainly on eukaryotic cells.

EUKARYOTES

In contrast to prokaryotes, eukaryotes (*eu*, good; *karyon*, nucleus) have internal membranes that surround subcellular material, organizing it into discrete compartments called organelles which have a variety of functions (Fig. 10.4). If cells are lysed by means that disrupt only the cell membrane, leaving the internal membranes intact, these subcellular structures may be isolated and studied (Fig. 10.5).

The following sections describe the various organelles and other subcellular components of animal cells. The aim of these descriptions is to outline the relationship of these subcellular structures to their biochemical function.

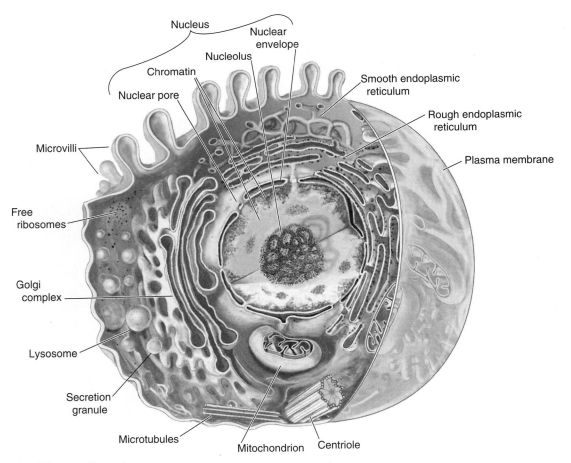

Fig. 10.4. An animal cell in three dimensions.

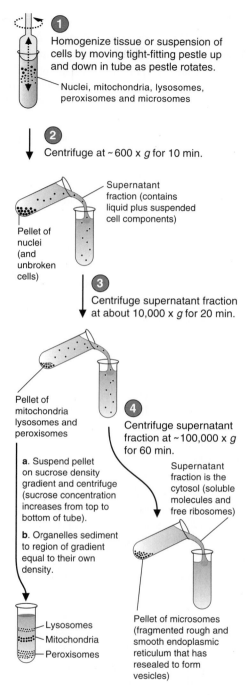

Fig. 10.5. Differential centrifugation.

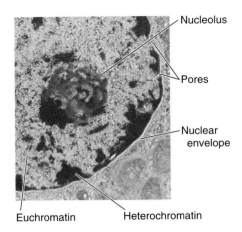

Euchromatin   Heterochromatin

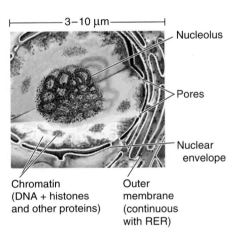

Chromatin
(DNA + histones
and other proteins)

Outer
membrane
(continuous
with RER)

Fig. 10.6. Nucleus. Electron micrograph (top); three-dimensional drawing (bottom).

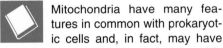

Mitochondria have many features in common with prokaryotic cells and, in fact, may have originated when primordial anaerobic eukaryotes engulfed ancient aerobic prokaryotes, establishing a symbiotic relationship. These prokaryotes provided eukaryotes with a more efficient mechanism for oxidizing fuels to obtain energy.

NUCLEUS

The largest of the subcellular organelles of animal cells is the nucleus (Fig. 10.6). It is separated from the rest of the cell (the cytoplasm) by the nuclear envelope, which consists of two membranes. The outer membrane of the nuclear envelope is continuous with the rough endoplasmic reticulum and contains ribosomes (subcellular components involved in protein synthesis). Pores through the two membranes of the nuclear envelope allow communication between the nuclear contents (the nucleoplasm) and the cytoplasm. Even large molecules such as RNA and proteins can pass through these pores.

Most of the genetic material of the cell is located in the chromosomes of the nucleus, which are composed of DNA, an equal weight of small, positively charged proteins known as histones, and a variable amount of other proteins. This nucleoprotein complex is called chromatin.

Genes, which are composed of DNA, direct the process of protein synthesis. Messenger RNA is transcribed from DNA and travels through the nuclear pores into the cytoplasm, where it is translated on the ribosomes by a process that produces proteins. Ribosomes are generated in the nucleolus and then travel through the nuclear pores to the cytoplasm. Replication, transcription, translation, and the regulation of these processes are the major focus of molecular biology (see Section III).

MITOCHONDRIA

Mitochondria are organelles that produce most of the chemical energy required by eukaryotic cells. Each mitochondrion is surrounded by an envelope composed of an outer and an inner membrane. The inner membrane has invaginations known as cristae, and the material enclosed by the inner membrane is known as the matrix (Fig. 10.7).

The final stages of fuel oxidation and most of the conversion of fuel energy to ATP occur in mitochondria. The enzymes of the TCA cycle, responsible for the final stages of fuel oxidation, are located solely in mitochondria, and the components of the electron transport chain are located in the inner mitochondrial membrane. The TCA cycle and electron transport chain are described in more detail in Section IV.

Mitochondria contain DNA. They can reproduce by replicating their DNA and then dividing in half. Mitochondrial division is not coupled to cell division. Mitochondrial DNA is used to synthesize proteins within the organelle. However, many mitochondrial proteins are encoded by nuclear genes, synthesized on cytoplasmic ribosomes, and subsequently imported into mitochondria by a complex process.

ENDOPLASMIC RETICULUM

The endoplasmic reticulum (ER) is a network of membranous tubules within the cell (Fig. 10.8). Some parts of this network are studded with ribosomes and are called the rough endoplasmic reticulum (RER). The remainder lacks ribosomes and is called the smooth endoplasmic reticulum (SER).

The RER and SER have a number of functions. They contain enzymes involved in lipid metabolism. Glycogen is stored in regions of liver cells that are rich in SER. The SER contains oxidative enzymes that use cytochrome P450 and are involved in the production of compounds, such as the steroid hormones, and in the metabolism of drugs and other toxic chemicals.

The RER is involved in the synthesis of certain types of proteins. Ribosomes, attached to the membranes of the RER, give them their "rough" appearance. Proteins, produced on these ribosomes, enter the lumen of the RER, travel to the Golgi complex in vesicles, and subsequently are either secreted from the cell, sequestered within membrane-bound organelles such as lysosomes, or embedded in cellular membranes.

GOLGI COMPLEX

The Golgi complex is involved in modifying proteins produced in the RER and in distributing these proteins to other regions of the cell or to the cell exterior. It consists of a curved stack of flattened vesicles in the cytoplasm (Fig. 10.9). Proteins that are produced on the RER travel in vesicles to the concave face (called the *cis* face) of the Golgi complex, entering the lumen where carbohydrates that were added in the RER may be modified or extended. These glycosylated proteins or glycoproteins are then packaged in vesicles. Glycolipids are also produced in the Golgi complex. Vesicles released from the convex face (the *trans* face) of the Golgi complex may travel to the cell membrane. After fusion of the vesicular and cell membranes, the proteins in the vesicles may be released into the extracellular space by a process known as exocytosis (Fig. 10.10). Glycoproteins or glycolipids that are anchored in the membrane of the vesicle remain in the cell membrane when the vesicular and cell membranes fuse.

Another function of Golgi vesicles is to carry the appropriate proteins, which were synthesized on the RER, to regions of the cell where they become part of organelles such as lysosomes.

LYSOSOMES

Lysosomes, cytoplasmic organelles similar in size to small mitochondria, are involved in intracellular digestion. They are enclosed by a single membrane that con-

Ron Templeton was examined and his ankle ligament sprain was judged to be minor. He was given a support bandage and crutches and told to avoid full weight bearing for 10 days.

An exercise physiologist reviewed the status of Ron's conditioning program and concluded that his rapid fatigue indicated that his endurance training schedule had to be stepped up. He was told that more frequent and longer periods of aerobic exercise would increase the rate at which new mitochondria developed in his skeletal muscle cells. As a result, he could produce ATP more rapidly and would be able to run longer before becoming exhausted.

The adjective "microsomal" is sometimes used for processes that occur in the endoplasmic reticulum (ER). This term is derived from experimental cell biology. When cells are ruptured in the laboratory, the ER is fragmented into vesicles called "microsomes." Microsomes are not actually present in cells.

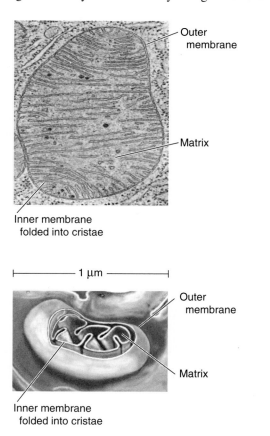

Outer membrane

Matrix

Inner membrane folded into cristae

|—— 1 µm ——|

Outer membrane

Matrix

Inner membrane folded into cristae

Fig. 10.7. Mitochondrion. Electron micrograph (top); three-dimensional drawing (bottom).

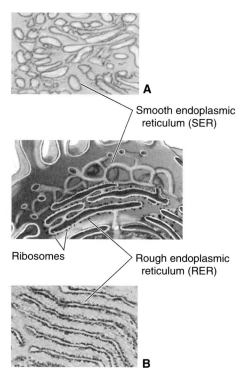

A

Smooth endoplasmic reticulum (SER)

Ribosomes

Rough endoplasmic reticulum (RER)

B

Fig. 10.8. A. Smooth endoplasmic reticulum. **B.** Rough endoplasmic reticulum. **A** and **B** are electron micrographs. A three-dimensional drawing is in the middle.

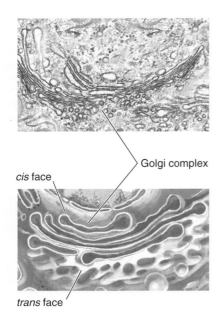

Fig. 10.9. Golgi complex. Electron micrograph (top); three-dimensional drawing (bottom).

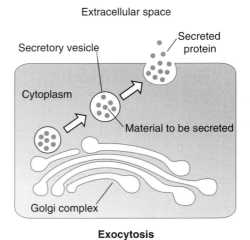

Fig. 10.10. Exocytosis.

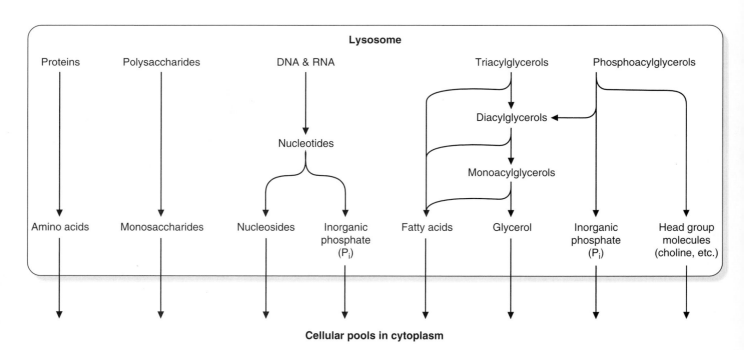

Fig. 10.11. Lysosomal digestion.

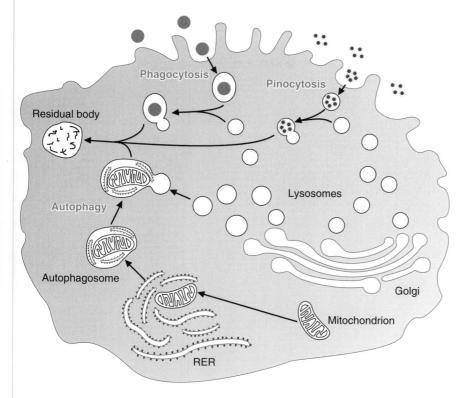

Fig. 10.12. Phagocytosis, pinocytosis, and autophagy.

The elevated level of uric acid in **Yves Topaigne's** blood led to the deposition of monosodium urate crystals in the joint space of his right great toe. Phagocytic cells attempted to digest these foreign bodies. However, the size and indigestibility of the crystals caused the phagocytes to rupture, releasing their lysosomal enzymes into the joint space. These enzymes, in turn, initiated an acute inflammatory reaction in the tissue of the joint capsule (synovitis), leading to the typical symptoms and signs of acute gouty arthritis.

tains proton pumps which keep the internal pH near 5. Lysosomes contain enzymes, called acid hydrolases, that act at an acid pH to digest all types of biomolecules, including lipids, proteins, polysaccharides, and nucleic acids (Fig. 10.11). Amino acids are produced from proteins, monosaccharides from polysaccharides, and nucleotides from nucleic acids. Acid phosphatases remove inorganic phosphate from organic compounds, such as nucleotides. Fatty acids are removed from mono-, di-, and triacylglycerols, and phosphate from phospholipids. The products of lysosomal digestion return to the cytosol. Lysosomes are thus involved in recycling the component parts of the large molecules of the cell, so that they may be reutilized.

The lysosomal membrane is impermeable both to the lysosomal enzymes and to the large molecules in the cytoplasm that serve as their substrates. Therefore, under normal conditions, the lysosomal membrane protects the cell from digesting itself. However, under certain adverse conditions, the membrane ruptures and enzymes leak from the lysosomes, causing autodigestion.

A number of mechanisms are involved in bringing the substrates and the lysosomal enzymes into contact (Fig. 10.12). Large extracellular particles, such as bacteria or yeast, may be engulfed and digested by the cell in a process known as phagocytosis (*phago*, to eat). The major phagocytic cells are macrophages and polymorphonuclear leukocytes. The process of phagocytosis starts when large particles approach the cell membrane. Many particles, such as bacteria and yeast, actually bind to receptors on the outer surface of the cell, and the receptor-particle (receptor-ligand) complexes move into coated pits (depressions on the cell surface that contain the protein clathrin underneath the membrane). In a process known as endocytosis, the cell membrane invaginates and pinches off, forming a phagocytic vesicle inside the cell. The membrane of this vesicle then fuses with the membrane of a lysosome, and the lysosomal

Ron Templeton's ankle healed because phagocytic cells entered the injured area and engulfed and digested the debris produced by the injury. Autophagy in damaged, but viable, cells permitted them to recover, regaining their normal appearance and function.

Phagocytes, located mainly in the spleen but also in the liver, remove 300,000 million (3×10^{11}) red blood cells from the circulation each day.

 Every hour, approximately four mitochondria in each liver cell are degraded by the process of autophagy.

Genetic defects in lysosomal enzymes may lead to an abnormal accumulation of residual bodies which may be so extensive that normal cellular function is compromised. Genetic diseases such as the mucopolysaccharidoses, Tay-Sachs disease, and Pompe's disease are caused by the absence or deficiency of specific lysosomal enzymes.

enzymes mix with the contents of the vesicle, now called a secondary lysosome, and digestion occurs. This fusion of the vesicular and lysosomal membranes ensures that the lysosomal enzymes remain safely inside a membrane-enclosed compartment within the cell. Many lysosomes may fuse with a single endocytic vesicle. The process has been filmed, and resembles a ground target being hit by a cluster of bombs.

A similar mechanism (see Fig. 10.12) results in the endocytosis and digestion of smaller extracellular particles, such as proteins. In this case, the process is called pinocytosis (*pino*, to drink).

Intracellular material may also be digested in a carefully controlled process known as autophagy ("self-eating") (see Fig. 10.12). In this case, the cell forms a membrane around the subcellular components that are to be digested, lysosomal membranes fuse with this membrane, and digestion occurs.

As shown in Table 10.1, lysosomes are central to a wide variety of body functions, all involved with eliminating unwanted material. Many of these functions involve phagocytes, cells specialized for phagocytosis and digestion. Phagocytes devour pathogenic microorganisms, such as bacteria and yeasts, and are thus involved in defense against infection. They also clean up wound debris and dead cells, thus aiding in repair. Cells that are damaged, but still viable, recover, in part, by using autophagy to eliminate damaged components.

Phagocytosis and autophagy are also involved in normal bodily processes, such as in the remodeling that occurs when a tissue assumes a new function and during involution, the process by which the tissue returns to its original state after the new function is no longer needed. For example, during pregnancy, the breast develops the capacity for lactation, and after weaning of an infant, the lactating breast returns to normal.

Phagocytosis plays a role in removing from the body cells that have a life span shorter than that of the whole organism.

After lysosomal enzymes have digested the contents of a secondary lysosome and the products have crossed the membrane and joined their respective pools in the cytoplasm of the cell, indigestible material may remain. The membrane-enclosed vesicles that contain this indigestible material are known as residual bodies. Some cells may expel this material by the process of exocytosis, but in many cells residual bodies accumulate with age.

PEROXISOMES

Peroxisomes are cytoplasmic organelles, similar in size to lysosomes, that are involved in oxidative reactions using molecular oxygen (Fig. 10.13). These reactions produce hydrogen peroxide (H_2O_2), a very toxic chemical, which fortunately is used in the peroxisome for other oxidative reactions or degraded by the enzyme catalase to water and molecular oxygen. One of the tasks of peroxisomes is to oxidize very long chain fatty acids (containing 20 or more carbons) to shorter chain fatty acids, which are then transferred to mitochondria for complete oxidation.

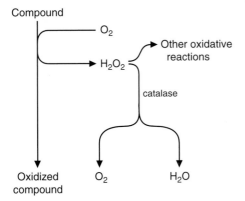

Fig. 10.13. Types of reactions in peroxisomes.

Table 10.1. Functions of Lysosomes

Destruction of infectious agents, such as bacteria and yeast
Recovery from injury
Tissue remodeling
Involution of tissues
Normal turnover of cells and organelles

NONMEMBRANOUS CYTOPLASMIC COMPONENTS

Cytoskeleton

The complex array of subcellular organelles is dispersed throughout the cell in an arrangement that is organized by a cytoskeleton composed of proteins. The major components of the cytoskeleton, actin filaments and microtubules (Fig. 10.14), are involved in maintaining the shape of the cell and in producing cellular and subcellular movements. Actin filaments combine with the protein myosin to produce movement, such as the contraction of skeletal muscles.

Microtubules consist of polymerized arrays of a protein called tubulin. The tubulin units add to or dissociate from the ends of microtubules, causing them to lengthen or shorten. Microtubules are responsible for the shape and the movement of cilia and flagella, hairlike cellular projections that move with a beating or whipping motion.

Microtubules are also responsible for the movements of organelles within the cell, including the distribution of transport vesicles from the Golgi complex. They are also essential for cell division, forming the spindle apparatus.

Polysomes

Polysomes are formed by the attachment of ribosomes to messenger RNA during the translation of proteins (Fig. 10.15). Many ribosomes may be attached to a single messenger RNA, and each ribosome produces a protein. These polysomes may be free in the cytoplasm or they may be attached to the RER.

Cytosol

The soluble material of the cytoplasm, which remains in solution after very high speed centrifugation ($100,000 \times g$ for 1 hour; see Fig. 10.5), is called the cytosol. It is not, however, simply an inert fluid; it contains many critical intermediates of metabolism and also the enzymes and cofactors for many important pathways such as glycolysis and fatty acid and protein biosynthesis.

TRANSPORT ACROSS MEMBRANES

Membranes form hydrophobic barriers around cells or cellular organelles that prevent polar substances from entering or escaping. Yet, in order to survive, cells and organelles must interact with a constantly changing environment, taking up external substances and releasing internal substances. These problems are resolved by means of transport mechanisms that selectively permit certain substances to cross membranes

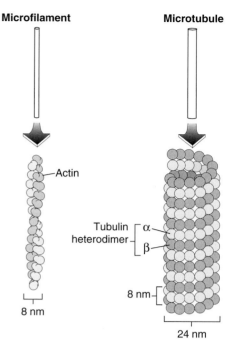
Fig. 10.14. Microfilaments and microtubules.

 Fluid or mucus is propelled over the surface of ciliated epithelial cells by the coordinated beating of cilia. A sperm cell swims by means of a flagellum.

Yves Topaigne was given colchicine, a drug that is frequently used to treat gout. One of its actions is to prevent phagocytic activity by binding to dimers of the α and β subunits of tubulin. When the tubulin dimer-colchicine complexes bind to microtubules, further polymerization of the microtubules is inhibited. Microtubules are constantly undergoing polymerization by addition of tubulin dimers and depolymerization by dissociation of dimers. If polymerization is inhibited by colchicine, depolymerization predominates, and the microtubules disassemble. Because microtubules are necessary for phagocytosis, colchicine inhibits this process and thus prevents the inflammatory response that results when phagocytes attempt to ingest urate crystals.

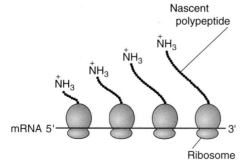
Fig. 10.15. A polysome.

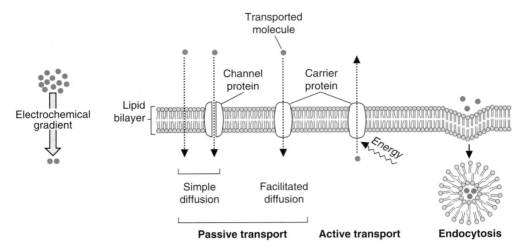

Fig. 10.16. Transport mechanisms.

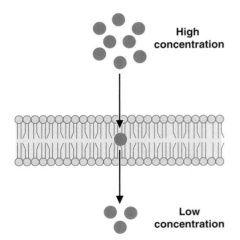

Fig. 10.17. Simple diffusion.

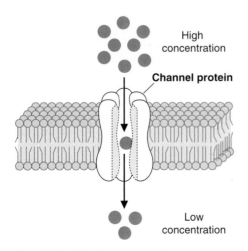

Fig. 10.18. Membrane channels.

(Fig. 10.16). These mechanisms involve simple diffusion, including the passage of substances, either directly through the membrane or through membrane channels or pores, and facilitated diffusion, involving carrier proteins known as transporters. Simple and facilitated diffusion are examples of passive transport. The substance travels down a chemical gradient from a region of higher concentration to one of lower concentration and/or down an electrical gradient from a region that is higher in substances of similar charge (or lower in substances of opposite charge) to a region that is lower in substances of similar charge (or higher in substances of opposite charge).

Active transport involves the movement of a substance against its electrochemical gradient by a process that requires energy. Very large molecules travel across membranes by the processes of endocytosis and exocytosis which were described previously.

Simple Diffusion

Small, uncharged molecules (such as O_2, CO_2, and H_2O) and lipid-soluble substances (such as steroid hormones) cross membranes by simple diffusion (Fig. 10.17). Channels formed by integral membrane proteins can selectively allow substances to pass, depending on their charge and size (Fig. 10.18). These channels may be gated, that is they may open or close in response to changes in voltage or to the binding of regulatory molecules.

Transporter Proteins

Transporter proteins involved in both passive and active transport function by binding a specific substance on one side of a membrane and undergoing a conformational change that allows the substance to be transported and released on the other side of the membrane. The transporter then resumes its original conformation and is ready for another round of transport (Fig. 10.19). Transporter proteins behave much like enzymes (Fig. 10.20). They have specific sites that selectively bind certain substances. When the binding sites on all of the transporter proteins in the membrane are occupied, the system is saturated and the rate of transport reaches a plateau (the maximum velocity). Inhibitors are substances that prevent transport by blocking the binding sites or by interacting with the transporter proteins, altering their conformation so that they are less functional.

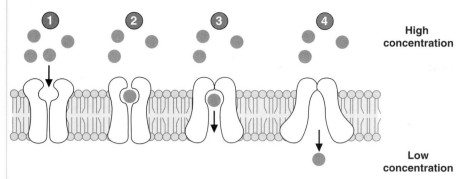

Fig. 10.19. Action of transporter proteins—passive transport.

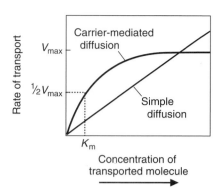

Fig. 10.20. Saturation of transporter proteins.

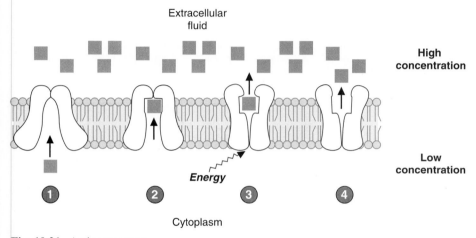

Fig. 10.21. Active transport.

Passive and Active Transport

Passive transport occurs when a substance crosses a membrane down an electrochemical gradient. This type of transport may or may not be mediated by a protein. In active transport, the cell uses energy to transport the substance and is able to pump it against an electrochemical gradient (Fig. 10.21). The energy may be provided by the hydrolysis of ATP or by the movement of electrons. Active transport is always mediated by proteins.

EXAMPLES OF PASSIVE AND ACTIVE TRANSPORT SYSTEMS

Most cells take up glucose by a passive mechanism. The concentration of glucose in the extracellular fluid is high compared to the concentration within the cell, where glucose is being rapidly metabolized. Therefore, glucose travels down its chemical gradient. ADP is passively transferred into mitochondria in exchange for ATP, and Cl^- into red blood cells in exchange for HCO_3^-.

The concentrations of Na^+ and K^+ in the intra- and extracellular fluid are maintained by an active transport system, the Na^+,K^+-ATPase (Fig. 10.22). The Na^+,K^+-ATPase is responsible for about one third of the basal energy requirement of the human.

SECONDARY ACTIVE TRANSPORT

Secondary active transport occurs when a substance is transported against its electrochemical gradient coupled to the transport of another substance down an electro-

The conduction of impulses along nerve cells is an example of a process that depends on the passive diffusion of ions through gated channels. For example, nerve cells have voltage-gated Na^+ channels, which open in response to a reduction of the electrical gradient across the membrane (depolarization). Some nerve cells also have Na^+ channels that are insensitive to voltage but open when they bind the neurotransmitter acetylcholine. The subsequent hydrolysis of acetylcholine causes these channels to close.

Di Beatty's insulin deficiency affects the transport of glucose into her muscle and adipose cells. Normally, insulin stimulates the synthesis of glucose transporters in muscle and adipose cells and recruits them to the cell membrane. If Di does not take her insulin, the concentration of glucose transporters in her muscle and adipose cell membranes will be low. The low rate of entry of glucose into these cells will cause Di's blood glucose levels to be elevated.

The cardiac glycoside (cardiotonic steroid) ouabain is a drug that inhibits the Na^+,K^+ pump by competing for the K^+ binding site.

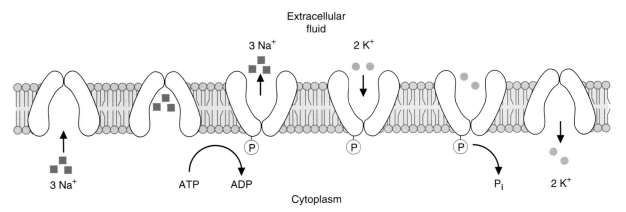

Fig. 10.22. Na⁺,K⁺-ATPase. Three sodium ions bind to the transporter protein on the cytoplasmic side of the membrane. When ATP is hydrolyzed to ADP, the carrier protein is phosphorylated and undergoes a change in conformation that causes the sodium ions to be released into the extracellular fluid. Two potassium ions then bind on the extracellular side. Dephosphorylation of the carrier protein produces another conformational change, and the potassium ions are released on the inside of the cell membrane. The transporter protein then resumes its original conformation, ready to bind more sodium ions.

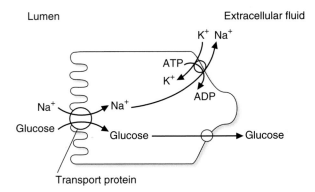

Fig. 10.23. Secondary active transport of glucose. One sodium ion binds to the carrier protein in the luminal membrane, stimulating the binding of glucose. After a conformational change, the protein releases Na⁺ and glucose into the cell and returns to its original conformation. Na⁺,K⁺-ATPase in the basolateral membrane pumps Na⁺ against its concentration gradient into the extracellular fluid. Thus, the Na⁺ concentration in the cell is low, and Na⁺ moves from the lumen down its concentration gradient into the cell and is pumped against its gradient into the extracellular fluid. Glucose, consequently, moves against its concentration gradient from the lumen into the cell by traveling on the same carrier as Na⁺. Glucose then passes down its concentration gradient into the extracellular fluid on a passive transporter protein.

chemical gradient established and maintained by primary active transport. An example is the transport of glucose into cells of the proximal kidney tubule or the intestinal epithelium in conjunction with sodium ions (Fig. 10.23). These cells create a gradient in Na⁺ and then use this gradient to drive the transport of glucose from the lumen into the cell against a concentration gradient.

Group Translocation

Group translocation occurs when the substance being transported is chemically modified by the transport system. The substance is bound more tightly by the transporter prior to its modification. After modification, it is bound less tightly and, thus, more readily released. The γ-glutamyl cycle that transports amino acids into certain types of cells is an example of a group translocation mechanism (Fig. 10.24).

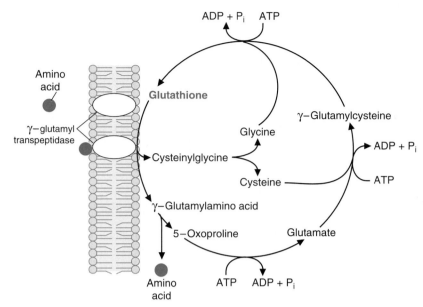

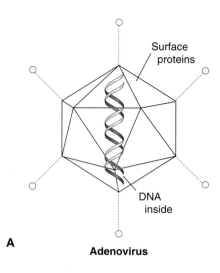

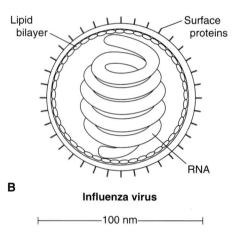

Fig. 10.24. γ-Glutamyl cycle. Glutathione is a tripeptide, γ-glutamylcysteinylglycine. It covalently binds the amino acid. The cysteine and glycine residues of the glutathione are released, and a γ-glutamylamino acid is produced, which is cleaved, forming the free amino acid and 5-oxoproline. 5-Oxoproline is converted to glutamate, which reacts with cysteine. The product, γ-glutamylcysteine, then reacts with glycine to reform glutathione, completing the cycle. The left side of the figure shows the transport of the amino acid, and the right side shows the resynthesis of glutathione. Note that this process consumes 3 ATP.

VIRUSES

Viruses are packets of genetic material that invade living cells. They are composed mainly of DNA or RNA surrounded by a protein coat or membrane, although some of the larger viruses have more complicated structures (Fig. 10.25). Viruses cannot reproduce by themselves. Instead, they inject their genetic material into cells, commandeering the DNA, RNA, and protein synthesizing machinery of the host cell, which they use to produce new virus particles. Even though viruses are not living cells, they are important medically because they cause many types of infections for which no specific therapy is available.

Fig. 10.25. Structure of viruses. **A.** Adenovirus, a DNA-containing virus. **B.** Influenza virus, an RNA-containing virus.

CLINICAL COMMENTS. **Di Beatty** responded well to the treatment of her diabetes mellitus. She is faithfully injecting insulin, which binds to insulin receptor molecules located in the plasma membranes of various cells. In skeletal muscle and adipose cells, this hormone-receptor interaction leads to a series of complex "post-receptor" steps which result in the mobilization of insulin-sensitive glucose transport molecules from an intracellular pool. They are translocated to the cell surface where they promote the transport of glucose from the blood into muscle and fat cells. This process helps to lower blood glucose levels.

  Yves Topaigne had a rapid and gratifying clinical response to the hourly administration of colchicine. Evidence suggests that this drug diminishes phagocytosis and the subsequent release of the lysosomal enzymes which initiate the inflammatory response in synovial tissue.

  In addition, phagocytic cells, known as leukocytes, associated with the inflammatory processes produce lactic acid, which causes a local decrease in pH that results in more rapid uric acid crystal deposition. Colchicine diminishes lactic acid production by leukocytes, decreasing uric acid crystal deposition and, thus, relieving the symptoms of acute gouty arthritis.

Ron Templeton's sprained ankle healed quickly, and he was able to gradually increase the frequency and duration of his exercise. His exercise endurance gradually improved, and he lost 6 lb over the next 2 months.

These positive changes resulted not only from the exercise-induced increase in the number and oxidative efficiency of his skeletal muscle mitochondria, but also from a variety of other adaptations which are part of the physiological response to exercise training. Among these are a greater capacity to extract oxygen from the inspired air, metabolically more efficient pumping action of heart muscle, and an enhanced ability of the vascular system to deliver fuels and oxygen to the exercising muscles.

BIOCHEMICAL COMMENTS. Different subcellular organelles contain different sets of enzymes. For instance, the nucleus contains the enzymes for DNA and RNA synthesis, while the enzymes for glycolysis and for fatty acid biosynthesis are located mainly in the cytosol. Mitochondria contain the enzymes for β-oxidation of fatty acids, the TCA cycle, the electron transport chain, and ketone body synthesis and degradation (Table 10.2).

Not all cells are alike, however. Different cell types contain different groups of organelles. Therefore, they have different sets of enzymes and, consequently, different functions. For example, red blood cells lack mitochondria. Therefore, they cannot produce ATP from reactions of the TCA cycle and the electron transport chain, and although they carry oxygen, they do not utilize it.

Sometimes the same type of organelle may contain slightly different sets of enzymes in one tissue versus another. For instance, liver mitochondria contain a key enzyme for synthesizing ketone bodies, but they lack a key enzyme for their utilization. The reverse is true in muscle mitochondria.

Cells are grouped into tissues and organs. The blood provides the fluid that bathes these cells, allowing them to exchange metabolites. Thus, cells can affect the metabolism of other cells by releasing molecules into the blood or by taking up molecules from the blood.

The organelles, the membrane receptors and membrane transporters, and the enzymes that the cells of a tissue contain determine which substances the cells can take up from the blood and metabolize and which metabolites the cells can release into the blood. Thus, an understanding of subcellular architecture is essential for understanding the metabolic activity of cells.

Table 10.2. Metabolic Capacities of Various Organelles

Process	Organelles Involved in Process
TCA cycle (acetyl CoA→CO_2 + H_2O)	Mitochondria
β-Oxidation of fatty acids	Mitochondria
Ketone body formation	Mitochondria (liver)
Ketone body utilization	Mitochondria (muscle, kidney — not liver)
Lipogenesis (glucose→fatty acids)	Cytosol and mitochondria (mainly liver)
Gluconeogenesis (lactate→glucose)	Cytosol and mitochondria (liver)
Glycogen metabolism (synthesis and degradation)	Cytosol
Lactate production (glucose→lactate)	Cytosol

Suggested Reading

For a more detailed review of cell biology, see

Alberts B, Bray D, Lewis J, et al. Molecular biology of the cell. New York: Garland, 1994.

PROBLEM

A consequence of a deficiency of the enzyme pyruvate kinase in red blood cells is a hemolytic anemia. Pyruvate kinase is a key enzyme in the glycolytic pathway, which produces ATP by converting glucose to pyruvate. This pathway is located in the cytosol. In a person with a pyruvate kinase deficiency, an anemia (a reduced number of red blood cells) occurs because of increased destruction of these cells by phagocytes in the spleen. Using your knowledge of cell biology and fuel metabolism, explain what happens to these cells.

ANSWER

Red blood cells do not contain mitochondria and therefore are totally dependent for energy production on glycolysis, the cytosolic pathway that converts glucose to pyruvate. Pyruvate kinase is a key glycolytic enzyme. If glycolysis cannot occur at a normal rate because of a deficiency of pyruvate kinase, the cells cannot produce an adequate amount of ATP. As a consequence, the cells cannot maintain the ion pumps in their cell membranes, and they gain Ca^{2+}, lose K^+ and water, and become rigid. They then undergo hemolysis (i.e., they are removed from the circulation by phagocytosis in the spleen).

Gene Expression and the Synthesis of Proteins

Currently, a major change in the biological sciences is beginning to have repercussions in medicine. New information about genes and new techniques that probe the human genome will completely revolutionize the way medicine is practiced in the 21st century. This revolution began in the middle of the 20th century with the identification of DNA as the genetic material and the determination of its structure. Using this knowledge, researchers discovered the mechanisms by which genetic information is inherited and expressed. During the last 20 years, our understanding of this critical area of science, known as molecular biology, has grown at an increasingly rapid pace.

The genome of a cell consists of all its genetic information, encoded in DNA (deoxyribonucleic acid). In eukaryotes, DNA is located mainly in nuclei, but small amounts are also found in mitochondria. Nuclear genes are packaged in chromosomes which contain DNA and protein in tightly coiled structures.

The molecular mechanism of inheritance involves a process known as replication, in which the strands of parental DNA serve as templates for the synthesis of DNA copies (Fig. 11.1). After DNA replication, cells divide and these DNA copies are passed to daughter cells. Alterations in genetic material occur by recombination (the exchange of genes between chromosomes), and by mutation (the result of alterations in DNA). DNA repair mechanisms correct much of the damage to DNA, but many gene alterations are passed to daughter cells.

The expression of genes within cells requires two processes, transcription and translation (see Fig. 11.1). DNA is transcribed to produce ribonucleic acid (RNA). Three major types of RNA are transcribed from DNA and, subsequently, participate in the process of translation (the synthesis of proteins). Messenger RNA (mRNA) carries the genetic information from the nucleus to the cytoplasm, where translation occurs on ribosomes, structures that contain proteins complexed with ribosomal RNA (rRNA). Transfer RNA (tRNA) carries amino acids to the ribosomes, where they are joined in peptide linkage to form proteins. During translation, the sequence of bases in mRNA is read in sets of three (each set of three bases constitutes a codon). The sequence of codons in the mRNA dictates the sequence of amino acids in the protein.

Proteins are involved in cell structure, and they function as enzymes, which determine the reactions that occur in cells. Thus, by producing proteins, genes determine the appearance and behavior of cells, and, consequently, the appearance and behavior of organisms. The regulation of gene expression in eukaryotic cells permits only a fraction of the genome to be expressed at any given time; therefore, cells can undergo development and differentiation.

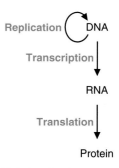

Fig. 11.1. Replication, transcription, and translation. Replication: DNA serves as a template for producing DNA copies. Transcription: DNA serves as a template for the synthesis of RNA. Translation: RNA provides the information for the process of protein synthesis.

Research in molecular biology has produced a host of new techniques which are known collectively as recombinant DNA technology, biotechnology, or genetic engineering. Although these techniques are just beginning to be applied to medicine, a number of genetic diseases can now be detected, which previously could be diagnosed only when full-blown or, in earlier stages, by relatively unreliable methods. Diagnosis of these diseases can now be made with considerable accuracy even before birth, and carriers of these diseases can also be identified.

Because of recent developments in the field of gene therapy, diseases which for centuries have been considered hopeless are now potentially curable. Although much of the therapy for these diseases is currently experimental, during the 21st century, physicians should be using genetic engineering techniques routinely, not only to diagnose but also to treat their patients.

11 Structure of the Nucleic Acids

The monomeric units of the nucleic acids are nucleotides. Each nucleotide contains a heterocyclic nitrogenous base, a sugar, and a phosphate. DNA contains the purine bases adenine (A) and guanine (G) and the pyrimidine bases cytosine (C) and thymine (T). RNA contains uracil (U) instead of thymine. In DNA, the sugar is deoxyribose, whereas in RNA it is ribose.

Polynucleotides such as DNA and RNA contain 3′- to 5′-phosphodiester bridges between the nucleotide monomers. The bases are not involved in the sugar-phosphate backbone and, therefore, are free to interact with other bases or with proteins.

DNA is composed of two antiparallel polynucleotide strands, joined by pairing between their bases. Adenine pairs with thymine, and guanine pairs with cytosine. The two DNA strands run in opposite directions. One strand runs 5′ to 3′ (that is, the 5′-carbon of the sugar is above the 3′-carbon), while the other chain runs 3′ to 5′. The two DNA strands wind around each other, forming a double helix.

In contrast to DNA, RNA is single-stranded. However, RNA strands may loop back on themselves, and bases in the portions of the strand that run in opposite directions can pair, guanine with cytosine and adenine with uracil.

The three major types of RNA are messenger RNA (mRNA), ribosomal RNA (rRNA), and transfer RNA (tRNA). Eukaryotic mRNA has a structure known as a cap at the 5′-end and a sequence of adenine nucleotides (a poly(A) tail) at the 3′-end. rRNA lacks these structures, but has extensive base pairing. tRNA is small compared to mRNA or the large rRNAs. There is at least one tRNA for each amino acid involved in protein synthesis. Although each of the tRNAs has a different base sequence and contains a number of unusual nucleotides, they all assume a similar cloverleaf structure. In addition, each tRNA contains a unique anticodon, a sequence of three bases that pairs with the codon on mRNA.

 A small amount of thymine is present in tRNA.

Colin Tuma had intestinal polyps at age 45 which were removed via a colonoscope. However, he did not return for annual colonoscopic examinations as instructed. At age 56, he reappeared, complaining of tar-colored stools (melena), which are caused by intestinal bleeding. The source of the blood loss was an adenocarcinoma growing from a colonic polyp of the large intestine. At surgery, it was found that the tumor had invaded the gut wall and perforated the visceral peritoneum. Several pericolic lymph nodes contained cancer cells, and several small nodules of metastatic cancer were found in the liver. Following resection of the tumor, the oncologist suggested palliative therapy with 5-fluorouracil (5-FU) combined with other chemotherapeutic agents.

Ivy Sharer is a 26-year-old intravenous (IV) drug abuser who admitted to sharing unsterile needles with another addict for several years. Five months before presenting to the hospital emergency department with soaking night sweats, she experienced a 3-week course of a flulike syndrome with fever, malaise, and muscle aches. Four months ago she noted generalized lymph node enlargement

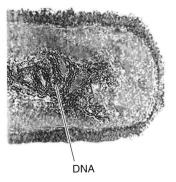

Fig. 11.2. DNA of a bacterial (prokaryotic) cell.

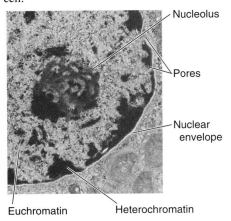

Fig. 11.3. Chromatin in an interphase nucleus of a eukaryotic cell.

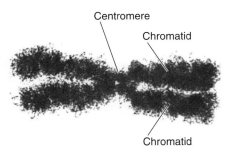

Fig. 11.4. Sister chromatids during mitosis. Every mitotic chromosome contains two identical sister chromatids.

 The genetic information in a human haploid nucleus in an egg or a sperm cell is contained in about 3×10^9 base pairs of DNA, whereas that in a mitochondrion is contained in less than 20,000 base pairs.

 Genetic engineers use plasmids as tools because segments of DNA can readily be incorporated into plasmids and, thus, plasmids can be used to transfer foreign genes into bacteria.

associated with chills and anorexia, followed by diarrhea which led to a 22-lb weight loss. An enzyme-linked immunosorbent assay (ELISA) and a Western blot assay were both positive for antibodies to the human immunodeficiency virus (HIV). Because her symptoms indicated that she had the acquired immunodeficiency syndrome (AIDS), therapy with azidothymidine (AZT) was initiated.

Arlyn Foma, a 68-year-old male, complained of fatigue, anorexia, and a low grade fever. He was found to have a generalized distribution of enlarged rubbery nontender lymph nodes. An open biopsy of a supraclavicular node revealed the presence of non-Hodgkin's lymphoma, follicular type. Noninvasive staging procedures, for example, computed tomography (CT) scans, as well as bone marrow biopsies, revealed a diffuse process with bone marrow involvement. Multiagent chemotherapy was planned including the use of doxorubicin (adriamycin).

Michael Sichel presented to the hospital emergency room just 2 months after he had been discharged following therapy for a sickle cell crisis. His current symptoms of severe back and leg pains had started 24 hours earlier and were not relieved by potent oral analgesics. Because of the severity of his symptoms and the discovery that his usual baseline hemoglobin of 7.5 g/dL had fallen to 5.9 g/dL, he was readmitted for hydration, blood transfusions, and pain relief with parenteral analgesics.

Thomas Appleman's weight reduction program is behind schedule. He returns complaining of a fever and cough, which produces a thick yellow-brown sputum. A stain of his sputum reveals many Gram-positive, bullet-shaped diplococci. A culture of his sputum confirms that his respiratory infection is caused by *Streptococcus pneumoniae*, sensitive to penicillin, erythromycin, tetracycline, and other antibiotics. Because of a history of penicillin allergy, he is started on oral erythromycin therapy.

DNA STRUCTURE

Location of DNA

DNA serves as the genetic material for cells, both prokaryotes and eukaryotes. Because prokaryotes lack internal membrane systems, their DNA is not separated from the rest of the cellular contents (Fig. 11.2). In eukaryotes, DNA is located in the nucleus, separated from the cytoplasm by the nuclear envelope (Fig. 11.3).

Eukaryotic DNA is bound to proteins, forming a complex known as chromatin. During interphase (when cells are not dividing), chromatin may be dense (heterochromatin) or diffuse (euchromatin), but no distinct structures can be observed. However, during mitosis (when cells are in the process of dividing), chromatin condenses into discrete, visible chromosomes, each consisting of two identical sister chromatids joined at their centromere regions (Fig. 11.4).

Mitochondria contain DNA, however, it is only a very small amount (less than 0.1% of the total DNA in the average cell).

The mitochondria of eukaryotic cells are similar to prokaryotic cells. The DNA and protein synthesizing systems in mitochondria more closely resemble the systems in bacteria than in the eukaryotic cytoplasm. It has been suggested that mitochondria were derived from ancient bacterial invaders of primordial eukaryotic cells.

Many viruses also contain DNA as their genetic material. In viruses, however, systems for replication, transcription, and translation are not present, and consequently, viruses must invade other cells and commandeer their DNA, RNA, and protein-synthesizing machinery in order to reproduce. Viruses can infect both eukaryotes and prokaryotes. Those that infect bacteria are known as bacteriophage (or more simply as phage).

Plasmids are small, circular DNA molecules that can enter bacteria and replicate autonomously, that is, outside the host genome. In contrast to viruses, plasmids are not infectious; they do not convert their host cells into factories devoted to plasmid production.

Determination of the Structure of DNA

In 1865, Frederick Meischer first isolated DNA, obtaining it from pus scraped from surgical bandages. Initially, scientists speculated that DNA was a cellular storage form for inorganic phosphate, an important but unexciting function that did not spark widespread interest in determining its structure. In fact, the details of DNA structure were not fully determined until 1953, almost 90 years after it had first been isolated, but only 9 years after it had been identified as the genetic material.

Early in the 20th century, the bases were identified as the purines adenine (A) and guanine (G), and the pyrimidines cytosine (C) and thymine (T) (Fig. 11.5). The sugar was found to be deoxyribose, a derivative of ribose, lacking a hydroxyl group on carbon 2 (Fig. 11.6).

Nucleotides, composed of a base, a sugar, and phosphate, were found to be the monomeric units of the nucleic acids (Table 11.1). The nitrogenous base is linked by an *N*-glycosidic bond to the anomeric carbon of the sugar, and inorganic phosphate forms an ester with a hydroxyl group of the sugar (Fig. 11.7).

 Watson and Crick's one-page paper, published in 1953, contained little more than 900 words. However it triggered a major revolution in the biological sciences and produced the conceptual foundation for the discipline of molecular biology.

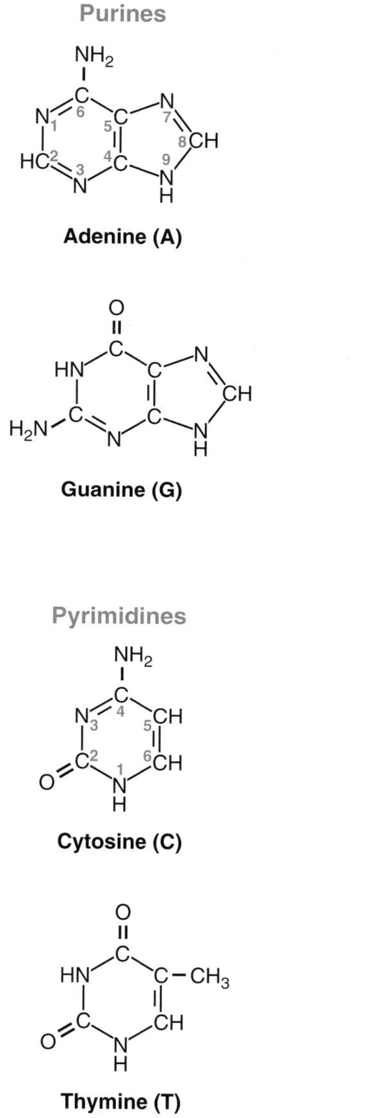

Purines

Adenine (A)

Guanine (G)

Pyrimidines

Cytosine (C)

Thymine (T)

Fig. 11.5. Nitrogenous bases of DNA. Adenine and guanine are purines and cytosine and thymine are pyrimidines.

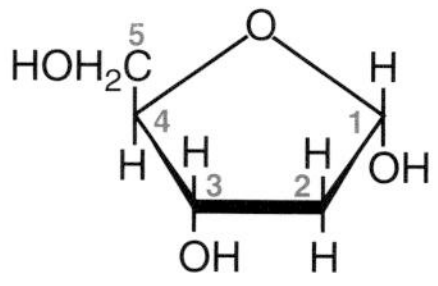

Fig. 11.6. Deoxyribose, the sugar of DNA. The carbon atoms are numbered from 1 to 5. When the sugar is attached to a base, the carbon atoms are numbered from 1′ to 5′.

Table 11.1. Names of Bases and Their Corresponding Nucleosides[a]

Base	Nucleoside
Adenine (A)	Adenosine
Guanine (G)	Guanosine
Cytosine (C)	Cytidine
Thymine (T)	Thymidine
Uracil (U)	Uridine
Hypoxanthine (I)	Inosine[b]

[a]If the sugar is deoxyribose rather than ribose, the nucleoside has "deoxy" as a prefix (e.g., deoxyadenosine). Nucleotides are given the name of the nucleoside plus mono-, di-, or triphosphate (e.g., adenosine triphosphate or deoxyadenosine triphosphate).

[b]The base hypoxanthine is not found in DNA or RNA but is produced during degradation of the purine bases. Its nucleoside, inosine, is produced during synthesis of the purine nucleotides (see Chapter 41).

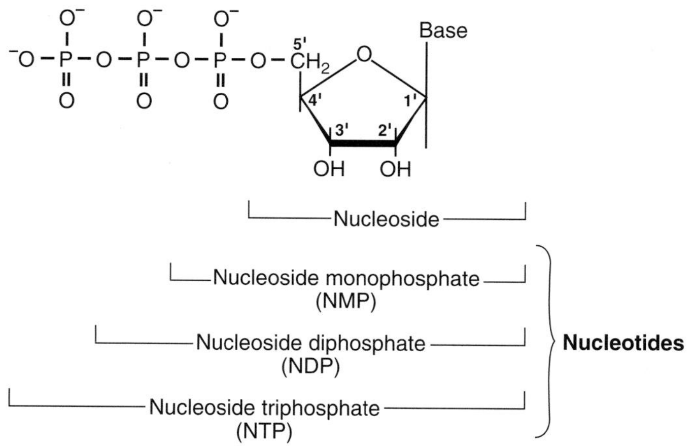

Fig. 11.7. Nucleoside and nucleotide structures. Shown with ribose as the sugar. The corresponding deoxyribonucleotides are abbreviated dNMP, dNDP, and dNTP. N = any base (A, G, C, U, or T).

Colin Tuma was treated with 5-FU for metastatic cancer related to a primary tumor of the colon. 5-FU is an analogue of the thymine base found in DNA.

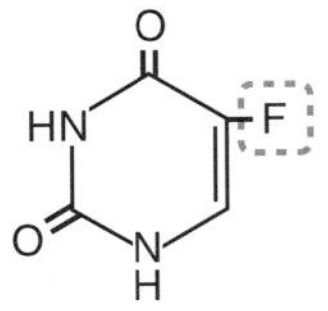

5–Fluorouracil,
an analogue of uracil or thymine

In 1944, after Oswald Avery's experiments establishing DNA as the genetic material were published, interest in determining the structure of DNA intensified. Digestion with enzymes of known specificity proved that inorganic phosphate joined the nucleotide monomers, forming a phosphodiester bond between the 3′-carbon of one sugar and the 5′-carbon of the next sugar along the polynucleotide chain (Fig. 11.8). Erwin Chargaff analyzed the base composition of DNA from various sources and concluded that, on a molar basis, the amount of adenine was always equal to the amount of thymine and the amount of guanine was equal to the amount of cytosine.

During this era, James Watson and Francis Crick joined forces and, using the information then available, including the x-ray diffraction data of Maurice Wilkins and Rosalind Franklin, they concluded that DNA consisted of two polynucleotide strands joined by pairing between their bases. In 1953, they published a brief paper, describing DNA as a double helix.

After **Ivy Sharer** was found to have AIDS, she was treated with AZT, an analogue of the thymine nucleotide found in DNA.

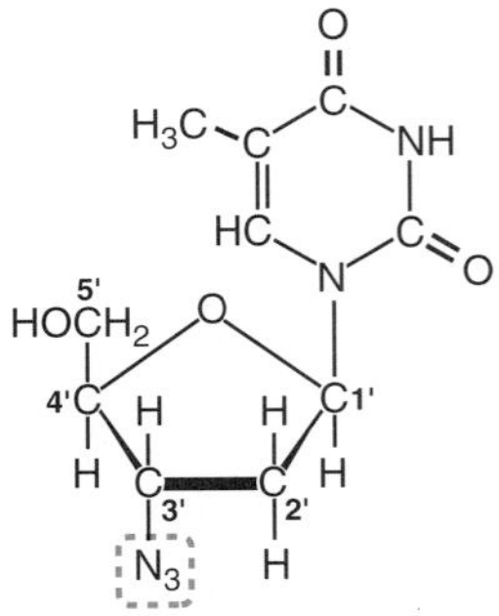

AZT,
an analogue of deoxythymidine

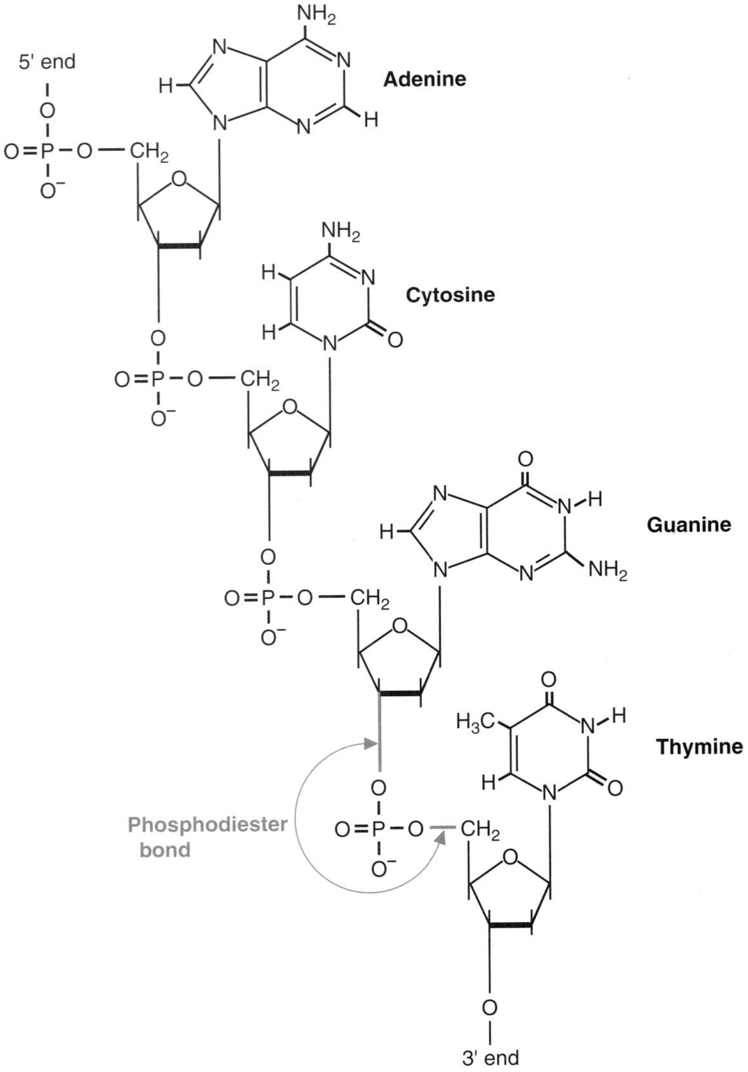

Fig. 11.8. A polynucleotide chain of DNA.

Concept of Base-Pairing

To explain Chargaff's data, Watson and Crick proposed that each DNA molecule consists of two polynucleotide chains joined by hydrogen bonds between the bases. Adenine on one strand forms a base pair with thymine on the other strand (Fig. 11.9). This base pair is stabilized by two hydrogen bonds. The second type of base pair in DNA, formed between guanine and cytosine, is stabilized by three hydrogen bonds. As a consequence of base-pairing, the two strands of DNA are complementary. Adenine on one strand is matched by thymine on the other strand, and guanine is matched by cytosine.

The concept of base-pairing proved to be essential for determining the mechanism of DNA replication (in which the copies of DNA are produced that are distributed to daughter cells) and the mechanisms of transcription and translation (in which mRNA is produced from genes and used to direct the process of protein synthesis). Obviously, as Watson and Crick suggested, base-pairing allows one strand of DNA to serve as a template for the synthesis of the other strand (Fig. 11.10). Base-pairing also allows a strand of DNA to serve as a template for the synthesis of a complementary strand of RNA.

DNA Strands Are Antiparallel

Watson and Crick concluded that the two complementary strands of DNA run in opposite directions. As shown in Figure 11.11, on one strand, the oxygen of each sugar ring is above the carbons, so that the 5′-carbon is above the 3′-carbon. This strand is said to run in a 5′ to 3′ direction. On the other strand, the oxygen of each ring is below the carbons, so that the 3′-carbon is above the 5′-carbon. This strand is said to run in a 3′ to 5′ direction. Thus, the strands are antiparallel, that is they run in opposite directions.

This concept of directionality of nucleic acid strands is essential for understanding the mechanisms of replication and transcription.

"It has not escaped our notice that the specific pairing we have postulated immediately suggests a possible copying mechanism for the genetic material."

J.D. Watson and F.H.C. Crick, *Nature*, April 25, 1953

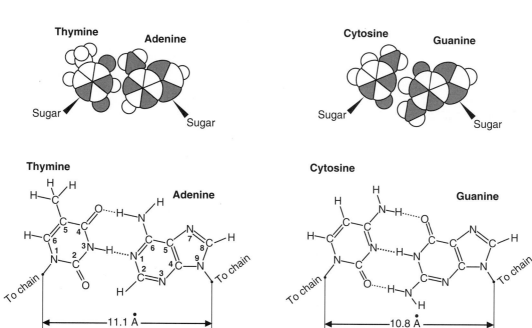

Fig. 11.9. Base pairs of DNA. Note that the pyrimidine bases are "flipped over" from the positions in which they are usually shown (see Fig. 11.5). The bases must be in this orientation to form base pairs.

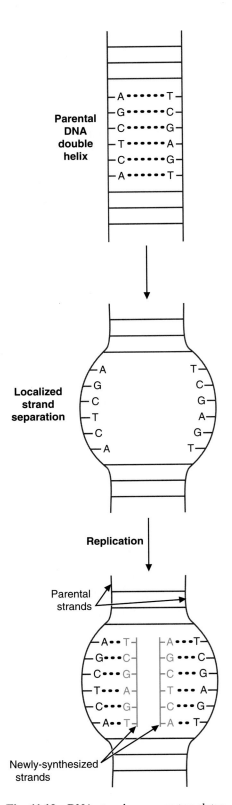

The Double Helix

Because each base pair contains a purine bonded to a pyrimidine, the distance across the base pairs, that is, the distance between the two phosphodiester backbones, is about 11 Å. If two strands that are equidistant from each other are twisted at the top and the bottom, they form a double helix (Fig. 11.12).

In the double helix of DNA, the base pairs that join the two strands are stacked like a spiral staircase along the central axis of the molecule. The electrons of the adjacent base pairs interact, generating stacking forces that, in addition to the hydrogen bonding of the base pairs, help to stabilize the helix.

The phosphate groups of the sugar-phosphate backbones are on the outside of the helix. Two of the acidic groups of each phosphate are involved in forming ester bonds with adjacent sugars. The third acidic group is free and dissociates a proton at physiological pH. Therefore, each DNA helix has negative charges coating its surface.

The helix contains grooves of alternating size, known as the major and minor grooves (Fig. 11.13). The bases in these grooves are exposed and, therefore, can interact with proteins or other molecules.

Watson and Crick described the B form of DNA, a right-handed helix, containing 3.4 Å between base pairs and 10 base pairs per turn. Although this form predominates in aqueous solution, other forms may also occur (Fig. 11.14). The A form, which predominates in DNA-RNA hybrids, is similar to the B form, but is more compact. In the Z form, the bases of the two DNA strands are positioned toward the periphery of a left-handed helix. This form of the helix was designated "Z" because, in each strand, a line connecting the phosphates "zigs" and "zags."

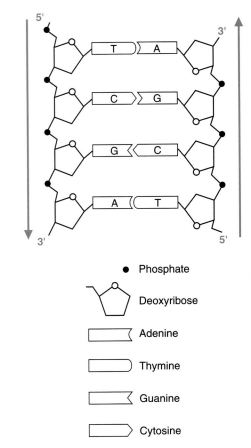

Fig. 11.11. Antiparallel strands of DNA.

Fig. 11.10. DNA strands serve as templates. During replication, the strands of the helix separate in a localized region. Each parental strand serves as a template for the synthesis of a new DNA strand.

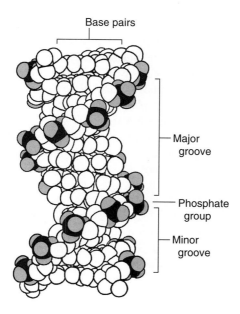

Fig. 11.13. DNA double helix.

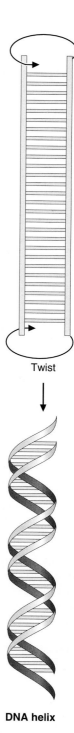

DNA helix

Fig. 11.12. Two DNA strands twisted to form a double helix.

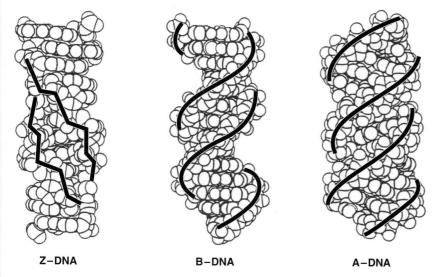

Z–DNA   **B–DNA**   **A–DNA**

Fig. 11.14. Z, B, and A forms of DNA. The solid black lines connect one phosphate group to the next. Modified from Saenger W. Principles of nucleic acid structure. New York: Springer Verlag, 1984:257–286.

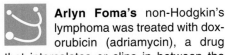

Arlyn Foma's non-Hodgkin's lymphoma was treated with doxorubicin (adriamycin), a drug that intercalates or slips in between the stacked base pairs of DNA.

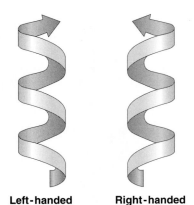

Doxorubicin

Left-handed   **Right-handed**

If you look up through the bottom of a helix along the central axis and the helix spirals away from you in a clockwise direction (toward the arrowhead in the drawing), it is a right-handed helix. If it spirals away from you in a counterclockwise direction, it is a left-handed helix.

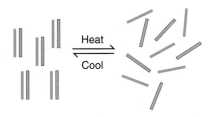

Fig. 11.17. Denaturation and renaturation of DNA strands. If a solution of DNA is heated, the strands separate (or denature). If the solution is slowly cooled, the strands reanneal (or renature).

Characteristics of DNA

Under certain laboratory conditions, the two strands of the DNA helix separate or denature. Many techniques employed to study DNA or to produce recombinant DNA molecules make use of this property.

Alkali causes the two strands of DNA to separate, but in contrast to its effect on RNA, alkali does not break the phosphodiester bonds of DNA (Fig. 11.15). Treatment with alkali is used to remove RNA from DNA and to separate DNA strands prior to or after electrophoresis on polyacrylamide or agarose gels.

Heat also can be used to convert double-stranded DNA to single-stranded DNA (Fig. 11.16). If the temperature is slowly decreased, complementary single strands can realign and base-pair, re-forming a double helix essentially identical to the original DNA (Fig. 11.17). This process is known as renaturation or reannealing.

Hybridization is the term used to refer to the process by which single-stranded DNA aligns and base-pairs with sequences on complementary strands of RNA (Fig. 11.18). Hybridization is used extensively in research and clinical testing. The term is also sometimes used to connote the reannealing of two complementary strands of DNA.

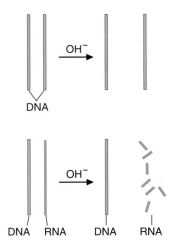

Fig. 11.15. Effect of alkali on DNA and RNA. DNA strands stay intact, but they separate. RNA strands are degraded to nucleotides.

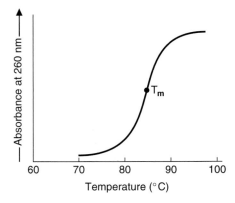

Fig. 11.16. A melting curve for DNA. As the temperature rises, the two strands of DNA separate which causes the absorbance at 260 nm to increase. The separation of strands ("melting") occurs over a very small temperature range. T_m is the midpoint of the melting curve.

STRUCTURE OF CHROMOSOMES

Size of DNA Molecules

A prokaryotic cell generally contains a single chromosome composed of double-stranded DNA that forms a circle (Fig. 11.19). These circular DNA molecules are extremely large. The entire chromosome of the bacterium *Escherichia coli*, composed of a single, circular double-stranded DNA molecule, contains over 4×10^6 base pairs. Its molecular weight is over $2{,}500 \times 10^6$. If this molecule were linear, its length would measure almost 2 mm.

The size of these DNA molecules can best be appreciated if they are compared with other molecules. Compared to glucose, which has a molecular weight of 180, DNA molecules are obviously enormous.

DNA from eukaryotic cells is even larger than that from bacterial cells (Fig. 11.20). The DNA of the longest human chromosome is over 7 cm in length. In fact, the DNA from all 46 chromosomes in a diploid human cell, placed end to end, would stretch for a distance of about 2 m (over 6 feet). This DNA contains 6×10^9 base pairs.

Packing of DNA in Cells

Because DNA molecules are so large, they require special packaging to enable them to reside within cells. In *E. coli*, the circular DNA is supercoiled and attached to an RNA-protein core.

Eukaryotes contain over 1,000 times the amount of DNA found in prokaryotes. Consequently, their method of packaging DNA is much more complex. Eukaryotic DNA interacts with an equal weight of small, basic proteins known as histones, which contain a large amount of arginine and lysine. There are five classes of histones: H1, H2A, H2B, H3, and H4.

When chromatin, the complex of DNA and proteins found in the nucleus, is extracted from cells, it has the appearance of beads on a string (Fig. 11.21). The beads with DNA protruding from each end are known as nucleosomes, and the beads themselves are known as nucleosome cores (Fig. 11.22). Two molecules of each of four histone classes (histones H2A, H2B, H3, and H4) form a core around which approximately 140 base pairs of double-stranded DNA are wound. The DNA wrapped around the nucleosome cores is continuous and joins one nucleosome core to the next. The DNA joining the cores is complexed with the fifth type of histone, H1.

 Heating and cooling cycles are used to separate and reanneal DNA strands in the polymerase chain reaction (PCR), a technique for obtaining large quantities of DNA from very small samples for research or for clinical or forensic testing.

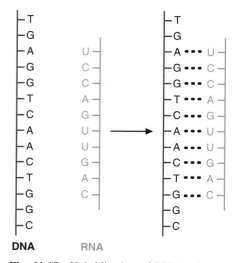

Fig. 11.18. Hybridization of DNA and complementary RNA.

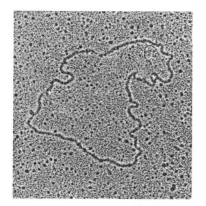

Fig. 11.19. *E. coli* DNA. The circular chromosome is 1.7 mm in length and contains about 4 $\times 10^6$ base pairs.

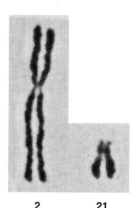

Fig. 11.20. Human chromosomes.

Q 11.1: If histones contain large amounts of arginine and lysine, will their net charge be positive or negative?

Michael Sichel has two alleles for the β-globin gene that each produce the mutated form of hemoglobin, HbS. His younger sister Amanda, a carrier for sickle cell trait, has one normal allele (that produces HbA) and one that produces HbS.

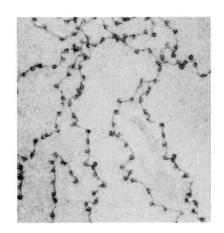

Fig. 11.21. Chromatin showing "beads on a string" structure.

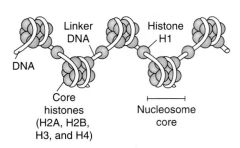

Fig. 11.22. A polynucleosome. Modified from Olins DE, Olins AL. Am Sci 1978;66:704.

Further compaction of chromatin occurs as the strings of nucleosomes wind into helical, tubular coils (often called solenoid structures) (Fig. 11.23).

Although complexes of DNA and histones form the nucleosomal substructures of chromatin, other types of proteins are also associated with DNA in the nucleus. These proteins were given the unimaginative name of "non-histone chromosomal proteins." The cells of different tissues contain different amounts and types of these proteins, which include enzymes that act on DNA and factors that regulate transcription.

The Human Genome

The genome, or total genetic content, of a human haploid cell (a sperm or an egg) is distributed in 23 chromosomes. The human genome contains 3 billion (3×10^9) base pairs. In diploid cells, each of the 22 autosomal chromosomes has a homologue. Homologous chromosomes contain a similar series of genes, i.e., they have similar DNA sequences. They are not necessarily identical, however, because one homologue comes from the haploid sperm of the father and one from the haploid egg of the mother when they unite to produce the diploid zygote. In addition, to the autosomal chromosomes, each diploid cell has two sex chromosomes, designated X and Y. A female has two X chromosomes, and a male has one X and one Y chromosome. The total number of chromosomes per diploid cell is 46 (Fig. 11.24).

Each gene on a chromosome in a diploid cell is matched by a corresponding allele on the homologous chromosome (Fig. 11.25). The alleles may be identical in base sequence or they may differ to some extent (one is derived from the mother and one from the father). If the alleles differ, the amino acid sequence of the proteins they produce may also differ.

The genomes of prokaryotic and eukaryotic cells differ in size. The genome of the bacterium *E. coli* contains about 3,000 genes. All of this DNA has a function. It either codes for proteins, rRNA, and tRNA or it serves to regulate the synthesis of these

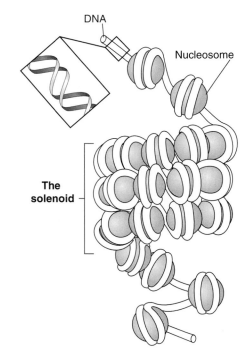

Fig. 11.23. Solenoid structure of chromatin.

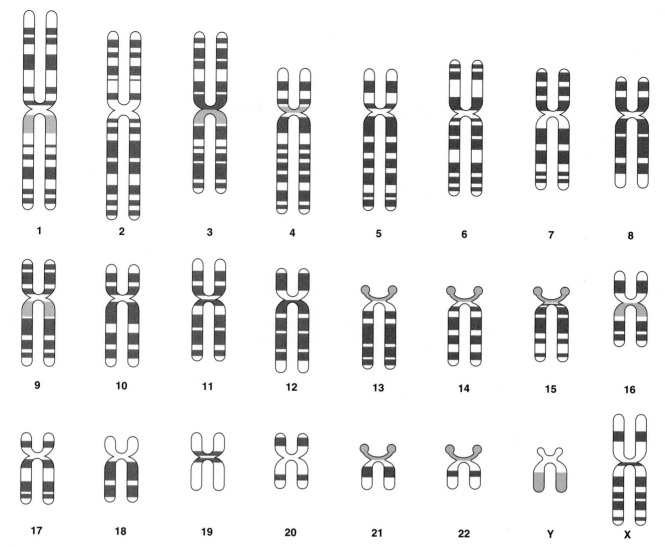

Fig. 11.24. Human chromosomes. Drawings of stained chromosomes are shown. Each haploid cell contains chromosomes 1 through 22 plus either an X or a Y. Each diploid cell contains two copies (homologues) of each of the numbered chromosomes plus two X chromosomes (female) or one X and one Y (male). From de Grouchy J, Turleau C. Clinical atlas of human chromosomes. New York: John Wiley & Sons, 1977:287.

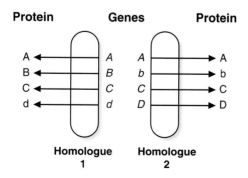

Fig. 11.25. Homologous chromosomes and their protein products. A set of homologous chromosomes is shown diagrammatically. (Of course, during interphase when they are producing their protein products, they cannot be visualized as discrete entities.) Four genes are shown as examples on each homologue. The genes of the homologues are alleles (e.g., *AA, Bb, CC, dD*). They may be identical (e.g., *AA, CC*), or they may differ (e.g., *Bb, dD*) in DNA sequence. Thus the corresponding protein products may be identical or they may differ in amino acid sequence.

A 11.1: At physiological pH, arginine and lysine carry positive charges on their side chains; therefore, histones have a net positive charge. The arginine and lysine residues are clustered in regions of the histone molecules. These positively charged regions of the histones can interact with the negatively charged DNA phosphate groups.

Haploid cells are used to compare the size of genomes. Haploid cells contain only one copy of each chromosome. Diploid cells contain two copies of each chromosome. Diploid cells, therefore, have two copies of each gene (two alleles)—one on each of the homologous chromosomes. These alleles may be identical or their DNA sequences may differ to some extent.

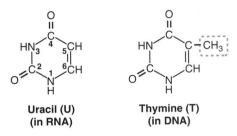

Uracil (U) (in RNA)   **Thymine (T) (in DNA)**

Fig. 11.26. Comparison of the structures of uracil and thymine.

Ribose (in RNA)

Deoxyribose (in DNA)

Fig. 11.27. Comparison of the structures of ribose and deoxyribose.

gene products. Human DNA, in contrast, contains between 50,000 and 100,000 genes, 10–30 times the number in *E. coli*. However, the genome of the human haploid cell is about 1,000 times larger than that of *E. coli*. The function of most of this extra DNA has not been determined, an issue that will be considered in more detail in Chapter 15.

RNA STRUCTURE

General Features of RNA Structure

RNA is similar to DNA in that it is composed of nucleotides joined by 3′ to 5′-phosphodiester bonds. RNA contains the purine bases adenine and guanine and the pyrimidine base cytosine. However, its other pyrimidine base is uracil rather than thymine. Thymine contains a methyl group at position 5; uracil does not. Otherwise, these bases are identical (Fig. 11.26).

In RNA, the sugar is ribose, which contains a hydroxyl group on the 2′-carbon (Fig. 11.27). The presence of this hydroxyl group allows RNA to be cleaved to its constituent nucleotides in alkaline solutions.

RNA chains are usually single-stranded and lack the continuously repeated structure of the double-stranded DNA helix. However, RNA still has considerable secondary and tertiary structure because base pairs can form in regions where the strand loops back on itself. As in DNA, pairing between the bases is complementary and antiparallel. But in RNA, adenine pairs with uracil rather than thymine (Fig. 11.28). Base-pairing in RNA may be extensive, and the irregular, looped structures that are generated are important for the binding of molecules, such as enzymes, that interact with specific regions of the RNA.

The three major types of RNA (mRNA, rRNA, and tRNA) participate in the process of protein synthesis. Other less abundant RNAs are involved in replication or in the processing of RNA, that is, in the conversion of RNA precursors to their mature forms.

Some RNA molecules are capable of catalyzing reactions. Thus, RNA, as well as protein, can have enzymatic activity. Certain rRNA precursors can remove internal segments of themselves, splicing the remaining fragments together. Because this RNA is changed by the reaction that it catalyzes, it is not truly an enzyme and, therefore, has been termed a "ribozyme." Other RNAs act as true catalysts, serving as ribonucleases, which cleave other RNA molecules, and as peptidyl transferase, the enzyme in protein synthesis that catalyzes the formation of peptide bonds.

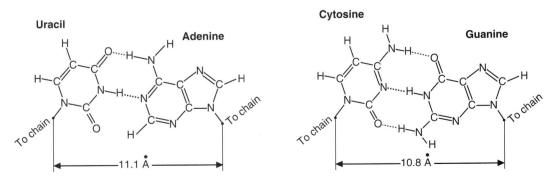

Fig. 11.28. Base pairing in RNA.

Structure of mRNA

In eukaryotes, messenger RNA (mRNA) is transcribed as a long primary transcript from regions of DNA that code for proteins. The primary transcript is processed to form mRNA in the nucleus. mRNA travels through nuclear pores to the cytoplasm, where it directs the sequential insertion of the appropriate amino acids into a polypeptide chain.

Eukaryotic mRNA contains a structure known as a cap at its 5'-end. The cap consists of a methylated guanosine triphosphate attached to the 5'-hydroxyl group of the ribose at the 5'-end of the mRNA (Fig. 11.29). The 2'-hydroxyl groups of the ribose moieties of the first and second nucleotides of the mRNA may also be methylated.

A poly(A) tail is attached to the 3'-end of eukaryotic mRNA (Fig. 11.30). This tail consists of a series of adenosine nucleotides joined by 3'- to 5'-phosphodiester bonds. As many as 200 adenine residues may be present in a poly(A) tail.

Structure of rRNA

Ribosomes are subcellular structures on which protein synthesis occurs. Different types of ribosomes are found in prokaryotes and in the cytoplasm and mitochondria of eukaryotic cells (Fig. 11.31). Prokaryotic ribosomes contain three types of rRNA molecules with sedimentation coefficients of 16, 23, and 5S. 16S rRNA complexes with proteins and forms the 30S ribosomal subunit, while 23S and 5S rRNAs complex with proteins and form the 50S ribosomal subunit. The 30S and 50S ribosomal subunits join to form the 70S ribosome (Fig. 11.32).

Cytoplasmic ribosomes in eukaryotes contain four types of rRNA molecules of 18, 28, 5, and 5.8S. 18S rRNA is complexed with proteins to form the 40S ribosomal subunit, and the 28, 5, and 5.8S rRNAs are complexed with proteins to form the 60S ribosomal subunit. The 40 and 60S ribosomal subunits combine to form the 80S ribosomes found in the cytoplasm of eukaryotes.

Mitochondrial ribosomes, with a sedimentation coefficient of 55S, are smaller than cytoplasmic ribosomes. Their properties are similar to those of the 70S ribosomes of bacteria.

 A sedimentation coefficient is a measure of the rate of sedimentation of a macromolecule in a high speed centrifuge (an ultracentrifuge). It is expressed in Svedberg units (S). Larger macromolecules have higher sedimentation coefficients than do smaller macromolecules.

Sedimentation coefficients are not additive. Because frictional forces acting on the surface of a macromolecule slow its migration through the solvent, the rate of sedimentation depends not only on the density of the macromolecule, but also on its shape.

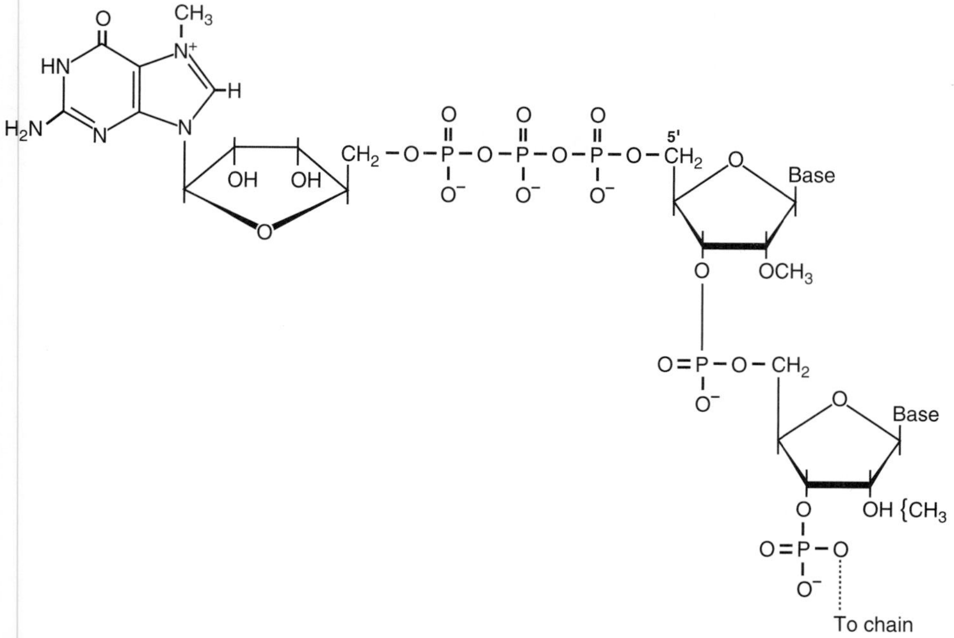

Fig. 11.29. The cap structure in eukaryotic mRNA.

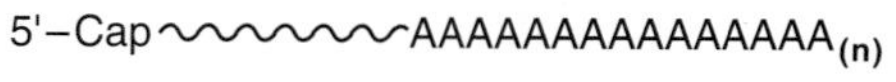

5'–Cap〰〰〰〰AAAAAAAAAAAAAAAA$_{(n)}$

Fig. 11.30. The poly(A) tail of eukaryotic mRNA.

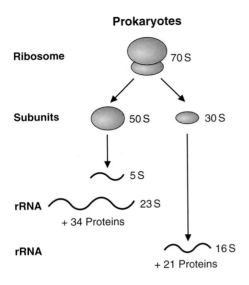

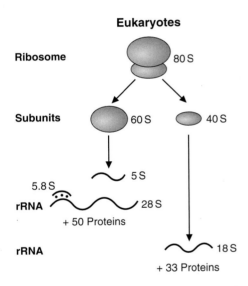

Fig. 11.31. Comparison of prokaryotic and eukaryotic ribosomes. The cytoplasmic ribosomes of eukaryotes are shown. Mitochondrial ribosomes are similar to prokaryotic ribosomes, but they are smaller (55S rather than 70S).

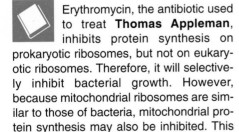

Erythromycin, the antibiotic used to treat **Thomas Appleman**, inhibits protein synthesis on prokaryotic ribosomes, but not on eukaryotic ribosomes. Therefore, it will selectively inhibit bacterial growth. However, because mitochondrial ribosomes are similar to those of bacteria, mitochondrial protein synthesis may also be inhibited. This fact is important in understanding some of the side effects of antibiotics that work by inhibiting bacterial protein synthesis.

Fig. 11.32. Details of prokaryotic ribosome structure.

rRNAs contain many loops and exhibit extensive base-pairing. The sequences of the rRNAs of the smaller ribosomal subunits have been compared for a number of different organisms. The secondary structures that they can form are similar in many different genera (Fig. 11.33).

Structure of tRNA

During protein synthesis, tRNA molecules carry amino acids to ribosomes and ensure that they are incorporated into the appropriate positions in the growing polypeptide chain. Therefore, cells contain at least 20 different tRNA molecules, one for each of the amino acids that is used in the synthesis of proteins. Many amino acids have more than one tRNA.

tRNA molecules contain not only the usual nucleotides, but also derivatives of these nucleotides that are produced by posttranscriptional modifications. In eukaryotic cells, 10–20% of the nucleotides of tRNA may be modified. Most tRNA molecules contain dihydrouridine (D), in which one of the double bonds of the base is reduced; ribothymidine (T), in which a methyl group is added to uracil to form thymine; and pseudouridine (ψ), in which uracil is attached to ribose by a carbon-carbon bond rather than a nitrogen-carbon bond (Fig. 11.34). The base at the 5′-end of the anticodon of tRNA, which base-pairs with the base at the 3′-end of the codon on mRNA, is frequently modified.

tRNA molecules are rather small compared to both mRNA and the large rRNA molecules. On average, tRNA molecules contain about 80 nucleotides and have a sedimentation coefficient of 4S. Because of their small size and high content of modified nucleotides, tRNAs were the first nucleic acids to be sequenced. Since 1965 when Robert Holley deduced the structure of the first tRNA, the nucleotide sequence of many different tRNAs has been determined. Although their primary sequences differ, all tRNA molecules can form a structure that resembles a cloverleaf (Fig. 11.35). The loop closest to the 5′-end is known as the D-loop because it contains dihydrouridine (D). The second, or anticodon, loop contains the anticodon that base-pairs with the codon on mRNA, and the third loop (the TψC loop) contains both ribothymidine (T) and pseudouridine (ψ). A fourth loop, known as the variable loop because it varies in size, is frequently found between the anticodon and TψC loops. Base-pairing occurs in the stem regions, and a CCA sequence at the 3′-end is the attachment site for the amino acid that is carried by the tRNA. The three-dimensional structure of tRNA has been determined and is shown in Figure 11.35.

Other Types of RNA

In addition to the three major types of RNA described above, other RNAs are present in cells. These RNAs include the oligonucleotides that serve as primers for DNA replication and the RNAs in the small nuclear ribonucleoproteins (snRNPs or snurps) that are involved in the splicing and modification reactions that occur during the maturation of RNA precursors (see Chapter 13).

RNA also serves as the genome for certain types of viruses, known as retroviruses, including the human immunodeficiency virus (HIV) that causes AIDS.

 CLINICAL COMMENTS. **Colin Tuma's** original benign adenomatous polyp was located in the ascending colon, where 10% of large bowel cancers eventually arise. Because his father died from a cancer of the colon, his physician had warned him that his risk for developing colon cancer was three times higher than for the general population. Unfortunately, Mr. Tuma neglected to have his annual colonoscopic examinations as prescribed.

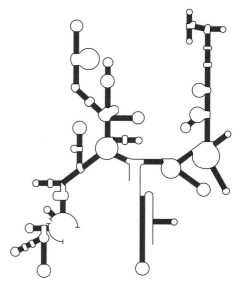

Fig. 11.33. Common features of the secondary structure of the 16S-type ribosomal RNA. Darkened areas are base-paired. Circles are unpaired loops. Reproduced with permission, from Annu Rev Biochem. 1984;53:137. © 1984, by Annual Reviews, Inc.

Ribothymidine (T)

Dihydrouridine (D)

Pseudouridine (ψ)

Fig. 11.34. Three modified nucleosides found in most tRNAs.

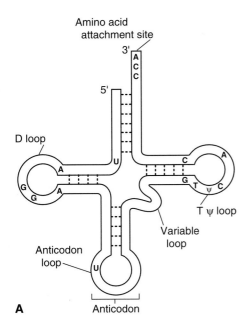

Amino acid
attachment site

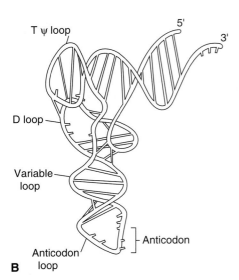

Fig. 11.35. Structure of tRNA. **A.** The tRNA cloverleaf. Bases that commonly occur in a particular position are indicated by letters. Base-pairing in stem regions is indicated by lines between the strands. **B.** The three-dimensional folding of tRNA. **B** reprinted with permission from Kim SH, et al. Science 1974;185:436. Copyright 1974 American Association for the Advancement of Science.

Ivy Sharer's clinical course was typical for the development of full-blown AIDS, in this case caused by the use of needles contaminated with HIV. The progressive immunological deterioration that accompanies this disease ultimately results in life-threatening opportunistic infections with fungi (e.g., *Candida*, cryptococcus), other viruses (e.g., cytomegalovirus, herpes simplex), and bacteria (e.g., *Mycobacterium*, *Pneumocystis carinii*, *Salmonella*). Certain neoplasms also frequently develop in this disorder of immunological incompetence (e.g., Kaposi's sarcoma, non-Hodgkin's lymphoma) as do meningitis, neuropathies, and neuropsychiatric disorders causing cognitive dysfunction. An intensive worldwide search is in progress to find a cure for this dread disease.

Arlyn Foma's non-Hodgkin's lymphoma appears to be progressing slowly and, therefore, is classified as a "low grade" malignancy of the immune system. Yet 75–90% of patients with "low grade" disease have involvement of more than one lymph node region, as is true for Mr. Foma. Such patients are ineligible for localized radiation therapy and may require single or multiagent chemotherapy combined with whole-body irradiation. Although disappearance of all discernible tumor may occur in up to 80% of such cases, remissions are usually limited to 1–5 years. The recent addition of interferon-α to the regimen promises to improve the prognosis.

Michael Sichel has had repeated hospital admissions related to the symptoms of small vessel vasoocclusive sickle cell crises. Fortunately, none of these vascular events has resulted in large vessel catastrophes such as a cerebrovascular accident (stroke), pulmonary artery occlusion (chest pain and shortness of breath), or hepatic crisis (marked upper abdominal pain associated with hyperbilirubinemia and abnormal liver function tests). Until a cure can be found for this relentless disease, Michael is a ticking time-bomb, waiting for some vascular "explosion" to occur.

Thomas Appleman's infection was treated with erythromycin, a macrolide antibiotic. Because this agent may inhibit mitochondrial protein synthesis in eukaryotic cells, it has the potential to alter host cell function leading to such side effects as epigastric distress, diarrhea, and, infrequently, cholestatic jaundice.

BIOCHEMICAL COMMENTS. Viruses must invade host cells in order to reproduce. They are not capable of reproducing independently. Some viruses that are pathogenic to humans contain DNA as their genetic material (Fig. 11.36A). Others contain RNA as their genetic material (Fig. 11.36B).

Some viruses that contain an RNA genome are known as retroviruses. HIV, the human immunodeficiency virus, is the retrovirus that causes AIDS. It invades cells of the immune system and prevents the affected individual from mounting an adequate immune response to combat infections.

According to the "central dogma" proposed by Francis Crick, information flows from DNA to RNA to proteins. For the most part, this concept holds true. However, retroviruses provided one violation of this rule. When retroviruses invade cells, their RNA genome is transcribed to produce a DNA copy. The enzyme that catalyzes this process is known as reverse transcriptase. This DNA copy integrates into the genome of the infected cell and is used to produce many copies of the viral RNA, as well as viral proteins, which can be packaged into new viral particles.

Suggested Readings

Watson JD. The double helix. New York: Atheneum, 1968.

Watson JD, Crick FHC. Molecular structure of nucleic acids. A structure for deoxyribose nucleic acid. Nature 1953;171:737–738.

PROBLEMS

1. For the following DNA sequence, determine the sequence and direction of the complementary strand.

5′ - A C C A A A G A T G C C T G C G G A A T C C - 3′

2. If the following DNA strand serves as a template for the synthesis of RNA, determine the sequence and direction of the RNA.

Template 3′ - T G G T T T C T A C G G A C G C C T T A G G -5′

ANSWERS

1. DNA Sequence

5′ - A C C A A A G A T G C C T G C G G A A T C C - 3′

Complementary Strand

3′ - T G G T T T C T A C G G A C G C C T T A G G - 5′

2. DNA Template

3′ - T G G T T T C T A C G G A C G C C T T A G G - 5′

RNA

5′ - A C C A A A G A U G C C U G C G G A A U C C - 3′

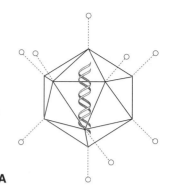

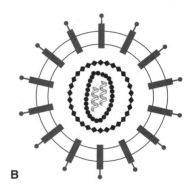

Fig. 11.36. Viruses that infect humans. **A.** A DNA virus that infects humans. The adenovirus contains 35–40 kb. **B.** The RNA virus that causes AIDS. HIV contains 7–10 kb.

12 Synthesis of DNA

DNA synthesis occurs by the process of replication. During replication, each of the two parental strands of DNA serves as a template for the synthesis of a complementary strand. Thus each DNA molecule generated by the replication process contains one intact parental strand and one newly synthesized strand (Fig. 12.1). In eukaryotes, DNA replication occurs during the S phase of the cell cycle. Then the cell divides during the M phase, and each daughter cell receives an exact copy of the DNA of the parent cell.

In both prokaryotes and eukaryotes, the site where replication is occurring at any given moment is called the replication fork. As replication proceeds, the two parental strands separate in front of the fork. Behind the fork, each newly synthesized strand of DNA base-pairs with its complementary parental template strand. Thus, the replication fork is Y-shaped.

A complex of proteins is involved in replication. Helicases and topoisomerases unwind the parental strands, and single-strand binding proteins prevent them from reannealing.

The major enzyme involved in the replication of DNA is a DNA polymerase that copies the parental template strands in the 3′ to 5′ direction, producing new strands in a 5′ to 3′ direction. Deoxyribonucleoside triphosphates serve as the precursors. One strand of newly synthesized DNA grows continuously, while the other strand is synthesized discontinuously in short segments known as Okazaki fragments. These fragments are subsequently joined by DNA ligase.

DNA polymerase cannot initiate the synthesis of new strands. Therefore, a short oligonucleotide composed of RNA is produced which serves as a primer. This RNA is subsequently removed and replaced by deoxyribonucleotides.

Errors that occur during replication could lead to deleterious mutations. However, many of them are corrected by enzymes associated with the complex at the replication fork. The error rate during replication is thus kept at a very low level.

Damage to DNA molecules can also cause mutations. Repair mechanisms correct DNA damage, usually by removing and replacing the damaged region. The intact, undamaged strand serves as a template for the DNA polymerase involved in the repair process.

Although cells have mechanisms to correct replication errors and to repair DNA damage, some genetic change is desirable. It produces new proteins or variations of proteins that may increase the survival rate of the species. Genetic change is produced by unrepaired mutations, and by a mechanism known as recombination in which portions of chromosomes are exchanged.

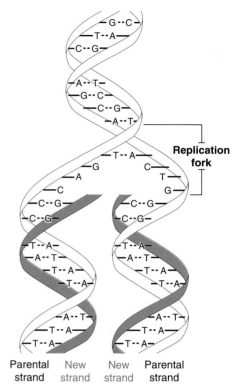

Fig. 12.1. A replicating DNA helix. The parental strands separate at the replication fork. Each parental strand serves as a template for the synthesis of a new strand.

Colin Tuma completed his first course of intravenous 5-fluorouracil (5-FU) in the hospital. He tolerated the therapy with only mild anorexia and diarrhea and a slight fall in his white blood cell count. Thirty days after the completion of the initial course, these symptoms have abated and he is about to start his second course of chemotherapy with 5-FU as an outpatient.

Ivy Sharer has tolerated azidothymidine (AZT) therapy reasonably well but her night sweats persist. She has heard that ddI and ddC are being used to treat acquired immunodeficiency syndrome (AIDS) and asks if she should try these agents.

Di Beatty responded to treatment for her diabetic ketoacidosis but subsequently developed a low grade fever, urinary urgency, frequency, and burning at the urethral opening with urination (dysuria). A urinalysis showed a large number of white blood cells and many Gram-negative bacilli. A urine culture revealed many colonies of *Escherichia coli*, which is sensitive to several antibiotics including the quinolone norfloxacin.

William Hartman saw his physician for regular examinations after his heart attack. On the third visit, while examining Mr. Hartman's lungs, his physician noted a superficial brownish-black 5-mm nodule with irregular borders in the skin overlying his right shoulder. He was scheduled for outpatient surgery at which time a wide excision biopsy was performed. Examination of the nodule revealed histological changes characteristic of a malignant melanoma reaching a thickness of only 0.7 mm from the skin surface (Stage I).

Nick O'Tyne is a 62-year-old electrician who has smoked two packs of cigarettes a day for 40 years. He recently noted that his chronic cough had gotten worse. His physician ordered a chest radiograph which showed a 2-cm nodule in the upper lobe of the right lung. Cytological study of the sputum by Papanicolaou technique revealed cells consistent with the presence of a well-differentiated adenocarcinoma of the lung.

DNA SYNTHESIS IN PROKARYOTES

Many of the basic features of the mechanism of DNA replication are best illustrated by the processes that occur in the bacterium *E. coli*, the bacillus that grows symbiotically in the human colon. This organism has been very extensively studied and serves as a model for the more complex and, consequently, less well-understood processes that occur in eukaryotic cells.

Replication Is Bidirectional

Replication of the circular, double-stranded DNA of the chromosome of *E. coli* begins with the binding of proteins (DnaA) at a single point of origin, designated *oriC* (Fig. 12.2). The two parental strands separate within this region, and both strands are copied simultaneously. Synthesis begins at the origin and occurs at two replication forks that move away from the origin bidirectionally (in both directions at the same time). Replication ends on the other side of the chromosome at a termination point. One round of synthesis, involving the incorporation of over 4 million nucleotides in each new strand of DNA, is completed in about 40 minutes.

Replication Is Semiconservative

Each daughter chromosome contains one of the parental DNA strands and one newly synthesized, complementary strand. Therefore, replication is said to be semiconservative, i.e., the parental strands are conserved but are no longer together. Each one is paired with a newly synthesized strand (see Figs. 12.1 and 12.2).

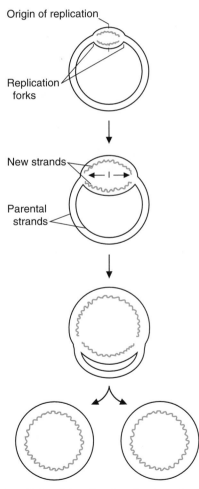

Fig. 12.2. Bidirectional replication of a circular chromosome. Replication begins at the point of origin and proceeds in both directions at the same time.

Origin of replication

Replication forks

New strands

Parental strands

Unwinding of Parental Strands

Replication requires separation of the parental DNA strands ahead of the replication fork. Helicases unwind the parental DNA, and single-strand binding proteins prevent the strands from reassociating and protect them from enzymes that cleave single-stranded DNA (Fig. 12.3). Topoisomerases, enzymes that can break and rejoin DNA strands, relieve the supercoiling produced by unwinding of the parental duplex. A major topoisomerase in bacterial cells is DNA gyrase.

Action of DNA Polymerase

Enzymes that catalyze the synthesis of DNA are known as DNA polymerases. *E. coli* has three DNA polymerases, Pol I, Pol II, and Pol III. Pol III is the replicative enzyme. All DNA polymerases that have been studied copy a DNA template strand in its 3′ to 5′ direction, producing a new strand in the 5′ to 3′ direction (Fig. 12.4). Deoxyribonucleoside triphosphates serve as precursors, molecules that act as substrates, for the addition of nucleotides to the growing chain.

The incoming nucleotide forms a base pair with the complementary nucleotide on the template strand, an ester bond is formed with the free 3′-hydroxyl group at the end of the growing chain, and pyrophosphate is released. The release of pyrophosphate and its subsequent cleavage by a pyrophosphatase provide the energy that drives the polymerization process.

DNA polymerases that catalyze the synthesis of new strands during replication exhibit processivity, that is, they remain bound to the parental template strand rather than dissociating and reassociating as each nucleotide is added to the growing chain. Consequently, synthesis is much more rapid than it would be with an enzyme that was not processive.

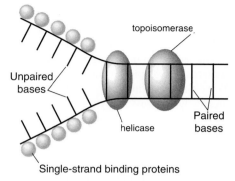

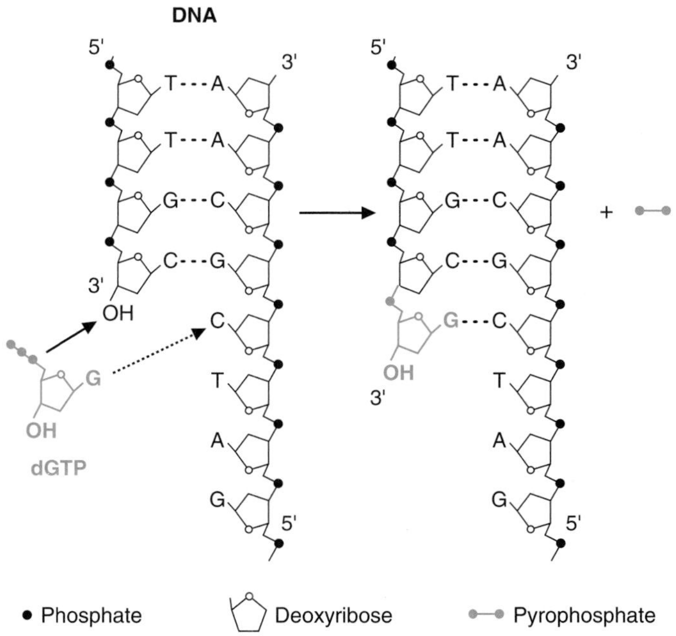

Fig. 12.3. Proteins involved in unwinding parental DNA strands at the replication fork in prokaryotes.

Fig. 12.4. Action of DNA polymerase. Deoxyribonucleoside triphosphates serve as precursors (substrates) used by DNA polymerase to lengthen the DNA chain. DNA polymerase copies the DNA template strand in the 3′ to 5′ direction. The new strand grows 5′ to 3′.

• Phosphate   ⬠ Deoxyribose   •—• Pyrophosphate

Di Beatty's urinary tract infection was treated with norfloxacin.

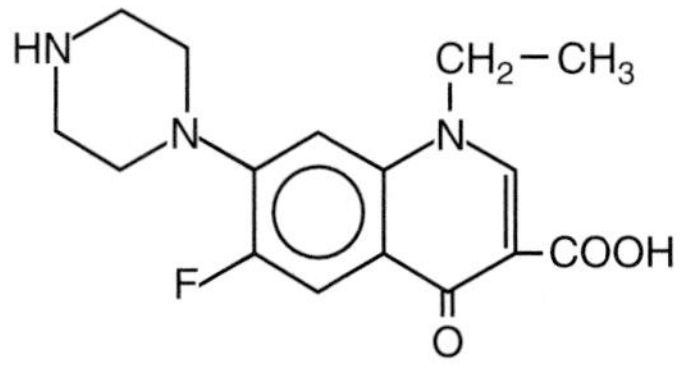

Norfloxacin

Norfloxacin is a fluorinated member of the quinolone family. This group of drugs inhibits bacterial DNA gyrase, an enzyme that unwinds DNA ahead of the replication fork, and thus inhibits bacterial DNA synthesis. Because eukaryotic cells do not contain DNA gyrase, they are not affected by quinolones at the normally prescribed dosage.

Colin Tuma is being treated with 5-fluorouracil (5-FU), a pyrimidine base that is structurally similar to uracil and thymine. DNA requires the base thymine for replication. Thymine is produced by a reaction catalyzed by thymidylate synthetase in which deoxyuridine monophosphate (dUMP) is converted to deoxythymidine monophosphate (dTMP). 5-FU can be converted in the body to the nucleotide F-dUMP. When bound to the cofactor on the enzyme, F-dUMP produces a complex that resembles the transition state complex ("X" in the diagram below). The complex containing F-dUMP causes inhibition of the reaction catalyzed by thymidylate synthetase. As a result, thymidine triphosphate is not produced for DNA synthesis, and the rate of cell proliferation decreases.

$$5\text{-FU} \rightarrow \text{F-dUMP}$$
$$\downarrow$$
$$\text{dUMP} \rightarrow \text{X} \blacksquare\!\!\rightarrow \text{dTMP} \rightarrow \text{dTTP} \rightarrow \text{DNA}$$

Ivy Sharer is being treated with AZT (azidothymidine), also called zidovudine, a nucleoside that contains an azido group on the 3'-carbon of the ribose.

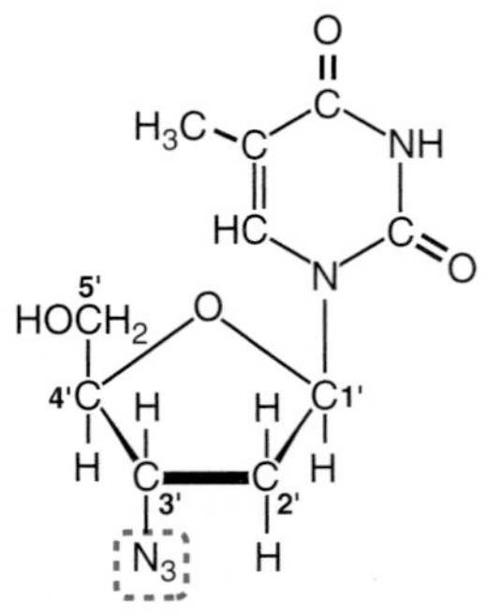

AZT

AZT can be phosphorylated in the body and added to the 3'-end of a growing DNA chain. However, further chain elongation cannot occur because polymerization of DNA chains requires a 3'-hydroxyl group.

Elimination of Base-Pairing Errors

In *E. coli*, the replicative enzyme Pol III also performs a proofreading or editing function. This enzyme has $3' \rightarrow 5'$-exonuclease activity in addition to its polymerase activity (Table 12.1). If the nucleotide at the end of the growing chain is incorrectly base-paired with the template strand, Pol III removes this nucleotide before continuing to lengthen the growing chain. This proofreading activity eliminates most base-pairing errors as they occur. Only about one base pair in a million is mismatched in the final DNA product; the error rate is about 10^{-6}. If this proofreading activity is experimentally removed from the enzyme, the error rate increases to about 10^{-3}.

After replication, other mechanisms can replace mismatched bases that escaped proofreading. These two processes of proofreading and postreplication mismatch repair result in an overall error rate of about 10^{-10}, that is, less than one mismatched base pair in 10 billion. Therefore, the fidelity of DNA replication is very high.

Function of RNA Primers

Because DNA polymerase cannot initiate synthesis of new strands, a primer is required. This primer is an RNA oligonucleotide. It is synthesized in a 5' to 3' direction by an RNA polymerase (primase) that copies the DNA template strand. DNA polymerase initially adds a deoxyribonucleotide to the 3'-hydroxyl group of the primer and then continues to add deoxyribonucleotides to the 3'-end of the growing strand.

DNA Synthesis at the Replication Fork

Both parental strands are copied at the same time in the direction of the replication fork, an observation difficult to reconcile with the known activity of DNA polymerase, which can produce chains only in a 5' to 3' direction. Because the parental strands run in opposite directions relative to each other, synthesis should occur in a 5' to 3' direction **toward** the fork on one template strand and in a 5' to 3' direction **away** from the fork on the other template strand.

Okazaki resolved this dilemma by showing that synthesis on one strand, called the leading strand, is continuous in the 5' to 3' direction toward the fork. The other strand, called the lagging strand, is synthesized discontinuously in short fragments (Fig. 12.5). These fragments, named for Okazaki, are produced in a 5' to 3' direction (away from the fork), but then joined together so that, overall, synthesis proceeds toward the replication fork. In *E. coli*, Okazaki fragments are between 1,000 and 2,000 nucleotides in length.

Function of DNA Ligase

As replication progresses, the RNA primers are removed from Okazaki fragments, probably by the combined action of DNA polymerase I (Pol I) and RNase H (see Fig.

Table 12.1. Functions of Bacterial DNA Polymerases

Polymerase	Functions[a]	Exonuclease Activity[b]
Pol I	Filling of gap after removal of RNA primer DNA repair Removal of RNA primer in conjunction with RNase H	5' to 3' and 3' to 5'
Pol II	DNA repair	3' to 5'
Pol III	Replication—synthesis of DNA	3' to 5'

[a]Synthesis of new DNA strands always occurs 5' to 3'.

[b]Exonucleases remove nucleotides from DNA strands and act at the 5'-end (cleaving 5' to 3') or at the 3'-end (cleaving 3' to 5').

12.5). Pol I fills in the gaps that are produced by removal of the primers. Because DNA polymerase cannot join two polynucleotide chains together, an additional enzyme, DNA ligase, is required to perform this function. The 3′-hydroxyl group at the end of a fragment is ligated to the phosphate group at the 5′-end of the next fragment (Fig. 12.6).

DNA SYNTHESIS IN EUKARYOTES

The process of replication in eukaryotes is similar to that in prokaryotes. Differences in the processes are related mainly to the vastly larger amount of DNA in eukaryotic cells (over 1,000 times the amount in *E. coli*) and the association of eukaryotic DNA with histones in nucleosomes. Enzymes with DNA polymerase, primase, ligase, helicase, and topoisomerase activity are all present in eukaryotes, although these enzymes differ in some respects from those of prokaryotes.

Eukaryotic Cell Cycle

The cell cycle of eukaryotic cells consists of four phases (Fig. 12.7). The first three phases constitute interphase. Cells spend most of their time in these three phases, carrying out their normal metabolic activities. The fourth phase is mitosis, the process of cell division. This phase is very brief.

The first phase of the cell cycle, G_1 (the first "gap" phase), is the most variable in length. Late in G_1, the cells prepare to duplicate their chromosomes (e.g., by producing nucleotide precursors). In the second or S phase, DNA replicates. Nucleosomes dissociate as the replication forks advance. Throughout S phase, the synthesis of histones and other proteins associated with DNA is markedly increased. The amount of DNA and histones both double, and chromosomes are duplicated. Histones complex with DNA, and nucleosomes are formed very rapidly behind the advancing replication forks.

During the third phase of the cell cycle, G_2 (the second "gap" phase), the cells prepare to divide, synthesizing tubulin for construction of the microtubules of the spindle apparatus. Finally, division occurs in the brief mitotic or M phase.

Following mitosis, cells may reenter G_1, repeatedly going through the phases of the cell cycle and dividing. Cells may also leave the cycle after mitosis, never to divide again, or they may enter an extended G_1 phase (sometimes called G_0), in which they may remain for long periods of time. Upon the appropriate signal, cells in G_0 may be stimulated to reenter the cycle and divide.

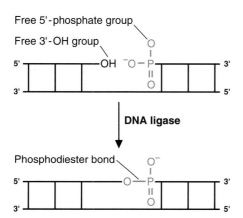

Fig. 12.6. Action of DNA ligase. Two polynucleotide chains, one with a free 3′-OH group and one with a free 5′-phosphate group, are joined by DNA ligase, which forms a phosphodiester bond.

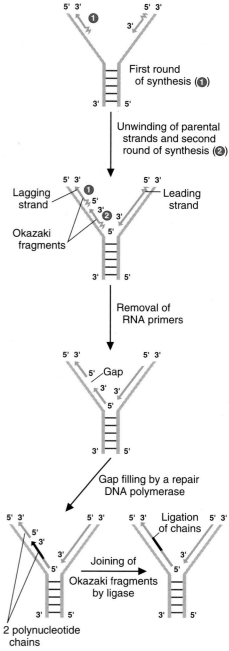

Fig. 12.5. Synthesis of DNA at the replication fork. (See Fig. 12.6 for the ligation reaction.)

 HeLa cells, derived from a human cervical carcinoma, are rapidly dividing cells that can be grown in culture flasks. Their cell cycle is about 20 hours in length. Only 1 hour of this time is spent in mitosis.

Cells within the body that divide less frequently, such as liver cells, may spend days, weeks, or months in interphase before going through a brief mitotic phase.

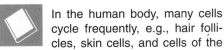

12.1: Although Prometheus was chained to a rock as punishment for his theft of fire from the gods, and a vulture pecked at his liver each day, he survived. Why?

In the human body, many cells cycle frequently, e.g., hair follicles, skin cells, and cells of the duodenal crypts. Other cells, such as the precursors of red blood cells, divide a number of times, then lose their nuclei and leave the cell cycle to form mature red blood cells. These cells transport oxygen and carbon dioxide between the lungs and other tissues for about 120 days, then they die. Other cells (e.g., hepatocytes) are normally quiescent (in G_0). However, they can be stimulated to divide. In many instances, the stimuli are growth factors or hormones. In the case of liver cells, the stimulus is produced by death of some of the cells.

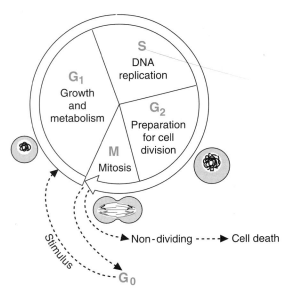

Fig. 12.7. Eukaryotic cell cycle.

Table 12.2. Functions of Eukaryotic DNA Polymerases

Polymerase	Functions[a]	Exonuclease Activity
α	Replication (with polymerase δ): synthesis of DNA DNA repair	None
β	DNA repair	None
γ	Replication in mitochondria	3′ to 5′
δ	Replication (with polymerase α): synthesis of DNA	3′ to 5′
ϵ	DNA repair	3′ to 5′

[a]DNA synthesis (in replication and repair) always occurs 5′ to 3′.

Points of Origin for Replication

In contrast to bacterial chromosomes, eukaryotic chromosomes have multiple points of origin at which replication begins. "Bubbles" appear at these points on the chromosomes, and bidirectional DNA synthesis proceeds from each point (Fig. 12.8). As the bubbles enlarge, they eventually merge, and replication is completed. Because eukaryotic chromosomes contain multiple points of origin of replication (and, thus, multiple replicons—units of replication), duplication of even the largest chromosomes can occur within a reasonable period of time. In the body, dividing cells complete the S phase of the cell cycle over a period of 10–14 hours.

Eukaryotic DNA Polymerases

At least five DNA polymerases exist in eukaryotic cells (α, β, γ, δ, and ϵ) (Table 12.2). DNA polymerases α and δ are the primary enzymes involved in replication. Polymerase δ produces the continuous, leading strand, while α produces the discontinuous, lagging strand (Fig. 12.9). Polymerase δ has an associated helicase.

Polymerase δ has high processivity. Polymerase α, on the other hand, has low processivity. It is released from DNA after the addition of only about 200 nucleotides, the length of Okazaki fragments in eukaryotes. In addition to low processivity, polymerase α has primase activity, required for the production of the RNA primers that initiate synthesis of Okazaki fragments.

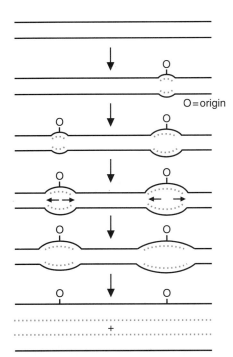

Fig. 12.8. Replication of a eukaryotic chromosome. Synthesis is bidirectional from each point of origin (O) and semiconservative, each daughter DNA helix contains one intact parental strand (solid line) and one newly synthesized strand (dashed line).

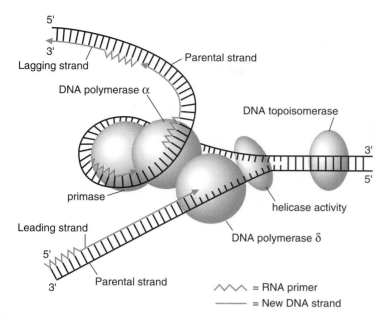

5'
3'
Lagging strand
Parental strand
DNA polymerase α
DNA topoisomerase
3'
5'
primase
helicase activity
Leading strand
DNA polymerase δ
5'
3'
Parental strand

∿∿∿ = RNA primer
——— = New DNA strand

Fig. 12.9. Replication complex in eukaryotes. The lagging strand is shown looped around the replication complex. Single strand binding proteins (not shown) are bound to the unpaired DNA.

Okazaki fragments are much smaller in eukaryotes than in prokaryotes (about 200 nucleotides versus 1,000). Because the size of eukaryotic Okazaki fragments are equivalent to the size of the DNA found in nucleosomes, it seems likely that one nucleosome at a time may release its DNA for replication.

Proofreading occurs in eukaryotes as well as in prokaryotes. Polymerase δ, which is part of the replication complex, has the $3' \rightarrow 5'$-exonuclease activity required for this function. Enzymes that catalyze repair of mismatched bases are also present. Consequently, eukaryotic replication occurs with high fidelity; approximately one mispairing occurs for every 10^9 to 10^{12} nucleotides incorporated into growing DNA chains.

Eukaryotic DNA polymerases β and ε, as well as polymerase α, appear to be involved in DNA repair. Polymerase γ is located in mitochondria, and, therefore, its function is most likely related to replication of mitochondrial DNA.

DNA REPAIR

Actions of Mutagens

Despite proofreading and mismatch repair during replication, some mismatched bases do persist. In addition, DNA can be damaged by mutagens produced in cells or inhaled or absorbed from the environment. Mutagens are agents that damage DNA, causing mutations that can have devastating effects on cells. Mutagens that cause normal cells to become cancer cells are known as carcinogens. Unfortunately, mismatching of bases and DNA damage produce thousands of potentially mutagenic lesions in each cell every day. Without repair mechanisms, we could not survive these assaults on our genes.

DNA damage can be caused by radiation and by chemicals (Fig. 12.10). These agents may directly affect the DNA or they may act indirectly. For example, x-rays, a type of ionizing radiation, act indirectly by exciting molecules in the cell that interact with DNA, altering the structure of the bases or cleaving DNA strands.

A 12.1: Liver cells are in G_0. Up to 90% of the human liver can be removed. The remaining liver cells are stimulated to re-enter the cell cycle and divide, regenerating a mass equivalent to the original mass of the liver within a few weeks.

The myth of Prometheus indicates that the capacity of the liver to regenerate was recognized even in ancient times.

Nick O'Tyne has been smoking for 40 years in spite of the warnings on cigarette packs that this habit can be dangerous and even deadly. The burning of tobacco, and, for that matter, the burning of any organic material, produces many different carcinogens, such as benzo[*a*]pyrene. These carcinogens coat the airways and lungs. They can cross cell membranes and interact with DNA, causing "damage" to bases that interferes with normal base pairing. If these DNA lesions cannot be repaired or if they are not repaired rapidly enough, a permanent mutation may be produced when the cells replicate. Some mutations cause abnormal cell growth, and cancer results.

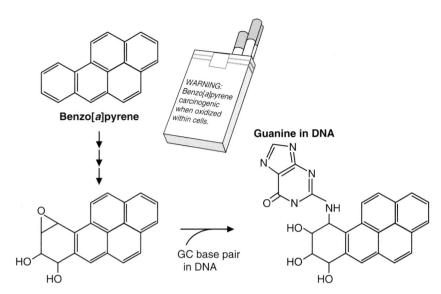

Fig. 12.10. Oxidation of benzo[*a*]pyrene and covalent binding to DNA. Benzo[*a*]pyrene is not carcinogenic until it is oxidized within cells. Then it can covalently bind to guanine residues in DNA, interrupting hydrogen bonding in G-C base pairs and producing distortions of the helix.

While exposure to x-rays is infrequent, it is more difficult to avoid exposure to cigarette smoke, and virtually impossible to avoid exposure to sunlight. Cigarette smoke contains carcinogens such as the aromatic polycyclic hydrocarbon benzo[*a*]pyrene (see Fig. 12.10). When this compound is oxidized by cellular enzymes, which normally act to make foreign compounds more water soluble and easy to excrete, it becomes capable of forming bulky adducts with guanine residues in DNA. Ultraviolet rays from the sun also produce distortions in the DNA helix. Ultraviolet light excites adjacent pyrimidine bases on DNA strands, causing them to form covalent dimers (Fig. 12.11).

Repair Mechanisms

The mechanisms used for the repair of DNA have many similarities (Fig. 12.12). First, a distortion in the DNA helix is recognized and the region containing the distortion is removed. The gap in the damaged strand is replaced by the action of a DNA polymerase that uses the intact, undamaged strand as a template. Finally, a ligase seals the nick in the strand that has undergone repair.

NUCLEOTIDE EXCISION REPAIR

Endonucleases that recognize local distortions of the DNA helix, such as mismatched bases or bulky adducts, cleave the abnormal chain and remove the distorted region (see Figs. 12.12 and 12.13). The gap is then filled by a DNA polymerase that adds deoxyribonucleotides, one at a time, to the 3′-end of the cleaved DNA, using the intact, complementary DNA strand as a template. The newly synthesized segment is joined to the 5′-end of the remainder of the original DNA strand by a DNA ligase.

BASE EXCISION REPAIR

DNA glycosylases recognize small distortions in DNA, involving lesions caused by damage to a single base. A glycosylase cleaves the *N*-glycosidic bond joining the

Melanomas develop because of exposure of the skin to the ultraviolet rays of the sun. This radiation causes pyrimidine dimers to form in DNA. Mutations can result which may produce melanomas that appear as dark brown growths on the skin.

Fortunately, **William Hartman's** melanoma was discovered at an early stage during a physical examination following his heart attack. The growth was excised surgically, and further recurrence of the cancer could be the least of his medical problems.

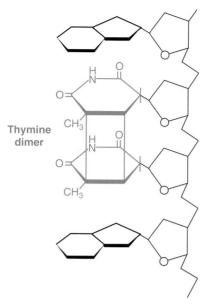

Fig. 12.11. A thymine dimer in a DNA strand. Ultraviolet light can cause two adjacent pyrimidines to form a covalent dimer.

 Pyrimidine dimers, most commonly thymine dimers, can be repaired by photoreactivating enzymes that cleave the bonds between the bases using energy from visible light. In this process, nucleotides are not removed from the damaged DNA. This repair process is used by bacteria and might serve as a very minor mechanism in human cells.

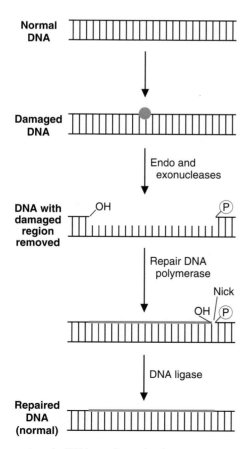

Fig. 12.12. Common steps in DNA repair mechanisms.

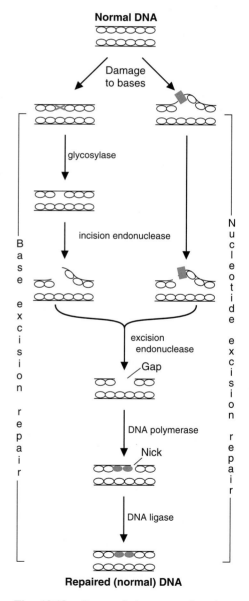

Fig. 12.13. Types of damage and various repair mechanisms.

Pyrimidine dimers occur frequently in the skin. Usually repair mechanisms correct this damage, and cancer rarely occurs. However, in individuals with xeroderma pigmentosum, cancers are extremely common. These individuals have been shown to have defects in their DNA repair systems. The first defect to be identified was a deficiency of the endonuclease involved in the removal of pyrimidine dimers from DNA. By scrupulously avoiding light, these individuals can reduce the number of skin cancers that develop.

Hereditary nonpolyposis colorectal cancer (a human cancer that does not arise from intestinal polyps) is caused by mutations in genes for proteins involved in mismatch repair (hMSH1, hMSH2, hPMS1, or hPMS2).

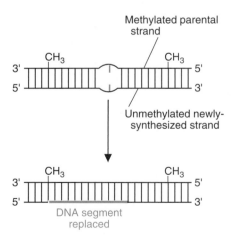

Fig. 12.14. Mismatch repair. Normal, undamaged but mismatched bases bind proteins of the mismatch repair system that replace a segment of DNA (including the mismatched base). Bacterial enzymes replace the mismatched base on the unmethylated strand. The mechanism for distinguishing between parental and newly synthesized strands in humans is not as well understood.

damaged base to deoxyribose (see Fig. 12.13). The sugar-phosphate backbone of the DNA now lacks a base at this site (known as an apurinic or apyrimidinic site, or an AP site). Then an AP endonuclease cleaves the sugar-phosphate strand at this site. Subsequently, the same types of enzymes involved in other types of repair mechanisms restore this region to normal.

MISMATCH REPAIR

Mismatched bases (bases that do not form normal Watson-Crick base pairs) are recognized by enzymes of the mismatch repair system. Because neither of the bases in a mismatch is damaged, these repair enzymes must be able to determine which base of the mispair to correct.

Errors that occur during replication are repaired by the mismatch repair enzyme complex (Fig. 12.14). In bacteria, parental DNA strands contain methyl groups on bases in specific sequences. During replication, the newly synthesized strands are not immediately methylated. Before methylation occurs, the proteins involved in mismatch repair can distinguish parental from newly synthesized strands. A region of the new unmethylated strand, including the mismatched base, is removed and replaced.

Human enzymes can also distinguish parental from newly synthesized strands and repair mismatches. However, the mechanisms have not yet been as clearly defined as those in bacteria.

TRANSCRIPTION-COUPLED REPAIR

Genes that are actively transcribed to produce mRNA are preferentially repaired. The RNA polymerase that is transcribing a gene (see Chapter 13 for a description of the process) stalls when it encounters a damaged region of the DNA template. Excision repair proteins are attracted to this site and repair the damaged region. Subsequently, RNA polymerase can resume transcription.

GENETIC REARRANGEMENTS

The exchange of segments between DNA molecules occurs quite frequently and is responsible for genetic alterations that may have beneficial or devastating consequences for the affected individuals and, in some instances, for their offspring. The DNA segments that are exchanged may be homologous (that is, of very similar sequence) or they may be totally unrelated. The size of the fragments may range from a few nucleotides to tens of thousands and may include many different genes or portions of genes. Many of the enzymes involved in these exchanges are the same as or similar to those used for replication and repair and include endonucleases, exonucleases, unwinding enzymes, topoisomerases, DNA polymerases, and ligases.

One type of genetic rearrangement that has been observed for many years is "crossing-over" between homologous chromosomes during meiosis. Another type occurs in stem cells as they differentiate into lymphocytes. Segments of the genes of stem cells are rearranged so that the mature cell is capable of producing only a single type of antibody. Other types of genetic exchanges involve transposable elements (transposons) that can move from one site in the genome to another or produce copies that can be inserted into new sites. Translocations occur when chromosomes break and portions randomly become joined to other chromosomes, producing gross changes that can be observed under the light microscope. Genetic exchanges can even occur between species, for example when foreign DNA is inserted into the human genome as a result of viral infection.

General or Homologous Recombination

Various models, supported by experimental evidence, have been proposed for the mechanism of recombination between homologous DNA sequences. Although these mechanisms are complex, a simplified scheme for one type of recombination is presented in Figure 12.15.

Initially, two homologous chromosomes or segments of double-helical (duplex) DNA that have very similar, but not necessarily identical, sequences become aligned (see Fig. 12.15). One strand of one duplex is nicked by an enzyme and invades the other DNA duplex, base-pairing with a region of complementary sequence. The match between the sequences does not have to be perfect, but a significant number of bases must pair so that the strand displaced from its partner can form a displacement (D) loop. This D loop is nicked, and the displaced strand now base-pairs with the former partner of the invading strand. Ligation occurs, and a Holliday structure is generated (see Fig. 12.15). The branch point of the Holliday structure can migrate and may move many thousands of nucleotides from its original position. The Holliday structure, named for the scientist who discovered it, is finally cleaved and then religated, forming two homologous chromosomes that have exchanged segments. In addition to enzymes similar to those used in DNA replication, enzymes for strand invasion, branch migration, and cleavage of the Holliday structure are required.

Transposable Elements

Movable (or transposable) genetic elements, "jumping genes," were first observed by Barbara McClintock in the 1940s. Her work, initially greeted with skepticism, was ultimately accepted, and she was awarded the Nobel Prize in 1983.

Transposons are segments of DNA found in all organisms including eukaryotes, which can move from their original position in the genome to a new location (Fig. 12.16). Transposons contain the gene for an enzyme called a transposase, which is involved in cleaving the transposon from the genome and moving it from one location to another.

Retroposons are similar to transposons except that they involve an RNA intermediate. Reverse transcriptase makes a single-stranded DNA copy of the RNA. A double-stranded DNA is then produced that is inserted into the genome at a new location.

Reverse Transcriptase

Reverse transcriptase is an enzyme that uses an RNA template and makes a DNA copy (Fig. 12.17). The RNA template can be transcribed from DNA by RNA polymerase or obtained from another source, such as an RNA virus. The DNA copy of the RNA produced by reverse transcriptase is known as cDNA. Retroviruses (RNA viruses) use reverse transcriptase. A double-stranded cDNA is produced, which can become integrated into the human genome. After integration, the viral genes may be inactive, adding to the "junk" DNA that accumulates in the human genome, or they may be transcribed, sometimes causing diseases such as AIDS and cancer. (See Chapter 17.)

Translocations

Breaks in chromosomes, caused by agents such as x-rays or chemical carcinogens, can result in gross chromosomal rearrangements (Fig. 12.18). If the free ends of the DNA at the break point reseal with the free ends of a different broken chromosome, a translocation is produced. These exchanges of large portions of chromosomes can have deleterious effects and are frequently observed in cancer cells.

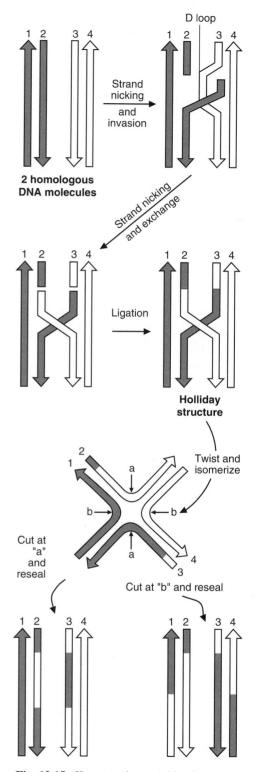

Fig. 12.15. Key steps in recombination.

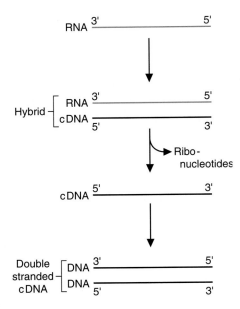

Fig. 12.17. Action of reverse transcriptase. This enzyme catalyzes the production of a DNA copy from an RNA template. The RNA of a DNA-RNA hybrid is degraded, and the single DNA strand is used as a template to make double-stranded DNA. This figure is a simplified version of a more complex process.

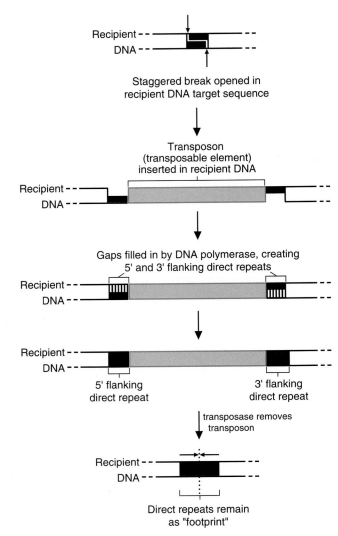

Fig. 12.16. Transposons. From Wolfe SL. Mol Cell Biol 1993:764.

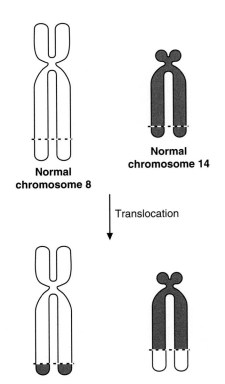

Fig. 12.18. Translocation. A portion of the long arm of chromosome 8 is exchanged for a portion of the long arm of chromosome 14. This chromosomal translocation is found in Burkitt's lymphoma.

CLINICAL COMMENTS. Although the malignant degeneration of an adenomatous polyp in **Colin Tuma's** large bowel was in part, at least, genetically determined, the increased fat and animal protein intake in the Western diet may increase the risk as well. This diet may favor bacterial flora capable of increasing the conversion of acid and neutral sterols to carcinogens (compounds that cause cancer). The feces produced from high beef diets also contain carcinogens such as nitrosamide.

Ivy Sharer contracted AIDS when she used needles contaminated with HIV to inject drugs intravenously. Intravenous drug abusers account for 15 to 20% of new AIDS cases in the United States. Parenteral transmission also occurs in hemophiliacs receiving clotting factor concentrates. But with the current practice of heat-treating factor VIII concentrates, HIV is inactivated, which should reduce the incidence of AIDS in the hemophiliac population dramatically. The use of factor VIII produced by recombinant DNA techniques may ultimately eliminate the risk of AIDS for this group of patients.

Di Beatty's poorly controlled diabetes mellitus predisposed her to a urinary tract infection because glucose in the urine serves as a "culture medium" for bacterial growth. The kidney glomerulotubular unit is capable of keeping glucose from entering the urine until the serum glucose level exceeds 175–185 mg/dL (the tubular threshold for glucose). In Di Beatty's case, blood glucose levels frequently exceed this threshold.

The average person has 20 moles on the body surface, yet only seven people out of every 100,000 develop a malignant melanoma. The incidence of malignant melanoma, however, is rising rapidly. Because 35–40% of patients with malignant melanoma die because of this cancer, the physician's decision to biopsy a pigmented mole with an irregular border and variation of color probably saved **William Hartman's** life.

Lung cancer currently accounts for one fifth of all cancers in men and one tenth in women. The overall 5-year survival rate is still less than 15%. For those who smoke two or more packs of cigarettes daily, as is true for **Nick O'Tyne**, the death rate is 265 per 100,000 population. Thankfully, cigarette smoking has declined in the United States. Whereas 50% of men and 32% of women smoked in 1965, these figures have currently fallen to 26% and 24%, respectively.

BIOCHEMICAL COMMENTS. Growth of human cells, which involves DNA replication and cell division, is regulated by agents such as growth factors and hormones. These agents, produced by certain sets of cells, promote growth in their target cell populations by mechanisms that are not understood in full detail. However, it is apparent that these mechanisms are important for understanding the abnormal growth of cancerous cells.

Growth factors are polypeptides that do not enter cells but bind to receptors on the cell surface, triggering events within the cell that stimulate growth and division. When the growth factor binds to the receptor, the receptor itself can act as a protein kinase, phosphorylating tyrosine residues of intracellular proteins. Other receptors activate enzymes in the cell membrane that produce "second messengers."

Steroid and thyroid hormones may also be involved in regulation of the cell cycle. These compounds cross the cell membrane and interact with receptors within the cell.

Ultimately, the hormone-receptor complex binds to chromatin, activating genes that encode proteins involved in regulating cell division.

Many steps in these growth-promoting mechanisms are beginning to be elucidated, mainly as a result of studies of oncogenes. Oncogenes are mutated forms of normal cellular genes that regulate cell growth. The protein products of oncogenes cause cells to divide without the restraints that limit normal cell growth.

Suggested Readings

Hanawalt P. Transcription-coupled repair and human disease. Science 1994;266:1957–1958.

Kunkel T. DNA replication fidelity. J Biol Chem 1992;267:18251–18254.

Modrich P. Mismatch repair, genetic stability, and cancer. Science 1994;266:1959–1960.

Sancar A. Mechanisms of DNA excision repair. Science 1994;266:1954–1956.

PROBLEM

Ivy Sharer asked her physician if she could be treated with ddI or ddC. These compounds are dideoxynucleosides.

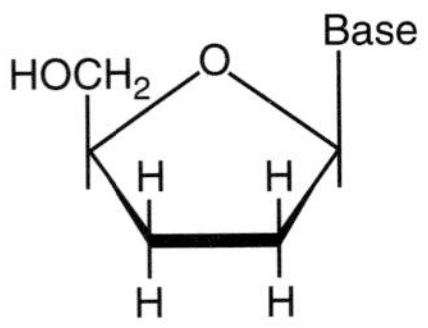

A dideoxynucleoside

How do these agents inhibit viral replication?

ANSWER

The dideoxynucleosides do not have a hydroxyl group on either the 2'- or 3'-carbon. They can be converted to nucleoside triphosphates in cells, and like AZT, they terminate DNA chain growth. It is currently recommended that AIDS patients on AZT be shifted to dideoxynucleosides as the disease progresses or if the patient becomes intolerant to AZT.

Dideoxynucleotides are also used as chain terminators in the Sanger method for DNA sequencing (see Chapter 16).

13 Transcription: Synthesis of RNA

Synthesis of RNA from a DNA template is called transcription. Transcription is catalyzed by enzymes known as RNA polymerases. The mechanisms of action of RNA and DNA polymerases are very similar, with one important difference: RNA polymerases can initiate the synthesis of new strands.

RNA polymerases copy a DNA template in the 3′ to 5′ direction and synthesize an RNA strand in the 5′ to 3′ direction. Because RNA is single-stranded, the mechanism of transcription is not as complex as that of replication.

In bacteria, a single RNA polymerase produces the precursors of mRNA, rRNA, and tRNA. Because bacteria do not contain nuclei, ribosomes bind to mRNA as it is being transcribed and protein synthesis occurs simultaneously with transcription.

Eukaryotic RNA is transcribed in the nucleus by three different RNA polymerases. The primary transcripts are modified and trimmed to produce the mature RNAs which travel to the cytoplasm to participate in translation. The precursors of mRNA undergo the most extensive processing. mRNA precursors have a "cap" added at the 5′-end and a poly(A) "tail" added at the 3′-end. Exons, the regions that form the mature mRNA, are separated in mRNA precursors by introns, regions that have no coding function and are removed by splicing reactions. During the splicing reactions, the exons are connected and the mature mRNA is produced. In eukaryotes, tRNA and rRNA precursors are also modified and trimmed, although not as extensively as mRNA precursors.

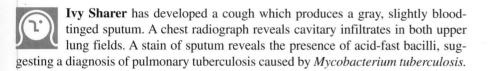

Ivy Sharer has developed a cough which produces a gray, slightly blood-tinged sputum. A chest radiograph reveals cavitary infiltrates in both upper lung fields. A stain of sputum reveals the presence of acid-fast bacilli, suggesting a diagnosis of pulmonary tuberculosis caused by *Mycobacterium tuberculosis*.

Annie Myck is a 4-year-old girl of Mediterranean ancestry whose height and body weight are below the 20th percentile for girls of her age. She is listless, tires easily, and complains of anorexia and shortness of breath on exertion. A dull pain has been present in her right upper quadrant for the last 3 months. Her complexion is slate-gray, and she appears pale. Initial laboratory studies reveal a severe anemia with a hemoglobin of 6.2 g/dL (reference range 12–16). A battery of additional hematological tests reveal that Annie has thalassemia, intermediate type.

Yves Topaigne, who has been free of gout symptoms since starting the xanthine oxidase inhibitor allopurinol, picked mushrooms in a wooded area near his home. A few hours after eating one small mushroom, he experienced mild nausea and diarrhea. He went to the hospital emergency room, where a poison expert identified the mushrooms as *Amanita phalloides* (the "death cap").

181

Sellie D'Souder, a 28-year-old computer programmer, notes increasing fatigue, pleuritic chest pain, and a nonproductive cough. In addition, she complains of joint pains, especially in her hands. A maculopapular erythematous rash on both cheeks and the bridge of her nose ("butterfly rash") has been present for the last 6 months. Initial laboratory studies reveal a subnormal white blood cell count, a mild reduction in hemoglobin, and proteinuria with a slight increase in serum creatinine.

ACTION OF RNA POLYMERASE

The action of RNA polymerase is very similar to that of DNA polymerase, except that RNA polymerase can initiate the synthesis of new chains (Fig. 13.1). A strand of DNA serves as the template, which is copied in the 3′ to 5′ direction. Synthesis occurs in the 5′ to 3′ direction. The ribonucleoside triphosphates ATP, GTP, CTP, and UTP serve as the precursors, which form base pairs with the complementary nucleotides on the DNA template. The phosphate attached to the 5′-hydroxyl of the precursor forms an ester bond with the 3′-hydroxyl at the end of the growing RNA chain. The release of pyrophosphate and its cleavage by a pyrophosphatase to form two inorganic phosphates provides energy that helps to drive the polymerization reaction.

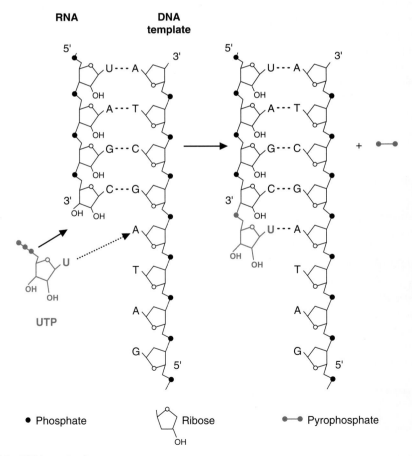

Fig. 13.1. RNA synthesis.

Because RNA is single-stranded, the mechanism of RNA transcription is not as complicated as that of DNA replication. However, the DNA template has two strands. Consequently, for every gene, RNA polymerase must be able to determine which strand to transcribe. Sequences on DNA determine where RNA polymerase binds, how frequently and tightly it binds, and where it begins to transcribe the gene (Fig. 13.2). These sequences, known as promoters, are usually located near the point at which transcription begins (the startpoint). Other sequences, known as enhancers, also affect the frequency of transcription, but may be located at considerable distances, sometimes thousands of nucleotides, from the startpoint.

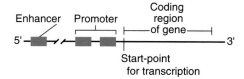

Fig. 13.2. Regions of the gene that regulate transcription. The coding region of a gene contains the information for the amino acid sequence of a protein.

TYPES OF RNA POLYMERASES

Bacterial cells have a single RNA polymerase that transcribes all types of RNA. The RNA polymerase of *Escherichia coli* contains four subunits ($\alpha_2\beta\beta'$), which form the core enzyme. The active enzyme (the holoenzyme) contains this core and a fifth subunit called a σ (sigma) factor (Fig. 13.3). The σ factor is required for binding of the polymerase to specific promoter regions of the DNA template. *E. coli* has a number of σ factors that recognize the promoter regions of different groups of genes. The primary σ factor is σ^{70}, a designation related to its molecular weight of 70,000.

In contrast to prokaryotes, eukaryotic cells have three RNA polymerases (Table 13.1). Polymerase I produces most of the rRNAs, polymerase II produces mRNA, and polymerase III produces small RNAs, such as tRNA and 5S rRNA. All of these RNA polymerases have the same mechanism of action. However, they recognize different types of promoters.

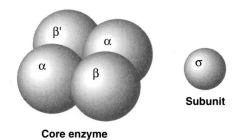

Fig. 13.3. *E. coli* RNA polymerase. The core enzyme contains two α-subunits, one β, and one β'. The σ-factor is a subunit that joins the core enzyme, enabling it to bind to promoter regions of specific genes.

SEQUENCES OF GENES

By convention, the nucleotide sequence of a gene is represented by the letters of the nitrogenous bases of the coding strand of the DNA duplex. It is written from left to right in the 5′ to 3′ direction (Fig. 13.4). The other strand of the DNA helix serves as the template strand that is actually used by RNA polymerase during the process of transcription. The DNA template strand is complementary and antiparallel both to the coding (nontemplate) strand of the DNA and to the RNA transcript produced from the template. Thus the coding strand of the DNA is identical in base sequence and direction to the RNA transcript, except, of course, that wherever this DNA strand contains a T, the RNA transcript contains a U (Fig. 13.4).

During translation, mRNA is read 5′ to 3′ in sets of three bases, called codons, that determine the amino acid sequence of the protein. Thus, the base sequence of the coding strand of the DNA can directly be used to determine the amino acid sequence of the protein.

The base in the coding strand of the gene serving as the startpoint for transcription is numbered +1 (Fig. 13.5). This nucleotide corresponds to the first nucleotide incorporated into the RNA at the 5′-end of the transcript. Subsequent nucleotides within the transcribed region of the gene are numbered +2, +3, etc., toward the 3′-end of the gene. Untranscribed sequences to the left of the startpoint, known as the 5′-flanking

Patients with acquired immune deficiency syndrome (AIDS) frequently develop tuberculosis. After **Ivy Sharer's** sputum stain suggested that she had tuberculosis, a multidrug antituberculous regimen, which includes an antibiotic of the rifamycin family (rifampin) was initiated. A culture of her sputum was taken to confirm the diagnosis.

Rifampin inhibits bacterial RNA polymerase, selectively killing the bacteria that cause the infection. The nuclear RNA polymerase from eukaryotic cells is not affected. Although rifampin can inhibit the synthesis of mitochondrial RNA, the dosage required is considerably higher than that used for treatment of tuberculosis.

Table 13.1. Eukaryotic RNA Polymerases

Enzyme	RNA Produced
RNA polymerase I	rRNA
RNA polymerase II	mRNA
RNA polymerase III	tRNA and other small RNAs
a

DNA coding strand 5' – A T G C C A G T A G G C C A C T T G T C A – 3'

DNA template strand 3' – T A C G G T C A T C C G G T G A A C A G T – 5'

mRNA 5' – AUG CCA GUA GGC CAC UUG UCA – 3'

Protein N – Met –Pro –Val –Gly –His –Leu –Ser – C

Fig. 13.4. Relationship between the coding strand of DNA, the DNA template strand, the mRNA transcript, and the protein produced from the gene. The bases in mRNA are used in sets of three (called codons) to specify the order of the amino acids inserted into the growing polypeptide chain during the process of translation.

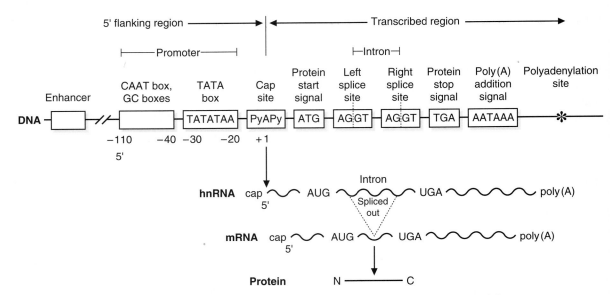

Fig. 13.5. Structure of a eukaryotic gene and its products. Py = pyrimidine.

region of the gene, are numbered –1, –2, –3, etc., starting with the nucleotide (–1) immediately to the left of the startpoint and moving from right to left. Comparing gene sequences to a river, the sequences to the left of the startpoint are said to be upstream from the startpoint and those to the right are said to be downstream.

Recognition of Genes by RNA Polymerase

In order for genes to be expressed, RNA polymerase must recognize the appropriate point to start transcription and the strand of the DNA to transcribe (the template strand). RNA polymerase must also recognize which genes to transcribe because transcribed genes are only a small fraction of the total and the genes that are transcribed differ from one type of cell to another and change with changes in physiological conditions. The signals in DNA that RNA polymerase recognizes are known as promoters. They are sequences in DNA (often called boxes or elements) that determine the startpoint and the frequency of transcription. Because they are located on the same molecule of DNA and near the gene they regulate, they are said to be *cis* acting. Proteins that bind to these DNA sequences and facilitate or prevent the binding of RNA polymerase are said to be *trans* acting because they are encoded by genes that are different from the ones they help to regulate.

Promoter Regions of Genes for mRNA

Promoter regions of genes that produce mRNA contain a number of consensus sequences (Fig. 13.6). When many genes are examined, the sequence most commonly found in a given region is called a consensus sequence. The one closest to the startpoint is usually rich in adenine and thymine residues. In *E. coli*, the consensus sequence for this promoter region, centered about –10, is TATAAT. It is known as the TATA or Pribnow box and is recognized by the primary sigma factor σ^{70}. A similar sequence in the –25 region of eukaryotic genes has a consensus sequence of TATA(A/T)A. The A/T in the fifth position indicates that either A or T occurs with equal frequency. This eukaryotic sequence is known as the TATA box. It is sometimes called the Hogness or Hogness-Goldberg box, named for its discoverers. The AT-rich region of the promoter binds proteins that facilitate the binding of RNA polymerase and determines the startpoint of transcription.

Other sequences involved in binding of RNA polymerase are found further upstream in the promoter region (see Fig. 13.6). Bacterial promoters contain a sequence TTGACA in the –35 region. Eukaryotes frequently have CAAT boxes and GC-rich sequences in the region between –40 and –110.

In bacteria, a number of protein-producing genes may be linked together and controlled by a single promoter. This genetic unit is called an operon (Fig. 13.7). Proteins bind to the promoter and either inhibit or facilitate transcription of the operon. Repressors are proteins that bind to a region in the promoter known as the operator and inhibit transcription by preventing the binding of RNA polymerase. Activators are proteins that stimulate transcription by binding within the –35 region or upstream from it, facilitating the binding of RNA polymerase. Operons are described in more detail in Chapter 15.

In eukaryotes, proteins known as transcription factors (or basal factors) bind to the TATA box and facilitate the binding of RNA polymerase II, the polymerase that transcribes mRNA (Fig. 13.8). This binding process involves at least six transcription fac-

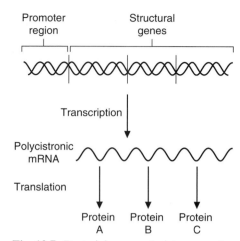

Fig. 13.7. Bacterial operon. A cistron encodes a single protein. In bacteria, a single promoter may control transcription of many cistrons. A single polycistronic mRNA is transcribed. Its translation produces a number of proteins.

Annie Myck has a form of thalassemia. The thalassemias are hereditary anemias that comprise the single most common gene disorders in the world, with a carrier rate of almost 7%. The disease is most prevalent in countries around the Mediterranean Sea. The mutations that cause the thalassemias affect the synthesis of either the α- or the β-chains of globin, causing a decreased production of hemoglobin and, consequently, an anemia. Mutations may occur in one or both of the alleles for the genes that produce the affected chain. Heterozygotes have only one mutant allele. Therefore, half of their globin chains will be normal and these "carriers" are asymptomatic. In homozygotes, both alleles have mutations. Depending on the severity of the effect of the mutation, they may produce some functional globin (β+ phenotype) or none at all (β0 phenotype).

Point mutations within the TATA box (A → G or A → C in the –28 to –31 region) produce a β+ phenotype. These mutations reduce the accuracy of the startpoint of transcription so that only 20–25% of the normal amount of β-globin is synthesized. Other mutations have been observed further upstream in the promoter region (–87 C → G and –88 C → T) that reduce the frequency of transcription and result in a decreased amount of normal β-globin (β+ phenotype).

Because **Annie Myck** produces some functional β-globin chains (her hemoglobin is 6.2 g/dL), she could be homozygous for a mutation within the promoter region of the β-globin gene.

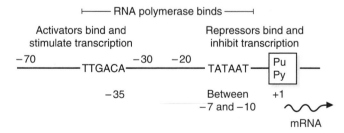

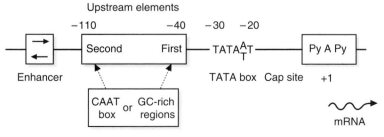

Fig. 13.6. Prokaryotic and eukaryotic promoters. Pu = purine; Py = pyrimidine.

Q 13.1: What property of an AT-rich region of a DNA double helix makes it suitable to serve as a recognition site for the startpoint of transcription?

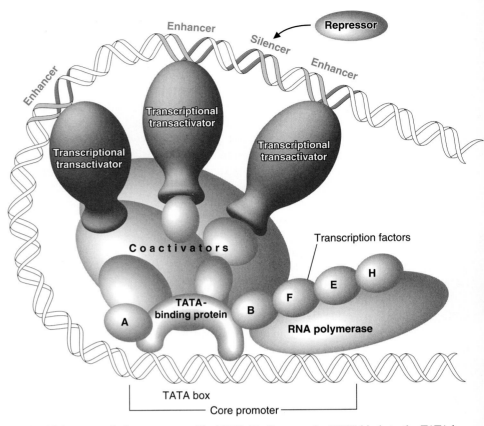

Fig. 13.8. Transcription apparatus. The TATA-binding protein (TBP) binds to the TATA box. Transcription factors A and B bind to TBP. RNA polymerase binds, then factors E, F, and H bind. This complex can transcribe at a basal level. When coactivator proteins bind to TBP and to transcriptional transactivator proteins attached to enhancers, the frequency of transcription is greatly increased. Binding of repressor proteins to silencers decreases the rate of transcription. Adapted from Tjian R. Molecular mechanisms that control genes. Copyright © 1995 by Scientific American, Inc. All rights reserved.

tors (labeled TFII, transcription factor for RNA polymerase II). The TATA-binding protein (TBP) initially binds to the TATA box. TFIIA and TFIIB interact with TBP. RNA polymerase II binds to the complex of transcription factors and to DNA, and is aligned at the startpoint for transcription. TFIIE, TFIIF, and TFIIH subsequently bind, cleaving ATP, and transcription of the gene is initiated. With only these transcription (or basal) factors and RNA polymerase II attached, the gene is transcribed at a low or basal rate.

Enhancers and Silencers

Enhancers and silencers are DNA elements that regulate the frequency of transcription of genes in eukaryotic cells. They dictate the rate at which the basal complex initiates transcription (see Fig. 13.8). They differ from promoters in that their sequences are dissimilar and they may be located thousands of base pairs from the startpoint of transcription. They are orientation independent (i.e., the sequence can run in either direction). They are also position independent (i.e., they can be experimentally moved to varying distances from the startpoint and still stimulate transcription).

Enhancers have been found upstream, downstream, and within genes. Their peculiar locations led to the suggestion, confirmed by experimental evidence, that they bind proteins (called transcriptional transactivators) which cause loops to form in the DNA. The enhancers are thus brought into proximity with the promoter region of the gene. Transcriptional transactivators bound to enhancer sequences are believed to stimulate transcription via coactivators which form protein:protein interactions between the transcriptional transactivators and the transcription factors bound in the region of the TATA box (see Fig. 13.8).

Silencers are DNA sequences which bind proteins that act to inhibit the rate of transcription.

TRANSCRIPTION OF BACTERIAL GENES

Binding of RNA polymerase to the promoter region of DNA causes DNA strands to unwind and separate within a region about 10–20 nucleotides in length. As the polymerase transcribes the DNA, the untranscribed region of the helix continues to separate, while the transcribed region of the DNA template rejoins its partner (Fig. 13.9). The sigma factor is released when the growing RNA chain is about 10 nucleotides long. The elongation reactions continue until the RNA polymerase encounters a transcription termination signal. One type of termination signal involves the formation of a hairpin loop in the transcript, preceding a number of U residues. The second type of mechanism for termination involves the binding of a protein, the rho factor, which causes release of the RNA transcript from the template.

A cistron is a region of DNA that encodes a single protein. In bacteria, mRNA is usually generated from an operon as a polycistronic transcript (one that contains the information to produce a number of different proteins). The polycistronic transcript is translated as it is being transcribed. This transcript is not modified and trimmed, and it does not contain introns (regions within the coding sequence of a transcript that are removed before translation occurs). Several different proteins are produced during translation of the polycistronic transcript, one from each cistron (see Fig. 13.7).

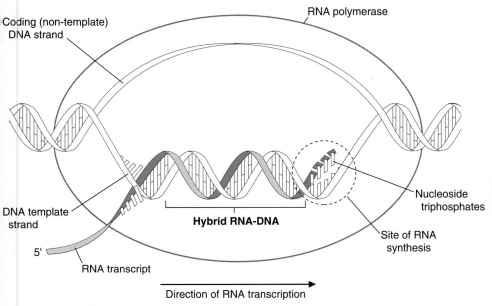

Fig. 13.9. Mechanism of transcription. From Wolfe SL. Mol Cell Biol 1993:579.

A 13.1: In regions where DNA is being transcribed, the two strands of the DNA must be separated. AT base pairs in DNA are joined by only two hydrogen bonds, while GC pairs have three hydrogen bonds. Therefore, in AT-rich regions of DNA, the two strands can be separated more readily than in regions that contain GC base pairs.

The mushrooms that **Yves Topaigne** picked contained a toxin, α-amanitin, that inhibits eukaryotic RNA polymerases. It is particularly effective at blocking the action of RNA polymerase II. This toxin initially causes gastrointestinal disturbances, then electrolyte imbalance and fever, followed by liver and kidney dysfunction. Between 40 and 90% of the individuals who ingest α-amanitin die within a few days.

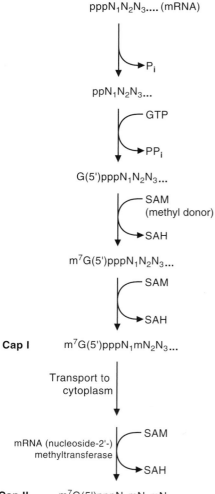

Fig. 13.11. Synthesis of the 5′-cap. The nucleotides at the 5′-end of mRNA (N_1, N_2, and N_3) are involved in formation of the cap. GTP provides the guanine residue that is methylated by *S*-adenosylmethionine (SAM), which becomes *S*-adenosylhomocysteine (SAH). The ribose of the first nucleotide (N_1) is methylated on the 2′-hydroxyl group to form the cap I structure. A second methylation (of the ribose of N_2) may also occur, forming cap II.

In prokaryotes, rRNA is produced as a single, long transcript that is cleaved to produce the 16S, 23S, and 5S ribosomal RNAs. tRNA is also cleaved from larger transcripts (Fig. 13.10). One of the cleavage enzymes, RNase P contains an RNA molecule that catalyzes the cleavage reaction.

TRANSCRIPTION OF EUKARYOTIC GENES

The process of transcription is similar in eukaryotes and prokaryotes. RNA polymerase binds to the transcription factor complex in the promoter region, the helix unwinds within a region near the startpoint of transcription, DNA strand separation occurs, synthesis of the RNA transcript is initiated, and the RNA transcript is elongated, copying the DNA template. The DNA strands separate as the polymerase approaches and rejoin as the polymerase passes. The major difference is that eukaryotes have more elaborate mechanisms for processing the transcripts, particularly the precursors of mRNA. Eukaryotes also have three polymerases, rather than one.

Other differences include the fact that eukaryotic mRNA usually contains the coding information for only one protein and that eukaryotic RNA is transcribed in the nucleus and migrates to the cytoplasm where translation occurs.

Synthesis of Eukaryotic mRNA

TRANSCRIPTION AND CAPPING OF mRNA

In eukaryotes, mRNA is produced by RNA polymerase II as a large transcript, heterogeneous nuclear RNA (hnRNA). "Capping" of this primary transcript occurs at its 5′-end as it is being transcribed. The cap (see Fig. 11.29) is produced from GTP, which is linked through three phosphate groups to the 5′-hydroxyl of the first nucleotide of the transcript (Fig. 13.11). The added guanine is methylated at position 7. Methylation also occurs on the 2′-hydroxyl of the ribose moieties of the first and sometimes the second transcribed nucleotides. This cap functions in the binding of the mature mRNA to the ribosome during protein synthesis.

ADDITION OF A POLY(A) TAIL

Although RNA polymerase continues to transcribe the DNA, the transcript is cleaved by enzymes about 10–20 nucleotides downstream from the polyadenylation sequence (AAUAAA) (Fig. 13.12). Following this cleavage, a poly(A) tail is added to the transcript. There is no poly(T) sequence in the DNA template that corresponds to this tail;

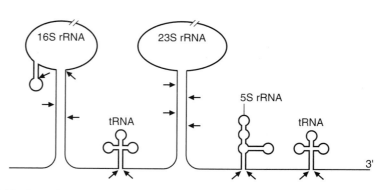

Fig. 13.10. Bacterial rRNA and tRNA transcripts. One large precursor is cleaved (at arrows) to produce 16S, 23S, and 5S rRNA and some tRNAs.

it is added posttranscriptionally. ATP serves as the precursor for addition of adenine nucleotides to the 3′-end of the transcript. They are added one at a time, with poly(A) polymerase catalyzing each addition (see Fig. 13.12).

REMOVAL OF INTRONS

Eukaryotic transcripts contain regions known as exons and introns. Exons appear in the mature mRNA. Introns are removed and are not found in the mature mRNA (Fig. 13.13). Introns, therefore, do not contribute to the amino acid sequence of the protein. Some genes contain 50 or more introns. These introns are carefully removed and the exons spliced together, so that the appropriate protein is produced from the gene.

The consensus sequences at the intron/exon boundaries of the hnRNA are AGGU (AGGT in the DNA). The sequences may vary to some extent on the exon side of the boundary, but almost all introns begin with a 5′ GU and end with a 3′ AG (Fig. 13.14). These sequences at the left splice site of the intron and the right splice site are, therefore, invariant. Since every 5′ GU and 3′ AG combination does not result in a functional splice site, clearly other features within the exon and/or intron help to define the appropriate splice sites. These features are currently unknown but probably do not involve specific base sequences. They may, however, prove to be regions of secondary structure.

A complex structure known as a spliceosome ensures that exons are spliced together with great accuracy (Fig. 13.15). Small nuclear ribonucleoproteins (snRNPs), called "snurps," are involved in formation of the spliceosome. Because snurps are rich in uracil, they are identified by numbers preceded by a U.

The U1 snurp binds near the first exon/intron junction, and U2 binds within the intron in a region containing an adenine nucleotide residue (see Fig. 13.15). Another group of snurps, U4, U5, and U6, binds to the complex, causing it to form a looped structure. The phosphate attached to the G at the 5′-end of the intron forms a 2′-5′ linkage with the 2′-hydroxyl group of the adenine nucleotide residue. Cleavage occurs at the end of the first exon, which continues to be held in place by the spliceosome. A second cleavage occurs at the 3′-end of the intron after the AG sequence. The intron, shaped like a lariat, is released and degraded to nucleotides. The exons are joined together (see Fig. 13.15).

Exons frequently code for separate functional or structural domains of proteins. A process known as exon shuffling has probably occurred throughout evolution, allowing new proteins to develop with functions similar to those of other proteins.

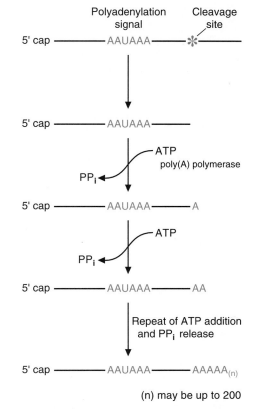

Fig. 13.12. Synthesis of the poly(A) tail. As RNA polymerase continues to transcribe the DNA, enzymes cleave the transcript (hnRNA) at a point 10–20 nucleotides beyond the polyadenylation site (AAUAAA). Adenine nucleotides are then added to the 3′-end of the hnRNA, one at a time, by poly(A) polymerase.

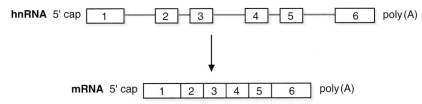

Fig. 13.13. Exons and introns in hnRNA. The introns are removed and the exons (numbered 1 to 6) are joined together to form mRNA.

Fig. 13.14. Splice junction sequences in hnRNA.

One type of β^+-thalassemia is caused by a point mutation (AATAAA → AACAAA) that changes the cleavage and polyadenylation signal in hnRNA from AAUAAA to AACAAA. Homozygous individuals with this mutation produce only one-tenth the amount of normal β-globin mRNA.

Because **Annie Myck** has a β^+-thalassemia, she could have a polyadenylation signal mutation.

Some types of thalassemia are caused by mutations in the splice junction sequences at intron/exon boundaries. In some individuals, mutations occur at the 5′-end of the first or second intron. An AT replaces a GT in the gene. Mutations also occur within the splice junction sequences at the 3′-end of introns. These splice junction mutations produce β^0-thalassemias. Because **Annie Myck** has a β^+-thalassemia, it is unlikely that she has a splice junction mutation.

Tests were performed on **Sellie D'Souder's** blood to determine if antibodies to a number of nuclear and cytoplasmic antigens were present. The tests were strongly positive and, in conjunction with her symptoms, lead to a diagnosis of systemic lupus erythematosus (SLE).

In this disorder, the body makes antibodies against many of its own components. snRNPs are one of the targets of these antibodies. In fact, snRNPs were discovered as a result of studies using antibodies obtained from patients with SLE.

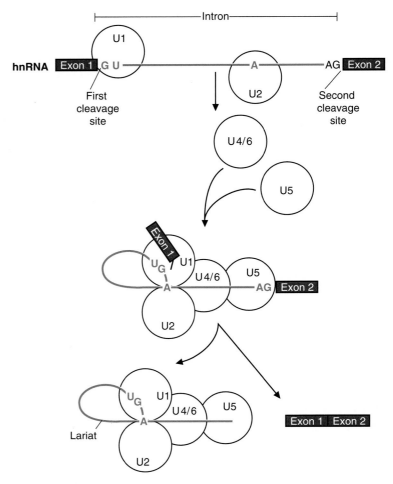

Fig. 13.15. Splicing process. Nuclear ribonucleoproteins (snRNPs U_1 to U_6) bind to the intron causing it to form a loop. Cleavage at the left splice site releases exon 1, which remains attached to the complex (the sliceosome). A 5′-2′ bond forms between the indicated G and A residues. A second cleavage releases exon 2, which is spliced to exon 1. The lariat-shaped intron is released.

MIGRATION OF mRNA TO THE CYTOPLASM

The mature, intronless mRNA, capped at the 5′-end and equipped with a poly(A) tail, complexes with proteins and travels through pores in the nuclear envelope into the cytoplasm (Fig. 13.16). There it combines with ribosomes and directs the incorporation of amino acids into proteins.

Synthesis of Eukaryotic rRNA

In eukaryotes, three of the four rRNAs are produced by RNA polymerase I in the nucleolus. Genes in the nucleolar organizer region produce a large, 45S transcript that is cleaved to produce the 18S, 28S, and 5.8S rRNAs. About 1,000 of these genes are present in the human genome. They are linked in tandem, separated by spacer regions that contain the termination signals for one gene and the promoter for the next (Fig. 13.17). Promoters for rRNA genes are located in the 5′-flanking region of the genes and extend into the region surrounding the startpoint.

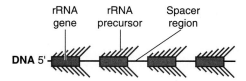

Fig. 13.17. rRNA genes undergoing transcription. rRNA genes, linked in tandem, are transcribed, producing rRNA precursors. Untranscribed spacer regions separate the genes.

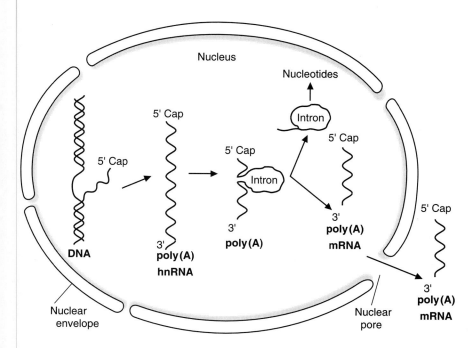

Fig. 13.16. Overview of mRNA synthesis. Transcription produces hnRNA from the DNA template. hnRNA processing involves addition of a 5′-cap and a poly(A) tail and splicing to join exons and remove introns. The product, mRNA, migrates to the cytoplasm.

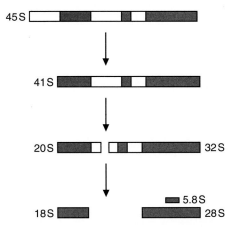

Fig. 13.18. Electron micrograph of the nucleolus. F = fibrous region. G = granular region.

rRNA genes caught in the act of transcription by electron micrographs show that many RNA polymerase I molecules may be attached to a gene at any given time. As the polymerase moves toward the 3′-end of the gene, the transcripts become longer. Thus, genes that are actively being transcribed resemble feathers (or in three dimensions, fir trees) with shorter branches emanating from one end that grow longer toward the other end.

Transcription of rRNA genes, located in the nucleolar organizer region of the genome, produces the fibrous regions of the nucleolus (Fig. 13.18). As the 45S rRNA precursor is released from the DNA, it complexes with proteins, forming ribonucleoprotein particles that generate the granular regions of the nucleolus. Processing of the transcript occurs in the granular regions.

5S rRNA, produced by RNA polymerase III from genes located outside the nucleolus in the nucleoplasm, migrates into the nucleolus and joins the ribonucleoprotein particles.

One to two percent of the nucleotides of the 45S precursor are methylated, primarily on the 2′-hydroxyl groups of ribose moieties. These methyl groups are conserved in the mature rRNA and may serve as markers for cleavage of the precursors.

The 45S precursor undergoes a number of cleavages. Most of the cleavages occur in regions that separate the sequences that become the mature rRNAs. Some precursors contain introns within the regions that become the mature rRNAs. These introns are removed by self-splicing reactions, and the rRNA precursors that catalyze their own splicing are known as ribozymes (see Chapter 11).

In the production of cytoplasmic ribosomes in human cells, one portion of the 45S rRNA precursor becomes the 18S rRNA that, complexed with proteins, forms the small ribosomal subunit (Fig. 13.19). Another segment of the precursor folds back on itself and is cleaved, forming 28S rRNA, hydrogen-bonded to the 5.8S rRNA. The 5S rRNA, transcribed from nonnucleolar genes, and a number of proteins join the 28S and 5.8S rRNAs to form the 60S ribosomal subunit.

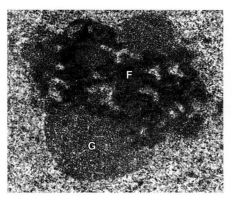

Fig. 13.19. Maturation of the 45S rRNA precursor. The clear regions are removed, and the shaded regions become the mature rRNAs. (The 5S rRNA is not produced from this precursor.)

The ribosomal subunits migrate through the nuclear pores. In the cytoplasm, they interact with mRNA, forming the 80S ribosomes on which protein synthesis occurs (Fig. 13.20).

Synthesis of Eukaryotic tRNA

At least 20 families of tRNAs occur in cells, one for every amino acid that is incorporated into growing polypeptide chains during the synthesis of proteins. tRNAs have a cloverleaf structure that folds into a three-dimensional L shape (see Fig. 11.35). Many of the bases are modified posttranscriptionally.

tRNA is produced by RNA polymerase III, which recognizes a split promoter within the coding region of the gene (Fig. 13.21). One segment of the promoter is located between +8 and +19. A second segment is 30–60 base pairs downstream from the first.

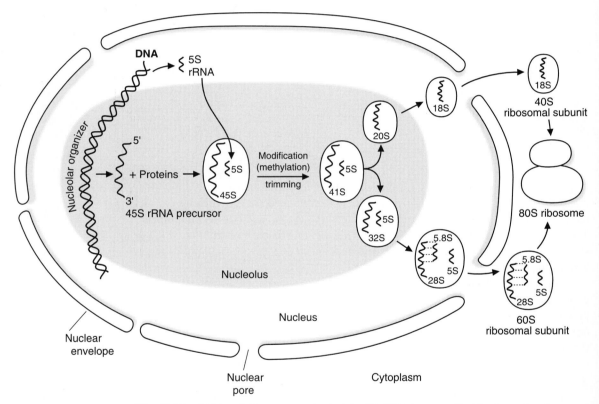

Fig. 13.20. rRNA and ribosome synthesis. The 5S rRNA is transcribed in the nucleoplasm and moves into the nucleolus. The other rRNAs are transcribed from DNA and mature in the nucleolus, forming the 40S and 60S ribosomal subunits, which migrate to the cytoplasm.

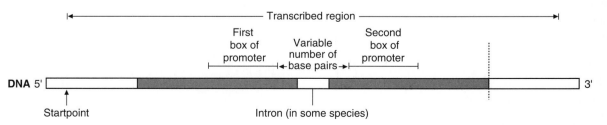

Fig. 13.21. Promoter for tRNA transcription. The segments of the genes from which the mature tRNA is produced are shaded. The two regions of the promoter lie within these segments.

A precursor about 100 nucleotides in length is generated. It assumes a cloverleaf shape and is subsequently cleaved at the 5′- and 3′-ends. The enzyme that acts at the 5′-end is RNase P, similar to the RNase P of bacteria. Both enzymes contain a small RNA (M1) that has catalytic activity, serving as an endonuclease.

The bases are modified at the same time the endonucleolytic reactions are occurring. Three modifications occur in most tRNAs: uracil is methylated by *S*-adenosylmethionine (SAM) to form thymine; one of the double bonds of uracil is reduced to form dihydrouracil; and a uracil residue (attached by an *N*-glycosidic bond) is rotated so that its linkage to ribose is converted to a carbon-carbon bond (pseudouridine). Other, more complex modifications also occur.

Some tRNA precursors contain introns that are removed (Fig. 13.22). This process has been most extensively studied in yeast, where the intron, less than 20 nucleotides

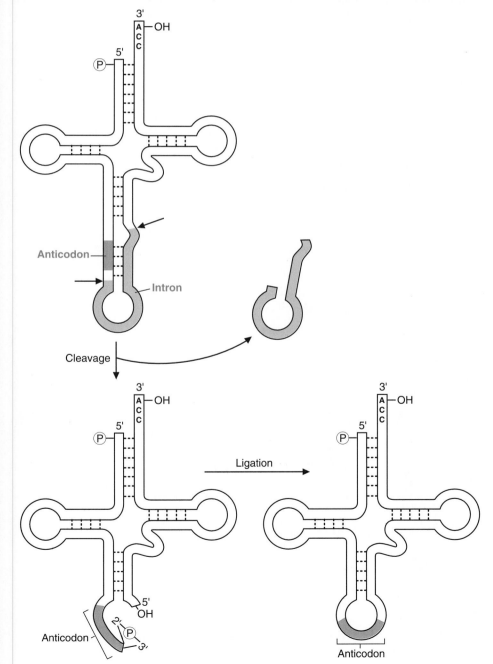

Fig. 13.22. Removal of introns from pretRNA. The intron, located at the 3′-end of the anticodon, is removed. Ligation produces the mature tRNA.

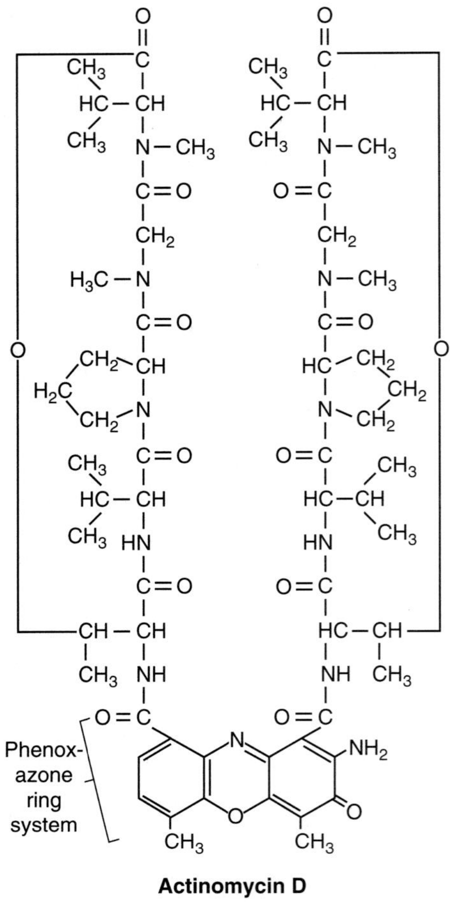

Actinomycin D

Fig. 13.24. Actinomycin D.

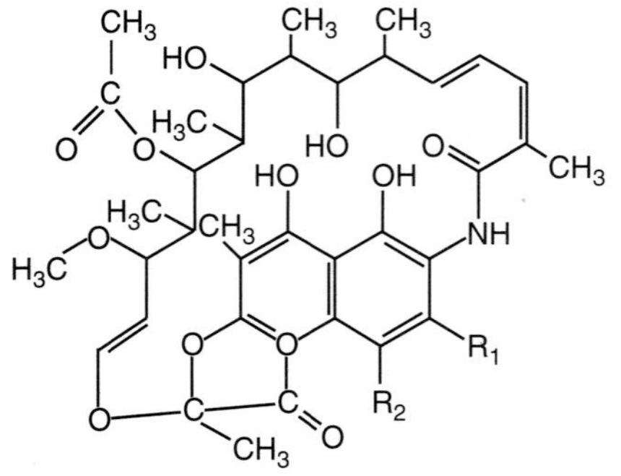

Rifamycin B (R$_1$ = H; R$_2$ = O−CH$_2$−COOH)

Rifampicin (R$_1$ = CH=N$^+$ N−CH$_3$; R$_2$ = OH)

Fig. 13.25. Rifampicin and rifamycin.

in length, is located within the anticodon loop. The intron is removed by endonucleases, leaving the two halves of the tRNA, which are held together by hydrogen bonds between base pairs in the stem regions. A 2′- or 3′-phosphate group is ligated to a 5′-hydroxyl by an RNA ligase.

In order to participate in protein synthesis, tRNA must have a CCA sequence added to its 3′-end. These nucleotides are added one at a time by nucleotidyltransferase. An amino acid forms an ester with a hydroxyl group on the adenine nucleotide residue at the 3′-end of the tRNA. The tRNA carries this amino acid to a ribosome, ensuring that the amino acid is inserted at the appropriate position in the growing polypeptide chain (Fig. 13.23).

INHIBITORS OF RNA SYNTHESIS

A number of compounds can inhibit RNA synthesis. Some bind to DNA and others to RNA polymerase. Those that inhibit RNA synthesis in bacteria under conditions that do not inhibit nuclear RNA synthesis in eukaryotes serve as antibiotics.

Agents That Bind to DNA

Actinomycin D inhibits RNA synthesis because it contains pentapeptide groups that fit into the grooves of DNA and a flat phenoxazone ring that intercalates or slips between the DNA base pairs (Fig. 13.24). DNA that interacts with actinomycin D cannot serve as a template for replication or for transcription. This compound is too toxic for clinical use, but it is used experimentally, for instance, to inhibit RNA synthesis so that the processing of previously synthesized RNA transcripts can be studied.

Agents That Bind to RNA Polymerase

Rifampin is a compound that binds to bacterial RNA polymerase and prevents initiation of RNA synthesis (the joining of more than the first few nucleotides) (Fig. 13.25). It does not prevent further elongation of RNA chains that are in the process of being transcribed.

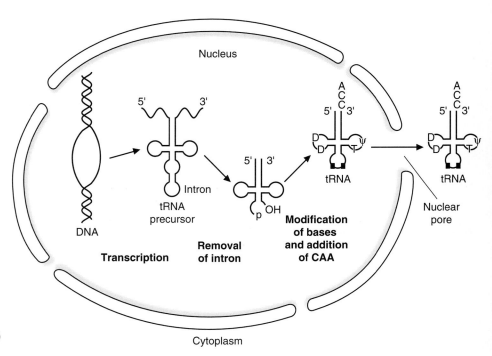

Fig. 13.23. Overview of tRNA synthesis. D, T, Ψ, and ■ indicate modified bases.

Streptolydigin binds to bacterial RNA polymerase and prevents elongation of RNA chains (Fig. 13.26).

α-Amanitin, a compound derived from the poisonous mushroom *Amanita phalloides*, inhibits eukaryotic RNA polymerases (Fig. 13.27). RNA polymerase II is more readily inhibited than polymerase III, and polymerase I is relatively insensitive to this compound.

Within a few days of initiation of treatment for tuberculosis, cultures of **Ivy Sharer's** sputum confirmed the diagnosis of pulmonary tuberculosis caused by *M. tuberculosis*. Therefore, the multidrug therapy, which included rifampin, was continued.

CLINICAL COMMENTS **Ivy Sharer** was treated with a multidrug regimen for tuberculosis because the microbes that cause the disease frequently become resistant to the individual drugs. Rifampin in combination with isoniazid is usually effective, but months of treatment are required.

Just as bacteria can become resistant to drugs, so can HIV. A great concern to physicians treating patients with AIDS is the appearance of resistant strains of HIV-1 in patients taking AZT (zidovudine) for 6 months or more. These resistant strains have remained relatively sensitive to drugs such as dideoxyinosine (didanosine, formerly called ddI) and dideoxycytidine (zalcitabine, formerly called ddC). Because her disease had been progressing in spite of AZT therapy, Ivy had been shifted to didanosine shortly before her symptoms of tuberculosis appeared.

Patients with β^+-thalassemia who maintain their hemoglobin levels above 6.0–7.0 g/dL may have thalassemia intermedia. People with this form of the disorder, such as

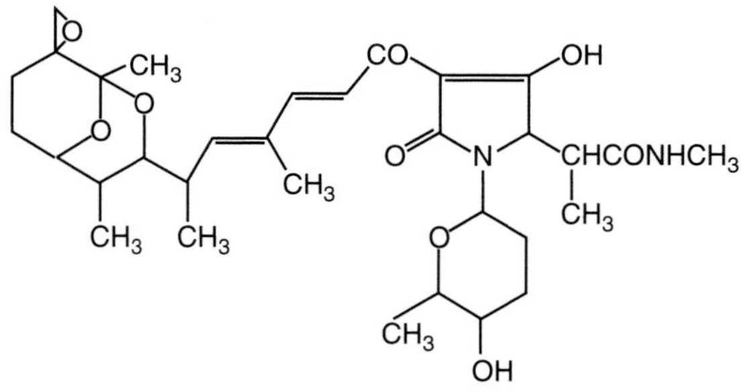

Streptolydigin

Fig. 13.26. Streptolydigin.

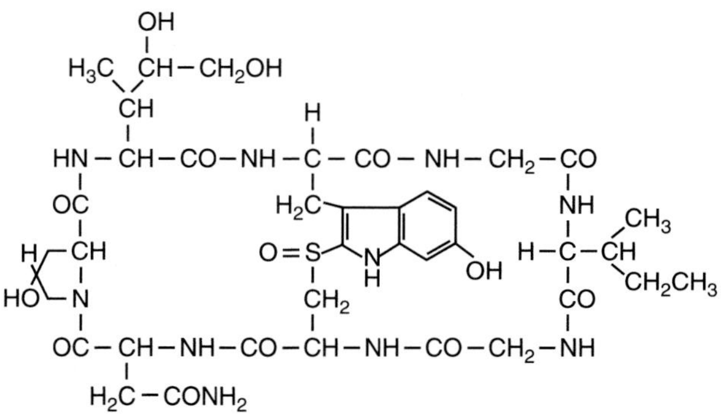

α–Amanitin

Fig. 13.27. α-Amanitin.

Q 13.2: Is **Yves Topaigne** likely to survive his mushroom poisoning? He weighs about 90 kg. An average-size mushroom weighs about 50 g and contains about 7 mg of α-amanitin. The LD_{50} (the oral dose that kills 50% of those who ingest the toxin) is 0.1 mg/kg body weight.

Annie Myck, may have inherited two different defective alleles, one from each parent. One parent may be a "silent" carrier, with one normal allele and one mildly affected allele. This parent produces enough functional β-globin so no symptoms of thalassemia appear. When this parent contributes the mildly defective allele and the other heterozygous parent contributes a more severely defective allele, thalassemia intermedia occurs in the child. The child is thus heterozygous for two defective alleles.

The toxin α-amanitin is capable of causing irreversible hepatocellular and renal dysfunction through inhibition of mammalian RNA polymerases. Fortunately, **Yves Topaigne's** toxicity proved to be mild. He developed only gastrointestinal symptoms and slight changes in his hepatic and renal function, which returned to normal within a few weeks. Treatment was primarily supportive, with fluid and electrolyte replacement for that lost via the gastrointestinal tract. No effective antidote is currently available for the *A. phalloides* toxin.

SLE is a multisystem disease of unknown etiology characterized by inflammation related to the presence of autoantibodies in the blood. These autoantibodies react with antigens normally found in the nucleus, cytoplasm, and plasma membrane of the cell. Such "self" antigen-antibody (autoimmune) interactions initiate an inflammatory cascade which produce the broad symptom profile of multiorgan dysfunction found in **Sellie D'Souder**.

Pharmacological therapy for SLE, directed at immunosuppression, includes corticosteroids, often in high doses. In refractory cases, cytotoxic agents such as azathioprine and cyclophosphamide, which, through their bone marrow toxicity, cause immunosuppression, have also been used.

BIOCHEMICAL COMMENTS AIDS is caused by the human immunodeficiency virus (HIV). Two forms of the virus have been discovered, HIV-1, which is prevalent in industrialized countries, and HIV-2, which is prevalent in Africa. Eight to ten years or more may elapse between the initial infection and development of the full-blown syndrome.

Proteins in the viral coat bind to receptors (CD4) in the membrane of the host cells, a class of helper T lymphocytes. The lipid in the viral coat fuses with the cell membrane, and the viral core enters the cell. The enzyme reverse transcriptase and the viral RNA are released from the viral core. Reverse transcriptase uses the viral RNA as a template to produce a single-stranded DNA copy, which then serves as a template for synthesis of a double-stranded DNA. An integrase enzyme, also carried by the virus, enables this DNA to integrate into the host cell genome as a provirus (Fig. 13.28).

In the initial stage of transcription of the provirus, the transcript is spliced, and three proteins are produced that stimulate transcription of the viral genes. As one of these proteins (Rev) accumulates, it allows unspliced viral RNA to leave the nucleus and to produce proteins of the viral envelope and proteins of the viral core, including reverse transcriptase. Two of the envelope proteins (gp41 and gp120) form a complex that embeds in the cell membrane. The other proteins combine with the full-length viral RNA to form core viral particles, which bud from the cell membrane. Thus, the virus obtains its lipid coat from the host cell membrane, and the coat contains viral proteins (gp41 and gp120). The surface protein of the virus, gp120, binds to CD4 receptors on other human helper T lymphocytes, and the infection spreads.

In an uninfected person, helper T lymphocytes usually number about 1,000/mL. Infection with HIV causes the number of these cells to decrease, which results in a deficiency of the immune system. When the number of T lymphocytes drops below

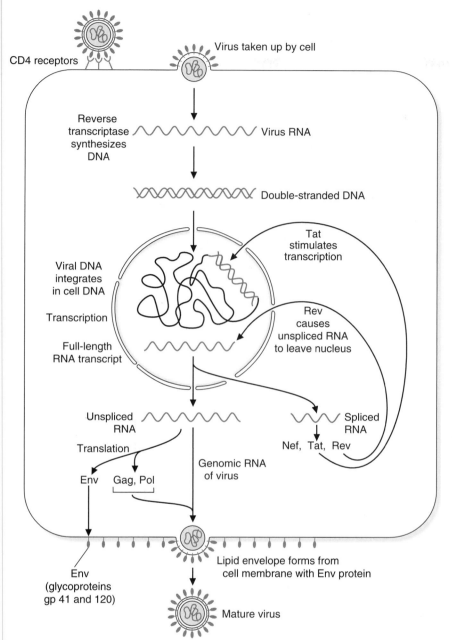

Fig. 13.28. Infection of a host cell by HIV. HIV binds to the CD4 receptor in the host cell membrane. The virus enters the cell and releases its RNA and the enzyme reverse transcriptase. This enzyme produces a double-stranded DNA copy that is integrated into the host cell genome. HIV is now a provirus. Before the Rev protein is produced, HIV transcripts are spliced and code for the proteins Tat, Rev, and Nef. Tat stimulates production of HIV-RNA, and Rev causes it to leave the nucleus unspliced. The unspliced RNA codes for proteins of the viral core and envelope. The envelope proteins (gp41 and gp120) enter the cell membrane. Viral particles form and bud from the cell membrane, carrying membrane lipid as a coat which contains gp41 and gp120. Nef is involved in maintaining the level of infection. From: Recombinant DNA 2/E by Watson, Gilman, Witkowski, and Zoller. Copyright © 1992 by James D. Watson, Michael Gilman, Jan Witkowski, and Mark Zoller. Used with permission of W.H. Freeman and Co.

A 13.2: Because **Yves Topaigne** weighs 90 kg, about 9 mg of α-amanitin would constitute an LD_{50} dose. Although he ate only one small mushroom, which probably contained less than 7 mg of the toxin, he has developed gastrointestinal symptoms and needs to be watched closely to see if further symptoms develop. He consumed enough of the poison to be near the dose that kills 50% of the time.

200/mL, the disease is in an advanced stage, and opportunistic infections, such as tuberculosis, occur. Macrophages and dendritic cells, which lack CD4 receptors, can also become infected with HIV and may carry the virus to the central nervous system.

The reverse transcriptase that copies the viral genome has a high error rate because it does not have proofreading capability. Because incorporation of mismatched bases leads to evolution of the virus, new populations develop rapidly in response to changes in the environment. Mutations in the viral reverse transcriptase gene cause the enzyme to become resistant to drugs such as AZT. Current vaccines developed experimentally against the gp120 surface protein may not be effective as this protein mutates. As a consequence of the rapid mutation rate of HIV, current treatments for AIDS have limited effectiveness, and a cure has proven elusive.

Suggested Readings

Lewin B. Genes V. Messenger RNA is the template. Oxford: Oxford University Press, 1994:378–411.

Lewin B. Genes V. Building the transcription complex: promoters, factors, and RNA polymerases. Oxford: Oxford University Press, 1994:847–877.

Tjian R. Molecular machines that control genes. Sci Am 1995;272:54–61.

PROBLEM

In some species of frogs, fertilized eggs are produced that do not form nucleoli. What would be the consequence of the absence of nucleoli?

ANSWER

An absence of nucleoli indicates that rRNA is not being transcribed and ribosomes are not being formed. Therefore, the only ribosomes in these cells are those derived from the original egg. After a few cell divisions, the number of ribosomes per cell will be too low to support the rate of protein synthesis required for further development, and the small mass of cells derived from the fertilized egg will die.

14   Translation: Synthesis of Proteins

Proteins are produced by a process known as translation, which occurs on ribosomes and is guided by mRNA. The genetic message encoded in DNA is first transcribed into mRNA, and the nucleotide sequence of the mRNA then determines the amino acid sequence of the protein.

The portion of mRNA that specifies the amino acid sequence of the protein is read in codons, which are sets of three nucleotides. Initiation of synthesis of a polypeptide chain begins with the codon AUG which specifies the amino acid methionine. The codons on mRNA are read sequentially in the 5′ to 3′ direction starting with the 5′-AUG that sets the reading frame and ending with a 3′-termination (or "stop") codon (UAG, UGA, or UAA). The protein is produced from its N-terminus to its C-terminus.

tRNA carries amino acids to the ribosomal site of protein synthesis. Base-pairing between the anticodon of the tRNA and the codon on the mRNA ensures that the amino acid carried by the tRNA is inserted into the growing polypeptide chain at the appropriate position.

Binding of the initial methionyl-tRNA to mRNA and the ribosome is called initiation and involves cytosolic proteins known as initiation factors (IFs) and GTP.

After initiation, the polypeptide chain elongates. Elongation involves three steps: (a) addition of an aminoacyl-tRNA to a site on the ribosome where it binds and base-pairs with the second codon on the mRNA, (b) formation of a peptide bond between the first and second amino acids, and (c) translocation, movement of the mRNA relative to the ribosome, so that an aminoacyl-tRNA can bind to the third mRNA codon and to the ribosome.

These three elongation steps are repeated until a termination codon aligns with the site on the ribosome where the next aminoacyl-tRNA would normally bind. Release factors bind instead of a charged tRNA, causing the completed protein to be released from the ribosome.

After one ribosome binds and moves along the mRNA, translating the polypeptide, another ribosome can bind and begin translation. The complex of a single mRNA with multiple ribosomes is known as a polysome.

Folding of the polypeptide into its three-dimensional configuration occurs as the polypeptide is being translated. This process involves proteins known as chaperones.

Modification of amino acid residues in a protein can occur during or following translation and may involve disulfide bond formation, glycosylation (the addition of carbohydrate groups), phosphorylation, cleavage of peptide bonds, and other types of alterations.

Some proteins are synthesized on cytosolic ribosomes and released into the cytosol. Others are transported into organelles, such as mitochondria. Proteins destined for lysosomes, for incorporation into cell membranes, or for secretion from the cell are synthesized on ribosomes attached to the rough endoplasmic reticulum (RER). These proteins are transferred from the RER to the Golgi complex, where they are modified and targeted to their ultimate location.

Michael Sichel returned to the hematology clinic 1 month after being discharged from the hospital for his last sickle crisis. He has had no further symptoms suggestive of acute hemolysis and his hemoglobin has stabilized at 7.4 g/dL.

 Annie Myck, on her second visit, was found to have no improvement in her symptoms. Her hemoglobin level was 6.0 g/dL (reference range = 12–16 g/dL).

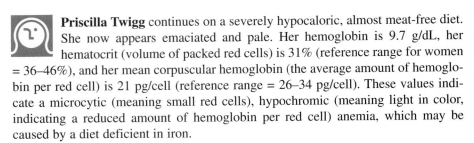 **Priscilla Twigg** continues on a severely hypocaloric, almost meat-free diet. She now appears emaciated and pale. Her hemoglobin is 9.7 g/dL, her hematocrit (volume of packed red cells) is 31% (reference range for women = 36–46%), and her mean corpuscular hemoglobin (the average amount of hemoglobin per red cell) is 21 pg/cell (reference range = 26–34 pg/cell). These values indicate a microcytic (meaning small red cells), hypochromic (meaning light in color, indicating a reduced amount of hemoglobin per red cell) anemia, which may be caused by a diet deficient in iron.

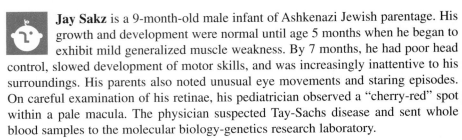 **Jay Sakz** is a 9-month-old male infant of Ashkenazi Jewish parentage. His growth and development were normal until age 5 months when he began to exhibit mild generalized muscle weakness. By 7 months, he had poor head control, slowed development of motor skills, and was increasingly inattentive to his surroundings. His parents also noted unusual eye movements and staring episodes. On careful examination of his retinae, his pediatrician observed a "cherry-red" spot within a pale macula. The physician suspected Tay-Sachs disease and sent whole blood samples to the molecular biology-genetics research laboratory.

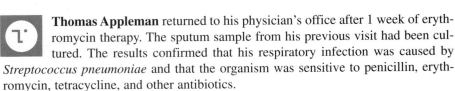 **Thomas Appleman** returned to his physician's office after 1 week of erythromycin therapy. The sputum sample from his previous visit had been cultured. The results confirmed that his respiratory infection was caused by *Streptococcus pneumoniae* and that the organism was sensitive to penicillin, erythromycin, tetracycline, and other antibiotics.

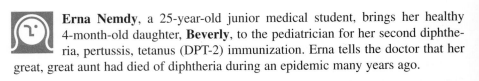 **Erna Nemdy**, a 25-year-old junior medical student, brings her healthy 4-month-old daughter, **Beverly**, to the pediatrician for her second diphtheria, pertussis, tetanus (DPT-2) immunization. Erna tells the doctor that her great, great aunt had died of diphtheria during an epidemic many years ago.

THE GENETIC CODE

Transcription, the transfer of the genetic message from DNA to RNA, is based on the rather simple concept of base-pairing. Translation, the transfer of the genetic message from the nucleotide language of the nucleic acids to the amino acid language of proteins, involves more complicated mechanisms, but also utilizes base-pairing as a key step.

In the late 1950s and early 1960s, molecular biologists attempting to decipher the process of translation recognized two problems. The first involved decoding the relationship between the "language" of the nucleic acids and the "language" of the proteins, and the second involved determining the molecular mechanism by which translation between these two languages occurred.

Twenty different amino acids are incorporated into proteins, and, therefore, there are 20 characters in the protein "alphabet." The nucleic acid alphabet has only four characters, corresponding to the four nucleotides of mRNA (A, G, C, and U). The cryptographers of molecular biology realized that if two nucleotides constituted the code for an amino acid, then only 4^2 or 16 amino acids could be specified. On the other hand, if four nucleotides constituted the code for an amino acid, vastly more amino acids (4^4 or 256) than actually occur in proteins could be specified. Therefore, the number of nucleotides that code for an amino acid was likely to be three, providing 4^3 or 64 possible combinations or "codons," more than required, but not overly excessive.

Scientists set out to determine the specific codons for each amino acid. The first crack in the genetic code (the collection of codons that specify all the amino acids found in proteins) was produced by Marshall Nirenberg in 1961. He showed that poly(U), a polynucleotide in which all the bases are uracil, produced polyphenylalanine in a cell-free protein-synthesizing system. Thus, UUU must be the codon for phenylalanine. As a result of experiments using synthetic polynucleotides in place of mRNA, other codons were identified by Nirenberg and also by H. Gobind Khorana.

The pioneering molecular biologists recognized that, because amino acids cannot bind directly to the sets of three nucleotides that form their codons, adapters are required. The adapters were found to be tRNA molecules. Each tRNA molecule contains an anticodon and covalently binds a specific amino acid at its 3'-end (see Chapters 11 and 13). The anticodon of a tRNA molecule is a set of three nucleotides that can interact with a codon on mRNA (Fig. 14.1). In order to interact, the codon and anticodon must be complementary (i.e., they must be able to form base pairs in an antiparallel orientation). Thus, the anticodon of a tRNA serves as the link between an mRNA codon and the amino acid that the codon specifies.

Obviously, each codon on mRNA must correspond to a specific amino acid. Nirenberg found that trinucleotides of known base sequence could bind to ribosomes and induce the binding of specific aminoacyl-tRNAs (i.e., tRNAs with amino acids covalently attached). As a result of these experiments and the earlier experiments by Nirenberg and Khorana, the relationship between all 64 codons and the amino acids they specify (the entire genetic code) was determined by the mid-1960s (Table 14.1).

Features of the Genetic Code

Three of the 64 possible codons (UGA, UAG, and UAA) were found to terminate protein synthesis and are known as "stop" or nonsense codons. The remaining 61

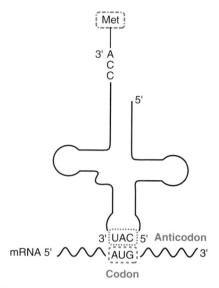

Fig. 14.1. Binding of tRNA to a codon on mRNA. The tRNA contains an amino acid at its 3'-end that corresponds to the codon on mRNA with which the anticodon of the tRNA can base-pair. Note that the codon-anticodon pairing is complementary and antiparallel.

Table 14.1. The Genetic Code

First Base (5')	Second Base				Third Base (3')
	U	C	A	G	
U	Phe	Ser	Tyr	Cys	U
	Phe	Ser	Tyr	Cys	C
	Leu	Ser	Stop	Stop	A
	Leu	Ser	Stop	Trp	G
C	Leu	Pro	His	Arg	U
	Leu	Pro	His	Arg	C
	Leu	Pro	Gln	Arg	A
	Leu	Pro	Gln	Arg	G
A	Ile	Thr	Asn	Ser	U
	Ile	Thr	Asn	Ser	C
	Ile	Thr	Lys	Arg	A
	Met	Thr	Lys	Arg	G
G	Val	Ala	Asp	Gly	U
	Val	Ala	Asp	Gly	C
	Val	Ala	Glu	Gly	A
	Val	Ala	Glu	Gly	G

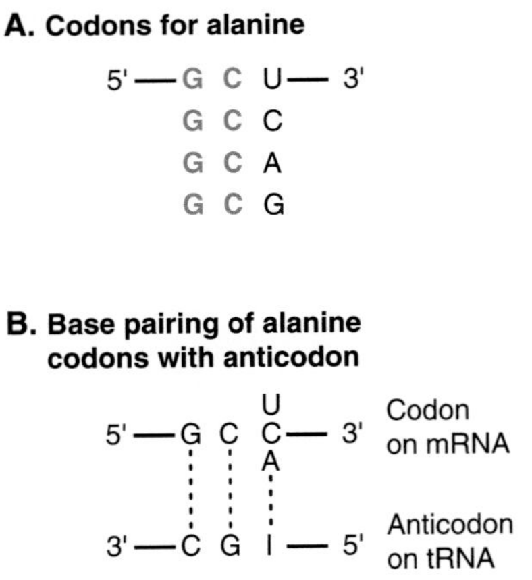

A. Codons for alanine

```
5' — G C U — 3'
    G C C
    G C A
    G C G
```

B. Base pairing of alanine codons with anticodon

```
          U
5' — G C  C — 3'   Codon
          A         on mRNA
     : : :
3' — C G  I — 5'   Anticodon
                    on tRNA
```

Fig. 14.2. Base-pairing of codons for alanine with 5′-IGC-3′. **A.** Note that the variation is in the third base. **B.** The first three of these codons can pair with a tRNA that contains the anticodon 5′-IGC-3′. Inosine (I) is an unusual nucleoside found in tRNA that can form base pairs with U, C, or A.

codons specify amino acids. Two amino acids each have only one codon (AUG = methionine; UGG = tryptophan). The remaining amino acids have multiple codons.

THE CODE IS DEGENERATE, BUT UNAMBIGUOUS

Because many amino acids are specified by more than one codon, the genetic code is described as "degenerate." The term "degenerate" is used in its precise mathematical sense. However, the more common term "redundant" might be more descriptive. Although an amino acid may have more than one codon, each codon specifies only one amino acid. Thus the genetic code is unambiguous.

Inspection of a codon table shows that in most instances of multiple codons for a single amino acid, the variation occurs in the third base of the codon (see Table 14.1). Crick noted that the pairing between the 3′-base of the codon and the 5′-base of the anticodon may not follow the strict base-pairing rules (i.e., A pairs with U, and G with C) that he and Watson had previously discovered. Crick called this concept the "wobble" hypothesis.

In eukaryotes, the 5′ position of the anticodon of tRNA often contains a modified base that is capable of pairing with more than one nucleotide. These modified bases provide an example of the wobble base-pairing rules. Inosine (I), one of the unusual nucleosides found in tRNA, can pair with U, C, or A. Three of the four codons for alanine (GCU, GCC, and GCA) can therefore pair with a single tRNA that contains the anticodon 5′-IGC-3′ (Fig. 14.2). Thus, fewer than 61 tRNA molecules are required to translate the genetic code, and, as a result of the degeneracy of the code, even if the last base in a codon pairs improperly, the correct amino acid is still often inserted into a growing polypeptide chain.

THE CODE IS ALMOST UNIVERSAL

All organisms studied so far use the same genetic code, with some rare exceptions. For example, in human mitochondria, UGA codes for tryptophan instead of serving as a stop codon, AUA codes for methionine instead of isoleucine, and CUA codes for threonine instead of leucine. Fewer than 10 exceptions to the code are known.

THE CODE IS NONOVERLAPPING AND WITHOUT PUNCTUATION

mRNA does not contain punctuation to separate one codon from the next, and the codons do not overlap. Each nucleotide is read only once. Beginning with a start codon (AUG) near the 5′-end of the mRNA, the codons are read sequentially, ending with a stop codon (UGA, UAG, or UAA) near the 3′-end of the mRNA.

RELATIONSHIP BETWEEN THE PROTEIN PRODUCT OF TRANSLATION AND THE mRNA

The start codon (AUG) sets the reading frame, the order in which the sequence of bases in the mRNA is sorted into codons (Fig. 14.3). The order of the codons in the mRNA determines the sequence in which amino acids are added to the growing polypeptide chain. Thus, the order of the codons in the mRNA determines the linear sequence of amino acids in the protein.

EFFECTS OF MUTATIONS

Mutations that result from damage to the nucleotides of DNA molecules or from unrepaired errors during replication (see Chapter 12) may be transcribed into mRNA, and, therefore, may result in the translation of a protein with an abnormal amino acid sequence. Various types of mutations can occur that have different effects on the encoded protein (Table 14.2).

Point Mutations

Point mutations occur when only one base in DNA is altered, producing a change in a single base of an mRNA codon.

SILENT MUTATIONS

Point mutations are said to be "silent" when they do not affect the amino acid sequence of the protein. For example, a codon change from CGA to CGG does not affect the protein because both of these codons specify arginine.

MISSENSE MUTATIONS

If the mutation causes one amino acid in the protein to be replaced by another, it is said to be a missense mutation. For example, a change from CGA to CCA causes arginine to be replaced by proline.

NONSENSE MUTATIONS

A nonsense mutation causes the premature termination of a polypeptide chain. For example, a codon change from CGA to UGA causes a codon for arginine to be replaced by a stop codon, and synthesis of the mutant protein terminates at this point.

Sickle cell anemia is caused by a missense mutation. In each of the alleles for β-globin, **Michael Sichel's** DNA has a single base change. In the sickle cell gene, GTG replaces the normal GAG. Thus, in the mRNA, the codon GUG replaces GAG and a valine residue replaces a glutamate residue in the protein.

Table 14.2. Types of Mutations

Type	Description	Example
Point	A single base change	
Silent	A change that specifies the same amino acid	CGA → CGG Arg → Arg
Missense	A change that specifies a different amino acid	CGA → CCA Arg → Pro
Nonsense	A change that produces a stop codon	CGA → UGA Arg → Stop
Insertion	An addition of one or more bases	
Deletion	A loss of one or more bases	

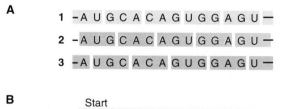

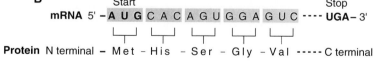

Fig. 14.3. Reading frame of mRNA. **A.** For any given mRNA sequence, there are three possible reading frames (1, 2, and 3). **B.** An AUG near the 5′-end of the mRNA (the start codon) sets the reading frame for translation of a protein from the mRNA. The codons are read in linear order, starting with this AUG. (The other potential reading frames are not used. They would give proteins with different amino acid sequences.)

Q 14.1: One type of thalassemia is caused by a nonsense mutation. Codon 17 of the β-globin chain is changed from UG**G** to UG**A**. This change results in the conversion of a codon for a tryptophan residue to a stop codon.

Is it likely that **Annie Myck** has this mutation in codon 17?

Q 14.2: Some types of thalassemia are caused by deletions in the globin genes. Patients have been studied who have large deletions in either the 5′ or the 3′ coding region of the β-globin gene, removing almost one third of the DNA sequence.

Is it likely that **Annie Myck** has a large deletion in the β-globin gene?

The results of tests performed in the molecular biology laboratory show that **Jay Sakz** has an insertion in exon 11 of the α-chain of the hexosaminidase A gene, the most common mutation found in patients of Ashkenazi Jewish background who have Tay-Sachs disease. (For more details, see the Problems section at the end of this chapter.)

Insertions

An insertion occurs when one or more nucleotides are added to DNA. If the insertion does not generate a stop codon, a protein with more amino acids than normal may be produced.

Deletions

When one or more nucleotides are removed from DNA, the mutation is known as a deletion. If the deletion does not affect the normal start and stop codons, a protein with fewer than the normal number of amino acids may be produced.

Frameshift Mutations

A frameshift mutation occurs when the number of inserted or deleted nucleotides is not a multiple of three (Fig. 14.4). The reading frame shifts after the insertion or deletion so that the bases are read in incorrect codons beyond that point.

FORMATION OF AMINOACYL-tRNA

A tRNA that contains an amino acid covalently attached to its 3′-end is called an aminoacyl-tRNA. Aminoacyl-tRNAs are named both for the amino acid and the tRNA that carries the amino acid (e.g., alanyl-tRNA^{Ala}). A particular tRNA recognizes only the AUG start codon that initiates protein synthesis and not other AUG codons that specify insertion of methionine within the polypeptide chain. This initiator methionyl-tRNA^{Met} is denoted by the subscript "i": methionyl-tRNA$_i^{Met}$.

Amino acids are attached to their tRNAs by highly specific enzymes known as aminoacyl-tRNA synthetases. Twenty different synthetases exist, one for each amino acid. Each synthetase recognizes a particular amino acid and all of the tRNAs that bind that amino acid.

The reaction catalyzed by an aminoacyl-tRNA synthetase occurs in two steps. In the first step, the amino acid is activated by reacting with ATP to form an enzyme/aminoacyl-AMP complex and pyrophosphate (Fig. 14.5). The pyrophosphate is cleaved by a pyrophosphatase, thus helping to drive the reaction by removing one of the products. In the second step, the activated amino acid is transferred to the 2′- or 3′-hydroxyl group of the CCA sequence at the 3′-end of the tRNA, and AMP is released.

A tRNA that carries an amino acid (an aminoacyl-tRNA) is said to be "charged." The energy in the aminoacyl-tRNA bond is subsequently used in the formation of a peptide bond during the process of protein synthesis.

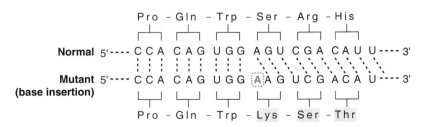

Fig. 14.4. A frameshift mutation. The insertion of a single nucleotide causes the reading frame to shift, so that the amino acid sequence of the protein translated from the mRNA is different after the point of insertion. A similar effect can result from the insertion or deletion of nucleotides if the number is not a multiple of 3.

Surprisingly, not all aminoacyl-tRNA synthetases use the anticodon of the tRNA as a recognition site during attachment of the amino acid to the tRNA (Fig. 14.6). Some recognize only bases at other positions in the tRNA. However, insertion of the amino acid into a growing polypeptide chain does depend solely on the bases of the anticodon, through complementary base-pairing with the mRNA codons.

PROCESS OF TRANSLATION

Translation of a protein involves three steps: initiation, elongation, and termination. It begins with the formation of the initiation complex. Subsequently, synthesis of the polypeptide occurs by a series of elongation steps that are repeated as each amino acid is added to the growing chain (Fig. 14.7). Termination occurs where the mRNA contains an in-frame stop codon, and the completed polypeptide chain is released.

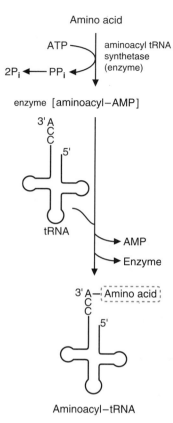

Fig. 14.5. Formation of aminoacyl-tRNA. The amino acid is first activated by reacting with ATP. The amino acid is then transferred from the aminoacyl-AMP to tRNA.

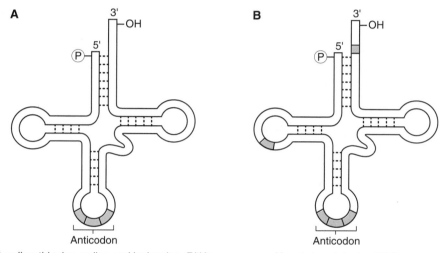

A E. coli methionine, valine and isoleucine tRNAs

B Yeast phenylalanine tRNA

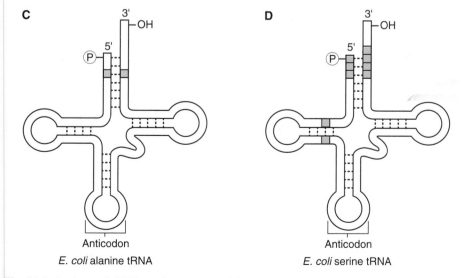

C E. coli alanine tRNA

D E. coli serine tRNA

Fig. 14.6. Aminoacyl-tRNA synthetase recognition sites on tRNA. The aminoacyl-tRNA synthetases recognize the indicated sites (blue). In some cases, the anticodon is a recognition site; in others, it is not.

A 14.1 and 14.2: A nonsense mutation at codon 17 would cause premature termination of translation. A nonfunctional peptide containing only 16 amino acids would result, producing a β^0-thalassemia if the mutation occurred in both alleles. A large deletion in the coding region of the gene could also produce a truncated protein. If **Annie Myck** has a nonsense mutation or a large deletion, it could only be in one allele. The mutation in the other allele must be milder. She produces some normal β-globin. Her hemoglobin is 6 g/dL, typical of thalassemia intermedia (a β^+-thalassemia).

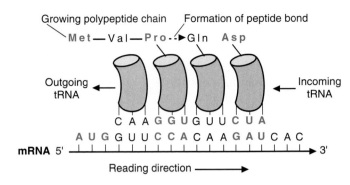

Fig. 14.7. Overview of the process of translation.

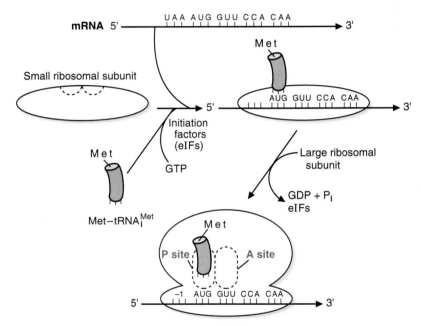

Fig. 14.8. Initiation of protein synthesis. P site = peptidyl site on the ribosome; A site = aminoacyl site on the ribosome.

Iron is required for the synthesis of heme, which regulates the synthesis of globin. In the absence of heme, the rate of initiation of globin synthesis decreases. Heme acts by inhibiting the phosphorylation of the initiation factor eIF2. When eIF2 is phosphorylated it is inactive, and protein synthesis is not initiated. Heme, by preventing phosphorylation of eIF2, keeps this initiation factor in its active state. Consequently, initiation can occur, and globin is synthesized. Globin combines with heme to form hemoglobin.

Priscilla Twigg has an iron deficiency anemia. Lack of iron in the diet causes a decrease in heme synthesis and, therefore, a decrease in globin synthesis. Consequently, blood levels of hemoglobin decrease, and an iron deficiency anemia results.

Initiation of Translation

In eukaryotes, initiation of translation involves formation of a complex composed of methionyl-tRNA$_i^{Met}$, mRNA, and a ribosome (Fig. 14.8). Methionyl-tRNA$_i^{Met}$ (also known as Met-tRNA$_i^{Met}$) initially forms a complex with an initiation factor (eukaryotic initiation factor 2 (eIF2)) and GTP. This complex then binds to the small (40S) ribosomal subunit. The cap at the 5′-end of the mRNA binds an initiation factor (eIF4E), known as the cap binding protein (CBP). Several other eIFs join, and the mRNA then binds to the 40S-Met-tRNA$_i^{Met}$ complex. In a reaction that requires hydrolysis of ATP, the small ribosomal subunit scans the mRNA until the first AUG codon is located. Other eIFs bind, GTP is hydrolyzed, the initiation factors are released, and the large ribosomal (60S) subunit binds. The ribosome is now complete. It contains one small and one large subunit. Two binding sites for tRNA, known as the P (peptidyl) and the A (aminoacyl) sites, are present on the ribosome. During initiation, Met-tRNA$_i^{Met}$ binds at the P site.

The initiation process differs for prokaryotes and eukaryotes (Table 14.3). In bacteria, the initiating methionyl-tRNA is formylated, producing a formyl-methionyl-$tRNA_f^{Met}$ that participates in formation of the initiation complex (Fig. 14.9). Only three IFs are required to generate this complex in prokaryotes, while eukaryotes require a dozen or more eIFs. The ribosomes also differ in size. Prokaryotes have 70S ribosomes, composed of 30S and 50S subunits, and eukaryotes have 80S ribosomes, composed of 40S and 60S subunits. Bacterial mRNA is not capped. Identification of the initiating AUG triplet in prokaryotes occurs as a consequence of binding of a sequence (known as the Shine-Dalgarno sequence) in the mRNA with a complementary sequence near the 3'-end of the 16S rRNA of the small ribosomal subunit.

Elongation of Polypeptide Chains

After the initiation complex is formed, addition of each amino acid to the growing polypeptide chain involves binding of an aminoacyl-tRNA to the A site on the ribosome, formation of a peptide bond, and translocation of the peptidyl-tRNA to the P site (Fig. 14.10). The peptidyl-tRNA contains the growing polypeptide chain.

BINDING OF AMINOACYL-tRNA TO THE A SITE

When $Met\text{-}tRNA_i$ (or a peptidyl-tRNA) is bound to the P site, the mRNA codon in the A site determines which aminoacyl-tRNA will bind to that site. An aminoacyl-tRNA binds when its anticodon is antiparallel and complementary to the mRNA codon. Before binding to the mRNA, the aminoacyl-tRNA first combines with GTP and an elongation factor (EF1α in eukaryotes and EF-Tu in prokaryotes) (Table 14.4). As the aminoacyl-tRNA binds to the A site, GTP is hydrolyzed, forming GDP.

The complex of GDP and the elongation factor (EF1α or EF-Tu) then binds another factor (EF1βγ in eukaryotes and EF-Ts in prokaryotes), allowing GDP to be released. GTP now binds, and the eukaryotic βγ or prokaryotic Ts dissociate, leaving the first elongation factor (EF1α in eukaryotes and EF-Tu in prokaryotes) bound to GTP, ready for another elongation cycle (Fig. 14.11).

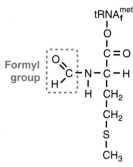

Fig. 14.9. Bacterial tRNA containing formyl-methionine. The initial methionine is not formylated in eukaryotic protein synthesis.

Many antibiotics that are used to combat bacterial infections in humans take advantage of the differences between the mechanisms for protein synthesis in prokaryotes and eukaryotes.

Streptomycin binds to the 30S ribosomal subunit of prokaryotes. It interferes with initiation of protein synthesis and causes misreading of mRNA.

Although the bacterium causing the infection was sensitive to streptomycin, this drug was not used to treat **Thomas Appleman** because it can cause permanent hearing loss. Its use is therefore confined mainly to the treatment of tuberculosis or other infections that do not respond adequately to other antibiotics.

Table 14.3. Differences between Eukaryotes and Prokaryotes in the Initiation of Protein Synthesis

	Eukaryotes	Prokaryotes
Binding of mRNA to small ribosomal subunit	Cap at 5'-end of mRNA binds to eIFs and 40S ribosomal subunit. mRNA is scanned for first AUG.	Shine-Dalgarno sequence upstream of initiating AUG binds to complementary sequence in 16S rRNA
First amino acid	Methionine	Formyl-methionine
Initiation factors	eIFs (12 or more)	IFs (3)
Ribosomes	80S (40 and 60S subunits)	70S (30 and 50S subunits)

Table 14.4. Differences between Eukaryotes and Prokaryotes in the Elongation of Polypeptide Chains

	Eukaryotes	Prokaryotes
First elongation factor	EF1α	EF-Tu
Factors involved in regenerating the first elongation factor	EFβγ	EF-Ts
Second elongation factor	EF2	EF-G

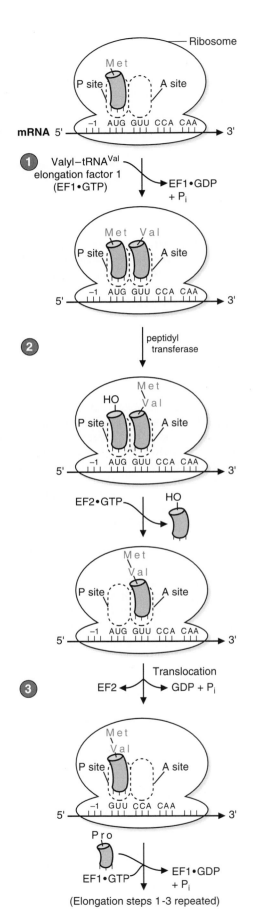

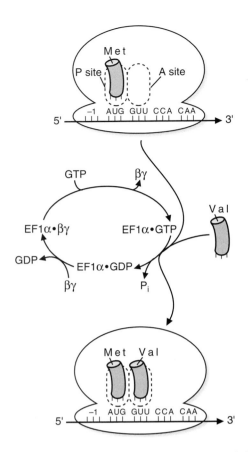

Fig. 14.11. Recycling of EF1. In prokaryotes, EF1α is EF-Tu and the protein corresponding to βγ is Ts.

Fig. 14.10. Elongation of a polypeptide chain. **1.** Binding of aminoacyl tRNA to the A site. **2.** Formation of a peptide bond. **3.** Translocation. The two steps shown in **3** occur simultaneously.

FORMATION OF A PEPTIDE BOND

The aminoacyl-tRNA in the A site now forms a peptide bond with the methionyl-tRNA in the P site in the first round of elongation (or the peptidyl-tRNA in subsequent rounds) (see Fig. 14.10). Peptidyltransferase, which is not a protein but the rRNA of the large ribosomal subunit, catalyzes the formation of the peptide bond. The tRNA in the A site now contains the growing polypeptide chain, and the tRNA in the P site is uncharged (i.e., it no longer contains any amino acids).

TRANSLOCATION

Translocation involves another elongation factor (EF2 in eukaryotes and EF-G in prokaryotes) that complexes with GTP and binds to the ribosome, causing a conformational change that moves the mRNA and its base-paired tRNAs with respect to the ribosome. The uncharged tRNA moves from the P site to a site known as the E (exit) site from which it is released from the ribosome. The peptidyl-tRNA moves into the P site and the next codon of the mRNA occupies the A site. During translocation, GTP is hydrolyzed to GDP, which is released from the ribosome along with the elongation factor (see Fig. 14.10).

Termination of Translation

The three elongation steps are repeated until a termination (stop) codon moves into the A site on the ribosome. Since no tRNAs with anticodons that can pair with stop codons normally exist in cells, release factors bind to the ribosome instead, causing peptidyltransferase to hydrolyze the bond between the peptide chain and tRNA. The newly synthesized polypeptide is released from the ribosome, which dissociates into its individual subunits, releasing the mRNA.

POLYSOMES

As one ribosome moves along the mRNA, producing a polypeptide chain, a second ribosome may bind to the vacant 5′-end of the mRNA. Many ribosomes can simultaneously translate a single mRNA, forming a complex known as a polysome (Fig. 14.12). A single ribosome covers about 80 nucleotides of an mRNA. Therefore, ribosomes are positioned on mRNA at intervals of about 100 nucleotides. The polypeptide chains attached to the ribosomes grow longer as each ribosome moves from the 5′-end toward the 3′-end of the mRNA.

POSTTRANSLATIONAL PROCESSING OF PROTEINS

As a polypeptide chain is produced on a ribosome, it travels through a tunnel in the ribosome. The tunnel can hold about 30 amino acid residues. As polymerization of the chain progresses, the amino acid residues at the N-terminal end begin to emerge from this protected region within the ribosome and to fold into the three-dimensional conformation of the polypeptide.

Proteins bind to a nascent polypeptide (i.e., a polypeptide that is in the process of being synthesized) and mediate the folding process. These mediators are called chaperones because they prevent improper interactions from occurring. Disulfide bond formation between cysteine residues may also be involved in producing the three-dimensional structure of the polypeptide.

Enzymes can act on the nascent polypeptide, modifying selected residues (Table 14.5). The N-terminal methionine is usually removed by proteases. Other cleavages may also occur.

The antibiotic tetracycline binds to the 30S ribosomal subunit of prokaryotes and inhibits binding of aminoacyl-tRNA to the A site of the ribosome.

The bacterium causing **Thomas Appleman's** infection was found to be sensitive to tetracycline.

Chloramphenicol is an antibiotic that interferes with the peptidyltransferase activity of the 50S ribosomal subunit of bacteria. It was not used to treat **Thomas Appleman** because it is very toxic to humans, in part as a consequence of its effect on mitochondrial protein synthesis.

Erythromycin binds to the 50S ribosomal subunit of bacteria and inhibits translocation. This antibiotic was used to treat **Thomas Appleman** because he had taken it previously without difficulty. Erythromycin has less serious side effects than many other antibiotics and is used as an alternative drug in patients, such as Mr. Appleman, who are allergic to penicillin. After 1 week of erythromycin therapy, Mr. Appleman recovered from his infection.

Diphtheria is a highly contagious disease caused by a toxin secreted by the bacterium *Corynebacterium diphtheriae*. Although the toxin is a protein, it is not produced by a bacterial gene, but by a gene brought into the bacterial cell by an infecting bacteriophage.

Diphtheria toxin is composed of two subunits. The B subunit binds to a cell surface receptor, facilitating the entry of the A subunit into the cell. After the A subunit of the toxin enters human cells, it catalyzes a reaction in which ADP-ribose (ADPR) from nicotinamide-adenine dinucleotide (NAD) covalently binds to EF2. ADPR is attached by this reaction to a modified histidine residue, known as diphthamide, in the protein EF2. This modification of EF2 inhibits protein synthesis, leading to cell death. Children, such as **Erna Nemdy's** daughter **Beverly**, are usually immunized against this often fatal disease at an early age.

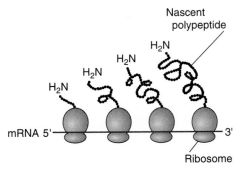

Fig. 14.12. A polysome. The complex of mRNA and multiple ribosomes, each of which is producing a polypeptide chain, is called a polysome.

Amino acid residues may be modified by the addition of various types of functional groups. The N-terminal amino acid is sometimes acetylated. Methyl groups may be added to lysine residues. Proline and lysine residues may be modified by hydroxylation, particularly in collagen. Carboxylations are important, particularly for the function of proteins involved in blood coagulation. Fatty acids may be added, providing hydrophobic regions that anchor the proteins in membranes. An ADPR group may be transferred from NAD to certain proteins. The addition and removal of phosphate groups (which bind covalently to serine, threonine, and tyrosine residues) serve to alter the activity of many proteins (e.g., the enzymes of glycogen synthesis and degradation). Glycosylation, the addition of carbohydrate groups, is a common modification that occurs mainly on proteins that are destined to be secreted or incorporated into membranes.

TARGETING OF PROTEINS TO SUBCELLULAR ORGANELLES, MEMBRANES, AND THE EXTRACELLULAR ENVIRONMENT

Many proteins are synthesized on polysomes in the cytosol. After they are released from ribosomes, they remain in the cytosol where they carry out their functions. Other proteins synthesized on cytosolic ribosomes enter mitochondria. These proteins have an amino acid sequence at the N-terminal end that facilitates their transport across the mitochondrial membranes.

Some proteins enter the RER as they are being synthesized (Fig. 14.13). These proteins have sequences composed of hydrophobic amino acid residues at the N-terminus known as signal sequences, 20–25 amino acids in length. A signal recognition particle (SRP) binds to the ribosome and to the signal sequence as the nascent polypeptide emerges from the tunnel in the ribosome, and translation ceases. When the SRP subsequently binds to an SRP receptor or docking protein on the RER, translation resumes, and the polypeptide begins to enter the lumen of the RER. The signal sequence is removed by a peptidase, and the remainder of the newly synthesized protein is transferred in small vesicles to the Golgi complex. Glycosylation of the protein may occur in the lumen of the RER and in the interior of the Golgi complex.

Proteins produced on the RER eventually appear within lysosomes and secretory vesicles (Fig. 14.14). A phosphomannose residue added to lysosomal enzymes targets them to lysosomes. Clusters of hydrophobic residues in proteins cause them to attach to cellular membranes. Proteins in secretory vesicles are ultimately extruded into the extracellular space from the cell by a process known as exocytosis. Those with hydrophobic regions may remain attached to the cell membrane, becoming cell membrane proteins.

Table 14.5. Some Common Posttranslational Modifications of Amino Acid Residues in Proteins

Acetylation	Fatty acylation
Methylation	ADP-ribosylation
Hydroxylation	Phosphorylation
Carboxylation	Glycosylation

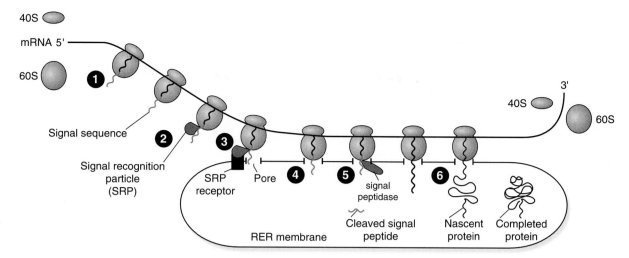

Fig. 14.13. Synthesis of proteins on the RER. **1.** Translation of the protein begins in the cytosol. **2.** As the signal sequence emerges from the ribosome, a signal recognition particle (SRP) binds to it and to the ribosome and inhibits further synthesis of the protein. **3.** The SRP binds to the SRP receptor in the RER membrane, docking the ribosome on the RER. **4.** The SRP is released and protein synthesis resumes. **5.** As the signal sequence moves through a pore into the RER, a signal peptidase removes the signal sequence. **6.** Synthesis of the nascent protein continues, and the completed protein is released into the lumen of the RER.

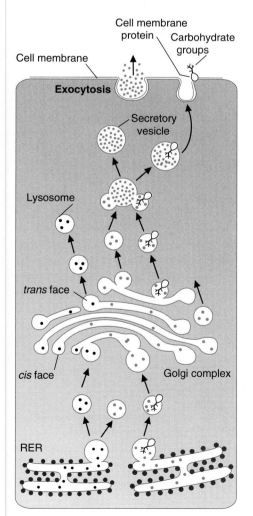

Fig. 14.14. Fate of proteins synthesized on the RER. Proteins synthesized on ribosomes attached to the ER travel in vesicles to the *cis* face of the Golgi complex. After the membranes fuse, the proteins enter the Golgi complex and bud from the *trans* face of the Golgi complex in vesicles. These vesicles may become lysosomes or secretory vesicles, depending on their contents. Secretory proteins are released from the cell when secretory vesicles fuse with the cell membrane (exocytosis). Proteins with hydrophobic regions embedded in the membrane of secretory vesicles may become cell membrane proteins. See Chapter 10 for descriptions of the endoplasmic reticulum, Golgi complex, lysosomes, and the cell membrane, and also for explanations of the process of exocytosis.

CLINICAL COMMENTS. The molecular biology-genetics research laboratory's report on **Jay Sakz's** white blood cells revealed that he had a deficiency of hexosaminidase A caused by a defect in the gene encoding the α subunit of this enzyme (variant B, Tay-Sachs disease). Hexosaminidases are lysosomal enzymes necessary for the normal degradation of glycosphingolipids, such as the gangliosides. Gangliosides are found in high concentrations in neural ganglia, although they are produced in many areas of the nervous system. Their function in cell membranes is not well established. When the activity of these degradative enzymes is absent or subnormal, partially degraded gangliosides accumulate in lysosomes in various cells of the central nervous system, causing a wide array of neurological disorders known collectively as gangliosidoses. When the enzyme deficiency is severe, symptoms appear within the first 3–5 months of life. Eventually symptoms include upper and lower motor neuron deficits, visual difficulties which may progress to blindness, seizures, and increasing cognitive dysfunction. By the second year of life, the patient may regress into a completely vegetative state, often succumbing to bronchopneumonia caused by aspiration or an inability to cough.

Priscilla Twigg has a moderately severe anemia, probably secondary to an inadequate dietary intake of iron, yet she is relatively asymptomatic. People can often tolerate even serious reductions in the oxygen transport capacity of the blood if the drop in hemoglobin has occurred over a long period of time. In symptomatic persons, however, fatigue, palpitations, shortness of breath on minimal exertion, and dizziness on standing upright may accompany an anemia of any etiology and are not characteristic of an iron deficiency anemia per se.

With the availability of diphtheria toxoid as part of the almost universal DPT immunization practices in the United States, fatalities due to infection by the Gram-positive bacillus *C. diphtheriae* are rare. Most children, as is the case with **Erna Nemdy's** daughter **Beverly**, are immunized. In unimmunized subjects, however, symptoms are caused by a bacterial exotoxin encoded by a phage that infects the bacterial cells. The toxin enters human cells, inhibiting protein synthesis and, ultimately, causing cell death. Complications related to cardiac and nervous system involvement are the major cause of morbidity and mortality. For documented cases of diphtheria, one of the mainstays of treatment is the use of equine diphtheria antitoxin.

BIOCHEMICAL COMMENTS. Many compounds have been discovered that serve as antibiotics by inhibiting protein synthesis. The processes of translation on bacterial ribosomes and on the cytoplasmic ribosomes of eukaryotic cells have many similarities, but there are a number of subtle differences. Many antibiotics act at steps where these differences occur (Table 14.6). Therefore, these compounds can be used selectively to prevent bacterial protein synthesis and inhibit bacterial proliferation, while having little or no effect on human cells. Caution

Table 14.6. Inhibitors of Protein Synthesis in Prokaryotes

Antibiotic	Mode of Action
Streptomycin	Binds to the 30S ribosomal subunit of prokaryotes, thereby preventing formation of the initiation complex. It also causes misreading of mRNA
Tetracycline	Binds to the 30S ribosomal subunit and inhibits binding of aminoacyl-tRNA to the A site
Chloramphenicol	Binds to the 50S ribosomal subunit and inhibits peptidyltransferase
Erythromycin	Binds to the 50S ribosomal subunit and prevents translocation

must be exercised in their use, however, because some of the antibiotics affect human mitochondria, which have a protein-synthesizing system similar to that of bacteria. Another problem with these drugs is that bacteria can become resistant to their action. Mutations in genes encoding the proteins or RNA of bacterial ribosomes can cause resistance. Resistance also results when bacteria take up plasmids carrying genes for inactivation of the antibiotic. Because of the widespread and often indiscriminate use of antibiotics, strains of bacteria are rapidly developing that are resistant to all known antibiotics.

Each of the major steps of protein synthesis can be inhibited by antibiotics. **Streptomycin** inhibits initiation by binding to three proteins and probably the 16S rRNA of the 30S ribosomal subunit of bacteria. Abnormal initiation complexes, known as streptomycin monosomes, accumulate. Streptomycin can also cause misreading of mRNA, resulting in the incorporation of incorrect amino acids into polypeptide chains that already have been initiated.

Tetracycline binds to the 30S ribosomal subunit of bacteria and prevents an aminoacyl-tRNA from binding to the A site on the ribosome. This effect of the drug is reversible, thus when the drug is removed, bacteria resume protein synthesis and growth, resulting in a rekindling of the infection. Furthermore, tetracycline is not absorbed well from the intestine and its concentration may become elevated in the contents of the gut, leading to changes in the intestinal flora. Because it has been used to treat human infections and, as an additive to animal feed, to prevent animal infections, humans have had extensive exposure to tetracycline. As a result, resistant strains of bacteria have developed.

Chloramphenicol binds to the 50S ribosomal subunit of bacteria and prevents binding of the amino acid portion of the aminoacyl-tRNA, effectively inhibiting peptidyltransferase action. This antibiotic is used only for certain extremely serious infections, such as meningitis and typhoid fever. Chloramphenicol readily enters human mitochondria where it inhibits protein synthesis. Cells of the bone marrow may fail to develop in patients treated with chloramphenicol, and use of this antibiotic has been linked to fatal blood dyscrasias, including an aplastic anemia.

Erythromycin binds to the 50S ribosomal subunit of bacteria near the binding site for chloramphenicol. Erythromycin prevents the translocation step, the movement of the peptidyl-tRNA from the "A" to the "P" site on the ribosome. Because its side effects are less severe and more readily reversible than those of many other antibiotics, erythromycin is often used to treat infections in persons who are allergic to penicillin, an antibiotic that inhibits bacterial cell wall synthesis.

Suggested Readings

Translation:

Lewin B. Genes V. Part 2. Translation: expressing genes as proteins. Oxford: Oxford University Press, 1994:161–276.

Tay-Sachs:

Gravel R, Clarke J, Kaback M, et al. The Gm_2 gangliosidoses. In: Scriver C, Beaudet A, Sly W, Valle D (eds): The metabolic and molecular bases of inherited disease. Vol II. New York: McGraw-Hill, 1995:2839–2879.

Thalassemia:

Weatherall D, Clegg J, Higgs D, Wood W. The hemoglobinopathies. In: Scriver C, Beaudet A, Sly W, Valle D (eds): The metabolic and molecular bases of inherited disease. Vol III. New York: McGraw-Hill, 1995:3417–3484.

Antibiotics that inhibit protein synthesis:

Gilman A, Rall T, Nies A, Taylor P. Goodman and Gilman's the pharmacological basis of therapeutics. New York: McGraw-Hill, 1990:1098–1145.

PROBLEMS

A ganglioside (G_{M2}) accumulates in Tay-Sachs disease because a lysosomal enzyme is defective. This enzyme is the β-hexosaminidase A that normally cleaves *N*-acetyl-galactosamine from the ganglioside. Because the G_{M2} ganglioside cannot be further degraded in Tay-Sachs disease, it accumulates in residual bodies (vacuoles that contain material that lysosomal enzymes cannot digest).

Normal cells contain some residual bodies. When a lysosomal enzyme is defective, however, large numbers of residual bodies accumulate, interfering with cell function. In Tay-Sachs disease, cells become packed with residual bodies, which ultimately cause death.

In 70% of the cases of Tay-Sachs disease in persons of Ashkenazi Jewish background, exon 11 of the gene for the α-chain of β-hexoaminidase A contains a mutation. Normally, this region of the gene would produce the amino acid sequence

Arg - Ile - Ser - Tyr - Gly - Pro - Asp

The normal gene sequence that codes for these amino acids is given below along with the gene sequence for the mutation.

```
         •      10      •      20
5′ C G T A T A T C C T A T G G C C C T G A C 3′      (Normal)

5′ C G T A T A T C T A T C C T A T G G C C C 3′      (Mutant)
```

(Dots mark every fifth base, and numbers every tenth base in this region of the gene.)

1. What kind of mutation causes Tay-Sachs disease?

2. What differences would be found in the amino acid sequences of proteins produced from the mutant gene and from the normal gene?

ANSWERS

1. In the mutant gene, a 4-base insertion occurs after the first 8 bases of the normal gene sequence. Note that positions 13–21 of the mutant sequence are the same as positions 9–17 of the normal gene. In fact, the only difference between the genes is the 4-base insert.

2. The normal gene encodes the amino acid sequence,

Arg - Ile - Ser - Tyr - Gly - Pro - Asp

while the mutant gene, because of the 4-base insert that causes a frameshift, encodes

Arg - Ile - Ser - Ile - Leu - Trp - Pro - [Stop]

Thus, the amino acid sequence encoded by the mutant differs from the normal gene in this region. Also, the mutant peptide is much shorter than the normal polypeptide because the 4-base insertion causes a premature stop codon to appear in the reading frame. (Positions 22, 23, and 24 of the Tay-Sachs gene are the same as positions 18, 19, and 20 of the normal gene.)

15 Regulation of Gene Expression

Gene expression is controlled by complex mechanisms. Prokaryotes regulate expression of genes mainly at the transcriptional level through genetic units known as operons. An operon consists of a set of genes that produce a series of proteins under the control of a single promoter (or regulatory region). Regulatory proteins bind to the promoter and facilitate or inhibit the binding of RNA polymerase.

Eukaryotic genes are not organized in operons. Instead, each gene for a polypeptide chain is controlled by its own promoter. Regulation of gene expression occurs at the level of DNA by chemical modification of bases, by gene loss or amplification, and by gene rearrangement. Regulation also occurs at the level of transcription, during the processing of RNA, or during RNA transport from the nucleus to the cytoplasm. Additional regulatory mechanisms operate in the cytoplasm at the level of translation.

Regulation can occur simultaneously at multiple levels for a specific gene, and many factors act in concert to stimulate or inhibit expression of a gene.

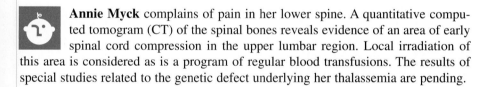

Annie Myck complains of pain in her lower spine. A quantitative computed tomogram (CT) of the spinal bones reveals evidence of an area of early spinal cord compression in the upper lumbar region. Local irradiation of this area is considered as is a program of regular blood transfusions. The results of special studies related to the genetic defect underlying her thalassemia are pending.

The course of **Arlyn Foma's** follicular lymphoma appears to be evolving into a more aggressive process. His disease is not responding well to his current multidrug chemotherapy which includes doxorubicin (adriamycin), vincristine, cyclophosphamide, and methotrexate (AV/CM). Because recombinant interferon α-2b has been reported to have synergistic or additive effects with these agents, it is added to the protocol. Although resistance to methotrexate is considered, the drug is continued as part of the combined therapeutic approach.

To determine the cause of **Priscilla Twigg's** hypochromic, microcytic anemia, a serum ferritin level (cellular storage form of iron) is ordered and is found to be subnormal (6 ng/mL, normal range = 12–150 ng/mL). The total plasma iron-binding capacity or transferrin level (transferrin is the iron transport protein in plasma) is greater than normal (510 mg/dL, reference range = 220–440 mg/dL). The transferrin iron saturation calculated from these values is less than 15% (normal = 20–55%). This laboratory profile is consistent with an iron deficiency state but does not establish whether or not the deficiency is the result of iron loss (e.g., bleeding) or of a deficient iron uptake. The history of anorexia nervosa strongly suggests a dietary deficiency of iron as the cause of anemia in this patient.

Q 15.1: Calculate the number of proteins, 300 amino acids in length, that could be produced from the *E. coli* genome (4 × 10⁶ base pairs of DNA).

Stem cells in the bone marrow normally differentiate and mature in a highly selective and regulated manner, becoming red blood cells or white blood cells. Various medical problems can affect this process. In patients such as **Annie Myck**, who have a deficiency of red blood cells, the conversion of precursor cells into mature cells is stimulated to compensate for the anemia. In patients such as **Mannie Weitzels**, who have a chronic myelogenous leukemia (CML), a single line of primitive myeloid cells produces leukemic cells that proliferate abnormally, causing a large increase in the number of white blood cells in the circulation.

Mannie Weitzels is a 56-year-old male who complains of headaches, weight loss related to a declining appetite for food, and a decreasing tolerance for exercise. He notes discomfort and fullness in the left upper quadrant of his abdomen. On physical examination he is noted to be pale and to have ecchymoses (bruises) on his arms and legs. His spleen is markedly enlarged.

Initial laboratory studies reveal a hemoglobin of 10.4 g/dL (normal = 13.5–17.5 g/dL) and a leukocyte (white blood cell) count of 86,000 cells/mm³ (normal = 4,500–11,000 cells/mm³). The majority of leukocytes are granulocytes, some of which have an "immature" appearance. The percentage of lymphocytes in the peripheral blood is decreased. A bone marrow aspiration and biopsy show the presence of an abnormal chromosome (the Philadelphia chromosome) in dividing marrow cells.

GENE EXPRESSION IS REGULATED FOR ADAPTATION, DEVELOPMENT, AND DIFFERENTIATION

Although most cells of an organism contain identical sets of genes, at any given time, only a small number of the total genes in a cell are expressed. The remaining genes are inactive. Organisms gain a number of advantages by regulating the activity of their genes. Both prokaryotic and eukaryotic cells adapt to changes in their environment by turning the expression of genes on and off. Because the process of RNA transcription and protein synthesis consumes a considerable amount of energy, cells conserve fuel by making proteins only when they are needed.

In addition to adapting to environmental changes, eukaryotic organisms regulate the expression of their genes during periods of development. As a fertilized egg becomes a multicellular organism, many different kinds of proteins are synthesized, in varying quantities. In the human, as the child progresses into adolescence and then into adulthood, the physical and physiological changes that occur are the result of variations in gene expression and, therefore, of protein synthesis. Even after an organism has reached the adult stage, regulation of gene expression enables certain cells to undergo differentiation in order to assume new functions.

REGULATION OF GENE EXPRESSION IN PROKARYOTES

Prokaryotes are single-celled organisms and, therefore, require less complex regulatory mechanisms than the multicellular eukaryotes (Fig. 15.1). The most extensively studied prokaryote is the bacterium *Escherichia coli*, an organism that thrives in the human colon, enjoying a symbiotic relationship with its host. All *E. coli* cells are morphologically similar and contain an identical circular chromosome.

In *E. coli* and other prokaryotes, DNA is not complexed with histones, and no nuclear envelope separates the genes from the contents of the cytoplasm. Gene transcripts do not contain introns, and mRNA does not contain a cap or a poly(A) tail. In fact, as mRNA is being synthesized, ribosomes bind and begin to produce proteins, so that transcription and translation occur simultaneously (Fig. 15.2).

Based on the size of its genome (4 × 10⁶ base pairs), *E. coli* should be capable of making several thousand proteins. However, under normal growth conditions, the cells are only making about 600–800 different proteins. Obviously, many genes are normally inactive.

Operons

In bacteria, the genes for proteins that are involved in performing a specific function are often grouped together in the genome in units known as operons. The genes in an

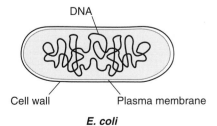

Fig. 15.1. *E. coli* cell. In prokaryotes, the DNA is not separated from the rest of the cellular contents by a nuclear envelope.

operon are coordinately expressed, that is, they are either all "turned on" or all "turned off." When an operon is expressed, all of its genes are transcribed. A single polycistronic mRNA is produced which codes for all the proteins of the operon. This polycistronic mRNA contains multiple sets of start and stop codons that allow a number of different proteins to be produced from this single transcript at the translational level (Fig. 15.3).

The genes for the proteins produced by an operon are called structural genes. The transcription of structural genes is regulated by a promoter which is located at the 5'-end of the operon, upstream from the genes for the proteins. Many of the mechanisms for regulation of protein synthesis affect the binding of RNA polymerase to the promoter and, thus, act at the level of initiation of transcription. Some regulatory proteins bind at or near the promoter and either stimulate or inhibit the binding of RNA polymerase. In positive control, regulatory proteins stimulate transcription. In negative control, regulatory proteins inhibit transcription.

Transcription of operons is also controlled by sigma (σ) factors that bind to RNA polymerase, causing it to recognize and bind more readily to certain promoters. Other mechanisms attenuate mRNA transcription that is already underway. Many of these regulatory mechanisms may be superimposed, acting on a single operon to allow it to respond rapidly to changing conditions.

Gene Control as a Response to Changes in the Environment

In order to grow, *E. coli* cells need a source of nitrogen and a source of carbon. Their normal carbon source is glucose, which serves as a precursor for the biosynthesis of all 20 amino acids required for protein synthesis. Glucose is also oxidized via glycolysis and the tricarboxylic acid (TCA) cycle to CO_2 and H_2O, producing energy in the form of ATP. The enzymes for oxidizing glucose are produced constitutively, that is, they are constantly being made.

If glucose in the growth medium is replaced by the milk sugar lactose, *E. coli* cells can adapt and begin to produce the enzymes required to convert lactose into compounds that can be oxidized via the pathways for glucose utilization. Synthesis of the enzymes for metabolism of lactose is turned on (Fig. 15.4).

A conceptually similar process occurs when the nitrogen source in the growth medium is replaced with a mixture of amino acids. Now *E. coli* cells no longer need to produce the enzymes required for the synthesis of the amino acids, so the synthesis of these enzymes is turned off. For instance, five enzymes are required for the synthesis of the amino acid tryptophan. When a ready-made source of tryptophan is available, *E. coli* cells save energy by no longer making the enzymes required for tryptophan biosynthesis.

Regulation by Proteins That Bind to the Operon

Proteins bind to regulatory regions of the operon and either prevent or facilitate the binding of RNA polymerase to the promoter, thereby inhibiting or stimulating transcription. When an operon is transcribed, the proteins it encodes are produced. When

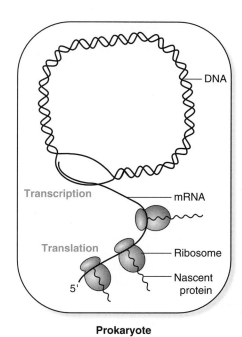

Prokaryote

Fig. 15.2. Simultaneous transcription and translation in bacteria. As transcription occurs, ribosomes bind to the mRNA and translation begins.

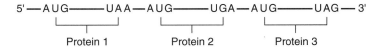

Fig. 15.3. Polycistronic mRNA of bacteria. The genes of an operon are transcribed as one long mRNA. During translation, start (AUG) and stop (UAA, UGA, UAG) codons cause a number of different proteins to be produced from this mRNA.

A 15.1: Four million base pairs contain $4 \times 10^6/3$ or 1.33 million codons. If each protein contained about 300 amino acids, *E. coli* could produce about 4,000 proteins (1.33 $\times 10^6/300$).

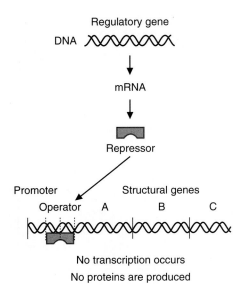

Fig. 15.5. Regulation of operons by repressors. When the repressor is bound to the operator, RNA polymerase cannot bind, and transcription, therefore, does not occur.

it is not transcribed, the proteins are not produced. (The proteins encoded by a gene are often called gene products.)

INHIBITION OF RNA POLYMERASE BINDING

Regulatory proteins known as repressors control operons by inhibiting the binding of RNA polymerase. A gene that is not part of the operon encodes the repressor. The repressor binds to a region of the operon it regulates known as an operator. The operator is located near the 3′-end of the promoter. When a repressor is bound to the operator, the operon is not transcribed because the repressor blocks the binding of RNA polymerase to the promoter (Fig. 15.5). Repressors act by two types of mechanisms: induction and repression.

Induction

Induction involves a small molecule, known as an inducer, that stimulates expression of the operon. In the absence of the inducer, an inducible operon binds its repressor, and the genes of the operon are not expressed. The genes are turned on when the inducer is present. The inducer binds to the repressor, changing the conformation of the repressor so that it does not bind very readily to the operator. When the repressor is not bound to the operator, the promoter is free and RNA polymerase can bind to it and transcribe the operon (Fig. 15.6).

Repression

Operons regulated by repression are expressed until small molecules known as corepressors enter the cell. The corepressor binds to the repressor, activating it. The repressor-corepressor complex then binds to the operator and prevents binding of RNA polymerase. As a result, the structural genes no longer produce proteins (Fig. 15.7).

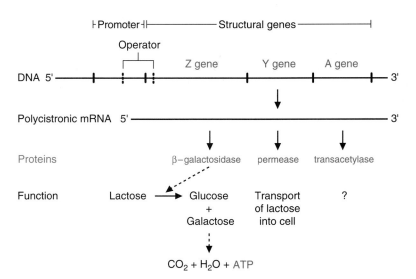

Fig. 15.4. The protein products of the *lac* operon. The permease causes the cell to take up lactose more readily, and the β-galactosidase cleaves lactose to glucose and galactose, which can be oxidized by the cell for energy. The function of the product of the A gene (the transacetylase) is unknown (?).

A. In the absence of inducer

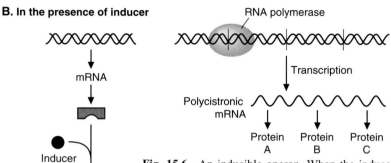

The lactose *(lac)* operon in *E. coli* is regulated by induction. When the cells are exposed to glucose and lactose is not present, the *lac* repressor has no inducer bound and, therefore, is active. The repressor binds to the operator, and the genes of the operon are not expressed. However, when the cells do not have a supply of glucose, but lactose is present, a metabolite of lactose (allolactose) serves as an inducer, binding to the repressor and inactivating it. The inactive repressor no longer binds to the operator. RNA polymerase now can bind to the promoter and transcribe the three structural genes of the operon (Z, Y, and A), producing a polycistronic mRNA that codes for three proteins (see Fig. 15.4).

B. In the presence of inducer

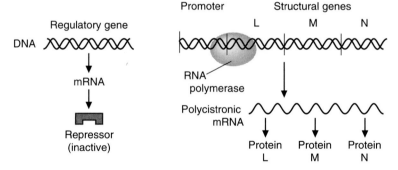

Fig. 15.6. An inducible operon. When the inducer is not present, the repressor binds to the operator. RNA polymerase cannot bind and transcription does not occur. When the inducer is present, the inducer binds to the repressor, inactivating it. The inactive repressor does not bind to the operator. Therefore, RNA polymerase can bind to the promoter region and transcribe the structural genes.

The protein product of the Z gene is a β-galactosidase that cleaves lactose, producing glucose and galactose. Glucose and galactose can then be oxidized by the cell for energy. The Y gene produces a lactose permease that increases the transport of lactose into the cell. The function of the transacetylase produced by the A gene has not yet been determined.

A. In the absence of the corepressor

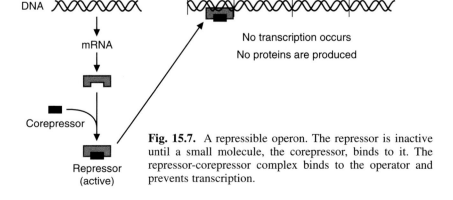

B. In the presence of the corepressor

Fig. 15.7. A repressible operon. The repressor is inactive until a small molecule, the corepressor, binds to it. The repressor-corepressor complex binds to the operator and prevents transcription.

The tryptophan *(trp)* operon is regulated by repression. Normally, when *E. coli* cells do not have a source of amino acids, the *trp* operon is expressed, producing enzymes that allow the cells to synthesize tryptophan. However, when tryptophan is supplied to the cells, this amino acid binds to the inactive repressor, causing it to change conformation so that it becomes active, binds to the operator, and inhibits expression of the operon. Because the cells have a supply of tryptophan, it would be a waste of energy to produce the enzymes for its synthesis.

STIMULATION OF RNA POLYMERASE BINDING

In addition to regulating transcription by means of repressors that prevent the binding of RNA polymerase to promoters, bacteria regulate transcription by means of proteins that stimulate the binding of RNA polymerase to promoters. For example, the *ara* operon is regulated by a protein (AraC) that binds to a region near the promoter of the operon. When glucose is absent but the sugar arabinose is present, arabinose binds to AraC. This complex of AraC and arabinose stimulates binding of RNA polymerase to the promoter of the ara operon. The operon is transcribed, and the enzymes that allow the cells to metabolize arabinose to obtain energy are produced (Fig. 15.8).

CATABOLITE REPRESSION

Some operons, particularly those that enable cells to produce enzymes that metabolize sugars other than glucose, cannot be turned on when glucose is present. In effect, glucose "represses" these operons by a process called catabolite repression (Fig. 15.9).

Changes in glucose concentration affect the cellular levels of cyclic AMP (cAMP) by a mechanism that is not well understood. However, as glucose levels decrease, cAMP levels rise. cAMP binds to a protein known as the cAMP receptor protein (CRP) (or the catabolite activator protein (CAP)). The cAMP-CRP complex binds to a regulatory region of the operon, stimulating the binding of RNA polymerase to the promoter, and transcription occurs.

When glucose is present, cAMP levels decrease. CRP assumes an inactive conformation if cAMP is not bound to it. Consequently, CRP does not bind to the operon, and transcription does not occur.

The *lac, ara,* and *gal* operons are subject to catabolite repression. The enzymes for metabolism of lactose, arabinose, and galactose are not produced if cells have an adequate supply of glucose even if these alternative energy sources are present at very high levels.

Regulation by Sigma Factors

E. coli has only one RNA polymerase. Sigma factors bind to this RNA polymerase, stimulating its binding to certain sets of promoters. The standard sigma factor in *E. coli* is σ^{70}, a protein with a molecular weight of 70,000 daltons. Another sigma factor,

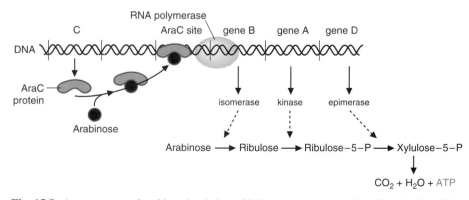

Fig. 15.8. An operon regulated by stimulation of RNA polymerase binding. The binding of the AraC-arabinose complex to the regulatory region of the operon stimulates binding of RNA polymerase to the promoter. RNA polymerase transcribes the structural genes of the operon, and proteins are produced that permit cells to oxidize arabinose to obtain energy.

A. In the presence of inducer and glucose

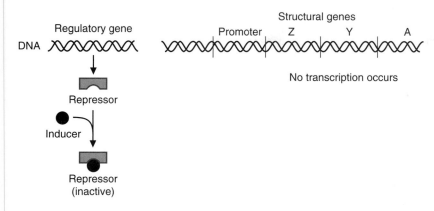

B. In the presence of inducer and absence of glucose

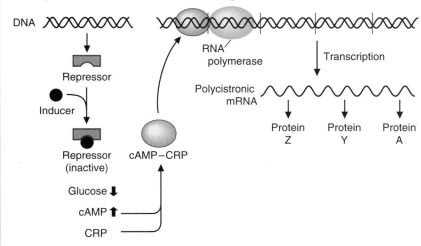

Fig. 15.9. Catabolite repression. The *lac* operon is used as an example. **A.** The inducer allolactose (a metabolite of lactose) inactivates the repressor. However, no transcription occurs unless glucose is absent. **B.** In the absence of glucose, cAMP levels rise. cAMP forms a complex with the cAMP receptor protein (CRP). The binding of the cAMP-CRP complex to a regulatory region of the operon permits the binding of RNA polymerase to the promoter. Now the operon is transcribed and the proteins are produced.

σ^{32}, helps RNA polymerase recognize promoters for the operons that encode "heat shock" proteins which are produced in response to elevated temperatures.

Attenuation

Some operons, particularly those encoding enzymes involved in the synthesis of amino acids, are regulated by a process that interrupts or attenuates transcription after it has been initiated (Fig. 15.10). As mRNA is being transcribed from an operon, such as the *trp* operon, that encodes enzymes for the synthesis of a particular amino acid, ribosomes bind and rapidly translate the mRNA transcript. If translation is rapid, a hairpin loop is generated in the mRNA that serves as a termination signal for RNA polymerase. Because the mRNA contains a number of codons for that amino acid near its 5′-end, rapid translation occurs only when levels of the aminoacyl-tRNA for the amino acid are relatively high in the cell, which occurs when levels of the amino

Near the 5'-end of the mRNA produced from the *trp* operon, two adjacent tryptophan codons are located. If tryptophan levels are high, trp-tRNA binds to these codons and translation proceeds rapidly, resulting in the formation of the hairpin loop in mRNA that terminates transcription. If tryptophan levels are low, translation stalls at these codons, the termination loop does not form in the mRNA, and transcription continues.

acid are high. Thus, attenuation terminates transcription when levels of the amino acid are high, preventing production of enzymes required for the synthesis of the amino acid. When levels of the amino acid are low, ribosomes stall at codons for that amino acid. A different hairpin loop forms in the mRNA. This loop does not terminate transcription, and the complete mRNA is transcribed. Translation of this mRNA produces enzymes that catalyze the synthesis of the amino acid.

The tryptophan, histidine, isoleucine, phenylalanine, and threonine operons are regulated by attenuation. Repressors and activators may also act on the promoters of these operons, allowing the levels of these amino acids to be very carefully regulated.

Stability of mRNA

mRNAs in *E. coli* have very short half-lives. They are degraded within a few minutes. Therefore, mRNA must be transcribed constantly in order to maintain protein synthesis. Because of the short half-life of mRNA, regulation of transcription, particularly at the level of initiation, is sufficient to regulate the level of proteins within the cell.

REGULATION OF PROTEIN SYNTHESIS IN EUKARYOTES

Multicellular eukaryotes are much more complex than single-celled prokaryotes. Although most of the cells in a multicellular eukaryotic organism contain the same complement of genes, different sets of these genes are active in different types of cells. As a consequence, the cells of the various tissues of the body exhibit different morphology and perform different functions.

A human being develops from a single cell, formed by the union of a sperm with

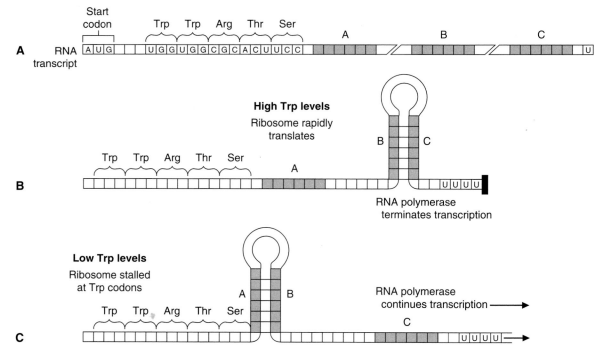

Fig. 15.10. Attenuation of the *trp* operon. Sequences A, B, and C in the mRNA transcript can form base pairs that generate hairpin loops (A-B or B-C). When tryptophan levels are high, translation is rapid. Ribosomes block formation of the A-B loop. Under these conditions, the B-C loop forms and terminates transcription. When tryptophan levels are low, the ribosome stalls at the adjacent trp codons, the A-B loop forms, and transcription continues.

an egg. The fertilized egg undergoes many divisions, producing a multitude of cells that continue to divide and differentiate until a complex organism composed of many different tissues and organs is produced. The developmental changes that occur are the result of alterations in gene activity. As the embryo develops, different sets of genes are turned on and different groups of proteins are produced. These changes in gene activity are programmed; that is, each new embryo repeats the same pattern of changes within a similar time frame.

Between childhood and adolescence and between adolescence and adulthood, other rapid developmental changes occur. Adults do not undergo rapid developmental changes except during a pregnancy. Even beyond the reproductive age, certain cells within the organism continue to differentiate, such as those that produce antibodies in response to an infection, renew the population of red blood cells, and replace digestive cells that have been sloughed into the intestinal lumen. All of these physiological changes are dictated by alterations in gene activity.

Because of the complexity in the morphology and behavior of eukaryotic cells, the mechanisms they employ for regulating gene activity, and thus for regulating protein synthesis, are much more complex than those used by prokaryotic cells.

Differences between Eukaryotic and Prokaryotic Cells

Eukaryotic cells contain nuclei. The process of transcription, which occurs in the nucleus, is separated by the nuclear membrane from the process of translation, which occurs in the cytoplasm. In contrast, because prokaryotes lack nuclei, the processes of transcription and translation occur simultaneously.

Within the nucleus of eukaryotic cells, DNA is complexed with histones. Prokaryotes do not contain histones.

The collection of genes that constitutes the human genome contains about 1,000 times more DNA (3×10^9 base pairs per haploid cell) than the genome of the bacterium *E. coli* (4×10^6 base pairs). Intuition immediately suggests that humans have more DNA than bacteria because they are more complex organisms. While some justification exists for such a conclusion, other factors need to be considered (Table 15.1).

Most Human Cells Are Diploid

Except for the germ cells, most normal human cells are diploid (Fig. 15.11). Therefore, they contain two copies of each chromosome, and each chromosome contains genes that are alleles of the genes on the homologous chromosome. Since one chromosome in each set of homologous chromosomes is obtained from each parent, the alleles may be identical, containing the same DNA sequence, or they may differ. A diploid human cell contains 2,000 times the amount of DNA in an *E. coli* cell.

Bacterial cells are usually haploid; they contain only one copy of a chromosome. Therefore, half of the difference between the DNA content of human and bacterial cells occurs because human cells have two copies of each chromosome.

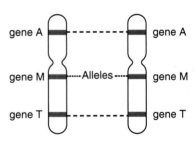

Homologous chromosomes

Fig. 15.11. Human cells are diploid. Haploid germ cells (the sperm and the egg), each containing 23 chromosomes, unite to form the diploid zygote (the fertilized egg), which, therefore, contains 46 chromosomes. The zygote divides and differentiates to form a new individual. Except for the haploid germ cells, each cell in the body is diploid. A diploid cell contains two copies of each chromosome, one derived from the father and one from the mother. The two copies of a chromosome are called homologues. Each chromosome contains thousands of genes in its DNA. The corresponding genes on two homologous chromosomes are known as alleles.

Table 15.1. Amount of DNA in the Genome of Various Organisms

Organism	Base Pairs per Haploid Genome
E. coli	4×10^6
Fruit fly	1×10^8
Bird	1×10^9
Human	3×10^9
Frog	4×10^9
Bean	2×10^{10}

Human Genes Contain Introns

In eukaryotic genes, introns (noncoding regions) occur within sequences that code for proteins. Because of these introns, the primary transcript, heterogeneous nuclear RNA (hnRNA), is about 10 times longer, on the average, than the mature mRNA produced when the introns are removed.

Bacterial genes do not contain introns. Therefore, some of the difference between bacteria and humans in the amount of DNA per cell is related to sequences such as introns that do not encode amino acid sequences in proteins.

Repetitive Sequences in Eukaryotic DNA

Although diploidy and introns may account for some of the difference between the DNA content of humans and bacteria, a large difference remains that may be related to the greater complexity of the human organism. An extension of this line of reasoning, however, would lead to the conclusion that frogs are more complex than humans because frogs have 8 feet of DNA per diploid nucleus compared to the 6 feet in a human cell. Logic, or perhaps vanity, suggests that the amount of DNA per cell does not necessarily reflect the complexity of the organism.

In fact, studies indicate that eukaryotic cells contain substantial amounts of DNA that do not code for proteins and that some genes that encode a protein are present in more than one copy. Bacterial cells, in contrast, have a single, or unique, copy of each gene, and they contain very little DNA that is not transcribed.

If the DNA from an organism is cleaved into relatively small fragments and then treated so that the strands dissociate, the process of reassociation of the strands can be measured and a curve (known as a C_0t curve) can be plotted. The rate of reassociation of a given sequence of bases within a sample of DNA depends upon the number of copies of that sequence that are present. When a large number of copies of a sequence are present, they readily find complementary sequences and reassociate rapidly. Conversely, a sequence present in only a small number of copies reassociates slowly. A single, smooth C_0t curve is produced by *E. coli* DNA, while mammalian DNA produces a curve with three segments as shown in Figure 15.12.

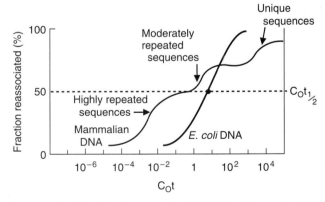

Fig. 15.12. C_0t curves for *E. coli* and mammalian DNA. Double-stranded DNA is cleaved into fragments and the strands are separated. The fraction that reassociates is measured over a period of time. This fraction is plotted against the initial DNA concentration (C_0) multiplied by the time (t) required for reassociation. The curve is called a C_0t curve. Bacterial DNA reassociates over a short period of time, producing a smooth curve. Mammalian DNA reassociates over a broad time span, producing a curve composed of three segments.

HIGHLY REPETITIVE DNA

The DNA that reassociates most readily is highly repetitive DNA, about 100 base pairs in length, present in hundreds of thousands to millions of copies, clustered within a few locations in the genome (Fig. 15.13). This DNA is not transcribed, and its function is unknown.

MODERATELY REPETITIVE DNA

DNA that reassociates at an intermediate rate is moderately repetitive, present in a few to tens of thousands of copies in the genome (see Fig. 15.13). This fraction contains DNA that is functional and transcribed to produce rRNA, tRNA, and also some mRNA. The histone genes, present in a few hundred copies in the genome, belong to this class. Moderately repetitive DNA also includes some gene sequences that are functional but not transcribed. Promoters and enhancers are examples of gene sequences in this category. Other groups of moderately repetitive gene sequences that have been found in the human are called the Alu sequences (about 300 base pairs in length) and the LINE (Long INterspersed Elements) sequences (6,000–7,000 base pairs in length). The function of the Alu and LINE sequences has not been determined.

UNIQUE DNA

About 64% of the DNA in the human genome is unique (Table 15.2). It consists of DNA sequences that are present in one or a very few copies in the genome (see Fig. 15.13). Therefore, this unique DNA reassociates very slowly in a mixture of DNA fragments from total genomic DNA. mRNA is transcribed from these unique DNA sequences and translated to produce proteins.

 Alu sequences were named for the enzyme AluI that cleaves them. They apparently were derived from a portion of the RNA component of the signal recognition particle (see Chapter 14). Alu sequences make up 6–8% of the human genome. In some cases of familial hypercholesterolemia, homologous recombination is believed to have occurred between two Alu repeats, resulting in a large deletion in the low density lipoprotein (LDL) receptor gene.

LINE (Long INterspersed Elements) make up about 5% of the human genome. In some cases of hemophilia, a LINE sequence has been found inserted into exon 14 of the gene for Factor VIII, a component of the blood-clotting system. The normal gene does not contain a LINE sequence.

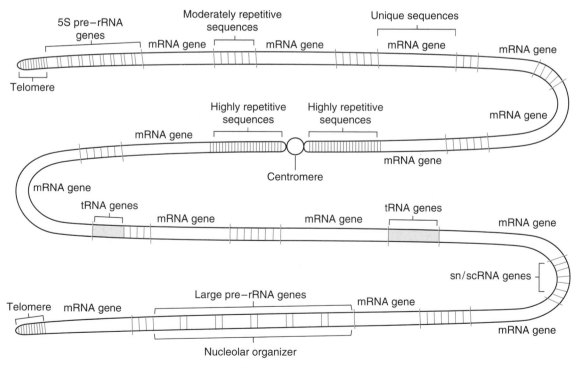

Fig. 15.13. Distribution of unique, moderately repetitive, and highly repetitive sequences in a hypothetical human chromosome. Unique genes encode mRNA. These genes occur in single copies. The genes for the large rRNA and the tRNA precursors occur in multiple copies that are clustered in the genome. The large rRNA genes form the nucleolar organizer. Moderately repetitive sequences are dispersed throughout the genome, and highly repetitive sequences are clustered around the centromere and at the ends of the chromosome (the telomeres). From Wolfe SL. Mol Cell Biol 1993:761.

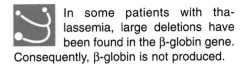 In some patients with thalassemia, large deletions have been found in the β-globin gene. Consequently, β-globin is not produced.

Bacterial DNA consists mainly of unique genes. The DNA reassociates relatively slowly, reflecting the complexity of the sequences, and only a single C_0t curve is produced.

Absence of Operons in Eukaryotes

Operons are not present in eukaryotes. The genes encoding proteins that function together are usually located on different chromosomes. For example, the gene for the α-globin chain of hemoglobin is on chromosome 16, while the gene for the β-globin chain is on chromosome 11. This situation is different from bacteria, where genes encoding proteins that function together are adjacent to each other in operons that are controlled by a single promoter (Table 15.3).

Mechanisms for Regulating Gene Expression in Eukaryotic Cells

Because of the differences between eukaryotic and prokaryotic cells (see Table 15.3), their mechanisms for regulating their protein content are different. Regulation of the types and quantities of proteins that are present in eukaryotic cells occurs at a number of different levels: transcriptional, posttranscriptional, translational, and posttranslational. First of all, alterations in the numbers or structures of genes can affect the amount or types of proteins produced in a cell. Genes can be lost from cells, increased in number (amplified), rearranged, or chemically modified. DNA can bind to other compounds (such as histones) and assume a conformation that is not readily transcribed.

Table 15.2. Percent of DNA That Is Unique, Moderately Repetitive, or Highly Repetitive in Various Organisms

Organism	Unique	Moderately Repetitive	Highly Repetitive
E. coli	100	0	0
Frog	22	67	9
Chick	70	24	6
Rat	65	19	9
Human	64	25	10

Table 15.3. Differences between Euraryotes and Prokaryotes

	Eukaryotes	Prokaryotes
Nucleus	Yes	No
Chromosomes		
Number	23 per haploid cell	1 per haploid cell
DNA	Linear	Circular
Histones	Yes	No
Genome		
Diploid	Somatic cells	No
Haploid	Germ cells	All cells
Size	3×10^9 base pairs per haploid cell	4×10^6 base pairs
Genes		
Unique	64%	100%
Repetitive		
Moderately	25%	None
Highly	10%	None
Operons	No	Yes
mRNA		
Polycistronic	No	Yes
Capped	Yes	No
Poly(A) tail	Yes	No
Introns	Yes	No
Translation	Separate from transcription	Simultaneous with transcription

At the level of transcription of specific genes, elements within the DNA sequence (called *cis* elements) bind other factors known as *trans* elements (usually proteins) that promote or inhibit the binding of RNA polymerase to the gene (see Chapter 14). Compounds, such as steroid hormones, can act as inducers, stimulating the binding of the *trans* elements to the *cis* elements of the DNA.

Regulation can occur during processing of the RNA transcript (hnRNA) into the mature mRNA. Alternative splicing sites or alternative sites for addition of the poly(A) tail (polyadenylation sites) can result in the production of different mRNAs from a single hnRNA and, consequently, in the production of different proteins from a single gene.

At the level of translation, regulatory factors can affect the initiation step. The stability of the mRNA also plays a role. mRNAs with long half-lives generate more proteins than those with shorter half-lives.

ALTERATIONS IN GENES

Gene Loss

If genes are deleted or partially deleted from cells, functional proteins cannot be produced. An extreme example of gene loss occurs during the development of the red blood cell. Immature cells (erythroblasts) contain nuclei that produce mRNA for the globin chains of hemoglobin. As the cells mature, the nuclei are extruded, so that the fully mature red blood cell has no nucleus and, therefore, no genes, so it can no longer produce mRNA.

Gene Amplification

In order to produce large numbers of specific proteins, many copies of genes can be generated. This process is known as gene amplification (Fig. 15.14). Genes are amplified in some species at certain stages of normal development. However, unscheduled amplification also occurs.

Gene Rearrangement

Segments of DNA may move from one location to another in the genome, associating with each other in various ways so that different proteins are produced.

The most thoroughly studied example of gene rearrangement occurs in cells that produce antibodies. Antibodies contain two light chains and two heavy chains, each of which contains both a variable and a constant region (see Chapter 8). Cells called B cells make antibodies. In the precursors of B cells, over 200 V_H sequences, 20 D_H sequences, and 6 J_H sequences are located in clusters within a long region of the chromosome. A series of recombinational events occur that join one V_H, one D_H, and one J_H sequence into a single exon that encodes the variable region of the heavy chain of the antibody (Fig. 15.15).

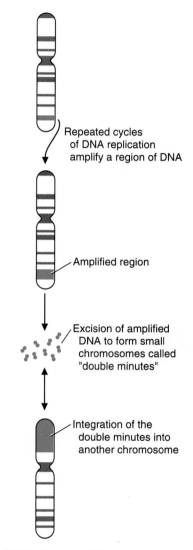

Repeated cycles of DNA replication amplify a region of DNA

Amplified region

Excision of amplified DNA to form small chromosomes called "double minutes"

Integration of the double minutes into another chromosome

Fig. 15.14. Gene amplification.

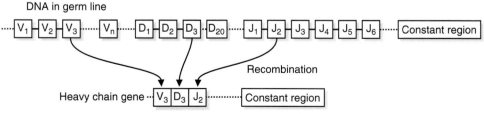

DNA in germ line

Recombination

Heavy chain gene

Fig. 15.15. Rearrangement of DNA. The heavy chain gene from which lymphocytes produce immunoglobulins is generated by combining specific segments from among a large number of potential sequences in the DNA of precursor cells. The variable and constant regions of immunoglobulins (antibodies) are described in Chapter 8.

Arlyn Foma has been treated with a combination of drugs that includes methotrexate. Because he has not been responding well, the possibility that he has become resistant to methotrexate was considered.

Methotrexate is an inhibitor of the enzyme dihydrofolate reductase (DHFR), which reduces dihydrofolate to tetrahydrofolate, a cofactor required for the synthesis of thymine nucleotides (see Chapter 40). If DHFR is inhibited, cells cannot produce adequate amounts of thymine nucleotides for DNA synthesis. Therefore, methotrexate inhibits the proliferation of cancer cells.

Sometimes, cells treated with methotrexate amplify the gene for DHFR, producing hundreds of copies in the genome. These cells generate large amounts of DHFR, and normal doses of methotrexate are no longer adequate to inhibit the DHFR reaction. Gene amplification is one of the mechanisms by which patients become resistant to a drug.

Although rearrangements of short DNA sequences are difficult to detect, major rearrangements have been observed for many years. Such major rearrangements, known as translocations, can be observed in metaphase chromosomes.

Mannie Weitzels has such a translocation, known as the Philadelphia chromosome because it was first observed in that city. The Philadelphia chromosome is produced by an exchange between chromosomes 9 and 22.

In a condition known as testicular feminization, patients produce androgens but cells fail to respond to these steroid hormones because they lack the appropriate intracellular receptors. Therefore, the genes responsible for masculinization are not activated. A patient with this condition has an XY (male) karyotype but looks like a female. External male genitalia do not develop, but testes are present usually in the inguinal region.

Later in development, during differentiation of mature B cells, recombinational events join a VDJ sequence to one of the five heavy chain elements. The result of all this gene rearrangement is that B cells subsequently produce one antibody containing only one variable and one constant region.

CHEMICAL MODIFICATION OF DNA

Cytosine residues in DNA can be methylated to produce 5-methylcytosine. In certain instances, genes that are methylated are less readily transcribed than those that are not methylated. For example, globin genes are more extensively methylated in nonerythroid cells than in the cells in which these genes are expressed.

REGULATION AT THE LEVEL OF TRANSCRIPTION

Condensation of Chromatin

A typical nucleus contains chromatin that is condensed (heterochromatin) and chromatin that is diffuse (euchromatin) (see Chapter 10). The genes in heterochromatin are inactive, while those in euchromatin produce mRNA. Long-term changes in the activity of genes occur during development as chromatin goes from a diffuse to a condensed state or vice versa.

For example, during maturation of the red blood cell, the hormone erythropoietin stimulates hemocytoblasts to divide and differentiate into erythroblasts. At this stage, the cells contain large amounts of euchromatin and are actively dividing and producing RNA. As the cells mature, their chromatin becomes more condensed, and RNA synthesis decreases (Fig. 15.16). Eventually, the nucleus is extruded from the cell.

Activation of Specific Genes

In eukaryotic cells, specific genes are activated within minutes to hours by inducers. The inducers are compounds, such as steroid hormones, that enter cells and bind to receptor proteins (Fig. 15.17). These receptors also contain domains that bind to specific response elements (*cis* elements, i.e., DNA sequences in the regulatory region of a gene). When the inducer-receptor complex is bound to DNA, the gene may be activated or, in some cases, inactivated. Other inducers that behave like steroid hormones include thyroid hormone, 1,25-dihydroxycholecalciferol (the active form of vitamin D), and retinoic acid (a form of vitamin A).

Polypeptide hormones and growth factors also regulate gene expression, although in these cases the compounds do not enter the cell. They react with receptors on the cell surface, stimulating reactions that generate second messengers inside the cell that ultimately activate genes.

The same inducer may activate many different genes if the genes each contain a common response element in their regulatory regions. In fact, a single inducer may activate sets of genes in an orderly, programmed manner. The inducer initially activates one set of genes. One of the protein products of this set of genes may then act as an inducer for another set of genes. If this process is repeated, the net result is that one inducer can set off a series of events that result in the activation of many different sets of genes (Fig. 15.18).

In addition to the sets of genes that respond to hormones, some sets of genes, called the heat shock genes, respond to elevated temperatures, producing proteins that protect cells from damage caused by heat.

Individual genes contain many different response elements in their regulatory regions. Thus each gene does not have a unique protein that regulates its transcrip-

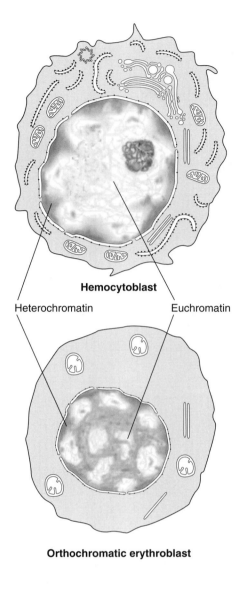

Hemocytoblast

Heterochromatin   Euchromatin

Orthochromatic erythroblast

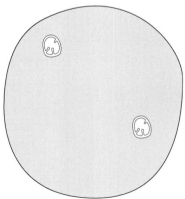

Reticulocyte

Fig. 15.16. Inactivation of genes during development of red blood cells. Diffuse chromatin (euchromatin) is active in RNA synthesis. Condensed chromatin (heterochromatin) is inactive. As red blood cell precursors mature, their chromatin becomes more condensed. Eventually, the nucleus is extruded.

Interferons are proteins that bind to cell surface receptors and, like polypeptide hormones, cause compounds that activate genes to be produced inside the cells. **Arlyn Foma** is being treated with interferon.

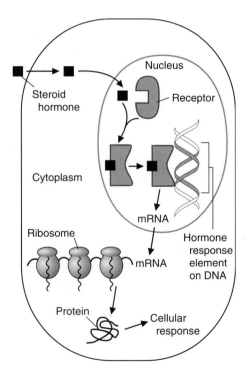

Fig. 15.17. Action of an inducer in mammalian cells. An inducer, such as a steroid hormone, binds to a receptor which is either located in the nucleus or enters the nucleus after binding to the hormone. The hormone-receptor complex binds to a response (*cis*) element on DNA and activates gene transcription. The mRNA is translated to produce the protein that causes the cellular response.

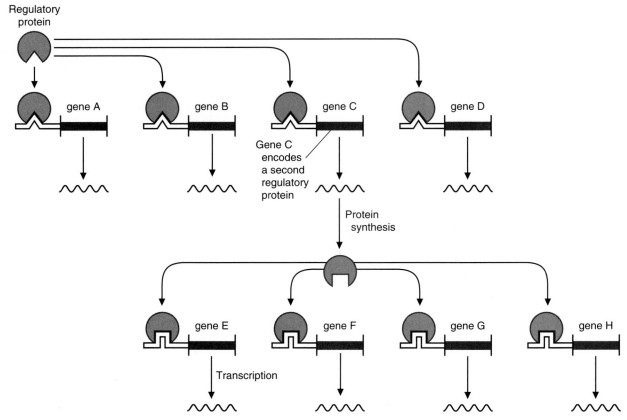

Fig. 15.18. Activation of sets of genes by a single inducer. Note that this process differs from the process that regulates bacterial operons. In eukaryotes, each gene has a separate promoter, and the genes may be located on different chromosomes. Each gene in a set has a common regulatory (*cis*) element, so one regulatory protein can activate all the genes in the set. One of the protein products of the first set of genes can activate a second set of genes by binding to a common *cis* element in their regulatory regions. From Wolfe SL. Mol Cell Biol 1993:700.

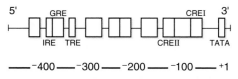

Fig. 15.19. Regulatory region of the PEPCK gene. Boxes represent various response elements in the 5′-flanking region of the gene. Not all elements are labeled. Regulatory proteins bind to these DNA elements and stimulate or inhibit the transcription of the gene. This gene encodes the enzyme phosphoenolpyruvate carboxykinase (PEPCK), which catalyzes a reaction of gluconeogenesis (the pathway for production of glucose) in the liver during fasting. Synthesis of the enzyme is stimulated by glucagon (by a cAMP-mediated process), by glucocorticoids, and by thyroid hormone. Synthesis of PEPCK is inhibited by insulin. CRE = cAMP response element; TRE = thyroid hormone response element; GRE = glucocorticoid response element; IRE = insulin response element.

tion. Rather a relatively small number of regulatory proteins acts in concert to generate a wide variety of responses from different genes.

Genes that encode different proteins contain different DNA response elements. Transcription of a gene is regulated by the various combinations of regulatory proteins that bind to its DNA response elements in response to different regulatory signals (Fig. 15.19). The net effect of positive and negative signals determines the extent of transcription of a gene.

A combination of signals may be required to achieve the configuration in the regulatory region required to maximally stimulate transcription. These signals promote binding of transactivators to the response elements of the gene. The transactivators are proteins that are joined by other proteins (coactivators) to the protein complex bound to the basal promoter at the TATA box. When the appropriate interactions between the transactivators, coactivators, and the basal promoter complex occur, RNA polymerase binds more frequently to the basal promoter and the rate of transcription of the gene is increased (see Fig. 13.8).

The interaction of these regulatory proteins with DNA involves structural features such as zinc fingers and helix-turn-helix motifs (see Fig. 8.11). These regulatory proteins also contain transactivation domains, regions that permit them to bind to other regulatory proteins. Many of these proteins form dimers through structural features such as leucine zippers.

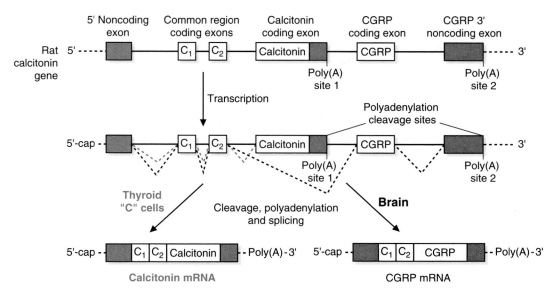

Fig. 15.20. Alternative splicing of the calcitonin gene. In thyroid cells, the transcript from the calcitonin gene is processed to form an mRNA that codes for calcitonin. Cleavage occurs at poly(A) site 1 and splicing along the blue dashed lines. In the brain, the transcript of this gene undergoes alternative splicing and polyadenylation to produce calcitonin gene-related protein (CGRP). Cleavage occurs at poly(A) site 2 and splicing along the black dashed lines.

POSTTRANSCRIPTIONAL REGULATION

Regulation can occur during processing of the primary transcript (hnRNA) and during the transport of mRNA from the nucleus to the cytoplasm.

Use of Alternative Splicing and Polyadenylation Sites

Processing of the primary transcript involves the addition of a cap to the 5′-end, removal of introns, and the addition of a poly(A) tail to the 3′-end (polyadenylation) to produce the mature mRNA (see Chapter 13). In certain instances, the use of alternative splicing and polyadenylation sites causes different proteins to be produced from the same gene. For example, in parafollicular cells of the thyroid gland, the calcitonin gene produces an mRNA that codes for calcitonin. In the brain, the same gene is spliced differently and uses a different polyadenylation site, so that the product is a protein which is involved in the sensation of taste (Fig. 15.20).

In addition to undergoing gene rearrangement, genes that code for antibodies are also regulated by alterations in splicing and polyadenylation. At an early stage of development, pre-B lymphocytes produce IgM antibodies that are bound to the cell membrane. These antibodies are produced from mRNA containing exons that code for a hydrophobic region at the C-terminus of the protein. This hydrophobic region anchors the IgM antibody in the cell membrane. Subsequently, during differentiation of the antibody-producing cells, an alternative polyadenylation site is utilized that eliminates these hydrophobic exons from the transcript. A shorter protein (IgD) is produced that no longer binds to the cell membrane, but rather is secreted from the cell (Fig. 15.21).

RNA Editing

In some instances, RNA is altered ("edited") after transcription. The sequence of the gene is the same in all tissues. However, the mRNAs transcribed from the gene dif-

In some types of thalassemia, mutations occur that affect the splicing of hnRNA to form mRNA. One example is a G to A mutation at the first base of the first intron (see figure on right). This mutation destroys the DNA sequence required for appropriate removal of this intron. Other sequences (cryptic splice sites) that do not normally function as splice sites are now recognized. Two of these sequences are located within the first exon, and the third is near the 5'-end of the first intron. Each of these cryptic splice sites contains a G followed by a GT. All three cryptic sequences are used as replacements for the mutated splice site at the start of the first intron. Consequently, three different mRNAs are produced, none of which produces functional β-globin. Hence, patients with this mutation have a β^0-thalassemia.

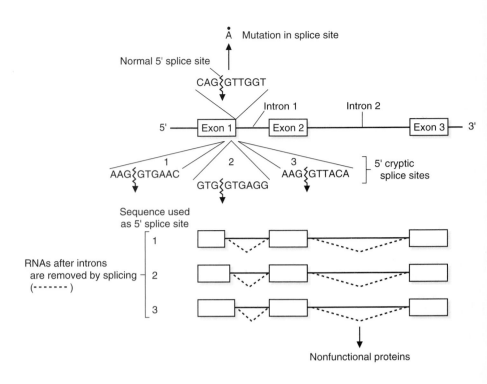

Interferons are proteins produced by cells that have been infected by a virus. One of the actions of the interferons is to inhibit synthesis of the proteins required for viral replication. Interferons stimulate synthesis of an enzyme that produces an oligonucleotide (2′-5′-oligo(A)) that activates a ribonuclease. This RNase degrades mRNA, thus inhibiting protein synthesis.

In addition to antiviral effects, interferons also have antitumor effects. The mechanisms of the antitumor effects are not as well understood as certain of the antiviral effects, but are probably related to the ability of interferons to bind to receptors on the cell surface and stimulate the production of compounds within the cell that activate genes.

Interferon-α, produced by recombinant DNA technology, has been used to treat patients, such as **Arlyn Foma**, who have certain types of nodular lymphomas. It has also been used to treat patients, such as **Mannie Weitzels**, who have chronic myelogenous leukemia.

fer. Although the mechanism is not fully understood, it appears to involve the alteration of a base or the addition or deletion of nucleotides after the transcript is synthesized.

An example of RNA editing occurs in the production of the B apoprotein (apoB) that is synthesized in liver and intestinal cells and serves as a component of the lipoproteins produced by these tissues (Fig. 15.22). Although these apoproteins are encoded by the same gene, the version of the protein made in the liver (B-100) contains 4,563 amino acid residues, while the one (B-48) made in intestinal cells has only 2,152 amino acids.

Within the genome, the sequence of codon 2,153 is CAA. In the liver, codon 2,153 of the fully processed mRNA is CAA, which specifies glutamine. In the intestine, the C of codon 2,153 in the RNA transcript is modified to a U, forming UAA in the fully processed mRNA. UAA is a stop codon that causes translation to terminate, producing a protein that is only 48% of the length of the protein produced from the same gene in the liver.

Transport of mRNA

In eukaryotes, mRNA must travel from the nucleus through the nuclear pores to the cytoplasm in order to be translated. Nucleases can degrade the mRNA, preventing the production of the proteins for which the mRNA codes. During transport, mRNA is bound to proteins that help to prevent its degradation.

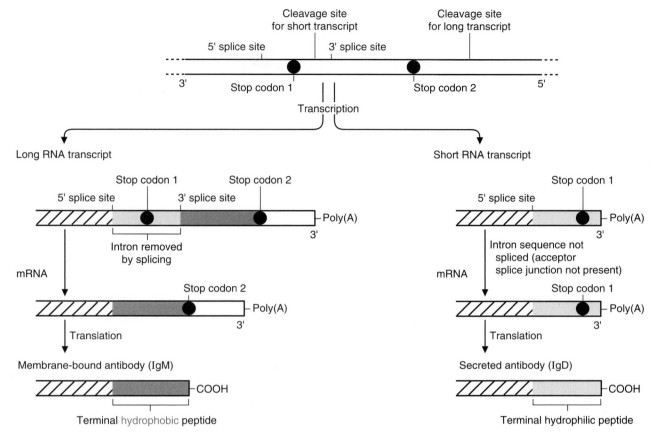

Fig. 15.21. Use of alternative polyadenylation and splicing sites in the production of the IgM and IgD antibodies. Initially, the lymphocytes produce a long transcript that is cleaved and polyadenylated after the second stop codon. The intron that contains the first stop codon is removed by splicing between the 5′- and 3′-splice sites. Therefore, translation ends at the second stop codon, and the protein contains a hydrophobic exon at its C-terminal end that becomes embedded in the cell membrane. After antigen stimulation, the cells produce a shorter transcript by using a different cleavage and polyadenylation site. This transcript lacks the 3′-splice site for the intron, so the intron is not removed. In this case, translation ends at the first stop codon. The IgD antibody does not contain the hydrophobic region at its C-terminus, so it is secreted from the cell.

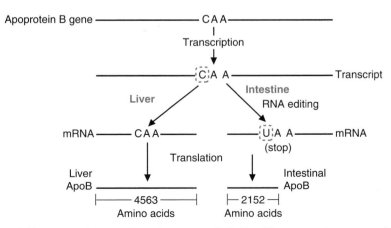

Fig. 15.22. RNA editing. In liver, the apoprotein B (ApoB) gene produces a protein that contains 4,563 amino acids. In intestinal cells, the same gene produces a protein that contains only 2,152 amino acids. Conversion of a C to a U in the RNA transcript generates a stop codon in the intestinal mRNA.

STABILITY OF mRNA

The mRNA of eukaryotes is much more stable (with half-lives measured in hours to days) than the mRNA of prokaryotes (with half-lives measured in minutes). Sequences at the 3′-end of the mRNA appear to be involved in determining its half-life. The poly(A) tail might protect the mRNA from attack by nucleases, prolonging its half-life and, thus, permitting it to produce larger amounts of protein.

Other sequences at the 3′-end also may be involved in protecting mRNA from degradation. For example, the transferrin receptor is a protein located in cell membranes that permits cells to take up transferrin, the protein that transports iron in the blood. The rate of synthesis of the transferrin receptor increases when iron levels are low, enabling cells to take up more iron (Fig. 15.23). Synthesis of the transferrin receptor is regulated by the binding of a protein to hairpin loops located at the 3′-end of the transferrin receptor mRNA. This protein has a high affinity for the hairpin loops of the mRNA when iron levels are low. Consequently, the protein binds to the mRNA, preventing its degradation. On the other hand, when iron levels are elevated,

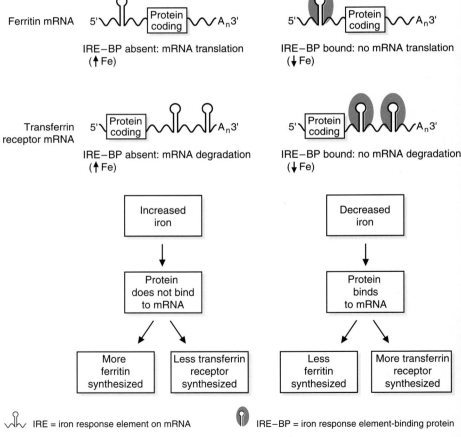

Fig. 15.23. Translational regulation of ferritin and transferrin receptor synthesis. When iron levels are elevated, iron binds to the IRE-BP. This protein then does not bind to the IRE on the mRNA. When IRE-BP is not bound to the mRNA, ferritin mRNA is translated and ferritin, the intracellular binding protein for iron, is synthesized. In contrast, transferrin receptor mRNA is degraded, so its protein is not synthesized. When iron levels are low, iron is not bound to the IRE-BP. This protein now binds to the IRE. Ferritin is not synthesized, but the transferrin receptor mRNA is stabilized and its protein is produced.

the protein binds iron and, as a result, has a low affinity for the mRNA. When the protein is not bound to the mRNA, the mRNA is rapidly degraded.

REGULATION AT THE LEVEL OF TRANSLATION

Most eukaryotic translational controls affect the initiation of protein synthesis. The initiation factors for translation, particularly eukaryotic initiation factor 2 (eIF2) (see Chapter 14), are the focus of these regulatory mechanisms. The action of eIF2 can be inhibited by phosphorylation.

Reticulocytes, which contain no nuclei and, therefore, no DNA for transcription, must regulate the synthesis of globin at the translational level. Globin is produced when heme levels in the cell are high, but not when they are low. Heme acts by preventing phosphorylation of eIF2. The kinase that phosphorylates eIF2 is inactive when heme is bound. Thus, when heme levels are high, eIF2 is not phosphorylated and, therefore, it is active in initiating the synthesis of globin. As heme levels decrease in the cell, eIF2 is phosphorylated and inactivated (Fig. 15.24).

Certain mRNAs contain hairpin loops at the 5'-end that can bind proteins that inhibit initiation of translation. For example, ferritin, the protein involved in the storage of iron within cells, is synthesized when iron levels increase. The mRNA for ferritin has a hairpin loop near its 5'-end that binds a regulatory protein when iron levels are low. When this protein is bound to the mRNA, translation does not occur. When iron levels increase, iron binds to the protein, which changes shape and no longer binds to the ferritin mRNA. Therefore, the mRNA is translated and ferritin is produced (see Fig. 15.23).

POSTTRANSLATIONAL REGULATION

After proteins are synthesized, their lifespan is regulated by proteolytic degradation. Proteins have different half-lives. Some last for hours or days. Others last for months or even years. Some proteins are degraded by lysosomal enzymes. The process of autophagy (see Chapter 10) allows subcellular material, including organelles, to be enclosed by a membrane and subjected to lysosomal action. Other proteins are degraded by proteases in the cytoplasm. Some of these proteins appear to be marked for degradation by attachment to a protein known as ubiquitin. Ubiquitin is a highly conserved protein. There is very little variation in its amino acid sequence between organisms that are widely separated on the phylogenetic tree.

 CLINICAL COMMENTS. **Annie Myck** is suffering from severe anemia. In cases of severe anemia, the production of red blood cell precursors (the erythroid mass) is stimulated. As a result of this stimulation, the bone marrow spaces may expand remarkably in all areas of the skeleton, leading to gross deformity of the facial and skull bones as well as expansion within the vertebral bodies. The latter may cause compression of the spinal cord itself, with back pain and eventually, paralysis. Local irradiation may bring immediate relief of these compression symptoms, but a regimen of regular blood transfusions to keep the hemoglobin at near normal levels may be required to suppress most of the disease manifestations, including those of bone marrow expansion.

Follicular lymphomas are the most common subset of non-Hodgkin's lymphomas (25–40% of cases). Patients with a more aggressive course, as seen in **Arlyn Foma**, die within 3–5 years after diagnosis if left untreated. In patients pretreated with multidrug chemotherapy (in this case AV/CM), a response rate of 50% has been reported

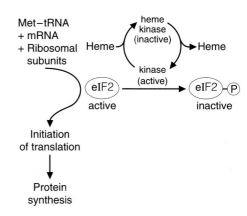

Fig. 15.24. Regulation of eIF2 activity by heme. eIF2 is a factor that is involved in initiation of the synthesis of proteins, including globin. When eIF2 is phosphorylated, it is inactive, and protein synthesis is not initiated. Heme acts by preventing phosphorylation of eIF2. When heme levels are elevated, globin is synthesized. When heme levels fall, globin is not produced.

 Priscilla Twigg has a hypochromic anemia, which means that her red blood cells are pale because they contain low levels of hemoglobin. Because of her iron deficiency, she is not producing adequate amounts of heme. Consequently, eIF2 is phosphorylated in her reticulocytes. Globin is not synthesized at a normal rate because phosphorylated eIF2 is not active in initiation of translation.

In addition to stimulating degradation of mRNA, interferon also causes eIF2 to become phosphorylated and inactive. This is a second mechanism by which interferon prevents synthesis of viral proteins.

Priscilla Twigg's ferritin levels are low, consistent with a diagnosis of iron deficiency anemia.

when interferon-α is added to this regimen. In addition, a significantly longer event-free survival has been reported using this approach.

Priscilla Twigg's iron stores are depleted. Normally, about 16–18% of total body iron is contained in a spherical protein (apoferritin), which is capable of storing as many as 4,000 atoms of iron in its center to form the protein ferritin. As expected, when an iron deficiency exists, serum and tissue ferritin levels fall. On the other hand, the levels of transferrin (the blood protein that transports iron) and the levels of the transferrin receptor (the cell surface receptor for transferrin) increase.

Mannie Weitzels has CML (chronic myelogenous leukemia), a hematological disorder in which the proliferating leukemic cells are believed to originate from a single line of primitive myeloid cells. Although classified as one of the myeloproliferative disorders, CML is distinguished by the presence of a specific cytogenetic abnormality of the dividing marrow cells known as the Philadelphia chromosome, found in over 90% of cases. In most instances, the etiology of CML is unknown but the disease occurs with an incidence of around 1.5 per 100,000 population in Western societies.

BIOCHEMICAL COMMENTS. The thalassemias are hemoglobinopathies caused by mutations in the globin genes. Two genes encode α-globin, both located on chromosome 16. Thus, a normal diploid cell has four copies of the α-globin gene. Only one gene encodes β-globin, located on chromosome 11. Thus, a normal diploid cell has two copies of this gene. Deficient production of α-globin leads to an α-thalassemia, and deficient production of β-globin leads to a β-thalassemia.

The mutations that cause the thalassemias have been studied extensively. Mutations in the β-globin gene have been found to occur within the promoter region and the cap site, within exons and introns, and at the splice junctions that occur at exon-intron boundaries. Mutations have also been found at the polyadenylation site, and large deletions have been observed in the 5′ and the 3′ regions of the gene (Table 15.4). Studies of the effects of these mutations have helped to uncover the mechanisms by which gene expression is regulated.

Suggested Readings

Regulation of gene expression in prokaryotic and eukaryotic cells:

Lewin B. Genes V. Oxford: Oxford University Press, 1994:414–489, 879–940.

Thalassemias:

Watson J, Gilman M, Witkowski J, Zoller M. Recombinant DNA. Scientific American Books. New York: WH Freeman, 1992:540–544.

Leukemias and Lymphomas:

Wyngaarden J, Smith L, Bennet J. Cecil textbook of medicine. Philadelphia: WB Saunders, 1992:933–955.

PROBLEM

As shown on the next page, a mutation has been found within the second intron in the β-globin gene in which a G replaces a C, creating a new 5′-splice site. A cryptic 3′-splice site within this intron is now recognized. It is located 5′ to the new splice site generated by the mutation. What effect would this mutation have on the mRNA and the protein produced from the gene?

Table 15.4. Some Examples of Mutations in β-Thalassemia

Type of Mutation	Phenotype	Origin
Nonsense		
Codon 17 (A → T)	β^0	Chinese
Codon 39 (C → T)	β^0	Mediterranean
Codon 121 (A → T)	β^0	Polish
Frameshift		
Codon 6 (−1 bp)	β^0	Mediterranean
Codon 16 (−1 bp)	β^0	Asian Indian
Codon 41/42 (−4 bp)	β^0	Asian Indian, Chinese
Codon 71/72 (+1 bp)	β^0	Chinese
Promoter		
Position −88 (C → T)	β^+	African American
Position −31 (A → G)	β^+	Japanese
Position −28 (A → C)	β^+	Kurdish
Cap site		
Position +1 (A → C)	β^+	Asian Indian
Splice junction		
Intron 1, position 1 (G → A)	β^0	Mediterranean
Intron 1, 3′-end (−25 bp)	β^0	Asian Indian
Intron 2, position 1 (G → A)	β^0	Mediterranean
Intron 2, 3′-end (A → G)	β^0	African American
Intron, internal		
Intron 1, position 5 (G → T)	β^+	Mediterranean
Intron 1, position 6 (T → C)	β^+	Mediterranean
Intron 2, position 110 (G → A)	β^+	Mediterranean
Intron 2, position 654 (C → T)	β^0	Chinese
Intron 2, position 745 (C → G)	β^+	Mediterranean
Exon, internal		
Codon 24 (T → A)	β^+	African American
Codon 26 (G → A)	β^E	Southeast Asian
Codon 27 (G → T)	$\beta^{Knossos}$	Mediterranean
RNA cleavage/polyadenylation		
AATAAA → AACAAA	β^+	African American

Data from Scriver CR, et al. The metabolic and molecular bases of inherited disease, Vol. III. New York: McGraw-Hill, 1995:3456–3457.

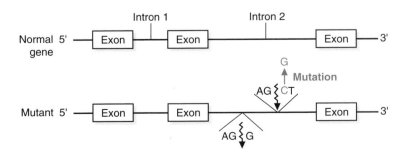

ANSWER

The intron is spliced out from the end of exon 2 (the beginning of intron 2) to the cryptic site. The region between the cryptic site and the mutation is no longer recognized as an intron, but as a "new" exon. The region between the mutation and the 5'-end of exon 3 is treated like an intron and removed. The result of these splices is that the mRNA now has four exons instead of the normal three, and therefore, it does not produce normal β-globin.

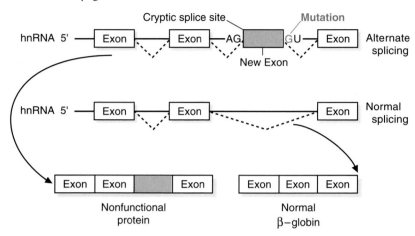

Individuals with this mutation have a β+-thalassemia because the correct splice sites are occasionally recognized by the splicing mechanism and a small amount of normal β-globin mRNA is produced. It is possible that **Annie Myck** has this mutation.

16   Use of Recombinant DNA Techniques in Medicine

As our knowledge of molecular biology has expanded over the last 20 years, it has become obvious that the development of this field is revolutionizing the practice of medicine. The potential uses of the techniques of molecular biology for the diagnosis and treatment of disease are vast.

Polymorphisms, inherited differences in DNA sequences, are found in abundance within the human population, and alterations in DNA sequences are associated with many diseases. Tests for DNA sequence variations are more sensitive than many other techniques (such as enzyme assays) and permit recognition of diseases at earlier and, therefore, potentially more treatable stages. These tests can also identify carriers of inherited diseases so they can receive appropriate counseling. Because genetic variations are so distinctive, DNA "fingerprinting" (analysis of DNA sequence differences) can be used to determine family relationships or to help identify the perpetrators of crimes.

Techniques of molecular biology are currently being used in the prevention and treatment of disease. For example, these techniques provide vaccines for the prevention of hepatitis, human insulin for the treatment of diabetes, and Factor VIII for the treatment of hemophilia. Although treatment of disease by gene therapy is in the experimental phase of development, the possibilities are limited only by the human imagination and, of course, by ethical considerations.

To recognize normal or pathological genetic variations, DNA must be isolated from the appropriate source and adequate amounts must be available for study. Techniques for isolating and amplifying genes and studying and manipulating DNA sequences involve the use of restriction enzymes, cloning, polymerase chain reaction (PCR), gel electrophoresis, blotting onto nitrocellulose paper, and the preparation of labeled probes which hybridize to the appropriate target DNA sequences. Gene therapy involves isolating normal genes and inserting them into diseased cells so that the normal genes are expressed, permitting the diseased cells to return to a normal state.

Students must have at least a general understanding of these techniques in order to fully appreciate their current use and the promise they hold for the future.

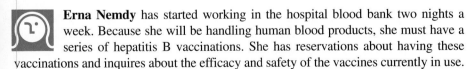

Erna Nemdy has started working in the hospital blood bank two nights a week. Because she will be handling human blood products, she must have a series of hepatitis B vaccinations. She has reservations about having these vaccinations and inquires about the efficacy and safety of the vaccines currently in use.

Sissy Fibrosa is a 3-year-old Caucasian female whose growth rate has been in the lower 30th percentile over the last year. Since birth, she has had occasional episodes of spontaneously reversible and minor small bowel obstruction. These episodes are superimposed on gastrointestinal symptoms that suggest a degree of dietary fat malabsorption, such as bulky, glistening, foul-smelling stools 2 or 3 times a day. She has experienced recurrent flare-ups of bacterial bronchitis in the last 10 months, each time caused by *Pseudomonas aeruginosa*. A quantitative pilocarpine iontophoresis sweat test was unequivocally positive (excessive sodium and chloride were found in her sweat on two occasions).

Based on these findings, her pediatrician informed her parents that Sissy probably has cystic fibrosis (CF). A sample of her blood was sent to the molecular biology and genetics research laboratory to determine specifically which one of the many potential genetic mutations known to cause CF was present in Sissy's cells.

 Anne Sulin's body weight has stabilized. Her fasting and 2-hour postprandial blood glucose levels remain in the acceptable range on an appropriate diabetic diet. She injects 24 units of synthetic human insulin subcutaneously each morning. The use of this insulin, prepared by recombinant DNA techniques, has not caused Anne to have any allergic reactions. A recent serum glycosylated hemoglobin (HbA$_{1c}$) level was in the mid-normal range. No evidence suggests the development of diabetic retinopathy, nephropathy, or peripheral neuropathy.

 Carrie Sichel, Michael's 19-year-old sister, is considering marriage. Her growth and development have been normal, and she is free of symptoms of sickle cell anemia. Because a younger sister, Amanda, was tested and found to have sickle trait, and because of Michael's repeated sickle crises, Carrie wants to know if she also has sickle trait. A hemoglobin electrophoresis is performed and reveals the composition of her hemoglobin to be HbA 52%, HbS 54%, and HbF 1%, a pattern consistent with the presence of sickle cell trait. The hematologist who saw her in the clinic on her first visit is studying the genetic mutations of sickle cell trait, and asks Carrie for permission to draw additional blood for more sophisticated analysis of the genetic disturbance which causes her to produce HbS.

Carrie Sichel informed her fiancé, **Willie Havet**, that she has sickle cell trait, and that she wants to delay their marriage until he is tested.

 Victoria Tim was a 21-year-old woman who drove to the local convenience store to buy several items she needed to prepare the evening meal for her parents. When she had not returned home an hour later, her father drove to the store, looking for Vicky. He found her car still parked in front of the store, but Vicky was not there. He called the police. A search was made in the area around the store, and Vicky's body was found in a wooded area behind the building. She had been sexually assaulted and strangled.

Medical technologists from the police laboratory collected a semen sample from vaginal fluid and took samples of dried blood found under the victim's fingernails.

 Ivy Sharer's cough is slightly improved on a multidrug regimen for pulmonary tuberculosis, but she continues to have night sweats. She is tolerating didanosine well, but complains of weakness and fatigue. The man with whom she has shared "dirty" needles to inject drugs accompanies Ivy to the clinic and requests that he be tested for the presence of HIV.

BASIS FOR THE USE OF RECOMBINANT DNA IN MEDICINE

Developments in the field of molecular biology are occurring at a rapid pace. Techniques for joining DNA sequences into new combinations (recombinant DNA) were originally developed as research tools to explore and manipulate genes, but they can also be used to identify defective genes associated with disease; eventually they will be used to correct genetic defects. Recombinant DNA technology is already being used to some extent in clinical laboratories, and even a cursory survey of the current literature leads to the conclusion that these techniques will soon replace many of the current clinical testing procedures.

RECOMBINANT DNA TECHNIQUES

In order to understand the ways in which genes differ from one individual to another and the use of these differences to diagnose disease, at least a basic appreciation of recombinant DNA techniques is required.

The first steps in determining individual variations in genes involve isolating the genes (or fragments of DNA) that contain variable sequences and obtaining adequate quantities for study. A number of techniques have been used to accomplish these goals.

Strategies for Obtaining Copies of Genes or Fragments of DNA

RESTRICTION FRAGMENTS

Enzymes called restriction endonucleases enable molecular biologists to cleave segments of DNA from the genome of various types of cells or to fragment DNA obtained from other sources.

A restriction enzyme is an endonuclease that recognizes a short sequence of DNA, usually 4–6 base pairs (bp) in length, and cleaves both DNA strands within this sequence. A key feature of restriction enzymes is their specificity. They always cleave at the same DNA sequence and only cleave at that particular sequence. Most of the DNA sequences recognized by restriction enzymes are palindromes, that is, both strands of DNA have the same base sequence when read in a 5′ to 3′ direction. The cuts made by these enzymes may be blunt (so that the products are double-stranded at the ends) or "sticky" (so that the products are single-stranded at the ends) (Fig. 16.1). Hundreds of restriction enzymes with different specificities have been isolated (Table 16.1).

Restriction endonucleases were discovered in bacteria in the late 1960s and 1970s. These enzymes were named for the fact that bacteria use them to "restrict" the growth of viruses (bacteriophage) that infect the bacterial cells.

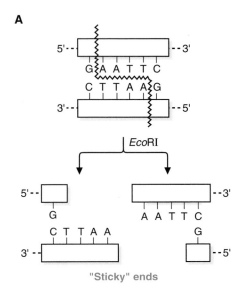

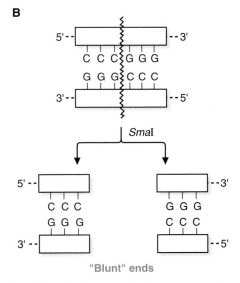

Fig. 16.1. Action of restriction enzymes. Note that each of the DNA sequences shown is a palindrome; each strand of the DNA, when read in a 5′ to 3′ direction, has the same sequence. Cleavage by *Eco*RI produces single-stranded (or "sticky") ends or tails and by *Sma*I produces double stranded (or "blunt") ends.

Table 16.1. Sequences Cleaved by Selected Restriction Enzymes

Restriction Enzyme	Source	Cleavage Site
*Alu*I	*Arthrobacter luteus*	5′ - A G C T - 3′ 3′ - T C G A - 5′
*Bam*HI	*Bacillus amyloliquefaciens* H	5′ - G G A T C C - 3′ 3′ - C C T A G G - 5′
*Eco*RI	*Escherichia coli* RY13	5′ - G A A T T C - 3′ 3′ - C T T A A G - 5′
*Hae*III	*Haemophilus aegyptius*	5′ - G G C C - 3′ 3′ - C C G G - 5′
*Hind*III	*Haemophilus influenzae* R_d	5′ - A A G C T T - 3′ 3′ - T T C G A A - 5′
*Msp*I	*Moraxella* species	5′ - C C G G - 3′ 3′ - G G C C - 5′
*Mst*II	*Microcoleus*	5′ - C C T N A G G - 3′ 3′ - G G A N T C C - 5′
*Not*I	*Nocardia otitidis*	5′ - G C G G C C G C - 3′ 3′ - C G C C G G C G - 5′
*Pst*I	*Providencia stuartii* 164	5′ - C T G C A G - 3′ 3′ - G A C G T C - 5′
*Sma*I	*Serratia marcescens* S_b	5′ - C C C G G G - 3′ 3′ - G G G C C C - 5′

In sickle cell anemia, the point mutation that converts a glutamate residue to a valine residue (**GAG** to **GTG**) occurs in a site that is cleaved by the restriction enzyme *Mst*II (recognition sequence CCTNAGG, where N may be any base) within the normal β-globin gene. The sickle cell mutation causes the β-globin gene to lose this *Mst*II restriction site. Therefore, neither of the two alleles of **Michael Sichel's** β-globin gene will be cleaved at this site.

Restriction fragments of DNA can base-pair with each other if they have sticky ends that are complementary. Therefore, two unrelated DNA fragments can base-pair with each other if they were cleaved by the same restriction enzyme. After the fragments have base-paired, the ends are covalently joined by the action of DNA ligase (Fig. 16.2). The use of restriction enzymes in conjunction with DNA ligase, therefore, can produce recombinant or chimeric DNA, that is, DNA molecules that have been recombined in vitro (in "glass"; i.e., in a test tube).

DNA PRODUCED BY REVERSE TRANSCRIPTASE

If mRNA transcribed from a gene is isolated, this mRNA can be used as a template by the enzyme reverse transcriptase, which produces a DNA copy (cDNA) of the RNA. In contrast to DNA fragments cleaved from the genome by restriction enzymes, DNA produced by reverse transcriptase, because it uses mRNA as a template, does not contain introns.

CHEMICAL SYNTHESIS OF DNA

Automated machines are now available for synthesizing oligonucleotides (fragments of single-stranded DNA) up to 100 nucleotides in length. These machines can be programmed to produce oligonucleotides with a specified base sequence. Although entire genes cannot yet be synthesized, oligonucleotides can be prepared that will base-pair with segments of genes. These oligonucleotides can be used in the process of identifying, isolating, and amplifying genes.

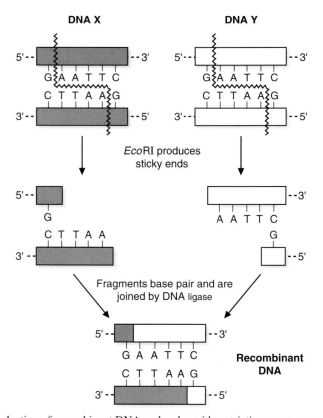

Fig. 16.2. Production of recombinant DNA molecules with restriction enzymes and DNA ligase.

Techniques for Identifying DNA Sequences

PROBES

A probe is a single strand of DNA that can form base pairs with a complementary sequence on another single-stranded polynucleotide composed of DNA or RNA. This process is known as reannealing or hybridization. In order to identify the target sequence, the probe must carry a label. If the probe has a radioactive label such as ^{32}P, it can be detected by autoradiography. An autoradiogram is produced by covering the material containing the probe with a sheet of x-ray film. Electrons emitted by disintegration of the radioactive atoms cause the film to be exposed in the region directly over the probe (Fig. 16.3).

Probes may be composed of cDNA (produced from mRNA by reverse transcriptase), fragments of genomic DNA (cleaved by restriction enzymes from the genome), chemically synthesized oligonucleotides, or, occasionally, RNA. There are a number of techniques for introducing labels into these probes. Not all probes are radioactive. Some are chemical adducts (compounds that bind covalently to DNA) that can be identified, for example, by fluorescence.

GEL ELECTROPHORESIS

Gel electrophoresis is a technique that uses an electrical field to separate molecules on the basis of size. Because DNA contains negatively charged phosphate groups, it will migrate in an electrical field toward the positive electrode (Fig. 16.4). Shorter molecules migrate more rapidly through the pores of a gel than longer molecules, so separation is based on length. Gels composed of polyacrylamide can separate DNA molecules that differ in length by only one nucleotide and are used to determine the base sequence of DNA. Agarose gels are used to separate DNA fragments that have larger size differences.

The bands of DNA in the gel can be visualized by various techniques. Staining with dyes such as ethidium bromide allows direct visualization under ultraviolet light of all DNA bands. Specific sequences are generally detected by means of a labeled probe.

DETECTION OF SPECIFIC DNA SEQUENCES

In order to detect specific sequences, DNA is usually transferred to a solid support, such as a sheet of nitrocellulose paper. For example, if bacteria are growing on an agar plate, cells from each colony will adhere to a nitrocellulose sheet pressed against the agar, and an exact replica of the bacterial colonies will be transferred to the nitrocellulose paper (Fig. 16.5). A similar technique is used to transfer bands of DNA from electrophoretic gels to nitrocellulose sheets. After bacterial colonies are transferred to nitrocellulose paper, the paper is treated with an alkaline solution. In the case where DNA is separated on agarose gels, the gel is treated with an alkaline solution. Alkaline solutions denature DNA, that is, separate the two strands of each double helix. The single-stranded DNA can be hybridized with a probe, and the regions on the nitrocellulose blot containing DNA that base-pairs with the probe can be identified.

E. M. Southern developed the technique, which bears his name, for identifying DNA sequences on gels. Southern blots are produced when DNA on a nitrocellulose blot of an electrophoretic gel is hybridized with a DNA probe. Molecular biologists decided to follow the compass as they named two additional techniques. Northern blots are produced when RNA on a nitrocellulose blot is hybridized with a DNA probe. A slightly different but related technique, known as a Western blot, involves separating proteins by gel electrophoresis and probing with labeled antibodies for specific proteins (Fig. 16.6).

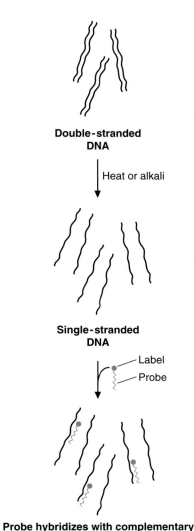

Double-stranded DNA

Heat or alkali

Single-stranded DNA

— Label
— Probe

Probe hybridizes with complementary sequence on DNA

Fig. 16.3. Use of probes to identify DNA sequences. The probe may be either DNA or RNA.

Western blots are currently being used as one of the tests for the AIDS virus. In this case, the presence of viral proteins in the blood is detected by antibodies. Tests performed on **Ivy Sharer's** friend, **Doug Bewser**, showed that he was HIV positive. Unlike Ivy, however, he has not yet developed the symptoms of AIDS.

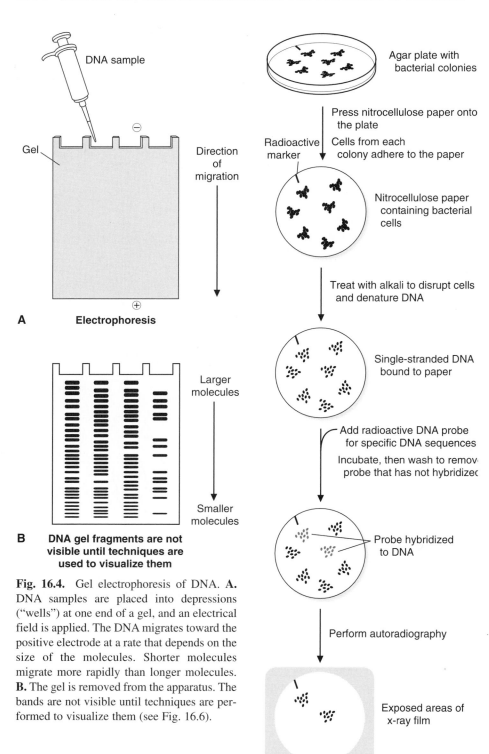

A Electrophoresis

B DNA gel fragments are not visible until techniques are used to visualize them

Larger molecules

Smaller molecules

Fig. 16.4. Gel electrophoresis of DNA. **A.** DNA samples are placed into depressions ("wells") at one end of a gel, and an electrical field is applied. The DNA migrates toward the positive electrode at a rate that depends on the size of the molecules. Shorter molecules migrate more rapidly than longer molecules. **B.** The gel is removed from the apparatus. The bands are not visible until techniques are performed to visualize them (see Fig. 16.6).

Fig. 16.5. Identification of bacterial colonies containing specific DNA sequences. The autoradiogram can be used to identify bacterial colonies on the original agar plate that contain the desired DNA sequence.

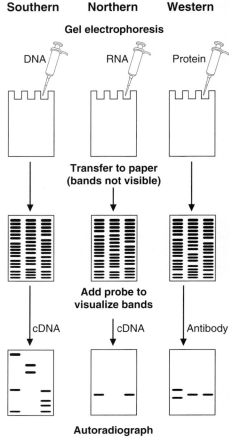

Fig. 16.6. Southern, Northern, and Western blots. In the Southern procedure, DNA molecules are separated by electrophoresis, denatured, transferred to nitrocellulose paper (by "blotting"), and hybridized with a cDNA probe. In the Northern procedure, RNA is electrophoresed and treated similarly except that alkali is not used. (Alkali hydrolyzes RNA.) In the Western procedure, proteins are electrophoresed and probed with a specific antibody. The probes are labeled to visualize the bands with which they hybridize.

DNA SEQUENCING

Although it was once considered an impossible task, the determination of the sequence of nucleotides in a DNA strand is now a routine laboratory technique. The most common procedure was developed by Frederick Sanger and involves the use of dideoxynucleotides (Fig. 16.7).

Four separate reactions are performed in which only one of the four dideoxynucleotides (ddNTPs) is added to each tube. Each tube contains a solution with all four normal deoxynucleotides (dNTPs), DNA polymerase, a primer, and a DNA template strand. The DNA polymerase catalyzes the polymerization of DNA strands complementary to the template. The dideoxynucleotide in each tube randomly adds to the 3′-ends of the growing strands, base-pairing with the corresponding nucleotide on the template strand. However, because a dideoxynucleotide does not contain a 3′-hydroxyl group, once the ddNTP is incorporated, further polymerization of the strand cannot occur, and synthesis is terminated. The ddNTPs compete with the normal dNTPs, and, therefore, chain termination is random but the base at which termination occurs corresponds to the particular ddNTP in the reaction mixture. For example, for a growing polynucleotide strand in which adenine (A) should add at positions 10, 15, and 17, competition between ddATP and dATP for each position results in some chains terminating at position 10, some at 15, and some at 17.

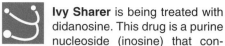

Ivy Sharer is being treated with didanosine. This drug is a purine nucleoside (inosine) that contains the base hypoxanthine attached via a glycosidic bond to dideoxyribose. In cells, didanosine is converted to a nucleoside triphosphate that adds to growing DNA strands. Because dideoxynucleotides lack both 2′- and 3′-hydroxyl groups, additional nucleotides cannot be added to the growing strands, and DNA synthesis is terminated. Reverse transcriptase, the enzyme that uses viral RNA as a template to produce a DNA copy, is more sensitive to the strand-terminating activity of didanosine than are cellular DNA polymerases.

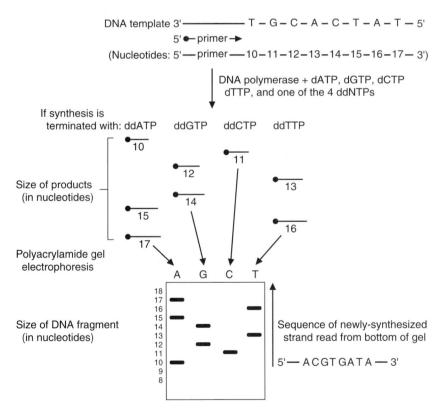

Fig. 16.7. DNA sequencing by the dideoxynucleotide method. Four tubes are used. Each one contains a DNA template hybridized to a primer, DNA polymerase, plus dATP, dGTP, dCTP, and dTTP. Either the primer or the nucleotides must have a radioactive label, so bands can be visualized on the gel by autoradiography. One of the four dideoxyribonucleotides (ddNTPs) is added to each tube. Termination of synthesis occurs where the ddNTP is incorporated into the growing chain. The template is complementary to the sequence of the newly synthesized strand.

Q 16.1: In the early studies on CF, DNA sequencing was used to determine the type of defect in patients. Buccal cells were obtained from washes of the mucous membranes of the mouth, DNA isolated from these cells was amplified by PCR, and DNA sequencing of the CF gene was performed. A sequencing gel for the region in which the normal gene differs from the mutant gene is shown below.

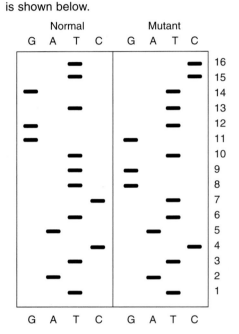

What is the difference between the normal and the mutant CF gene sequence shown on the gel, and what effect would this difference have on the protein produced from this gene?

 A "library" in molecular biologists' terms is a set of host cells that collectively contain all the DNA sequences from the genome of another organism.

As a consequence of random termination, DNA strands of varying lengths are produced from a template. The shortest strands are closest to the 5'-end of the growing DNA strand because the strand grows in a 5' to 3' direction. If these strands are subjected to gel electrophoresis, the sequence of the DNA strand can be determined from the positions of the bands on the gel.

Techniques for Amplifying DNA Sequences

In order to study genes or other DNA sequences, adequate quantities of material must be obtained. It is often difficult to isolate significant quantities of DNA from the original source. For instance, an individual cannot usually afford to part with enough tissue to provide the amount of DNA required for clinical testing. Therefore, the available quantity of DNA has to be amplified.

CLONING OF DNA

The first technique developed for amplifying the quantity of DNA is known as cloning (Fig. 16.8). A fragment of DNA from one organism ("foreign" DNA) is inserted into a vector (or carrier) composed of DNA, and the chimera (vector containing recombinant DNA) is used to transform host cells. As the host cells divide, in addition to replicating their own DNA, they also replicate the DNA of the vector, which includes the foreign DNA. Subsequently, relatively large quantities of the foreign DNA can be isolated.

If the host cells are bacteria, the first step in the cloning procedure is to insert the foreign DNA into a vector which can then carry this DNA into the bacteria. The most commonly used vectors are bacteriophage (viruses that infect bacteria), plasmids (extrachromosomal pieces of circular DNA that are taken up by bacteria), or cosmids (plasmids that contain DNA sequences from the lambda phage).

A segment of the foreign DNA and the DNA vector are usually cleaved with the same restriction enzyme. The simplest process uses an enzyme that produces complementary sticky ends in both the foreign DNA and the DNA vector. Complementary single-stranded regions can form base pairs, and the molecules can be covalently joined by DNA ligase.

When eukaryotic cells are used as the host, vectors are often unnecessary because techniques are available that allow foreign DNA to enter the host cells. The foreign DNA can then integrate into the host cell genome by recombinational events that are not well understood.

Host cells that contain recombinant DNA are often called transformed cells if they are bacteria, or transfected cells if they are eukaryotes. Markers in the vector DNA are used to identify cells that have been transformed, and probes for the foreign DNA are used to determine that the host cells actually contain the foreign DNA. This process is called screening (Fig. 16.9)

The host cells containing the foreign DNA are incubated under conditions in which they replicate rapidly. The foreign DNA is then isolated from the cells. If the host cells are grown under conditions permitting expression of the foreign DNA, the protein produced from this DNA can be isolated.

POLYMERASE CHAIN REACTION (PCR)

PCR is an in vitro method that can be used for rapid production of very large amounts of DNA. It is particularly suited for amplifying DNA for clinical or forensic testing procedures because only a very small sample of DNA is required as the starting material. DNA can be amplified by PCR from a single strand of hair or a single drop of blood or semen.

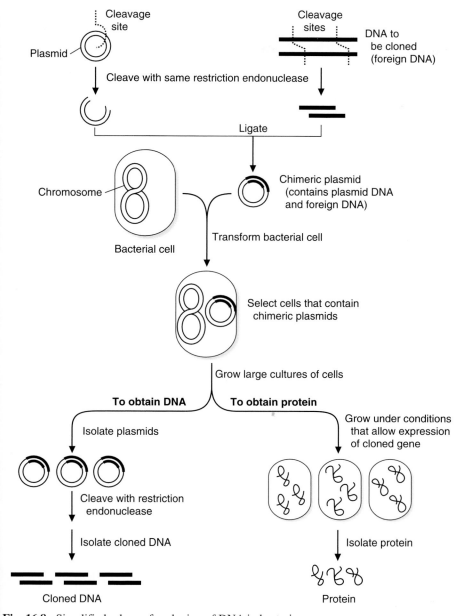

Fig. 16.8. Simplified scheme for cloning of DNA in bacteria.

Although only small amounts of semen were obtained from **Vicky Tim's** body, the quantity of DNA in these specimens could be amplified by PCR.

First, a sample of DNA containing the segment to be amplified must be isolated. Large quantities of primers, the four deoxyribonucleoside triphosphates, and a heat-stable DNA polymerase are added to a solution in which the DNA is heated to separate the strands. The primers are two synthetic oligonucleotides. Each oligonucleotide is complementary to a short sequence in one strand of the DNA to be amplified. As the solution is cooled, the oligonucleotides form base pairs with the DNA and serve as primers for the synthesis of DNA strands catalyzed by the heat-stable DNA polymerase. The four deoxyribonucleoside triphosphates serve as precursors for synthesis of the new DNA strands. The process of heating, cooling, and new DNA synthesis is repeated many times until a large number of copies of the DNA is obtained. The process can be automated so that each round of replication takes only a few minutes (Fig. 16.10). In 20 heating and cooling cycles, the DNA is amplified over a million fold.

16.1: In individuals of northern European descent, 70% of the cases of cystic fibrosis (CF) are caused by a deletion of 3 bases in the CF gene.

In the region of the gene shown on the gels, the base sequence (read from the bottom to the top of the gel) is the same for the normal and mutant gene for the first 6 positions, and the bases in positions 10–16 of the normal gene are the same as the bases in positions 7–13 of the mutant gene. Therefore, a 3-base deletion in the mutant gene corresponds to bases 7–9 of the normal gene.

Normal sequence: T A T C A T C T T T G G T (Ile Ile Phe Gly)
CF sequence: T A T C A T – – – T G G T (Ile Ile Gly)

Loss of 3 bp (indicated by the dashes) maintains the reading frame, so only the single amino acid phenylalanine (F) is lost. Phenylalanine would normally appear as residue 508 in the protein. Therefore, the deletion is referred to as ΔF_{508}. The rest of the amino acid sequence of the normal and the mutant proteins is identical.

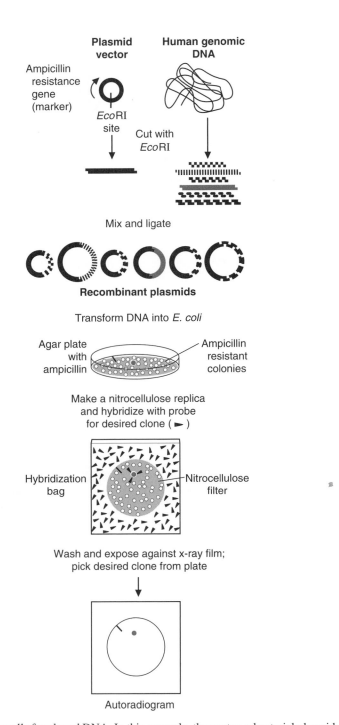

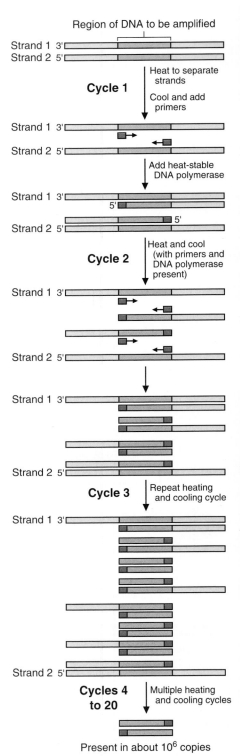

Region of DNA to be amplified

Fig. 16.9. Screening cells for cloned DNA. In this example, the vector, a bacterial plasmid carrying an ampicillin resistance gene, is cut with the restriction enzyme *Eco*RI, as is the genomic DNA, which contains within it the desired fragment. The sticky ends can be ligated together to generate a series of recombinant molecules, in which different genomic fragments have been inserted into the vector. This mixture is then transfected into ampicillin-sensitive *E. coli* which have been treated with calcium chloride to promote their uptake of DNA. Only those bacteria that have taken up a plasmid with an ampicillin resistance gene will form colonies when plated in the presence of ampicillin. Other bacterial cells will be killed. To identify the specific recombinant carrying the desired genomic fragment, hybridization is performed. A nitrocellulose filter replica is made of the plate and incubated in a hybridization bag with radiolabeled "probe," which contains at least part of the DNA sequence of interest. The probe will selectively bind to DNA from the colony that harbors the desired plasmid and therefore can be identified by placing the filter against x-ray film. Modified from Gelehrter T, Collins F. Principles of medical genetics. Baltimore: Williams & Wilkins, 1990:74.

Fig. 16.10. Polymerase chain reaction (PCR). Strand 1 and strand 2 are the original DNA strands. The short blue fragments are the primers. After multiple heating and cooling cycles, the original strands remain, but most of the DNA consists of amplified copies of the segment (shown in lighter blue) synthesized by the heat-stable DNA polymerase.

USE OF RECOMBINANT DNA TECHNIQUES FOR DIAGNOSIS OF DISEASE

DNA Polymorphisms

Polymorphisms in the genome serve as the basis for using recombinant DNA techniques in the diagnosis of disease. Polymorphisms are variations in DNA sequences. There may be millions of different polymorphisms in the human genome. The first to be identified involved point mutations, the substitution of one base for another. Subsequent studies have shown that deletions and insertions are also responsible for variations in DNA sequences. Some polymorphisms occur within the coding region of genes. Others are found in noncoding regions closely linked to genes involved in the etiology (cause) of inherited disease.

Detection of Polymorphisms

RESTRICTION FRAGMENT LENGTH POLYMORPHISMS

Occasionally, a point mutation occurs in a recognition site for a restriction enzyme. The enzyme, therefore, can cut at other recognition sites but not at the site of the mutation. Consequently, the restriction fragment produced by the enzyme is larger for a person with the mutation than for a normal person. Mutations can also create restriction sites that are not present in the normal gene. In this case, restriction fragments will be smaller for the person with the mutation than for the normal individual. These variations in the length of restriction fragments are known as restriction fragment length polymorphisms (RFLPs).

In some cases, the mutation that causes the disease affects a restriction site within the coding region of a gene. However, in most cases, the mutation affects a restriction site that is outside the coding region but tightly linked (i.e., physically close on the DNA molecule) to the abnormal gene that causes the disease.

DETECTION OF MUTATIONS BY ALLELE-SPECIFIC OLIGONUCLEOTIDE PROBES

Because many mutations associated with genetic diseases do not occur within restriction sites, other techniques have been developed to detect mutations.

Oligonucleotide probes can be synthesized that are complementary to a short DNA sequence that includes a mutation. Different probes are produced for alleles that contain mutations and for those that have a normal DNA sequence. The region of the genome that contains the abnormal gene is amplified by PCR, and the samples of DNA are placed in narrow bands on nitrocellulose paper ("slot blotting"). The paper is then treated with the probe for either the normal or the mutant sequence. Autoradiograms indicate whether the normal or mutant probe has preferentially base-paired with the DNA, that is, whether the alleles are normal or mutated. Carriers, of course, have two different alleles, one that binds to the normal probe and one that binds to the mutant probe.

This test can also be performed using gel electrophoresis and Southern blotting. However, the slot blotting method is simpler and more amenable for use as a screening test.

TESTING FOR MUTATIONS BY PCR

If the DNA sequence in a region containing a mutation is known, an oligonucleotide complementary to this region can be synthesized. The oligonucleotide will base-pair only with DNA obtained from an individual with that mutation. This oligonucleotide can be used as a primer for PCR. If DNA is amplified by PCR, the DNA used as the

 The DNA polymerase used for PCR is isolated from *Thermus aquaticus*, a bacterium that grows in hot springs. This polymerase can withstand the heat required for separation of DNA strands.

The mutation that causes sickle cell anemia abolishes a restriction site for the enzyme *Mst*II in the β-globin gene. The consequence of this mutation is that the restriction fragment produced by *Mst*II that includes the 5′-end of the β-globin gene is larger (1.3 kilobases (kb)) for individuals with sickle cell anemia than for normal individuals (1.1 kb). Analysis of restriction fragments provides a direct test for the mutation. In **Michael Sichel's** case, both alleles for β-globin lack the *Mst*II site and produce 1.3-kb restriction fragments.

Carriers have both a normal and a mutant allele. Therefore, their DNA will produce both the larger and the smaller *Mst*II restriction fragments.

When Michael Sichel's sister **Carrie Sichel** was tested, she was found to have both the small and the large restriction fragments, and her status as a carrier of sickle cell anemia, initially made on the basis of protein electrophoresis, was confirmed.

A

gene A (normal) — C C T — G A G — G ——
                        *Mst*II site

gene S (sickle) — C C T — G T G — G ——
                        (no *Mst*II site)

B

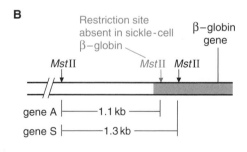

C

Southern blot of DNA cut with *Mst*II and hybridized with β-globin probe

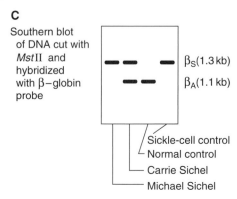

Q 16.2: Testing for CF by DNA sequencing is time-consuming and expensive. Therefore, another technique that utilizes allele-specific oligonucleotide probes has been developed. **Sissy Fibrosa** and her family were tested by this method. Oligonucleotide probes, complementary to the region where the 3-base deletion is located, have been synthesized. One probe binds to the mutant (ΔF_{508}) gene, and the other to the normal gene.

DNA was isolated from Sissy, her parents, and two siblings and amplified by PCR. Samples of the DNA were spotted on nitrocellulose paper, treated with the oligonucleotide probes, and the following results were obtained. (Dark spots indicate binding of the probe.)

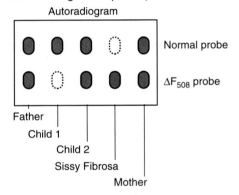

Autoradiogram

Which members of Sissy's family have CF, which are normal, and which are carriers?

PCR template must contain the mutation. If the DNA is normal, the primer will not bind to it and the DNA will not be amplified. This concept can be used for clinical testing.

Oligonucleotides that selectively bind to regions of genomic DNA containing various mutations can be synthesized. These oligonucleotides, each specific for a different mutation and each containing a different label, can be used as primers in a single PCR reaction. The oligonucleotides that function as primers and are amplified are those that correspond to the mutations present in the individual's DNA used as the template for PCR.

DETECTION OF MUTATIONS THAT CONTAIN HIGHLY VARIABLE REGIONS

Human DNA contains many sequences that are repeated in tandem a variable number of times at certain loci in the genome. These regions are called hypervariable regions because they contain a variable number of tandem repeats (VNTR). Digestion with restriction enzymes that recognize sites which flank the VNTR region produces fragments containing these loci, which differ in size from one individual to another, depending on the number of repeats that are present. Probes used to identify these restriction fragments bind to or near the sequence that is repeated (Fig. 16.11).

The restriction fragment patterns produced from these loci can be used to identify individuals as accurately as the traditional fingerprint. In fact, this restriction fragment technique has been called "DNA fingerprinting" and is gaining widespread use

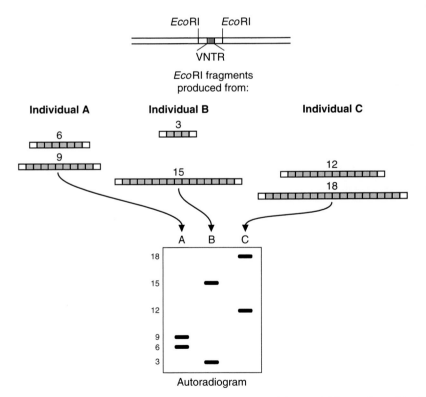

Fig. 16.11. Restriction fragments produced from a gene with a variable number of tandem repeats (VNTR). Each individual has two homologues of every somatic chromosome and thus two genes that each contain this region with a VNTR. Cleavage of each individual's genomic DNA with a restriction enzyme produces two fragments containing this region. The length of the fragments depends on the number of repeats they contain. Electrophoresis separates the fragments, and a labeled probe that binds to the fragments allows them to be visualized.

Witnesses identified three men who spoke to **Vicky Tim** during the time she spent purchasing food at the convenience store. DNA samples were obtained from these suspects and used for DNA fingerprinting. The samples were compared with DNA from semen taken from the victim and with her own DNA. The results, using a probe for one of the repeated sequences in human DNA, are shown below to illustrate the process. For more positive identification, a number of different restriction enzymes and probes were used.

The DNA from suspect 2 produced the same restriction pattern as the DNA from the semen obtained from the victim. If the other restriction enzymes and probes corroborate this finding, suspect 2 can be identified by DNA fingerprinting as the rapist/murderer.

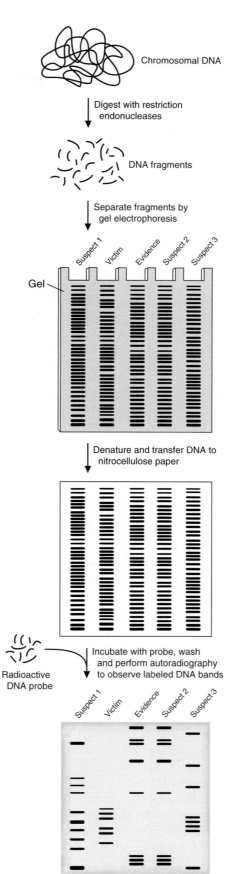

16.2: Obviously, the father and mother are both carriers of the defective allele, as is one of the two older siblings (Child 2). Sissy has the disease, and the other sibling (Child 1) is normal.

in forensic analysis. Family relationships can be determined by this method, and it can be used to help acquit or convict suspects in criminal cases.

Individuals who are closely related genetically will have restriction fragment patterns (DNA fingerprints) that are more similar than those who are more distantly related. Only monozygotic twins will have identical patterns.

USE OF RECOMBINANT DNA TECHNIQUES FOR THE PREVENTION AND TREATMENT OF DISEASE

Vaccines

Before the advent of recombinant DNA technology, vaccines were made from infectious agents which were either killed or attenuated (altered so that they can no longer multiply in an inoculated individual). Both types of vaccines were potentially dangerous because they could be contaminated with the live, infectious agent. In fact, in a small number of instances, disease has actually been caused by vaccination.

Because the human immune system responds to antigenic proteins on the surface of an infectious agent, the possibility of producing these antigens by recombinant DNA techniques was very attractive. By recombinant DNA techniques, the proteins could be produced, completely free of the infectious agent, and used in the vaccine. Thus, any risk of infection could be eliminated. The first successful recombinant DNA vaccine to be produced was for the hepatitis B virus (Fig. 16.12).

Production of Therapeutic Proteins

INSULIN AND GROWTH HORMONE

Recombinant DNA techniques are currently being used to produce proteins that have therapeutic properties. One of the first such proteins to be produced was human insulin. Because this protein is not glycosylated, it could be produced in *E. coli*. DNA corresponding to the A and B chains of human insulin was prepared and inserted into plasmids that were used to transform *E. coli* cells. The bacteria then synthesized the insulin chains which were purified and allowed to fold and form disulfide bonds, producing active insulin molecules (Fig. 16.13).

Human growth hormone has also been produced in *E. coli*. It can be used to treat children with growth hormone deficiencies.

COMPLEX HUMAN PROTEINS

More complex proteins have been produced in mammalian cell culture. The gene for Factor VIII, a protein involved in blood clotting, is defective in individuals with hemophilia. Before genetically engineered Factor VIII became available, many hemophiliacs died of AIDS or hepatitis which they contracted from transfusions of contaminated blood or from Factor VIII isolated from contaminated blood.

Tissue plasminogen activator (TPA) is a protease in blood which converts plasminogen to plasmin, a protease that cleaves fibrin, thereby dissolving blood clots. Recombinant TPA, produced in mammalian cell cultures, is frequently administered during or immediately after a heart attack to dissolve the thrombi that occlude coronary arteries, preventing oxygen from reaching the heart muscle.

Hematopoietic growth factors have also been produced in mammalian cell cultures by recombinant DNA techniques. Erythropoietin can be used in certain types of anemias to stimulate the production of red blood cells. Colony-stimulating factors (CSFs) and interleukins (ILs) can be used after bone marrow transplants and after chemotherapy to stimulate white blood cell production and decrease the risk of infection.

Erna Nemdy received her hepatitis B vaccine, and in addition was given the following information by the physician who administered the inoculation.

The hepatitis B virus (HBV) infects the liver, causing severe damage. The virus contains a surface antigen (HBsAg) or coat protein for which the gene has been isolated. However, because the protein is glycosylated, it could not be produced in *Escherichia coli*. (Bacteria, because they lack subcellular organelles, cannot produce glycosylated proteins.) Therefore, a yeast (eukaryotic) expression system was used which produced a glycosylated form of the protein. The viral protein, separated from the small amount of contaminating yeast protein, is used as a vaccine for immunization against HBV infection.

Ann Sulin had no further allergic reactions after she began using genetically engineered human insulin rather than beef insulin.

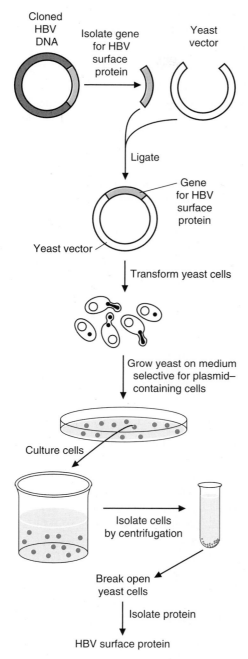

Fig. 16.12. Production of a hepatitis B vaccine by recombinant DNA techniques.

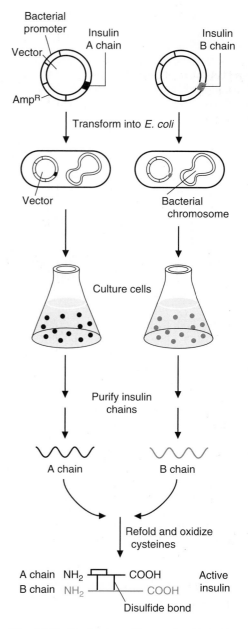

Fig. 16.13. Production of human insulin in *E. coli*. Amp^R = the gene for ampicillin resistance.

Carrie Sichel's fiancé, **Willie Havet**, decided to be tested for the sickle cell gene. He was found to have both the 1.3-kb and the 1.1-kb *Mst*II restriction fragments that include a portion of the β-globin gene. Therefore, like Carrie, he also is a carrier for the sickle cell gene.

 A defect in the adenosine deaminase (ADA) gene causes severe combined immunodeficiency syndrome (SCIDS). When ADA is defective, adenosine accumulates and indirectly causes decreased production of the deoxyribonucleotides required for DNA synthesis. Cells of the immune system, therefore, cannot proliferate at a normal rate, and children with SCIDS usually die at an early age because they cannot combat infections. In order to survive, they must be confined to a sterile, environmental "bubble." When an appropriate donor is available, bone marrow transplantation can be performed with a reasonable degree of success.

In 1990, a 4-year-old girl, for whom no donor was available, was treated with infusions of her own lymphocytes that had been treated with a retrovirus containing a normal ADA gene. Although she had not responded to previous therapy, she improved significantly after this attempt at gene therapy. Since this time, two other children have begun similar treatment for SCIDS.

A method for producing human proteins that is presently being tested involves transgenic animals. These animals have been genetically engineered to produce human proteins that are secreted into milk (Fig. 16.14).

Genetic Counseling

One means of preventing disease is to avoid passing defective genes to offspring. Testing for genetic diseases, particularly in families known to carry a defective gene, allows individuals to decide in advance whether or not to marry and/or to have children.

Screening tests, based on the recombinant DNA techniques outlined in this chapter, have been developed for many inherited diseases. Although these tests are currently rather expensive, particularly if entire families have to be screened, the cost may be trivial compared to the burden of raising children with severe disabilities. Obviously, ethical considerations must be taken into account, but recombinant DNA technology has provided individuals with the opportunity to make choices.

Screening can be performed on the prospective parents prior to conception. If they decide to conceive, the fetus can be tested for the genetic defect. If the fetus has the defect, treatment can be instituted at an early stage, even in utero. For certain diseases, early therapy leads to a more positive outcome.

Gene Therapy

The ultimate cure for genetic diseases is to introduce normal genes into individuals who have defective genes. Currently, gene therapy is being attempted at an experimental level in cell cultures or in animals and, in a few cases, in human subjects.

Transgenic Animals

The introduction of normal genes into somatic cells with defective genes corrects the defect only in the treated individuals, not in their offspring. In order to eliminate the defect for future generations, the normal genes must be introduced into the germ cell line (the cells that produce sperm in males or eggs in females). Experiments with animals indicate that gene therapy in germ cells is feasible. Genes can be introduced into fertilized eggs from which transgenic animals develop, and these transgenic animals can produce normal offspring.

Obviously, these experiments raise many ethical questions that will be difficult to answer.

 CLINICAL COMMENTS. In reading about the development of the hepatitis B vaccine, **Erna Nemdy** learned that the first vaccine available for HBV, marketed in 1982, was a purified and "inactivated" vaccine, containing HBV virus that was chemically killed. The virus was derived from the blood of known HBV carriers. Later, "attenuated" vaccines were used in which the virus remained live but was altered so that it no longer multiplied in the inoculated host. Both the inactivated and the attenuated vaccines are potentially dangerous because they can be contaminated with live infectious HBV.

The modern "subunit" vaccines, first marketed in 1987, were made by recombinant DNA techniques described earlier in this chapter. Since this vaccine consists solely of the viral surface protein or antigen to which the immune system responds, there is no risk for infection with HBV.

CF is a genetically determined autosomal recessive disease which can be caused by a variety of mutations within the CF gene located on chromosome 7. **Sissy**

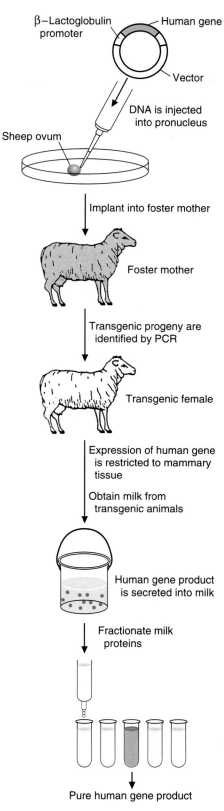

Fig. 16.14. Transgenic animals used to produce human proteins. The gene is inserted into a vector so that it is under the control of the β-lactoglobulin promoter, which is active only in mammary cells. Transgenic progeny (those that carry the human gene) are identified by PCR using primers for the human gene sequence. Milk proteins from these animals are fractionated to yield the pure human protein. From: Recombinant DNA 2/E by Watson, Gilman, Witkowski, and Zoller. Copyright © 1992 by James D. Watson, Michael Gilman, Jan Witkowski and Mark Zoller. Used with permission of W.H. Freeman and Co.

Fibrosa was found to have a 3-bp deletion at residue 508 of the CF gene (present in about 70% of Caucasian patients with CF in the United States) which is associated with a more severe clinical course than many other mutations causing the disease.

The normal CF protein probably serves as a chloride ion channel. Its absence in the tissues of patients with CF causes changes in sweat composition and, in addition, causes obstruction and dilatation of exocrine glands and their ducts. In patients with CF, sweat contains excessive sodium and chloride (the basis of the sweat test), and mucus is not cleared from the tracheobronchial tree. This excess mucus blocks the airways, markedly diminishing air exchange and predisposing the patient to stasis of secretions with resultant secondary infection. Pancreatic duct obstruction leads to decreased secretion of pancreatic enzymes into the small bowel lumen causing malabsorption of fat and other foodstuffs. Abnormal small bowel secretion leads to increased viscosity of the luminal contents causing varying degrees of small bowel obstruction. Liver and gallbladder secretions may be similarly affected.

CF is a relatively common genetic disorder in the United States, with a carrier rate of about 5% in Caucasians. The disease occurs in 1 per 1,600–2,000 Caucasian births in the country (1 per 17,000 in African Americans and 1 per 100,000 in Asians).

After learning the results of their tests for the sickle cell gene, **Carrie Sichel** and **Willie Havet** consulted a genetic counselor. The counselor informed them that, because they were both carriers of the sickle cell gene, their chance of having a child with sickle cell anemia was fairly high (about 1 in 4). She told them that prenatal testing was available with fetal DNA obtained from cells by amniocentesis or chorionic villus sampling. If these tests indicated that the fetus had sickle cell disease, abortion was a possibility. Carrie, because of her religious background, was not sure that abortion was an option for her. But having witnessed her brother's sickle cell crises for many years, she also was not sure that she wanted to risk having a child with the disease. **Willie Havet**, her fiancé, also felt that, at 25 years of age, he was not ready to deal with such difficult problems. They mutually agreed to cancel their marriage plans.

DNA fingerprinting has been an important advance in forensic medicine. Prior to development of this technique, identification of criminals was far less scientific. The suspect in the rape and murder of **Vicky Tim** was arrested and convicted mainly on the basis of the results of DNA fingerprint analysis.

It should be noted, however, that this technique has been challenged in some courts because of technical problems including the statistical interpretation of the data. It is absolutely necessary for all the appropriate controls to be run, including samples from the victim's DNA as well as the suspect's DNA. Another challenge to the fingerprinting procedure has been raised because PCR is such a powerful technique that it can amplify minute amounts of contaminating DNA from a source unrelated to the case.

BIOCHEMICAL COMMENTS. Efforts are currently underway to map the entire human genome. The Human Genome Project officially began in 1990 and is expected to be completed by the year 2005. Although funding is being provided mainly by the United States government, many laboratories around the world are participating.

The human genome contains over 3×10^9 (3 billion) bp. A large percentage of this genome (>95%) does not code for the amino acid sequences of proteins or for functional RNA (such as rRNA or tRNA), but is composed of repetitive sequences, introns, and other noncoding elements of unknown function. The human genome is estimated to contain only between 50,000 and 100,000 genes. Controversy about the wisdom of mapping so much "junk" DNA at so enormous a cost (estimated at between $1 and $10 per base pair, or a total of $3 to $30 billion) initially stalled the human genome mission. But, the lure of exploring the unknown, with the hope of unanticipated and vast rewards, triumphed over caution and frugality. Ultimately, the pessimists may be forced to admit that the optimists were right, but in the short term disappointment and turmoil will undoubtedly prevail.

As announcements of the identification of wayward genes appear in the morning newspaper, the average citizen expects the cure for the genetic disease to be described in the evening edition. Progress in treating genetic disease will not be that easy. In addition to solving the molecular puzzles involved in gene therapy, we will have to deal with many unanswerable questions.

Is it appropriate to replace defective genes in somatic cells to relieve human suffering? Many people may agree with this goal. But there is a related question: is it appropriate to replace defective genes **in the germ cell line** to relieve human suffering? Fewer people may agree with this goal. Genetic manipulation of somatic cells affects only one generation; these cells die with the individual. Germ cells, however, live on, producing each successive generation.

The techniques developed to explore the human genome could be used for many purposes. What are the limits for the application of the knowledge gained by advances in molecular biology? Who should decide what the limits are, and who should serve as the genetic police?

If we permit experiments that involve genetic manipulation of the human germ cell line, however nobly conceived, could we, in our efforts to "improve" ourselves, genetically engineer the human race into extinction?

Suggested Readings

Housman D. DNA on trial—the molecular basis of DNA fingerprinting. N Engl J Med 1995;332:534–535.

Trent RJ. Molecular medicine. New York: Churchill Livingstone, 1993.

Watson JD, Gilman M, Witkowski J, Zoller M. Recombinant DNA. 2nd ed. Scientific American Books. New York: WH Freeman, 1992.

PROBLEM

Two female infants (C_x and C_y) were born on the same day in the same hospital. Because of concern that the infants had been switched in the hospital nursery, genetic tests were performed based on a DNA restriction fragment that exhibits polymorphism because it contains a variable number of tandem repeats. Blood was drawn from the parents and the infants, the DNA extracted, and PCR performed. The DNA was then treated with the restriction enzyme *Ban*I, and the fragments were separated by gel electrophoresis. The results of a Southern blot are shown on the right. A radioactive probe was used that bound to a sequence within the *Ban*I fragments that exhibited polymorphism. Based on this test alone, who are most likely to be the parents of Child X and who are most likely to be the parents of Child Y? (M_A is one of the mothers and H_A is her husband. M_B is the other mother and H_B is her husband.)

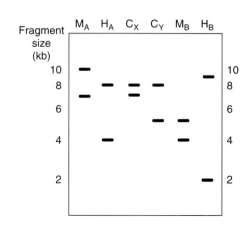

ANSWER

Child C_x could be the offspring of mother M_A and her husband, H_A. The child could have received the chromosome containing the 8-kb fragment from the father H_A and the homologous chromosome containing the 7-kb fragment from the mother M_A.

Child C_y could have received the 5-kb fragment from the mother M_B, but the 8-kb fragment could not have come from either mother M_B or her husband, H_B. In fact, it is unlikely that H_B is the father of either child. (H_A could be the father of C_y, but further testing would be required to establish a relationship.)

17 Oncogenes and the Molecular Biology of Cancer

The term "cancer" applies to a group of diseases in which cells grow abnormally and can become malignant. Malignant cells can invade nearby tissues and travel to other sites in the body, where they establish secondary areas of growth. In humans, the known causes of cancer are radiation, chemical carcinogens, and viruses.

Studies of viruses that cause cancer have led to the oncogene theory that has provided a coherent explanation for the mechanism by which various agents, including chemical carcinogens and radiation, cause normal cells to become transformed into cancer cells.

Mannie Weitzels has recently complained of pain and tenderness in various areas of his skeleton possibly stemming from the expanding mass of myeloid cells within his bone marrow. Because of the expansile process within this limited space, the normal platelet precursor cells (the megakaryocytes) in the marrow are "squeezed" or crowded and fail to develop into mature platelets, which would subsequently be released into the bloodstream. As a consequence, the number of mature platelets (thrombocytes) in the circulation falls and a thrombocytopenia develops. Because the platelets normally participate in the process of clot formation, patients with leukemia may experience a spectrum of hemorrhagic manifestations including ecchymoses (bruises), petechia (small red spots caused by extravasation of red cells into the skin), and bleeding gums.

Nick O'Tyne underwent anatomic staging procedures (bronchoscopy with transbronchial biopsy of the right upper lung nodule, a computed tomogram (CT) of the chest, mediastinoscopy, etc.). As a result of these tests, he was considered a candidate for surgical resection of the primary tumor aimed at cure. He survived the surgery and was recovering uneventfully when 6 months later he complained of an increasingly severe right temporal headache. A CT scan of his brain was performed.

Colin Tuma completed his second course of chemotherapy with 5-fluorouracil (5-FU) and had no serious side effects. He assured his physician at his most recent checkup that, this time, he intended to comply with any instructions his physicians gave him. He ruefully commented that he wished he had returned for regular examinations after his first round of surgery for benign intestinal polyps.

CANCER

Cancer is the term applied to a group of diseases in which cells are not responsive to the normal restraints on growth. A single cell that divides abnormally eventually

259

The results of **Nick O'Tyne's** CT scan indicated that the cancer, which originated in his lung, had metastasized to his brain.

An abnormal chromosome, known as the Philadelphia chromosome (named for the city in which it was first observed), could be seen in dividing cells from **Mannie Weitzels'** bone marrow.

$$H_2C = CH - Cl$$

Vinyl chloride

• Used to make plastics

**Benzo[a]pyrene
(3,4–benzpyrene)**

• Found in cigarette smoke

$$CH_3CH_2$$
$$\diagdown$$
$$N - N = O$$
$$CH_3CH_2$$

Diethylnitrosamine

• Found in whisky and new car interiors

Aflatoxin B$_1$

• Produced by a fungus that grows on peanut butter

Fig. 17.2. Examples of chemical carcinogens. Some of these compounds are not carcinogenic until they are oxidized by enzymes in cells (see benzo[a]pyrene in Chapter 12). The normal function of these enzymes is to make compounds more water soluble so they can be excreted more readily. Unfortunately, they also convert certain compounds into potent carcinogens.

forms a mass called a tumor. A benign tumor and a cancer differ in that cancer cells can invade surrounding tissues. Cancer cells can also metastasize, separating from the growing mass and traveling, through the blood or lymph, to unrelated organs, where they establish new growths of cancer cells. More than 20% of the deaths in the United States each year are caused by cancer, with tumors of the lung, large intestine, and the breast being the most common (Fig. 17.1).

Causes of Cancer

Although evidence for the disease has been found in dinosaur bones and Egyptian mummies, links between causative agents and cancer were not recognized until the late 1770s. One of the first associations was made by Sir Percival Pott, who observed that chimney soot was responsible for the scrotal cancer that affected chimney sweeps in London. Around the same time, the use of snuff was associated with nasal cancer and pipe smoking with lip cancer.

As the list of chemical carcinogens (compounds that cause cancer) continued to grow (Fig. 17.2), associations with other agents, particularly radiation and viruses, were made in the early part of the 20th century. A hereditary tendency to develop cancer was also noted, and chromosomal abnormalities were frequently observed when cancer cells were examined under the light microscope.

After DNA was established as the genetic material in the 1940s, it was found to be a major cellular target of chemical carcinogens and radiation. These agents cause damage to DNA, altering the structure of bases or causing breaks in DNA strands. Although DNA repair mechanisms can fix damaged regions of DNA (see Chapter 12), if the damage is not repaired properly or if it is not repaired before replication occurs, mutations can result. If the mutations occur in genes that control growth and development, cells can begin to divide abnormally and develop into cancerous growths.

Scientists began to identify the genes involved in normal growth and development as they used recombinant DNA techniques to study cancer-causing viruses. In recent years, this work has led to a clearer understanding of cancer, a disease that has frustrated scientists and caused enormous suffering for humankind.

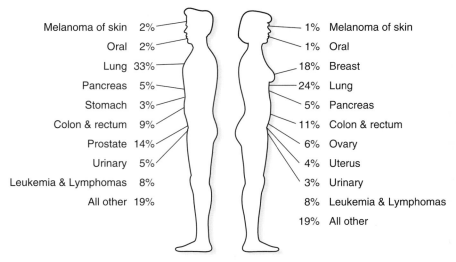

1995 Estimated cancer deaths, United States percent distribution of sites by sex

Male			Female	
Melanoma of skin	2%		1%	Melanoma of skin
Oral	2%		1%	Oral
Lung	33%		18%	Breast
Pancreas	5%		24%	Lung
Stomach	3%		5%	Pancreas
Colon & rectum	9%		11%	Colon & rectum
Prostate	14%		6%	Ovary
Urinary	5%		4%	Uterus
Leukemia & Lymphomas	8%		3%	Urinary
All other	19%		8%	Leukemia & Lymphomas
			19%	All other

Fig. 17.1. Estimated cancer deaths by site and sex. From Murphy GP. CA Cancer J Clin 1995;45:11.

Viruses that produce tumors (tumor viruses) contain genes that can cause infected cells to grow abnormally. These viral genes are similar to cellular genes that control normal growth and development.

 The term oncogene is derived from the Greek word "onkos" meaning bulk or tumor.

Tumor Viruses

In 1910, Peyton Rous was the first to show that extracts from tumor cells (cell-free extracts) could induce new tumors in healthy, uninfected animals. At the time, scientists were not ready for this concept. It literally took decades for the idea to be accepted that viruses could cause cancer. Finally, in 1966 at age 85, Rous won the Nobel Prize.

The molecular details of the carcinogenic effects of viruses were not uncovered until recombinant DNA techniques became available in the mid-1970s. Studies of the Rous sarcoma virus showed that it is a retrovirus: it has an RNA genome. It contains a gene named "*src*" in addition to the three genes usually found in the virus, *gag*, *pol*, and *env*, which encode viral core proteins, reverse transcriptase and integrase, and viral surface glycoproteins, respectively (Fig. 17.3). When the *src* gene was isolated and inserted into normal cells growing in culture, the cells were transformed (Fig. 17.4). Normal cells grow in flat monolayers that stop dividing when they come into contact with each other (a phenomenon known as contact inhibition). Transformed cells lack contact inhibition. They became round and grow in piles. Genes such as *src* that transform cells, causing them to develop a pattern of growth typical of cancer cells, are called oncogenes (Fig. 17.5).

When labeled *src* genes were incubated with DNA from healthy, uninfected chickens, annealing (base-pairing) occurred between the viral *src* DNA and the cellular DNA (Fig. 17.6). Obviously, a normal cellular gene (called c-*src*) was present in the chicken genome that was related to the viral *src* gene (called v-*src*). This normal gene and others that were subsequently discovered are called proto-oncogenes.

Proto-oncogenes regulate normal growth and development. When these genes are mutated, they become oncogenes, which cause cells to grow abnormally. Inappropriate or excessive expression of proto-oncogenes can also cause abnormal growth.

Tumor viruses probably obtained their oncogenes from the cells they infect. After viral genes integrate into the host genome, viral genes may be dormant for a period of time. When these genes are later expressed and new viruses are produced, the new viruses may carry genes from the host cell along with the viral genome. By infecting other cells, these viruses can transform the target cells. The genes that cause transformation (the oncogenes) are those the virus obtained from the host cell and transferred to the target cell.

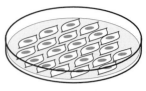

Normal cells

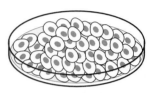

Transformed cells

Fig. 17.4. Normal versus transformed cells. Normal cells grow as flat monolayers. They exhibit contact inhibition, i.e., they stop growing when they touch each other. Transformed cells do not exhibit contact inhibition. They have a round shape and grow in disorganized piles.

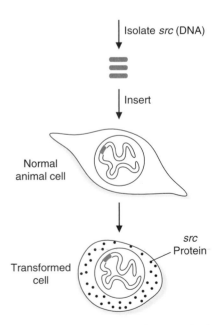

Fig. 17.5. Transformation of cells by isolated oncogenes. If cells growing in culture are exposed to an isolated oncogene, the oncogene can be incorporated into the cell's genome. Expression of the oncogene can cause the cells to be transformed.

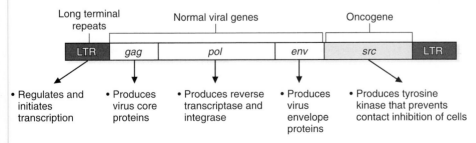

Long terminal repeats	Normal viral genes			Oncogene	
LTR	*gag*	*pol*	*env*	*src*	LTR

- Regulates and initiates transcription
- Produces virus core proteins
- Produces reverse transcriptase and integrase
- Produces virus envelope proteins
- Produces tyrosine kinase that prevents contact inhibition of cells

Fig. 17.3. Rous sarcoma virus genome. This is a retrovirus; it has an RNA genome. The RNA is copied by reverse transcriptase to produce a double-stranded cDNA that can integrate into the host cell genome. The virus has four genes. Three of these genes (*gag, pol*, and *env*) produce viral proteins, and the fourth (*src*) produces a protein that causes cells to be transformed. The long terminal repeats (LTR) contain promoters that regulate expression of the genes.

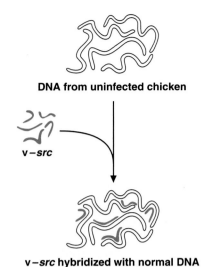

DNA from uninfected chicken

v—src

v—src hybridized with normal DNA

Fig. 17.6. Oncogenes hybridize with normal cellular genes (proto-oncogenes).

Although viruses are not a common cause of human cancer, they have greatly increased our understanding of this group of diseases. Virus research was useful because it would have taken much longer to find oncogenes in the human genome, where they represent a few genes among tens of thousands, than in viruses, where they represent one in a very small number of genes.

Normal Control of Growth

Proto-oncogenes control normal cell growth and division. These genes encode growth factors, growth factor receptors, transcription factors, or other proteins involved in promoting cell growth (Fig. 17.7).

Growth factors regulate growth by serving as ligands that bind to cellular receptors. In some cases, the receptors are proteins on the cell surface. Binding of ligands to these receptors stimulates a cascade of events within the cell. In other cases, the growth factors cross the cell membrane and bind to intracellular receptors. In both cases, the net result is that genes are activated and produce proteins. By processes that have not yet been defined in full detail, these events promote cell growth and division.

Oncogenes and Abnormal Growth

Oncogenes, inserted into normal cells by viruses or produced by the mutagenic effects of chemical carcinogens or radiation on proto-oncogenes, cause cells to grow abnormally when these oncogenes are expressed.

The protein products of oncogenes have been found to be mutated versions of growth factors, receptors in the cell membrane, proteins known as transducers that transmit the signal from the ligand-bound receptor to intracellular proteins, or regulatory proteins that stimulate gene expression in the cell nucleus (Table 17.1).

The Oncogene Theory

The oncogene concept unifies many of the present theories of the causes of cancer. The following points summarize these current ideas.

1. Normal cells contain proto-oncogenes that encode proteins involved in normal growth and development.
2. If an oncogenic virus infects a cell, its oncogene may integrate into the host cell genome, permitting production of the abnormal oncogene protein. The cell may be transformed and exhibit an abnormal pattern of growth (Fig. 17.8).

Table 17.1. Some Oncogenes and Their Protein Products[a]

Oncogene	Protein Product	
	Location	Structurally and Functionally Related to
sis	Secreted from cell	Growth factor
erbB	Cell membrane	Growth factor receptor
fms	Cell membrane	Growth factor receptor
trk	Cell membrane	Growth factor receptor
src	Cytoplasm	Protein kinase (tyrosine)
abl	Cytoplasm	Protein kinase (tyrosine)
raf	Cytoplasm	Protein kinase (serine)
ras	Cytoplasm	GTP binding protein
jun	Nucleus	Transcription factor
fos	Nucleus	Transcription factor
myc	Nucleus	DNA binding protein

[a]The proteins produced by oncogenes are related to growth factors, receptors for growth factors, proteins involved in signal transduction (e.g., protein kinases that phosphorylate tyrosine or serine residues, GTP binding proteins), or proteins involved in regulating gene expression in the nucleus.

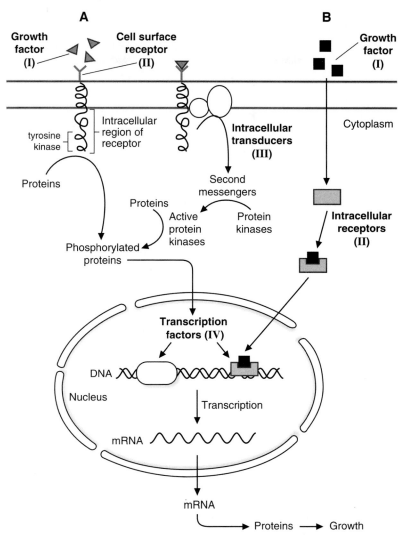

Fig. 17.7. Actions of growth factors. Growth factors bind to receptors that may be located on the cell surface or inside the cell. **A.** Cell surface receptors are proteins that often have intracellular domains with tyrosine kinase activity. When the growth factor binds to these receptors, they are activated and may directly phosphorylate proteins. Other cell surface receptors act through transducers that cause the production of second messengers, compounds that activate protein kinases. These protein kinases phosphorylate proteins. Phosphorylated proteins, produced by either mechanism, activate transcription factors, causing genes to be transcribed. The protein products of these genes promote growth. **B.** Other types of growth factors enter the cell and bind to intracellular receptors. These growth factor-receptor complexes activate genes that promote growth. Proto-oncogenes produce growth factors (I), their receptors (II), transducers (III), and transcription factors (IV). Mutated proto-oncogenes (oncogenes) produce altered versions of I, II, III, or IV that cause abnormal growth. Excessive expression or inappropriate expression of proto-oncogenes can also cause abnormal growth.

The first experiments to show that oncogenes were mutant forms of proto-oncogenes involved cells cultured from a human bladder carcinoma. The DNA sequence of the *ras* oncogene cloned from these cells differed from the normal c-*ras* proto-oncogene. Similar mutations were subsequently found in the *ras* gene of lung and colon tumors.

Colin Tuma's malignant polyp had a mutation in the *ras* oncogene (see the Problem at end of this chapter).

The oncogene N-*myc* is amplified in some neuroblastomas, and amplification of the *erb*-B-2 oncogene is associated with several breast carcinomas.

3. Rather than inserting an oncogene, a virus may simply insert a strong promoter into the host cell genome. This promoter may cause an increased or untimely expression of a normal proto-oncogene (see Fig. 17.8).

4. Radiation and chemical carcinogens act (*a*) by causing a mutation in the regulatory region of a gene, increasing the rate of production of the proto-oncogene protein, or (*b*) by producing a mutation in the coding portion of the oncogene that results in the synthesis of a protein of slightly different amino acid composition capable of transforming the cell (Fig. 17.9).

5. The entire proto-oncogene or a portion of it may be transposed or translocated, i.e., moved from one position in the genome to another (Fig. 17.10). In its new location, the proto-oncogene may be controlled by a more active promoter and, therefore, overexpressed (increased amounts of the protein product may be produced). If only a portion of the proto-oncogene is translocated, it may be expressed as a truncated protein with altered properties, or it may fuse with another gene and produce a fusion protein, which contains portions of what normally were two separate proteins. The truncated or fusion protein causes inappropriate cell growth (Fig. 17.11).

6. The proto-oncogene may be amplified, so that multiple copies of the gene are produced in a single cell. If more genes are active, more proto-oncogene protein will be produced, increasing the growth rate of the cells (Fig. 17.12).

In summary, the various agents that cause cancer may all act through their effects on oncogenes. Radiation and chemical carcinogens may cause mutations in proto-oncogenes or in their regulatory regions. These genes may begin to produce abnormal proteins or they may produce normal proteins, but at an inappropriate time.

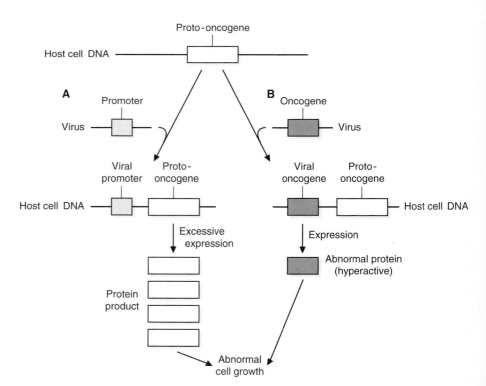

Fig. 17.8. Transformation of a host cell by insertion of a viral promoter (**A**) or a viral oncogene (**B**). Insertion of a viral promoter causes inappropriate expression of the normal proto-oncogene. The protein produced by the gene can be made in excessive amounts or at an inappropriate time, causing abnormal growth. Insertion of a viral oncogene can result in production of an abnormal protein that can cause abnormal growth.

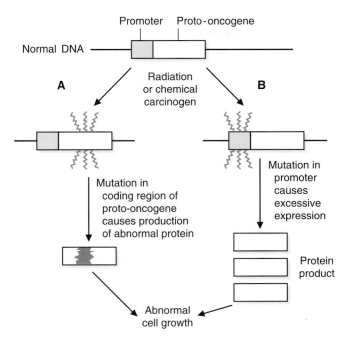

Fig. 17.9. Effect of radiation or chemial carcinogens on proto-oncogenes (**A**) or their promoters (**B**). The mutations may be point mutations, deletions, or insertions.

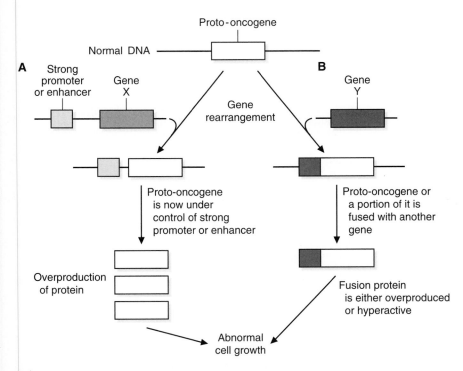

Fig. 17.10. Transposition or translocation of a proto-oncogene. A gene rearrangement causes the proto-oncogene to be regulated by a strong promoter or enhancer (**A**) or to fuse with another gene (**B**).

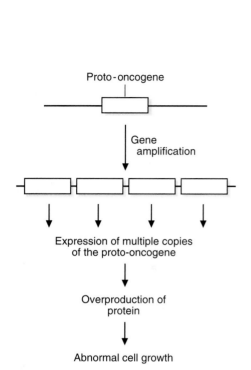

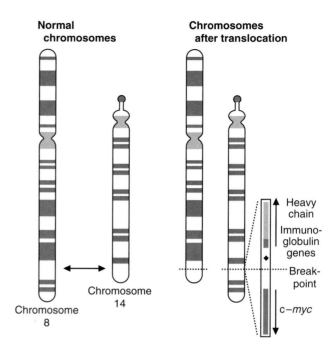

Fig. 17.11. Example of a chromosome translocation involving an oncogene. As a result of this translocation, the proto-oncogene c-*myc* comes under the control of the regulatory region of the immunoglobulin heavy chain genes. This translocation is seen in Burkitt's lymphoma.

Fig. 17.12. Amplification of a proto-oncogene. Gene amplification produces multiple copies of the proto-oncogene. More copies of the gene allow more protein to be produced.

Mannie Weitzels' bone marrow cells contain the Philadelphia chromosome, typical of chronic myelogenous leukemia (CML). The Philadelphia chromosome is produced by a recombinational event that involves an exchange of DNA between chromosomes 9 and 22. A portion of the *abl* oncogene is translocated during this exchange. The portion of c-*abl* that is translocated to chromosome 22 inserts into the *bcr* gene. The hybrid gene *bcr-abl* produces a single fusion protein derived from both the *bcr* and *abl* genes. This fusion protein promotes the growth of leukemic cells.

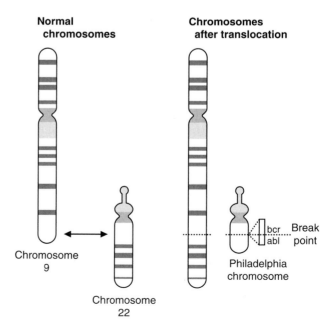

These proteins cause the cells to be transformed. Viruses may introduce oncogenes into cells, or they may introduce promoters into regions of the genome that regulate proto-oncogene expression, causing these genes to lose their normal controls.

Tumor Suppressors

In normal cells, some genes produce proteins called tumor suppressors that prevent abnormal growth. Examples of tumor suppressor proteins include the retinoblastoma protein (RB) and a protein called p53 because of its molecular weight of 53,000 (Fig. 17.13).

DNA tumor viruses do not contain oncogenes, but these viruses add genes to host cells that produce proteins capable of inactivating tumor suppressor proteins. Therefore, the DNA viruses, rather than directly stimulating abnormal growth (like the RNA tumor viruses), act by interfering with the processes that normally limit cell growth.

Cancer Requires Multiple Mutations

Cancer takes a long time to develop because multiple genetic alterations are required to transform normal cells into malignant cells (Fig. 17.14). A single change in one oncogene or tumor suppressor gene in an individual cell is not adequate for transformation. For example, if cells derived from biopsies of normal cells are not already "immortalized," that is, able to grow in culture indefinitely, addition of the *ras* oncogene to the cells is not sufficient for transformation. However, addition of a combination of oncogenes, for example *ras* and *myc*, can result in transformation. Epidemiologists have estimated that between four and six mutations are required for normal cells to be transformed.

Cells accumulate mutations during their lifespans. After a few mutations, a cell may begin to proliferate abnormally, but additional mutations are required for a cell to become malignant. Subsequent genetic changes lead to more uncontrolled growth and finally to metastasis.

 CLINICAL COMMENTS. The treatment of a symptomatic patient such as **Mannie Weitzels** with CML whose white blood cell count is in excess of 50,000 cells/mL^3 is usually initiated with busulfan. Alkylating agents such as cyclophosphamide have been used alone or in combination with busulfan. Purine and pyrimidine antagonists and hydroxyurea (an inhibitor of the enzyme ribonucleotide reductase, which converts ribonucleotides to deoxyribonucleotides for DNA synthesis) are sometimes effective in CML as well. In addition, trials with both α- and γ-interferon have shown promise in increasing survival in these patients. Interestingly, the latter agents have been associated with the disappearance of the Philadelphia chromosome in dividing marrow cells of some patients treated in this way.

Surgical resection of the primary lung cancer with an attempt at cure was justified in **Nick O'Tyne** who had a T_1,N_1,M_0 staging classification preoperatively. Without some evidence of spread to the central nervous system at that time, a preoperative CT scan of the brain would not have been justified. This conservative approach would require scanning of all of the potential sites for metastatic disease from a non-small cell cancer of the lung in all patients who present in this way. In an era of runaway costs of health care delivery, such an approach could not be considered cost-effective.

Unfortunately, Mr. O'Tyne developed a metastatic lesion in the right temporal cortex of his brain. Since metastases were almost certainly present in other organs, Mr. O'Tyne's brain tumor was not treated surgically. In spite of palliative radiation ther-

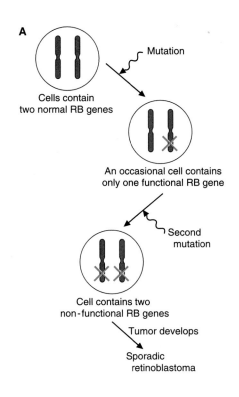

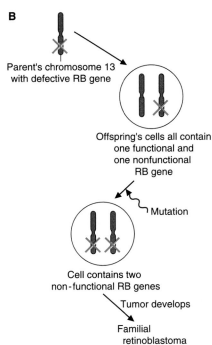

Fig. 17.13. Example of a tumor suppressor gene. RB = retinoblastoma. From: Recombinant DNA 2/E by Watson, Gilman, Witkowski and Zoller. Copyright © 1992 by James D. Watson, Michael Gilman, Jan Witkowski and Mark Zoller. Used with permission of W.H. Freeman and Co.

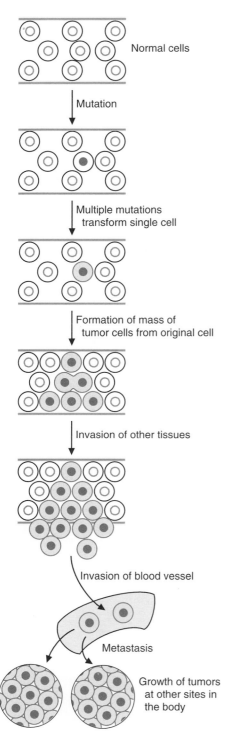

Fig. 17.14. Development of cancer. Accumulation of mutations in a number of genes results in transformation. The cancer cells can invade other tissues and metastasize.

Nick O'Tyne had been smoking for 40 years before he developed lung cancer. The fact that cancer takes so long to develop has made it difficult to prove that the carcinogens in cigarette smoke cause lung cancer. Studies in England and Wales show that cigarette consumption by men began to increase in the early 1900s. Followed by a 20-year lag, the incidence in lung cancer in men also began to rise. Women began smoking later, in the 1920s. Again the incidence of lung cancer began to increase after a 20-year lag.

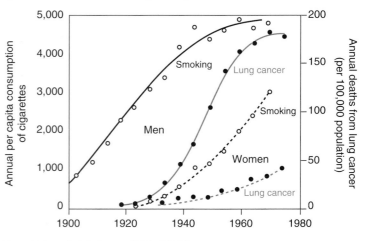

From Cairns J. Sci. Amer. 1975; 233:72

apy to the brain, Mr. O'Tyne succumbed to his disease just 9 months after its discovery, an unusually virulent course for this malignancy. On postmortem examination, his body was found to be riddled with metastatic disease.

BIOCHEMICAL COMMENTS. The development of cancer requires multiple mutations that cause normal cells to proliferate and ultimately to progress to malignancy. These mutations may involve both oncogenes and tumor suppressor genes. Some families have a strong predisposition to cancer. The genes in these individuals probably already have undergone some of the early mutations, and only a few additional somatic mutations cause the cancer to develop. These familial cancers include familial retinoblastoma, familial adenomatous polyps of the colon, and multiple endocrine neoplasia, one form of which involves tumors of the thyroid, parathyroid, and adrenal medulla (MEN type II).

Studies of benign and malignant polyps of the colon show that these tumors have a number of different genetic abnormalities. The incidence of these mutations increases with the level of malignancy. In the early stages, normal cells of the intestinal epithelium proliferate and polyps develop. This change is associated with a mutation in the *ras* proto-oncogene that converts it to an active oncogene. Progression to the next stage is associated with a deletion or alteration of a tumor suppressor gene on chromosome 5. Subsequently, mutations occur in chromosome 18, inactivating a gene that may be involved in cell adhesion, and in chromosome 17, inactivating the p53 tumor suppressor gene. The cells become malignant, and further mutations result in more aggressive growth and metastasis (Fig. 17.15). This sequence of mutations is not always followed precisely, but an accumulation of mutations in these genes is found in a large percentage of colon carcinomas.

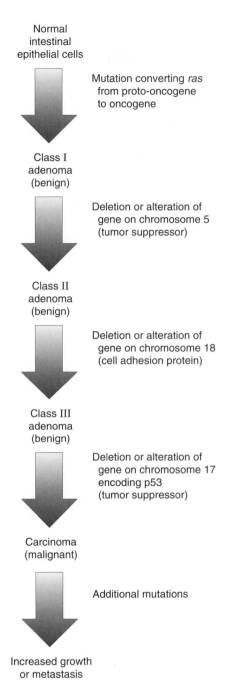

Normal
intestinal
epithelial cells

Mutation converting *ras*
from proto-oncogene
to oncogene

Class I
adenoma
(benign)

Deletion or alteration of
gene on chromosome 5
(tumor suppressor)

Class II
adenoma
(benign)

Deletion or alteration of
gene on chromosome 18
(cell adhesion protein)

Class III
adenoma
(benign)

Deletion or alteration of
gene on chromosome 17
encoding p53
(tumor suppressor)

Carcinoma
(malignant)

Additional mutations

Increased growth
or metastasis

Colin Tuma initially had the type of benign intestinal polyps that may transform into malignant tumors. Because he did not have routine checkups as instructed, one of the polyps he subsequently developed became malignant. If he had returned for regular colonoscopy, this polyp could have been detected at an earlier, premalignant stage and surgically removed.

Fig. 17.15. Possible steps in the development of colon cancer. The changes do not always occur in this order, but the most benign tumors have the lowest frequency of mutations and the most malignant have the highest frequency. From Wolfe SL. Mol Cell Biol 1993:943.

Suggested Readings

Culotta E, Koshland D, Jr. Molecule of the year. p53 sweeps through cancer research. Science 1993;262:1958–1959.

Darnell J, Lodish H, Baltimore D. Cancer. In: Molecular cell biology. Scientific American Books. New York: W.H. Freeman, 1990:955–1002.

Vogelstein B, Fearon ER, Hamilton SR, et al. Genetic alterations during colorectal tumor development. N Engl J Med 1988;319:525.

PROBLEMS

The *ras* oncogene in **Colin Tuma's** malignant polyp differs from the c-*ras* proto-oncogene only in the region that encodes the N-terminus of the protein. This portion of the normal and mutant sequences is shown below:

```
              .      10      .      20      .      30       .
Normal ATGACGGAATATAAGCTGGTGGTGGTGGGCGCCGGCGGT
Mutant ATGACGGAATATAAGCTGGTGGTGGTGGGCGCCGTCGGT
```

This mutation is similar to the mutation found in the *ras* oncogene in various tumors. What type of mutation converts the *ras* proto-oncogene to an oncogene? What effect does this mutation have on the protein product of the gene?

ANSWERS

The *ras* oncogene has a point mutation in codon 12 (position 35 in the DNA sequence). T replaces G, causing a valine residue to replace a glycine in the encoded protein.

The protein produced by the *ras* gene is one of the transducer proteins known as G proteins because they bind GTP. Ras (the protein produced by the *ras* gene) helps to transmit the signal from growth factors to intracellular proteins. When Ras is activated, it binds GTP. Ras hydrolyzes the GTP to GDP and inorganic phosphate, returning to its inactive state. The mutations that convert *ras* to an oncogene affect the ability of Ras to hydrolyze GTP. Thus the mutant Ras remains active, inappropriately continuing to stimulate growth.

Generation of ATP from Metabolic Fuels

All the processes of living cells are processes of energy transformation. The chemical bond energy of carbon-carbon and carbon-hydrogen bonds is converted into other forms: the information content held in the complex chemical structure of DNA, an electrochemical potential gradient which can create an intracellular environment different from the surrounding milieu, or the organized movement of groups of cells. The energy transformations involved in utilizing the chemical bond energy of fuels for energy-requiring processes in cells can be divided into three phases: (1) derivation of energy from the oxidation of fuels, (2) conversion of this energy into the biologically useful form found in the high energy phosphate bonds of ATP, and (3) utilization of ATP phosphate bond energy to drive energy-requiring processes (Fig. 18.1).

The first two phases of energy transformation are part of the process of cellular respiration, the utilization of O_2 to derive ATP from oxidizing fuels to CO_2 (Fig. 18.2). Cellular respiration is a mitochondrial process and the pathways reside, for the most part, in mitochondria (see Chapter 10).

In phase 1 of respiration, energy is derived from the oxidation of fuels by enzymes that transfer electrons from the fuels to the electron-accepting coenzymes NAD^+ and FAD. These two coenzymes are reduced to NADH and FAD(2H), respectively. The pathways for the oxidation of glucose, fatty acids, ketone bodies, and many amino acids converge in the generation of the activated 2-carbon acetyl group in acetyl CoA. The complete oxidation of the acetyl group to CO_2 occurs in the tricarboxylic acid (TCA) cycle, which collects the energy mostly as NADH and FAD(2H).

Phase 2 of cellular respiration occurs in mitochondria. The energy derived from fuel oxidation is converted to the high energy phosphate bonds of ATP by the process of oxidative phosphorylation. Electrons are transferred from NADH and FAD(2H) to O_2 by the mitochondrial electron transport chain. This process generates an electrochemical potential in the form of a transmembrane proton gradient which can be used to drive the synthesis of ATP from ADP and P_i.

The free energy available from ATP hydrolysis is then utilized for energy-requiring processes by altering the conformation of enzymes and other proteins which facilitate these processes. In general, the rates of reactions involved in the oxidation of fuels are tightly coordinated with the rate of ATP utilization by feedback regulation. Feedback regulation results in the storage of fuels which are not immediately required for ATP synthesis.

Although ATP generation from oxidative phosphorylation is essential to life, oxygen is also potentially toxic to cells. Oxygen has a tendency to form oxygen

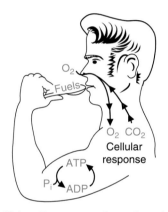

Fig. 18.1. Energy transformations in fuel metabolism.

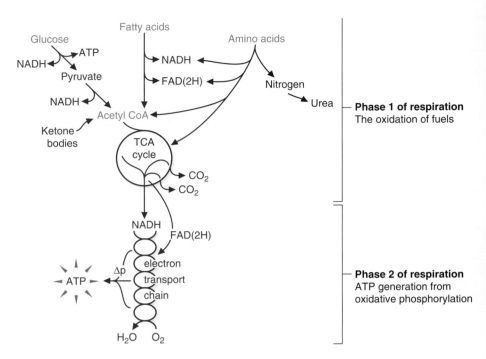

Fig. 18.2. Cellular respiration. Δp = the proton gradient.

radicals and other reactive oxygen species (ROS). The ROS can initiate free radical chain reactions, damage DNA, denature proteins, and degrade membrane lipids. Cells are protected against oxygen toxicity by enzymatic defense mechanisms and antioxidant vitamins, such as vitamin E.

The only pathway of fuel metabolism which can generate ATP without oxygen is anaerobic glycolysis. In glycolysis, 1 mole of glucose is converted to 2 moles of pyruvate by reactions that occur in the cytosol. ATP is generated by transfer of phosphate to ADP from a high energy phosphorylated intermediate of the pathway through a process termed substrate level phosphorylation. If the pyruvate is reduced to lactate by NADH, this generation of ATP does not require oxygen and is termed anaerobic glycolysis (Fig. 18.3). Anaerobic glycolysis enables tissues with a limited access to oxygen, or with few or no mitochondria, to generate enough ATP for their needs. However, in most tissues, glycolysis generates pyruvate which enters mitochondria and is converted to acetyl CoA for oxidation in the TCA cycle.

Fatty acids are the major fuels in the body. After a high carbohydrate meal, carbohydrate in excess of immediate need is stored as glucosyl units in glycogen or converted to triacylglycerol (fat) for storage in adipose tissue. Fatty acids from dietary fat are also stored as adipose triacylglycerol. Between meals, fatty acids are released from adipose tissue stores, circulate in blood as fatty acid-albumin, and are oxidized to acetyl CoA in muscle, liver, and many other tissues by the pathway of β-oxidation. The acetyl CoA enters the TCA cycle and is completely oxidized to CO_2 and H_2O. In the liver, the acetyl CoA can also be converted to the ketone bodies acetoacetate and β-hydroxybutyrate. The ketone bodies are oxidized in muscle and other tissues, and can become a major fuel for the brain during prolonged fasting. The pathways of fatty acid and ketone body oxidation use NAD^+ and FAD to collect electrons and oxidative phosphorylation to generate ATP.

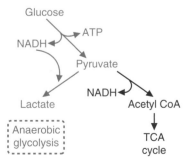

Fig. 18.3. Anaerobic glycolysis. The conversion of glucose to lactate is anaerobic. If the pyruvate derived from glucose is converted to acetyl CoA and oxidized in the TCA cycle, the process is aerobic.

All cells continuously use ATP and require a constant supply of fuels to provide energy for the generation of ATP. The constant availability of fuels despite variations in dietary supply and rates of utilization is termed metabolic homeostasis. Metabolic homeostasis is accomplished by hormonal regulation of the pathways of fuel storage and mobilization, principally by insulin and the insulin counterregulatory hormones glucagon, epinephrine, and cortisol.

Glucose has a special role in metabolic homeostasis because the brain and many other tissues require glucose for all, or a part, of their energy needs. Blood glucose levels are therefore maintained at about 80 mg/dL. Inadequate levels of insulin, or a resistance in tissues to the effects of insulin, result in the hyperglycemia characteristic of diabetes mellitus.

18 Bioenergetics of the Cell

The ATP-ADP cycle refers to the continuous utilization of ATP chemical bond energy to do the work required for life, and the continuous oxidation of fuels to regenerate this ATP (Fig. 18.4). Most of the energy-requiring processes in the body utilize the high energy phosphate bonds of ATP (or UTP, GTP, or CTP) to provide this energy. Active transport, mechanical work, and biosynthetic reactions are all energy-requiring processes in which ATP is converted to ADP and P_i. In order to regenerate ATP, energy is provided by catabolic reactions, reactions in which foodstuffs (fuels) are oxidized. The endproducts of fuel oxidation are CO_2, which we exhale, ATP, and heat. The synthesis of the high energy phosphate bonds of ATP from the oxidation of fuels requires O_2 and accounts for about 95% of the oxygen we inhale. The overall process utilizing O_2 for the generation of ATP from the oxidation of fuels to CO_2 is termed cellular respiration.

The term bioenergetics refers to the energy transformations which take place in the reactions of the ATP-ADP cycle. The energy changes in biological systems, like those in the rest of the universe, obey the first and second laws of thermodynamics (Table 18.1). An expression for the amount of useful energy available from any reaction or series of reactions, ΔG, has developed from these thermodynamic principles. $\Delta G^{0'}$, the change in free energy under standard conditions, can be used to compare the amount of energy available from various fuels. It can also be used to calculate the efficiency of various processes in transforming chemical bond energy into ATP high energy phosphate bonds, or to determine whether an energy-requiring process will proceed in the forward direction.

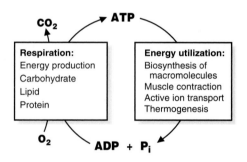

Fig. 18.4. ATP-ADP cycle.

Table 18.1. Thermodynamic Expressions, Laws, and Constants

Definitions

ΔG	Change in free energy, or Gibbs free energy
ΔG^0	Standard free enrgy change, ΔG at 1 M concentrations of substrates and products
$\Delta G^{0'}$	Standard free energy change at 25°C, pH 7.0
ΔH	Change in enthalpy, or heat content
ΔS	Change in entropy, or increase in disorder
K'_{eq}	Equilibrium constant at 25°C, pH 7.0, incorporating $[H_2O] = 55.5$ M and $[H^+] = 10^{-7}$ M in the constant
$E^{0'}$	Reduction potential
~P	Biochemical symbol for a high energy phosphate bond, i.e., a bond which is hydrolyzed with the release of more than about 7 kcal/mole of heat

Laws of thermodynamics

First law of thermodynamics, the conservation of energy: In any physical or chemical change, the total energy of a system, including its surroundings, remains constant.

Second law of thermodynamics: The universe tends toward disorder. In all natural processes, the total entropy of a system always increases.

Constants

Units of ΔG and ΔH = cal/mole or J/mole: 1 cal = 4.18 J
T, Absolute temperature: K, Kelvin = 273 + °C (25°C = 298 K)
R, Universal gas constant: 1.99 cal/mole•K or 8.31 J/mole•K
F, Faraday constant: F = 96,500 J/V•mole
Units of $E^{0'}$, volts

Formulas

$\Delta G = \Delta H - T\Delta S$
$\Delta G^{0'} = -RT \ln K'_{eq}$
$\Delta G^{0'} = -n F \Delta E_0'$
$\ln \times = 2.303 \log \times$

The BMR is really a measure of the ATP-ADP cycle of a resting individual. It is the amount of fuel that must be oxidized, in kilocalories, to provide ATP for the work performed by our tissues. The increased caloric expenditure of exercise is the increased oxidation of fuels to supply the increased ATP required for the increased mechanical work.

Thomas Appleman recovered from his streptococcal pneumonia uneventfully. He discovered that he had lost 6 lb during his illness, and was back to his original weight of 264 lb. This was his weight when he first came to his physician complaining of shortness of breath (see Chapter 1). His physician had estimated his basal metabolic rate (BMR) at 2,880 kcal/day. Because Mr. Appleman was sedentary, his physical activity was estimated at 30% of his BMR, and his daily energy expenditure at 3,744 kcal/day. Unfortunately, in the subsequent 2 weeks, he regained the weight. He calculated the caloric content of his food from tables his physician had recommended, and estimated that he was taking in far less than 3,744 kcal/day. So he returned to his physician for another visit.

A dietary history reveals Mr. Appleman has continued his habit of drinking scotch and soda each evening while watching TV, but has not added the ethanol calories to his dietary intake. He justifies this calculation on the basis of a comment he heard on a radio program that calories from alcohol ingestion "don't count" because they are empty calories that do not cause weight gain. He also explains to his physician that he really hasn't had time to start an exercise program.

Ahot Goyta is a 26-year-old male who noted heat intolerance with heavy sweating, heart palpitations, and tremulousness. Over the past 4 months he has lost weight in spite of a good appetite. He is sleeping poorly and describes himself as feeling "jittery inside."

On physical examination, his heart rate is rapid (116 beats/min) and he appears restless and fidgety. His skin feels warm, and he is perspiring profusely. A fine hand tremor is observed as he extends his arms in front of his chest. His thyroid gland appears to be diffusely enlarged and on palpitation is approximately 3 times normal size. His physician strongly suspects that Mr. Goyta's thyroid gland is secreting excessive amounts of thyroid hormone and orders a battery of thyroid function tests.

Cora Nari is a 64-year-old woman who had a myocardial infarction 8 months ago. Although she managed to lose 6 lb since that time, she remains overweight and has not reduced the fat content of her diet adequately. The graded aerobic exercise program she initiated 5 weeks after her infarction is now followed irregularly and falls far short of the cardiopulmonary conditioning intensity prescribed for her by the cardiologist. She is readmitted to the hospital cardiac care unit (CCU) after experiencing a severe viselike "pressure" pain in the mid-chest area while cleaning ice from the windshield of her car. The electrocardiogram (ECG) shows evidence of a new posterior wall myocardial infarction. Signs and symptoms of left ventricular failure are present.

UTILIZATION OF THE HIGH ENERGY PHOSPHATE BONDS OF ATP TO DO WORK

Energy Available from the High Energy Phosphate Bonds of ATP

The bonds between the phosphate groups of ATP are referred to as high energy phosphate bonds because they are so readily cleaved in hydrolysis and other reactions. The phosphate groups carry negative charges that repel each other and "strain" the bonds between them; it takes energy to make the phosphate groups stay together. When water is added to the bond between the terminal (β and γ) phosphate groups, ATP is hydrolyzed into ADP and phosphate (Fig. 18.5). The phosphate which is formed is very stable because it exists in several resonance forms; the electrons of the

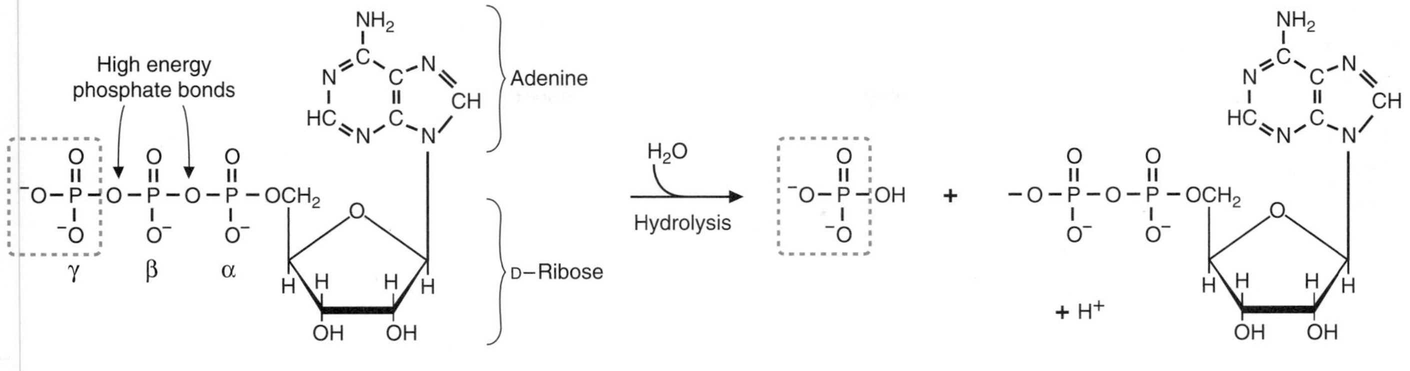

Fig. 18.5. Hydrolysis of ATP. The reaction is exothermic and has a negative ΔG^0. The value for ΔG^0 is strongly affected by pH because there are so many ionizable oxygens involved. It is also affected by the Mg^{2+} concentration because the terminal two phosphate groups of ATP (β and γ) are bound to Mg^{2+} in the cell. A value for $\Delta G^{0'}$ of -7.3 kcal/mole is often used for both standard and intracellular conditions. The hydrolysis of ADP to AMP and P_i has the same $\Delta G^{0'}$. However, the hydrolysis of the α-phosphate of AMP to form adenosine and P_i releases only 3.4 kcal, and consequently, the phosphate-adenosine bond is not considered a high energy phosphate bond.

oxygen double bond are shared by all the oxygen atoms. As a consequence, the products of ATP hydrolysis have a lower free energy than the reactants, and this reaction proceeds in the forward direction with the release of energy as heat. In the cell, the energy from cleaving the high energy phosphate bonds of ATP is coupled to energy-requiring processes.

CHANGE IN FREE ENERGY, ΔG, DURING A REACTION

The amount of energy from ATP hydrolysis and other chemical reactions which is available to do work is known as the ΔG, the change in Gibbs free energy of the reaction. The ΔG of a reaction depends on the difference in chemical bond energy between the products and substrates (the enthalpy, or ΔH), the amount of energy unavailable for work because it has gone into an increased disorder of the system (the increase of entropy, or ΔS), and the initial concentration of substrates and products. The value of ΔG for a reaction in which the concentration of substrates and products are equimolar (and equal to 1 M) is ΔG^0. Under biochemically defined standard conditions of temperature, pressure, and pH, the ΔG^0 is the $\Delta G^{0'}$ (see Table 18.1). In the hydrolysis of ATP, the products of the reaction are more stable and have a lower chemical bond energy than the reactants, and the change in disorder during the reaction is probably small. As a consequence, the $\Delta G^{0'}$ for ATP hydrolysis is negative, about -7 to -8 kcal/mole. A value of -7.3 kcal/mole is generally used.

RELATIONSHIP BETWEEN ΔG⁰′ AND THE CONCENTRATIONS OF SUBSTRATES AND PRODUCTS

The negative value of $\Delta G^{0'}$ for the hydrolysis of ATP indicates that at 1 M concentrations of substrates and products, the reaction proceeds in the forward direction, and ATP is hydrolyzed to ADP and P_i. The substrate concentrations will decrease and the product concentrations will increase until equilibrium is reached. The exact ratio of products to substrates at equilibrium depends on the value for $\Delta G^{0'}$, and is dictated principally by the differences in chemical bond energy of the products and reactants.

Reactions that release heat are called exothermic, or exergonic. Those which consume energy are called endothermic, or endergonic.

ΔG is the change in free energy (Gibbs free energy) during a reaction.

$$\Delta G = \Delta H - T\,\Delta S$$

where ΔH = the change in enthalpy. At constant temperature and pressure, ΔH is equivalent to the chemical bond energy of the products minus that of the reactants. T is the temperature of the system in Kelvin, and ΔS is the change in entropy, or increased disorder of the system. ΔG represents the maximum amount of useful energy that can be obtained from a reaction.

Adenosine 5'-triphosphate

ATP

Phosphate

P_i

Adenosine 5'-diphosphate

ADP

18.1: What is the $\Delta G^{0\prime}$ for the synthesis of ATP from ADP and P_i?

 18.2: Consider a reaction in which a substrate, S, is converted to a product, P: S ↔ P. At equilibrium, there is no net flux in either direction. Thus, the concentrations of substrate and product do not change with time. The relationship between the concentrations of substrates and products and $\Delta G^{0\prime}$ is given by the formula
$$\Delta G^{0\prime} = -RT \ln K'_{eq} = -RT \ln[P]_{eq}/[S]_{eq}$$
where R is the gas constant, T is the temperature in degrees Kelvin, and K'_{eq} is the equilibrium constant under standard conditions. Under standard conditions, RT is about 0.6 kcal/mole. $[P]_{eq}$ and $[S]_{eq}$ are the concentrations of product and substrate, respectively, at equilibrium. If $[P]_{eq}/[S]_{eq}$ is greater than 1, will $\Delta G^{0\prime}$ be positive or negative?

18.3: In muscle cells, [ATP] = 8.1 mM; [ADP] = 0.93 mM; and $[P_i]$ = 8.1 mM. Assume for this calculation that ΔG^0 at pH 7.4 and 37°C is −7.7 kcal/mole. R = 1.99 cal/mol•K. How much energy is available from the hydrolysis of ATP in the muscle cell?

The heart is a specialist in the transformation of ATP chemical bond energy into mechanical work. Each single heartbeat uses about 2% of the ATP in the heart. If the heart were not able to regenerate ATP, all its ATP would be hydrolyzed in less than 1 minute. Because the amount of ATP required by the heart is so high, the heart must rely on the pathway of oxidative phosphorylation for generation of this ATP. In the absence of oxygen, or at low oxygen tensions, the amount of ATP generated is inadequate.

A heart attack is caused by blockage of a coronary artery which prevents blood from bringing oxygen to the heart muscle cells beyond the block. These cells cannot produce an adequate amount of ATP, and cell death results.

Cora Nari has suffered two heart attacks in 8 months and has a significant reduction in the amount of functional heart muscle.

If the $\Delta G^{0\prime}$ is positive, the products have more energy than the reactants, and the reaction at 1 M concentrations of substrate and product will proceed in the reverse direction, with substrate accumulating at the expense of product.

The $\Delta G^{0\prime}$ is not an indicator of the velocity of the reaction, or the rate at which equilibrium can be reached. In the cell, the velocity of the reaction depends on the amount of enzyme available to catalyze the reaction, and the activation energy of the reaction—the energy required to reach the transition state. The velocity of the reaction is not directly related to the energy difference between substrates and products.

FREE ENERGY AVAILABLE FOR WORK IN CELLS

The $\Delta G^{0\prime}$ of a reaction is a measure of the maximum amount of work available from the reaction when substrates and products are present at 1 M concentrations. However, this situation does not usually occur in our cells. If a reaction has a negative $\Delta G^{0\prime}$, but the concentration of substrates is higher than 1 M and the product concentration is less than 1 M, more energy is available from proceeding to equilibrium. The further a reaction is from the equilibrium values for substrate and product concentrations, the larger the amount of energy required or released as the reaction proceeds to equilibrium. If a reaction is closer to equilibrium than it would be at a 1 M concentration of substrates and products, less energy is required or released to reach equilibrium. Consequently, the expression for the difference in free energy of the reaction at any concentration of substrate or product, ΔG, has two terms: the energy change for a 1 M concentration of substrate and product to reach equilibrium ($\Delta G^{0\prime}$), and the energy change to reach a 1 M concentration of substrates and products (+RT ln[P]/[S]). As a result,

$$\Delta G = \Delta G^{0\prime} + RT \ln[P]/[S]$$

where [P] and [S] are any concentration of substrate and product. For the general form of this equation, see Table 18.2.

Although the free energy available in cells from the cleavage of the high energy phosphate bond of ATP may vary somewhat with different concentrations of ADP, P_i, and ATP, it is usually greater than −8 kcal/mole in living human cells. Cells use this −8 kcal for mechanical work, transport work, and for energy-requiring biosynthetic reactions.

Energy Transformations to Do Work

The utilization of the 8 kcal available from ATP hydrolysis for work has to involve a mechanism for transforming the chemical bond energy of ATP into the movement of a muscle fiber or the formation of a new chemical bond. These transformations usually involve intermediate steps in which cleavage of the high energy phosphate bonds of ATP while it is bound to an enzyme is accompanied by conformational changes in the enzyme.

Table 18.2. A General Expression for ΔG

To generalize the expression for ΔG, consider a reaction in which
$$aA + bB \rightleftarrows cC + dD$$
The small letters denote a moles of A will combine with b moles of B to produce c moles of C and d moles of D.

$$\Delta G^{0\prime} = -RT \ln K'_{eq} = -RT \ln \frac{[C]^c_{eq}\,[D]^d_{eq}}{[A]^a_{eq}\,[B]^b_{eq}}$$

and

$$\Delta G = \Delta G^{0\prime} + RT \ln \frac{[C]^c\,[D]^d}{[A]^a\,[B]^b}$$

MECHANICAL WORK

In mechanical work, the high energy phosphate bond of ATP is converted into movement by changing the conformation of a protein. For example, in contracting muscle fibers, the hydrolysis of ATP while it is bound to myosin ATPase changes the conformation of the enzyme so that it dissociates and associates with the sliding actin filament (Fig. 18.6).

TRANSPORT WORK

In transport work, called active transport, the high energy phosphate bond of ATP is utilized to transport compounds against a concentration gradient. For example, Na^+,K^+-ATPase, uses ATP energy to pump Na^+ out of the cell. The chemical bond energy of ATP is converted into a Na^+ concentration gradient through conformational changes of Na^+,K^+-ATPase which occur when the enzyme phosphorylates itself by cleaving ATP (see Chapter 10). The inward movement of Na^+ drives the uptake of many compounds into the cell on cotransport proteins. Thus Na^+ must be continuously transported back out. The expenditure of ATP for Na^+ transport occurs even while we sleep. It is estimated that the energy required for active transport accounts for between 10 and 30% of our BMR.

BIOSYNTHETIC WORK

The high energy phosphate bonds of ATP are also used for biosynthetic work. The body synthesizes large molecules, such as DNA, glycogen, triacylglycerols, and proteins from smaller compounds. These biosynthetic pathways are called anabolic pathways. Reactions in the body involving the formation of peptide bonds (protein synthesis), —C—C— bonds (fatty acid synthesis), —C—N— bonds (urea synthesis), C—O— bonds (triacylglycerol formation), are all thermodynamically unfavorable. These processes acquire the energy from ATP, either directly or indirectly.

Biosynthetic processes are energy-requiring because the products have a higher chemical bond energy than the reactants, and because the system has become more ordered. The energy for anabolic pathways is supplied by ATP cleavage, either in a single enzymatic step, or in a sequence of several enzyme steps in which other activated compounds are formed. In general, the amount of ATP phosphate bond energy utilized is sufficient to provide the pathway with an overall negative $\Delta G^{0'}$. Glycogen, for example, is composed of glucosyl units linked by glycosidic bonds (see Figs. 20.19 and 20.20). The formation of glycosidic bonds from glucose requires energy, which is provided by the cleavage of four high energy phosphate bonds derived from ATP (one in ATP, a similar high energy phosphate bond in UTP, one in pyrophosphate (PP_i), and one in UDP-glucose (Fig. 18.7).

Phosphorylation of Glucose by ATP

Glycogen synthesis begins with the phosphorylation of glucose by ATP, catalyzed by hexokinase. This reaction is an example of the utilization of the high energy phosphate bond of ATP to drive a chemical reaction. If ATP were not part of the reaction, the phosphorylation of glucose from inorganic phosphate would have a positive $\Delta G^{0'}$ of 3.3 kcal. At equilibrium, the concentration of substrates in the cell would be much higher than the concentration of products. However, the phosphorylation of glucose is coupled to ATP hydrolysis by hexokinase, which transfers the phosphate from a bound ATP to a bound glucose molecule. The overall free energy change, which can be calculated from the sum of the energy required to make glucose 6-phosphate and that provided by the hydrolysis of ATP, is **negative** 4.0 kcal/mole (Table 18.3).

The thyroid function tests on **Ahot Goyta** confirmed the diagnosis of hyperthyroidism. In this disease, the thyroid gland excretes excessive amounts of thyroid hormones T_4 (thyroxine or tetraiodothyronine) and T_3 (triiodothyronine), the major thyroid hormone present in blood. These hormones accelerate oxidative metabolism and increase the BMR through mechanisms which have not yet been elucidated. One of their effects is a stimulation of ATP utilization by Na^+,K^+-ATPase. The increased rate of ATP utilization results in an acceleration of oxidative metabolism and a much greater rate of heat production. The hyperthyroid patient, therefore, complains of constantly feeling hot (heat intolerance) and sweaty. (Perspiration allows dissipation of excess heat through evaporation from the skin surface.)

A 18.1: If the $\Delta G^{0'}$ for the hydrolysis of ATP is −7.3 kcal/mole, the $\Delta G^{0'}$ for the reverse reaction, the synthesis of ATP from ADP and P_i, is +7.3 kcal/mole. The minus sign indicates that energy is released from cleavage of the high energy phosphate bond, and the positive sign indicates that energy is required for its synthesis.

A 18.2: If $[P]_{eq}/[S]_{eq}$ is greater than 1, the log of this value will be positive, and $\Delta G^{0'}$ will be negative, i.e., a negative value of $\Delta G^{0'}$ favors the forward direction. If $[P]_{eq}/[S]_{eq}$ is less than 1, the log of this value will be negative, and $\Delta G^{0'}$ will be positive.

A 18.3: The reaction for ATP hydrolysis is: $ATP + H_2O \rightarrow ADP + P_i$. The ΔG for the reaction is given by $\Delta G = \Delta G^0 + RT \ln[ADP][P_i]/[ATP]$. The term for H_2O has been incorporated into the constants and does not appear in the equation. At the body temperature of 37°C (310 K) with the concentrations expressed as M, $[ADP][P_i]/[ATP] = 0.93 \times 10^{-3}$ M, and $\Delta G = -7.7$ kcal + (−4.2 kcal) = −12 kcal. The real energy cost of synthesizing ATP in the muscle cell under these conditions is, therefore, +12 kcal/mole.

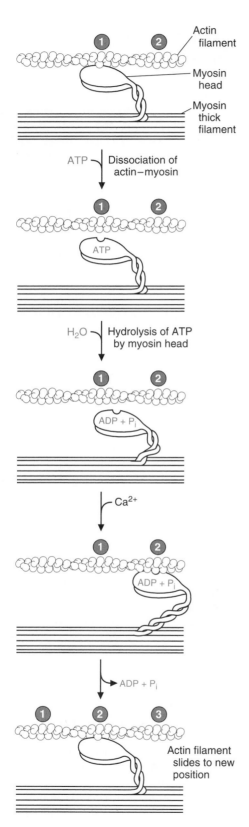

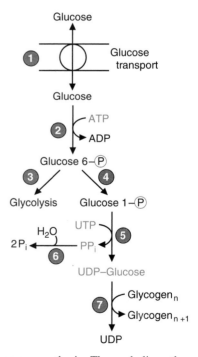

Fig. 18.6. Myosin ATPase. Muscle fiber is made of thick filaments composed of bundles of the protein myosin, and thin filaments composed of the protein actin. At many positions along the actin filament, a terminal domain of a myosin molecule, referred to as the "head," binds to a specific site on the actin. The myosin head has an ATP binding site and is an ATPase; it can hydrolyze ATP to ADP and P_i. As ATP binds to myosin, the conformation of myosin changes and it dissociates from the actin and hydrolyzes the ATP. Myosin then binds Ca^{2+}, changes its conformation, and reassociates with the actin filament at a new position. As the ADP and P_i dissociate, the myosin again changes conformation, or tightens. This change of conformation at multiple association points between actin and myosin slides the actin filament forward.

Fig. 18.7. Energetics of glycogen synthesis. The anabolic pathway of glycogen synthesis involves several compounds with high energy bonds: ATP, UTP, UDP-glucose, and PP_i. These are shown in blue. **1.** Glucose transport is facilitated diffusion, and not energy-requiring. **2.** The phosphorylation of glucose, catalyzed by hexokinase and glucokinase, utilizes the high energy phosphate bond (~P) of ATP. **3.** Glucose 6-phosphate can enter the pathway for glycolysis. **4.** The conversion of glucose 6-phosphate to glucose 1-phosphate by phosphoglucomutase initiates the pathway of glycogen synthesis. **5.** UDP-Glucose pyrophosphorylase cleaves a ~P bond in UTP, releasing pyrophosphate. **6.** The pyrophosphate is hydrolyzed, releasing additional energy. **7.** UDP-Glucose also has a high energy bond, which is cleaved in the addition of a glucosyl unit onto the end of a glycogen polysaccharide chain.

Table 18.3. $\Delta G^{0\prime}$ for the Transfer of a Phosphate from ATP to Glucose

	Glucose + P_i → glucose-6-P + H_2O	$\Delta G^{0\prime}$ = +3.3 kcal/mole
	ATP + H_2O → ADP + P_i	$\Delta G^{0\prime}$ = −7.3 kcal/mole
Sum:	glucose + ATP → glucose-6-P + ADP	$\Delta G^{0\prime}$ = −4.0 kcal/mole

The negative $\Delta G^{0\prime}$ helps the cell trap glucose inside as the phosphorylated sugar and prevents glucose 6-phosphate from being converted back to glucose by hexokinase. All cells can transport glucose through the plasma membrane via transport proteins, but cells do not transport glucose 6-phosphate because of the large negatively charged phosphate group. Thus, once glucose 6-phosphate is formed, it is committed to formation of glycogen, glycolysis, or another pathway in that cell. During strenuous exercise when a muscle cell derives glucose 6-phosphate from its own glycogen stores, there will be little tendency for this glucose 6-phosphate to be converted back to glucose by this reaction and leave the cell.

Additive Nature of Free Energy Changes within a Pathway

In the next step in the pathway for glycogen synthesis, glucose 6-phosphate is isomerized to glucose 1-phosphate. The new phosphate bond in glucose 1-phosphate has a slightly higher energy than the old bond, so the $\Delta G^{0\prime}$ of the reaction is positive, but small (+1.6 kcal). Within metabolic pathways, whether they are anabolic or catabolic, a single step with a positive $\Delta G^{0\prime}$ can be driven forward by preceding or subsequent steps with negative values of $\Delta G^{0\prime}$. The overall $\Delta G^{0\prime}$ for a sequence of reactions is obtained by adding the free energy changes of the individual reactions. Consequently, the $\Delta G^{0\prime}$ for the conversion of glucose to glucose 1-phosphate is (−4.0 kcal) + (+1.6 kcal) = −2.4 kcal/mole.

Formation of Activated Intermediates

To convert glucose 1-phosphate to glycogen, an activated pathway intermediate, UDP-glucose is formed (Fig. 18.8). UTP, GTP, or CTP are usually used for the activation of sugars, rather than ATP. The phosphate bond energy for these different nucleotides is essentially identical to that of ATP. The high energy phosphate bond of UTP is formed by an enzyme that transfers a phosphate from ATP to UDP:

$$ATP + UDP \rightleftarrows ADP + UTP$$

There are a number of other enzymes in the cell which transfer high energy phosphate bonds between nucleotides.

The synthesis of UDP-glucose is coupled to the cleavage of two high energy phosphate bonds, one in UTP and one in pyrophosphate. The glucosyl-phosphate bond of UDP-glucose is a high energy bond containing about 7.7 kcal/mole. The hydrolysis of the pyrophosphate bond (PP_i), which provides an additional −7.3 kcal, therefore, gives the two steps a net negative $\Delta G^{0\prime}$. The energy derived from cleavage of the glucosyl-phosphate bond is used in the formation of the new glycosidic bond in glycogen.

Reversibility of Individual Steps

Many metabolic pathways, such as glycogen synthesis, occur with individual steps which have positive values for $\Delta G^{0\prime}$. It is theoretically possible to increase the substrate concentration high enough or to keep the product concentration low enough so that the reaction will proceed in the forward direction regardless of how large and positive the value for $\Delta G^{0\prime}$. The more unfavorable the free energy difference between the products and the substrates, the higher the cell must raise the ratio of substrate to

Q 18.4: Assume that the hexokinase reaction is at equilibrium in the muscle cell.

$$\Delta G^{0\prime} = -RT \ln K'_{eq}$$
$$= -RT \ln \frac{[Glucose\text{-}6\text{-}P][ADP]}{[Glucose][ATP]}$$

Using values of 0.002 kcal/mole for R, 298° K for T, 0.010 M for ATP, and 0.001 M for ADP, calculate the ratio of glucose 6-phosphate to glucose in a muscle cell.

A 18.4: If the hexokinase reaction reached equilibrium, the ratio of glucose 6-phosphate to glucose would be about 8,000.

RT = (0.002)(298) = 0.596

ln × = 2.303 log ×

$$\Delta G^{0\prime} = -RT\ln \frac{[G6P][ADP]}{[G][ATP]}$$

$$-4 = -(0.596)(2.303) \log \frac{[G6P][0.001]}{[G][0.01]}$$

$$+2.9 = +\log \frac{[G6P](0.1)}{[G]}$$

$$8 \times 10^2 = \frac{[G6P](0.1)}{[G]}$$

$$8 \times 10^3 = \frac{[G6P]}{[G]}$$

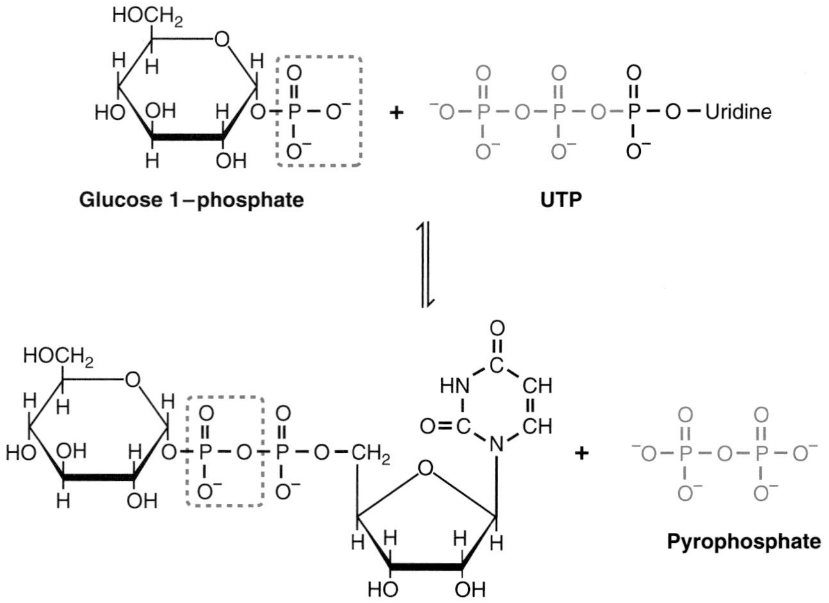

Fig. 18.8. Formation of UDP-glucose. The activated sugar, UDP-glucose, is formed from glucose 1-phosphate and UTP by the enzyme UDP-glucose pyrophosphorylase. UDP-Glucose retains a high energy pyrophosphate bond. (Uridine is uracil bonded to ribose.)

The $\Delta G^{0\prime}$ for the conversion of glucose 6-phosphate to glucose 1-phosphate is +1.65 kcal, and the ratio of glucose 6-phosphate to glucose 1-phosphate is 94 to 6. If the glucose 6-phosphate concentration is increased and the glucose 1-phosphate concentration is decreased slightly, so that the ratio is 95 to 5, the ΔG is negative (−0.1), and the forward reaction is thermodynamically favored. The capacity of the enzyme that catalyzes this reaction, phosphoglucomutase, is high enough so that this reaction is readily reversible in the cell and can participate in both the pathways for glycogen synthesis and glycogen degradation.

Compounds are oxidized in the human in three ways: direct combination with oxygen, transfer of electrons as part of a hydrogen atom, and direct transfer of electrons. In all of these, oxidation is the loss of electrons. The compound which gains electrons is reduced.

product concentrations to get the reaction to go forward. For example, the reversible isomerization of glucose 6-phosphate to glucose 1-phosphate is part of both glycogen synthesis and degradation.

Reactions with a negative $\Delta G^{0\prime}$ become irreversible under physiological conditions only if the products never accumulate to a sufficiently high level (thermodynamically irreversible), or if the enzymatic rate for the reverse reaction is very slow (kinetically irreversible).

ENERGY FOR GENERATION OF ATP

Energy Transformations in Respiration

The energy for the formation of ATP high energy phosphate bonds comes from the oxidation of fuels by the process of respiration. When a piece of wood is oxidized by lighting a match to it, the carbon-hydrogen bonds in that wood combine directly with O_2 to form CO_2 and H_2O and the energy is released as heat. Respiration, instead, transforms much of the energy in the —C—H and C—C bonds of fuels into a form which can be used for ATP synthesis (Fig. 18.9).

In the body, energy from fuel oxidation is conserved by the transfer of electrons with hydrogen from the fuel to electron-accepting coenzymes, principally NAD^+ and FAD. The fuel gains oxygen relative to the hydrogens it contains, but the oxygen is added from H_2O. The endproduct of fuel oxidation, CO_2, is formed principally from the oxidation of the acetyl group of acetyl CoA in the TCA cycle (see Fig. 18.1).

The electron-accepting coenzymes donate the electrons from fuel oxidation to O_2 via the electron transport chain, a series of proteins in the inner mitochondrial membrane. The electron transport chain transforms the energy obtained from the transfer of electrons from reduced NAD^+ and reduced FAD to O_2 into an electrochemical

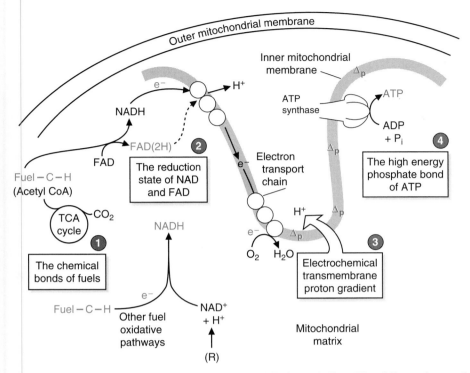

Fig. 18.9. Energy transformations in mitochondrial fuel metabolism. The different forms of energy are shown in blue. **1.** The energy in fuels is present in the chemical form of —C—H and C—C bonds. **2.** As the fuels are oxidized and electrons are transferred to the electron-accepting coenzymes, NAD^+ and FAD, these coenzymes are reduced. The change in energy for the electron transfer is quantitatively described by their reduction potential. The electrons are transferred to O_2 by the electron transport chain. **3.** The electron transport chain transforms the energy in the reduction potential of NADH and FAD(2H) into the form of an electrochemical potential across the inner mitochondrial membrane, the transmembrane proton gradient. **4.** The energy from the transmembrane proton gradient is utilized by ATP synthase to form the ~P bond of ATP, the biologically useful form of chemical bond energy.

transmembrane proton gradient across the inner mitochondrial membrane, Δp (see Fig. 18.9). This electrochemical gradient is then used for the synthesis of the high energy phosphate bond of ATP by the process known as oxidative phosphorylation. These reactions occur principally in the mitochondria, which are the engines of the cell.

Energy of Oxidation-Reduction Reactions

ELECTRON-ACCEPTING COENZYMES

NAD^+ and FAD accept electrons as the hydrogen atom (FAD) or as the hydride ion (NAD^+), and are reduced in the reaction (Figs. 18.10 and 18.11). The energy from the chemical bonds of the fuel is then present in the reduced form of the electron carriers. As the reduced coenzymes donate these electrons to the electron transport chain, they are reoxidized. Which coenzyme is used depends principally on the properties of the functional groups donating electrons and, of course, on the enzyme catalyzing the reaction.

$NADP^+$, which is NAD^+ with an extra phosphate added to the ribose moiety in the adenosine, can also accept electrons in oxidation-reduction reactions (see Fig. 18.10). NADPH does not, however, donate these electrons directly to the electron transport chain. Instead, the electrons are usually donated to a biosynthetic or detoxification pathway in the cell.

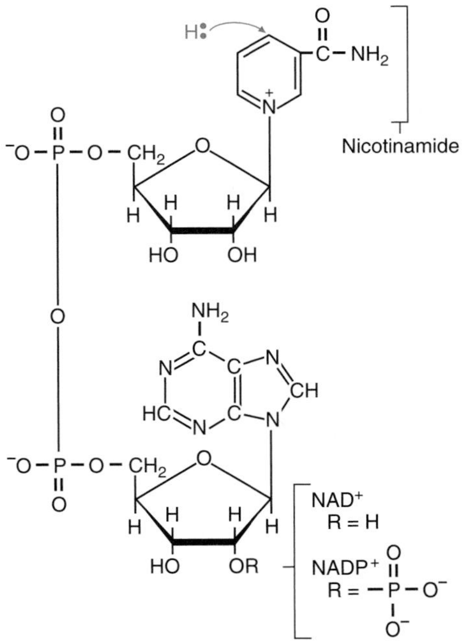

Fig. 18.10. Reduction of NAD^+ and $NADP^+$. These structurally related coenzymes are reduced by accepting 2 electrons as a hydride ion, $H:^-$. NAD^+ is synthesized in the human from the vitamin niacin. Niacin is converted in the body to nicotinamide by the addition of an —NH_2 to form the amide bond.

Q 18.5: **Thomas Appleman** has the mistaken impression that ethanol has no calories. However, it is a fuel with an oxidation state and, therefore, a caloric content. Compare the structure of ethanol to that of glucose and fatty acids (below). On the basis of their oxidation state, which compound provides the most energy (calories) per gram? Which compound gives the most ATP per gram?

$$HOH_2C - (HC-OH)_4 - \overset{\displaystyle O}{\overset{\|}{C}} - H$$

Glucose

$$CH_3CH_2OH$$

Ethanol

$$CH_3 - (CH_2)_{16} - \overset{\displaystyle O}{\overset{\|}{C}} - OH$$

A fatty acid

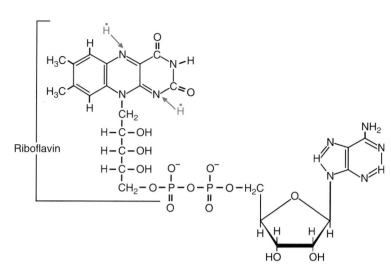

Fig. 18.11. Reduction of FAD. FAD accepts 2 electrons as 2 hydrogen atoms and is reduced to FAD(2H). FAD is synthesized from the vitamin riboflavin.

Table 18.4. Reduction Potentials of Some Oxidation-Reduction Half-Reactions

Reduction Half-Reactions	$E^{0'}$ at pH 7.0
$1/2\ O_2 + 2H^+ + 2\ e^- \rightarrow H_2O$	0.816
Cytochrome a-Fe^{3+} +1$e^- \rightarrow$ cytochrome a-Fe^{2+}	0.290
$CoQ + 2H^+ + 2e^- \rightarrow CoQH_2$	0.060
Dehydroascorbic acid +2H^+ + 2 $e^- \rightarrow$ ascorbic acid	0.050
Ox. glutathione + 2H^+ + 2 $e^- \rightarrow$ 2 red. glutathione	0.040
Fumarate + 2H^+ + 2 $e^- \rightarrow$ succinate	0.030
Oxalacetate + 2H^+ + 2 $e^- \rightarrow$ malate	−0.102
Acetaldehyde + 2H^+ + 2 $e^- \rightarrow$ ethanol	−0.163
Pyruvate + 2H^+ + 2 $e^- \rightarrow$ lactate	−0.190
Riboflavin + 2H^+ + 2 $e^- \rightarrow$ riboflavin-H_2	−0.200
1,3-Bisphosphoglycerate + 2H^+ + 2 $e^- \rightarrow$ glyceraldehyde 3-phosphate	−0.320
NAD^+ + 2H^+ + 2 $e^- \rightarrow$ NADH + H^+	−0.320
Acetate + 2H^+ + 2 $e^- \rightarrow$ acetaldehyde	−0.468

Ox. = oxidized; red. = reduced.

 The direct relationship between the energy changes in oxidation-reduction reactions and $\Delta G^{0'}$ is expressed by the equation

$$\Delta G^{0'} = -n\ F\ \Delta E_o'$$

where n is the number of electrons transferred and F is Faraday's constant (23 kcal/volt). $\Delta E_o'$ for the net oxidation-reduction reaction is calculated from the reduction potentials of the half-reactions shown in Table 18.1, rearranged in a way to give the appropriate net reaction. This equation simply shows how to convert the free energy available from electron transfer, expressed as volts, to $\Delta G^{0'}$.

REDUCTION POTENTIAL

The energy available for ATP synthesis from oxidation-reduction reactions is often expressed as the $\Delta E_o'$ (the difference in reduction potentials of the oxidation-reduction pair) rather than the $\Delta G^{0'}$. The reduction potential, E_o', of a compound is a measure in volts of energy released when that compound accepts electrons. It can be considered an expression of the willingness of the compound to accept electrons. Some examples of reduction potentials are shown in Table 18.4.

In metabolic pathways, electrons are generally transferred from compounds with a low reduction potential to compounds with a high reduction potential. Oxygen, which is the best electron acceptor, has the greatest reduction potential (i.e., is the most willing to accept electrons and be reduced). The more negative the reduction potential of a compound, the greater the energy available when this compound passes its electrons to oxygen. For instance, the reduction potential for NAD^+ is more negative (−0.320 volt) than riboflavin (−0.200 volt), and thus the $\Delta G^{0'}$ for oxidation of NADH by O_2 is usually greater than the $\Delta G^{0'}$ for oxidation of riboflavin-containing proteins. This value for NADH is about −53 kcal, and for FAD(2H) is about −41 kcal.

ATP Generation

OXIDATIVE PHOSPHORYLATION.

The major pathways for the oxidation of fuels are glycolysis, fatty acid oxidation, ketone body oxidation, the citric acid cycle (TCA cycle), the pentose phosphate pathway, and the individual pathways for oxidation of each of the amino acids. In all these pathways, the oxidation of fuels occurs by the donation of electrons to NAD^+, $NADP^+$, and FAD. ATP synthesis from these pathways depends upon the energy released by transfer of the electrons from the reduced carriers to O_2 and on oxidative phosphorylation—these are therefore all **aerobic pathways** (Fig. 18.12). They account for almost all of the O_2 we breathe in.

The thyroid hormones modulate cellular energy production and utilization at several steps involving energy transformations. Some of the effects of thyroid hormones arise from an increased transcription of the genes for the enzymes/proteins involved. For example, there is an increased synthesis of mitochondrial proteins; all the enzymes in the TCA cycle and the proteins of oxidative phosphorylation are increased in amount. An excess of thyroid hormones can also affect the efficiency of ATP production; less ATP is produced for a given O_2 consumption. The efficiency of ATP utilization is also altered. Because **Ahot Goyta** has hyperthyroidism, the increased thyroid hormone levels cause him to oxidize fuels more rapidly than normal.

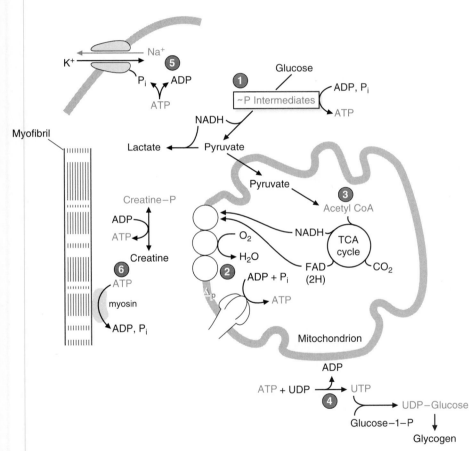

A 18.5: Remember **LEO GER**:
Loss of **E**lectrons = **O**xidation;
Gain of **E**lectrons = **R**eduction.
The reduced compounds have more hydrogen relative to oxygen than the oxidized compounds, and in a C—O bond, the electrons are counted with the oxygen. Consequently, aldehydes are more reduced than acids, and alcohols are more reduced than ketones. In fatty acids such as palmitate, the average carbon is more reduced than in glucose or ethanol (more of the carbons have electrons in carbon-hydrogen bonds). Therefore, fatty acids have the greatest caloric content/gram, 9 kcal. In glucose, the carbons have already formed bonds with oxygen, and fewer electrons in C—H bonds are available to generate energy. Thus, the complete oxidation of glucose gives about 4 kcal/g. The "average" carbon in ethanol is in an oxidation state intermediate between glucose and fatty acids, and ethanol thus has 7 kcal/g. The efficiency of converting the energy in the reduction state of each of these compounds to the high energy phosphate (~P) of ATP is about the same. Thus, the ATP generated from oxidative phosphorylation is highest for palmitate, intermediate for ethanol, and lowest for glucose.

Fig. 18.12. Utilization of high energy bonds in the cell. **1.** Glycolysis converts glucose to intermediates with high energy phosphate bonds, such as phosphoenolpyruvate. The ~P bond is transferred to ADP to form ATP in substrate level phosphorylation. **2.** The energy of the high energy phosphate bond of ATP (~P) is derived from oxidative phosphorylation. **3.** In order to oxidize fatty acids, pyruvate, and other compounds to CO_2, these compounds are converted to acetyl CoA, which has a high energy thioester bond. **4.** The ~P bond can be transferred from ATP to other nucleotides, such as UDP or AMP, to be used in biosynthetic processes. **5.** The energy of the ~P bond of ATP is converted into a conformational change of Na^+,K^+-ATPase, which transforms the energy into a Na^+ gradient. **6.** The relative movement of actin and myosin filaments utilizes ~P bond energy of ATP. ATP can be generated directly at the site of contraction from the ~P bond energy of creatine phosphate.

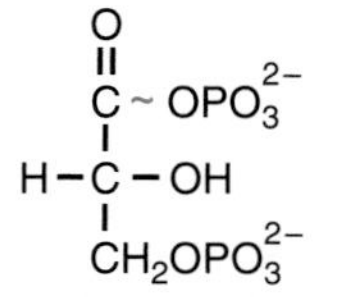

O
‖
C ~ OPO₃²⁻
|
H – C – OH
|
CH₂OPO₃²⁻

1,3–Bisphosphoglycerate

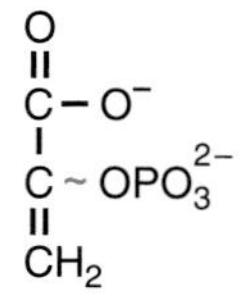

O
‖
C – O⁻
|
C ~ OPO₃²⁻
‖
CH₂

Phosphoenolpyruvate

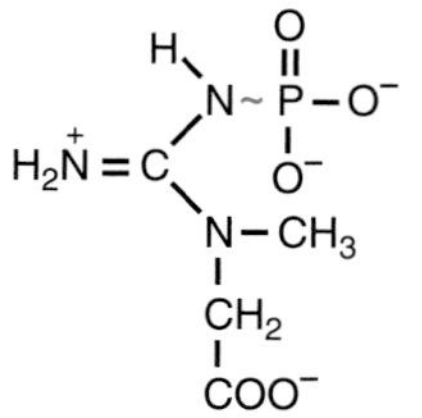

H   O
 \   ‖
  N ~ P – O⁻
 / |
H₂N⁺= C   O⁻
  \
   N – CH₃
   |
   CH₂
   |
   COO⁻

Creatine phosphate

O
‖
CH₃ – C ~ SCoA

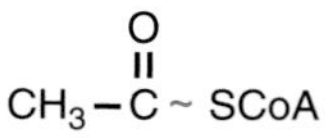

Acetyl CoA

Fig. 18.13. Some compounds with high energy bonds. 1,3-Bisphosphoglycerate and phosphoenolpyruvate are intermediates of glycolysis which contain high energy phosphate bonds. Creatine phosphate transfers a ~P bond to ADP in nervous tissue and muscle. Acetyl CoA contains a high energy thioester bond.

In general, those compounds which have free energies of hydrolysis approximately equal to or higher than that of ATP are termed "high energy" compounds. Charge repulsion in the substrate and stabilization of the product by resonance forms or ionization contributes to their large negative $\Delta G^{0'}$ of hydrolysis.

SUBSTRATE LEVEL PHOSPHORYLATION

One other way of forming the high energy phosphate bond of ATP from fuel metabolism exists—substrate level phosphorylation. Substrate level phosphorylation is the formation of a high energy phosphate bond where none previously existed without the use of molecular O_2. For example, in the glycolytic pathway between glucose and lactate, ATP is generated from the transfer of high energy phosphate from intermediates of the glycolytic pathway to ADP (see Fig. 18.12). One of the intermediates of the glycolytic pathway containing a high energy phosphate bond, phosphoenolpyruvate, has a $\Delta G^{0'}$ for hydrolysis of –14 kcal (Fig. 18.13). An enzyme transfers the phosphate from phosphoenolpyruvate to ADP to generate an ATP in an exothermic reaction. The conversion of glucose to lactate has no net transfer of electrons to NAD^+ or FAD, and consequently no use for O_2 as an electron acceptor. It is therefore termed **anaerobic glycolysis**. Anaerobic glycolysis is the only pathway available for converting fuel energy to ATP in tissues which lack mitochondria, such as erythrocytes (red blood cells).

OTHER HIGH ENERGY PHOSPHATE BONDS

Energy transfer from the high energy phosphate bond of ATP into other chemical bonds is also involved in the utilization of energy for work. An example is the utilization of the high energy phosphate bond of UTP for glycogen synthesis. Another example is the transfer of the high energy phosphate of creatine phosphate to ADP for rapid formation of ATP at the site of ATP utilization in muscle and brain (see Fig. 18.12).

REGULATION OF FUEL METABOLISM

All of these pathways of fuel oxidation are feedback regulated by ATP levels, or by compounds related to the concentration of ATP. In general, the less ATP utilized, the less fuel will be oxidized to generate ATP. Thus an intake of calories in excess of those expended results in storage of excess fuels. The simple statement, "If you eat too much and don't exercise, you will get fat" is really a summary of the bioenergetics of the ATP-ADP cycle.

CLINICAL COMMENTS. Thomas Appleman has the impression that ethanol has only "empty calories." However, it is a fuel that can be oxidized in the body, providing 7 calories (kcal) per gram. The phrase "empty calories" is used by nutritionists to refer to foods like table sugar, or sucrose, because they contain only calories and no vitamins or other essential nutrients. It means that the food has no nutritional value other than its caloric content.

When alcohol makes up less than 15% of the total calories in the diet in healthy nonalcoholic individuals, it is used as efficiently to produce ATP as isocaloric amounts of carbohydrate or fat and, therefore, is not "empty."

Ahot Goyta exhibited the classical signs and symptoms of hyperthyroidism, including a goiter (enlarged thyroid gland). Thyroid function tests confirmed this diagnosis.

Thyroid hormone modulates cellular energy production and utilization through its many actions on intermediary metabolism. Many of these metabolic effects are the result of thyroid hormone's gene-regulating actions which result in the synthesis of a wide variety of proteins, among which are enzymes which catalyze the oxidative metabolism of carbohydrates, fats, and proteins. The loss of weight experienced by Ahot Goyta in spite of a very good appetite reflects the increased rate of fuel oxidation in hyperthyroidism. The result is an enhanced oxidation of adipose tissue stores as well as a catabolic effect on muscle and other protein-containing tissues. Through mechanisms which are not well understood, increased levels of thyroid hormone in the blood also increase the activity or "tone" of the sympathetic (adrenergic) nervous system. An activated sympathetic nervous system leads to a more rapid and forceful heartbeat (tachycardia and palpitations), increased nervousness (anxiety and insomnia), tremulousness (a sense of shakiness or jitteriness), and other symptoms.

Cora Nari was in left ventricular heart failure (LVF) when she presented to the hospital with her second heart attack in 8 months. The diagnosis of LVF was based on the following information:

1. Her heart rate was rapid at 104 beats/min. This "tachycardia" resulted from a reduced capacity of her ischemic, failing left ventricular muscle to eject a normal amount of blood into the arteries leading away from the heart with each contraction. The resultant drop in intra-arterial pressure signaled a reflex response in the central nervous system which, in turn, caused an increase in heart rate in an attempt to bring the total amount of blood leaving the left ventricle each minute—the cardiac output—back toward a more appropriate level to maintain systemic blood pressure.

2. Her resting respiratory rate was rapid. The weakened pumping action of the ischemic left ventricular heart muscle caused back pressure to increase in the vessels which bring oxygenated blood from the lungs to the left side of the heart. The pressure inside these pulmonary vessels eventually reached a critical level above which water from the blood moves down a "pressure gradient" from the capillary lumen into alveolar air spaces of the lung (transudation), producing a condition known as congestive heart failure. Subjectively, the patient experiences shortness of breath as the fluid in the air spaces interferes with oxygen exchange from the inspired air into the arterial blood causing hypoxia. The latter then stimulates the respiratory center in the central nervous system leading to a more rapid respiratory rate in an effort to increase the oxygen content of the blood.

Objectively, the physician will hear gurgling sounds (known as inspiratory rales) with a stethoscope placed over the posterior lung bases as the patient inhales deeply. These sounds represent the bubbling of inspired air as it enters the fluid-filled pulmonary alveolar air spaces.

Treatment of Cora's congestive heart failure will include efforts to reduce the workload of the heart with diuretics and other "load reducers," attempts to improve the force of left ventricular contraction with digitalis and other "inotropes," and the administration of oxygen by nasal cannula to reduce the insult caused by lack of blood flow (ischemia) to the viable heart tissue in the vicinity of the infarction.

BIOCHEMICAL COMMENTS. The major pathway for oxidation of ethanol in the human occurs in the liver (Fig. 18.14). Ethanol is oxidized by alcohol dehydrogenase to acetaldehyde, which is further oxidized to acetate (see Chapter 9). Most of the acetate enters the blood and is taken up by skeletal muscles, where it is converted to acetyl CoA. The acetyl CoA enters the TCA cycle. When ethanol consumption is low (less than 15% of the calories in the diet), it is efficiently used to produce ATP.

In individuals with a chronic consumption of large amounts of ethanol, the caloric content of ethanol is not converted to ATP as effectively. Several factors may contribute to this decreased efficiency. At high doses of ethanol, 10–30% of the ethanol is oxidized to acetaldehyde by a microsomal oxidizing system (MEOS) in the liver

The rate of ATP utilization controls its rate of synthesis. As the demand for ATP increases, the rate of fuel oxidation increases to keep the ATP levels of the cell constant. The result of an increased daily energy expenditure is, therefore, an increased oxidation of fat, carbohydrate, and protein.

Excessive production of thyroid hormone results in an increase in basal metabolic processes that require ATP. An increased BMR was used for a presumptive diagnosis of hyperthyroidism prior to development of the tests to measure T_3 and T_4. Since **Ahot Goyta** did not fully compensate for his increased ATP requirements with an increased caloric intake, he was in negative caloric balance and lost weight.

In the absence of an adequate oxygen supply, **Cora Nari**'s heart is still able to synthesize some ATP. However, the amount synthesized from substrate level phosphorylation is inadequate to meet the high ATP requirements of the heart.

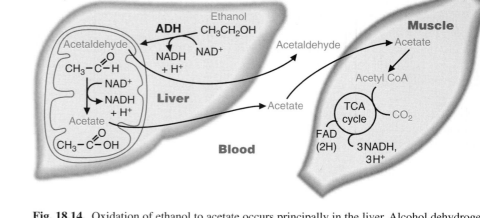

Fig. 18.14. Oxidation of ethanol to acetate occurs principally in the liver. Alcohol dehydrogenase (ADH) oxidizes ethanol to acetacetaldehyde in the cytosol. Acetaldehyde is oxidized to acetate principally by a mitochondrial acetaldehyde dehydrogenase. ATP is generated from the NADH by oxidative phosphorylation. Some of the acetaldehyde enters the blood, where it is transported to other tissues. Some acetate is oxidized in the TCA cycle, but most of it enters the blood and is taken up by muscle tissues, where it is converted to acetyl CoA and oxidized completely to CO_2 in the TCA cycle. Except at very high levels of ethanol, there is a rather efficient conversion of its caloric content to the ~P bond of ATP.

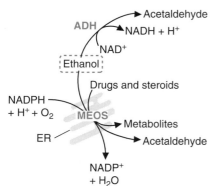

Fig. 18.15. At very high intakes of ethanol, some ethanol is oxidized to acetaldehyde by the microsomal ethanol-oxidizing system (MEOS) in the endoplasmic reticulum. This is one of the reactions in which the oxidation of fuels is not coupled to energy production. O_2 accepts electrons from the fuel and NADPH, and is reduced to H_2O. The reaction utilizes energy in the form of the reduction potential of NADPH.

(Fig. 18.15). This system utilizes reducing equivalents in the form of NADPH, rather than generating them as NADH. However, ATP is still generated from the subsequent oxidation of acetate.

Mitochondrial damage and the re-cycling of metabolites from fuel oxidation are two additional factors which might also contribute to a less efficient utilization of ethanol calories at high levels of ethanol intake. In contrast to normal mitochondria, the mitochondria from tissues of chronic alcoholics may not be able to maintain the transmembrane proton gradient necessary for normal rates of ATP synthesis. Consequently, a greater proportion of the energy in ethanol would be converted to heat. Ethanol oxidation interferes with the normal pathways of fatty acid and glucose oxidation. The cycling of intermediates between pathways to complete the oxidative process might also make fuel oxidation less efficient when ethanol is present.

Suggested Reading

Mezey E. Metabolic effects of alcohol. Fed Proc 1985;44:134–138.

PROBLEMS

1. Table 18.5 shows the metabolic rates of various tissues in the body. For each tissue, its rate of oxygen consumption has been calculated as an equivalent glucose consumption. In actuality, each tissue oxidizes various amounts of the different fuels. Overall, the caloric consumption of these tissues accounts for almost all of the BMR. The total amount of ATP produced by the average person, calculated from the sum of the ATP requirement of these tissues, amounts to almost 100 lb of ATP per day. For each tissue listed, explain why its ATP requirement is so high.

2. Different tissues can have different values of ΔG for hydrolysis of ATP. In muscle cells, [ATP] = 8.1 mM; ADP = 0.93 mM; and [P_i] = 8.1 mM. In erythrocytes, [ATP]

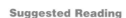

Because **Al Martini** has been an alcoholic for many years, his MEOS system has been induced and is very active, and the acetaldehyde present in his liver and circulating in his blood has damaged his tissues.

Table 18.5. Oxygen Consumption, Equivalent Glucose[a] Consumption, and ATP Turnover Rates by Human Tissues

Tissue	Approximate Oxygen Consumption		Equivalent Glucose Uptake		Equivalent ATP Turnover	
	mol/day^{-1}	µmol/g tissue/min	g/day	µmol/g tissue/min	mol/day	µmol/g tissue/min
Brain	3.4	1.7	103	0.3	20.4	10.2
Heart	1.9	4.5	57	0.7	11.4	27.0
Kidneys	2.9	7.1	88	1.1	17.4	42.6
Liver	3.6	1.6	108	0.3	21.6	9.6
Skeletal muscle (rest)	3.3	0.08	98	0.01	19.8	0.5
Skeletal muscle (marathon running)	257	6.4	7710	1.1	1542	
Lactating mammary gland			86[b]		38.4	

From Newsholme EA, Leach AR.
Biochemistry for the medical sciences. New York: John Wiley & Sons, 1983:146.

[a]The equivalent glucose uptake is the amount of glucose required to account for the oxygen consumption if it was the sole fuel. The equivalent ATP turnover is the ATP that would be produced under those circumstances. Summation of the values for the oxygen consumption of tissues at rest gives the total consumption of oxygen per day as 14.7 moles or 329 L. Since 1 L of oxygen is equivalent to 21 kJ of energy when glucose is oxidized, this represents 6,909 kJ of energy expenditure each day, which is only slightly less than that measured for a sedentary human subject. This indicates that other tissues contribute little to the magnitude of the metabolic rate. Not all of the tissues listed will use glucose; for example, under normal dietary conditions, liver and muscle (at rest) will obtain considerable energy from oxidation of amino acids, and during starvation most tissues will obtain energy from oxidation of fatty acids or ketone bodies.

[b]Calculated on the basis that all the lactose and 50% of the lipid secreted by the gland are produced from glucose. If some of the energy for biosynthesis and secretion is obtained from glucose, the rate of glucose utilization will be higher than shown in the table.

= 2.3 mM; [ADP] = 0.3 mM; [P_i] = 1.7 mM. Which tissue requires the most energy to synthesize ATP and derives the most energy from hydrolysis of ATP?

3. Why did **Thomas Appleman's** physician recommend that he exercise to lose weight?

ANSWERS

1. For each tissue, the oxygen consumption is related to the amount of ATP produced, which is related to the amount of ATP used. The brain utilizes high amounts of ATP for biosynthesis of neurotransmitters, regeneration of nervous tissue, and maintaining the Na^+ gradients required for conduction of the nerve impulse. The heart is, of course, constantly pumping and doing mechanical work. The kidneys are engaged in active transport, utilizing ATP energy to reabsorb metabolites that would otherwise be lost in the urine. The liver synthesizes glycogen, triacylglycerols, proteins (for example, most of the plasma proteins, such as serum albumin and the blood clotting proteins), and other compounds. Resting skeletal muscle uses very little ATP per gram of tissue. However, during exercise the mechanical work of contraction uses much more ATP and results in much greater rates of oxygen consumption. The large contribution of our muscles to our BMR results from our large muscle mass.

2. The synthesis of ATP is the reverse of hydrolysis. The ΔG for the synthesis of ATP is $\Delta G = \Delta G^{0\prime} + RT \ln[\text{ATP}]/[\text{ADP}][P_i]$, with the concentrations expressed as M. $[\text{ATP}]/[\text{ADP}][P_i] = 1.07 \times 10^3$ for muscle cells, and 4.5×10^3 for erythrocytes. Consequently, the ln of this value for erythrocytes is a larger positive number, and more energy would be required for synthesis of ATP in the erythrocyte.

3. A 50% increase in caloric expenditure during exercise represents a 50% increase in the rate of ATP hydrolysis, a 50% increase in the rate of ATP formation, and a 50% increase in the rate of fuel oxidation to provide the energy. The increased rate of fuel oxidation requires us to breathe more rapidly during exercise to increase our oxygen uptake and release the CO_2 produced in the oxidative pathways.

19 Tricarboxylic Acid Cycle

In most of the pathways of fuel oxidation, fats, carbohydrates, proteins, and ketone bodies are degraded to the activated 2-carbon acetyl portion of acetyl coenzyme A (acetyl CoA) (Fig. 19.1). In the tricarboxylic acid cycle (TCA cycle), this acetyl fragment is further oxidized to CO_2. The oxidation occurs in four reactions that transfer electrons to the electron-accepting coenzymes NAD^+ or FAD. Other reactions in the TCA cycle rearrange electrons to facilitate this transfer. Initially, the acetyl portion of acetyl CoA combines with the 4-carbon intermediate oxaloacetate to form citrate (6 carbons). A subsequent rearrangement of bonds in citrate is followed by two oxidative decarboxylation reactions. These reactions transfer electrons to NAD^+ and release 2 carbons as electron-depleted CO_2. In the next step of the TCA cycle, a high energy phosphate bond in GTP is generated from substrate level phosphorylation. In the remaining portion of the TCA cycle, two additional electron transfer reactions occur and oxaloacetate is regenerated. The overall process occurs with conservation of most of the energy in the chemical bonds of the acetyl group as 3 NADH, 1 FAD(2H), and 1 GTP.

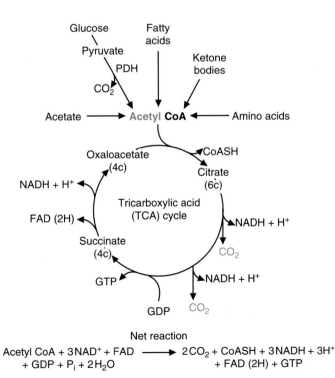

Net reaction

Acetyl CoA + 3 NAD⁺ + FAD $\longrightarrow$ 2 CO_2 + CoASH + 3 NADH + 3H⁺
+ GDP + Pᵢ + 2 H₂O   + FAD (2H) + GTP

Fig. 19.1. Summary of the TCA cycle. The major pathways of fuel oxidation generate acetyl CoA. In the TCA cycle, the 2-carbon acetyl group is oxidized to 2 CO_2. The net reaction of the TCA cycle is the sum of the equations for individual steps.

The TCA cycle is frequently called the Krebs cycle because its reactions were formulated into a cycle by Sir Hans Krebs. It is also called the "citric acid cycle" because citrate was one of the first compounds known to participate. The most common name for this pathway, the tricarboxylic acid or TCA cycle, denotes the involvement of the tricarboxylates citrate and isocitrate.

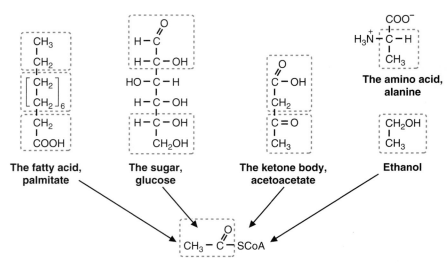

Fig. 19.2. Origin of the acetyl group in various fuels. Acetyl CoA is derived from the oxidation of fuels. The portions of fatty acids, glucose, ketone bodies, ethanol, and the amino acid alanine which are converted to the acetyl group of acetyl CoA are shown in blue.

The acetyl group which is the fuel, or source of electrons, for the TCA cycle is derived from the other pathways of fuel metabolism: fatty acid oxidation, glycolysis, ketone body oxidation, ethanol oxidation, and the oxidative pathways of the individual amino acids (Fig. 19.2). Approximately two thirds of the NADH and FAD(2H) generated from fuel oxidation arises from the oxidation of acetyl CoA in the TCA cycle.

The rate of the TCA cycle is tightly coordinated to the rate at which ATP is utilized through regulation of individual enzymes by ATP-related compounds, by the reduction state of NAD^+, and by Ca^{2+} concentration.

Ron Templeton has recovered completely from his ankle sprain and has faithfully followed his diet and aerobic exercise program of daily tennis and jogging. He has lost a total of 23 lb and is just 10 lb from his college weight of 154 lb. His exercise capacity has markedly improved; he can run for a longer time at a faster pace before noting shortness of breath or palpitations of his heart. Even his test scores in his medical school classes have improved.

Al Martini was discharged from the hospital after he completed an alcohol detoxification program. His alcohol-related neurological and cardiac manifestations of thiamine deficiency had partially cleared. He enrolled in a local Alcoholics Anonymous (AA) group and was given an appointment to see the same psychologist who had worked with him in the hospital. In spite of these support efforts and repeated attempts by his social worker to provide follow-up, he dropped out of his AA group meetings, failed to keep his appointment with the psychologist, and began drinking excessive amounts of alcohol again while eating poorly. Three weeks later he was readmitted with symptoms of "high output" heart failure.

OXIDATION OF ACETYL CoA IN THE TCA CYCLE

In the TCA cycle, the 2-carbon acetyl group of acetyl CoA is oxidized to 2 CO_2 (see Fig. 19.1). The function of the cycle is to conserve the energy from this oxidation in the form of the reduced electron-transferring coenzymes NADH and FAD(2H). The net reaction of the TCA cycle shows that the acetyl group serves as the source of the carbon for CO_2 and the source of electrons for transfer to NAD^+ and FAD. Acetyl CoA is, therefore, the fuel for the TCA cycle. The oxidation of the acetyl moiety does not directly involve O_2, and the oxidation is carried out by removing electrons as part of the hydrogen or hydride ion, and adding back H_2O. The 4 oxygens on the 2 CO_2 are derived from the carbonyl group of acetyl CoA, 2 H_2O, and the addition of a PO_4^{2-} to GDP. However, the individual steps of the TCA cycle rearrange the carbon and electrons donated by the acetyl group, so that the same carbon atoms and electrons do not enter and leave within a single turn of the cycle.

The overall yield of energy-containing compounds from the TCA cycle is 3 NADH, 1 FAD(2H), and 1 GTP. The oxidation-reduction reactions are catalyzed by 4 dehydrogenases: isocitrate dehydrogenase, α-ketoglutarate dehydrogenase, succinate dehydrogenase, and malate dehydrogenase (Fig. 19.3). The high energy phos-

 Enzymes which remove electron-containing hydrogen atoms from a substrate and transfer them to an electron-accepting coenzyme such as NAD^+ or FAD are called dehydrogenases.

Succinate thiokinase is also known as succinyl CoA synthetase. Both names refer to the reverse direction of the reaction, i.e., the conversion of succinate to the thioester, utilizing energy from GTP.

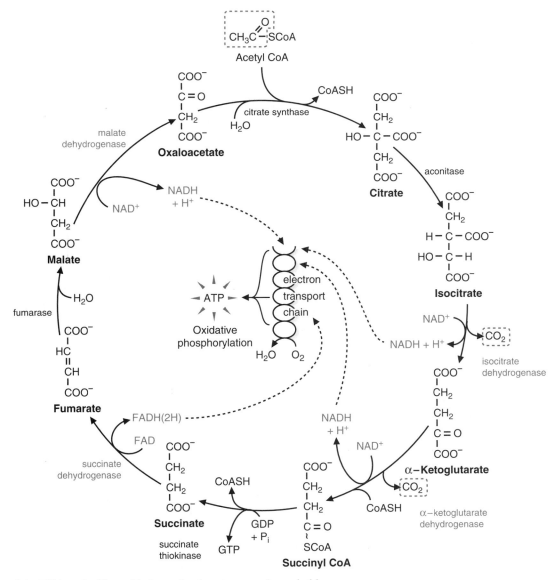

Fig. 19.3. Reactions of the TCA cycle. The oxidation-reduction steps are shown in blue.

Q   19.1:   From Figure 19.3, which enzymes in the TCA cycle release CO_2? How many moles of oxaloacetate are consumed in the TCA cycle for each mole of CO_2 produced?

The conversion of citrate to isocitrate is an isomerization, a reaction in which atoms/electrons are rearranged, but neither is removed or added in the net reaction. The enzyme that catalyzes this reaction, aconitase, is named for an intermediate in the reaction, aconitic acid (aconitate).

phate bond of GTP is generated from substrate level phosphorylation catalyzed by succinate thiokinase. As the NADH and FAD(2H) are reoxidized in the electron transport chain, about 3 ATP are generated for each NADH, and 2 ATP for each FAD(2H). Consequently, the net energy yield from the TCA cycle and oxidative phosphorylation is 12 high energy phosphate bonds for each acetyl group oxidized.

Formation and Oxidation of Isocitrate

The TCA cycle begins with the condensation of the activated acetyl group and oxaloacetate to form the 6-carbon intermediate citrate, catalyzed by the enzyme citrate synthase (see Fig. 19.3). In the next step of the TCA cycle, isocitrate is formed by moving the hydroxyl group of citrate to an adjacent carbon which has a C—H bond. Now the alcohol group can be oxidized to a keto group by isocitrate dehydrogenase (Fig. 19.4). Once the dehydrogenation step of the reaction has been carried out, the electrons rearrange and CO_2 is released, forming α-ketoglutarate.

Oxidative Decarboxylation of α-Ketoglutarate

The next step of the TCA cycle is the oxidative decarboxylation of α-ketoglutarate to succinyl CoA, catalyzed by the α-ketoglutarate dehydrogenase complex (Fig. 19.5). Five coenzymes are required for the overall reaction: thiamine pyrophosphate, lipoic acid, CoASH, FAD, and NAD+.

The decarboxylation of α-ketoglutarate and the oxidation of the keto group to the level of an acid release an enormous amount of energy. This energy is conserved principally in the reduction state of NADH, with a smaller amount present in the thioester bond of succinyl CoA. The energy from the succinyl CoA thioester bond is used for the generation of GTP in the subsequent step of the TCA cycle.

α-KETOGLUTARATE DEHYDROGENASE COMPLEX

The α-ketoglutarate dehydrogenase complex is a huge multisubunit enzyme complex composed of at least three different enzymes: α-ketoglutarate dehydrogenase (sometimes called α-ketoglutarate decarboxylase), transsuccinylase, and lipoamide dehydrogenase. Multiple subunits of each of these enzymes are present, resulting in a molecular weight for the complex of several million daltons. The α-ketoglutarate dehydrogenase complex is just one of a family of similar enzyme complexes which oxidatively decarboxylate α-ketoglutarate, pyruvate, α-ketobutyrate, and the α-keto acids of the branched chain amino acids (valine, leucine, and isoleucine).

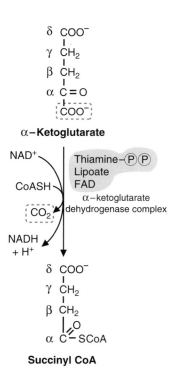

Fig. 19.5. Oxidative decarboxylation of α-ketoglutarate. The α-ketoglutarate dehydrogenase complex oxidizes α-ketoglutarate to succinyl CoA. The enzyme utilizes the coenzymes thiamine-PP, FAD, lipoate, NAD+ and CoA. The abbreviation CoASH, indicating the presence of a sulfhydryl group, is normally used for unacylated CoA. The α, β, γ, and δ on succinyl CoA refer to the atoms of α-ketoglutarate from which they are derived.

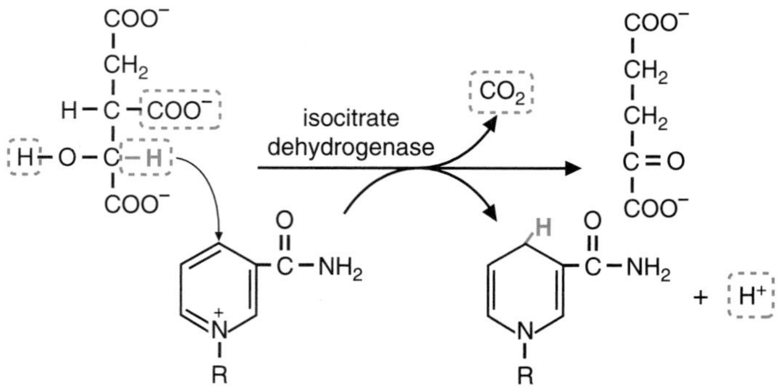

Fig. 19.4. Oxidative decarboxylation of isocitrate. The alcohol group (C—OH) is oxidized to a ketone, with the C—H electrons donated to NAD+ as the hydride ion. The H of the OH group dissociates into water as a proton. NAD+, the electron acceptor, is reduced.

The first enzyme of the α-ketoglutarate dehydrogenase complex, which is also called α-ketoglutarate dehydrogenase, contains thiamine pyrophosphate and carries out the decarboxylation step of the reaction (Fig. 19.6). The next enzyme in the complex, transsuccinylase, transfers the remaining 4-carbon portion of α-ketoglutarate from thiamine pyrophosphate to CoASH, forming succinyl CoA (Fig. 19.7). In this process, lipoic acid is reduced. The third enzyme of the complex, lipoamide dehydrogenase, transfers electrons from reduced lipoic acid to FAD, and then to NAD⁺. The NADH which is produced contains most of the free energy available from the oxidative decarboxylation of α-ketoglutarate to succinyl CoA. A smaller amount of energy remains in the thioester bond of succinyl CoA.

GENERATION OF GTP

The energy of the succinyl CoA thioester bond is used to generate GTP from GDP and P_i in the reaction catalyzed by succinate thiokinase, also called succinyl CoA synthetase (see Fig. 19.3). This reaction is an example of substrate level phosphorylation. By definition, substrate level phosphorylation is the formation of a high energy phosphate bond where none previously existed without the use of molecular O_2.

Oxidation of Succinate to Oxaloacetate

Up to this stage of the TCA cycle, 2 carbons have been stripped of their available electrons and released as CO_2. Two pairs of these electrons have been transferred to

The pyruvate dehydrogenase complex oxidatively decarboxylates pyruvate, which is a 3-carbon α-keto acid, to acetyl CoA. The pyruvate dehydrogenase complex is similar to the α-ketoglutorate dehydrogenase complex. It is composed of a thiamine-containing pyruvate dehydrogenase, a transacylase, and lipoamide dehydrogenase. Glucose is converted to pyruvate by glycolysis, and it can, therefore, be completely oxidized to CO_2 following this route: glycolysis → pyruvate dehydrogenase → TCA cycle.

In **Al Martini's** heart failure, which is caused by a dietary deficiency of the vitamin thiamine, pyruvate dehydrogenase, α-ketoglutarate dehydrogenase, and the other α-keto acid dehydrogenases are less functional than normal. Because heart and nervous tissue have a high rate of ATP production from the NADH produced by the oxidation of pyruvate to acetyl CoA and of acetyl CoA in the TCA cycle, these tissues are affected in thiamine deficiency.

Thiamine is one of the vitamins required in the diet. It turns over very rapidly in the human, and deficiency symptoms can develop after only 2 weeks on a thiamine-free diet. In Western societies, gross thiamine deficiency is most often associated with alcoholism. The mechanism for active absorption of thiamine is strongly and directly inhibited by alcohol. However, impairment of absorption may persist for several months after alcohol consumption has ceased. Marginal deficiency may also be common.

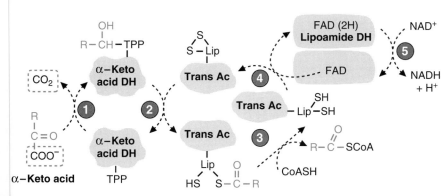

Fig. 19.6. Mechanism of α-keto acid dehydrogenase complexes. The individual steps in the oxidative decarboxylation of α-keto acids are catalyzed by three enzymes: an α-keto acid dehydrogenase (α-keto acid DH), a transacylase (Trans Ac), and lipoamide dehydrogenase (Lipoamide DH). Each α-keto acid dehydrogenase and each transacylase has a specific name corresponding to the specific α-keto acid which is the substrate (e.g., α-ketoglutarate dehydrogenase is specific for α-ketoglutarate). **1.** Thiamine pyrophosphate (TPP) on the α-keto acid DH forms a covalent bond with the α-carbon, which contains the keto group, thereby releasing the carboxyl group as CO_2. **2.** Lipoamide (Lip) on Trans Ac picks up the remaining fragment of the α-keto acid from TPP. The fragment is converted to an acyl group by this process. **3.** CoASH binds to the Trans Ac, forms a thioester bond with the acyl group, and the acyl CoA (e.g., succinyl CoA) is released. During steps 2 and 3, the lipoamide on the Trans Ac enzyme has accepted electrons from the α-keto acid fragment and been reduced from a disulfide (S—S) to two sulfhydryl (SH) groups. **4.** The electrons are transferred from Lip(SH)₂ to an FAD-lipoamide DH complex, thereby regenerating the disulfide. **5.** The electrons are transferred to NAD⁺, which is reduced to NADH. The structure of TPP and the mechanism of this reaction are shown in Figure 9.14. For the structure of lipoamide, see Figure 19.7. For the structure of CoA, see Figure 9.15.

19.1: Isocitrate dehydrogenase releases the first CO_2, and α-ketoglutarate dehydrogenase releases the second CO_2. There is no net consumption of oxaloacetate in the TCA cycle—the first step utilizes an oxaloacetate, and the last step produces one. The utilization and regeneration of oxaloacetate is the "cycle" part of the TCA cycle.

Q 19.2: One of **Ron Templeton's** tennis partners told him that he had heard about a health food designed for athletes that contained succinate. The advertisement made the claim that succinate would provide an excellent source of energy during exercise because it could be metabolized directly without oxygen. Do you see anything wrong with this statement?

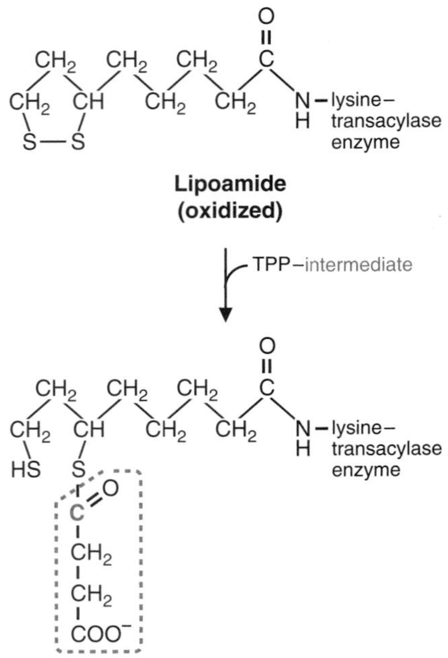

Lipoamide (oxidized)

TPP–intermediate

Fig. 19.7. Lipoic acid. Lipoic acid forms an amide bond with the amino group of a lysine residue on the transacylase enzyme and, therefore, is often referred to as lipoamide. Lipoic acid is one of the few coenzymes which does not require a vitamin precursor. It can be totally synthesized from carbohydrate and protein. In the reaction, the long side-chain arm created by lipoate and the lysine swings from the transacylase enzyme to the thiamine pyrophosphate to pick up the decarboxylated group of the α-keto acid. The succinyl group of α-ketoglutarate is shown here.

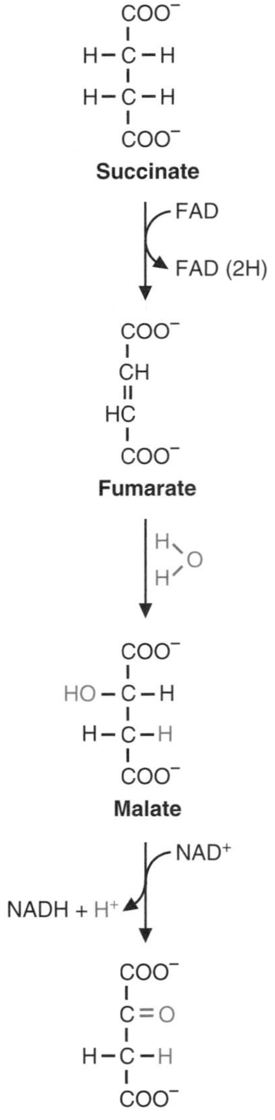

Succinate

FAD

FAD (2H)

Fumarate

H_2O

Malate

NAD^+

$NADH + H^+$

Oxaloacetate

Fig. 19.8. Oxidation of succinate to oxaloacetate.

2 NAD^+, and one GTP has been generated. However, two additional pairs of electrons arising from acetyl CoA still remain in the TCA cycle as part of succinate. The remaining steps of the TCA cycle transfer these two pairs of electrons to FAD and NAD^+ and add H_2O, thereby regenerating oxaloacetate.

The sequence of reactions converting succinate to oxaloacetate begins with the oxidation of succinate to fumarate (Fig. 19.8). Single electrons are transferred from the two adjacent $-CH_2-$ methylene groups of succinate to an FAD bound to succinate dehydrogenase, thereby forming the double bond of fumarate. From the reduced enzyme-bound FAD, the electrons are passed into the electron transport chain. An OH^- group and a proton from water add to the double bond of fumarate, converting it to malate. In the last reaction of the TCA cycle, the alcohol group of malate is oxidized to a keto group through the donation of electrons to NAD^+. This sequence of reactions—oxidation through formation of a double bond, addition of water to the double bond, and oxidation of the resultant alcohol to a ketone—is found in many oxidative pathways in the cell, such as the pathways for the oxidation of fatty acids, and of the branched chain amino acids.

COENZYMES OF THE TCA CYCLE

The enzymes required for the oxidation of acetyl CoA to CO_2 in the TCA cycle utilize NAD^+, FAD, thiamine pyrophosphate, lipoate, and CoA as coenzymes.

Differences between NAD⁺ and FAD

In the oxidation of succinate to fumarate and the oxidation of reduced lipoate to lipoate disulfide, FAD is the electron acceptor. In the other oxidation reactions of the TCA cycle, NAD⁺ is the electron acceptor. Why do some reactions utilize FAD and some NAD⁺? The two different electron-accepting coenzymes in the TCA cycle have different properties, and therefore perform somewhat different functions. FAD is able to accept single electrons (H•), and forms a half-reduced single electron intermediate (Fig. 19.9). It thus participates in reactions in which single electrons are transferred independently from two different atoms, such as the two adjacent —C—H bonds in succinate or the two —SH groups of dihydrolipoic acid. NAD⁺ accepts a hydride ion (H:), in reactions such as in the conversion of an alcohol to a ketone.

The difference in chemical structure of the two coenzymes results in different physiological roles. The free radical, single-electron forms of FAD are very reactive, and FADH might lose its electron through exposure to water or the initiation of chain reactions. FAD, thus, remains attached very tightly, sometimes covalently, to its enzyme while it accepts and transfers electrons to another group bound on the enzyme. The FAD(2H) in succinate dehydrogenase, for instance, is covalently bound and does not dissociate from the enzyme (Fig. 19.10). The enzyme resides in the inner mitochondrial membrane where the electrons on FAD are donated to coenzyme Q, which is part of the electron transport chain. All the other enzymes of the TCA cycle are found in the mitochondrial matrix.

> **A** 19.2: The claim that succinate oxidation could produce energy without oxygen is wrong. It was probably based on the fact that succinate is oxidized to fumarate by the donation of electrons to FAD. However, ATP can only be generated from this process when these electrons are donated to oxygen in the electron transport chain. The energy generated by the electron transport chain is used for ATP synthesis in the process of oxidative phosphorylation. After the covalently bound FAD(2H) is oxidized back to FAD by the electron transport chain, succinate dehydrogenase can oxidize another succinate molecule.

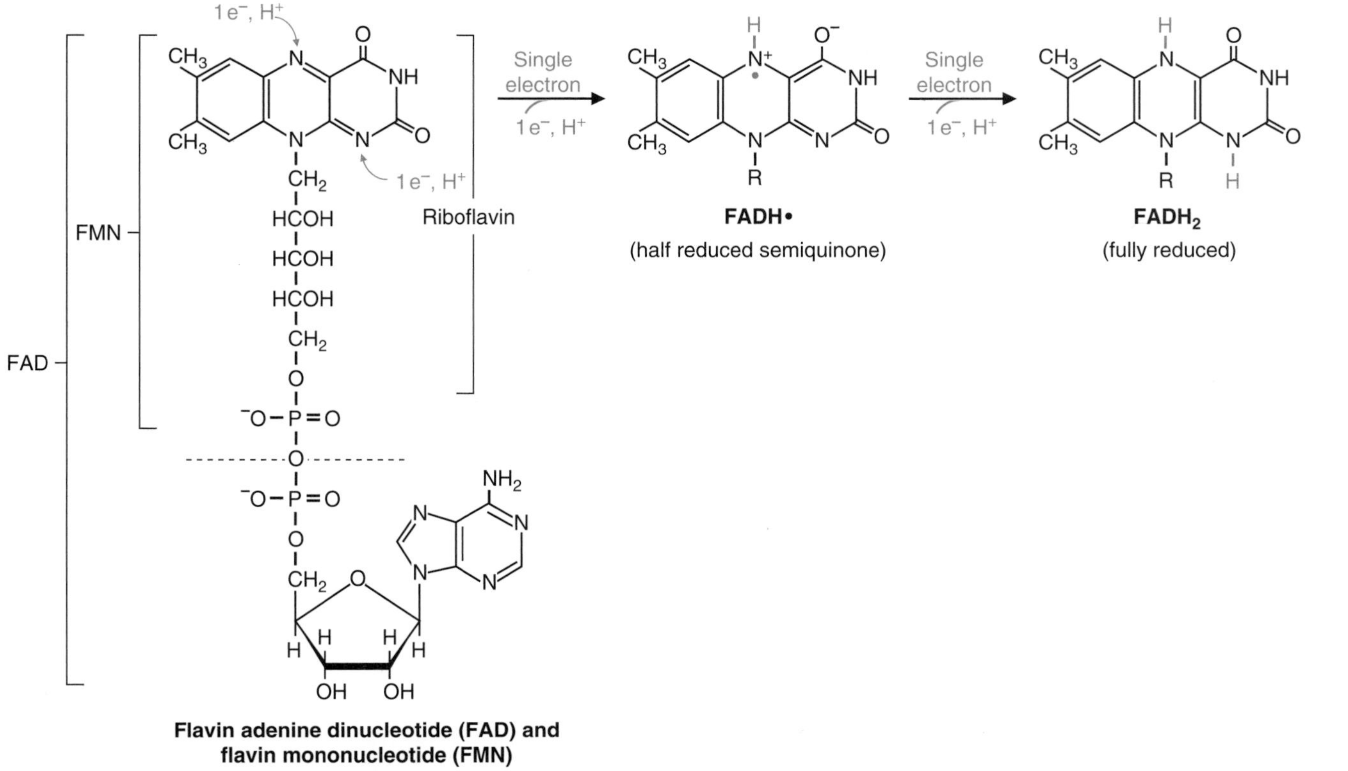

Flavin adenine dinucleotide (FAD) and flavin mononucleotide (FMN)

Fig. 19.9. One-electron steps in the reduction of FAD and FMN. FAD is formed from the vitamin riboflavin. FAD and FMN are reduced to a semistable single electron form when they accept one electron to form the half reduced semiquinone. They can also accept 2 electrons to form the fully reduced form, FADH₂. In many of the dehydrogenases, FADH₂ is never formed. Instead, the one electron is shared with a group on the protein as the next electron is transferred. Consequently, the FAD acceptance of 2 electrons has been denoted by the more general abbreviation, FAD(2H).

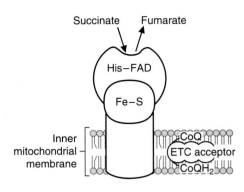

**Succinate
dehydrogenase**

Fig. 19.10. Succinate dehydrogenase. This enzyme is located in the inner mitochondrial membrane where it transfers electrons to the electron transport chain through the electron transporter, coenzyme Q (CoQ). Other components of the electron transport chain also use CoQ (see Chapter 20).

CoA is synthesized from the vitamin pantothenate in a sequence of reactions which phosphorylate pantothenate, add the sulfhydryl portion of CoA from cysteine, and then add AMP and an additional phosphate group from ATP (see Fig. 9.15). Although CoA is required in approximately 100 different reactions in mammalian cells, no Recommended Daily Allowance (RDA) has been established for pantothenate, in part because indicators have not yet been found which specifically and sensitively reflect a deficiency of this vitamin in the human. The reported symptoms of fatigue, nausea, and loss of appetite are characteristic of vitamin deficiencies in general.

Ethanol is oxidized to acetate in the liver. The acetate is carried in the blood to muscles, where it is activated to acetyl CoA. Thus, most of the 7 kcal/g that **Thomas Appleman** consumed in his ethanol (see Chapter 18) arose from oxidation of acetyl CoA to CO$_2$ in the TCA cycle.

Acetate is also supplied by the diet. Vinegar, which is a dilute solution of acetate in the form of acetic acid, was carried by Roman soldiers. The acidity of the vinegar made it a relatively safe source of drinking water because many kinds of pathogenic bacteria do not grow well in acid solutions. The acetate also provided an excellent fuel for muscular exercise.

NAD$^+$, in contrast, is usually free in the medium, binds to the dehydrogenase and accepts electrons, then is released and diffuses away. NAD$^+$ and NADH are, thus, much more like substrates and products than coenzymes. (For the mechanism, see Fig. 18.10.) This characteristic allows NADH to become a regulator of cell function. The NADH generated by one dehydrogenase can inhibit another dehydrogenase if the electrons are not utilized in the electron transport chain for ATP synthesis. The regulation of the TCA cycle by the NADH/NAD$^+$ ratio is part of the mechanism for coordinating the rate of fuel oxidation to the rate of ATP utilization.

Role of Coenzyme A in the TCA Cycle

CoA, the acylation coenzyme, participates in reactions through the formation of a thioester bond with an acyl group (e.g., acetyl CoA, succinyl CoA) (Fig. 19.11). The carbonyl carbon, the α-carbon, and the β-carbons of the acyl group are activated for different types of reactions by formation of the acyl thioester bond with the sulfhydryl group of CoA.

The acyl CoA thioester bonds of acetyl CoA and succinyl CoA, like the high energy phosphate bond of ATP, have large negative values for the $\Delta G^{0'}$ of hydrolysis (approximately -13 kcal). The thioester bond is far less stable than an oxygen ester bond because S, unlike O, does not share its electrons and participate in resonance formations. The energy released from cleavage of acetyl CoA and succinyl CoA in the TCA cycle serves two functions: it provides the energy for generation of GTP and makes the entry of acetyl CoA into the TCA cycle more thermodynamically favorable (Fig. 19.12).

In the condensation of the acetyl portion of acetyl CoA and oxaloacetate to form citrate, the cleavage of the acetyl CoA thioester bond results in a large negative $\Delta G^{0'}$ of -7.7 kcal/mole for the reaction. When this negative value for the citrate synthase-catalyzed reaction is added to the large positive $\Delta G^{0'}$ for the preceding malate dehydrogenase reaction, a net value of $\Delta G^{0'}$ near 0 is obtained for the overall conversion of malate to citrate. Thus the entry of acetyl CoA into the TCA cycle is facilitated by the energy released from cleavage of acetyl CoA.

Since the acetyl CoA thioester bond has a negative $\Delta G^{0'}$ of -13 kcal, the formation of acetyl CoA requires energy. When the acetyl CoA is formed from glucose oxidation, the energy is supplied by the oxidative decarboxylation of pyruvate in the reaction catalyzed by the pyruvate dehydrogenase complex. When acetyl CoA arises from fatty acid, ketone body, or amino acid degradation pathways, the energy comes from oxidation reactions and splitting —C—C— bonds. Acetate can also be converted directly to acetyl CoA using the energy supplied by ATP (see Fig. 19.11).

Energetics of the TCA Cycle

OVERALL EFFICIENCY OF THE TCA CYCLE

The reactions of the TCA cycle are extremely efficient in converting the energy in the chemical bonds of acetate to other forms. The total amount of energy in acetate is 243 kcal/mole. This amount of energy is released as heat from the complete combustion of 1 mole of acetate to CO$_2$ in a bomb calorimeter. To activate acetate to acetyl CoA requires the equivalent of two high energy phosphate bonds, or about 15 kcal/mole, so only about 228 kcal/mole is available from the oxidation of acetyl CoA. The products of the TCA cycle (NADH, FAD(2H), and GTP) contain about 206 kcal (Table 19.1). Thus, the TCA cycle reactions are able to conserve about 90% of the energy available from the oxidation of acetyl CoA.

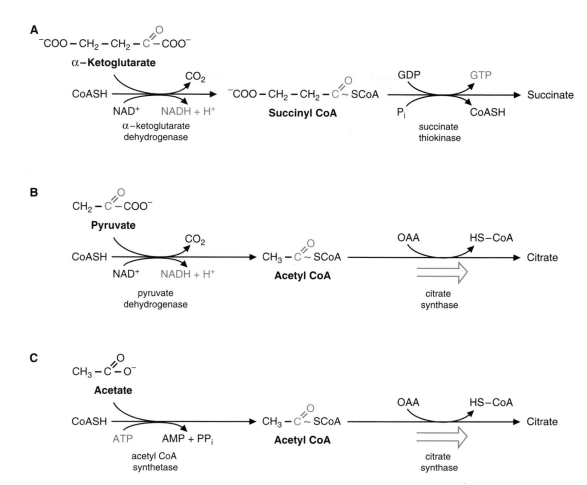

Fig. 19.11. Formation and utilization of the thioester bond of acyl CoA. Energy transformations are shown in blue. **A.** The energy from the oxidative decarboxylation of α-ketoglutarate is used for the formation of the acyl CoA-thioester bond of succinyl CoA in the reaction catalyzed by α-ketoglutarate dehydrogenase. The energy of the succinyl CoA-thioester bond is used for the synthesis of the high energy phosphate bond of GTP. **B.** The energy from the oxidative decarboxylation of pyruvate is used for the synthesis of the high energy thioester bond of acetyl CoA in the reaction catalyzed by pyruvate dehydrogenase. The energy released by hydrolysis of this thioester bond in the citrate synthase reaction contributes a large negative $\Delta G^{0\prime}$ to the forward direction of the TCA cycle. **C.** Acetyl CoA can also be synthesized from the activation of acetate by acetyl CoA synthetase. The energy is derived from the cleavage of the high energy phosphate bond of ATP.

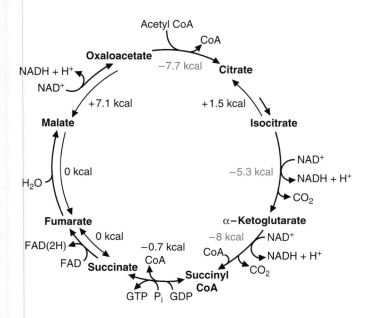

Fig. 19.12. Approximate $\Delta G^{0\prime}$ values for the reactions in the TCA cycle. The reactions with large negative $\Delta G^{0\prime}$ values are shown in blue. These reactions are both thermodynamically and kinetically irreversible in the cell. The reaction catalyzed by malate dehydrogenase is the only reaction with a large $+\Delta G^{0\prime}$, but it is both kinetically and thermodynamically reversible under physiological conditions.

Q 19.3: The difference between the 228 kcal available from oxidation of acetyl CoA and the 206 kcal conserved as products of the TCA cycle is 22 kcal/mole. This energy is lost as heat. It should be approximately equal to the sum obtained by adding together the $\Delta G^{0'}$ values for the individual reactions in the TCA cycle. What is the value for the net $\Delta G^{0'}$ obtained by this summation?

When NADH and FAD(2H) are reoxidized in the electron transport chain, the energy from transfer of their electrons to O_2 is utilized in oxidative phosphorylation for the generation of ATP. A maximum of 3 ATP are generated for each NADH oxidized and 2 ATP for each FAD(2H). Thus, the overall yield of high energy phosphate bonds from oxidation of acetyl CoA in the TCA cycle is 3 (NADH × 3 ATP) + 1(FAD(2H) × 2 ATP) + 1 GTP, for a total of 12.

Table 19.1. Energy Yield of the TCA Cycle

	kcal/mole
3 NADH: 3 × 53 =	159
1 FAD(2H) =	40
1 GTP =	7
Sum: =	206

Three reactions in the TCA cycle have large negative values for $\Delta G^{0'}$: the reactions catalyzed by citrate synthase, isocitrate dehydrogenase, and α-ketoglutarate dehydrogenase. These reactions are irreversible under physiological conditions—both because of the large negative $\Delta G^{0'}$ values, and because the enzymes involved catalyze the reverse reaction very slowly. These reactions make the major contribution to the overall negative $\Delta G^{0'}$ for the TCA cycle.

EFFLUX OF INTERMEDIATES FROM THE TCA CYCLE

The equilibrium constants of the reactions catalyzed by malate dehydrogenase and aconitase favor the accumulation of citrate and malate, which efflux from the TCA cycle (Fig. 19.13). Two steps within the TCA cycle have positive $\Delta G^{0'}$ values—the reactions catalyzed by malate dehydrogenase and aconitase. The enzymatic capacity for both these reactions is high enough to maintain equilibrium values for the concentrations of substrates and products. As a consequence, the concentration of malate is much greater than that of oxaloacetate, and the concentration of citrate is much greater than isocitrate. The rapid rate of malate dehydrogenase in both directions facilitates the reversibility of the malate dehydrogenase reaction. In the liver during fasting, gluconeogenic precursors are converted to malate, which leaves the mitochondria to enter the pathway of gluconeogenesis in the cytosol. The high concentration of citrate in mitochondria also results in its transport to the cytosol. In the liver (after a meal), cytosolic citrate is converted to acetyl CoA, thereby providing the precursor for fatty acid synthesis and other cytosolic reactions requiring acetyl CoA.

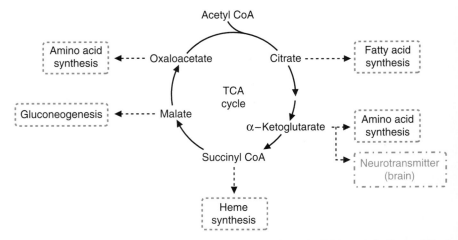

Fig. 19.13. Efflux of 4-carbon containing intermediates from the TCA cycle in liver and brain. In the liver, TCA cycle intermediates are continuously withdrawn into the pathways of fatty acid synthesis, amino acid synthesis, gluconeogenesis, and heme synthesis. In nervous tissue, α-ketoglutarate is converted to glutamate and GABA, both neurotransmitters.

CATALYTIC NATURE OF THE TCA CYCLE AND THE NEED FOR ANAPLEROTIC REACTIONS

In order for the TCA cycle to keep running, tissues have to supply enough 4-carbon intermediates to compensate for their removal by other pathways, such as gluconeogenesis or fatty acid synthesis (Fig. 19.14). In every tissue, metabolic pathways intersect the TCA cycle and remove intermediates, such as citrate and malate, which contain the 4-carbon unit of oxaloacetate. In nervous tissue, α-ketoglutarate is converted to glutamate and then to γ-aminobutyric acid (GABA), a neurotransmitter. Succinyl CoA is removed for heme synthesis in the liver. Carbon skeletons of some of the amino acids are also derived from intermediates of the TCA cycle. Oxaloacetate, which brings acetyl CoA into the TCA cycle, is always regenerated in the cycle. During each cycle, 2 carbons enter as the acetyl group, and 2 leave as CO_2; the 4-carbon unit, present as succinate, fumarate, malate, and oxaloacetate, stays. However, if

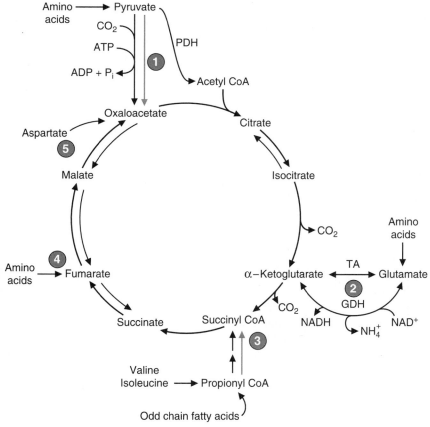

Fig. 19.14. Major anaplerotic pathways of the TCA cycle. **1.** Pyruvate carboxylase, which converts pyruvate to oxaloacetate, is present in both liver and muscle. Pyruvate dehydrogenase (PDH) is an alternate route of pyruvate utilization. **2.** Glutamate is reversibly converted to α-ketoglutarate by transaminases (TA) and glutamate dehydrogenase (GDH) in many tissues. **3.** The carbon skeletons of valine and isoleucine, a 3-carbon unit from odd chain fatty acids, the carbon skeleton of thymine, and a number of other compounds enter the TCA cycle at the level of succinyl CoA. This pathway is present in almost all tissues. The degradation of valine and isoleucine is probably the major anabolic route in tissues which do not contain pyruvate carboxylase. Other amino acids are also degraded to fumarate (**4**) and oxaloacetate (**5**), principally in the liver. 1 and 3 (blue arrows) are the two major anabolic pathways.

A 19.3: Summation of the $\Delta G^{0\prime}$ values for the individual reactions of the TCA cycle (see Fig. 19.12) yields a net $\Delta G^{0\prime}$ of about −13 kcal/mole. This value is in reasonable agreement with the value of −22 kcal/mole obtained by comparing the free energies of TCA cycle substrates and products.

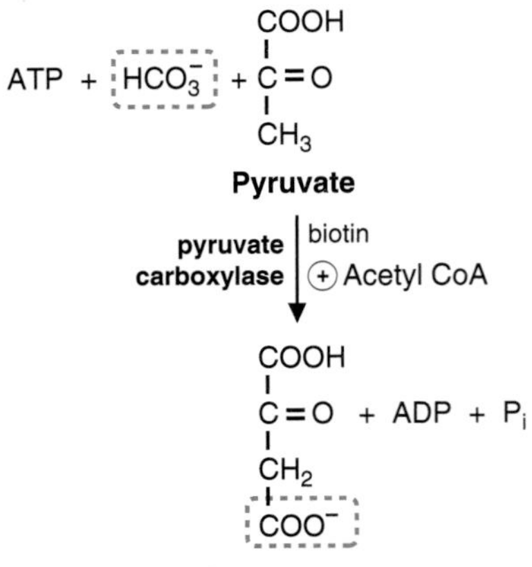

$$ATP + \boxed{HCO_3^-} + \begin{array}{c} COOH \\ | \\ C=O \\ | \\ CH_3 \end{array}$$

Pyruvate

pyruvate carboxylase | biotin, (+) Acetyl CoA

$$\begin{array}{c} COOH \\ | \\ C=O \\ | \\ CH_2 \\ | \\ \boxed{COO^-} \end{array} + ADP + P_i$$

Oxaloacetate

Fig. 19.15. Pyruvate carboxylase reaction. Pyruvate carboxylase adds a carboxyl group from bicarbonate (which is in equilibrium with CO_2) to pyruvate to form oxaloacetate. Biotin is used to activate and transfer the CO_2. The energy to form the covalent biotin-CO_2 complex is provided by the high energy phosphate bond of ATP. The enzyme is activated by acetyl CoA. As the concentration of oxaloacetate is depleted through the efflux of compounds containing the 4-carbon unit, the rate of the citrate synthase reaction decreases, resulting in the accumulation of acetyl CoA. The acetyl CoA then activates pyruvate carboxylase to synthesize more oxaloacetate.

Biotin is a vitamin. A deficiency of biotin is very rare in humans because it is required in such small amounts, and is synthesized by intestinal bacteria. However, an interesting case of biotin deficiency arose in a person eating a diet composed principally of peanuts and raw egg whites. Eggs contain a biotin binding protein, avidin. Since this protein was not denatured by cooking, it depleted his diet of biotin.

a TCA cycle intermediate containing this 4-carbon unit leaves the TCA cycle and enters another pathway, the level of 4-carbon intermediates must be restored.

Reactions which supply 4-carbon intermediates to the TCA cycle are called "anaplerotic" or "filling up" reactions. One of the major anaplerotic reactions is the conversion of pyruvate and CO_2 to oxaloacetate by pyruvate carboxylase. This enzyme contains biotin, which, in the presence of ATP and Mg^{2+}, forms a covalent intermediate with CO_2. (For the structure and mechanism of biotin, see Fig. 9.15.) The CO_2 is then added as a carboxyl group to pyruvate to form oxaloacetate (Fig. 19.15). The carboxylases in other metabolic pathways are also biotin-requiring enzymes and work by a similar mechanism.

Pyruvate carboxylase is found in high concentration in the liver and in nervous tissue because these tissues have a constant efflux of TCA cycle intermediates. Like most anaplerotic pathways, pyruvate carboxylase forms part of an overall pathway intersecting the TCA cycle. For instance, in liver, pyruvate carboxylase is part of the gluconeogenic pathway for converting alanine and lactate to glucose.

Amino acids form another source of 4-carbon intermediates. The pathway which converts isoleucine, valine, methionine, and other compounds to succinyl CoA is a major anaplerotic route. Most tissues, including the brain, skeletal muscle, and heart degrade isoleucine and valine to succinyl CoA via this route. In the liver, the TCA cycle is part of the pathway converting valine and isoleucine to glucose; in skeletal muscle, the TCA cycle is part of the pathway converting these amino acids to glutamine.

REGULATION OF THE TCA CYCLE

The oxidation of acetyl CoA and the conservation of this energy as reduced NAD^+ and FAD is essential for the generation of ATP in all tissues containing mitochondria. The rate of ATP utilization is, therefore, the primary physiological driving force for the TCA cycle (Fig. 19.16). Two major messengers feed information on the rate of ATP utilization back to the TCA cycle: (a) the phosphorylation state of ATP, as reflected in ATP and ADP levels, and (b) the reduction state of NAD^+, as reflected in the ratio of $NADH/NAD^+$. Within the cell, even within the mitochondrion, the adenine nucleotide pool (AMP, ADP, and ATP) and the NAD pool (NAD^+ and NADH) are relatively constant. However, the rate of interconversion of the adenine nucleotides varies considerably as does the rate of oxidation and reduction of NADH and NAD^+. Thus, an increased rate of ATP utilization results in a small decrease of ATP concentration and an increase of ADP. Likewise, increased NADH oxidation to NAD^+ by the electron transport chain would increase NAD^+ and decrease NADH levels, if the TCA cycle and other pathways of fuel oxidation were not stimulated.

A number of generalizations can be made about the regulation of metabolic pathways which are applicable to the TCA cycle (Table 19.2). One of these generalizations is that the regulation of metabolic pathways occurs at enzymes which catalyze the rate-limiting, or slowest steps in a pathway (Fig. 19.17). Pathways which must maintain a constant level of endproduct, such as ATP, are feedback regulated by the endproduct of the pathway or a related metabolite. In this case, ATP, ADP, NADH, and NAD^+ all participate in feedback regulation.

ALLOSTERIC REGULATION OF ISOCITRATE DEHYDROGENASE

Two of the major sites of regulation in the TCA cycle are isocitrate dehydrogenase and α-ketoglutarate dehydrogenase. The capacity of both these enzymes is relatively low under physiological conditions, and thus they constitute rate-limiting steps. Isocitrate dehydrogenase is a multisubunit enzyme which is allosterically activated by ADP and inhibited by NADH (Fig. 19.18). In the absence of ADP, the enzyme

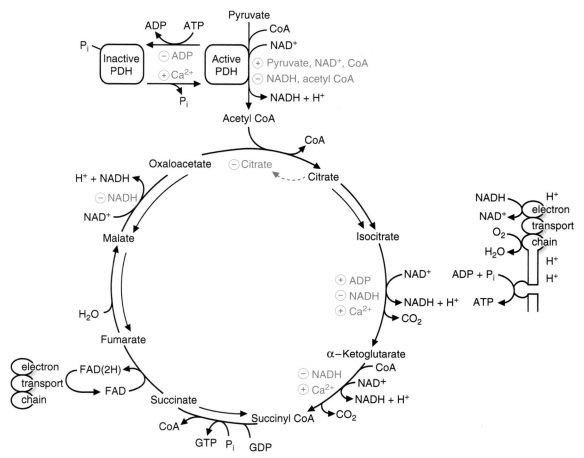

Fig. 19.16. Major regulatory interactions in the TCA cycle. The rate of ATP hydrolysis controls the rate of ATP synthesis, which controls the rate of NADH oxidation in the electron transport chain. All NADH produced by the cycle donates electrons to this chain (shown on the right). The oxidation of acetyl CoA in the TCA cycle can go only as fast as electrons from NADH and FAD(2H) enter the electron transport chain. The rate of the TCA cycle is adjusted to the rate of oxidative phosphorylation, and thus most cells are able to maintain constant levels of NADH/NAD$^+$ and ATP. The ADP and NADH concentrations feed information on the rate of oxidative phosphorylation back to the TCA cycle. Isocitrate dehydrogenase, α-ketoglutarate dehydrogenase, and pyruvate dehydrogenase (PDH) are inhibited by increased NADH concentration. The NADH/NAD$^+$ ratio changes the concentration of oxaloacetate. Citrate is a product inhibitor of citrate synthase. ADP is an allosteric activator of isocitrate dehydrogenase, and an inhibitor of pyruvate dehydrogenase kinase. During muscular contraction, increased Ca^{2+} concentrations activate PDH, α-ketoglutarate dehydrogenase, and isocitrate dehydrogenase.

Table 19.2. Generalizations on the Regulation of Metabolic Pathways

1. Regulation of metabolic pathways occurs at rate-limiting steps, the slowest steps, in the pathway. These are reactions where a small change of rate will affect the flux through the whole pathway.
2. Regulation usually occurs at the first committed step of a pathway or at metabolic branchpoints. In human cells, most pathways are interconnected with other pathways and have regulatory enzymes for every branchpoint.
3. Regulatory enzymes often catalyze physiologically irreversible reactions. These are also the steps which will differ in biosynthetic and degradative pathways.
4. Many pathways have "feedback" regulation, that is, the endproduct of the pathway controls the rate of its own synthesis. Feedback regulation can involve inhibition of an early step in the pathway (feedback inhibition) or regulation of gene transcription.
5. Human cells utilize compartmentation to control access of substrate and activators or inhibitors to different enzymes.
6. Hormonal regulation integrates responses in pathways requiring more than one tissue. Hormones generally regulate fuel metabolism by
    a. changing the phosphorylation state of enzymes
    b. inducing or repressing enzyme synthesis, or changing the rate of translation
    c. changing the concentration of an activator or inhibitor
7. Regulation matches function. The type of regulation utilized depends on the function of the pathway. Tissue-specific isozymes allow the features of regulatory enzymes to match the function of different tissues.

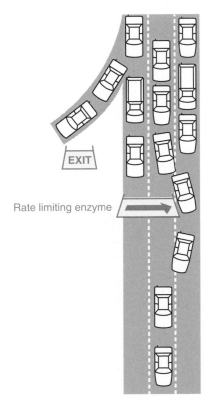

Fig. 19.17. Rate-limiting enzymes are like highway barriers. Enzymatic pathways are like highways. A rate-limiting enzyme like isocitrate dehydrogenase is similar to an obstruction in a three-lane highway that restricts traffic to just one lane. The steady-state concentration of cars before the barrier is increased, and the concentration of cars after the barrier is decreased. The barrier affects traffic for miles in either direction. The traffic jam may back up all the way to the entry ramp. Some of the cars will move into an alternate route (follow a different metabolic branch of the pathway). Moving the barrier just a little to open an additional lane is like activating the rate-limiting enzyme. The traffic will increase enormously, the car concentration before the barrier will decrease, and the car concentration after the barrier will increase.

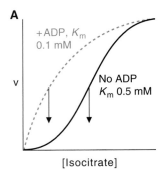

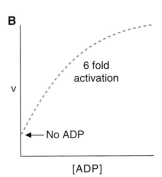

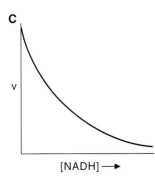

Fig. 19.18. Allosteric regulation of isocitrate dehydrogenase (ICDH). Isocitrate dehydrogenase has 8 subunits, and two active sites. Isocitrate, NAD^+, and NADH bind in the active site; ADP and Ca^{2+} are activators and bind to separate allosteric sites. **A.** A graph of velocity versus substrate concentration shows positive cooperativity in the absence of ADP. The allosteric activator ADP changes the curve into one closer to a rectangular hyperbola, and decreases the K_m ($S_{0.5}$) for isocitrate. **B.** The allosteric activation by ADP is not an all-or-nothing response. The extent of activation by ADP depends on its concentration. **C.** Increases in the concentration of product, NADH, decrease the velocity of the enzyme.

exhibits positive cooperativity; as isocitrate binds to the first subunit, other subunits are converted to an active conformation. In the presence of ADP, the conformation of all the subunits is changed so that isocitrate binds more readily, and the $K_{m,app}$ (the $S_{0.5}$, see Chapter 9) shifts to a much lower value. Thus, at the concentration of isocitrate found in the mitochondrial matrix, a small change in the concentration of ADP can produce a large change in flux. Small changes in the concentration of the product, NADH, and of the cosubstrate, NAD^+, also affect the rate of the enzyme more than they would a nonallosteric enzyme.

REGULATION OF α-KETOGLUTARATE DEHYDROGENASE

α-Ketoglutarate dehydrogenase, although not an allosteric enzyme, is product-inhibited by NADH and succinyl CoA. Thus, both α-ketoglutarate dehydrogenase and isocitrate dehydrogenase respond directly to changes in the phosphorylation state of ADP or the reduction state of NAD^+. Both of these enzymes are also activated by Ca^{2+}. In contracting heart muscle, and possibly other muscle tissues, the release of Ca^{2+} from the sarcoplasmic reticulum during muscle contraction may provide an additional activation of these enzymes when ATP is being rapidly hydrolyzed.

REGULATION OF ACETYL CoA ENTRY INTO THE TCA CYCLE

Neither isocitrate dehydrogenase nor α-ketoglutarate dehydrogenase are present at the first step of the TCA cycle. Therefore, these enzymes do not directly control the entry of acetyl CoA into the cycle. Citrate synthase, which is the first enzyme of the TCA cycle, is a simple enzyme in mammalian tissues, and has no allosteric regulators. Its rate is controlled principally by the concentration of citrate, a product inhibitor, and oxaloacetate, its substrate. When isocitrate dehydrogenase is activated, the concentration of citrate decreases, thus relieving the product inhibition of citrate synthase and increasing its rate. Because the malate-oxaloacetate equilibrium favors malate, the oxaloacetate concentration is very low inside the mitochondrion—below the $K_{m,app}$ of citrate synthase. When the NADH/NAD^+ ratio decreases, the ratio of oxaloacetate to malate increases. The increased oxaloacetate concentration accelerates citrate synthase. In the liver, the NADH/NAD^+ ratio helps determine whether acetyl CoA enters the TCA cycle or goes into the pathway for ketone body synthesis.

There are a number of additional regulatory interactions in the TCA cycle. These may function to control the levels of TCA intermediates and their flux into pathways which adjoin the TCA cycle.

REGULATION OF PYRUVATE DEHYDROGENASE

One of the major sources of acetyl CoA for the TCA cycle is pyruvate formed from glucose in the glycolytic pathway. Pyruvate is oxidized to acetyl CoA by the pyruvate dehydrogenase complex. Although the pyruvate dehydrogenase complex belongs to the same family of enzyme complexes as the α-ketoglutarate dehydrogenase complex, it contains additional regulatory subunits that remain bound to the enzyme. One of the regulatory subunits is a protein kinase, pyruvate dehydrogenase kinase, which phosphorylates the pyruvate dehydrogenase enzyme at a specific serine residue. This phosphorylation converts pyruvate dehydrogenase to an inactive form. Another regulatory protein subunit is a phosphatase, which removes this phosphate residue (Fig. 19.19).

Acetyl CoA formation by the pyruvate dehydrogenase complex is coordinated with the rate of ATP utilization by the concentrations of ADP, pyruvate, CoASH, NAD^+, acetyl CoA, and intramitochondrial Ca^{2+}. All of these compounds affect the amount of enzyme in the phosphorylated inactive form. Pyruvate dehydrogenase

As **Ron Templeton** exercises, his myosin ATPase hydrolyzes ATP to provide the energy for movement of myofibrils. The decrease of ATP and increase of ADP stimulates the electron transport chain to oxidize more NADH and FAD(2H). The TCA cycle is stimulated to provide more NADH and FAD(2H) to the electron transport chain. The activation of the TCA cycle occurs through decreases of the NADH/NAD^+ ratio, an increase of ADP concentration, and an increase of Ca^{2+}.

ADP is a true feedback regulator. It is directly related to ATP concentration, and ATP is the endproduct of oxidative metabolism. Feedback regulation often utilizes an allosteric regulator. It is the only regulatory mechanism in which a compound that does not resemble the substrate or the product of a reaction can directly interact with an enzyme. Allosteric regulators bind at allosteric sites, which are separate from the catalytic site where the substrate and product bind. A small change in the concentration of the allosteric regulator can cause a large change in the activity of the enzyme.

Kinases transfer phosphate from ATP to an –OH group on the substrate, releasing ADP. The substrate for a protein kinase is another protein, and a protein kinase phosphorylates a serine, threonine, or tyrosine –OH group. Pyruvate dehydrogenase kinase is specific for the pyruvate dehydrogenase complex and is a subunit of the complex.

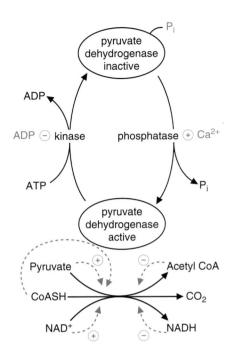

Fig. 19.19. Regulation of pyruvate dehydrogenase. The regulation of pyruvate dehydrogenase occurs through phosphorylation and dephosphorylation. Pyruvate dehydrogenase kinase, a subunit of the enzyme, phosphorylates pyruvate dehydrogenase at a specific serine residue, thereby converting it to an inactive form. This kinase is inhibited by ADP. Pyruvate dehydrogenase phosphatase, another subunit of the enzyme, removes the phosphate, thereby activating the enzyme. The phosphatase is activated by Ca^{2+}. The products, acetyl CoA and NADH, inhibit pyruvate dehydrogenase and increase activity of the kinase. When the substrates, pyruvate and CoASH are bound to the enzyme, the kinase activity is decreased, and pyruvate dehydrogenase is active.

As **Ron Templeton** exercises, the ADP concentration in his muscle cells increases as ATP is hydrolyzed to ADP and P_i during muscular contraction. NADH is more rapidly oxidized to NAD_+ by the electron transport chain. Acetyl CoA enters the TCA cycle more rapidly, and releases CoASH. The result is that pyruvate dehydrogenase kinase does not phosphorylate pyruvate dehydrogenase, which, therefore, is active and produces more acetyl CoA for the TCA cycle.

kinase is inhibited by ADP. When rapid ATP utilization is signaled by an increase of ADP, pyruvate dehydrogenase remains in the active, nonphosphorylated form. This action is aided in some tissues by the increased intramitochondrial Ca^{2+}, which stimulates the phosphatase.

The products of pyruvate dehydrogenase, acetyl CoA and NADH, inhibit the pyruvate dehydrogenase complex by stimulating phosphorylation to the inactive form. The substrates of the enzyme, pyruvate, CoASH, and NAD^+ oppose the phosphorylation. Thus, the buildup of acetyl CoA and NADH under conditions in which an ample supply of substrates for the TCA cycle is already available dramatically decreases the rate of the pyruvate dehydrogenase complex.

Pyruvate dehydrogenase is also activated through a mechanism involving insulin. The effect of insulin binding to its receptor on the plasma membrane is transmitted to the mitochondrial matrix. It is not yet clear how this is accomplished, but it may involve increased levels of mitochondrial Ca^{2+}. As a result, pyruvate dehydrogenase phosphatase is activated, and the pyruvate dehydrogenase complex is rapidly converted to the nonphosphorylated form. This mechanism is particularly effective in adipocytes. A slower, long term, hormonally directed mechanism may also be involved in adipocytes and other cell types.

CLINICAL COMMENTS. **Ron Templeton** is experiencing the benefits of physical conditioning. A variety of functional adaptations in the heart, lungs, vascular system, and skeletal muscle occur in response to regular graded exercise. The pumping efficiency of the heart increases, allowing a greater cardiac output with fewer beats per minute and at a lower rate of oxygen utilization. The lungs extract a greater percentage of oxygen from the inspired air, allowing fewer respirations per unit of activity. The vasodilatory capacity of the arterial beds in skeletal muscle increases, promoting greater delivery of oxygen and fuels to exercising muscle. Concurrently, the venous drainage capacity in muscle is enhanced, ensuring that lactic acid will not accumulate in contracting tissues. These adaptive changes in physiological responses are accompanied by intracellular changes in the content of respiratory enzymes. The number, size, and activity of skeletal muscle mitochondria increase, along with the content of TCA cycle enzymes. These changes markedly enhance the oxidative capacity of exercising muscle. In histological cross-sections of the muscles of trained athletes, this increased oxidative capacity appears as an increase in the content of slow twitch oxidative fibers relative to fast twitch glycolytic fibers.

Al Martini presents a second time with an alcohol-related high output form of heart failure sometimes referred to as "wet" beriberi, or as the "beriberi heart" (see Chapter 9). The term "wet" refers to the fluid retention which may eventually occur when left ventricular contractility is so compromised that cardiac output, although initially relatively "high," cannot meet the "demands" of the peripheral vascular beds which have been dilated in response to the thiamine deficiency.

The cardiomyopathy is directly related to a reduction in the normal biochemical function of the vitamin thiamine in heart muscle. If a thiamine deficiency is present, keto acids accumulate in heart muscle (and, to some extent, enter the blood), causing a chemically induced cardiomyopathy. In addition, thiamine pyrophosphate serves as the coenzyme for transketolase in the pentose phosphate pathway. In its absence, the pentose phosphates accumulate, possibly contributing to the cardiomyopathy.

Immediate treatment with large doses (50–100 mg) of intravenous thiamine may produce a measurable decrease in cardiac output and increase in peripheral vascular resistance as early as 30 minutes after the initial injection. Dietary supplementation of thiamine is not as effective because ethanol consumption interferes with thiamine absorption. Ethanol also affects the absorption and/or conversion to the coenzyme form of most other vitamins.

BIOCHEMICAL COMMENTS. **Mitochondrial Compartment.** The mitochondrion forms a structural, functional, and regulatory compartment within the cell. The inner mitochondrial membrane is impermeable to anions and cations, and compounds can cross the membrane only on specific transport proteins. The enzymes of the TCA cycle, therefore, have a more direct access to products of the previous reaction in the pathway than they would if these products were able to diffuse throughout the cell. Complex formation between enzymes further restricts access to pathway intermediates. Malate dehydrogenase and citrate synthetase may form a loosely associated complex in which citrate synthase is able to utilize oxaloacetate directly provided by the malate dehydrogenase. The multienzyme pyruvate dehydrogenase and α-ketoglutarate dehydrogenase complexes are examples of substrate channeling by tightly bound enzymes; only the transacylase enzyme has access to the thiamine-bound intermediate of the reaction, and only lipoamide dehydrogenase has access to reduced lipoic acid.

Compartmentation plays an important role in regulation. NAD^+, NADH, CoASH, and acyl CoA derivatives have no transport proteins. Therefore, these compounds cannot cross the mitochondrial membrane, and the concentration of the total NAD pool and the total CoA pool within the mitochondrion can change only very slowly. The accumulation of acyl CoA derivatives, such as acetyl CoA or succinyl CoA, within the mitochondrial matrix inhibits other CoA utilizing reactions, either by competing at the active site of the enzyme or decreasing the limited availability of CoASH. The regulatory mechanisms for the TCA cycle enzymes are specifically related to the content of the regulator in the mitochondrial matrix. The close association between the rate of the electron transport chain and the rate of the TCA cycle is maintained by their access to the same pool of NAD^+ and NADH.

Import of Nuclear Encoded Proteins. Because the inner mitochondrial membrane is impermeable to proteins, proteins synthesized in the nucleus must be imported into mitochondria by special mechanisms. Although mitochondria have DNA and the capacity for protein synthesis, most of the mitochondrial enzymes, including all enzymes of the TCA cycle, are encoded by the nuclear genome.

The process of importing these protein subunits synthesized on cytoplasmic ribosomes into the mitochondrion is complex, and requires both the expenditure of energy in the form of ATP or the transmembrane electrochemical potential and heat shock proteins (hsp), otherwise known as "chaperones" (Fig. 19.20). The newly synthesized precursor protein bearing an N-terminal sequence which targets it for the mitochondrial matrix or the inner mitochondrial membrane interacts with cytosolic "antifolding" proteins, hsp70, and precursor binding factor (PBF) in the cytosol. These proteins prevent premature tight folding of the protein before it can be imported into the mitochondria. In a process which requires ATP hydrolysis for energy, the precursor protein is released from hsp70 and binds to a receptor on the outer mitochondrial membrane. The receptor brings the protein to a junction point in the inner and outer membrane where it is driven through a channel with energy provided by the electrochemical potential across the inner mitochondrial membrane. It is pulled into the matrix, refolded, and the N-terminal targeting sequence is cleaved by a protease.

Lactic acid (lactate) is produced from the glycolytic pathway when ATP demand stimulates glycolysis and the rate of pyruvate production exceeds the capacity of the muscle to metabolize pyruvate in the TCA cycle. The capacity of the electron transport chain to transfer electrons from NADH to oxygen is exceeded, and excess pyruvate is converted to lactate in the pathway of anaerobic glycolysis (see Fig. 18.2). Because lactate is an acid, its accumulation affects the muscle and causes pain.

Suggested Readings

Behal RH, Buxton DB, Robertson JG, Olson MS. Regulation of the pyruvate dehydrogenase multienzyme complex. Annu Rev Nutr 1993;13:497–520.

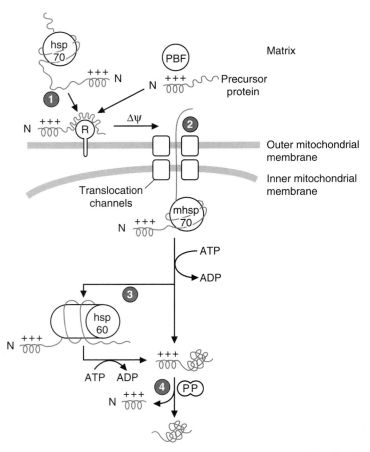

Fig. 19.20. Model for the import of a precursor protein into the mitochondrial matrix. The protein has an N-terminal target sequence for the matrix. **1.** The precursor protein interacts with heat shock protein 70 (hsp70), which is a chaperone protein, and precursor binding protein (PBF) in the cytosol. PBF facilitates binding to a receptor, R, on the outer mitochondrial membrane. **2.** The receptor brings the protein to translocation channels at junctions between the inner and outer membranes. As it enters the matrix, the protein attaches to a mitochondrial heat shock protein (mhsp 70) to prevent improper folding. **3.** Another mitochondrial heat shock protein, hsp 60, helps with the proper unfolding. **4.** In the final step, a protease cleaves off the targeting sequence. Reproduced, with permission, from the Annual Review of Genetics, Volume 25, © 1991, by Annual Reviews, Inc.

Glover LA, Lindsay JG. Targeting proteins to mitochondria: a current overview. Biochem J 1992;284:609–620.

Patel MS, Roche TE. Molecular biology and biochemistry of pyruvate dehydrogenase complexes. FASEB J 1990;4:3223–3224.

PROBLEMS

1. Sir Hans Krebs discovered in 1937 that the reactions which produced CO_2 from the oxidation of "active acetate" were arranged in a cyclical series which regenerated oxaloacetate. At the time of this experiment, pyruvate had not been characterized. It was called "active acetate." Coenzyme A and NAD had not been discovered. Now that you know the reactions of the TCA cycle, can you explain the results from which he was able to propose this sequence of reactions?

Krebs found that ground pigeon breast muscle (which contains intact mitochondria and pyruvate as a source of 2-carbon units for the TCA cycle) incubated in buffer consumed a total of 1,187 µL of O_2.

a. In the presence of pyruvate, an amount of citrate was added which should have required 302 µL of O_2 for its oxidation. It actually caused the consumption of a total of 2,080 µL of O_2. How do you explain this excess O_2 consumption?

	O_2 Consumption (µL)
Pyruvate (observed)	1,187
Citrate (theoretical)	302
Pyruvate + citrate (theoretical)	1,489
Pyruvate + citrate (observed)	2,080

b. Malonate, an inhibitor of succinate dehydrogenase, dramatically decreased O_2 consumption. Addition of citrate did not then stimulate O_2 use above that expected. Explain.

c. Addition of fumarate, instead of citrate, to malonate-poisoned tissue extract also caused a large increase in O_2 utilization. Explain.

2. Dietary deficiencies of pantothenate, riboflavin, niacin, and thiamine all result in fatigue. Why?

ANSWERS

Krebs knew that:

$$\text{Citrate} \xrightarrow[\;\;O_2\;\; \nearrow\;\; CO_2]{} \alpha\text{-Ketoglutarate} \xrightarrow[\;\;O_2\;\; \nearrow\;\; CO_2]{} \text{Succinate} \xrightarrow[\;\;O_2\;\;]{} \text{Fumarate}$$

Krebs also knew that:

$$\text{"active acetate"} \xrightarrow[\;\;O_2\;\;]{} 2\ CO_2$$

so he concluded that something from citrate, probably fumarate, was increasing the amount of "active acetate" which could be oxidized to CO_2. He drew a cycle similar to that shown in Figure 19.3. Later, oxaloacetate was discovered.

1b. When malonate was added, citrate would not stimulate "active acetate" oxidation, since there was no source of fumarate (oxaloacetate) for citrate formation.

1c. When fumarate was added, there was again an increase of O_2 consumption because he had added back a source of oxaloacetate. Fumarate "bypassed" the block.

2. These vitamins are all precursors of coenzymes used in the TCA cycle and other pathways of fuel metabolism. Riboflavin is the precursor of FAD, niacin is the precursor of NAD^+, pantothenate of CoA, and thiamine of thiamine pyrophosphate. Because the TCA cycle accounts for such a large percentage of our fuel metabolism, decreased TCA cycle activity due to decreased levels of coenzymes as a consequence of vitamin deficiencies affects ATP production, which causes fatigue.

20 Oxidative Phosphorylation and the Electron Transport Chain

The energy from oxidation of fuels is converted to the high energy phosphate bonds of ATP by the process of oxidative phosphorylation. Most of the energy from the oxidation of fuels in the TCA cycle and other oxidative pathways is conserved in the form of the reduced electron-accepting coenzymes, NADH and FAD(2H). The electron transport chain oxidizes NADH and FAD(2H), and donates the electrons to O_2, which is reduced to H_2O. The energy from the reduction of O_2 is utilized for the phosphorylation of ADP to ATP by ATP synthase. The overall process is, therefore, referred to as oxidative phosphorylation. The net yield of oxidative phosphorylation is about 3 moles of ATP per mole of NADH oxidized, or 2 moles of ATP per mole of FAD(2H) oxidized.

Oxidative phosphorylation is a mitochondrial process (Fig. 20.1). The ATP which is synthesized is released into the mitochondrial matrix. It is actively transported to the cytosol by a transport protein, ATP/ADP translocase.

Mitochondria are generally located near the major sites of ATP utilization, and the amount and type of mitochondria are correlated with the demand for ATP and the physical properties of the tissue (Fig. 20.2).

The chemiosmotic theory explains how the energy from the transport of electrons to O_2 is transformed into the high energy phosphate bond of ATP. Basically, the transport of electrons in the electron transport chain generates an electrochemical potential across the inner mitochondrial membrane by pumping protons from the mitochondrial matrix to the cytosolic side of the membrane. ATP synthase, which is activated by the transmembrane electrochemical gradient, provides a transmembrane pore or channel through which the protons enter and stimulate the formation of ATP from PO_4^{2-} and ADP. Inhibitors of the electron transport chain, such as cyanide, prevent the generation of the transmembrane proton gradient and, therefore, the synthesis of ATP.

The coupling of ATP synthesis to electron transport through the transmembrane proton gradient provides a regulatory mechanism by which the rate of ATP synthesis can control the rate of electron flow. As a consequence, the rate of oxygen consumption is coordinated with the rate of ATP utilization. When ATP synthesis and electron transport become "uncoupled" in brown adipose tissue or in the presence of chemical compounds, the energy from the electron transport chain is converted to heat.

Genetic diseases and other problems with the electron transport chain result in increased levels of NADH. The increased NADH concentration inhibits the TCA cycle and the entry of pyruvate and fatty acids into the cycle. As a consequence, pyruvate is converted to lactate, which appears in the blood, and fatty acids accumulate in the tissue as triacylglycerols.

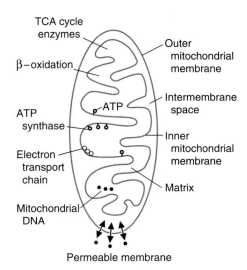

Fig. 20.1. Oxidative metabolism in mitochondria. The outer mitochondrial membrane is permeable to anions and small molecules. The inner mitochondrial membrane is impermeable to almost everything, including protons. The protein complexes of the electron transport chain and ATP synthase are embedded in the inner mitochondrial membrane. The electron transport chain accepts electrons from NADH in the mitochondrial matrix, or from flavin-containing proteins (flavoproteins) embedded in the membrane. ATP synthase projects into the matrix, where it generates ATP.

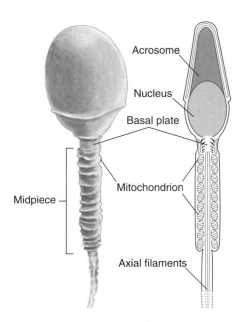

Fig. 20.2. A single mitochondrion encircles the midpiece of the mammalian sperm tail. The spiral shape of the mitochondrion accommodates the wavelike whipping motion of the sperm tail as it propels the sperm. The densely packed cristae of the mitochondrion contain the components of oxidative phosphorylation. While the sperm is in an aerobic environment, an estimated 60–85% of the ATP required for movement arises from oxidative phosphorylation. The rest of the ATP is formed from substrate level phosphorylation in anaerobic glycolysis.

ATP synthesis depends upon the structural integrity of the inner mitochondrial membrane. In Reye's syndrome, a disease caused by aspirin ingestion after a viral infection, the mitochondria are enlarged, swollen, and have disrupted membranes. The impaired energy metabolism results in an inability to incorporate ammonia into urea and consequent hepatic coma.

Cora Nari was recovering uneventfully from her heart attack 1 month earlier when she was attacked by her neighbor's vicious dog. As friends pulled the animal from her, she experienced crushing chest pain, grew short of breath, and passed out. She regained consciousness as she was being rushed to the hospital emergency room.

On initial examination, her blood pressure was extremely high and her heart rhythm irregular. An electrocardiogram showed unequivocal evidence of severe lack of oxygen (ischemia) in the muscles of the anterior and lateral walls of her heart. Life-support measures including nasal oxygen were initiated. An intravenous drip of nitroprusside, a vasodilating agent, was started in an effort to reduce her hypertension. After her blood pressure was well-controlled, a decision was made to administer intravenous tissue plasminogen activator (TPA), in an attempt to break up any intracoronary artery blood clots in vessels supplying the ischemic myocardium (thrombolytic therapy).

A ^{123}I thyroid uptake and scan performed on **Ahot Goyta** confirmed that his hyperthyroidism was the result of Graves' disease. Graves' disease, also known as diffuse toxic goiter, is an autoimmune genetic disorder caused by the generation of human thyroid-stimulating immunoglobulins (HTSIs). Mr. Goyta's heat intolerance and sweating were growing worse with time. His physician described the therapeutic alternatives for this disease to Mr. Goyta.

Arlyn Foma continued his multidrug chemotherapy with adriamycin, vincristine, cyclophosphamide, and methotrexate (AV/CM) and interferon α-2b (see Chapters 11 and 15). Although the response of his lymphoma was favorable, he complained of increasing shortness of breath on exertion associated with palpitations and growing fatigue.

CHEMIOSMOTIC THEORY OF OXIDATIVE PHOSPHORYLATION

Respiration begins with the oxidation of fuels in metabolic pathways which transfer electrons to NAD^+ and FAD. In the second phase of respiration, the energy available from the reoxidation of NADH and FAD(2H) by O_2 is converted to the high energy phosphate bonds of ATP by the process of oxidative phosphorylation. Our current understanding of this process is based on the chemiosmotic theory, which proposes that the energy for ATP synthesis is provided by a proton gradient across the inner mitochondrial membrane.

Overview of Oxidative Phosphorylation

The energy for the synthesis of the high energy phosphate bond of ATP is provided from the oxidation of NADH and FAD(2H) by the electron transport chain, which transfers electrons in a stepwise fashion from NADH and FAD(2H) to O_2 (Fig. 20.3). The electron transport chain is a sequence of electron-transfer carriers which are principally bound to proteins embedded in the inner mitochondrial membrane. They accept electrons from their reduced neighbor and pass them on to their oxidized neighbor, until the electrons are finally accepted by O_2. Each subsequent electron acceptor exists at a lower energy level (more positive reduction potential) so that energy is released as electrons pass down the chain.

The electron transport carriers that oxidize NADH are principally organized into three large membrane-spanning complexes: Complex I, NADH dehydrogenase;

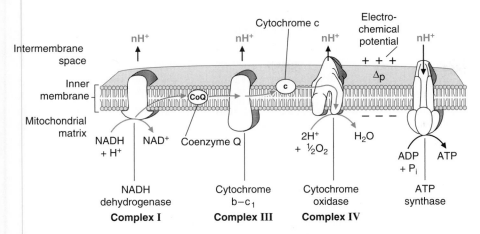

Fig. 20.3. Components of oxidative phosphorylation. The major complexes of the electron transport chain, NADH dehydrogenase, b-c_1 complex, and cytochrome oxidase, span the inner mitochondrial membrane. As electrons are passed through the chain to oxygen (along the route shown in blue), protons are pumped from the matrix side to the intermembrane space (the cytosolic side of the inner membrane). n, which denotes the number of protons, is about 4. The protons are dissociating from H_2O in the matrix. An electrochemical potential is generated by the transmembrane proton gradient (Δp). The return of protons to the matrix through the ATP-synthase pore drives ATP synthesis. Complex II (not present in this figure) is described in the text and in Figure 20.7.

Complex III, the cytochrome b-c_1 complex; and Complex IV, cytochrome oxidase. Coenzyme Q (CoQ), a lipid-soluble nonprotein component of the chain, and cytochrome c, a small protein located on the outer surface of the mitochondrial membrane, transport electrons between complexes. As the first complex, NADH dehydrogenase, accepts electrons from NADH, it is reduced; as it passes the electrons to CoQ, it is reoxidized. CoQ passes the electrons to the b-c_1 complex. The electrons are then picked up by cytochrome c and transported to cytochrome oxidase, which contains the binding site for O_2. O_2 accepts 4 electrons as it is reduced to H_2O.

The stepwise oxidation sequence is essential for conversion of the energy from the oxidation of NADH into a form which can be used for the generation of ATP. As the electrons are transferred through each of the three membrane-spanning complexes, protons are pumped from the mitochondrial matrix to the cytosolic side of the inner mitochondrial membrane. The energy drop of about 16 kcal in reduction potential as electrons pass through each of these membrane-spanning carriers provides the energy for the pumping of protons. The transmembrane movement of protons generates an electrochemical potential across the inner mitochondrial membrane.

ATP synthase, the enzyme that generates ATP, also spans the inner mitochondrial membrane. It contains a pore, or channel, through which the protons can reenter the matrix. Conformational changes in ATP synthase associated with the entry of protons activate the enzyme so that it catalyzes the addition of phosphate to ADP to form ATP.

TENETS OF THE CHEMIOSMOTIC THEORY

The chemiosmotic theory states that the energy available from oxidation generates the electrochemical potential by the pumping of protons, and that the energy in this electrochemical potential can be converted into the high energy phosphate bond of ATP. There are three basic tenets to the theory.

1. The major electron carriers are organized into three complexes which span the

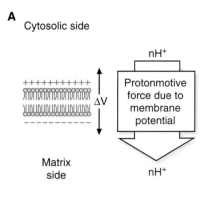

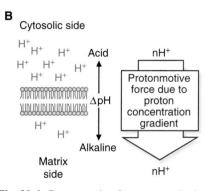

Fig. 20.4. Protonmotive force across the inner mitochondrial membrane, created by pumping protons from the matrix across the inner membrane. **A.** Protonmotive force, or electrochemical potential, due to the membrane potential. **B.** Protonmotive force, or electrochemical potential, due to the concentration gradient.

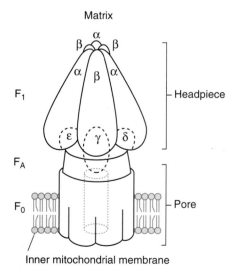

Fig. 20.5. ATP synthase. The F_0 subunits form a pore or channel through the inner mitochondrial membrane, shown in blue. The F_1 headpiece projects into the matrix. The subunits of the F_1 headpiece form three α,β pairs which each have a binding site for ADP and P_i.

inner mitochondrial membrane and have a vectorial arrangement within the membrane. This structural feature of the electron transport chain allows protons to be pumped across the inner mitochondrial membrane from the matrix to the intermembrane space while electrons are passed from one carrier to another.

2. The inner mitochondrial membrane is impermeable to protons, so that their pumping results in the generation of the electrochemical potential. Protons, once pumped to the cytosolic side of the membrane, cannot diffuse back through the membrane into the matrix. Thus, the pumping of protons builds up a much higher concentration of protons outside of the mitochondrion than inside, resulting in a transmembrane electrochemical potential gradient that is sometimes referred to as the protonmotive force. The pH of the cytosol is about one pH unit lower than the mitochondrial matrix (Fig. 20.4).

The electrochemical potential, or protonmotive force, exists in two forms: a membrane potential (the "electro" part), and a proton concentration gradient (the chemical part). The accumulation of positively charged protons on the outside of the inner mitochondrial membrane gives the membrane a positive charge relative to the inside, thereby forming the membrane potential. A protonmotive force (the force which tends to push the protons back in) results from repulsion of the positive charges.

The chemical potential is the force associated with a greater concentration of a substance, the protons, on the outside of the membrane relative to the inside. This force would become zero if the protons could diffuse back across the membrane until their concentration is equal on both sides of the membrane.

3. The electrochemical potential can drive ATP synthesis through the return of protons to the matrix via the ATP synthase channel. This step of the energy transformation occurs in another membrane-spanning complex, ATP synthase (also called F_0F_1-ATPase) (Fig. 20.5). This huge protein complex has a number of subunits which form a pore or channel through the inner mitochondrial membrane (F_0), and an ATP-forming headpiece which sticks into the matrix (F_1). The protons enter through the pore, and return to the matrix. The headpiece catalyzes the addition of PO_4^{2-} to ADP, a process that requires protons and splits out water. In the absence of the transmembrane proton gradient, ATP synthase catalyzes the reverse process, the hydrolysis of ATP, hence the name, F_0F_1-ATPase.

BINDING CHANGE MODEL OF ATP SYNTHESIS

According to the "binding change" mechanism, the energy from the transmembrane proton gradient is used to change the conformation of ATP synthase so that ATP dissociates from one subunit binding site while ADP and P_i bind to another. The headpiece consists of three sets of α,β-subunit pairs which make a cap over the γ-, δ-, and ε-subunits. As protons enter through the pore, the energy is converted into conformational changes in the headpiece subunits (a "binding change"). The α,β pairs rotate relative to the $\gamma,\delta,\varepsilon$ stalk and change their conformation so that a bound ATP dissociates, and an ADP and P_i bind to a different α,β-reaction site. Once tightly bound, the ADP and P_i spontaneously combine to form ATP (Fig. 20.6).

ENTRY OF ELECTRONS FROM FLAVOPROTEINS

After FAD accepts electrons and is reduced, it must transfer those electrons to an electron acceptor that is bound to the enzyme (see Chapter 19). Neither the single electron or 2-electron forms of FAD dissociate from the enzyme. As a consequence, flavoprotein enzymes are also protein complexes embedded in the inner mitochondrial membrane, and succinate dehydrogenase has acquired the name of Complex II. The flavoproteins transfer electrons to CoQ and contain CoQ binding sites (Fig. 20.7). There is no proton pumping associated with this transfer and, consequently, no generation of a proton gradient or ATP synthesis.

ENERGY YIELD FROM THE ELECTRON TRANSPORT CHAIN

Approximately 53 kcal are available for ATP synthesis from the oxidation of NADH by O_2 in the electron transport chain. Electron transport through each of the proton pumping spans of the electron transport chain is associated with a 13–20 kcal decrease in the energy content of the carriers (less negative reduction potential) and the pumping of about 4 protons. A maximum of one ATP is synthesized from the proton pumping at each of the three membrane-spanning complexes.

Approximately 40 kcal is available for ATP synthesis from the oxidation of FAD(2H). Between reduced FAD in succinate dehydrogenase (and other flavoproteins) and O_2, there are only two proton pumping sites to form the electrochemical gradient, and consequently only a maximum of 2 ATP can be generated from the oxidation of reduced flavin coenzymes.

About 40–45% of the energy available from NADH and FAD(2H) oxidation by O_2 is used for ATP synthesis. Some of the remaining energy in the electrochemical potential is used for the transport of anions and Ca^{2+} into the mitochondrion. The remainder of the energy is released as heat. The free energy drop through oxidative phosphorylation is large enough so that the overall process is irreversible under physiological conditions. The large negative $\Delta G^{0'}$ helps to pull the oxidative reactions in the TCA cycle and other metabolic pathways in the direction of oxidation and ATP synthesis.

ELECTRON TRANSPORT CHAIN

The carriers in the electron transport chain convert the energy in the reduction potential of the electron donors into the electrochemical potential gradient across the inner mitochondrial membrane while accepting electrons and passing them on to the next carrier in the chain. The compounds in the protein complexes which are actually reduced are FMN, Fe-S centers, Fe-heme, and Cu^{2+} (Table 20.1). Transport through the chain must be sequential, and inhibition of the chain at any point results in cell death for oxygen-dependent cells.

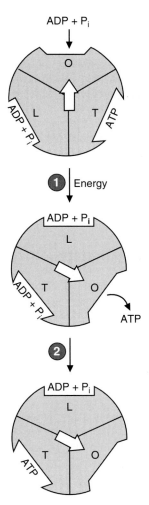

Fig. 20.6. Binding change mechanism for ATP synthesis. The three α,β-subunit pairs of the ATP synthase headpiece have binding sites which can exist in an open (O), tight (T), or loose (L) configuration. ADP and P_i are bound to the loose site, and ATP to the tight. **1.** In the presence of the high concentration of protons, ADP + P_i bind to the open site, the headpiece rotates relative to the stalk, and conformational changes occur. The O site becomes an L site and the tight ATP site opens (becomes an O site), releasing the ATP. **2.** The initial L site becomes a T site, where ATP forms spontaneously from ADP and P_i. The white arrow indicates the movement of the stalk (F_0) relative to the headpiece (F_1) that contains the three α,β subunits, which undergo conformational changes, producing O, T, and L sites. Reprinted from Cross RL. The reaction mechanism of F_0F_1-ATP synthases. In: Ernster L, ed. Molecular mechanisms in bioenergetics, 1992:321, with kind permission of Elsevier Science NL, Sara Burgerhartstraat 25, 1055 KV, Amsterdam, Netherlands.

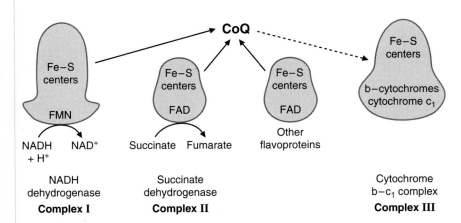

Fig. 20.7. Transfer of electrons to coenzyme Q. NADH dehydrogenase, succinate dehydrogenase, and other flavoproteins in the inner mitochondrial membrane donate electrons to CoQ. The electrons are transferred from the flavin to an Fe-S center, and then to CoQ, which is reduced. The other flavoproteins include L-glycerol 3-phosphate dehydrogenase and an electron-transferring flavoprotein which is involved in the transfer from the acyl CoA dehydrogenase of fatty acid oxidation.

20.1: Does the transfer of electrons from succinate to CoQ under standard conditions provide enough energy for the generation of a high energy phosphate bond in ATP? How does this compare with the energy of electron transfer from NADH to CoQ? (The values for the standard reduction potentials of these compounds can be found in Table 18.4.)

FMN, like FAD, is synthesized from the vitamin riboflavin. It contains the electron-accepting flavin ring structure, but not the adenosine monophosphate (AMP) portion of FAD (see Fig. 18.11). A severe deficiency of riboflavin decreases the ability of mitochondria to generate ATP from oxidative phosphorylation. In severe riboflavin deficiency induced in experimental animals, tissues develop megamitochondria almost as large as the nucleus. In general, impairment of Complex I results in the formation of mitochondria with unusual structures.

Table 20.1. Components of the Electron Transport Chain

Names	Prosthetic Groups	e⁻ Donor → e⁻ Acceptor	Inactivated by
NADH dehydrogenase Complex I NADHQ reductase	FMN Fe-S	NADH→CoQ	Rotenone Riboflavin deficiency
CoQ Coenzyme Q Ubiquinone	CoQ	NADH dehydrogenase → b-c_1 complex	Generation of free radicals Doxorubicin
Cytochrome b-c_1 complex Complex III Ubiquinone-cytochrome c oxidoreductase	Fe-S Heme b_{562} Heme b_{566} Heme c_1	CoQ → cytochrome c	Antimycin Demerol Fe deficiency
Cytochrome c	Heme c	b-c_1 complex → cytochrome oxidase	Fe deficiency
Cytochrome oxidase Complex IV Cytochrome aa_3	Heme a Heme a_3 Cu_A, Cu_B	Cytochrome c → O_2	Cyanide Carbon monoxide Ischemia Fe and Cu deficiency
Succinate dehydrogenase Complex II	FAD Fe-S	Succinate → CoQ	Malonate

Components of the Chain

NADH DEHYDROGENASE

The transfer of electrons from NADH to O_2 starts with the donation of 2 electrons from NADH to the first protein complex in the chain, NADH dehydrogenase. This enormous complex, consisting of many protein subunits, contains flavin mononucleotide (FMN) and iron-sulfur (Fe-S) centers (Fig. 20.8). FMN accepts the electrons from NADH and is able to pass single electrons to Fe-S centers. NADH is oxidized back to NAD^+ which can return to the TCA cycle or another metabolic pathway to accept electrons. Fe-S centers, which are able to delocalize electrons and give them very large orbitals, are involved in the transfer of electrons to and from CoQ (see Fig 20.7).

COENZYME Q

The next acceptor of electrons is CoQ, frequently called ubiquinone. CoQ is the only component of the electron transport chain that is not protein bound. The large hydrophobic side chain confers lipid solubility, and CoQ is able to diffuse through the lipids of the inner mitochondrial membrane (Fig. 20.9). The oxidation and reduction of CoQ and its associated transmembrane movement is part of the proton pumping mechanism for both the NADH dehydrogenase complex and the cytochrome b-c_1 complex.

b-c_1 COMPLEX AND CYTOCHROME c

The remainder of the components in the electron transport chain are cytochromes (Fig. 20.10). Each cytochrome is a protein that contains a bound heme (i.e., a Fe atom bound to a porphyrin nucleus similar in structure to the heme in hemoglobin). Thus, the flow of electrons from one cytochrome to another continues toward cytochromes of a lower energy level. The iron atoms in the cytochromes are in the Fe^{3+} state. As they accept an electron, they are reduced to Fe^{2+}. As they are reoxidized to Fe^{3+}, the electrons pass to the next component of the electron transport chain.

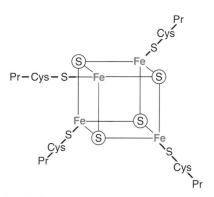

Fig. 20.8. Fe_4S_4 center. In Fe-S centers, the Fe is chelated to free sulfur (S) atoms, and to cysteine sulfhydryl groups on proteins. Other Fe-S centers contain Fe_2S_2. The protein subunits are sometimes called non-heme iron proteins. When these proteins are treated with acid, the free sulfur produces hydrogen sulfide (H_2S)—the familiar smell of rotten eggs.

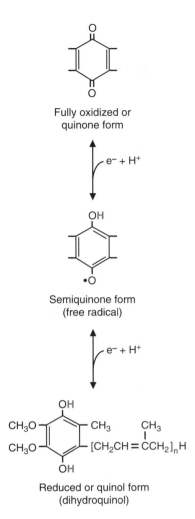

Fully oxidized or
quinone form

$e^- + H^+$

Semiquinone form
(free radical)

$e^- + H^+$

Reduced or quinol form
(dihydroquinol)

Fig. 20.9. Coenzyme Q contains a quinone with a long lipophilic isoprenoid side chain. CoQ can be synthesized in the human from precursors derived from carbohydrates and fat. The long side chain, which has an isoprenoid structure, is formed by the same series of reactions which produce cholesterol precursors. CoQ can accept one electron (e^-) to become the half-reduced form, or 2 e^- to become fully reduced.

The *b* and c_1 cytochromes are arranged with other protein subunits into the large, membrane-spanning *b*-c_1 complex. Cytochrome *c* is a much smaller separate protein located on the outer side of the inner mitochondrial membrane.

CYTOCHROME OXIDASE AND THE OXYGEN BINDING SITE

The last cytochrome complex is cytochrome oxidase, which passes electrons from cytochrome *c* to O_2. It contains cytochromes *a* and a_3 and the oxygen binding site. A whole oxygen molecule, O_2, must accept 4 electrons to be reduced to 2 H_2O. Bound copper (Cu^{2+}) ions in the cytochrome oxidase complex facilitate the collection of the 4 electrons and the reduction of O_2. Cytochrome oxidase has a much lower K_m for O_2 than myoglobin (the heme-containing intracellular oxygen carrier) or hemoglobin (the heme-containing oxygen transporter in the blood). Thus, O_2 is "pulled" from the erythrocyte to its site of reduction.

Electron Transport Chain

Transferring 2 electrons
To Coenzyme Q
Takes Fe-S proteins
And riboflavin, too.

Transferring an electron
Down the E.T. chain
Takes Fe 3 to Fe 2
And back to 3 again.

Transferring 4 electrons
To an oxygen
Takes some Cu ions
And Fe porphyrin.

C.M. Smith

A 20.1: From Table 18.4, the $\Delta E_0'$ for reduction of fumarate to succinate is +0.03 V, and for reduction of CoQ is 0.06 V. The value for the oxidation of succinate is therefore −0.03 V. The $\Delta E_0'$ for the oxidation of succinate by CoQ is the sum of these two values (−0.03 V + 0.06 V = 0.03 V). $\Delta G^{0'} = -nF\Delta E_0' = -1.38$ kcal/mole. The energy released by this oxidation-reduction step is far less than that required for formation of a high energy phosphate bond of ATP. In contrast, about −17.5 kcal are available from the oxidation of NADH by CoQ.

Although iron deficiency anemia is characterized by decreased levels of hemoglobin and other iron-containing proteins in the blood, the iron-containing cytochromes and Fe-S centers of the electron transport chain are affected as well. Fatigue in iron deficiency anemia, in patients such as **Priscilla Twigg** (see Chapters 14 and 15), results in part from the lack of electron transport for ATP production.

Intravenous nitroprusside rapidly lowers elevated blood pressure through its direct vasodilating action. Fortunately, it was only required in **Cora Nari's** case for several hours. During prolonged infusions of 24–48 hours or more, nitroprusside is converted to cyanide, an inhibitor of the cytochrome oxidase complex. Because small amounts of cyanide are detoxified in the liver by conversion to thiocyanate, which is excreted in the urine, the conversion of nitroprusside to cyanide can be monitored by following blood thiocyanate levels.

Cyanide has been used for years to commit murder, and is used in gas chambers to enact the death penalty. In acid solution the gas, HCN, is volatile and readily absorbed through the lungs. Cyanide is also deadly when ingested, and the oral LD_{50} is only 50 mg. Cyanoglycosides are present in high concentrations in the pits of fruits like apricots, cherries, and peaches. When the pit is broken, enzymes hydrolyze the glycosidic bond and release a cyanide-containing benzaldehyde derivative which spontaneously releases cyanide. The cyanoglycoside derivative laetrile was used for treating cancer on the basis that it would preferentially destroy ATP production by cells which had high ATP requirements for rapid proliferation. It was never approved for use in the U.S., but several accidental deaths resulted from the illegally obtained drug.

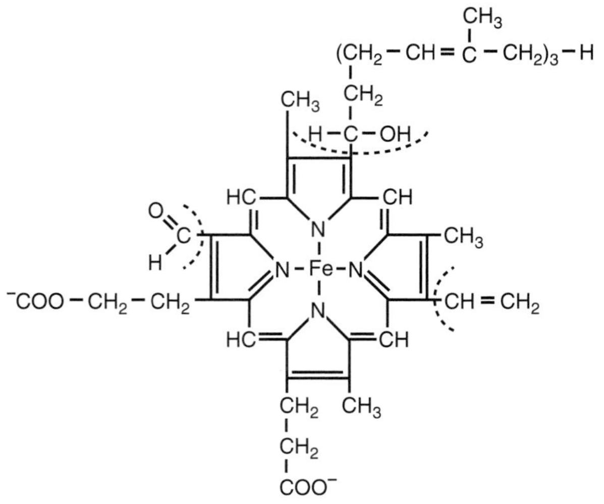

Fig. 20.10. Heme A. Heme A is found in cytochromes a and a_3. Cytochromes are proteins containing a heme chelated with an iron atom. Hemes are derivatives of protoporphyrin IX. Each cytochrome has different modifications of the side chains (indicated with dashed lines), resulting in a slightly different reduction potential and, consequently, a different position in the sequence of electron transfer.

The cytochrome oxidase complex is the site of cyanide inhibition. Cyanide (—C—N) is highly toxic in the human. It binds to the Fe^{3+} in the heme of the cytochrome oxidase complex and prevents transfer of the electrons to O_2. Cytochrome oxidase is also the site of CO (carbon monoxide) poisoning.

Proton Pumps

The mechanisms for the transmembrane "pumping" of protons by the span of the electron transport chain between NADH and CoQ (NADH dehydrogenase) and between CoQ and cytochrome c (cytochrome b-c_1 complex) are called Q cycles. In these cycles CoQ picks up electrons from a component of the electron transport chain, and picks up protons from the matrix side of the membrane. The protons are delivered to the opposite side of the membrane, together with an electron which is accepted by an electron transport chain component located on the cytosolic side of the membrane. Proton pumping by the b-c_1 complex involves a double cycle of CoQ reduction and oxidation. In each cycle, CoQ accepts 2 protons at the matrix side together with 2 electrons; it then releases protons into the intermembrane space while donating one electron back to another component of the cytochrome b-c_1 complex and one to cytochrome c. The mechanism for coupling transmembrane proton movement to transfer of protons through the third complex, cytochrome oxidase, may involve one of the Cu^{2+} ions. The overall stoichiometry is that transfer of 2 electrons through each of the complexes pumps about 4 protons.

Importance of Uninterrupted and Sequential Transfer

In the cell, electron flow in the electron transport chain must be sequential from NADH or a flavoprotein all the way to O_2 to generate ATP. Even though there are three spans of the electron transport chain which pump protons, and each of these complexes is associated with the generation of one ATP, the three complexes do not function independently in the body. Blocking the chain at any point prevents the formation of any ATP. This is because the pumping of protons is associated with the movement of electrons from one carrier to the next. If the movement is blocked any-where in the chain, the carriers on the oxidized side of the block have no source of electrons, and the carriers on the reduced side of the block have nowhere to donate their electrons. For example, Antimycin A, an inhibitor of the cytochrome b-c_1 complex can inhibit all of ATP generation from oxidative phosphorylation (see Table 20.1). Electrons that enter from NADH cannot be passed to CoQ, because CoQ already has the electrons it could not pass on to the b-c_1 complex. Physiologically, the only acceptor for electrons in the electron transport chain is O_2.

COUPLING OF ELECTRON TRANSPORT AND ATP SYNTHESIS

Regulation

The rate of ATP synthesis is tightly coordinated with the rate of ATP utilization, and the rate of ATP synthesis regulates the rate of electron flow. The coupling is accomplished through the proton gradient. As ATP chemical bond energy is utilized by energy-requiring reactions, ADP, PO_4^{2-} and heat are produced. The substrate concentrations for ATP synthase have increased, and the product concentration has decreased, favoring ATP synthesis. As a consequence of proton utilization for ATP synthesis, more protons enter through the ATP-synthase channel. The entry of protons from the cytosolic side relieves the proton "back-pressure" on the electron transport chain (i.e., as energy in the transmembrane electrochemical potential is utilized, more is generated). Since the electron flow must be accompanied by the pumping of protons, the flow of electrons from NADH or FAD(2H) to O_2 is accelerated to maintain the proton gradient. The increased reoxidation of NADH in the electron transport chain and the increased concentration of ADP stimulate oxidative pathways such as the TCA cycle. ATP synthase may also be directly activated under certain conditions by ADP binding or by activator proteins (Fig. 20.11).

The system is poised to maintain very high levels of ATP at all times. In most tissues, the rate of ATP utilization is nearly constant over time. However, in skeletal muscles the rates of hydrolysis change dramatically as the muscle goes from rest to rapid contraction. Even under these circumstances ATP concentration decreases by only about 20% because it is so rapidly regenerated. The electron transport chain has a very high capacity, and can respond very rapidly to any increase in ATP utilization.

Uncoupling ATP Synthesis from Electron Transport

If the proton gradient across the mitochondrial membrane is dissipated, the ability of ATP and ADP concentrations to control the rate of electron transport is lost. This loss is referred to as "uncoupling" oxidative phosphorylation. It occurs with chemical compounds, known as uncouplers, and it occurs physiologically in brown adipose tissue.

CHEMICAL UNCOUPLERS

Chemical uncouplers, also known as proton ionophores, rapidly transport protons from the cytosolic to the matrix side of the inner mitochondrial membrane. They are lipid soluble and have an acidic group which has a pK_a near 7.2. Since the proton concentration is higher in the intermembrane space than in the matrix, uncouplers pick up protons on the cytosolic side of the membrane. Their lipid solubility enables them to diffuse through the inner mitochondrial membrane carrying protons, and release the protons on the matrix side. At high enough concentrations, they can bring protons back into the mitochondrial matrix as rapidly as they are pumped out by the electron transport chain. The rapid influx of protons prevents the formation of an electro-

On physical examination, **Arlyn Foma** was found to have a rapid heart rate, increased respirations, fluid in the air spaces of his lungs (causing a sound called rales during inspiration), and swelling of his lower extremities. A diagnosis of biventricular heart failure was made. The most likely cause for decompensation of Arlyn's cardiac muscle is the dose-related cardiotoxic effect of long term doxorubicin (adriamycin) therapy.

Anthracyclines, such as doxorubicin, are highly effective anticancer agents against a wide variety of human tumors. The clinical use of doxorubicin is limited by a specific, cumulative, dose-dependent cardiotoxicity. It has been suggested that impairment of mitochondrial function plays a major role in this toxicity. The hearts of experimental animals treated with doxorubicin have decreased ATP levels, and the mitochondria are mildly swollen. Doxorubicin binds to cardiolipin, a lipid component of the inner membrane of heart mitochondria, where it might directly affect components of oxidative phosphorylation. It inhibits succinate oxidation, inactivates cytochrome oxidase, interacts with CoQ, affects the ion pumps and inhibits ATP synthase. It decreases the ability of the mitochondria to sequester Ca^{2+}. It forms free radicals (highly reactive single electron forms) which may damage the mitochondrial membrane (see Chapter 21). It might also affect heart function indirectly via prostaglandins or histamine.

In addition to its effects on transcription of genes for enzymes involved in energy metabolism, thyroid hormone also influences bioenergetics through its poorly delineated but potent actions on mitochondrial oxidative phosphorylation. In hyperthyroidism, the efficiency with which energy is derived from the oxidation of these fuels is significantly less than normal. The precise mechanisms that lead to this putative "uncoupling" of oxidative phosphorylation by thyroid hormone excess are poorly understood. The net result, however, is a marked increase in heat production which causes patients with hyperthyroidism, such as **Ahot Goyta**, to complain of constantly feeling hot and sweaty.

Q 20.2: How does exercise generate heat?

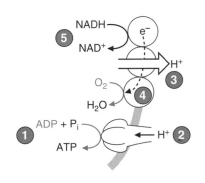

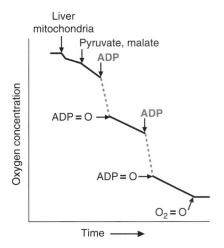

Fig. 20.11. Rate of oxygen consumption is controlled by the concentration of ADP, or by the phosphate potential ($[ATP]/[ADP][P_i]$). Isolated mitochondria are incubated in a closed chamber with an isosmotic phosphate buffer, pyruvate, and malate. Once ADP is added, the oxygen concentration rapidly falls until the ADP has been converted to ATP and its concentration is near 0. The upper diagram shows the sequence of events. **1.** ADP is phosphorylated to ATP. **2.** The phosphorylation pulls protons through ATP synthase into the matrix. **3.** The use of protons from the cytosolic side for ATP synthesis decreases the proton gradient. **4.** As a result, the electron transport chain pumps more protons and oxygen is reduced to H_2O thereby decreasing the oxygen concentration in the chamber. **5.** As NADH donates electrons to the electron transport chain, NAD^+ is regenerated and returns to the TCA cycle.

chemical potential across the inner mitochondrial membrane. As a consequence, the mitochondria are unable to synthesize ATP, and the oxidation of NADH and FAD(2H) is extremely rapid. The energy is lost as heat (Fig. 20.12).

BROWN ADIPOSE TISSUE AND THERMOGENESIS

In brown adipose tissue, the naturally occurring protein uncoupler thermogenin is used to activate heat production in response to norepinephrine (Fig. 20.13). In the presence of cold or other stimuli, norepinephrine is released from sympathetic nerve endings. In brown fat cells, norepinephrine activates a lipase which releases fatty acids to provide a fuel for oxidation. Norepinephrine also stimulates GTP hydrolysis. The GDP which is formed activates thermogenin, a protein which spans the inner mitochondrial membrane. Thermogenin transports protons back into the mitochondrion. The tissue thus becomes partially "uncoupled" and generates additional heat from the oxidation of NADH and FAD(2H) by the electron transport chain.

Although human infants have large brown fat deposits around vital organs (Fig. 20.14), most adult humans have only very small amounts of brown adipose tissue. It is thought that certain individuals or genetically predisposed groups might have larger amounts. Brown adipose tissue can also be stimulated by overeating, and uncoupling of brown adipose tissue may convey an ability to eat greater than average amounts of food without weight gain. In contrast to humans, hibernating mammals maintain relatively large amounts of brown adipose tissue on their shoulders, which they use to generate heat when they are physically inactive.

TRANSPORT OF IONS THROUGH THE INNER MITOCHONDRIAL MEMBRANE

The process of oxidative phosphorylation depends upon the continuous transport of anions such as ADP, PO_4^{2-}, and pyruvate across the inner mitochondrial membrane (Fig. 20.15). Compounds that contain negative or positive charges cannot readily diffuse through a plasma membrane, and are transported by proteins called translocases which balance charge during the transport process. This exchange transport is a form of active transport which utilizes some of the energy from the electrochemical potential.

The translocases are either symports or antiports. ATP-ADP translocase is an example of a transport protein which is an antiport; it balances charge by exchanging an anion on one side of the membrane for an anion of similar charge on the opposite side of the membrane. ATP formed in the mitochondrial matrix is translocated to the cytosol in exchange for ADP produced by energy-requiring reactions. Because ATP contains four negative charges and ADP only 3, the exchange is promoted by the positive charge on the outside of the inner mitochondrial membrane, and by the proton gradient. Pyruvate, in contrast, is transported together with a proton to balance the charge. This type of translocase is called a symport. Because one of the cytosolic protons is used to bring pyruvate into the mitochondrial matrix, this transport system also requires energy. Specific energy-requiring transport proteins also exist for Ca^{2+} and other compounds which must enter the mitochondrial matrix.

MAINTENANCE OF ATP LEVELS IN THE HEART

Cardiac muscle, because of its high ATP demand, has a higher content of mitochondria than most tissues. The densely packed cristae of heart mitochondria contain a high content of electron transport chain proteins, ATP synthase, ATP-ADP translocase, enzymes of the TCA cycle, and other components of energy metabolism (Fig. 20.16).

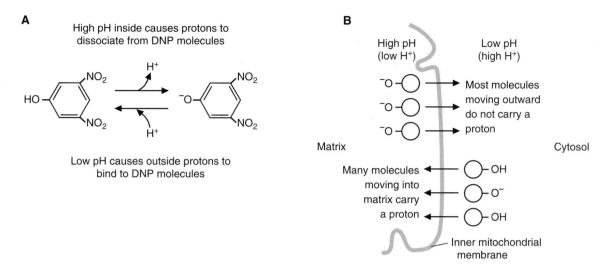

Fig. 20.12. Chemical uncouplers are proton ionophores which equilibrate the pH across the inner mitochondrial membrane. **A.** Dinitrophenol (DNP) has a dissociable proton with a pK_a near 7.2. **B.** On the cytosolic side of the inner mitochondrial membrane, the pH is low ([H$^+$] is high), and DNP picks up a proton which it carries across the membrane. At the lower proton concentration of the matrix, the H$^+$ dissociates.

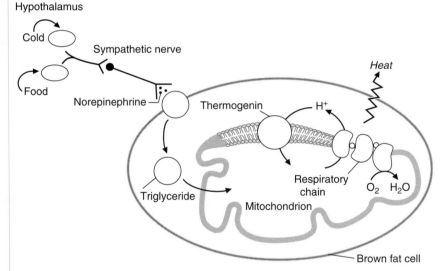

Fig. 20.13. Brown fat is a tissue specialized for thermogenesis. Cold or excessive food intake stimulates the release of norepinephrine from the sympathetic nerve endings. As a result, a lipase is activated which releases fatty acids for oxidation. The proton conductance protein, thermogenin, is activated, and protons are brought into the matrix. This stimulates the electron transport chain, which increases its rate of NADH and FAD(2H) oxidation and produces more heat.

Salicylate, which is a degradation product of aspirin in the human, is lipid soluble and has a dissociable proton. In high concentrations, as in salicylate poisoning, salicylate is able to partially uncouple mitochondria. The decline of ATP concentration in the cell and consequent increase of AMP in the cytosol stimulate glycolysis. The overstimulation of the glycolytic pathway (see Chapter 22) results in increased levels of lactic acid in the blood and a metabolic acidosis. Fortunately, **Dennis Livermore** did not develop this consequence of aspirin poisoning (see Chapter 4).

20.2: During exercise, the rate of ATP hydrolysis is increased. As a consequence of the increased rate of ATP synthesis by ATP synthase, protons enter the matrix, and the electron transport chain is stimulated. Oxygen consumption increases, as does the amount of energy lost as heat by the electron transport chain. The stimulation of the electron transport chain from uncoupling oxidative phosphorylation and the electron transport chain also increases O$_2$ consumption and produces heat, but no ATP is generated.

Q 20.3: Investigators reported finding antibodies against cardiac ATP-ADP translocase in an individual who died from a viral cardiomyopathy. How could these antibodies result in death?

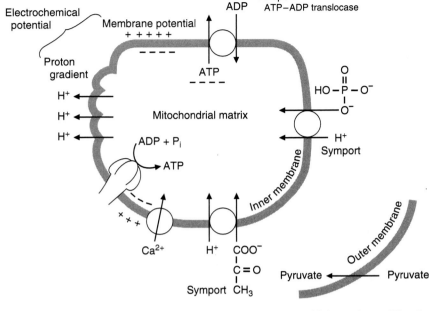

Fig. 20.15. Transport of compounds across the inner mitochondrial membrane. The electrochemical potential gradient drives the transport of charged compounds. The antiport ATP-ADP translocase exchanges an ATP for an ADP. Phosphate enters together with a proton on a symport translocator. Pyruvate is also transported into the matrix on a symporter. One of the transporters for Ca^{2+} is driven by the membrane potential. Pyruvate and other compounds can diffuse through the outer mitochondrial membrane.

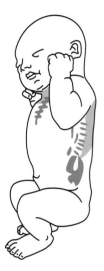

Fig. 20.14. Brown adipose tissue is present in infants along the neck, the breastplate, between the scapulae, and around the kidneys. It serves an important function in babies, who have little control over their environment and kick their blankets off in the middle of the night. From Dawkins MJR, Hull D. Sci Am 1965;213:63.

Cardiac tissue also contains a high content of creatine kinase, the enzyme which transfers the high energy phosphate bond of ATP to creatine (Fig. 20.17). The role of creatine phosphate in heart (as well as brain and skeletal) muscle is that of an energy buffer and an energy shuttle. The mitochondrial creatine kinase isozyme is located on the outside of the inner mitochondrial membrane. Here it rapidly uses ATP for creatine phosphate formation and regenerates ADP at a site near the ATP-ADP translocase. The creatine phosphate and ATP both diffuse to the plasma membrane and the site of ATP utilization by myosin ATPase, Na^+,K^+-ATPase, and other enzymes. At the myofibril, the MB and MM creatine kinase isozymes regenerate ATP (see Chapter 9).

The heart (as well as the brain) is particularly sensitive to the effects of ischemia, anoxia, and a number of compounds which interfere with energy metabolism. The loss of ATP at the cellular membrane results in the influx of ions, such as Na^+ and Ca^{2+}, and swelling of the tissue. Cardiac mitochondria can sequester Ca^{2+}, which in low amounts stimulates the TCA cycle and other reactions in oxidative metabolism. In high amounts, it activates a phospholipase which degrades membrane lipids. The result is swelling of mitochondria and leakage of adenine and nicotinamide nucleotides.

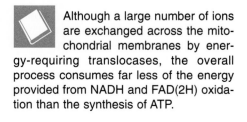

Although a large number of ions are exchanged across the mitochondrial membranes by energy-requiring translocases, the overall process consumes far less of the energy provided from NADH and FAD(2H) oxidation than the synthesis of ATP.

CLINICAL COMMENTS. Thrombolysis stimulated by intravenous recombinant tissue plasminogen activator (TPA) successfully decreased the extent of ischemic damage to **Cora Nari's** heart muscle. The rationale for the use of TPA within 4–6 hours after the onset of a myocardial infarction relates to the function of the normal intrinsic fibrinolytic system (see Chapter 9). This system is designed to dissolve unwanted intravascular clots through the action of the enzyme

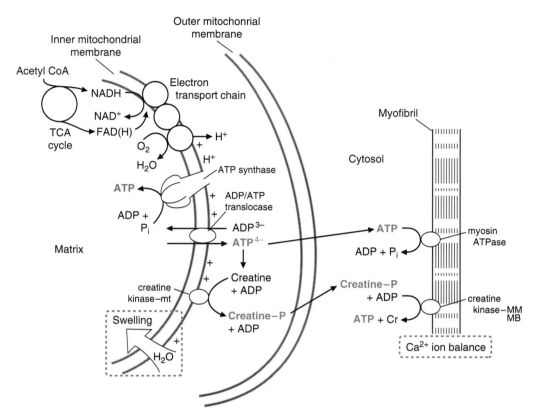

Fig. 20.16. Energy metabolism in the heart. A high rate of ATP utilization for muscular contraction requires a high rate of oxidative metabolism, ATP synthesis, and ATP transport. The transfer of high energy phosphate compounds is shown in blue. During a myocardial infarction, ATP levels cannot be maintained and there is an increase of Ca^{2+}.

Although small increases of Ca^{2+} concentration stimulate the TCA cycle, high concentrations result in mitochondrial (mt) swelling and damage (shown in the blue box). MM and MB are isozymes of creatine kinase. M = muscle; B = brain; Cr = creatine.

plasmin, a protease that digests the fibrin matrix within the clot. TPA stimulates the conversion of plasminogen to its active form, plasmin. The result is a lysis of the thrombus and improved blood flow through the previously obstructed vessel, allowing fuels and oxygen to reach the heart cells. The human TPA protein used in Mrs. Nari is produced by recombinant DNA technology (see Chapter 16).

Before the advent of precise and accurate radioimmunoassays to determine the amount of thyroid hormone in the blood, a "presumptive" diagnosis of the presence of a hypermetabolic state in patients such as **Ahot Goyta** was made using such nonspecific measures of the rate of oxygen utilization as the basal metabolic rate (BMR).

Mr. Goyta could be treated with antithyroid drugs, by subtotal resection of the thyroid gland, or with radioactive iodine. Successful treatment normalizes thyroid hormone secretion, and all of the signs, symptoms, and metabolic alterations of hyperthyroidism quickly subside.

Because **Arlyn Foma** was suffering from cardiotoxicity related to long term treatment with doxorubicin, this drug was discontinued and appropriate therapy for heart failure was initiated. He was advised to return for regular check-ups to determine whether his symptoms of heart failure subsided and to determine the effect of discontinuing this drug on the course of his lymphoma.

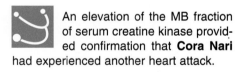 An elevation of the MB fraction of serum creatine kinase provided confirmation that **Cora Nari** had experienced another heart attack.

A 20.3: As ATP is hydrolyzed during muscular contraction, ADP is formed. This ADP must exchange into the mitochondria on ATP-ADP translocase to be converted back to ATP. Inhibition of ATP-ADP translocase results in rapid depletion of the cytosol ATP levels and loss of cardiac contractility.

Q 20.4: A decreased activity of the electron transport chain can result from inhibitors as well as from mutations in mtDNA and nuclear DNA. Why does an impairment of the electron transport chain result in lactic acidosis?

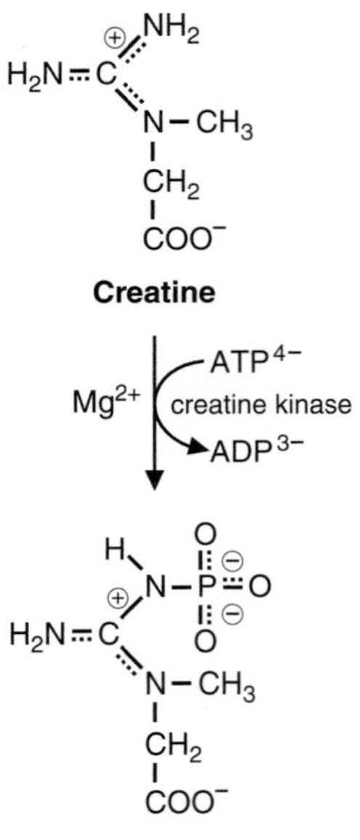

BIOCHEMICAL COMMENTS. OXPHOS Diseases. Clinical diseases involving components of oxidative phosphorylation (referred to as OXPHOS diseases) are among the most commonly encountered degenerative diseases. Although the clinical pathology may be caused by gene mutations in either mitochondrial DNA (mtDNA) or nuclear DNA, to date most of the defects have been identified as deletions, duplications, or point mutations in mtDNA. The mtDNA encodes seven subunits of the electron transport chain Complex I (NADH dehydrogenase complex), one subunit of Complex III (cytochrome b-c_1 complex), three subunits of Complex IV (cytochrome oxidase), and two subunits of the ATP synthase complex (Fig. 20.18). In addition, mtDNA encodes the necessary components for its translation—a large and small rRNA gene and 22 tRNAs. In contrast, nuclear DNA encodes over 70 subunits of proteins involved in oxidative phosphorylation.

OXPHOS Diseases Caused by Mutations in Mitochondrial DNA. The genetics of mutations in mtDNA are defined by maternal inheritance, replicative segregation, threshold expression, a high mtDNA mutation rate, and the accumulation of somatic mutations with age. Mutations in mtDNA are maternally inherited because almost all of the mitochondrial genes in the zygote are contributed by the ovum. Usually, some mitochondria are present with the mutant mtDNA and some with wild-type DNA. The mitotic and meiotic segregation of the heteroplasmic (mutant and wild-type) mtDNA mutation results in variable oxidative phosphorylation deficiencies between patients with the same mutation, and even among a patient's own tissues. The disease pathology usually becomes worse with age because a small amount of normal mitochondria might confer normal function and exercise capacity while the patient is young. As the patient ages, somatic mutations in mtDNA accumulate from the generation of free radicals within the mitochondria (see Chapter 21). These mutations frequently become permanent because mtDNA does not have access to the same repair mechanisms available for nuclear DNA. Even in normal individuals, somatic mutations result in a decline of oxidative phosphorylation capacity with age. At some stage, the ATP-generating capacity of a tissue falls below the tissue-specific threshold for normal function.

Other Genetic Disorders of Mitochondrial Function. Genetic mutations have also been reported for mitochondrial proteins encoded by nuclear DNA, including each of the enzymes of the TCA cycle, and many of the nuclear encoded subunits of the electron transport chain and the ATP synthase complex. These mutations do not show a pattern of maternal inheritance. In general, symptoms of these defects would appear in one or more of the tissues with the highest ATP demands: nervous tissue, heart, skeletal muscle, and kidney.

Creatine

Mg^{2+} | ATP^{4-}
creatine kinase
→ ADP^{3-}

Creatine phosphate

Fig. 20.17. Creatine phosphate has a high energy phosphate bond which allows it to serve as an energy buffer in brain, skeletal muscle, and the heart. The negative $\Delta G^{0\prime}$ of hydrolysis arises from the resonance stabilization of creatine and the phosphate anion. This high energy phosphate is transferred into and from ATP by creatine kinase. When ATP is rapidly utilized during muscular contraction or some other ATP-requiring process, there is a net transfer of high energy phosphate from creatine phosphate to ADP to form ATP. As the ATP levels return to resting levels, creatine phosphate is regenerated.

Suggested Readings

Boyer PD. A perspective of the binding change mechanism for ATP synthesis. FASEB J 1989;3:2164–2178.

Brown GC. Control of respiration and ATP synthesis in mammalian mitochondria and cells. Biochem J 1992;284:1–11.

Carafoli E. Mitochondrial pathology: an overview. Ann NY Acad Sci 1986;488:1–18.

Lactic acidosis and mitochondrial myopathy in a young woman. Nutr Rev 1988;46:157–163.

Lander ES, Lodish H. Mitochondrial diseases: gene mapping and gene therapy. Cell 1990;61:925–926.

Muhammed H, Ramasarma T. Inhibition of mitochondrial oxidative phosphorylation by adriamycin. Biochim Biophys Acta 1982;722:43–50.

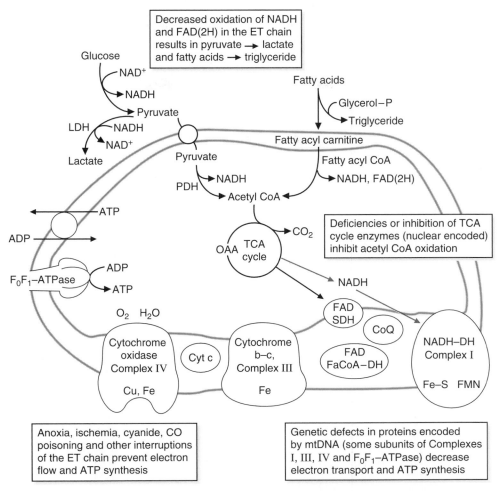

Fig. 20.18. Dysfunctional mitochondria. Genetic deficiencies or other problems in oxidative metabolism result in accumulation of lactate in the blood, and incorporation of fatty acids into triglycerides (triacylglycerols). ET = electron transport.

Olson RD, Mushlin PS. Doxorubicin cardiotoxicity: analysis of prevailing hypotheses. FASEB J 1990;4:3076–3086.

Pedersen PL, Amzel LM. ATP synthases. J Biol Chem 1993;268:9937–9940.

Shaffner JM, Wallace DC. Oxidative phosphorylation diseases. In: Scriver C, Beaudet AL, Sly WS, Valle D (eds): The metabolic and molecular bases of inherited disease. Vol I. 7th ed. New York: McGraw-Hill, 1995:1535–1609.

PROBLEMS

1. Rotenone, an inhibitor of NADH dehydrogenase, was originally used for fishing. When it was sprinkled on a lake, fish would absorb it through their gills and die. It is currently being used in the U.S. as an organic pesticide and is frequently recommended for tomato plants. It is considered nontoxic to mammals and birds, who cannot readily absorb it. What effect would rotenone have on ATP production by heart mitochondria, if it could be absorbed?

2. J.S. was born after a 34-week gestation period. In the first 24 hours of life, he developed respiratory distress. At 3 weeks, he became dependent on a ventilator, which he required for the rest of his life. By 6 weeks, he had developed neurological

A 20.4: The effect of inhibition of electron transport is an impaired oxidation of pyruvate, fatty acids, and other fuels (see Fig. 20.18). In many cases, the inhibition of mitochondrial electron transport results in higher than normal levels of lactate and pyruvate in the blood and an increased lactate/pyruvate ratio. NADH oxidation requires the completed transfer of electrons from NADH to O_2, and a defect anywhere along the chain will result in the accumulation of NADH and decrease of NAD^+. The increase in $NADH/NAD^+$ inhibits pyruvate dehydrogenase and causes the accumulation of pyruvate. It also increases the conversion of pyruvate to lactate, and elevated levels of lactate appear in the blood. A large number of genetic defects of the proteins in respiratory chain complexes have, therefore, been classified together as "congenital lactic acidosis."

A patient experienced spontaneous muscle jerking (myoclonus) in her mid-teens, and her condition progressed over 10 years to include debilitating myoclonus, mitochondrial myopathy with ragged-red fibers and abnormal mitochondria, neurosensory hearing loss, dementia, hypoventilation, and mild cardiomyopathy. Energy metabolism was affected in the central nervous system, heart, and skeletal muscle, resulting in lactic acidosis. The symptoms of the patient are those of myoclonic epileptic ragged red fiber disease (MERRF). The affected tissues (central nervous system and muscle) are two of the tissues with the highest ATP requirements.

A history revealed that the patient's mother, her grandmother, and two maternal aunts had symptoms involving either nervous or muscular tissue (clearly a case of maternal inheritance). However, no other relative had identical symptoms.

Most of the cases of MERRF are caused by a point mutation in mitochondrial tRNA^{Lys} (mtRNA^{Lys}). The symptoms are similar to those of mitochondrial encephalomyopathy, lactic acidosis, and stroke-like episodes (MELAS), which is also caused by a point mutation in a gene for mtRNA. A mutation in a mtRNA would have a generalized effect on the formation of complexes in the electron transport chain and of ATP synthase, thus decreasing the ability of the tissue to generate ATP. In cases of MERRF, mitochondria can be obtained from the patient by muscle biopsy. The mitochondria are enlarged and show abnormal patterns of cristae. The muscle tissue also shows ragged red fibers.

problems. A heart murmur was observed, and tests revealed a cardiomyopathy. Between 5 and 16 weeks, he developed progressive lacticacidemia (an increased ratio of lactate to pyruvate in the blood) and an elevation of serum pyruvate. The lacticacidemia persisted until the child died of cardiopulmonary arrest at 16 weeks of age.

Tests performed on the infant showed normal levels of glycolytic and gluconeogenic enzymes. Pyruvate dehydrogenase activity was also normal.

After the infant's death, mitochondria were prepared from his heart. The rate of oxygen consumption by these mitochondria was measured with succinate as a substrate. It was normal, both in the presence and absence of ADP. When the mitochondria were incubated with pyruvate plus malate, however, the rate of oxygen consumption was extremely low. It was still far below normal when ADP was added. Electron paramagnetic resonance (EPR) measurements showed a lower than normal content of iron, and were able to pinpoint the complex and type of iron involved.

Determine whether each of the statements below is true (T) or false (F).

1. The muscle weakness and neurological problems could be explained by an inability to generate ATP from pyruvate oxidation.
2. The infant did not have a problem with pyruvate metabolism because the levels of the major enzymes of pyruvate metabolism were normal.
3. The data obtained with isolated mitochondria rule out a genetic defect that inactivates a key protein in the b-c_1 complex.
4. The data obtained with isolated mitochondria suggest that the patient has an inability to transfer electrons from NADH to CoQ.
5. The data obtained with isolated mitochondria suggest that the mitochondria are uncoupled.
6. The most likely site of the defect was an Fe-S center in Complex I (NADH dehydrogenase complex) in the electron transport chain.
7. The most likely site of the defect was an Fe-cytochrome protein in the NADH dehydrogenase complex.

ANSWERS

1. Because rotenone inhibits the oxidation of NADH, it would completely block the generation of the electrochemical potential gradient in vivo and, therefore, it would block ATP generation. In the presence of rotenone, NADH would accumulate, and NAD$^+$ concentrations would decrease, Although the mitochondria might still be able to oxidize compounds like succinate, which transfer electrons to FAD, no succinate would be produced in vivo if the NAD$^+$-dependent dehydrogenases of the TCA cycle were inhibited.

2. (1)T; (2)F; (3)T; (4)T; (5)F; (6)T; (7)F.

Succinate was oxidized normally by mitochondria isolated from the infant's heart, but pyruvate was not. Therefore, the problem was not between succinate and the end of the electron transport chain, but in the NADH dehydrogenase complex (Complex I). Because the iron content of his mitochondria was low, the problem was most likely in an Fe-S center in Complex I. (This complex does not contain a cytochrome.) The problem in Complex I caused NADH/NAD$^+$ to increase, which resulted in an inhibition of pyruvate dehydrogenase, the accumulation of pyruvate, and its conversion to lactate. Consequently, the levels of pyruvate and lactate increased in the blood.

21   Oxygen Metabolism and Oxygen Toxicity

The electron transport chain accounts for over 90% of our total oxygen consumption, and all the other oxygen-requiring reactions in the body account for only 5–10%. In the electron transport chain, O_2 accepts electrons from NADH and FAD(2H) which are derived from the oxidation of fuels. In this pathway, the powerful oxidizing power of the oxygen molecule is ultimately converted into the high energy phosphate bond of ATP. The remainder of the oxygen we consume is utilized by other oxidases (enzymes that reduce oxygen to water or hydrogen peroxide) and by oxygenases (enzymes that directly incorporate oxygen into the molecules being oxidized). Although these latter oxidations are not coupled to the generation of ATP, they are important for specific metabolic pathways, such as the catabolism of amino acids, the detoxification of drugs, and the synthesis of steroid hormones.

As a result of the electronic structure of oxygen, both the physiological oxidation reactions and the toxicological reactions of oxygen occur through single electron transfers. Molecular oxygen (O_2 or dioxygen) has two unpaired electrons with parallel spin states (Fig. 21.1). The antibonding parallel spins prevent C—H organisms, such as humans, from spontaneously igniting in an O_2 atmosphere. Instead, oxidation can occur by the transfer of single electrons to O_2 via enzymes containing transition metals (e.g., Fe^{2+} and Cu^+ in cytochrome oxidase). However, another consequence of the biradical nature of O_2 is that O_2 has a tendency to form highly reactive oxygen species (ROS) which can initiate free radical (single electron) chain reactions and damage cellular components.

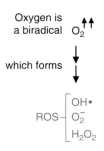

Fig. 21.1. O_2 is a biradical. It has a tendency to form toxic reactive oxygen species (ROS), such as the hydroxyl radical ($OH^\bullet$), superoxide (O_2^-), and hydrogen peroxide (H_2O_2). It has 2 antibonding electrons with parallel spins, denoted by the parallel arrows.

Oxygen radicals and their derivatives can be deadly to cells. The hydroxyl radical causes oxidative damage to proteins, DNA, membrane lipids containing polyunsaturated bonds, and other cellular components. In some cases, oxygen free radicals are the direct cause of a disease state (e.g., tissue damage initiated by exposure to ionizing radiation). In other cases, such as rheumatoid arthritis, ROS may perpetuate the cellular damage caused by another process. Granulomatous cells such as macrophages and neutrophils use ROS to destroy foreign organisms during phagocytosis.

Cells have a number of mechanisms to protect themselves against damage from the naturally occurring continuous generation of ROS. Superoxide dismutase (SOD) removes the superoxide free radical and catalase and glutathione peroxidase remove hydrogen peroxide and lipid peroxides. Vitamins E and C act as antioxidants. Cells are also protected by compartmentalization of the processes which result in generation of highly reactive oxygen species. Oxidative stress occurs when the rate at which the ROS are generated exceeds the capacity of the cell for their removal (Fig. 21.2).

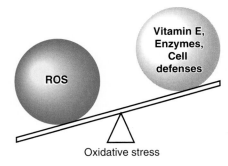

Fig. 21.2. Oxidative stress. Oxidative stress occurs when ROS are produced faster than they can be removed by the cellular defense mechanisms. These defense mechanisms include a number of enzymes and antioxidant vitamins, such as vitamin E.

 Two years ago, **Les Dopaman**, a 62-year-old male, noted an increasing tremor of his right hand when sitting quietly. The tremor disappeared if he actively used this hand to do purposeful movement. As this symptom progressed, he also complained of stiffness in his muscles which slowed his movements. His wife noticed a change in his gait; he had begun taking short, shuffling steps and leaned forward as he walked. He often appeared to be staring ahead with a rather immobile facial expression. She noted a tremor of his eyelids when he was asleep and, recently, a tremor of his legs when he was at rest. Because of these progressive symptoms and some subtle personality changes (anxiety and emotional lability), she convinced Les to see their family doctor.

The physician recognized the signs and symptoms of a relatively early movement disorder probably caused by neuronal loss in the basal ganglia. Since Mr. Dopaman's medical history and physical examination did not suggest any of the secondary causes of dysfunction of these brainstem nuclei (e.g., postencephalitic destruction, drug toxicity, cerebrovascular accident, trauma), the doctor concluded that the patient probably had "primary" or "idiopathic" parkinsonism, i.e., Parkinson's disease, and referred Mr. Dopaman to a neurologist.

 Cora Nari had done well since the successful lysis of blood clots in her coronary arteries with the use of intravenous recombinant tissue plasminogen activator (TPA). This therapy had quickly relieved the crushing chest pain (angina) she experienced after she was attacked by her neighbor's dog. At her first office visit to her cardiologist following her discharge from the hospital, Cora was told that she had developed multiple premature contractions of the ventricular muscle of her heart as the clots in her coronary arteries were being lysed. At times, these premature beats occurred in "runs" of 7 or 8 in a row. This process could have led to a life-threatening arrhythmia known as ventricular fibrillation, a condition in which these rapid, premature beats occur at a very rapid rate, compromising cardiac output and eventually causing death. However, Cora's arrhythmia responded quickly to pharmacological suppression and did not recur during the remainder of her hospitalization. The doctor explained that the arrhythmia could have simply resulted from severe ischemia (lack of blood flow) in her heart muscle caused by vascular obstruction from clots at the site of atherosclerotic coronary plaques. However, because the rapid beats began during the infusion of TPA, they were more likely the result of reperfusion of a previously ischemic area of her heart's ventricular muscle with oxygenated blood as the clot was lysed. This phenomenon is known as ischemia-reperfusion injury. Reperfusion injury is believed to be caused by the generation of cytotoxic ROS derived from molecular oxygen in the blood which reperfuses previously hypoxic cells.

PROPERTIES OF O₂ AND ROS

Oxygen is both necessary to human life and toxic. The electronic structure of oxygen (O_2, dioxygen) is responsible for this paradox because it favors the reduction of oxygen in single electron steps. This stepwise reduction slows the direct combination of oxygen with organic compounds (spontaneous combustion) and allows the cell to oxidize fuels through the action of dehydrogenases, which eventually couple the reducing power of oxygen to ATP generation in the electron transport chain. On the other hand, the structure of oxygen also results in the generation of oxygen radicals and other ROS which are capable of causing cell injury (Fig. 21.3). The role of oxygen in cell injury is reflected in events that occur during ischemia (a condition caused by a decreased supply of oxygen that diminishes ATP production), and in other conditions that increase the conversion of oxygen to ROS.

Oxygen and the Spin Restriction

The characteristic of O_2 which is responsible for the evolutionary development of life in an oxygen-rich environment is its two unpaired electrons with parallel spins.

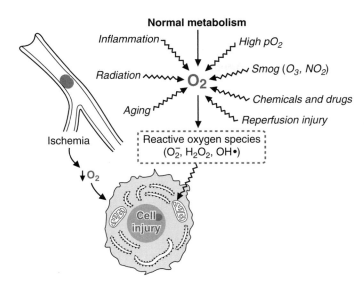

Normal metabolism

A radical, by definition, is an atom that has an unpaired electron in an outer orbital. It is highly reactive, and can initiate chain reactions by extracting an electron from a neighboring molecule to complete its own orbital. In contrast, the transition metals such as Fe, Cu, and Mo are more stable and are not considered free radicals.

O_2 is really a biradical; it has two unpaired electrons. Because the 2 electrons have parallel spins, they cannot form a thermodynamically stable pair, and reside in separate orbitals.

Fig. 21.3. Role of oxygen in cell injury. O_2 is necessary for the generation of ATP from oxidative phosphorylation, but it is also toxic. Normal oxygen metabolism continuously converts O_2 to ROS, which can cause cell injury. Various stimuli, such as radiation, inflammation, aging, and a higher than normal partial pressure of O_2 (pO_2), increase the formation of ROS. Ozone (O_3) and nitrous oxide (NO_2) are air pollutants that form free radicals in the cells of the lungs, resulting in pulmonary emphysema and pulmonary fibrosis. A lack of O_2 due to decreased blood flow from a clot (ischemia) also causes cell injury. The reintroduction of oxygen (reperfusion) enhances cellular injury due to ROS. Modified from Cotran RS, Robbins SL, Kumar V. Robbins pathologic basis of disease. Philadelphia:WB Saunders, 1994:5.

Typical organic molecules that serve as substrates for oxidation (such as the —CH—OH portion of malate or isocitrate) contain no unpaired electrons; their bonds are in the stable form of 2 electrons with antiparallel spins. For O_2 to accept a pair of electrons from a substrate, one of the electrons on O_2 or one of the electrons from the incoming pair on the substrate would have to spin invert. There is a large thermodynamic barrier to spin inversion, and it would have to occur through a multistep process with a high activation energy. The kinetic barrier resulting from this spin restriction slows down direct oxidation of —C—H bonds in organic molecules and deters the spontaneous combustion of fuels.

One-electron reductions of O_2 are not subject to the kinetic barrier imposed by spin restriction, and occur in the presence of one-electron donors. The O_2 molecule, which can accept a total of 4 electrons to be reduced to 2 molecules of H_2O, can be reduced one electron at a time (Fig. 21.4). However, the first step, the formation of superoxide, is not thermodynamically favorable and requires a moderately strong reducing agent which can donate single electrons. Enzymes that catalyze the reduction of oxygen, such as cytochrome oxidase in the electron transport chain, must have mechanisms that get around the spin restriction and/or the energy requirement of the first electron transfer. In addition, they must have active sites that prevent the interaction of these partially reduced forms of oxygen with other cellular components. Before considering how oxidases and oxygenases function, let us examine some of the consequences of formation of these highly reactive one-electron intermediates of oxygen reduction.

Reactive Oxygen Species

The major oxygen metabolites produced by one-electron reduction of oxygen are ROS: superoxide (O_2^-), the hydroxyl free radical (OH•), and the partially reduced

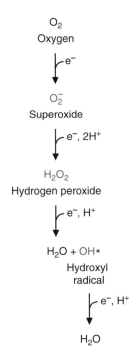

Fig. 21.4. One-electron reduction steps of oxygen. The one-electron reduction steps of O_2 generate superoxide, hydrogen peroxide, and the hydroxyl radical. Superoxide is a free radical, and is sometimes written $O_2^{-•}$. However, superoxide has only one unpaired electron and is, therefore, less of a radical than O_2, which has 2 unpaired electrons. H_2O_2, the half-reduced form of O_2, has accepted 2 electrons and is, therefore, not an oxygen radical. However, it is considered a ROS because it is readily converted to the hydroxyl radical.

The Fenton reaction

$$Fe^{2+}$$
$$+$$
$$\boxed{H_2O_2}$$
$$\downarrow$$
$$Fe^{3+}$$
$$+$$
$$\boxed{OH\bullet}$$
$$+$$
$$OH^-$$

The Haber–Weiss reaction

$$\boxed{O_2^-}$$
$$+$$
$$\boxed{H_2O_2}$$
$$\bigg\downarrow H^+$$
$$O_2$$
$$+$$
$$H_2O$$
$$+$$
$$\boxed{OH\bullet}$$

Fig. 21.5. Generation of the hydroxyl radical by the Fenton and Haber-Weiss reactions. In the simplified versions of these reactions shown here, the transfer of single electrons generates the hydroxyl radical. ROS are shown in blue. Other metals, such as Cu^+, can also serve as single-electron donors in the Fenton reaction.

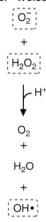 The toxicity of oxygen is related to the production of oxygen free radicals which, through their interaction with lipids, proteins, carbohydrates, and DNA, produce cellular dysfunction. Evidence of free radical damage has been described in over 100 disease states (some of these are listed in Table 21.2). The free radical damage could be the primary cause of the disease, could enhance complications of the disease, or could be the consequence of cell damage caused by other agents.

form of oxygen, hydrogen peroxide (H_2O_2) (Table 21.1). The free radicals are capable of reacting indiscriminately with any molecules with which they come in contact, extracting electrons, and generating new free radicals in cytotoxic oxidative chain reactions. The hydroxyl radical is probably the most potent of the ROS, and the probable initiator of the chain reactions which form lipid peroxides and organic radicals. Hydrogen peroxide, although not actually a radical, is an oxidizing agent and, in the presence of Fe^{2+} or another transition metal, generates the hydroxyl radical by the Fenton reaction (Fig. 21.5). Because hydrogen peroxide is lipid soluble, it can create damage at localized Fe^{2+}-containing membranes far from its site of formation. The superoxide anion, which can be formed from free O_2 by donation of an electron to another free radical, is highly reactive but has limited lipid solubility and cannot diffuse far. However, O_2^- can also generate the more reactive hydroxyl and hydroperoxy radicals by reaction with hydrogen peroxide in the Haber-Weiss reaction. HOCl, or hypochlorous acid, is the major reactive component of household bleach. In the human, it is formed by neutrophils and other granulomatous cells from H_2O_2 during the destruction of foreign organisms in a response called the respiratory burst.

Formation of Lipid and Lipid Peroxy Radicals

The formation of lipid free radicals and lipid peroxides is considered an important feature of the cellular injury brought about by ROS (Fig. 21.6). This type of reaction, termed free radical autoxidation, requires an initiator (such as the hydroxyl radical) to begin the chain reaction. Like the one-electron reduction steps of O_2, free radical auto-oxidation is not subject to the kinetic barriers of spin restriction. Peroxidation usually begins with the extraction of hydrogen atoms containing one electron from conjugated double bonds in fatty acids. The local production of the hydroxyl radical from hydrogen peroxide, mediated by Fe^{2+}, can initiate the chain reaction. It is propagated by the addition of oxygen to form lipid peroxyl radicals and lipid peroxides (see Fig. 21.6). The major fatty acids that undergo lipid peroxidation in the cell membranes are all polyunsaturated fatty acids. Eventually degradation of the lipid occurs, forming such products as malondialdehyde (from fatty acids with three or more double bonds) and ethane and pentane (from the ω-terminal carbons of ω3 and ω6 fatty acids, respectively). Malondialdehyde appears in the blood and urine and is used as an indicator of free radical damage.

Table 21.1. Reactive Oxygen Species

Origin and Characteristics	
O_2^- Superoxide anion	Produced by the electron transport chain and at other sites. Generates other reactive oxygen species, but cannot diffuse far from the site of origin.
H_2O_2 Hydrogen peroxide	Not a free radical, but can generate free radicals by reaction with a transition metal (e.g., Fe^{2+}). Can diffuse into and through cell membranes.
$OH\bullet$ Hydroxyl radical	The most reactive species in attacking biological molecules. Produced by H_2O_2 in the presence of Fe^{2+}.
$R\bullet$ Organic radicals	An organic free radical produced from RH by $OH\bullet$ attack. RH can be the carbon of a double bond in a fatty acid (resulting in $-C^\bullet=C-$) or RSH (resulting in $R-S\bullet$).
$RCOO\bullet$ Organic peroxide radical	An organic peroxide radical, such as occurs during lipid degradation.
HOCl Hypochlorous acid	Produced in bacteria during the respiratory burst to destroy invading organisms.
$O2^{\uparrow\downarrow}$ Singlet oxygen	Oxygen with antiparallel spins. Produced at high oxygen tensions from the absorption of energy. Decays with the release of light.

Table 21.2. Some of the Disease States Associated with Free Radical Injury

Atherogenesis
Emphysema/bronchitis
Parkinson's disease
Duchenne-type muscular dystrophy
Pregnancy/preeclampsia
Cervical cancer
Alcoholic liver disease
Hemodialysis patients
Diabetes
Acute renal failure
Down syndrome
Aging
Retrolental fibroplasia
Cerebrovascular disorders
Ischemia/reperfusion injury

REACTIVE OXYGEN SPECIES AND CELLULAR DAMAGE

Proteins, membrane lipids, carbohydrates, and nucleic acids are subject to cellular damage caused by oxygen radicals (Fig. 21.7). This free radical damage is thought to contribute to the complications of many chronic diseases (see Table 21.2). In proteins, the amino acids proline, histidine, arginine, cysteine, and methionine are particularity susceptible to hydroxyl radical attack and oxidative damage. The oxidation of amino acids in proteins leads to fragmentation of the protein, cross-linking and aggregation, and susceptibility to proteolytic digestion.

Peroxidation of lipid molecules invariably changes or damages lipid molecular structure. In addition to the self-destructive nature of membrane lipid peroxidation, the aldehydes that are formed can cross-link proteins. When the damaged lipids are the constituents of biological membranes, the cohesive lipid bilayer arrangement and structural organization is disrupted (see Fig. 21.7).

Oxygen-derived free radicals are also a major source of DNA damage. Approximately 20 types of oxidatively altered DNA molecules have been identified. The nonspecific binding of Fe^{2+} to DNA facilitates localized production of the hydroxyl radical, which can cause strand breaks and base alterations in the DNA. To some extent, this DNA damage can be repaired by the cell (see Chapter 12).

ENZYME-CATALYZED REACTIONS USING O_2

The enzymes for which oxygen is a substrate must reduce oxygen in a controlled manner without releasing highly reactive free radical intermediates into the surrounding medium. These enzymes utilize metal ions, flavins, and other cofactors to overcome the kinetic barrier imposed by spin restrictions and the energy barrier to the first step in the one-electron reduction pathway. The reactive oxygen intermediates which are formed usually remain tightly bound in the active sites of the enzymes, usually as metallo-oxygen complexes, until the reaction is finished. With a few exceptions, the only ROS that is released during the course of the normal reaction is hydrogen peroxide.

The enzymes which catalyze reactions involving O_2 can be classified as oxidases or oxygenases (Fig. 21.8). The oxidases transfer electrons to O_2, which is reduced to H_2O or H_2O_2. Oxygenases incorporate oxygen into the substrate; monooxygenases

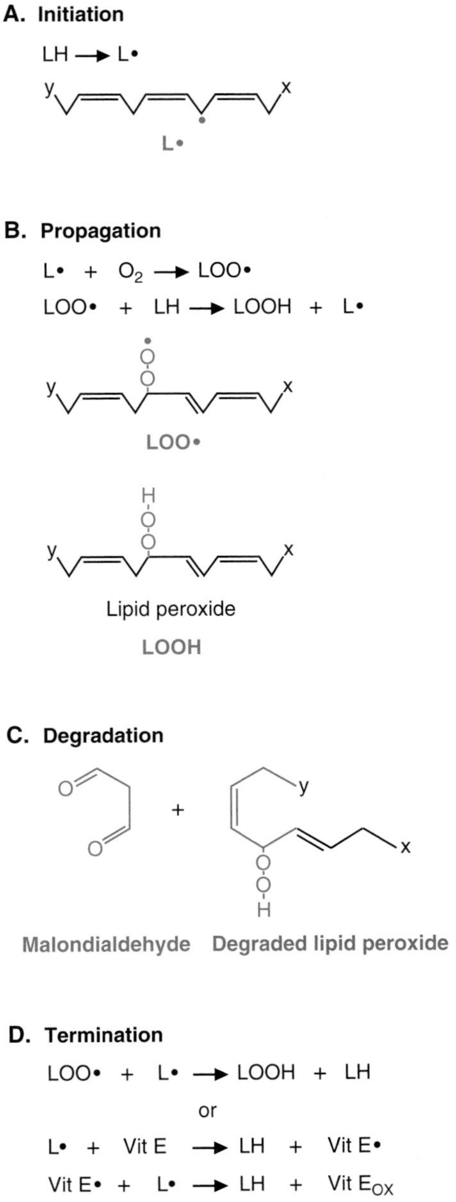

Fig. 21.6. Lipid peroxidation: a free radical chain reaction. **A.** Lipid peroxidation is initiated by a free radical compound, such as the hydroxyl radical, which extracts a hydrogen from a polyunsaturated lipid (LH), resulting in the formation of a lipid radical (L•). **B.** The free radical chain reaction is propagated by the addition of O_2, which forms the lipid peroxy radical (LOO•) and lipid peroxide (LOOH). **C.** Rearrangements of the single electron result in degradation of the lipid. Malondialdehyde, one of the compounds formed, is soluble and appears in the blood. **D.** The chain reaction can be terminated by antioxidants, such as vitamin E, which donate single electrons in two subsequent steps to form a stable oxidized compound.

The pathological hallmark of patients with Parkinson's disease, such as **Les Dopaman**, is a gradual loss of dopamine-producing nerve cells in the basal ganglia of the brainstem. The neurotransmitter dopamine trips off a cascade of signals which regulate normal movement or motor activity.

In Parkinson's disease, the cellular damage is postulated to result, in part, from excess oxygen free radical formation and/or diminished inactivation of the free radicals within the nuclei of the basal ganglia. Since the caudate nucleus of the striatum is also involved in emotional and cognitive function, deficient neurotransmitter synthesis caused by oxygen free radical-induced cell damage to this nucleus may explain the personality changes and disorders of mentation seen in some patients with advanced parkinsonism. The presence of elevated levels of lipid peroxides and malondialdehyde (see Fig. 21.6) in these regions of the brain provides evidence that ROS are involved in the pathogenesis of this disease.

 In patients with unstable hemoglobin and hemolytic anemia, oxidation damage to the red blood cells results in the formation of protein aggregates called Heinz bodies (see Chapter 28). In patients with cataracts, the proteins of the lens of the eye also show signs of free radical damage, and contain methionine sulfoxide residues and tryptophan degradation products.

 The appearance of age pigments (liver spots), commonly found in the skin of the dorsum of the hands and traditionally considered hallmarks of aging, suggests a link between free radical injury and progressive lipid damage. The pigment lipofuscin (from the Greek "lipos" referring to lipids and the Latin "fuscus" meaning dark) consists of a heterogeneous mixture of cross-linked polymerized lipids and some undigested protein products formed from malondialdehyde and other products of lipid peroxidation. These are presumably derived from peroxidatively damaged cell organelles that were autophagocytized but unable to be digested by lysosomes.

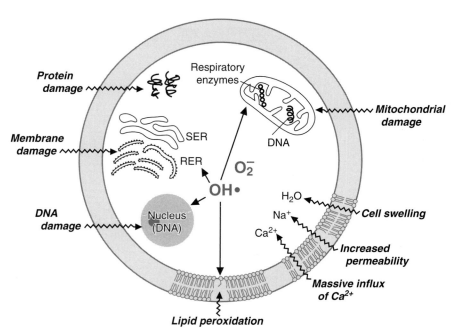

Fig. 21.7. Free radical-mediated cellular injury. Superoxide and the hydroxyl radical initiate lipid peroxidation in the cellular, mitochondrial, nuclear, and endoplasmic reticulum membranes. The increase in cellular permeability results in an influx of Ca^{2+}, which causes further mitochondrial damage. The cysteine sulfhydryl groups and other amino acid residues on proteins are oxidized and degraded. Nuclear and mitochondrial DNA are oxidized, resulting in strand breaks and other types of damage.

incorporate one atom of oxygen into the substrate and reduce the other to H_2O. Dioxygenases incorporate both atoms of oxygen into the substrate.

Oxidases

Cytochrome c oxidase, the terminal electron transport complex of the electron transport chain (cytochrome aa_3) is an example of an oxidase. It catalyzes the 4-electron reduction of O_2 to H_2O. In the reaction, O_2 is bound to 2 paramagnetic metal ions (one Cu^+ and one heme-Fe) in the active site, thus overcoming the spin restriction. O_2 is then reduced in a 2-electron step to provide peroxide, thus bypassing the unfavorable one-electron reduction that would form free superoxide. An additional 2 electrons reduce the reactive oxygen intermediate, resulting in the formation of 2 moles of H_2O per mole of O_2 reduced. This mechanism allows the reaction to occur in a very controlled fashion without an interaction between oxygen free radicals and adjacent mitochondrial components.

Most of the oxidases in the cell form hydrogen peroxide (H_2O_2) instead of H_2O. These enzymes are generally confined to peroxisomal or mitochondrial sites, where the hydrogen peroxide is removed by two of the cellular defense enzymes, catalase or glutathione peroxidase.

Oxygenases

In contrast to oxidases, oxygenases incorporate one or two of the atoms of oxygen into the substrate. Monooxygenases, enzymes that incorporate one atom of O_2 into the substrate and the other into H_2O, are often named hydroxylases (e.g., phenylalanine hydroxylase, which adds a hydroxyl group to phenylalanine to form tyrosine). Monooxygenases require an electron donor-substrate such as NADPH, a coenzyme such as FAD which can transfer single electrons, and a metal or similar compound to form a reactive oxygen complex.

CYTOCHROME P450 ENZYMES

Cytochrome P450 enzymes are a superfamily of structurally related monooxygenases which hydroxylate many physiological compounds, such as steroids and fatty acids, and many xenobiotic compounds, such as drugs, carcinogens, and environmental agents (Fig. 21.9). Like other monooxygenases, they incorporate one atom of O_2 into the substrate, which is usually hydroxylated in this process, and one into H_2O. The electrons are usually donated by NADPH. There are about 100 different P450 isoenzymes in the human, with different, but overlapping, specificities. They all have two major components: an electron-donating reductase system which transfers electrons from NADPH, and a cytochrome P450 which binds the substrate and O_2 and carries out the reaction.

DIOXYGENASES

Dioxygenases, enzymes that incorporate both atoms of oxygen into the substrate, are found in the pathways for converting arachidonate into prostaglandins, thromboxanes, and leukotrienes (see Chapter 35). The lipoxygenases, for instance, form organic peroxides as intermediates in the pathway for leukotriene synthesis. Dioxygenases are also used in carbon-carbon cleavage in the degradation of amino acids.

SOURCES OF REACTIVE OXYGEN SPECIES IN THE CELL

ROS are constantly being formed in the cell through normal metabolic pathways (see Fig. 21.3). Free radical intermediates of enzymatic reactions "leak" from the active

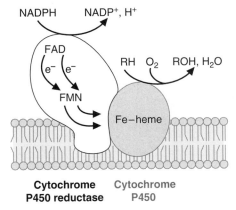

Fig. 21.9. Cytochrome P450 enzymes. Microsomal cytochrome P450 enzymes are composed of two functional units embedded in the membrane of the endoplasmic reticulum: cytochrome P450 and cytochrome P450 reductase, an NADPH-dependent electron-donating system. Cytochrome P450 contains the binding sites for O_2 and the substrate (RH), and an Fe-heme similar to that found in hemoglobin. The "P450" denotes a pigment, the heme, which absorbs visible light at a wavelength of 450 nm. O_2 binds to the P450 heme-Fe in the active site, and is activated to a reactive form by accepting electrons. The electrons are donated by the cytochrome P450 reductase, which contains an FAD plus an FMN or Fe-S center to facilitate the transfer of single electrons from NADPH to O_2.

Cora Nari was initially confused by her physician's statement that the lysis of the intracoronary clots may have induced the cardiac arrhythmia which developed after TPA was administered. Many studies have confirmed that, although timely restoration of blood flow to underperfused cells is crucial to the prevention of ischemic cell death, this same reexposure to oxygenated arterial blood may be responsible for acute anatomic and functional alterations in the newly perfused tissues. Of the many hypotheses regarding the mechanism for reperfusion injury, the generation of oxygen free radicals is among the most plausible. Another mechanism, calcium overload of cells exposed to ischemic stress, suggests that an increase in cytosolic free calcium (which occurs during ischemia and increases further with reperfusion) activates phospholipases and other degradative enzymes which lead to cellular injury. These two hypotheses are related. For example, the generation of oxygen free radicals results in peroxidation of polyunsaturated fatty acids in the plasma membrane as well as in the membranes of subcellular organelles. These changes increase the flux of free calcium ions into the cytosol of involved cells, thereby increasing cellular damage by enhancing the activity of degradative enzymes.

Oxidases

$$O_2 + 4e^-, 4H^+ \longrightarrow 2H_2O$$

$$O_2 + SH_2 \longrightarrow S + H_2O_2$$

Monooxygenases

$$O_2 + S + \text{Electron donor–}XH_2 \longrightarrow H_2O + \text{Electron donor–}X + S{-}OH$$

Dioxygenases

$$S + O_2 \longrightarrow SO_2$$

Fig. 21.8. Oxidases, monooxygenases, and dioxygenases. Enzymes that utilize oxygen to oxidize an organic substrate (shown in the diagram as S) can be classified as oxidases, monooxygenases, and dioxygenases. Oxidases reduce both atoms of O_2 to H_2O or to H_2O_2. Monooxygenases incorporate one atom of O_2 into the substrate and one into water. Dioxygenases incorporate both atoms of O_2 into the substrate.

Q 21.1: Could an enzyme be designed which is capable of transferring electrons directly from NADH to O_2?

Q 21.2: Most monooxygenases utilize NADPH, rather than NADH, as a source of electrons. Why is NADPH the coenzyme of choice?

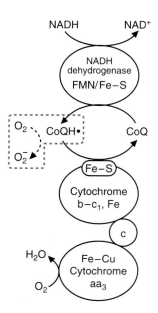

Fig. 21.10. Generation of superoxide by the electron transport chain. Reduced CoQ in the mitochondrial electron transport chain is a major source of oxygen free radicals. Some of the electrons which are being transported from NADH and other compounds to O_2 "escape" when CoQH$^\bullet$ interacts with O_2 to form the superoxide radical. In contrast, the binuclear Fe-Cu center of cytochrome oxidase prevents the release of free oxygen radicals.

The self-perpetuating mechanism of radical release by neutrophils during inflammation and immune complex formation may explain some of the features of chronic inflammation in patients with rheumatoid arthritis. As a result of free radical release, the immunoglobulin G (IgG) proteins present in the synovial fluid are partially oxidized, which improves their binding with the rheumatoid factor antibody. This binding, in turn, stimulates the neutrophils to release more free radicals.

site of enzymes through accidental interactions with O_2 or other compounds. Hydrogen peroxide, formed by some of the oxidases described above, is released into the surrounding medium and generates hydroxyl radicals at iron-containing sites in the cell. Drugs, natural ultraviolet radiation, air pollutants, and other chemicals can also act in the cell to increase formation of free radicals.

Coenzyme Q Generates Superoxide

One of the major sites of superoxide generation is the electron transport chain, which "leaks" free radicals at coenzyme Q (CoQ) (Fig. 21.10). Although the free radicals produced by cytochrome oxidase are tightly bound to the enzyme in a carefully controlled reaction, the one-electron form of CoQ is free within the membrane. An accidental nonspecific interaction between CoQH$^\bullet$ and O_2 results in the formation of superoxide. In a similar way, enzyme-bound intermediates of oxidases and monooxygenases may accidentally extract an electron from some other molecule and initiate a chain reaction.

Respiratory Burst during Phagocytosis

ROS are released during phagocytosis. The respiratory burst produced in granulomatous cells in response to infectious agents and other stimuli is a major source of superoxide anion, hydrogen peroxide, the hydroxyl radical, and hypochlorite (HOCl), nitric oxide (NO), and other free radicals (Fig. 21.11). This process is central to the human antimicrobial defense system, and is intended to damage the membranes and other cellular components of the invading organism.

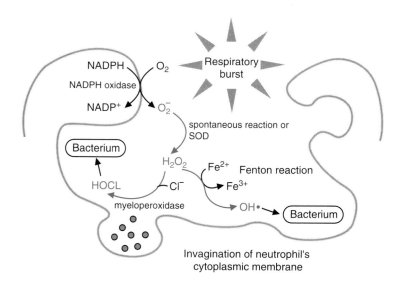

Fig. 21.11. Production of reactive oxygen species during the phagocytic respiratory burst by activated macrophages, neutrophils, and eosinophils. Activation of NADPH oxidase, presumably located on the outer side of the plasma membrane, initiates the respiratory burst with the generation of superoxide. During phagocytosis, the plasma membrane invaginates, so superoxide is released into the vacuole space. The superoxide anion (either spontaneously or enzymatically via SOD) generates the other reactive species, including H_2O_2 and the hydroxyl radical. Myeloperoxidase, an Fe-heme containing enzyme present in granules in the neutrophils, is secreted into the vacuole, where it generates HOCl and other halides. The result is an attack on the membranes and other components of the bacterial cell, and eventual lysis. The whole process is referred to as the respiratory burst because it lasts only 30–60 minutes, and consumes O_2.

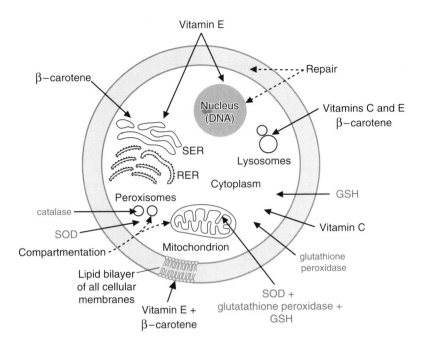

Fig. 21.12. A summary of cellular defense mechanisms. Cellular defenses against ROS include enzymatic reduction of the ROS, removal of ROS by antioxidant vitamins, enzymatic repair of damaged membranes and DNA, and compartmentation—the location of the repair processes in the same subcellular compartments in which most of the ROS are generated. The enzymes SOD and glutathione peroxidase are present as isozymes in the different compartments. The antioxidant vitamins, vitamins E, C, and β-carotene, are also compartmentalized; vitamin E and β-carotene are lipid soluble and found in membranes, and vitamin C is water soluble and present in the cytosol. Modified from Bertini I, et al. Bioinorganic chemistry. Sausalito, CA: University Science Books, 1994:263.

CELLULAR DEFENSES AGAINST OXYGEN TOXICITY

Cellular defenses against oxygen toxicity fall into the categories of antioxidant enzymes for the removal of ROS, antioxidant free radical scavengers and vitamins, cellular compartmentation, and repair (Fig. 21.12). The antioxidant scavenging enzymes remove superoxide and hydrogen peroxide. Vitamin E, vitamin C, and possibly carotenoids, generally referred to as the antioxidant vitamins, can terminate the free radical chain reactions. The defense mechanism of compartmentation refers to separation of species and sites involved in ROS generation from the rest of the cell. For instance, iron, which promotes the nonenzymatic formation of the hydroxyl ion, is tightly bound to its storage protein, ferritin, and cannot react with ROS. Many of the enzymes that produce hydrogen peroxide are sequestered in peroxisomes with a high content of antioxidant enzymes (see Chapter 10). Repair mechanisms for DNA, and for removal of oxidized fatty acids from membrane lipids, are available to the cell. Oxidized amino acids on proteins are repaired through protein degradation and resynthesis of new proteins.

Antioxidant Scavenging Enzymes

The enzymatic defense against ROS includes superoxide dismutase, catalase, and glutathione peroxidase (see Fig. 21.13).

The dopaminergic neurons involved in Parkinson's disease in patients like **Les Dopaman** are particularly susceptible to the cytotoxic effects of ROS. Degradation of dopamine (the neurotransmitter for these neurons) produces H_2O_2, which can be transformed into the hydroxyl radical by the iron-mediated Fenton reaction.

The doxorubicin (adriamycin) with which **Arlyn Foma** was treated (see Chapter 20) has the potential to cause cardiac problems as a result of oxidative damage to the mitochondria in myocardial cells. A toxic hydroxyl radical is generated when this drug interacts with the electron transport chain at the site between coenzyme Q and oxygen.

A 21.1: The enzyme could not achieve any catalytic power because it has no means of overcoming the spin restriction. NAD^+ accepts and transfers an electron pair as the hydride ion. These electrons are coming from a substrate —C—H bond and have 2 electrons with antiparallel spins. Because the 2 electrons of O_2 have parallel spins, one electron from NADH or O_2 would have to spin invert (the spin restriction). Consequently, enzymes which reduce oxygen such as oxidases or monooxygenases usually use FAD as an intermediate to accept electrons from NADH (or NADPH) and transfer them as single electrons to O_2 or to a metal and then to O_2. Some of the metals involved in oxidation-reduction reactions include Fe, Cu, and Mo.

A 21.2: Monooxygenases need a source of electrons and normally utilize NADPH as a substrate. The reaction is favored by high reduction states of NADP in the cell, i.e., a high $NADPH/NADP^+$ ratio. The $NADH/NAD^+$ ratio in the cell is much lower because NADH generated from fuel oxidation rapidly transfers electrons to O_2 in the electron transport chain.

21.3: Why does the cell need such a high content of mitochondrial SOD?

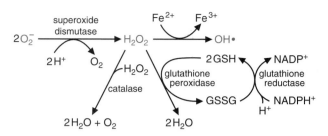

Fig. 21.13. Enzymatic defenses against free radical injury. The highest activities of the antioxidant scavenging enzymes are found in the liver, adrenal gland, and kidney, where mitochondrial and peroxisomal contents are high, and cytochrome P450 enzymes are found in abundance.

Xanthine oxidase, an enzyme that reduces O_2 to H_2O_2 in the cytosol, is thought to be a major factor in ischemia/reperfusion injury especially in intestinal mucosal cells. In undamaged tissues, xanthine oxidase exists as a dehydrogenase which can utilize NAD^+ rather than O_2 as an electron acceptor in the pathway for degradation of purines (hypoxanthine $\rightarrow$ xanthine $\rightarrow$ uric acid (see Chapter 41)). As phosphorylation of ADP to ATP decreases due to lack of oxygen, ADP is degraded and the base is converted to hypoxanthine. In the process, xanthine dehydrogenase is converted to an oxidase. As long as O_2 levels are below the high K_m of the enzyme for O_2, little damage is done. However, once O_2 levels are returned to normal (during the reperfusion), the enzyme generates H_2O_2 and O_2^- at the site of injury.

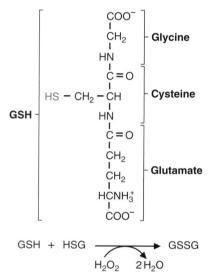

$$GSH + HSG \xrightarrow[H_2O_2 \quad 2H_2O]{} GSSG$$

Fig. 21.14. Oxidation of glutathione. Glutathione contains a sulfhydryl group, shown in blue, which is oxidized to a disulfide when H_2O_2 is reduced to H_2O.

Carbon tetrachloride, used as a solvent in the dry-cleaning industry, is converted by cytochrome P450 to a highly reactive free radical which can cause hepatocellular necrosis. It "escapes" from the enzyme active site. Carbon tetrachloride (CCl_4) accepts an electron and dissociates to $CCl_3^\bullet$ and $Cl^\bullet$. The $CCl_3^\bullet$, which cannot continue through the P450 reaction sequence, initiates chain reactions in the polyunsaturated lipids of the ER. These reactions spread into the plasma membrane and to proteins, eventually resulting in cell swelling, accumulation of lipids, and cell death.

SUPEROXIDE DISMUTASE

Dismutation of superoxide anion to hydrogen peroxide and O_2 by SOD is often called the primary defense against oxidative stress because superoxide is a strong initiator of chain reactions. Different SOD isozymes are present in the cytosol and the mitochondria of the cell. The activity of SOD is increased through enzyme induction by chemicals or conditions which increase the production of superoxide.

CATALASE

Hydrogen peroxide, once formed, must also be removed to prevent generation of the hydroxyl radical. The major routes involve decomposition of hydrogen peroxide to water by catalase and glutathione peroxidase (Fig. 21.13). Catalase is found principally in peroxisomes, and to a lesser extent in the cytosol and microsomal fraction of the cell. In granulomatous cells, catalase serves to protect the cell against its own respiratory burst.

GLUTATHIONE REDUCTASE AND GLUTATHIONE PEROXIDASE

Glutathione peroxidase is one of the body's principal means of protecting against oxidative damage (see Fig. 21.13). It catalyzes the reduction of hydrogen peroxide and lipid peroxides (LOOH) by glutathione (γ-glutamylcysteinylglycine) (Fig. 21.14). The sulfhydryl groups of glutathione (GSH) serve as electron donors, and are oxidized to the disulfide form (GSSG) during the reaction. The cell has two glutathione peroxidases, one of which requires selenium for activity (thus accounting for our dietary requirement for selenium) and acts principally with organic hydroperoxides such as those produced during lipid peroxidation in membranes.

Once the disulfide is formed, it must be reduced back to the sulfhydryl form by glutathione reductase. Glutathione reductase requires electrons from NADPH, which are usually generated from the pentose phosphate pathway (see Chapter 28).

Vitamin Antioxidants

Vitamin E (tocopherol), the most widely distributed antioxidant in nature, is a lipophilic free radical scavenger which functions principally to protect against lipid peroxidation in membranes. Of the three vitamins with the ability to act as antioxidants and terminate free radical chain reactions (vitamin E, vitamin C, and carotenoids), it is the only one whose sole physiological role is to quench free radical reactions.

Vitamin E consists of tocopherol structures, with various methyl groups attached, and a phytyl side chain (Fig. 21.15). Among these, α-tocopherol is the most potent antioxidant. Vitamin E is an efficient terminator of free radical propagation reactions in membrane lipids because the free radical form is stabilized by resonance. Therefore, the vitamin E radical has little tendency to extract a hydrogen atom from another compound and propagate the reaction. Instead, the vitamin E radical can interact directly with lipid peroxy radicals to lose another hydrogen atom, and become the fully oxidized tocopheryl quinone.

Ascorbate, in contrast to vitamin E, is hydrophilic and functions best in an aqueous environment. As a free radical scavenger, it can directly react with the superoxide and the hydroxyl anion, as well as various lipid hydroperoxides (Fig. 21.16). However, its role as a chain-breaking antioxidant is probably to regenerate the reduced form of vitamin E. Deficiency symptoms, such as scurvy, are related to its other role as an oxidation-reduction coenzyme.

It has also been hypothesized that carotenoids can prevent or slow the progression of cancer and degenerative diseases by acting as chain-breaking antioxidants. The carotenoids are a group of compounds related in structure to β-carotene, the precursor of vitamin A (Fig. 21.17). Although much of β-carotene is converted to vitamin A in intestinal mucosal cells, carotenoids are also absorbed and circulate in the blood in lipoproteins. Carotenoids may protect lipids against peroxidation by reacting with lipid hydroperoxyl radicals.

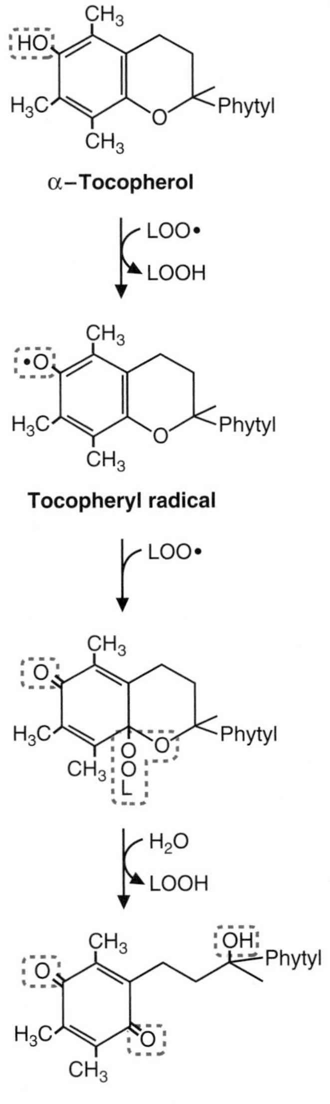

CLINICAL COMMENTS. Because the pathogenesis of "primary" parkinsonism is not well-established and because it may be multifactorial, therapy remains relatively nonspecific and with limited long term efficacy. For patients such as **Les Dopaman**, maintenance of optimal general health and neuromuscular efficiency through formal programs of exercise and rest are an essential part of the treatment plan. Drug therapy is based upon the severity of the disease. In the early phases of the disease, a monoamine oxidase β-inhibitor is used. Monoamine oxidase is a copper-containing enzyme which produces H_2O_2 from the oxidative

Fig. 21.15. Vitamin E. Vitamin E terminates free radical lipid peroxidation by donating single electrons to form the stable, fully oxidized tocopheryl quinone. Of the eight or more different tocopherols that comprise vitamin E, α-tocopherol, shown here, is the most common in the diet.

A 21.3: Mitochondria are major sites for generation of ROS, such as superoxide from the interaction of O_2 and CoQ. Mitochondria also have a high content of SOD and glutathione peroxidase, and can thus convert superoxide to H_2O_2 and then to H_2O.

Premature infants with low levels of lung surfactant (see Chapter 33) require oxygen therapy. The level of oxygen must be closely monitored to prevent retinopathy and subsequent blindness (the retinopathy of prematurity) and to prevent bronchial pulmonary dysplasia. The tendency for these complications to develop is enhanced by the possibility of low levels of SOD and vitamin E in the premature infant.

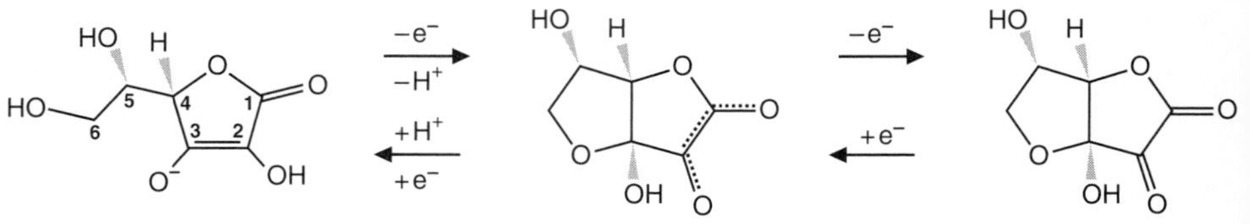

Fig. 21.16. Oxidation and reduction of vitamin C. L-Ascorbate (ascorbic acid) is an efficient free radical scavenger in an aqueous environment. It accepts single electrons from superoxide, hydrogen peroxide, hypochlorite, and the hydroxyl and peroxyl radicals. It can react with NO_2, one of the toxic pollutants in automobile emissions and cigarette smoke. It also reacts with the vitamin E radical to regenerate vitamin E.

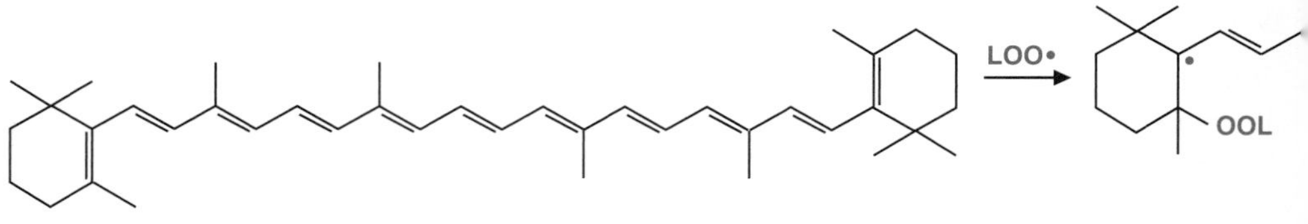

Fig. 21.17. Carotenoids such as β-carotene can also act as chain-breaking antioxidants. Carotenoids are a group of compounds which can serve as precursors of vitamin A. They are related in structure to β-carotene. Carotenoids inhibit lipid peroxidation principally by acting as chain-breaking antioxidants; they accept an electron from lipid peroxy radicals to form a free radical intermediate.

Vitamin E is found in the diet in the lipid fractions of some vegetable oils and in liver, egg yolks, and cereals. It is absorbed together with lipids, and symptomatic deficiencies are associated with fat malabsorption. Vitamin E circulates in the blood in lipoprotein particles. Deficiency of vitamin E results in a neurological syndrome.

degradation of dopamine and other catecholamines, and the drug was originally administered to inhibit dopamine degradation. The current theory suggests that the effectiveness of the drug is also related to the decrease of free radical formation within the cells of the basal ganglia. The application of the antioxidant vitamins such as β-carotene, vitamin C, and vitamin E has theoretical, but unsubstantiated, potential usefulness in these patients. In later stages of the disease, patients are treated with levodopa (L-dopa), a precursor of dopamine (see Chapter 41).

In patients such as **Cora Nari**, who experience ischemia (a limitation in blood flow and, consequently, oxygen supply to tissues), ATP production is compromised. In many cases, the damage appears to accelerate when the oxygen is first reintroduced (reperfused) into the tissue. Ischemia might also arise during surgery or during transplantation of tissues. In support of the role of oxygen radicals in ischemia-reperfusion injury, it has been observed that antioxidants protect against reperfusion injury to ischemic tissue.

Currently, an intense study of ischemic insults to a variety of animal organ models is underway in an effort to discover ways of preventing reperfusion injury. These include methods designed to increase endogenous antioxidant activity, to reduce the generation of free radicals, and, finally, to develop exogenous antioxidants that, when administered prior to reperfusion, would prevent its injurious effects. Each of these approaches has met with some success, but their clinical application awaits further refinement. With the growing number of invasive procedures aimed at restoring arterial blood flow through partially obstructed coronary vessels, such as clot lysis, balloon or laser angioplasty, and coronary artery bypass grafting, development of methods to prevent ischemia-reperfusion injury will become increasingly urgent.

Epidemiological evidence suggests that individuals with a higher intake of foods containing vitamin E, β-carotene, and vitamin C have a somewhat lower risk of cancer and certain other ROS-related diseases than do individuals on diets deficient in these vitamins. However, studies in which well-nourished populations were given supplements of these antioxidant vitamins found either no effects or harmful effects compared to the beneficial effects from eating foods containing a wide variety of antioxidant compounds.

BIOCHEMICAL COMMENTS. The cytochrome P450 enzymes are one of the major groups of enzymes which oxidize xenobiotic agents such as administered drugs and naturally occurring chemicals. There are about 100 different P450 isozymes with varying degrees of specificity for different substrates. It is not known whether the evolutionary development of so many P450 isozymes is related to the need to oxidize physiological compounds, the need to dispose of xenobiotic chemicals in plants and the environment, or both.

The P450 enzymes are inducible both by their most specific substrate and by substrates for some of the other cytochrome P450 enzymes. For instance, phenobarbital, a barbiturate long used as a sleeping pill or for treatment of epilepsy, is converted to an inactive metabolite by cytochrome P450 monooxygenases P450 2B1 and 2B2. Following treatment with phenobarbital, P450 2B2 is increased 50–100-fold, but some of the other P450s from the same subfamily, from different subfamilies, and even from different gene families are increased 2–4-fold. The induction of 2B1 and 2B2 occurs through the binding of phenobarbital or another compound to an intracellular receptor (PBR) and binding of the activated receptor to a phenobarbital response element (PBRE) in the target gene. Phenobarbital treatment also results in a general proliferation of the microsomal endoplasmic reticulum, and a general stabilization of microsomal proteins.

The P450 enzymes involved in steroidogenesis are quite different from the microsomal enzymes. The P450 protein is embedded in the mitochondrial membrane. The electron-donating system consists of a soluble NADPH-oxidizing protein and Fe–S-containing protein which can shuttle electrons between the electron-donating system and the P450 enzyme. The Fe-S protein has been named adrenodoxin for its high concentration in the adrenal cortex.

Accidental ROS generation by cytochrome P450 enzymes in the cell is decreased by two protective mechanisms: ordered substrate binding prior to O_2 binding, and induction/repression of P450 synthesis. The ordered binding in many of the P450 enzymes prevents highly reactive oxygen intermediates from being generated until substrate is present in the active site. Induction and repression of the synthesis of P450 enzymes in response to increased presence of substrate is also protective; it prevents the accumulation of unnecessary iron-containing proteins in the cell which might generate oxygen free radicals.

The cytochrome P450 superfamily has at least 27 distinct gene families, of which at least 10 are found in mammals. Within these 10 gene families are over 100 different cytochrome P450 isozymes. Each isozyme has a distinct classification according to its structural relationship with other isozymes. For example, the activity of the microsomal ethanol-oxidizing system (MEOS) referred to in Chapter 18, is comprised principally of P450 2E1. The "2" refers to the gene family, which is comprised of isozymes with greater than 40% amino acid sequence identity. The "E" refers to the subfamily, a grouping of isozymes with greater than 55–60% sequence identity, and the "1" refers to the individual enzymes within this subfamily.

The overlapping specificity in catalytic activity and in induction/repression of gene transcription is responsible for several types of drug interactions. For example, individuals who take phenobarbital for prolonged periods develop a drug tolerance as the P450 2B2 is induced and the drug is metabolized to an inactive metabolite more rapidly. Consequently, these individuals utilize progressively higher doses of phenobarbitol. Ethanol, which is a substrate for the P450 MEOS, is an inhibitor of the phenobarbitol-oxidizing P450 system. When large amounts of ethanol are consumed, the inactivation of phenobarbital is directly or indirectly inhibited. Therefore, when high doses of phenobarbital and ethanol are consumed at the same time, toxic levels of the barbiturate can accumulate in the blood.

Suggested Readings

Forster RE, Estabrook RW. Is oxygen an essential nutrient? Annu Rev Nutr 1993;13:383–403.

Guengerich FP. Reactions and significance of cytochrome P450 enzymes. J Biol Chem 1993;266:10019–10022.

Gutteridge JMC, Halliwell B. Antioxidants in nutrition, health and disease. Oxford: Oxford University Press, 1994.

Herber V. The antioxidant supplement myth. Am J Clin Nutr 1994;60:157–158.

Role of iron and oxidant stress in the normal and parkinsonian brain. Ann Neurol 1992;32:S1–S145.

Shigenaga MK, Hagen TM, Ames BN. Oxidative damage and mitochondrial decay in aging. Proc Natl Acad Sci USA 1994;92:10771–10778.

Waxman DJ, Azaroff L. Phenobarbital induction of cytochrome P-450 gene expression. Biochem J 1992;281:23–38.

Yu BP. Cellular defenses against damage from reactive oxygen species. Physiol Rev 1994;74:139–162.

PROBLEMS

1. Why is vitamin E referred to as an antioxidant?

2. What would be the benefit of administering therapeutic drugs or steroid derivatives which are free radical scavengers immediately after injury to tissues, such as occurs in a car accident?

3. The levels of oxidative damage to mitochondrial DNA are at least 10-fold higher than to nuclear DNA, and increase with a person's age. What accounts for the different levels of oxidative damage in mitochondrial and nuclear DNA?

ANSWERS

1. When vitamin E acts as a "free radical scavenger," it is not terminating chain reactions by "absorbing" single electrons. Instead, it donates a single electron ($H^•$) to the free radical, which is thereby reduced to a stable form (e.g., $LOO^•$ is converted to LOOH). The vitamin radical then loses another single electron ($H^•$) to become fully oxidized. Thus, vitamin E is oxidized by the reaction, the free radicals in the cell are reduced, and the spread of oxidative damage is diminished.

2. Tissue injury, especially that involving the brain or spinal cord, disrupts the cellular and compartmental structures that organize defense enzymes near the site of ROS formation. Iron and iron-containing proteins are released into the injured site where they can accelerate ROS formation by the Fenton reaction. Invading macrophages, which respond to the injury, generate additional ROS as part of the inflammatory response.

3. There is a high rate of free radical generation from the mitochondrial electron transport chain at CoQ. Mitochondrial DNA is located near the inner mitochondrial membrane where the electron transport chain is located. Mitochondrial DNA has a lack of protective histones, and there are few DNA repair enzymes in mitochondria. The consequence has been described as mitochondrial aging.

22 Generation of ATP from Glucose: Glycolysis

Glucose is the universal fuel for human cells. Every cell type in the human is able to generate ATP from glycolysis, the pathway in which glucose is oxidized and cleaved to form pyruvate. Glycolysis, which occurs in the cytosol, directly generates ATP by transfer of high energy phosphate from intermediates of the pathway to ADP (substrate level phosphorylation). In this process, NAD^+ is reduced to NADH. If a cell has a sufficiently high oxidative capacity (an adequate amount of mitochondria, mitochondrial enzymes, and oxygen), the reducing equivalents in NADH can be transferred to the mitochondrial electron transport chain and the pyruvate can be oxidized completely to CO_2 in the tricarboxylic acid (TCA) cycle. Because the inner mitochondrial membrane is impermeable to NADH, this transfer of reducing equivalents from the cytosol into the mitochondrion requires a shuttle system, either the malate-aspartate shuttle or the glycerol 3-phosphate shuttle. The aerobic oxidation of glucose to pyruvate and the subsequent oxidation of pyruvate to CO_2 generates 36–38 moles of ATP per mole of glucose.

Under conditions in which the oxidative capacity of cells is limited by mitochondrial capacity or oxygen availability, the NADH generated from glycolysis is reoxidized by conversion of pyruvate to lactate by lactate dehydrogenase. The conversion of glucose to lactate is called anaerobic glycolysis, which means that the process does not require molecular oxygen. The energy yield from anaerobic glycolysis (2 moles of ATP per mole of glucose) is much lower than the yield from aerobic oxidation.

Many cell types are partially or totally dependent on glucose as a fuel. In some cases, anaerobic glycolysis must generate all, or a major portion, of the cell's ATP requirements. Other cell types that oxidize glucose aerobically, such as the brain, are glucose dependent because they have a limited ability to oxidize fatty acids, the body's other major fuel.

The principal function of the glycolytic pathway is the generation of ATP, and the pathway is feedback regulated by ATP and its related metabolite, AMP. The rate-limiting enzyme of the glycolytic pathway is phosphofructokinase-1 (PFK-1). This enzyme is allosterically activated by AMP, which increases in the cytosol as ATP is hydrolyzed by energy-requiring reactions. In many cells, the rate of PFK-1 influences the rate of glucose entry into the cell and its phosphorylation by hexokinase to glucose 6-phosphate.

Glycolysis has functions other than ATP production. In liver and adipose tissue, this pathway provides pyruvate as a precursor for fatty acid biosynthesis. The hormonal regulators of glucose homeostasis, insulin and glucagon, regulate glycolysis in these two tissues. Glycolysis also provides precursors for the synthesis of compounds such as amino acids and 5-carbon sugars (pentoses).

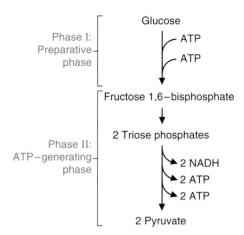

Fig. 22.1. Phases of the glycolytic pathway.

The ATP expenditure at the beginning of the glycolytic pathway is sometimes called "priming the pump" because it gets the pathway going. The subsequent steps of the pathway regenerate this ATP and provide an additional 2 moles of ATP per mole of glucose.

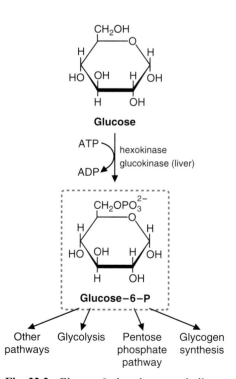

Fig. 22.2. Glucose 6-phosphate metabolism.

 Although **Thomas Appleman** hated going to the dentist, he made an appointment because every time he ate ice cream, he felt excruciating, throbbing pain in his teeth. He really liked sweets and always kept hard candies in his pocket. He knew that one or two would not contribute much to his caloric intake and found they decreased his appetite. The dentist noted that Thomas had always had dental problems, and had dental caries (cavities) even in his baby teeth. At this visit, the dentist found caries in two of Mr. Appleman's teeth.

Lopa Fusor is a 68-year-old woman who is admitted to the hospital emergency room with very low blood pressure (80/20 mm Hg) caused by an acute hemorrhage from a previously diagnosed ulcer of the stomach. She is known to have chronic obstructive pulmonary disease (COPD) as a result of 42 years of smoking two packs of cigarettes a day. Her respiratory rate is rapid and labored, her skin is cold and clammy, and her lips are slightly blue in color (cyanotic). She appears anxious and moderately confused.

As appropriate emergency measures are taken to stop the bleeding and to reverse her hypotension, a battery of laboratory tests are ordered, including venous hemoglobin, hematocrit, and lactate levels, and arterial blood pH, partial pressures of oxygen (pO_2) and carbon dioxide (pCO_2), and oxygen saturation. Venous blood is also sent for immediate blood type and cross-matching (for the likelihood that blood transfusions would be necessary).

REACTIONS OF GLYCOLYSIS

The glycolytic pathway cleaves one mole of glucose to 2 moles of the 3-carbon compound pyruvate. In the initial preparative phase of glycolysis, glucose is phosphorylated by ATP and cleaved into 2 triose phosphates (Fig. 22.1). In the second or ATP-generating phase, a triose phosphate (glyceraldehyde 3-phosphate), is oxidized by NAD^+ and phosphorylated in a reaction that uses inorganic phosphate. This and subsequent reactions rearrange the phosphates into high energy bonds so that they can be transferred to ADP to form ATP. The result is a net yield of 2 moles of ATP, 2 moles of NADH, and 2 moles of pyruvate per mole of glucose.

Conversion of Glucose to Glucose 6-Phosphate

Glucose metabolism begins with the phosphorylation of glucose to glucose 6-phosphate by transfer of a phosphate from ATP. Phosphorylation commits glucose to metabolism within the cell because glucose 6-phosphate cannot be transported out of cells and the high negative $\Delta G^{0'}$ of the reaction prevents a net conversion back to glucose under physiological conditions.

Hexokinases, the enzymes that catalyze this reaction, are a family of isoenzymes with slightly different kinetic properties and amino acid sequences in different tissues. The isoenzyme found in liver and B cells of the pancreas has a much higher K_m than other hexokinases and is called glucokinase. Glucose 6-phosphate is an intermediate in almost every pathway that uses glucose, including glycolysis, the pentose phosphate pathway, and the pathway for glycogen synthesis (Fig. 22.2). Hexokinases catalyze the first step in glycolysis (Fig. 22.3).

Conversion of Glucose 6-Phosphate to the Triose Phosphates

In the next three steps of the glycolytic pathway, glucose 6-phosphate is isomerized to fructose 6-phosphate, which is phosphorylated to fructose 1,6-bisphosphate and

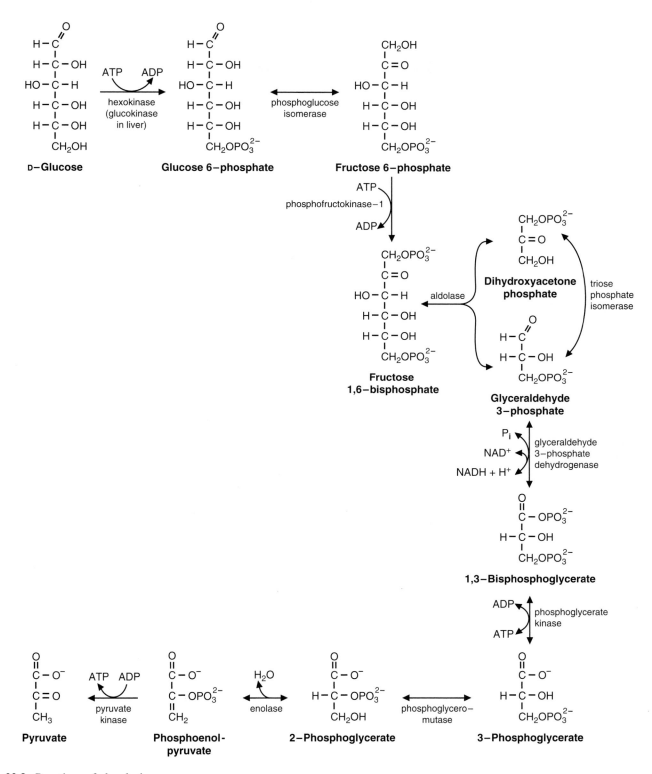

Fig. 22.3. Reactions of glycolysis.

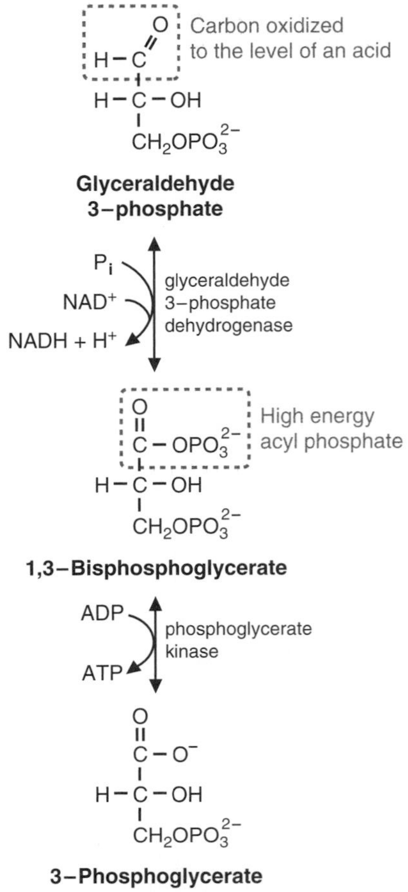

Glyceraldehyde 3-phosphate

1,3-Bisphosphoglycerate

3-Phosphoglycerate

Fig. 22.5. Generation of the first ATP. The aldehyde group of an enzyme-bound glyceraldehyde 3-phosphate is oxidized by NAD$^+$ to an acid, which accepts a phosphate group from inorganic phosphate (P$_i$). This high energy phosphate group is transferred to ADP to form ATP.

 The bisphosphoglycerate shunt is a "side reaction" of the glycolytic pathway in which 1,3-bisphosphoglycerate is converted to 2,3-bisphosphoglycerate (2,3-BPG, formerly called 2,3-diphosphoglycerate (2,3-DPG)). 2,3-BPG functions as a conenzyme in the conversion of 2-phosphoglycerate to 3-phosphoglycerate by the glycolytic enzyme phosphoglyceromutase. Since 2,3-BPG is not depleted by its rtole in this catalytic process, most cells need only very small amounts. Red blood cells (erythrocytes) are an exception, and form 2,3-BPG in higher amounts to serve as an allosteric inhibitor of oxygen binding to hemoglobin (see Chapter 8). 2,3-BPG reenters the glycolytic pathway via dephosphorylation to 3-phosphoglycerate.

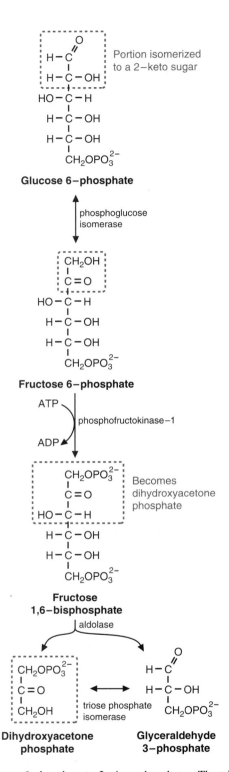

Glucose 6-phosphate

Fructose 6-phosphate

Fructose 1,6-bisphosphate

Dihydroxyacetone phosphate

Glyceraldehyde 3-phosphate

Fig. 22.4. Conversion of glucose 6-phosphate to 2 triose phosphates. The triose phosphates, glyceraldehyde 3-phosphate and dihydroxyacetone phosphate, are interconverted by triose phosphate isomerase.

cleaved into two phosphorylated 3-carbon compounds (triose phosphates) (Fig. 22.4). The isomerization, which positions a keto group next to carbon 3, is essential for the subsequent cleavage of the bond between carbons 3 and 4.

In the phosphorylation of fructose 6-phosphate to fructose 1,6-bisphosphate by the enzyme PFK-1, energy from cleavage of ATP is again expended. This reaction is thermodynamically and kinetically irreversible and, therefore, irrevocably commits glucose to the glycolytic pathway. Regulation of PFK-1 controls the entry of glucose into glycolysis.

Fructose 1,6-bisphosphate is cleaved into dihydroxyacetone phosphate and glyceraldehyde 3-phosphate by aldolase, an enzyme named for the mechanism of the forward and reverse reactions, aldol cleavage and aldol condensation. Dihydroxyacetone phosphate is isomerized to glyceraldehyde 3-phosphate, so that for every mole of glucose entering glycolysis, 2 moles of glyceraldehyde 3-phosphate continue through the pathway.

Conversion of Glyceraldehyde 3-Phosphate to Pyruvate

In the next part of the glycolytic pathway, the glyceraldehyde 3-phosphate undergoes oxidation, formation of a high energy phosphate bond from inorganic phosphate, and rearrangement so that the phosphate can be transferred to ADP to form ATP (Fig. 22.5). The first reaction in this sequence is really the key to the pathway because it provides the high energy phosphate for net ATP synthesis. In this reaction, the enzyme-bound aldehyde group of glyceraldehyde 3-phosphate is oxidized to an enzyme-bound carboxyl group that immediately accepts an inorganic phosphate to form a high energy acyl phosphate bond. The enzyme that catalyzes the reaction, glyceraldehyde 3-phosphate dehydrogenase, transfers the electrons to NAD^+ to form NADH. The formation of the acyl phosphate is termed substrate level phosphorylation, the formation of a high energy phosphate bond where none previously existed—without the utilization of oxygen. The free energy of hydrolysis of phosphate in this bond is sufficiently high so that the transfer of the phosphate to ADP to form ATP by 3-phosphoglycerate kinase in the next step of the pathway is a thermodynamically favorable reaction.

To transfer the remaining phosphate on 3-phosphoglycerate to ADP, the phosphoester bond must be converted into a high energy phosphate bond. This conversion is accomplished by moving the phosphate to the 2 position (forming 2-phosphoglycerate), and then removing water to form phosphoenolpyruvate (PEP). The enolphosphate bond contains about 14 kcal. The subsequent transfer of this phosphate from PEP to ADP by pyruvate kinase is now energetically favorable (Fig. 22.6). In this reaction, PEP is converted to pyruvate.

Summary of the Glycolytic Pathway

The overall net reaction in the glycolytic pathway is:

Glucose + $2NAD^+$ + $2P_i$ + 2ADP → 2Pyruvate + 2NADH + $4H^+$ + 2ATP + $2H_2O$

The pathway occurs with an overall negative $\Delta G^{0'}$ of about −22 kcal. It is, therefore, not readily reversible. Reversal in the direction of glucose production (gluconeogenesis) requires an input of energy.

Oxidation of Cytosolic NADH

For the glycolytic pathway to operate continuously, the NADH produced by glyceraldehyde 3-phosphate dehydrogenase must be reoxidized to NAD^+ (Fig. 22.7). This

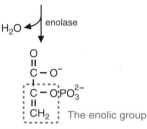

3−Phosphoglycerate

phosphoglycero−mutase

2−Phosphoglycerate

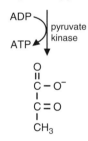

Phosphoenolpyruvate

Pyruvate

Fig. 22.6. Generation of the second ATP. Rearrangement of the phosphate group and removal of water produce an enolic group containing a high energy phosphate, which is transferred to ADP to form ATP.

Hexokinases, other kinases, and many other enzymes that catalyze reactions involving the hydrolysis of ATP require Mg^{2+}. The Mg^{2+} forms a complex with the phosphate groups of ATP. Kinases also require K^+.

Kinases transfer a phosphate from ATP to another compound. For instance, hexokinase transfers a phosphate to glucose or another hexose to form a hexose phosphate. 3-Phosphoglycerate kinase is, therefore, named for the direction of the reaction which reverses glycolysis—transfer of a phosphate from ATP to 3-phosphoglycerate to form 1,3-bisphosphoglycerate. Pyruvate kinase is also named for the reverse of the glycolytic direction, although phosphorylation of pyruvate to phosphoenolpyruvate by ATP does not occur under physiological conditions.

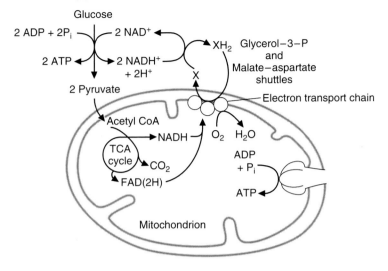

A. Aerobic glycolysis

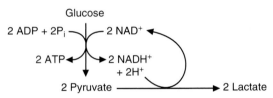

B. Anaerobic glycolysis

Fig. 22.7. Alternate routes of glycolysis. **A.** The pyruvate produced by glycolysis enters mitochondria and is oxidized to CO_2 and H_2O. The reducing equivalents in NADH enter mitochondria via a shuttle system. **B.** Pyruvate is reduced to lactate in the cytosol, thereby utilizing the reducing equivalents in NADH.

The constant sucrose medium **Thomas Appleman** created in his mouth by sucking on hard candy was ideal for the growth of the bacteria responsible for dental caries. Many strains of *Streptococcus mutans* and lactobacilli, major contributors to dental caries, are able to generate sufficient ATP from the glycolytic pathway for high growth rates.

Fluoride is able to kill these bacteria by inhibiting enolase, the glycolytic enzyme that converts 2-phosphoglycerate to PEP. However, this inhibition is weak and does not occur at the concentrations of fluoride present in fluoridated water. Fluoride in water helps to prevent dental caries by decreasing the demineralization of tooth enamel at acid pH and promoting remineralization.

reoxidation can be accomplished in two ways: (*a*) the electrons can be transferred into mitochondria via the glycerol 3-phosphate or the malate-aspartate shuttle and ultimately passed to oxygen via the electron transport chain, or (*b*) NADH can be reoxidized to NAD^+ by the reaction catalyzed by lactate dehydrogenase which converts pyruvate to lactate.

In tissues with mitochondria, reoxidation of NADH is accomplished completely, or in part, by the glycerol 3-phosphate and malate-aspartate shuttles. These shuttle systems are a series of reactions which transfer reducing equivalents from NADH to the electron transport chain. The inner mitochondrial membrane is impermeable to NADH, and no transport protein exists that can directly translocate NADH across this membrane. Instead, the reducing equivalents (in the form of H:, a hydride ion) are transferred by a cytosolic oxidation-reduction reaction to a compound that has a transport protein in the inner mitochondrial membrane. Thus, in the initial step of this process, NAD^+ is regenerated in the cytosol and returned to the glycolytic pathway. The electrons are ultimately transferred to the electron transport chain, where approximately 2 moles of ATP per mole of NADH are generated from the glycerol 3-phosphate shuttle, and 3 moles of ATP per mole of NADH are generated from the malate-aspartate shuttle.

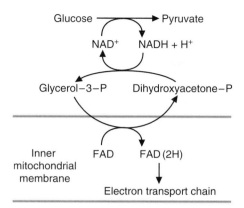

Fig. 22.8. Glycerol 3-phosphate shuttle. Because NAD$^+$ and NADH cannot cross the mitochondrial membrane, shuttles transfer the reducing equivalents into mitochondria. Dihydroxyacetone phosphate (DHAP) is reduced to glycerol 3-phosphate by the NADH produced in the cytosol by glycolysis. Glycerol 3-phosphate reacts in the inner mitochondrial membrane with an enzyme that transfers the electrons to FAD. These electrons are passed by FAD(2H) to the electron transport chain, which generates approximately 2 ATP for each FAD(2H) that is reoxidized. DHAP is regenerated and returns to the cytosol.

GLYCEROL 3-PHOSPHATE SHUTTLE

The glycerol 3-phosphate shuttle is the predominant shuttle in tissues (Fig. 22.8). In the cytosol, electrons are transferred from the NADH produced in glycolysis to dihydroxyacetone phosphate (DHAP) to form glycerol 3-phosphate. This compound is transported into the inner mitochondrial membrane where the electrons are donated to an FAD-containing glycerophosphate dehydrogenase which passes electrons to coenzyme Q. This pathway, like other FAD-containing pathways that donate electrons to coenzyme Q, generates approximately 2 ATP by transfer of these electrons to oxygen. The dihydroxyacetone phosphate returns to the cytosol.

MALATE-ASPARTATE SHUTTLE

The malate-aspartate shuttle is more complex than the glycerol-3-P shuttle, but follows the same principles (Fig. 22.9). NAD$^+$ is regenerated from NADH in the cytosol by reduction of oxaloacetate to malate by the cytosolic malate dehydrogenase. Malate is translocated by a transport protein into the mitochondrial matrix, where NADH is regenerated by the mitochondrial malate dehydrogenase. Reoxidation of this NADH by NADH dehydrogenase and the electron transport chain generates approximately 3 ATP. Oxaloacetate, which cannot cross the inner mitochondrial membrane, is transaminated to aspartate in the mitochondrion. Aspartate is translocated out of the mitochondrion and transaminated back to oxaloacetate in the cytosol (Fig. 22.10). The translocators exchange compounds in such a way that the shuttle is completely balanced and is driven by the unidirectional energy-requiring transport of aspartate from the mitochondrion to the cytosol.

Tissues with mitochondria have both these shuttle systems in varying amounts. The presence of two shuttles provides a "safety net" for tissues with high ATP demands. Reoxidation of NADH by a shuttle allows pyruvate to enter the TCA cycle and generate an additional 15 ATP. In contrast, if the NAD$^+$ must be regenerated by reduction of pyruvate to lactate, the ATP yield from oxidation of both the NADH and pyruvate is lost.

Q 22.1: Aminoxyacetate inhibits the transamination step in the malate-aspartate shuttle. What effect would this compound have on glucose metabolism?

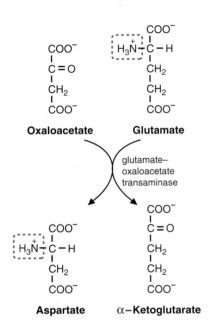

Fig. 22.10. Transamination of oxaloacetate to aspartate. In transamination reactions, an α-keto acid is converted to its corresponding α-amino acid. The amino group is supplied by glutamate, which is converted to its corresponding α-keto acid, α-ketoglutarate. These reactions are readily reversible and require pyridoxal phosphate as a cofactor (see Chapter 38). Glutamate-oxaloacetate transaminase is also called aspartate transaminase.

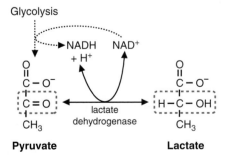

Fig. 22.11. Lactate dehydrogenase reaction. Pyruvate, which may be produced by glycolysis, is reduced to lactate. The reaction, which occurs in the cytosol, requires NADH and is catalyzed by lactate dehydrogenase. This reaction is readily reversible.

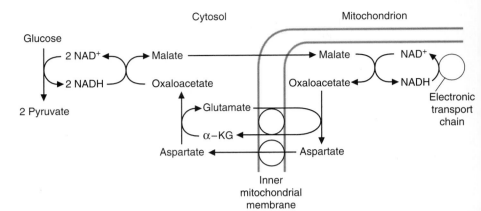

Fig. 22.9. Malate-aspartate shuttle. NADH produced by glycolysis reduces oxaloacetate (OAA) to malate, which crosses the mitochondrial membrane and is reoxidized to OAA. NADH produced by this reaction in the mitochondrion is reoxidized by the electron transport chain, and 3 ATPs are generated for each NADH. Because OAA cannot cross the mitochondrial membrane, it is transaminated to aspartate, which can cross the membrane. In the cytosol, aspartate is transaminated to regenerate OAA. α-KG = α-ketoglutarate.

ANAEROBIC GLYCOLYSIS

The NADH produced in glycolysis by the glyceraldehyde 3-phosphate dehydrogenase reaction can also be reoxidized in the cytosol by the reduction of pyruvate to lactate. This reaction is catalyzed by lactate dehydrogenase (Fig. 22.11). Because lactate production from glucose occurs without the need for oxygen to reoxidize the NADH, it is termed anaerobic glycolysis. The net equation for anaerobic glycolysis is:

$$\text{Glucose} + 2\ \text{ADP} + 2\ P_i \rightarrow 2\ \text{Lactate} + 2\ \text{ATP} + 2\ H_2O + 2\ H^+$$

Pyruvic acid and lactic acid are formed in the glycolytic pathway. At the intracellular pH of 7.4, these acids each release a proton to form pyruvate and lactate, respectively. Glycolysis is therefore an acid-producing pathway. Subsequent oxidation of pyruvate in the TCA cycle utilizes this proton. However, when lactate cannot be metabolized further in the cells which produce it, it crosses the plasma membrane accompanied by a proton (or in exchange for a hydroxide ion) on a transport protein. Pyruvate can also cross the plasma membrane, but the equilibrium of the lactate dehydrogenase reaction favors lactate, so that the levels of pyruvate in the cell and in the blood are always much lower than those of lactate.

Many tissues, such as erythrocytes, lymphocytes, white blood cells, the kidney medulla, the tissues of the eye, and skeletal muscles, rely on anaerobic glycolysis for at least a portion of their ATP requirements. The relative proportion of glucose metabolized by oxidation to CO_2 versus anaerobic glycolysis depends on the mitochondrial oxidative capacity of the tissue and its oxygen supply. Tissues which must rely on anaerobic glycolysis have a low ATP demand and compensate for the low yield of anaerobic glycolysis with higher levels of glycolytic enzymes. For example, the mature erythrocyte, which has no mitochondria, relies totally on anaerobic glycolysis for ATP production. The skin also has a high rate of anaerobic glycolysis. Some of the lactic acid produced is secreted in sweat, where it acts as an antibacterial agent.

The tissues of the eye are also partially dependent on anaerobic glycolysis (Fig. 22.12). They have cells that transmit or focus light and that cannot, therefore, be filled with opaque structures like mitochondria, or densely packed capillary beds. The corneal epithelium generates most of its ATP aerobically from its few mitochondria, but still metabolizes some glucose anaerobically. Oxygen is supplied by diffusion from the air. The lens of the eye is composed of fibers which must remain birefringent to transmit and focus light, so mitochondria are nearly absent. The small amount of ATP required (principally for ion balance) can readily be generated from anaerobic glycolysis even though the energy yield is low. The lens is able to pick up glucose and release lactate into the vitreous body and aqueous humor. It does not need oxygen and has no use for capillaries. Regions of the retina also use anaerobic glycolysis for a portion of their ATP requirement.

In skeletal muscles, lactate production occurs when the need for ATP exceeds the capacity of the mitochondria for oxidative phosphorylation, and increased lactate production accompanies an increased rate of the TCA cycle. The extent to which skeletal muscles utilize aerobic versus anaerobic glycolysis to supply ATP varies with the type of muscle fiber, its mitochondrial capacity for oxidative phosphorylation, the length of time from the onset of exercise, and the intensity of exercise. In skeletal muscles, anaerobic glycolysis is closely associated with the utilization of muscle glycogen stores (see Chapter 26).

Most of the lactate released from tissues undergoing anaerobic glycolysis is taken up by other tissues which have an excess mitochondrial capacity. For instance, the heart, with its huge mitochondrial content, is able to utilize lactate released from other tissues during exercise. Lactate is transported into the tissue, oxidized to pyruvate by lactate dehydrogenase, and enters the TCA cycle.

The other major fate of lactate is conversion to glucose by the process of gluconeogenesis. Lactate produced from skeletal muscles and other tissues is taken up by the liver and converted to glucose. The cycling of lactate between muscle and liver is called the Cori cycle (Fig. 22.13).

FUNCTIONS OF GLYCOLYSIS

The glycolytic pathway, in addition to providing ATP, generates precursors for biosynthetic pathways. Intermediates of the pathway may be converted to ribose 5-phosphate, which forms the sugar of nucleotides (see Chapter 28), and to the amino acids serine, glycine, and cysteine (see Chapter 39). Pyruvate may be transaminated to alanine. In the liver, and to a lesser extent in adipose tissue, pyruvate provides substrate for fatty acid biosynthesis. Glycerol 3-phosphate, which forms the backbone of the triacylglycerols, is derived from the glycolytic pathway (see Chapter 33).

REGULATION OF GLYCOLYSIS BY THE NEED FOR ATP

Because the principal function of the glycolytic pathway is the generation of ATP, flux through the pathway must be regulated so that the rate of ATP generation corre-

 The overall ATP yield for the complete oxidation of one mole of glucose to 6 moles of CO_2 is 36–38 moles; approximately 2 moles of ATP are produced by the glycolytic pathway, 4–6 by the shuttles, and 30 from the oxidation of 2 moles of pyruvate via pyruvate dehydrogenase and the TCA cycle. In contrast, the ATP yield from anaerobic glycolysis is only 2. Thus, anaerobic glycolysis must occur about 19 times as fast as aerobic glucose oxidation to produce the same amount of ATP per unit time.

 The dental caries in **Thomas Appleman's** mouth were caused principally by the low pH generated from lactic acid produced from anerobic glycolysis in the oral bacteria. Below a pH of 5.5, decalcification of tooth enamel and dentine occurs. Lactobacilli and *S. mutans* are major contributors to this process because almost all of their energy is derived from the conversion of glucose or fructose to lactic acid, and they are able to grow well at the low pH generated by this process. Mr. Appleman's dentist explained that bacteria in his dental plaque could convert the sugar in his candy into acid in less than 20 minutes. Since saliva production decreases in the evening, he would have less saliva to buffer and remove the lactic acid, which would dissolve the hydroxyapatite in his tooth enamel during the night.

A 22.1: Although inhibitors of the malate-aspartate shuttle decrease the capacity of the cells to reoxidize cytosolic NADH, they do not completely block glycolysis. Like many inhibitors of other pathways, inhibitors of this shuttle increase the flux through alternative pathways. In this case, more of the NADH is reoxidized in the glycerol 3-phosphate shuttle, and reoxidation of NADH by conversion of pyruvate to lactate may also increase.

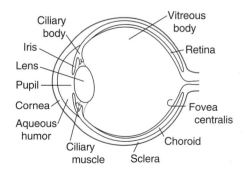

Fig. 22.12. Tissues of the eye.

22.2: The kidney is composed of two different tissues, the cortex and the medulla. The cortex contains the proximal convoluted tubules, where metabolites are reabsorbed by active transport. It is well vascularized. The medulla, which reabsorbs ions from the loops of Henle, has a lower ATP requirement, and a much smaller blood supply. Which tissue utilizes anaerobic glycolysis?

The laboratory values for the blood drawn from **Lopa Fusor** in the emergency room were: hemoglobin (Hb), 5.6 g/dL (reference range = 12–16); hematocrit (Hct), 17% (reference range = 36–46 for a female); arterial pH, 7.18 (reference range = 7.35–7.45); pO₂, 51 mm Hg (reference range = 83–100); pCO₂, 65 mm Hg (reference range = 36–48); oxygen saturation, 51% (reference range = 95–99); and plasma lactate, 5.6 mM (reference range = 0.4–1.8). Lopa Fusor has a lactic acidosis. The other laboratory values provide clues to the cause of her problem (see Clinical Comments).

Lactic acidosis, the accumulation of lactic acid in the blood to levels that significantly affect the pH, results from production of lactate in excess of its metabolism. This pathological state (lactate levels greater than 5 mM and a decrease of blood pH below 7.2) results from such metabolic problems as: (a) impaired oxidation of pyruvate via pyruvate dehydrogenase and the TCA cycle—usually related to an inability to reoxidize NADH in the electron transport chain at adequate rates (e.g., MERRF, see Chapter 20); (b) excessive NADH production (e.g., ethanol intoxication) (see Chapter 27); (c) pyruvate carboxylase deficiency; (d) impaired pyruvate dehydrogenase activity, e.g., severe thiamine deficiency (see Chapter 19); (e) inhibition of lactate utilization for gluconeogenesis (e.g., hereditary fructose intolerance); (f) and enhanced glycolysis promoted by the blockage of another pathway (e.g., glucose 6-phosphatase deficiency). In the absence of disease, elevated lactate levels in the blood are associated with anaerobic glycolysis during exercise.

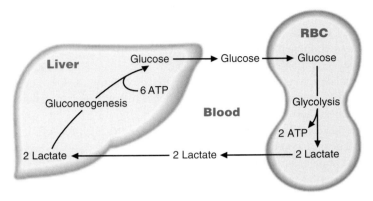

Fig. 22.13. Cori cycle. Glucose, produced in the liver by gluconeogenesis, is converted via glycolysis in red blood cells (or exercising muscle cells) to lactate. Lactate returns to the liver and is reconverted to glucose by gluconeogenesis.

sponds to its rate of utilization. The allosteric activation of PFK-1 by AMP and its inhibition by ATP is a type of feedback regulation in which ATP is controlling its own rate of synthesis. PFK-1 is the rate-limiting step in the glycolytic pathway, and thus regulation of PFK-1 changes flux through the entire pathway. AMP, an allosteric activator of PFK-1, is a sensitive indicator of the rate of ATP utilization.

The AMP levels within the cytosol provide a better indicator of the rate of ATP utilization than the ATP concentration itself (Fig. 22.14). The concentration of AMP in the cytosol is determined by the equilibrium position of the adenylate kinase reaction.

adenylate kinase

$$2 \text{ ADP} \longleftrightarrow \text{AMP} + \text{ATP}$$

The equilibrium is such that hydrolysis of ATP to ADP in energy-requiring reactions increases both the ADP and AMP contents of the cytosol. However, ATP is present in much higher quantities than AMP or ADP, so that a small decrease of ATP concentration in the cytosol causes a much larger percentage increase in the small AMP pool. In skeletal muscles, for instance, ATP levels are between 5 and 10 mM, and decrease by no more than 20% during strenuous exercise (see Fig. 22.14). At the same time ADP levels may increase by 50%, and AMP levels, which are in the micromolar range, increase by 300%.

The allosteric activation of PFK-1 by AMP is shown in Figure 22.15. Allosteric activators, which bind at a site separate from the catalytic site, change the conformation at the active site. The binding of AMP increases the affinity of the enzyme for fructose-6-P, so that the velocity of the reaction is much greater at low fructose-6-P concentrations, and a small change of AMP concentration in the critical range causes a large increase in velocity. The effect of ATP on PFK-1 is biphasic because there are two ATP binding sites: the substrate binding site and the allosteric binding site. At low concentrations of ATP, an increase of ATP will increase the velocity of PFK-1 because ATP is acting as a substrate and binding at the catalytic site. Under physiological conditions in the cell, the ATP concentration is always higher than this range, and the substrate binding site is saturated. Thus, in the cell, increases of ATP concentration decrease flux through PFK-1 by increasing the allosteric inhibition. The inhibition by ATP is opposed by the binding of AMP at the AMP allosteric activation site (Fig. 22.15).

In most tissues, the regulation of PFK-1 contributes to regulation of the rate of glucose phosphorylation by hexokinase (Fig. 22.16). The hexokinases found in almost all tissues (with the exception of liver and pancreatic B cells) are product-inhibited by glucose 6-phosphate at the concentrations found in the cell. As flux through PFK-1 decreases, fructose 6-phosphate and glucose 6-phosphate accumulate, and glucose 6-phosphate inhibits hexokinase. Glucose 6-phosphate is also the substrate for glycogen synthesis and other pathways of glucose metabolism, and the rate at which glucose 6-phosphate is used in these pathways also affects the rate of hexokinase.

PFK-1 is allosterically inhibited by citrate. The inhibition by citrate may play a role in decreasing glycolytic flux in the heart during the oxidation of fatty acids. However, citrate levels in the liver and human skeletal muscle are decreased under conditions in which fatty acid oxidation is elevated, so that the physiological role of this regulation is uncertain.

Other Regulators of Glycolysis

Fructose 2,6-bisphosphate is an important regulator of PFK-1 in liver and adipose tissue, where it mediates the effects of insulin and glucagon on the glycolytic pathway. The concentration of fructose 2,6-bisphosphate is increased under conditions which increase the insulin/glucagon ratio, and this compound, like AMP, acts as an allosteric

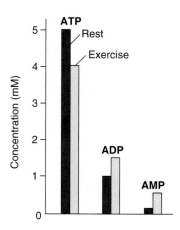

Fig. 22.14. Changes in ATP, ADP, and AMP concentrations in skeletal muscle during exercise. The concentration of ATP decreases by only about 20% during exercise, and the concentration of ADP rises. The concentration of AMP, produced by the adenylate kinase reaction, increases manyfold and serves as a sensitive indicator of decreasing ATP levels.

During **William Hartman's** myocardial infarction (see Chapter 20), his heart had a limited supply of oxygen and blood-borne fuels. The absence of oxygen for oxidative phosphorylation would decrease the levels of ATP and increase those of AMP, an activator of PFK-1. Acceleration of glycolysis could provide more ATP, but with low levels of oxygen, glucose would be converted to lactate, causing a decrease of intracellular pH. At very low pH levels, PFK-1 is inhibited, further decreasing the rate at which ATP can be generated.

A 22.2: The kidney cortex has high ATP demands, a good oxygen supply through the blood, a high mitochondrial content, and oxidizes glucose completely to CO_2. The kidney medulla relies principally on anaerobic glycolysis to meet its much smaller ATP demand. Both its oxygen supply and its mitochondrial content are much lower than those of the cortex.

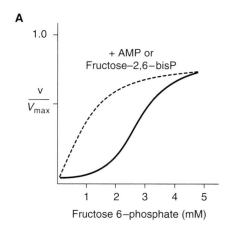

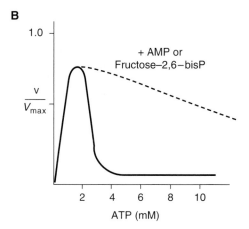

Fig. 22.15. Regulation of PFK-1 by AMP and ATP. **A.** AMP and fructose 2,6-bisphosphate activate PFK-1. **B.** ATP increases the rate of the reaction at low concentrations, but allosterically inhibits the enzyme at high concentrations.

22.3: How do the principles of regulation (see Table 19.2) apply to the glycolytic pathway?

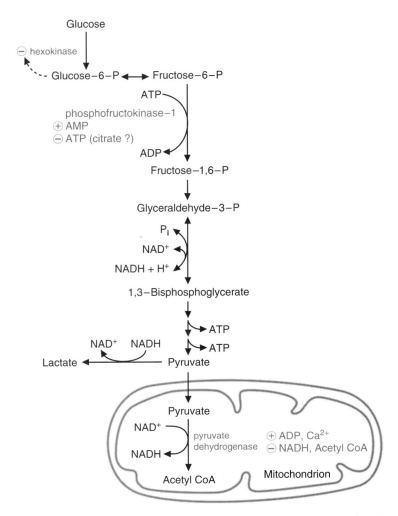

Fig. 22.16. Major sites of regulation in the glycolytic pathway. Hexokinase and phosphofructo-kinase-1 are the major regulatory enzymes in skeletal muscle. The activity of pyruvate dehydrogenase in the mitochondrion determines whether pyruvate is converted to lactate or to acetyl CoA.

activator (see Fig. 22.15). In these tissues, glycolysis functions as a source of carbon for the synthesis of fatty acids and glycerol 3-phosphate, precursors for triacylglycerol formation. In liver, biosynthetic processes, such as plasma protein synthesis, are also stimulated by insulin. Thus the need for ATP production from the glycolytic pathway coincides with the other roles of glycolysis, and AMP and fructose 2,6-bisphosphate provide a complementary activation. During fasting, when fructose 2,6-bisphosphate levels decrease, the glycolytic pathway is inhibited and the gluconeogenic pathway is activated.

The regulation of glycolysis in various tissues is coordinated with the regulation of glycogen metabolism, pyruvate oxidation in the TCA cycle, gluconeogenesis, fatty acid synthesis, and other pathways. The regulation of glycolysis in liver is covered in more detail in Chapter 27.

CLINICAL COMMENTS. **Thomas Appleman** had two sites of dental caries: one was on a smooth surface, and the other was in a fissure. Fissure decay is thought to be caused principally by the decreased pH resulting from lactic acid production by lactobacilli. *S. mutans* plays a major role in smooth surface caries because it secretes dextran, an insoluble polysaccharide, which forms the base for plaque.

S. mutans contains dextran-sucrase, a glucosyltransferase that transfers glucosyl units from dietary sucrose (the glucose-fructose disaccharide in sugar and sweets) to form the (1→6) and (1→3) linkages between the glucosyl units in dextran (Fig. 22.17). Dextran-sucrase is specific for sucrose and does not catalyze the polymerization of free glucose, or glucose from other disaccharides or polysaccharides. Thus sucrose is responsible for the cariogenic potential of candy. The sticky water-insoluble dextran mediates the attachment of *S. mutans* and other bacteria to the tooth surface. Fructose from sucrose is converted to intermediates of glycolysis and is rapidly metabolized to lactic acid. The decrease in pH that results initiates demineralization of the hydroxyapatite of the tooth enamel.

Lopa Fusor was admitted to the emergency room with a lactic acidosis. Her plasma lactic acid level was elevated and her arterial pH was low. The underlying mechanism for Ms. Fusor's derangement in acid-base balance is a severe reduction in the amount of oxygen delivered to her tissues for cellular respiration (hypoxia). Several concurrent processes contributed to this oxygen lack. The first was her severely reduced blood pressure caused by a brisk hemorrhage from a bleeding gastric ulcer. The blood loss led to hypoperfusion and, therefore, reduced delivery of oxygen to her

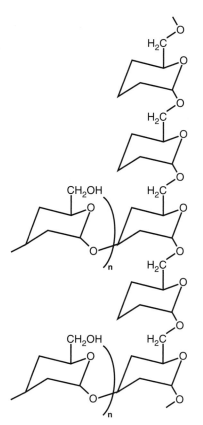

Fig. 22.17. General structure of dextran. Glucosyl residues are linked by α-1,3, α-1,6, and some α-1,4 bonds.

A 22.3: 1. Regulation by AMP and ATP corresponds to the function of glycolysis, the generation of ATP.
2. Additional regulators match the additional functions of glycolysis in cells, such as those in liver and adipose tissue.
3. PFK-1 is the major regulatory enzyme. A regulated enzyme usually catalyzes the slowest step in a pathway. Although phosphoglucoisomerase catalyzes an earlier step in glycolysis, the reaction is not slow and is freely reversible. Inhibition at PFK-1 decreases the concentration of substrates for the remainder of the pathway.
4. ATP is the necessary product of the pathway, both the ATP generated by substrate level phosphorylation and from oxidative phosphorylation. ATP feeds back to control its own rate of synthesis, both directly and through AMP.
5. Small changes of AMP generate large changes in flux.

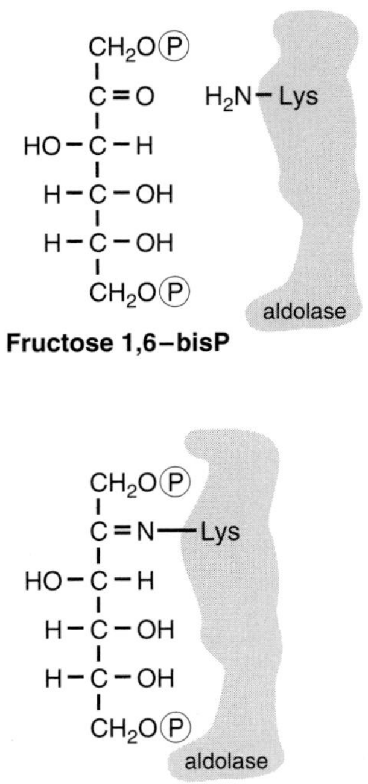

Fig. 22.18. Aldolase-fructose 1,6-bisphosphate complex. The substrate covalently binds to the enzyme by forming a Schiff base with a lysine residue.

tissues. The marked reduction in the number of red blood cells in her circulation caused by blood loss further compromised oxygen delivery. The preexisting chronic obstructive pulmonary disease (COPD) added to her hypoxia by reducing her capacity to extract oxygen from the inspired air and transfer it to the arterial blood (low pO_2). In addition, her COPD led to a retention of carbon dioxide (high pCO_2), which caused a respiratory acidosis because the retained CO_2 interacted with water to form carbonic acid (H_2CO_3).

Processes such as hypoxia, which impair cell respiration, lead to an accumulation of lactate. Hypoxic cells regenerate cytosolic NAD^+ by reducing pyruvate to lactate, a process which can result in lactic acidosis.

BIOCHEMICAL COMMENTS. **Enzymes of Glycolysis.** The reactions catalyzed by aldolase and glyceraldehyde 3-phosphate dehydrogenase provide examples of formation of covalent bonds between the substrate and the enzyme which contribute to the catalytic efficiency of the enzyme. With aldolase, the covalent bond is in the form of a Schiff base between the keto group of the substrate and the $\in$-amino group of a lysine residue in the active site of the enzyme (Fig. 22.18). Formation of the covalent bond, as with other types of substrate bonding, positions and orients the substrate in the active site and stabilizes the transition state. The Schiff base also participates in the aldol cleavage and condensation reactions. Transaldolase, an enzyme in the pentose phosphate pathway, operates by a similar reaction mechanism.

In the oxidation and phosphorylation catalyzed by glyceraldehyde 3-phosphate dehydrogenase, a thiohemiacetal is formed between the aldehyde carbon on glyceraldehyde 3-phosphate and the sulfhydryl group of a cysteine in the active site (Fig. 22.19). The cysteines within the active site are extremely reactive. Enzyme activity is lost if they are oxidized by O_2 or if they are complexed with heavy metals, such as the mercury found in organic mercurials.

Tissue-Specific Isozymes. The enzymes of the glycolytic pathway are common to all tissues. However, many of the enzymes exist as tissue-specific isoenzymes with differences in amino acid composition between the forms found in different tissues. Hexokinase, for instance, exists as at least four different isozymes. Of these isozymes, only one, the form found in liver and pancreas, has properties which are very different from the others. Aldolase has at least three isoenzymes, aldolase A, present in muscle and most tissues, aldolase B, present in liver, and aldolase C, present in brain. Only aldolase B catalyzes the cleavage of fructose 1-phosphate at significant rates. Lactate dehydrogenase differs in skeletal muscle and heart, containing 4 M and 4 H subunits, respectively. Liver has a form composed of 2 M and 2 H subunits. (M represents skeletal muscle type subunits, and H, heart type.) Glyceraldehyde 3-phosphate dehydrogenase and phosphoglucomutase also have tissue-specific isoforms.

For some glycolytic enzymes, the isoforms do not appear to differ significantly in their kinetic properties in a way that can be related to tissue function. The properties of the regulatory enzymes, however, do differ in different tissues. Liver hepatic pyruvate kinase, for instance, is allosterically inhibited by alanine, so that alanine influx during fasting inhibits glycolysis and stimulates the gluconeogenic pathway. The existence of tissue-specific isoforms also permits genetic mutations to affect the activity in one tissue without affecting all tissues.

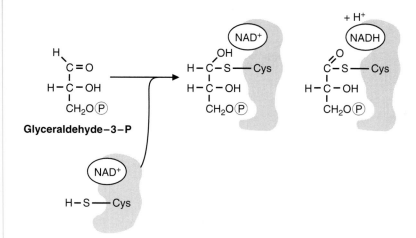

Fig. 22.19. Role of cysteine in the formation of a covalent intermediate in the glyceraldehyde 3-phosphate dehydrogenase reaction.

Suggested Reading

Cole AS, Eastoe JE. Biochemistry and oral biology. 2nd ed. Boston: Butterworth, 1988:490–519.

Newsholme EA, Leech AR. Biochemistry for the medical sciences. New York: John Wiley & Sons, 1983:178–235.

PROBLEMS

1. Why does exercise training cause muscles to produce less lactate than untrained muscles produce for the same amount of exercise?

2. A deficiency of the isozyme of pyruvate kinase found in red blood cells results in a hemolytic anemia. Predict the biochemical consequences of this enzyme deficiency.

ANSWERS

1. Endurance training causes the number of mitochondria, the capacity of the mitochondrial enzymes, and the content of myoglobin to increase in the exercised muscles. Therefore, a trained muscle converts less glucose to lactate and more to CO_2 and H_2O than an untrained muscle.

2. Pyruvate kinase is a key enzyme in glycolysis. It catalyzes the final step and is one of the two enzymes that produce ATP. A deficiency in red blood cells causes accumulation of the intermediates of glycolysis including 2,3-BPG. Elevated levels of 2,3-BPG decrease the affinity of hemoglobin for oxygen, and partially compensate for the decreased oxygen-carrying capacity of blood due to the decreased number of red blood cells. The number of red blood cells decreases because decreased ATP production affects the cation pumps in the cell membrane. Ca^{2+} enters cells, while K^+ and H_2O leave. The cells become dehydrated and are phagocytosed by cells in the spleen. As the number of red blood cells decreases, the number of reticulocytes increases. The reticulocytes develop into new red blood cells.

23 Generation of ATP from Fatty Acids and Ketone Bodies

Fatty acid oxidation is the major source of energy for ATP synthesis in the human. Fatty acids are oxidized mainly in mitochondria by a process known as β-oxidation. This process generates acetyl CoA and energy in the form of ATP. Oxidation of the acetyl CoA in the tricarboxylic acid (TCA) cycle produces additional ATP. Tissues, such as muscle, oxidize fatty acids to CO_2 and H_2O. However, fatty acids are not a significant source of fuel for the brain and other nervous tissue, and they cannot be utilized by red blood cells, which have no mitochondria.

The liver obtains energy from β-oxidation of fatty acids, but, in this tissue, much of the acetyl CoA is converted within mitochondria to the ketone bodies acetoacetate and β-hydroxybutyrate, which are released into the blood. A small amount of acetone is also produced by spontaneous decarboxylation of acetoacetate.

Ketone bodies serve as fuels for tissues such as muscle and kidney. They also are used by the brain and other nervous tissue, but only when the concentration in the blood is elevated (after 3–5 days of starvation). Liver does not use ketone bodies because it does not produce the enzyme for their activation. Red blood cells cannot oxidize ketone bodies because they lack mitochondria.

Tissues oxidize fatty acids whenever their concentration increases in the blood. Fatty acids are the predominant fuel during fasting when they are released from adipose triacylglycerols. The need for energy in the form of ATP controls the rate of fatty acid oxidation.

After fatty acids enter cells, they are activated by conversion to their CoA derivatives. Activation of long chain fatty acids (containing 12 or more carbons) occurs on the outer mitochondrial membrane and other cytoplasmic membranes. Long chain fatty acids cross the inner mitochondrial membrane on a carnitine carrier. Because long chain fatty acids predominate in the body, inhibition of this carrier system serves as a mechanism for regulating fatty acid oxidation and ketone body synthesis. Malonyl CoA, a key intermediate in fatty acid synthesis, inhibits the carnitine acyltransferase that attaches the fatty acyl group to the carnitine carrier.

Fatty acids that are saturated or unsaturated and that contain an even or an odd number of carbon atoms (even chain or odd chain fatty acids) can undergo β-oxidation. The 3 carbons at the ω-end of an odd chain fatty acid produce propionyl CoA.

Although β-oxidation is the major process for obtaining energy from fatty acids, α-, ω-, and peroxisomal oxidation also occur. In α-oxidation, one-carbon units are released from the carboxyl end as CO_2. In ω-oxidation, the ω-carbon is oxidized to a carboxyl group. Peroxisomal fatty acid oxidation is similar to mitochondrial β-oxidation except that it directly uses molecular oxygen and does not produce ATP via the electron transport chain.

Al Martini was found lying semiconscious at the bottom of the stairs by his landlady when she returned from an overnight visit with friends. His face had multiple bruises and his right forearm was grotesquely angulated. Nonbloody dried vomitus stained his clothing. Mr. Martini was rushed by ambulance to the emergency room at the nearest hospital. In addition to multiple bruises and the compound fracture of his right forearm, he had deep and rapid (Kussmaul) respirations and was moderately dehydrated.

Initial laboratory studies showed a relatively large anion gap of 34 (reference range = 9–15). The anion gap is calculated by subtracting the sum of the value for serum chloride and for the serum CO_2 content from the serum sodium concentration. If the gap is greater than normal, it suggests that anions such as ketone bodies are present in the blood in increased amounts. An arterial blood gas analysis confirmed the presence of a metabolic acidosis. Mr. Martini's blood alcohol level was only slightly elevated. His serum glucose was 68 mg/dL (low normal).

The admitting physician suspected an alcohol-induced ketoacidosis superimposed on a starvation ketoacidosis and requested β-hydroxybutyrate levels. Although the urinary test for acetone was negative, the plasma free fatty acid level was elevated and the β-hydroxybutyrate concentration was 40 times the upper limit of normal.

Rehydration with intravenous fluids containing glucose and potassium was initiated. His initial potassium was low, possibly secondary to vomiting. An orthopedic surgeon was consulted regarding the compound fracture of his right forearm.

Lofata Burne is a 16-year-old female who since age 14 months has experienced recurrent episodes of profound fatigue associated with vomiting and increased perspiration, which usually occurred after an overnight fast. During more severe episodes, she had to be admitted to the hospital where she improved within hours of initiating an intravenous infusion of glucose.

These episodes occurred only if she fasted for more than 8 hours. Because her mother gave her food late at night and woke her early in the morning for breakfast, Lofata's physical and mental development had progressed normally. On the day of admission, she had missed breakfast and by noon became extremely fatigued, nauseated, sweaty, and limp. She was unable to hold any food in her stomach and was rushed to the hospital where an infusion of glucose was started intravenously. Her symptoms responded dramatically to this therapy.

Her initial serum glucose level was low at 38 mg/dL (reference range = 80–100). Her blood urea nitrogen (BUN) level was slightly elevated at 26 mg/dL (reference range = 8–25) as a result of vomiting which led to a degree of dehydration. Her blood levels of liver transaminases (AST, formerly called SGOT, and ALT, formerly called SGPT) were slightly elevated although her liver was not palpably enlarged. There was evidence of decreased ketogenesis (0.3 mM β-hydroxybutyrate) despite elevated levels of free fatty acids (4.3 mM) in the blood.

FATTY ACIDS AS FUELS

The body oxidizes more fatty acids each day than any other fuel (Table 23.1). Fatty acids are derived from the diet or synthesized mainly in the liver from glucose. The sets of enzymes that act on the fatty acids and the location of the pathways for fatty acid metabolism differ depending on the number of carbons in the fatty acid chain. The fatty acids are divided into four groups: short chain with 2 or 3 carbons (acetate and propionate), medium chain with 4–12 carbons, long chain with 12–20 carbons, and very long chain with more than 20 carbons (Table 23.2). Long chain fatty acids with 14–20 carbons predominate in the body. (See Chapter 6 for nomenclature of fatty acids.)

Table 23.1. Turnover of Fuels in Blood[a]

Fuel	Amount in the Circulation (blood, extracellular fluid)		Amount Used (12 hr, basal state)	
	g	Cal	g	Cal
Fatty acids	0.3	3	60	540
Glucose	20	80	70	280
Amino acids	0.3	1	20	80

[a]Fatty acids are the major fuel in the human; 540 calories are used in a 12-hr period in the basal state versus 280 calories of glucose or 80 calories of amino acids. There are only 3 calories of fatty acids in the blood at any given time. Therefore, fatty acids must constantly be released from triacylglycerols to provide the 540 calories required. Thus, fatty acids in the blood "turn over" (i.e, are replaced by being released from triacylglycerols) 540/3 or 180 times during 12 hours in the basal state. Glucose turns over 280/80 or 3.5 times, and amino acids turn over 80/1 or 80 times in the 12-hr period. So, although there is more glucose than fatty acids in the blood at any given time, the glucose is not used and replaced as rapidly as the fatty acids. The glucose does not turn over as rapidly as the fatty acids. (These calories are nutritional calories, i.e., kcal.)

Table 23.2. Size Classes of Fatty Acids

Class	Chain Length (no. carbons)
Short chain	2–3
Medium chain	4–12
Long chain	12–20
Very long chain	More than 20

Because of their hydrophobicity, fatty acids with more than about 4 carbons are usually bound to proteins. They travel in the blood complexed with albumin, the major serum protein, and when they enter cells they form complexes with fatty acid binding proteins.

ACTIVATION OF FATTY ACIDS

Fatty acids must be activated before they can be oxidized (Fig. 23.1). The process of activation involves an acyl CoA synthetase (also called a thiokinase) that utilizes ATP to produce a high energy fatty acyl-AMP and pyrophosphate. Cleavage of the pyrophosphate produces energy that helps to drive the reaction. The AMP attached to the fatty acyl group is exchanged for coenzyme A (CoA), a fatty acyl CoA is formed, and AMP is released. Overall, the activation process consumes two high energy phosphate bonds, one in the formation of the fatty acyl-AMP and the second in the cleavage of pyrophosphate.

Short chain acids (2–3 carbons in length, including acetate and propionate) may be activated in the cytosol or in mitochondria. Medium chain fatty acids (4–12 carbons in length) cross the mitochondrial membrane and are activated in the matrix. The long chain fatty acids, 12 or more carbons in length, which predominate in the body, are activated by enzymes in the endoplasmic reticulum, the outer mitochondrial membrane, and peroxisomal membranes. After activation, long chain fatty acids destined for β-oxidation travel on the carnitine carrier system into mitochondria where the enzymes for β-oxidation are located.

Acetate, produced by oxidation of ethanol or ingested as vinegar, is activated, forming acetyl CoA.

TRANSPORT OF LONG CHAIN FATTY ACYL CoA INTO MITOCHONDRIA

Carnitine serves as the carrier that transports the long chain fatty acyl groups across the inner mitochondrial membrane (Fig. 23.2). Carnitine is obtained from the diet or

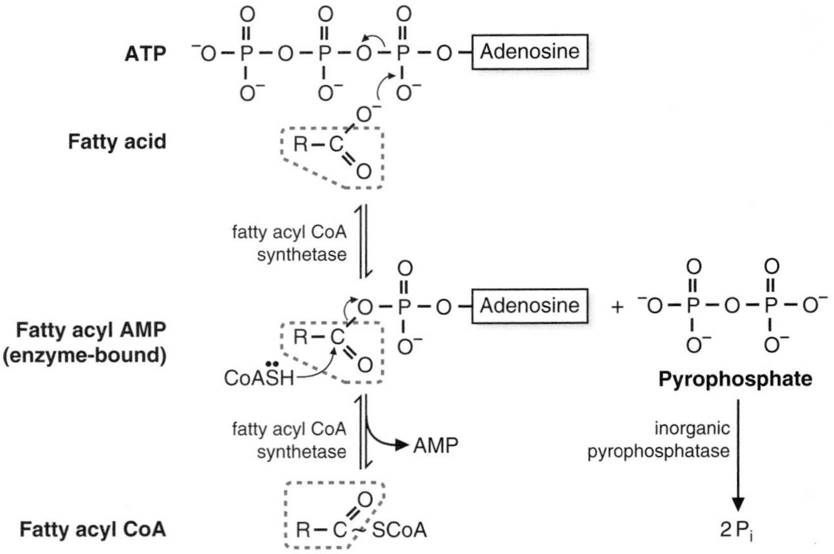

Fig. 23.2. Structure of carnitine.

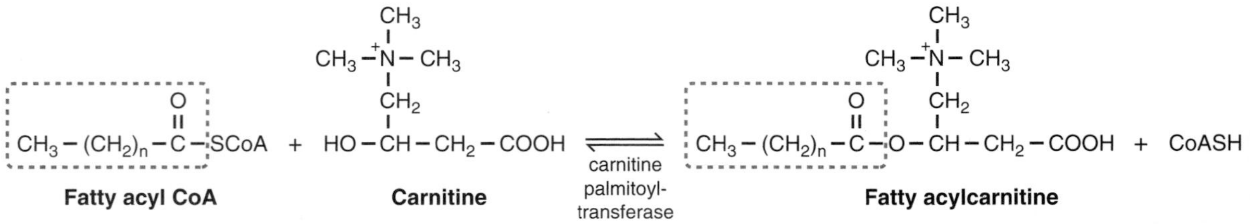

Fig. 23.1. Activation of a fatty acid. The fatty acid is activated by reacting with ATP to form a high energy fatty acyl AMP and pyrophosphate. The AMP is then exchanged for CoA. These reactions are catalyzed by fatty acyl CoA synthetase (also called fatty acid thiokinase). Pyrophosphate is cleaved by a pyrophosphatase.

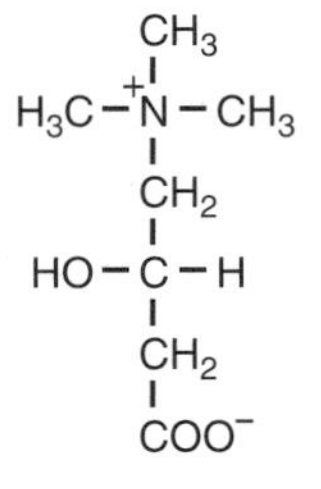

Fig. 23.3. Formation of fatty acylcarnitine. In the forward direction, the reaction, catalyzed by carnitine:palmitoyltransferase I (CPTI), occurs on the outer mitochondrial membrane. In the reverse direction, the reaction is catalyzed by carnitine:palmitoyltransferase II (CPTII) and occurs on the inner mitochondrial membrane. The enzymes, also called carnitine:acyltransferases I and II, act only on long chain fatty acids.

synthesized from the amino acid lysine by reactions that include the transfer of methyl groups from *S*-adenosylmethionine and oxidation reactions that require vitamin C (ascorbate).

An enzyme associated with the outer mitochondrial membrane, carnitine:palmitoyltransferase I (CPTI, also called carnitine:acyltransferase I) catalyzes the transfer of the fatty acyl group from CoA to carnitine (Fig. 23.3). Malonyl CoA, an intermediate in fatty acid synthesis, inhibits this enzyme (see Chapter 33). Therefore, newly synthesized long chain fatty acids are not immediately transported into mitochondria for oxidation.

Fatty acylcarnitine crosses the inner mitochondrial membrane with the aid of a translocase. The fatty acyl group is transferred back to CoA by a second enzyme, carnitine:palmitoyltransferase II (CPTII, or carnitine:acyltransferase II). Carnitine, released in this reaction, returns to the cytosolic side of the mitochondrial membrane by the same translocase that brings fatty acylcarnitine to the matrix side (Fig. 23.4). Long chain fatty acyl CoA, now located within the mitochondrial matrix, is a substrate for β-oxidation.

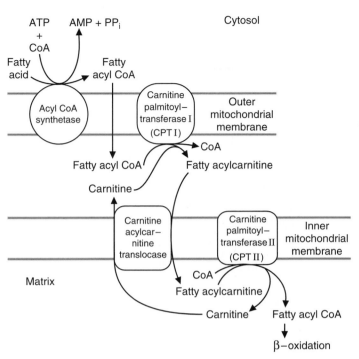

 The process for mitochondrial oxidation of fatty acids is called β-oxidation because all the reactions involve the β-carbon.

Fig. 23.4. Transport of long chain fatty acids into mitochondria. After activation, the fatty acyl CoA crosses the outer mitochondrial membrane and reacts with carnitine to form a fatty acylcarnitine. This compound is translocated into the mitochondrial matrix as carnitine moves out. The fatty acyl group is then transferred back to CoA.

OXIDATION OF FATTY ACIDS

β-Oxidation of Fatty Acids

The first three of the four steps of β-oxidation are similar to those in the TCA cycle between succinate and oxaloacetate. The four steps, which produce FAD(2H), NADH, and acetyl CoA, are repeated until all the carbons of a linear even chain fatty acyl CoA are converted to acetyl CoA. Each set of reactions results in the shortening of the chain by 2 carbon atoms, which are released as acetyl CoA. Thus, β-oxidation can be viewed as a spiral of reactions that remove 2 carbons at a time from the fatty acyl chain (Fig. 23.5).

In the first step, as 2 hydrogens with their electrons are transferred to an enzyme-bound FAD, a double bond in the *trans* configuration forms between the α- and β-carbons (a Δ^2-*trans* double bond), and the fatty acyl chain becomes an enoyl CoA (Fig. 23.6). The enzyme-bound FAD(2H), produced by this reaction, transfers the electrons to electron transfer flavoproteins (ETF) that pass them through iron-sulfur centers to coenzyme Q in the electron transport chain. This electron transfer, therefore, produces ATP by the process of oxidative phosphorylation. Every FAD(2H) that is reoxidized by the electron transport chain generates approximately 2 ATP.

In the next step, H_2O adds across the double bond in a reaction catalyzed by an enoyl hydratase. The β-hydroxyacyl CoA which forms is then oxidized by NAD^+ to a β-ketoacyl CoA by a β-hydroxyacyl CoA dehydrogenase. Oxidation via the electron transport chain of the NADH produced by this reaction generates approximately 3 ATP.

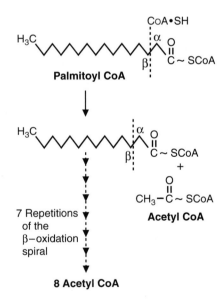

Fig. 23.5. Overall process of β-oxidation. Oxidation at the β-carbon is followed by cleavage of the α—β bond, which forms acetyl CoA and a fatty acyl CoA that is 2 carbons shorter than the original. Successive spirals of β-oxidation completely cleave an even chain fatty acyl CoA to acetyl CoA. The dashed line indicates the bond that is cleaved.

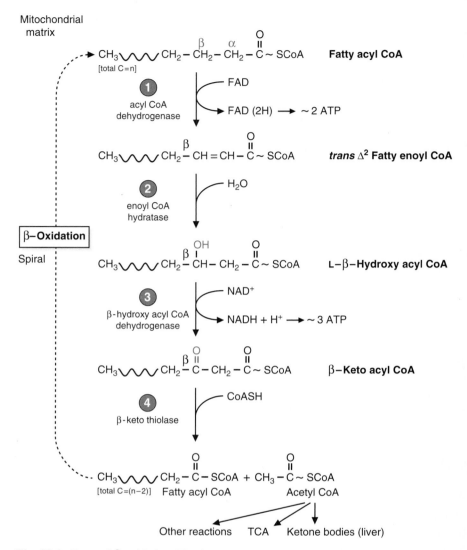

Fig. 23.6. Steps of β-oxidation. The four steps are repeated until an even chain fatty acid is completely converted to acetyl CoA. The FAD(2H) and NADH are reoxidized by the electron transport chain, producing ATP. Note that the first three steps are similar to those in the TCA cycle which convert succinate to oxaloacetate.

In the last reaction of the sequence, the bond between the α- and β-carbons is cleaved by a thiolytic reaction catalyzed by β-ketothiolase, an enzyme that requires CoA. The release of 2 carbons from the carboxyl end of the original fatty acyl CoA produces acetyl CoA and a fatty acyl CoA that is 2 carbons shorter than the original.

The shortened fatty acyl CoA repeats these four steps until all of its carbons are converted to acetyl CoA. β-Oxidation is, thus, a spiral rather than a cycle. Although the steps are repeated, the substrate for each spiral is shorter by 2 carbons than the substrate for the previous spiral. In the last spiral, cleavage of the 4-carbon fatty acyl CoA (butyryl CoA) produces 2 acetyl CoA. Thus, an even chain fatty acid such as palmitoyl CoA, which has 16 carbons, is cleaved 7 times, producing 7 FAD(2H), 7 NADH, and 8 acetyl CoA. Approximately 14 ATP are generated by the FAD(2H), 21 by the NADH, and 96 by oxidation of the acetyl CoA in the TCA cycle.

A 16-carbon fatty acyl CoA, therefore, generates approximately 131 ATP. If activation, which consumes the equivalent of 2 ATP, is considered, the net energy yield is about 129 ATP.

Many tissues, such as muscle and kidney, oxidize fatty acids completely to CO_2 and H_2O. In these tissues, the acetyl CoA produced by β-oxidation enters the TCA cycle. The FAD(2H) and the NADH from β-oxidation and the TCA cycle are reoxidized by the electron transport chain and ATP is generated. The process of β-oxidation is regulated by the cells' requirements for energy, i.e., by the levels of ATP and NADH.

The four reactions of β-oxidation are catalyzed by sets of enzymes that are specific for fatty acids of different chain lengths. For example, the enzymes that catalyze the first reaction in the liver include a very long chain acyl CoA dehydrogenase (VLCAD) that acts on acyl chains that range in length from over 20 to 14 carbons, a long chain acyl CoA dehydrogenase (LCAD) that acts on chains from 18 to 12 carbons long, a medium chain acyl CoA dehydrogenase (MCAD) that acts on chains from 12 to 4 carbons long, and a short chain acyl CoA dehydrogenase (SCAD) that acts only on 6- and 4-carbon chains. Although these enzymes are structurally distinct, their specificity overlaps to some extent. As the fatty acyl chains are shortened by β-oxidation, they are probably transferred from enzymes that act on longer chains to those that act on shorter chains.

Tissues that lack mitochondria, such as red blood cells, cannot oxidize fatty acids by β-oxidation. Fatty acids also do not serve as a significant fuel for the brain and other nervous tissue.

OXIDATION OF ODD CHAIN FATTY ACIDS

Fatty acids containing an odd number of carbon atoms undergo β-oxidation, producing acetyl CoA, until the last spiral, when 5 carbons remain in the fatty acyl CoA. In this case, cleavage by thiolase produces acetyl CoA and a 3-carbon fatty acyl CoA, propionyl CoA (Fig. 23.7).

Carboxylation of propionyl CoA yields methylmalonyl CoA, which is converted to succinyl CoA, an intermediate of the TCA cycle (Fig. 23.8). These 3 carbons at the ω-end of an odd chain fatty acid, therefore, can form glucose in the liver via the process of gluconeogenesis (see Chapter 27). No other fatty acid carbons can produce significant amounts of glucose because the other carbons form acetyl CoA. Acetyl CoA cannot form pyruvate, a substrate for gluconeogenesis, because pyruvate dehydrogenase is physiologically irreversible. As the 2 carbons of acetyl CoA traverse the TCA cycle, 2 carbons are lost as CO_2. Therefore, although malate, which can be converted to glucose, is formed in the TCA cycle, no *net* production of malate (and, thus, of glucose) occurs from acetyl CoA.

OXIDATION OF UNSATURATED FATTY ACIDS

About one half of the fatty acids in humans are unsaturated. The double bonds of these fatty acids must be moved into the proper positions so that β-oxidation can occur. This process requires two enzymes, an isomerase and a reductase, in addition to the enzymes that catalyze the four reactions of the β-oxidation spiral.

β-Oxidation of a monounsaturated fatty acid occurs until the double bond is between carbons 3 and 4 near the carboxyl end of the fatty acyl chain. An isomerase moves the double bond so that it is between the α- and β-carbons (carbons 2 and 3) in a *trans* configuration (Fig. 23.9). Then β-oxidation resumes, but at the second step because a Δ^2,*trans* double bond is already present.

A research scientist in the metabolism section at the nearby university hospital was notified of **Lofata Burne's** admission. After reviewing Lofata's previous hospital records, she suspected that a disorder in fatty acid metabolism was the cause of Lofata's medical problems. The researcher performed a battery of special analyses on Lofata's urine and blood.

A urine specimen showed an increase in organic acid metabolites of medium chain fatty acids containing from 6 to 10 carbons and increased levels of dicarboxylic acids. The profile of acylcarnitine species in the urine was characteristic of a genetically determined medium chain acyl CoA dehydrogenase (MCAD) deficiency.

Lofata's blood contained elevated levels of several partially oxidized medium chain fatty acids, such as octanoic acid (8:0) and 4-decenoic acid (10:1,Δ4).

Finally, the specific enzyme deficiency was demonstrated in cultured fibroblasts from Lofata's skin as well as in her circulating monocytic leukocytes.

In LCAD deficiency, fatty acylcarnitines accumulate in the blood. Those containing 14 carbons predominate. In MCAD deficiency, shorter acylcarnitines that are 6 to 10 carbons in length accumulate. These shorter compounds can pass into the urine.

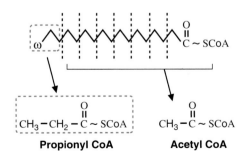

Fig. 23.7. Formation of propionyl CoA from odd chain fatty acids. Successive spirals of β-oxidation cleave each of the bonds marked with dashed lines, producing acetyl CoA except for the 3 carbons at the ω-end, which produce propionyl CoA.

Q 23.1: Calculate the amount of ATP produced when one molecule of oleic acid is oxidized to CO_2 and H_2O.

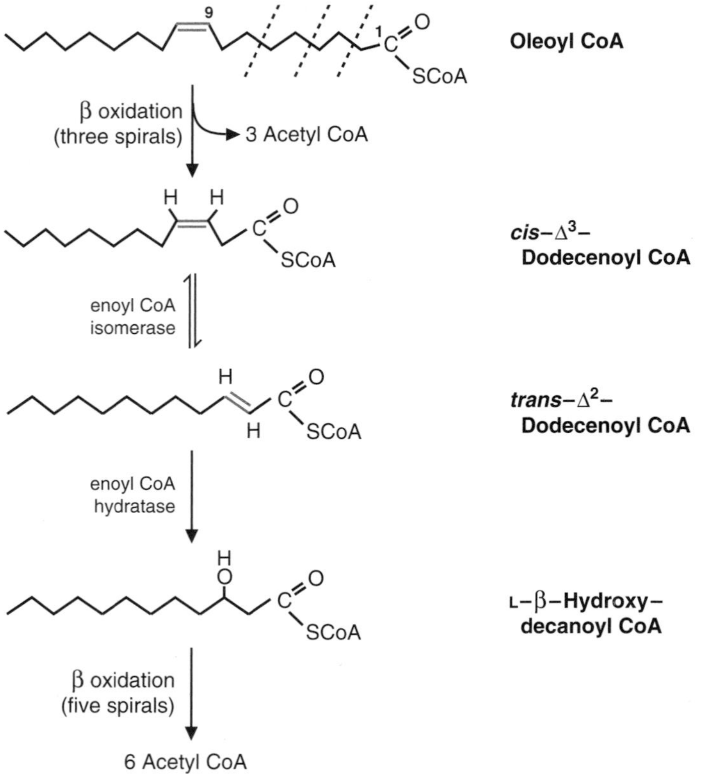

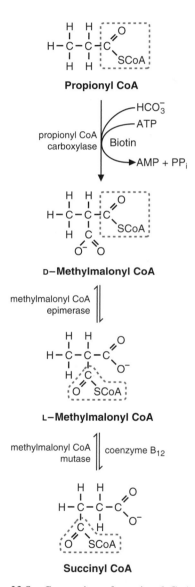

Propionyl CoA

propionyl CoA carboxylase

HCO_3^-
ATP
Biotin
$AMP + PP_i$

D−Methylmalonyl CoA

methylmalonyl CoA epimerase

L−Methylmalonyl CoA

methylmalonyl CoA mutase | coenzyme B_{12}

Succinyl CoA

Fig. 23.8. Conversion of propionyl CoA to succinyl CoA. Succinyl CoA, an intermediate of the TCA cycle, can form malate, which can be converted to glucose in the liver via the process of gluconeogenesis. Certain amino acids also form glucose by this route (see Chapter 39).

Oleoyl CoA

β oxidation (three spirals) → 3 Acetyl CoA

***cis*−Δ³−Dodecenoyl CoA**

enoyl CoA isomerase

***trans*−Δ²−Dodecenoyl CoA**

enoyl CoA hydratase

L−β−Hydroxydecanoyl CoA

β oxidation (five spirals)

6 Acetyl CoA

Fig. 23.9. Oxidation of a fatty acid with a single double bond. After three spirals of β-oxidation (dashed lines), the 3,4-*cis* double bond is isomerized to a 2,3-*trans* double bond, which is in the proper configuration for the normal enzymes of β-oxidation to act. β-Oxidation resumes at the second step, bypassing the first step, because a double bond in the appropriate configuration is already present.

Polyunsaturated fatty acids, such as linoleic acid (18:2,$\Delta^{9,12}$), undergo β-oxidation until one double bond is between carbons 3 and 4 and another is between carbons 6 and 7 (Fig. 23.10). The isomerase shifts the 3,4-double bond to a 2,3-*trans* position, and one spiral of β-oxidation occurs plus the first step of a second spiral. A reductase that uses NADPH now converts these two double bonds (between carbons 2 and 3 and carbons 4 and 5) to one double bond between carbons 3 and 4 in a *trans* configuration. The isomerase (which can act on double bonds that are in either the *cis* or the *trans* configuration) moves this double bond to the 2,3-*trans* position, and β-oxidation can resume.

Oxidation of Very Long Chain Fatty Acids in Peroxisomes

Very long chain fatty acids, which contain 20–26 carbons, are oxidized in peroxisomes by a process very similar to β-oxidation (Fig. 23.11). The first enzyme differs, however, in that it donates electrons directly to molecular oxygen and produces hydrogen peroxide (H_2O_2), which can generate oxygen free radicals (see Chapter 21). Catalase, an enzyme located in peroxisomes, converts H_2O_2 to water and molecular oxygen.

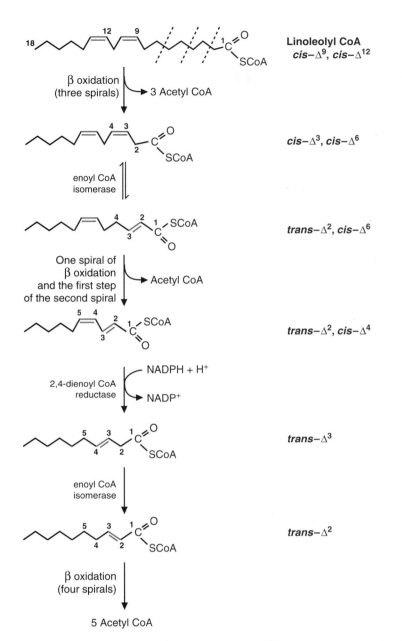

Fig. 23.10. Oxidation of a polyunsaturated fatty acid. In addition to an isomerase (see Fig. 23.9), a reductase is required to shift the double bonds so that β-oxidation can proceed.

Another difference between β- and peroxisomal oxidation is that the process in peroxisomes does not produce ATP by oxidative phosphorylation. The very long chain fatty acids are converted to octanoyl CoA, which contains 8 carbons in its fatty acyl chain. The acyl groups produced by peroxisomal oxidation (octanoyl CoA and acetyl CoA) are transferred to carnitine and transported into mitochondria, where they can undergo β-oxidation coupled to oxidative phosphorylation.

ω-Oxidation of Fatty Acids

Fatty acids may be oxidized at the ω-carbon of the chain by enzymes in the endoplasmic reticulum (Fig. 23.12). The ω-methyl group is first oxidized to an alcohol by

People with a rare inherited absence of peroxisomes (Zellweger's syndrome) accumulate very long chain fatty acids, particularly in the brain.

Clofibrate, a drug used to treat certain types of hyperlipoproteinemias (high blood lipid levels associated with heart attacks and strokes), stimulates the proliferation of peroxisomes and causes induction of the peroxisomal fatty acid oxidation system.

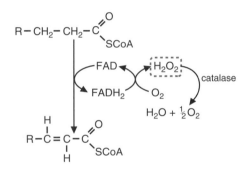

Fig. 23.11. Oxidation of fatty acids in peroxisomes. The first reaction is shown in which hydrogen peroxide (H_2O_2) is generated. H_2O_2 is converted to water and molecular oxygen by catalase, a peroxisomal enzyme. The remainder of the reactions are similar to those of β-oxidation.

A 23.1: Oleic acid ($18:1,\Delta^9$) undergoes eight cleavages, producing 9 acetyl CoA and 8 NADH. However, only 7 FAD(2H) are formed because a double bond is already present in oleic acid, which is moved into the appropriate trans position by an isomerase. Therefore, only 146 ATP are generated: 108 from the acetyl CoA, 24 from the NADH, and 14 from the FAD(2H). If 2 ATP are subtracted for activation, the total is 144 ATP.

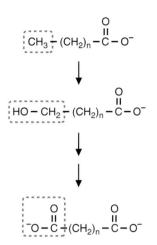

Fig. 23.12. ω-Oxidation of fatty acids. The methyl group at the ω-end is converted to a carboxyl group. Thus, a dicarboxylic acid is generated.

Normally, ω-oxidation is a minor process. However, in conditions that interfere with β-oxidation (such as a carnitine deficiency or a deficiency in an enzyme of β-oxidation), ω-oxidation produces dicarboxylic acids in increased amounts. These dicarboxylic acids are excreted in the urine.

Lofata Burne was excreting dicarboxylic acids in her urine, particularly adipic acid (which has 6 carbons) and suberic acid (which has 8 carbons).

$^-OOC-CH_2-CH_2-CH_2-CH_2-COO^-$ Adipic acid

$^-OOC-CH_2-CH_2-CH_2-CH_2-CH_2-COO^-$ Suberic acid

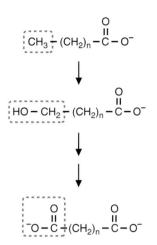

Fig. 23.14. Oxidation of phytanic acid. α-Oxidation removes the carbon at the carboxyl end of the fatty acid. Then β-oxidation at the dashed lines can produce propionyl CoA and acetyl CoA in alternate spirals.

In Refsum's disease, a rare neurological disorder, phytanic acid accumulates because of a defect in α-oxidation.

an enzyme that uses cytochrome P450, molecular oxygen, and NADPH. Dehydrogenases convert the alcohol group to an acid. The dicarboxylic acids produced by ω-oxidation undergo β-oxidation in mitochondria, forming compounds with 6–10 carbons, which are excreted in the urine.

α-Oxidation of Fatty Acids

Very long chain fatty acids may be oxidized by a process that involves the α-carbon. Oxidation of this carbon facilitates the release of the carboxyl group as CO_2 (Fig. 23.13). This process occurs mainly in brain and other nervous tissue and oxidizes fatty acids with 20 or more carbons, removing one carbon at a time.

A similar process is involved in the oxidation of branched chain fatty acids, such as phytanic acid, obtained from plants in the diet. Phytanic acid is produced by oxidation of phytol, a 20-carbon alcohol derived from chlorophyll. This 20-carbon acid, which contains a number of methyl groups, appears to be degraded in mitochondria by α-oxidation followed by spirals of β-oxidation that produce both propionyl CoA and acetyl CoA (Fig. 23.14).

METABOLISM OF KETONE BODIES

Synthesis of Ketone Bodies

The ketone bodies include acetoacetate, β-hydroxybutyrate (3-hydroxybutyrate), and acetone, which is a degradation product of acetoacetate. Ketone body synthesis occurs whenever fatty acid levels are elevated in the blood, that is, during fasting, starvation, or as a result of a high fat, low carbohydrate diet. The enzymes for ketone body synthesis are located mainly in liver mitochondria.

When blood fatty acid levels are elevated, fatty acids enter liver cells. Within liver mitochondria, the process of β-oxidation generates acetyl CoA, NADH, and ATP. Under these conditions (fasting or a high fat, low carbohydrate diet), the glucagon/insulin ratio is high, and the liver is synthesizing glucose by the process of gluconeogenesis. Pyruvate, produced from lactate or alanine, is converted to oxaloacetate, which leaves the mitochondrion either as aspartate or malate to participate in gluconeogenesis in the cytosol (see Chapter 27). The NADH produced by β-oxidation helps to drive oxaloacetate to malate. Less oxaloacetate is available for the reaction catalyzed by citrate synthase, and acetyl CoA accumulates.

Two molecules of acetyl CoA react to form acetoacetyl CoA by a reversal of the thiolase reaction (or by a reaction catalyzed by an isozyme of the thiolase of β-oxidation). Another acetyl CoA reacts with the acetoacetyl CoA, producing 3-hydroxy-3-methylglutaryl CoA (HMG-CoA) and releasing free, unacylated coenzyme A

Fig. 23.13. α-Oxidation of fatty acids. Oxidation occurs at the α-carbon (carbon 2). One carbon is removed from the carboxyl end of the fatty acid chain and released as CO_2. The remaining carbons of the fatty acid can repeat the process.

(CoASH). The enzyme that catalyzes this reaction is HMG-CoA synthetase. It is induced during fasting and inhibited by one of its products, CoASH. In the next reaction, HMG-CoA lyase catalyzes the cleavage of HMG-CoA to form acetyl CoA and acetoacetate (Fig. 23.15).

Acetoacetate has three fates (Fig. 23.16). It can directly enter the blood or it can be reduced by an NAD-dependent dehydrogenase to a second ketone body, β-hydroxybutyrate, which enters the blood. This dehydrogenase reaction is readily reversible and serves to interconvert these two ketone bodies, which both enter the blood and travel from the liver to other tissues where they are oxidized for energy. The third fate of acetoacetate is spontaneous decarboxylation, in which a nonenzymatic reaction releases CO_2 and produces acetone. Further metabolism of acetone does not readily occur. Because acetone is volatile, it is expired by the lungs.

The NADH/NAD$^+$ ratio determines the relative amounts of acetoacetate and β-hydroxybutyrate that are produced. Humans usually produce more β-hydroxybutyrate than acetoacetate.

The most plausible explanation for alcohol-related ketoacidosis involves several metabolic consequences of excessive alcohol ingestion. First, alcoholics often do not eat well. In effect, Al Martini was starving because he had a chronically poor appetite, he had been vomiting, and he may have been lying at the foot of the stairs for many hours since his last intake of food. When hepatic glycogen stores are low, they may be depleted in a few hours. The depletion of glycogen plus the reduction in gluconeogenesis caused by the oxidation of ethanol (see Chapter 27) leads to a relative hypoglycemia. This "metabolic stress" plus the "stress" of fluid depletion due to lack of intake and increased urination causes secretion of epinephrine and other hormones which stimulate the breakdown of adipose triacylglycerols (lipolysis). Adipose cells release large amounts of free fatty acids which travel to the liver, undergo β-oxidation, and produce ketone bodies. The ketone bodies enter the blood, causing a ketoacidosis. A high NADH/NAD$^+$ ratio results from the oxidation of ethanol (see Chapter 27) and drives ketone body production toward β-hydroxybutyrate.

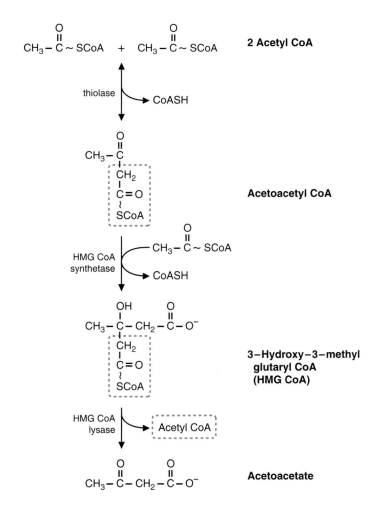

Fig. 23.15. Synthesis of the ketone body acetoacetate. The portion of HMG-CoA shown in blue is released as acetyl CoA, and the remainder of the molecule forms acetoacetate.

Patients in diabetic ketoacidosis and other patients who are producing large amounts of ketone bodies smell of acetone.

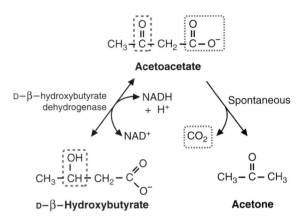

Fig. 23.16. Fates of acetoacetate. Acetoacetate is reduced to β-hydroxybutyrate or decarboxylated to acetone. Note that the dehydrogenase that interconverts acetoacetate and β-hydroxybutyrate is specific for the D-isomer. Thus, it differs from the dehydrogenase of β-oxidation, which acts on 3-hydroxy acyl CoA derivatives and is specific for the L-isomer.

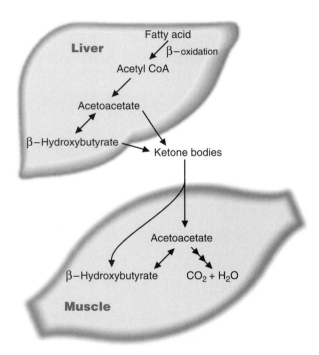

Fig. 23.17. Transfer of ketone bodies from liver to other tissues.

Oxidation of Ketone Bodies

Ketone bodies provide fuel for tissues particularly during fasting. When fatty acids are released from adipose triacylglycerols, the liver uses them to produce ketone bodies which travel to tissues, such as muscle and kidney, where they are oxidized (Fig. 23.17). During starvation, ketone bodies rise to a level in the blood that enables them to enter brain cells, where they are oxidized, reducing the amount of glucose required by the brain (Fig. 23.18).

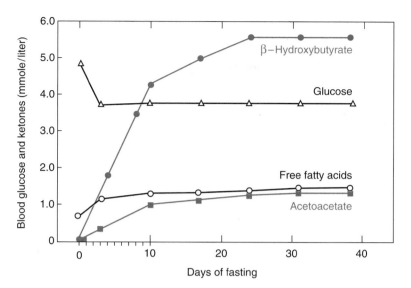

Fig. 23.18. Levels of ketone bodies in the blood at various times during fasting. Glucose levels remain relatively constant, as do levels of fatty acids. Ketone body levels, however, increase markedly, rising to levels at which they can be utilized by the brain and other nervous tissue. From Cahill GF Jr, Aoki TT. Med Times 1970;98:109.

Acetoacetate may enter cells directly, or it may be produced within cells by oxidation of β-hydroxybutyrate. This reaction, catalyzed by β-hydroxybutyrate dehydrogenase, produces NADH which generates ATP by oxidative phosphorylation. Therefore, more energy is derived from β-hydroxybutyrate than from acetoacetate.

The activation of acetoacetate occurs in mitochondria and is catalyzed by succinyl CoA:acetoacetate CoA transferase. As the name suggests, CoA is transferred from succinyl CoA, a TCA cycle intermediate, to acetoacetate. Acetoacetyl CoA and succinate are the products of this reaction (Fig. 23.19). Although the liver produces ketone bodies, it does not utilize them because this thiotransferase enzyme is not present in sufficient quantity.

β-Ketothiolase, the same enzyme involved in β-oxidation, catalyzes the cleavage of acetoacetyl CoA. One molecule of acetoacetyl CoA produces 2 molecules of acetyl CoA, which enter the TCA cycle.

GTP, the equivalent of ATP, is normally produced when succinyl CoA is converted to succinate in the TCA cycle. However, when succinyl CoA transfers CoA to acetoacetate, GTP is not produced. Therefore, although the 2 acetyl CoA derived from acetoacetate generate 24 ATP via the TCA cycle and oxidative phosphorylation, the net yield is only 23 ATP because the equivalent of one ATP is used in the activation of acetoacetate.

Overall, fatty acids released from adipose triacylglycerols serve as the major fuel for the body during fasting. These fatty acids are completely oxidized to CO_2 and H_2O by some tissues. The liver oxidizes fatty acids, converting most of the acetyl CoA to ketone bodies, which are shipped to other tissues via the blood. In these tissues, the remaining energy is used to generate ATP as the ketone bodies are oxidized to CO_2 and H_2O.

The total amount of energy derived by partially oxidizing fatty acids in the liver and sending ketone bodies to other tissues for completion of the oxidation process is almost the same as the energy derived by oxidizing fatty acids all the way to CO_2 and H_2O within a single tissue. The advantages gained by the formation of ketone bodies

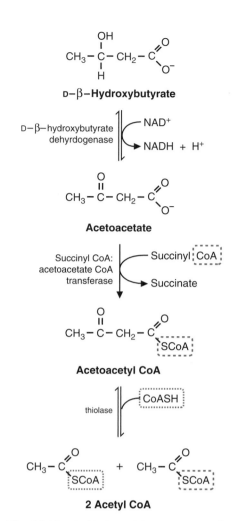

Fig. 23.19. Oxidation of ketone bodies. β-Hydroxybutyrate is oxidized to acetoacetate, which is activated by accepting a CoA group from succinyl CoA. Acetoacetyl CoA is cleaved to 2 acetyl CoA which enter the TCA cycle and are oxidized.

are that: (*a*) the liver derives the energy required to drive processes, such as gluco-neogenesis, by only partially oxidizing fatty acids and forming ketone bodies; (*b*) other tissues use the ketone bodies as fuel; and (*c*) during starvation, the brain can oxidize ketone bodies, reducing its need for glucose. Consequently, during starvation gluconeogenesis decreases, and muscle protein, which provides amino acids as a carbon source for glucose production in the liver, is spared.

REGULATION OF FATTY ACID OXIDATION AND KETONE BODY UTILIZATION

Fatty acid oxidation is regulated by the mechanisms that control the reoxidation of FAD(2H) and NADH by the electron transport chain, that is, by the demand for ATP.

Muscle preferentially uses fatty acids as a fuel. When fatty acids are plentiful, glucose oxidation in muscle is inhibited. β-Oxidation produces NADH and acetyl CoA which cause pyruvate dehydrogenase to be phosphorylated and inactivated. Therefore, pyruvate produced from glucose by glycolysis cannot be converted to acetyl CoA for entry into the TCA cycle. Thus, intermediates of glycolysis accumulate if ATP production from fatty acids is adequate to meet the needs of the cell. Glucose 6-phosphate inhibits hexokinase, decreasing the rate of entry of glucose into the glycolytic pathway, and other mechanisms may operate to slow glycolysis. For instance, citrate can inhibit phosphofructokinase-1. However, the physiological importance of this mechanism in humans, which was once thought to be a major explanation for the preferential use of fatty acids by muscle, is currently being questioned (see Chapter 22).

After a high carbohydrate meal, when fatty acids are being synthesized in the cytosol of liver cells, their immediate oxidation in liver mitochondria is prevented by malonyl CoA, an intermediate in fatty acid synthesis (see Chapter 32). Malonyl CoA inhibits the carnitine:acyltransferase I involved in the transport of fatty acids into mitochondria where the enzymes of β-oxidation are located. Thus, in the fed state, fatty acids are neither oxidized in liver nor converted to ketone bodies.

During fasting, fatty acid synthesis and, thus, malonyl CoA levels decrease in the liver. The mobilization of fatty acids from adipose triacylglycerols occurs as a result of the high glucagon/insulin ratio. The liver can now take up these fatty acids and transport them into mitochondria. Because the flow of oxaloacetate and malate is toward glucose during fasting (i.e., gluconeogenesis is occurring), acetyl CoA accumulates and is used for ketone body synthesis. As fasting progresses, HMG-CoA synthetase, the key enzyme in ketone body synthesis, is induced.

 CLINICAL COMMENTS. Although ketoacidosis can occur in alcoholics, such as **Al Martini**, diabetic ketoacidosis (DKA) is more common. (See the case of **Di Beatty** in Chapters 4 and 5.) DKA occurs because of an increased rate of fatty acid release from adipose triacylglycerols and subsequent hepatic ketone body production due to a lack of insulin.

The cause of the ketosis of prolonged starvation is reduced caloric intake, which, of course, leads to decreased blood glucose and insulin levels and, consequently, to increased hepatic ketogenesis. Thus, in a general sense, DKA, starvation ketosis, and alcohol-induced ketoacidosis, as described for **Al Martini**, share the common metabolic abnormalities of accelerated lipolysis (which delivers more fatty acids to the liver) and enhanced ketogenesis, secondary to low levels of circulating insulin.

More than 25 enzymes and specific transport proteins participate in mitochondrial fatty acid metabolism. At least 15 of these have been implicated in human disease.

Recently, MCAD deficiency, the cause of **Lofata Burne's** problems, has emerged as one of the most common of the inborn errors of metabolism with a carrier frequency ranging from 1 in 40 in northern European populations to less than 1 in 100 in Asians. Overall, the predicted disease frequency for MCAD deficiency is 1 in 15,000 persons, a prevalence equal to or greater than that of phenylketonuria, a genetic disorder for which newborn infants are screened in the United States.

MCAD deficiency is an autosomal recessive disorder caused by the substitution of a T for an A at position 985 of the MCAD gene. This mutation causes a lysine to replace a glutamate residue in the protein, resulting in the production of an unstable dehydrogenase.

The most frequent manifestation of MCAD deficiency is intermittent hypoketotic hypoglycemia (low levels of ketone bodies and low levels of glucose in the blood). The hypoglycemia is more likely to occur after prolonged fasting when hepatic glycogen stores have been depleted and available glucose is rapidly being utilized. Fatty acids normally would be oxidized to CO_2 and H_2O under these conditions. In MCAD deficiency, however, fatty acids of medium chain length cannot be further oxidized. As a result, the body must rely to a greater extent on glucose oxidation to meet its energy needs, and hypoglycemia occurs. Because the full complement of energy (ATP) required to drive gluconeogenesis in the liver is not available and because accumulation of unoxidized fatty acyl CoA results in inhibition of gluconeogenesis, glucose levels fall still further. The decrease in fatty acid oxidation results in less acetyl CoA for ketone body synthesis. These circumstances produce a hypoketotic hypoglycemia.

Some of the symptoms once ascribed to hypoglycemia are now believed to be due to the accumulation of toxic fatty acid intermediates, especially in those patients with only mild reductions in blood glucose levels. **Lofata Burne's** mild elevation in the blood of liver transaminases may reflect an infiltration of her liver cells with unoxidized medium chain fatty acids.

The management of MCAD-deficient patients includes the intake of a relatively high carbohydrate diet and the avoidance of prolonged fasting.

 BIOCHEMICAL COMMENTS. The unripe fruit of the akee tree produces a toxin, hypoglycin, which causes a condition known as Jamaican vomiting sickness. The victims of the toxin are usually unwary children who eat this unripe fruit and develop a severe hypoglycemia, which is often fatal.

Although hypoglycin causes hypoglycemia, it acts by inhibiting an acyl CoA dehydrogenase of β-oxidation that has specificity for short and medium chain fatty acids. Because more glucose must be oxidized to compensate for the decreased ability of fatty acids to serve as fuel, blood glucose levels may fall extremely low. Fatty acid levels, however, rise because of decreased β-oxidation. As a result of the increased fatty acid levels, ω-oxidation increases, and dicarboxylic acids are excreted in the urine. The diminished capacity to oxidize fatty acids in liver mitochondria results in decreased levels of acetyl CoA, the substrate for ketone body synthesis.

Suggested Readings

Balasse EO, Fery F. Ketone body production and disposal: effects of fasting, diabetes, and exercise. Diabetes Metab Rev 1989;5:247–270.

Fery F, Balasse EO. Ketone body production and disposal in diabetic ketosis. A comparison with fasting ketosis. Diabetes 1985;34:326–332.

Halperin ML, Cheema-Dhadli S. Renal and hepatic aspects of ketoacidosis: a quantitative analysis based on energy turnover. Diabetes Metab Rev 1989;5:321–336.

Roe CR, Coates PM. Mitochondrial fatty acid oxidation disorders. In: Scriver CR, Beaudet AL, Sly WS, Valle D, eds. The metabolic and molecular bases of inherited disease. 7th ed. Vol I. New York: McGraw-Hill, 1995:1501–1533.

PROBLEM

A person with a deficiency of an enzyme in the pathway for carnitine synthesis is not eating adequate amounts of carnitine in the diet. During fasting, which of the following substances would you expect to be elevated or decreased in this person's blood compared to the levels in a normal person's blood?

Substance in blood	Elevated	Decreased
Glucose		
Fatty acids		
Ketone bodies		

ANSWER

Because of decreased levels of carnitine, the rate of transport of long chain fatty acids (the predominant fatty acids) into liver mitochondria for β-oxidation and ketone body synthesis would be lower than normal in this person. Therefore, fatty acid levels would be increased in the blood and ketone body levels would be decreased. Glucose oxidation would be increased to compensate for the decreased ability to oxidize fatty acids, and hypoglycemia (low blood glucose) would result.

24 Basic Concepts in the Regulation of Fuel Metabolism by Insulin, Glucagon, and Other Hormones

All cells continuously use ATP and require a constant supply of fuels to provide energy for ATP generation. Insulin and glucagon are the two major hormones that regulate fuel mobilization and storage (Fig. 24.1). Their function is to ensure that cells have a constant source of glucose, fatty acids, and amino acids for ATP generation and for cellular maintenance.

Because most tissues are partially or totally dependent on glucose for ATP generation and for production of precursors of other pathways, insulin and glucagon maintain blood glucose levels near 80–100 mg/dL despite the fact that carbohydrate intake varies considerably over the course of a day. The maintenance of constant blood glucose levels (glucose homeostasis) requires these two hormones to regulate carbohydrate, lipid, and amino acid metabolism in accordance with the needs and capacities of individual tissues. Basically, the dietary intake of all fuels in excess of immediate need is stored, and the appropriate fuel is mobilized when a demand occurs. For example, when dietary glucose is not available in sufficient quantities so that all tissues can use it, fatty acids are mobilized and made available to skeletal muscle for use as a fuel (see Chapters 2 and 31). Fatty acids spare glucose for use by the brain and other glucose-dependent tissues.

The concentrations of insulin and glucagon in the blood regulate fuel storage and mobilization (Fig. 24.2). Insulin, released in response to carbohydrate ingestion, promotes glucose utilization as a fuel and glucose storage as fat and glycogen. Insulin is the major anabolic hormone of the body. It increases protein synthesis and cell growth in addition to fuel storage. Blood insulin levels decrease as glucose is taken up by tissues and utilized. Glucagon, the major counterregulatory hormone of insulin, is decreased in response to a carbohydrate meal and elevated during fasting. Its concentration in the blood signals the absence of dietary glucose, and it promotes glucose production via glycogenolysis (glycogen degradation) and gluconeogenesis (glucose synthesis from amino acids and other noncarbohydrate precursors). Increased levels of glucagon relative to insulin also stimulate the mobilization of fatty acids from adipose tissue. Epinephrine (the fight or flight hormone) and cortisol (a glucocorticoid released in response to fasting and chronic stress) have effects on fuel metabolism which oppose those of insulin. These two hormones are therefore also considered insulin counterregulatory hormones.

Insulin and glucagon are polypeptide hormones synthesized as prohormones in the B and A cells, respectively, in the islets of Langerhans in the pancreas. Proinsulin is cleaved into mature insulin and C-peptide in vesicles and precipitated

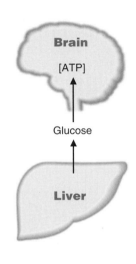

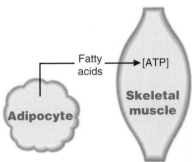

Fig. 24.1. Maintenance of fuel supplies to tissues.

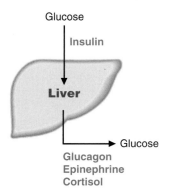

Fig. 24.2. Insulin and the insulin counterregulatory hormones.

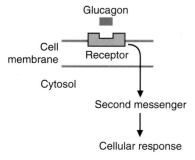

Fig. 24.3. Cellular response to glucagon.

 Fatty acids provide an example of the influence of the level of a compound in the blood on its own rate of metabolism. The concentration of fatty acids in the blood is the major factor determining whether skeletal muscles will use fatty acids or glucose as a fuel (see Chapter 23). In contrast, hormones are (by definition) carriers of messages between tissues. Insulin and glucagon, two hormonal messengers, are carrying messages about dietary intake. Epinephrine, on the other hand, is a flight-or-fight hormone which carries a message about an increased need for fuel. Its level is regulated principally through the sympathetic nervous system.

with Zn^{2+}. Although insulin secretion is regulated principally by blood glucose levels, its secretion can also be stimulated by certain amino acids and inhibited by epinephrine. Glucagon is also synthesized as a prohormone and cleaved into mature glucagon within storage vesicles. Its release is regulated principally through suppression by glucose and by insulin. However, amino acids and epinephrine stimulate its release.

Glucagon exerts its effects on cells by binding to a receptor on the cell surface, which stimulates the synthesis of the intracellular second messenger, cAMP (Fig. 24.3). cAMP activates protein kinase A, which phosphorylates key regulatory enzymes, activating some and inhibiting others. Changes of cAMP levels also induce or repress the synthesis of a number of enzymes.

Insulin binds to a receptor on the cell surface, but the postreceptor events which follow differ from those stimulated by glucagon. Insulin binding activates both autophosphorylation of the receptor and the phosphorylation of other enzymes by the receptor's tyrosine kinase domain. The complete routes for signal transduction between this point and the final effects of insulin on the regulatory enzymes of fuel metabolism have not yet been established.

 Ann Sulin returned to her physician for her monthly office visit. She still weighed 198 lb, despite her insistence that she had adhered strictly to her diet. Her blood glucose level at the time of the visit, 3 hours after lunch, was 180 mg/dL (reference range = 80–100).

 Bea Selmass is a 46-year-old woman who 6 months earlier began noting episodes of fatigue and confusion as she finished her daily pre-breakfast jog. These episodes were occasionally accompanied by blurred vision and an unusually urgent hunger. The ingestion of food relieved all of her symptoms within 25–30 minutes. In the last month, these "attacks" have occurred more frequently throughout the day and she has learned to diminish their occurrence by eating between meals. As a result, she has recently gained 8 lb.

A random serum glucose level done at 4:30 PM during her first office visit was subnormal at 46 mg/dL. Her physician, suspecting she had a form of fasting hypoglycemia, ordered a series of fasting serum glucose levels. In addition, he asked Bea to keep a careful daily diary of all of the symptoms that she experienced when her attacks were most severe.

METABOLIC HOMEOSTASIS

Living cells require a constant source of fuels from which to derive ATP for the maintenance of normal cell function and growth. Therefore, a balance must be achieved between carbohydrate, fat, and protein intake, their storage when present in excess of immediate need, and their mobilization and synthesis when in demand. The balance between need and availability is referred to as metabolic homeostasis (Fig. 24.4). There are three principal ways the intertissue integration required for metabolic homeostasis is achieved:

- the concentration of nutrients or metabolites in the blood affects the rate at which they are utilized and stored in different tissues
- hormones carry messages to individual tissues about the physiological state of the body and nutrient supply or demand

• the central nervous system uses neural signals to control tissue metabolism, directly or through the release of hormones.

Insulin and glucagon are the two major hormones that regulate fuel storage and mobilization (see Fig. 24.2). Insulin is the major anabolic hormone of the body. It promotes the storage of fuels and the utilization of fuels for growth. Glucagon is the major hormone of fuel mobilization. Other hormones, such as epinephrine, are released as a response of the central nervous system to hypoglycemia, exercise, or other types of physiological stress. Epinephrine and other stress hormones also increase the availability of fuels (Fig. 24.5).

The special role of glucose in metabolic homeostasis is dictated by the fact that many tissues (e.g., the brain, red blood cells, the lens of the eye, the kidney medulla, exercising skeletal muscle) are dependent on glycolysis for all or a portion of their energy needs and require uninterrupted access to glucose on a second-to-second basis to meet their rapid rate of ATP utilization. In the adult, a minimum of 190 g of glucose are required per day; about 150 g for the brain and 40 g for other tissues. Significant decreases of blood glucose below 60 mg/dL limit glucose metabolism in the brain and elicit hypoglycemic symptoms, presumably because the overall process of glucose flux through the blood-brain barrier, into the interstitial fluid, and subsequently into the neuronal cells, is slow and has a relatively high K_m (see Chapter 25).

The continuous movement of fuels into and out of storage depots is necessitated by the high amounts of fuel required each day to meet the need for ATP. Disastrous results would occur if even a day's supply of glucose, amino acids, and fatty acids were left circulating in the blood. Glucose and amino acids would be at such high concentrations that the hyperosmolar effect would cause coma. The concentration of glucose and amino acids would be above the renal threshold (the maximal concentration in the blood at which the kidney can completely resorb metabolites), and some of these compounds would be wasted as they spilled over into the urine. Nonenzymatic glycosylation of proteins would increase at higher blood glucose levels. Triacylglycerols circulate in cholesterol-containing lipoproteins, and the levels of these lipoproteins would be chronically elevated, increasing the likelihood of atherosclerotic vascular disease. Consequently, glucose and other fuels are continuously moved in and out of storage depots as needed.

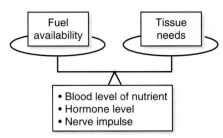

Fig. 24.4. Metabolic homeostasis. The balance between fuel availability and the needs of tissues for different fuels is achieved by three types of messages: the level of the fuel or nutrients in the blood, the level of one of the hormones of metabolic homeostasis, or nerve impulses which affect tissue metabolism or the release of hormones.

The consequences of having high blood glucose levels (hyperglycemia) are manifested in patients with untreated diabetes mellitus. Extremely high levels of glucose can cause nonketotic hyperosmolar coma. Hyperglycemia also produces pathological effects through the nonenzymatic glycosylation of a variety of proteins. Hemoglobin (HbA), one of the proteins that becomes glycosylated, forms HbA$_{1c}$ (see Chapter 8). **Ann Sulin's** high levels of HbA$_{1c}$ (14% of the total HbA, compared to the reference range of 5.2–7.8%) indicate that her blood glucose has been very elevated over the last 6–8 weeks.

All membrane and serum proteins exposed to high levels of glucose in the blood or interstitial fluid are candidates for glycosylation, which distorts protein structure and generally affects function. Nonenzymatic glycosylation of other membrane and serum proteins contributes to the long term complications of diabetes mellitus which include diabetic retinopathy, nephropathy, and neuropathy, in addition to other vascular complications of the disease.

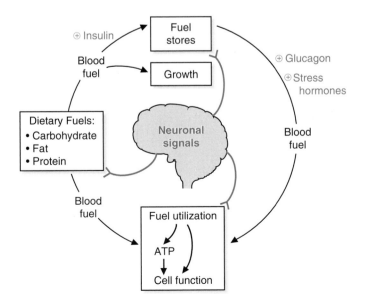

Fig. 24.5. Signals that regulate metabolic homeostasis. The major stress hormones are epinephrine and cortisol.

Bea Selmass's studies confirmed that her fasting serum glucose levels were below normal. She continued to experience the fatigue, confusion, and blurred vision she had described on her first office visit. These symptoms are called neuroglycopenic (neurological symptoms resulting from an inadequate supply of glucose to the brain for the generation of ATP).

Bea also noted the symptoms that are part of the adrenergic response to hypoglycemic stress. Stimulation of the sympathetic nervous system (because of the low levels of glucose reaching the brain) results in the release of epinephrine, a stress hormone, from the adrenal medulla. Elevated epinephrine levels cause tachycardia, palpitations, anxiety, tremulousness, pallor, and sweating.

In addition to the symptoms described by Bea Selmass, individuals may experience confusion, lightheadedness, headache, aberrant behavior, blurred vision, loss of consciousness, or seizures.

Ms. Selmass's doctor explained that the general diagnosis of "fasting" hypoglycemia was now established and that a specific cause for this disorder must be found.

MAJOR HORMONES OF METABOLIC HOMEOSTASIS

The hormones of metabolic homeostasis respond to changes in dietary intake and physiological state in a way that adjusts the availability of fuels. Insulin and glucagon are considered the major hormones of metabolic homeostasis because they continuously fluctuate in response to our daily eating pattern. We will describe the release and action of these two hormones in preparation for the section on carbohydrate metabolism. They provide good examples of the basic concepts of hormonal regulation. Certain features of the release and action of other insulin counterregulatory hormones, epinephrine, norepinephrine, and cortisol, will be described and compared to insulin and glucagon. These hormones will be considered in more detail in Section VIII.

Insulin is the major anabolic hormone that promotes the storage of nutrients: glucose storage as glycogen in liver and muscle, conversion of glucose to triacylglycerols in liver and their storage in adipose tissue, and amino acid uptake and protein synthesis in skeletal muscle (Fig. 24.6). It also increases the synthesis of albumin and other blood proteins by the liver. Insulin promotes the utilization of glucose as a fuel by stimulating its transport into muscle and adipose tissue. At the same time, insulin acts to inhibit fuel mobilization.

Glucagon acts to maintain fuel availability in the absence of dietary glucose by stimulating the release of glucose from liver glycogen, by stimulating gluconeogenesis from lactate, glycerol, and amino acids, and, in conjunction with decreased insulin, by mobilizing fatty acids from adipose triacylglycerols to provide an alternate source of fuel (Fig. 24.7). Its sites of action are principally the liver and adipose tissue; it has no influence on skeletal muscle metabolism.

The release of insulin is dictated primarily by the blood glucose level, and the highest levels of insulin occur approximately 30–45 minutes after a high carbohydrate meal (Fig. 24.8). They return to basal levels as the blood glucose concentration falls, about 120 minutes after the meal. The release of glucagon, on the other hand, is controlled principally through suppression by glucose and insulin. Therefore, the lowest levels of glucagon occur after a high carbohydrate meal. Because all of the effects of glucagon are opposed by insulin, the simultaneous stimulation of insulin

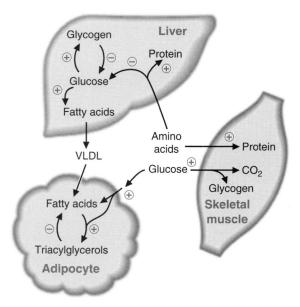

Fig. 24.6. Major sites of insulin action on fuel metabolism. $\oplus$ = stimulated by insulin; $\ominus$ = inhibited by insulin.

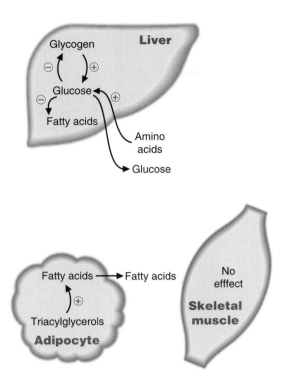

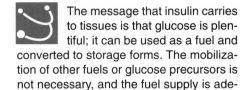

The message that insulin carries to tissues is that glucose is plentiful; it can be used as a fuel and converted to storage forms. The mobilization of other fuels or glucose precursors is not necessary, and the fuel supply is adequate for growth.

Because insulin stimulates the uptake of glucose into tissues and its storage and oxidation, it lowers blood glucose levels. Therefore, one of the possible causes of **Bea Selmass's** hypoglycemia is an insulinoma, a tumor that produces excessive insulin.

The message carried by glucagon is that "glucose is gone," i.e., the current supply of glucose is inadequate to meet the immediate fuel requirements of the body.

Fig. 24.7. Major sites of glucagon action in fuel metabolism. ⊕ = pathways stimulated by glucagon; ⊖ = pathways inhibited by glucagon.

Table 24.1. Physiological Actions of Insulin and Insulin Counterregulatory Hormones

Hormone	Function	Major Metabolic Pathways Affected
Insulin	• Promotes fuel storage after a meal • Promotes growth	• Stimulates glucose storage as glycogen (muscle and liver) • Stimulates fatty acid synthesis and storage after a high carbohydrate meal • Stimulates amino acid uptake and protein synthesis
Glucagon	• Mobilizes fuels • Maintains blood glucose levels during fasting	• Activates gluconeogenesis and glycogenolysis (liver) during fasting • Activates fatty acid release from adipose tissue
Epinephrine	• Mobilizes fuels during acute stress	• Stimulates glucose production from glycogen (muscle and liver) • Stimulates fatty acid release from adipose tissue
Cortisol	• Provides for changing requirements over the long-term	• Stimulates amino acid mobilization from muscle protein • Stimulates gluconeogenesis • Stimulates fatty acid release from adipose tissue

release and suppression of glucagon secretion by a high carbohydrate meal provides an integrated control of carbohydrate, fat, and protein metabolism.

Insulin and glucagon are not the only regulators of fuel metabolism. The intertissue balance between the utilization and storage of glucose, fat, and protein is also accomplished by the circulating levels of metabolites in the blood, by neuronal signals, and by the other hormones of metabolic homeostasis (epinephrine, norepinephrine, cortisol, and others) (Table 24.1). These hormones, which will be described in more detail in Section VIII, oppose the actions of insulin by mobilizing fuels. Like glucagon, they are called insulin counterregulatory hormones (Fig. 24.9). Of all these hormones, only insulin and glucagon are synthesized and released in direct response

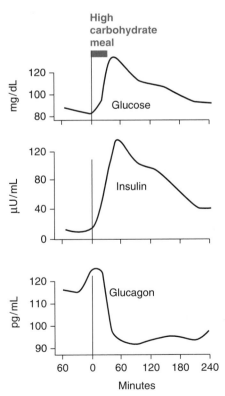

Fig. 24.8. Blood glucose, insulin, and glucagon levels after a high carbohydrate meal.

Whenever an endocrine gland continues to release its hormone in spite of the presence of signals which normally would suppress secretion of the hormone its release is said to be "autonomous." Secretory neoplasms of endocrine glands generally produce their hormonal product autonomously.

Autonomous hypersecretion of insulin from a suspected pancreatic B-cell tumor (an insulinoma) can be demonstrated in several ways. The most simple test is to simultaneously draw blood for the measurement of both glucose and insulin at a time when the patient is spontaneously experiencing the characteristic adrenergic and/or neuroglycopenic symptoms of hypoglycemia. During such a test, **Bea Selmass's** glucose levels fell to 45 mg/dL (normal = 80–100), and her ratio of insulin to glucose was far higher than normal.

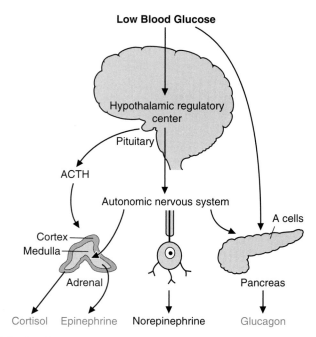

Fig. 24.9. Major insulin counterregulatory hormones. The stress of a low blood glucose level mediates the release of the major insulin counterregulatory hormones through neuronal signals. Hypoglycemia is one of the stress signals which stimulates the release of cortisol, epinephrine, and norepinephrine. Adrenocorticotropic hormone (ACTH) is released from the pituitary, and stimulates the release of cortisol (a glucocorticoid) from the adrenal cortex. Neuronal signals stimulate the release of epinephrine from the adrenal medulla and norepinephrine from nerve endings. Neuronal signals also play a minor role in the release of glucagon. Although norepinephrine and growth hormone have counterregulatory actions, they are not major counterregulatory hormones.

to a changing level of a circulating fuel in the blood. The release of cortisol, epinephrine, and norepinephrine is mediated by neuronal signals.

Rising levels of the insulin counterregulatory hormones in the blood, reflect, for the most part, a current increase in the demand for fuel. As you proceed through the chapters on carbohydrate and lipid metabolism and the section on endocrinology, the mechanisms by which these hormones regulate the individual pathways of fuel metabolism will be explained.

SYNTHESIS AND RELEASE OF INSULIN AND GLUCAGON

Endocrine Pancreas

Insulin and glucagon are synthesized in different cell types of the endocrine pancreas, which consists of microscopic clusters of small glands, the islets of Langerhans, scattered throughout the exocrine pancreas. The A (or α) cells secrete glucagon and the B (or β) cells secrete insulin into the hepatic portal vein via the pancreatic veins.

Synthesis and Secretion of Insulin

Di Beatty has insulin-dependent diabetes mellitus (IDDM), which is usually caused by autoimmune destruction of the B cells of the pancreas. Susceptibility to IDDM is generally conferred by a genetic defect in the human leukocyte antigen (HLA) region which codes for the major histocompatibility complex II (MHC II), a protein which presents antigen on the cell surface for "self-recognition" by the cells involved in the immune response. Because of this defective protein, a cell-mediated immune response, initiated by a viral infection or some other factor, does not recognize the B cells as "self" and destroys them.

Insulin is a polypeptide hormone. The active form of insulin is composed of two polypeptide chains (the A-chain and the B-chain) linked by two interchain disulfide bonds (see Chapter 8). The A-chain has an intrachain disulfide bond (Fig. 24.10).

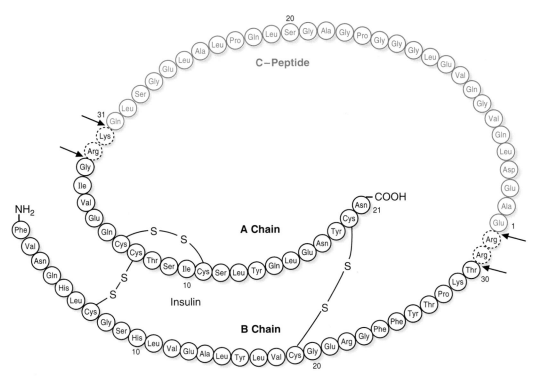

Fig. 24.10. Cleavage of proinsulin to insulin. Proinsulin is converted to insulin by proteolytic cleavage, which removes the C-peptide and a few additional amino acid residues. Cleavage occurs at the arrows. From Murray RK, et al. Harper's biochemistry, 23rd ed. Stanford, CT: Appleton & Lange, 1993:560.

Insulin, like many other polypeptide hormones, is synthesized as a preprohormone which is converted in the rough endoplasmic reticulum (RER) to proinsulin. The "pre" sequence, a short hydrophobic signal sequence at the N-terminal end, is cleaved as it enters the lumen of the RER. Proinsulin folds into the proper conformation and disulfide bonds are formed between the cysteine residues. It is then transported in microvesicles to the Golgi complex. It leaves the Golgi complex in storage vesicles, where a protease removes the C-peptide (a fragment with no hormonal activity) and a few small remnants, resulting in active insulin (see Fig. 24.10). Zinc ions are transported into these storage vesicles. Cleavage of the C-peptide region decreases the solubility of the resulting insulin, which then coprecipitates with zinc.

Stimulation of the B cells by glucose causes exocytosis of the insulin storage vesicles, a process dependent on K^+, ATP, and Ca^{2+} ions. The phosphorylation of glucose in the B cells and its subsequent metabolism initiate the release of insulin through an intracellular mobilization of Ca^{2+}.

Stimulation and Inhibition of Insulin Release

Blood insulin levels rise rapidly in response to increases in blood glucose levels (see Fig. 24.8). The release of insulin occurs within minutes after the pancreas is exposed to a high glucose concentration. The threshold for insulin release is about 80 mg of glucose/dL. Above 80 mg/dL, the rate of insulin release is not an all-or-nothing response, but is proportional to the glucose concentration up to about 300 mg/dL glucose. As insulin is secreted, the synthesis of new insulin molecules is stimulated, so that secretion is maintained until blood glucose levels fall. Insulin is rapidly removed from the circulation and degraded by the liver (and, to a lesser extent, by kidney and skeletal muscle), so that blood insulin levels fall rapidly once the rate of secretion slows.

Ann Sulin is taking a sulfonylurea compound known as glipizide to treat her diabetes. The sulfonylureas act on specific receptors on the surface of the pancreatic B cells. The ensuing activation of these receptors closes K^+ channels which, in turn, increases Ca^{2+} movement into the interior of the cell. The calcium modulates the interaction of the storage vesicles with the plasma membrane, resulting in insulin release.

Measurements of proinsulin and C-peptide in **Bea Selmass's** blood during her hospital fast provided confirmation that she had an insulinoma. Insulin and C-peptide are secreted in approximately equal proportions, but C-peptide is not cleared from the blood as rapidly as insulin. Therefore, it provides a measure of the rate of insulin secretion.

Plasma C-peptide measurements are also potentially useful in treating patients with diabetes mellitus because they provide a way to estimate the degree of endogenous insulin secretion in patients who are receiving exogenous insulin.

Patients with IDDM, like **Di Beatty**, have almost no circulating insulin. Patients with NIDDM, like **Ann Sulin**, have near-normal levels of insulin; however, the level of insulin in their blood is low relative to their elevated blood glucose concentration. In NIDDM, skeletal muscle, liver, and other tissues exhibit insulin resistance and insulin has a smaller effect on glucose and fat metabolism than normal. As a result, levels of insulin must be higher than normal to maintain normal blood glucose levels.

In fasting subjects the average level of immunoreactive glucagon in the blood is 75 pg/mL, and does not vary as much as insulin during the daily fasting-feeding cycle. However, only 30–40% of the measured immunoreactive glucagon is pancreatic glucagon. The rest is composed of larger immunoreactive fragments also produced in the pancreas or in the intestinal L cells.

A number of factors other than the blood glucose concentration can modulate insulin release (Table 24.2). The pancreatic islets are innervated by the autonomic nervous system, including a branch of the vagus nerve, which helps to coordinate insulin release with the act of eating. However, signals from the central nervous system are not required for insulin secretion. Certain amino acids can also stimulate insulin secretion, although the amount of insulin released during a high protein meal is very much lower than that released by a high carbohydrate meal. Gastric inhibitory polypeptide (a gut hormone released after the ingestion of food) also aids in the onset of insulin release. Epinephrine, secreted in response to fasting, stress, trauma, and vigorous exercise, decreases the release of insulin.

Synthesis and Secretion of Glucagon

Glucagon is synthesized in the A cells (Fig. 24.11) of the pancreas by cleavage of the much larger preproglucagon, a 160 amino acid peptide. Like insulin, preproglucagon is produced on the RER and is converted to proglucagon as it enters the lumen. Proteolytic cleavage at various sites produces the mature 29 amino acid polypeptide glucagon (molecular weight 3,500) and larger glucagon-containing fragments. Glucagon is rapidly metabolized, primarily in the liver and kidneys, and its plasma half-life is only about 3–5 minutes.

Glucagon secretion is regulated principally by glucose and insulin, both of which inhibit glucagon release. Glucose probably has both a direct suppressive effect on the A cell and an indirect effect mediated by its ability to stimulate the release of insulin. The direction of blood flow in the pancreas carries insulin from the B cells in the center of the islets to the peripheral A cells, where it suppresses glucagon secretion.

Certain hormones stimulate glucagon secretion. Among these are the catecholamines (including epinephrine), cortisol, and certain gastrointestinal (gut) hormones (Table 24.3).

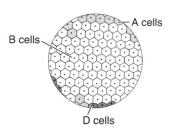

Fig. 24.11. B and A cells in pancreatic islets. Throughout the pancreas, the islets are composed of about 70–80% B cells. The highest concentration of A cells is in the tail, body, and part of the head of the pancreas. The D cells, which secrete other hormones, comprise about 5% of the total pancreatic cells. White = B cells (produce insulin); grey = A cells (produce glucagon); dark = D cells.

Table 24.2. Regulators of Insulin Release[a]

Major	
Glucose	+
Minor	
Amino Acids	+
Neural Input	+
Gut hormones	+
Epinephrine	−
(−adrenergic)	

[a] + = stimulates
− = inhibits

Table 24.3. Regulators of Glucagon Release[a]

Major	
Glucose	−
Insulin	−
Amino acids	+
Minor	
Cortisol	+
Neural (stress)	+
Epinephrine	+
Gut hormones	+

[a] + = stimulates
− = inhibits

Many amino acids also stimulate glucagon release (see Fig. 24.12). Thus, the high fasting levels of glucagon do not decrease after a high protein meal. In fact, glucagon levels may increase, stimulating gluconeogenesis in the absence of dietary glucose. The relative amounts of insulin and glucagon in the blood after a mixed meal are dependent on the composition of the meal.

MECHANISMS OF HORMONE ACTION

For a hormone to affect the flux of substrates through a metabolic pathway, it must be able to change the rate at which that pathway proceeds by increasing or decreasing the rate of the slowest step(s). Either directly or indirectly, hormones affect the activity of specific enzymes or transport proteins which limit the flux through a pathway. Thus, ultimately the hormone must either cause the amount of the substrate for the enzyme to increase (if substrate supply is a rate-limiting factor), change the conformation at the active site by phosphorylating the enzyme, change the concentration of an allosteric effector of the enzyme, or change the amount of the protein by inducing or repressing its synthesis or by changing its turnover rate or location. Insulin, glucagon, and other hormones utilize all of these regulatory mechanisms to change the rate of flux in metabolic pathways. The effects mediated by phosphorylation or changes in the kinetic properties of an enzyme occur rapidly, within minutes. In contrast, it may take hours for induction or repression of enzyme synthesis to change the amount of an enzyme in the cell.

The physiological importance of insulin's usual action of mediating the suppressive effect of glucose on glucagon secretion is apparent in patients with IDDM and NIDDM. Despite the hyperglycemia present in such patients, glucagon levels initially remain elevated (near fasting levels) either due to the absence of insulin or to the resistance of the A cells to insulin's suppressive effect. Thus, these patients have inappropriately high glucagon levels.

During the "stress" of hypoglycemia, the autonomic nervous system stimulates the pancreas to secrete glucagon, which tends to restore the serum glucose level to normal. The increased activity of the adrenergic nervous system (through epinephrine) also alerts a patient, like **Bea Selmass**, to the presence of a worsening hypoglycemia so that the patient will eat simple sugars or other carbohydrates. Bea Selmass gained 8 lb because these signals urged her to eat.

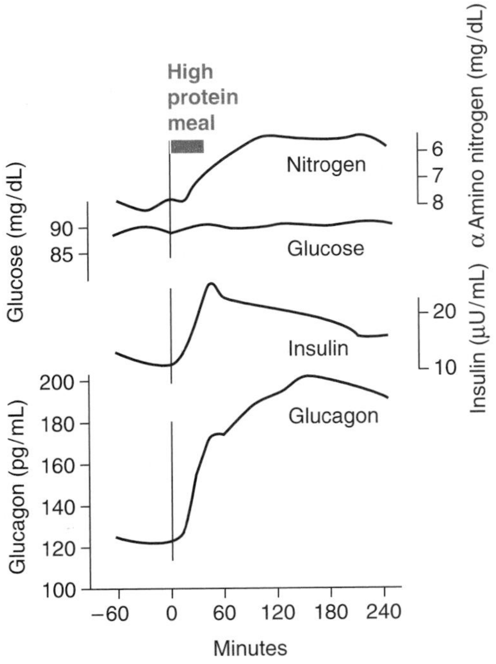

Fig. 24.12. Release of insulin and glucagon in response to a high protein meal. This figure shows the increase of insulin and glucagon after a person who has fasted overnight ingests 100 g of protein (equivalent to a slice of roast beef). Insulin levels do not increase nearly as much as they do after a high carbohydrate meal. However, glucagon increases above fasting levels.

Q 24.1: Phosphodiesterase is inhibited by methylxanthines, a class of compounds which includes caffeine. Would the effect of a methylxanthine on fuel metabolism be similar to fasting or to a high carbohydrate meal?

Signal Transduction by Hormones That Bind to Plasma Membrane Receptors

Hormones initiate their actions on target cells by binding to specific receptors or binding proteins. In the case of polypeptide hormones (such as insulin and glucagon), and catecholamines (epinephrine and norepinephrine), the action of the hormone is mediated through binding to a specific receptor on the plasma membrane (Fig. 24.13). The "message" of the hormone is transmitted to intracellular enzymes by the receptor and an intracellular second "messenger"; the hormone does not need to enter the cell to exert its effects. (In contrast, steroid hormones like cortisol and the thyroid hormone triiodothyronine (T_3) move into the cell nucleus to exert their effects.)

The mechanism by which the message carried by the hormone ultimately affects the rate of the regulatory enzyme in the cell is called signal transduction. The three basic types of signal transduction for hormones binding to receptors on the plasma membrane are (*a*) receptor coupling to adenylate cyclase which produces cAMP, (*b*) receptor kinase activity, and (*c*) receptor coupling to hydrolysis of phosphatidylinositol bisphosphate (PIP_2). The hormones of metabolic homeostasis provide examples of each of these mechanisms (see Fig. 24.13). In addition, some hormones and neurotransmitters act through receptor coupling to gated ion channels (see Fig. 24.13).

SIGNAL TRANSDUCTION BY GLUCAGON

The pathway for signal transduction by glucagon is one common to a number of hormones; the glucagon receptor is coupled to adenylate cyclase and cAMP production (Fig. 24.14). Glucagon, through G proteins, activates the membrane-bound adenylate cyclase, increasing the synthesis of the intracellular second messenger 3′,5′-cyclic AMP (cAMP) (Fig. 24.15). cAMP activates protein kinase A (cAMP-dependent protein kinase), which changes the activity of enzymes by phosphorylating them at specific serine residues. Phosphorylation activates some enzymes and inhibits others.

The G proteins, which couple the glucagon receptor to adenylate cyclase, are proteins in the plasma membrane that bind GTP and have dissociable subunits that interact with both the receptor and adenylate cyclase. In the absence of glucagon, the stimulatory G_s protein complex binds GDP, but cannot bind to the unoccupied receptor or adenylate cyclase (Fig. 24.16). Once glucagon binds to the receptor, the receptor also binds the G_s complex, which then releases GDP and binds GTP. The α-subunit then dissociates from the βγ-subunits and binds to adenylate cyclase, thereby activating it. As the GTP on the α-subunit is hydrolyzed to GDP, the subunit dissociates and recomplexes with the β- and γ-subunits. Only continued occupancy of the glucagon receptor can keep adenylate cyclase active.

Although glucagon works by activating adenylate cyclase, a few hormones inhibit adenylate cyclase. In this case, the inhibitory G protein complex is called a G_i complex.

The hormonal activation of adenylate cyclase through G proteins controls the concentration of cAMP in the cell. cAMP is very rapidly degraded to AMP by a membrane-bound phosphodiesterase. The concentration of cAMP is thus very low in the cell so that changes in its concentration can occur rapidly in response to changes in the rate of synthesis. The amount of cAMP present at any time is a direct reflection of hormone binding and the activity of adenylate cyclase. It is not affected by ATP, ADP, or AMP levels in the cell.

cAMP transmits the hormone signal to the cell by activating protein kinase A (cAMP-dependent protein kinase). As cAMP binds to the regulatory subunits of protein kinase A, these subunits dissociate from the catalytic subunits, which are thereby activated (see Fig. 24.14). Activated protein kinase A phosphorylates serine residues of key regulatory enzymes in the pathways of carbohydrate and fat metabolism. Some

cAMP is the intracellular second messenger for a number of hormones which regulate varied responses. The specificity of the message of each hormone results from the presence of receptors for that hormone in only certain target tissues. For example, glucagon activates glucose production from glycogen in liver, but not in skeletal muscle because glucagon receptors are present in liver, but absent in skeletal muscle. However, skeletal muscle has adenylate cyclase, cAMP, and protein kinase A, which can be activated by epinephrine binding to the $β_2$ receptors in the membrane of muscle cells. Liver cells also have epinephrine receptors.

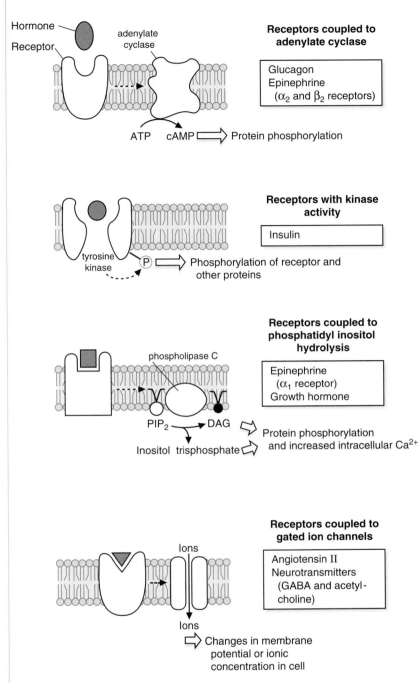

Receptors coupled to adenylate cyclase

Glucagon
Epinephrine
(α_2 and β_2 receptors)

ATP cAMP ⟹ Protein phosphorylation

Receptors with kinase activity

Insulin

tyrosine kinase (P) ⟹ Phosphorylation of receptor and other proteins

Receptors coupled to phosphatidyl inositol hydrolysis

Epinephrine
(α_1 receptor)
Growth hormone

PIP_2 ⟶ DAG ⟹ Protein phosphorylation and increased intracellular Ca^{2+}
Inositol trisphosphate ⟹

Receptors coupled to gated ion channels

Angiotensin II
Neurotransmitters
(GABA and acetyl-choline)

Ions ⟹ Changes in membrane potential or ionic concentration in cell

Fig. 24.13. Signal transduction by hormones which bind to receptors in the plasma membrane. Most of the hormones of metabolic homeostasis (glucagon, insulin, epinephrine, norepineph-rine, and growth hormone) exert their effects by binding to a receptor on the plasma membrane. This binding affects intracellular events by producing an intracellular second messenger such as cAMP, diacylglycerol (DAG), or inositol trisphosphate (IP_3), by catalyzing phosphorylation, or by opening/closing gated ion channels. These basic mechanisms of signal transduction are employed by many other hormones and by neurotransmitters (which also have cell surface receptors).

A 24.1: Inhibition of phosphodi-esterase by methylxanthine would increase cAMP and have the same effects on fuel metabolism as an increase of glucagon and epinephrine. Increased fuel mobilization would occur (glycogenolysis, the release of glucose from glycogen, and lipolysis, the release of fatty acids from triacylglycerols).

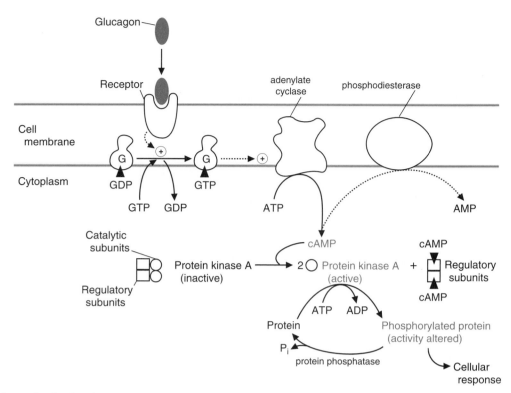

Fig. 24.14. Signal transduction by glucagon.

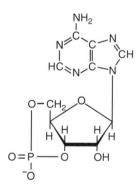

Fig. 24.15. Structure of cAMP.

Protein kinases are a class of enzymes that change the activity of other enzymes by phosphorylating them at serine or tyrosine residues and are referred to as serine or tyrosine kinases, respectively. Serine kinases also phosphorylate some enzymes at threonine residues. Protein kinase A phosphorylates many of the enzymes in the pathways of fuel metabolism.

enzymes are activated and others are inhibited by this change in phosphorylation state. The message of the hormone is terminated by the action of semi-specific protein phosphatases which remove phosphate groups from the enzymes. The activity of the protein phosphatases is also controlled through hormonal regulation.

Changes in the phosphorylation state of proteins which bind to cAMP response elements (CREs) in the promoter region of genes contribute to the regulation of gene transcription by a number of cAMP-coupled hormones (see Chapter 15). For instance, cAMP response element binding protein (CREB) is directly phosphorylated by protein kinase A, a step essential for its activation of transcription. Other phosphorylations may also play a role.

The mechanism for signal transduction by glucagon illustrates some of the important principles of hormonal signaling mechanisms. The first is that specificity of action in tissues is conferred by the receptor; in general, the major actions of glucagon occur in liver, adipose tissue, and certain cells of the kidney because these are the cells that contain glucagon receptors. The second is that the system involves amplification of the message. Glucagon and other hormones are present in very small amounts in the blood. The binding of one molecule of glucagon at one receptor ultimately activates many protein kinase A molecules which each phosphorylate hundreds of enzyme molecules. The third is integration of metabolic responses. For instance, the glucagon-stimulated phosphorylation of enzymes simultaneously activates glycogen degradation, inhibits glycogen synthesis, and inhibits glycolysis in the liver. The fourth is augmentation and antagonism of signals. For example, glucagon and epinephrine (which is released during exercise) bind to different receptors, but both can increase cAMP and stimulate glycogen degradation by phosphorylation. A fifth principle is rapid signal termination. In the case of glucagon, both the mechanism of the G proteins and the rapid degradation of cAMP contribute to signal termination.

Signal Transduction by Insulin

Insulin initiates its action by binding to a receptor on the plasma membrane of the target cell (Fig. 24.17). The insulin receptor has two types of subunits, the α-subunits to which insulin binds, and the β-subunits, which span the membrane and protrude into the cytosol. The cytosolic portion of the β-subunit has tyrosine kinase activity. On binding of insulin, the tyrosine kinase phosphorylates tyrosine residues on the β-subunit (autophosphorylation) as well as on several other enzymes within the cytosol. A principal substrate for phosphorylation by the receptor, insulin receptor substrate (IRS-1), then recognizes and binds to various signal transduction proteins in regions referred to as SH_2 domains. IRS-1 is involved in many of the physiological responses to insulin, but the mechanisms of insulin action between this point and the final effect on the enzymes and transport proteins of carbohydrate metabolism have not been well-defined. The net result of insulin action is a number of tissue-specific cellular responses which can be grouped into five categories: (*a*) insulin reverses glucagon-stimulated phosphorylation, (*b*) insulin works through a phosphorylation cascade which stimulates the phosphorylation of several enzymes, (*c*) insulin induces and represses the synthesis of specific enzymes, (*d*) insulin acts as a growth factor and has a general stimulatory effect on protein synthesis, and (*e*) insulin stimulates glucose and amino acid transport into cells.

A number of mechanisms have been proposed for the action of insulin in reversing glucagon-stimulated phosphorylation of the enzymes of carbohydrate metabolism. From the student's point of view, the ability of insulin to reverse glucagon-stimulated phosphorylation occurs as if it were lowering cAMP and stimulating phosphatases which could remove those phosphates added by protein kinase A. In reality, the mechanism must be much more complex.

Signal Transduction by Cortisol and Other Hormones with Intracellular Receptors

Signal transduction by the glucocorticoid cortisol and other steroids involves intracellular receptors or binding proteins which interact with chromatin and change the rate of gene transcription (see Section VIII). Thus, these hormones mediate changes in fuel metabolism that occur over long periods of time, as in starvation or septic stress (a whole-body response to infection).

The effects of cortisol on gene transcription are usually synergistic to those of certain other hormones. For instance, the rates of gene transcription for some of the enzymes in the pathway for glucose synthesis from amino acids (gluconeogenesis) are induced by glucagon and also by cortisol.

Signal Transduction by Epinephrine and Norepinephrine

Epinephrine and norepinephrine are catecholamines (Fig. 24.18). They can act as neurotransmitters or as hormones, compounds released into the blood that act on cells of a target organ. The general effects of these hormones prepare us for fight or flight, that is they increase fuel mobilization, cardiac output, blood flow, etc.

Epinephrine and norepinephrine bind to four different types of receptors: α_1, α_2, β_1, and β_2 (Table 24.4). The two receptors that have direct effects on fuel metabolism are the β_2 and β_1 receptors. The β_2 receptor works through the adenylate cyclase-cAMP system. This receptor is present in liver, skeletal muscle, and other tissues, and is involved in the mobilization of fuels (such as glucose from glycogen). It also mediates vascular, bronchial, and uterine smooth muscle contraction. Epinephrine is a much more potent agonist for this receptor than norepinephrine, which acts more as

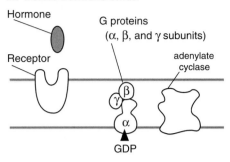

A. Before hormone binds

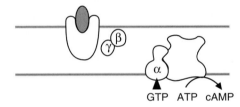

B. After hormone binds

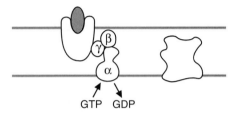

C. G proteins dissociate

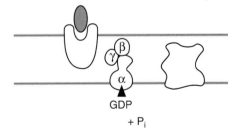

D. GTPase cleaves GTP to GDP and P_i

Fig. 24.16. G proteins in signal transduction. **A.** Before hormone binds. **B.** After hormone binds. GDP on G protein α is exchanged for GTP. **C.** G proteins dissociate. α-Subunit with GTP activates adenylate cyclase, which converts ATP to cAMP. **D.** The GTPase activity of the α-subunit cleaves GTP to GDP and P_i. Adenylate cyclase is no longer active. α-, β-, and γ-subunits of G protein reassociate. Hormone dissociates from the receptor. In G_i protein complexes, the α_i subunits inhibit adenylate cyclase, and cAMP decreases.

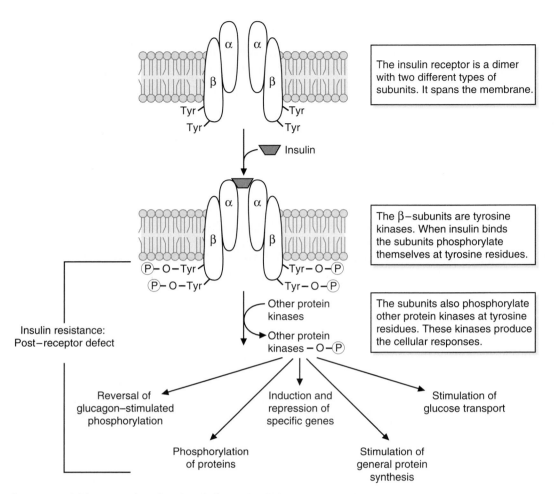

Fig. 24.17. Insulin receptor initiates tyrosine phosphorylation and cellular responses to insulin.

The insulin receptor is a dimer with two different types of subunits. It spans the membrane.

The β–subunits are tyrosine kinases. When insulin binds the subunits phosphorylate themselves at tyrosine residues.

The subunits also phosphorylate other protein kinases at tyrosine residues. These kinases produce the cellular responses.

Table 24.4. Adrenergic Responses of Selected Tissues

Organ or Tissue	Receptor	Effect
Heart (myocardium)	β_1	Increased force of contraction Increased rate of contraction
Blood vessels	α β_2	Vasoconstriction Vasodilation
Gut	α,β	Decreased motility and increased sphincter tone
Liver	α,β	Increased glycogenolysis
Adipose tissue	β	Increased lipolysis
Skin (apocrine glands on hands, axillae, etc.)	α	Increased sweating
Bronchioles	β_2	Dilation

Priscilla Twigg, in order to stay thin, frequently fasts for prolonged periods of time, but jogs every morning (see Chapter 2). The release of epinephrine and norepinephrine and the increase of glucagon and fall of insulin during her exercise provide coordinated and augmented signals that stimulate the release of fuels above the fasting levels. Fuel mobilization will occur, of course, only as long as she has fuel stored as triacylglycerols.

a neurotransmitter. The α_1 receptors, which are postsynaptic receptors, mediate vascular and smooth muscle contraction. They work through the phosphatidylinositol bisphosphate system (see Fig. 24.13 and Section VIII). This receptor also mediates glycogenolysis in liver. Some of the adrenergic responses of various tissues are summarized in Table 24.4.

CLINICAL COMMENTS. **Di Beatty** and **Ann Sulin** have two different types of diabetes mellitus, IDDM and NIDDM, respectively. The defining and diagnostic criterion for both types of diabetes is hyperglycemia. As the pancreatic B cells are gradually destroyed and insulin secretion falls below a critical level, the symptoms of IDDM develop rapidly. In NIDDM, the symptoms may develop more gradually over the course of years, and go undiagnosed. About 80–85% of NIDDM patients are obese and, like **Thomas Appleman**, have a high abdominal fat to hip ratio (are apple rather than pear shape). Many of these patients improve as they lose weight, and the insulin resistance declines.

Bea Selmass underwent a high resolution ultrasonographic (ultrasound) study of her upper abdomen which demonstrated a 2.6-cm mass in the midportion of her pancreas. With this finding, her physicians decided that further noninvasive studies would not be necessary before surgical exploration of her upper abdomen was performed. At the time of surgery, a yellow-white 2.8-cm mass was resected from her pancreas. No evidence of malignant behavior by the tumor (such as local metastases) was found. Bea had an uneventful immediate and long term postoperative course.

BIOCHEMICAL COMMENTS. One of the important cellular responses to insulin is the reversal of glucagon-stimulated phosphorylation of enzymes. Mechanisms proposed for this action include the inhibition of adenylate cyclase, a reduction of cAMP levels, the stimulation of phosphodiesterase, the production of a specific protein (insulin factor), the release of a second messenger from a bound glycosylated phosphatidylinositol, and the phosphorylation of enzymes at a site which antagonizes protein kinase A phosphorylation. None of these mechanisms seems to be universally applicable to all of the metabolic effects of insulin in all tissues.

Insulin is also able to antagonize the actions of glucagon at the level of specific induction or repression of key regulatory enzymes of carbohydrate metabolism. For instance, the rate of synthesis of mRNA for phosphoenolpyruvate carboxykinase, a key enzyme of the gluconeogenic pathway, is increased severalfold by glucagon (via cAMP), and decreased by insulin. Thus all the effects of glucagon, even the induction of certain enzymes, can be reversed by insulin. This antagonism is exerted through an insulin-sensitive hormone response element (IRE) in the promoter region of the genes. Insulin causes repression of the synthesis of enzymes that are induced by glucagon.

The general stimulation of protein synthesis by insulin (its growth effect) appears to occur through both a general increase in rates of mRNA translation and pronounced increases in the translation of certain mRNAs. The increases of translation occur through a phosphorylation cascade initiated by the insulin receptor and ending in the phosphorylation of subunits of proteins that bind to and inhibit eukaryotic initiation factors (eIFs). When phosphorylated, the subunits are released and the eIFs become active and initiate translation. In this respect, the actions of insulin are similar to those of hormones that act as growth factors and also have receptors with tyrosine kinase activity.

In addition to signal transduction, the insulin receptor mediates the internalization of insulin and its subsequent degradation. Although unoccupied receptors can recycle to the membrane, the receptor itself is degraded after prolonged stimulation of the cell by insulin. The result of this process, referred to as "down-regulation," is an attenuation of the insulin signal. The physiological role of receptor internalization in metabolic responses to insulin is unknown.

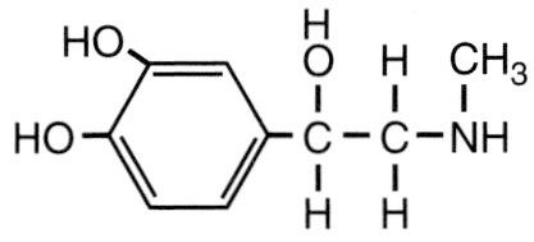

Ann Sulin is experiencing insulin resistance. Her levels of circulating insulin are normal, although inappropriately low for her level of blood glucose. However, her insulin target cells do not respond adequately to this level of insulin. For most NIDDM patients, the site of insulin resistance is subsequent to binding at the receptor, i.e., the number of receptors and their affinity for insulin is near normal. However, the binding of insulin at these receptors does not elicit the normal intracellular effects on the activity of regulatory proteins. Consequently, there is little stimulation of glucose metabolism and storage after a high carbohydrate meal and little inhibition of hepatic gluconeogenesis.

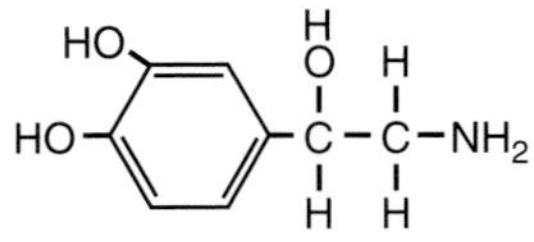

Fig. 24.18. Structure of epinephrine and norepinephrine. Epinephrine and norepinephrine are both hormones and neurotransmitters. They are catecholamines. Catechol refers to the ring structure containing two –OH groups. They are synthesized from tyrosine.

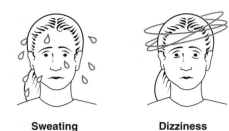

Sweating   **Dizziness**

Fig. 24.19. Symptoms of hypoglycemia.

Suggested Readings

O'Brien C. Missing link in insulin's path to protein production. Science 1994;266:542–543.

White MF, Kahn CR. The insulin signaling system. J Biol Chem 1994;269:1–4.

PROBLEMS

1. Figure 24.19 shows two of the symptoms of hypoglycemia experienced by **Bea Selmass**. Can you account for her symptoms?

2. Both **Di Beatty** and **Ann Sulin** experienced fatigue before they were diagnosed. Can you account for their fatigue?

ANSWERS

1. **Bea Selmass** experienced neuroglycopenia symptoms related to an inadequate amount of glucose reaching brain cells. Because the brain is dependent on glucose for ATP generation, totally under normal conditions and partially during prolonged starvation, she could have experienced dizziness and light-headedness from a lack of ATP. She also experienced adrenergic symptoms, which included sweating. Hypoglycemia stimulates the autonomic nervous system, which stimulates the release of epinephrine from the adrenal medulla. Thus hypoglycemia increases fuel mobilization (e.g., β_2 receptors stimulate glycogenolysis) and increases sweating by stimulating α receptors in the apocrine glands of the skin (see Table 24.4).

2. Although both **Di Beatty** and **Ann Sulin** had hyperglycemia, they experienced fatigue from an inability to generate ATP from glucose (and other fuels). Insulin stimulates glucose transport into muscle. Therefore, little glucose was available for the glycolytic pathway in skeletal muscle both in the case of Di Beatty (whose pancreatic B cells were destroyed by an autoimmune response and could not produce insulin) and of Ann Sulin (whose tissues exhibited insulin resistance and did not respond normally to insulin).

Carbohydrate Metabolism

Glucose is central to all of metabolism. It is the universal fuel for human cells and the source of carbon for the synthesis of most other compounds. Every human cell type uses glucose to obtain energy. Other dietary sugars (mainly fructose and galactose) are converted to glucose or to intermediates of glucose metabolism.

Glucose is the precursor for the synthesis of an array of other sugars required for the production of specialized compounds, such as lactose, cell surface antigens, nucleotides, or glycosaminoglycans. Glucose is also the fundamental precursor of noncarbohydrate compounds; it can be converted to lipids (including fatty acids, cholesterol, and steroid hormones), amino acids, and nucleic acids. Only those compounds that are synthesized from vitamins, essential amino acids, and essential fatty acids cannot be synthesized from glucose in humans.

More than 50% of the calories in the typical diet in the United States are obtained from starch, sucrose, and lactose. These dietary carbohydrates are converted to glucose, galactose, and fructose in the digestive tract (Fig. 25.1). Monosaccharides are absorbed from the intestine, enter the blood, and travel to the tissues where they are metabolized.

After glucose is transported into cells, it is phosphorylated by a hexokinase to form glucose 6-phosphate. Glucose 6-phosphate can then enter a number of metabolic pathways. The three that are common to all cell types are glycolysis, the pentose phosphate pathway, and glycogen synthesis (Fig. 25.2). In tissues, fructose and galactose are converted to intermediates of glucose metabolism. Thus, the fate of these sugars parallels that of glucose (Fig. 25.3).

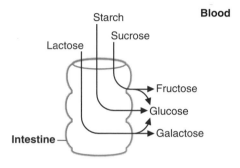

Fig. 25.1. Overview of carbohydrate digestion. The major carbohydrates of the diet (starch, lactose, and sucrose) are digested to produce monosaccharides (glucose, fructose, and galactose), which enter the blood.

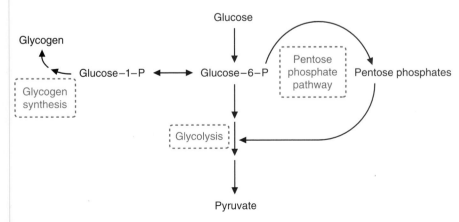

Fig. 25.2. Major pathways of glucose metabolism.

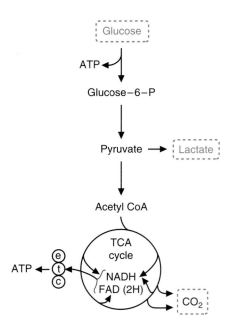

Fig. 25.4. Conversion of glucose to lactate or to CO_2. etc = electron transport chain.

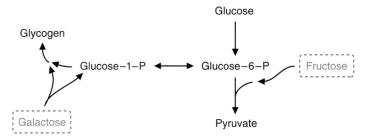

Fig. 25.3. Overview of fructose and galactose metabolism. Fructose and galactose are converted to intermediates of glucose metabolism.

The major fate of glucose 6-phosphate is oxidation via the pathway of glycolysis (see Chapter 22), which provides a source of ATP for all cell types. Cells that lack mitochondria cannot oxidize other fuels. They produce ATP from anaerobic glycolysis (the conversion of glucose to lactate). Cells that contain mitochondria oxidize glucose to CO_2 and H_2O via glycolysis and the TCA cycle (Fig. 25.4). Some tissues, such as the brain, depend on the oxidation of glucose to CO_2 and H_2O for energy because they have a limited capacity to use other fuels.

Glucose produces the intermediates of glycolysis and the TCA cycle that are used for the synthesis of amino acids and both the glycerol and fatty acid moieties of triacylglycerols (Fig. 25.5).

Another important fate of glucose 6-phosphate is oxidation via the pentose phosphate pathway, which generates NADPH. The reducing equivalents of NADPH are used for biosynthetic reactions and for the prevention of oxidative damage to cells. In this pathway, glucose is oxidatively decarboxylated to 5-carbon sugars (pentoses), which may reenter the glycolytic pathway. They may also be used for nucleotide synthesis (Fig. 25.6).

Glucose 6-phosphate is also converted to UDP-glucose, which has many functions in the cell (Fig. 25.7). The major fate of UDP-glucose is the synthesis of glycogen, the storage polymer of glucose. Although most cells have glycogen to provide emergency supplies of glucose, the largest stores are in muscle and liver. Muscle glycogen is used to generate ATP during muscle contraction. Liver glycogen is used to maintain blood glucose during fasting and during exercise or periods of enhanced need. UDP-Glucose is also used for the formation of other sugars, and galactose and glucose are interconverted while attached to UDP. UDP-Galactose is used for lactose synthesis in the mammary gland. In the liver, UDP-glucose is oxidized to UDP-glucuronate, which is used to convert bilirubin and other toxic compounds to glucuronides for excretion (see Fig. 25.7).

Nucleotide sugars are also used for the synthesis of proteoglycans, glycoproteins, and glycolipids (see Fig. 25.7). Proteoglycans are major carbohydrate components of the extracellular matrix, cartilage, and extracellular fluids (such as the synovial fluid of joints). Most extracellular proteins are glycoproteins, i.e., they contain covalently attached carbohydrates. For both cell membrane glycoproteins and glycolipids, the carbohydrate portion extends into the extracellular space.

All cells are continuously supplied with glucose; the body maintains a constant glucose level in the blood (about 80–100 mg/dL) in spite of the changes in dietary supply and tissue demand as we eat, sleep, and exercise. This process is called glucose homeostasis. Low blood glucose levels (hypoglycemia) are prevented by a release of glucose from the large glycogen stores in the liver (glycogenolysis);

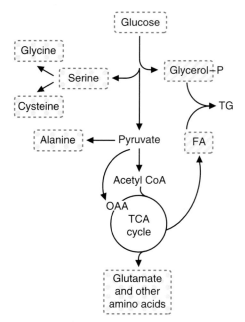

Fig. 25.5. Conversion of glucose to amino acids and to the glycerol and fatty acid (FA) moieties of triacylglycerols (TG). OAA = oxaloacetate.

by synthesis of glucose from lactate, glycerol, and amino acids in liver (gluco-neogenesis) (Fig. 25.8); and by a release of fatty acids from adipose tissue stores (lipolysis) to provide an alternate fuel when glucose is in short supply. High blood glucose levels (hyperglycemia) are prevented both by the conversion of glucose to glycogen and by its conversion to triacylglycerols in liver. Thus, the pathways for glucose utilization as a fuel cannot be considered as totally separate from pathways involving amino acid and fatty acid metabolism (Fig. 25.9).

Intertissue balance in the utilization and storage of glucose during fasting and feeding is accomplished principally by the actions of the hormones of metabolic homeostasis—insulin and glucagon. However, cortisol, epinephrine, norepineph-rine, and other hormones are also involved in intertissue adjustments of supply and demand in response to changes of physiological state.

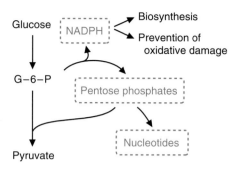

Fig. 25.6. Overview of the pentose phosphate pathway.

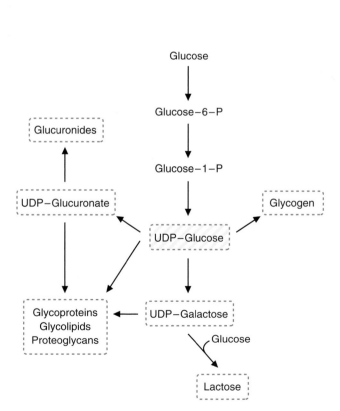

Fig. 25.7. Products derived from UDP-glucose.

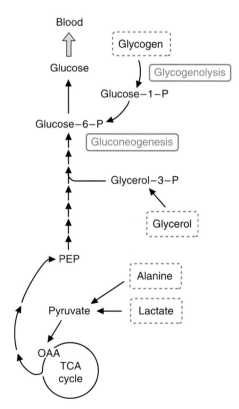

Fig. 25.8. Production of blood glucose from glycogen (by glycogenolysis) and from ala-nine, lactate, and glycerol (by gluconeogene-sis). PEP = phosphoenolpyruvate; OAA = oxaloacetate.

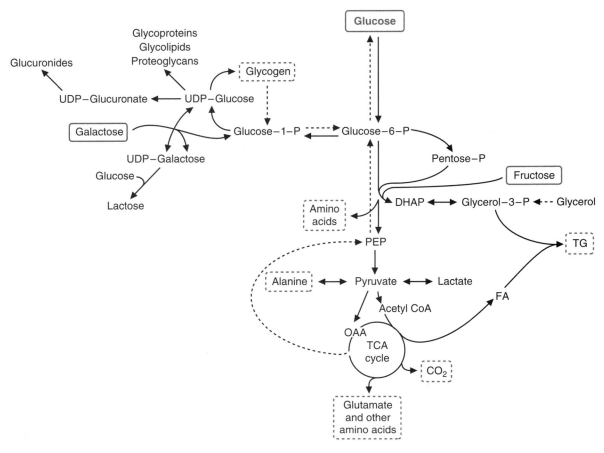

Fig. 25.9. Overview of the major pathways of glucose metabolism. Pathways for production of blood glucose are shown by dashed lines. FA = fatty acids; TG = triacylglycerols; OAA = oxaloacetate; PEP = phosphoenolpyruvate; UDP-G = UDP-glucose; DHAP = dihydroxyacetone phosphate.

25 Digestion, Absorption, and Transport of Carbohydrates

Carbohydrates are the largest source of dietary calories for most of the world's population. The major carbohydrates in the American diet are starch (a polysaccharide composed of glucosyl units), lactose (a disaccharide composed of glucose and galactose), and sucrose (a disaccharide composed of glucose and fructose).

The digestive process converts the dietary carbohydrates to monosaccharides by hydrolyzing the glycosidic bonds between the sugars. The major enzymes involved are pancreatic and salivary α-amylase and semispecific disaccharidase complexes in the brush-border membrane of intestinal mucosal cells. In human infants, the activity of the mucosal disaccharidase lactase is high, but this activity decreases during childhood in every population group but Northern Europeans. Dietary fiber, composed principally of polysaccharides, cannot be digested by the enzymes of the human intestinal tract. Some types of fiber may have beneficial effects.

Glucose, galactose, and fructose formed by the digestive enzymes are transported into the absorptive epithelial cells of the small intestine via Na^+-dependent active transport and facilitated diffusion. The facilitated transport of these monosaccharides is mediated by a family of glucose transport proteins (GLUT). Monosaccharides enter the capillaries of the splanchnic bed, circulate to the liver and peripheral tissues, and are transported into cells via one of the tissue-specific glucose transporters. The type of transporter found in each tissue reflects the role of glucose metabolism in that tissue.

 Pectins are found in fruits, such as apples. Could this be the basis for the saying "An apple a day keeps the doctor away"?

Deria Voider is a 20-year-old exchange student from Nigeria who has noted gastrointestinal bloating, abdominal cramps, and intermittent diarrhea ever since arriving in the United States 6 months earlier. A careful history reveals that these symptoms occur most commonly about 45 minutes to 1 hour after eating breakfast but may occur after other meals as well. Dairy products, not a part of Deria's diet in Nigeria, were identified as the probable offending agent since her gastrointestinal symptoms disappeared when milk and milk products were eliminated from her diet.

Ann Sulin's fasting and postprandial blood glucose levels are frequently above the normal range in spite of good compliance with insulin therapy. Her physician has referred her to a dietician skilled in training diabetic patients in the successful application of an appropriate American Diabetes Association diet. As part of the program, Mrs. Sulin is asked to incorporate foods containing fiber into her diet such as whole grains (e.g., wheat, oats, corn), legumes (e.g., peas, beans, lentils), tubers (e.g., potatoes, peanuts), and fruits.

Nona Melos is a 7-month-old baby girl, the second child born to unrelated parents. Her mother had a healthy, full-term pregnancy, and Nona's birth weight was normal. She did not respond well to breastfeeding and was changed entirely to a formula based on cow's milk at 4 weeks. Between 7 and 12

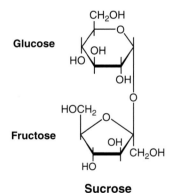

Fig. 25.10. Major dietary carbohydrates. Amylose and amylopectin are components of starch. Milk sugar is lactose, and table sugar is sucrose.

weeks of age, she was admitted to the hospital twice with a history of screaming after feeding, but was discharged after observation without a specific diagnosis. Elimination of cow's milk from her diet did not relieve her symptoms; Nona's mother reported that the screaming bouts were worse after Nona drank juice and that Nona frequently had gas and a distended abdomen. At 7 months she was still thriving (weight above 97th percentile) with no abnormal findings on physical examination. A stool sample was taken.

DIETARY CARBOHYDRATES

Carbohydrates are the largest source of calories in the average American diet and usually comprise 40–45% of our caloric intake. Most of these calories (60%) are present in grains, tubers, and vegetables in the form of the plant starches amylopectin and amylose (Fig. 25.10). These polysaccharides contain 10,000 to 1 million glucosyl units. Table sugar is sucrose, a disaccharide of glucose and fructose. Sucrose and small amounts of the monosaccharides glucose and fructose are the major natural sweeteners found in fruit, honey, and vegetables. Foods derived from animals, such as meat or fish, contain very little carbohydrate except for small amounts of glycogen. The major dietary carbohydrate of animal origin is lactose, a disaccharide composed of glucose and galactose found exclusively in milk and milk products. Dietary fiber, that portion of the diet which cannot be digested by human enzymes of the intestinal tract, is also composed principally of polysaccharides.

Specific sugars are not required in the diet. Glucose can be obtained in the diet or synthesized from certain amino acids found in dietary protein. Fructose, galactose, xylose, and all the other sugars required for metabolic processes in the human can be synthesized from glucose.

DIGESTION OF STARCH

In the digestive tract, the dietary polysaccharides and disaccharides are converted to monosaccharides by enzymes (glycosidases) that hydrolyze the glycosidic bonds between the sugars. These enzymes exhibit some specificity for the sugar, the glycosidic bond (α or β), and the number of saccharide units in the chain. Monosaccharides are transported across the intestinal mucosal cells into the interstitial fluid from which they enter the bloodstream (Fig. 25.11).

The conversion of starch (amylopectin and amylose) to glucose begins in the mouth. The salivary gland secretes about 1 liter of liquid per day containing salivary mucin and salivary α-amylase. Salivary mucin is a slippery glycoprotein important for lubrication and for dispersion of the polysaccharides. α-Amylase randomly hydrolyzes internal α-1,4 bonds between glucosyl residues within amylopectin, amylose, and glycogen, converting the large polysaccharides to smaller polysaccharides called dextrins. α-Amylase acts on internal bonds at scattered sites in the polysaccharide chain. For this reason, α-amylase is called an endoglycosidase. In contrast, exoglycosidases act sequentially from one end of a carbohydrate chain. The food moves from the mouth through the esophagus into the stomach, where the action of α-amylase is terminated by the acid pH, which denatures enzymes (Fig. 25.12).

The digestive process continues as food moves from the stomach into the upper part of the small intestine (duodenum). The exocrine pancreatic secretions (about 1.5 liters/day) contain bicarbonate ion (HCO_3^-), which neutralizes the acid (HCl) from the stomach. It also contains pancreatic α-amylase, which continues to hydrolyze the α-1,4 bonds in the starch. The products of the digestive process at this stage are disaccharides containing glucosyl units connected by α-1,4 bonds (maltose) and α-1,6

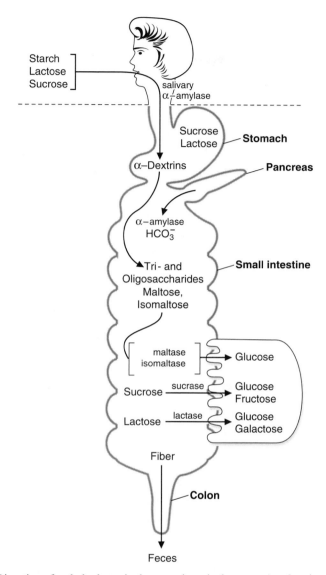

Fig. 25.11. Digestion of carbohydrates in the gastrointestinal tract. α-Amylase is an enzyme produced by the salivary glands and the pancreas. Maltase, isomaltase, sucrase, and lactase are enzymatic activities located in enzyme complexes on the brush border of intestinal epithelial cells.

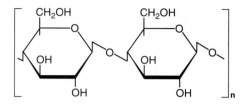

 25.1:

Can the glycosidic bonds of the structure shown above be hydrolyzed by α-amylase?

Sweeteners, in the form of sucrose and high fructose corn syrup (starch, partly hydrolyzed and isomerized to fructose), also appear in the diet as additives to processed foods. On average, a person in the U.S. consumes 65 lb of added sucrose and 40 lb of high fructose corn syrup solids per year.

bonds (isomaltose), and oligosaccharides (limit dextrins) containing from 3 to about 8 glucosyl residues, including the α-1,6 branching bond (see Fig. 25.12).

GLYCOSIDASES OF THE INTESTINAL BRUSH-BORDER MEMBRANE

Conversion of dietary disaccharides and the di- and oligosaccharides formed from starch to monosaccharides is carried out by glycosidases in the brush-border membrane of absorptive cells in the intestinal villi (Fig. 25.13). The glycosidases (enzymes that hydrolyze glycosidic bonds) are present as four large glycoprotein complexes that protrude from the membrane toward the intestinal lumen: the sucrase-isomaltase complex, glucoamylase complex, lactase or β-glycosidase complex, and trehalase. The major complexes all have more than one type of substrate or activity.

25.1: No. This polysaccharide is cellulose. The glucosyl units are joined by β-1,4 glycosidic bonds, and pancreatic and salivary α-amylase cleave only α-1,4 bonds between glucosyl units.

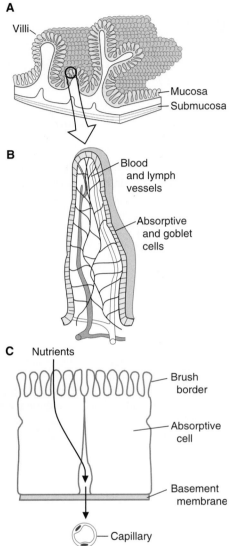

Fig. 25.13. Absorptive cells of the intestine **A.** The villi of the mucosa. **B.** A villus. **C.** Flow of nutrients through the microvilli, the cell, and into the blood.

Q 25.2:

Which of the bonds are hydrolyzed by the sucrase-isomaltase complex? Which by glucoamylase?

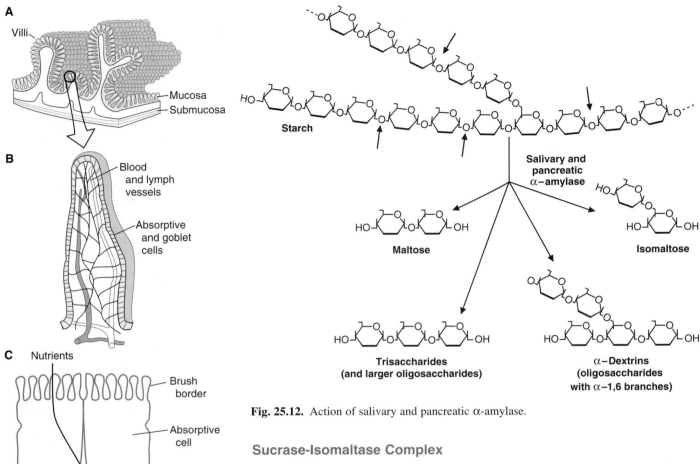

Fig. 25.12. Action of salivary and pancreatic α-amylase.

Sucrase-Isomaltase Complex

The sucrase-isomaltase complex hydrolyzes maltose, sucrose, and isomaltose (Fig. 25.14). Its concentration is highest in the jejunum and lower at the proximal and distal ends of the small intestine. The major portion of the sucrase-isomaltase complex, containing the catalytic sites, protrudes from the absorptive cells into the lumen of the intestine. Other domains of the protein form a connecting segment (stalk), and an anchoring segment which extends through the membrane into the cell. The complex is synthesized as a single polypeptide chain which is split into its two enzyme subunits (sucrase and isomaltase) extracellularly. Both enzyme subunits have high maltase and maltotriase activity and hydrolyze α-1,4-glucosyl bonds. The maltase activity cleaves the disaccharides, and the maltotriase activity cleaves the trisaccharides formed from starch (Figs. 25.15 and 25.16). Together, sucrase and isomaltase account for about 80% of the maltase activity in the intestine. In spite of their maltase activity, these enzymes are named for their specific actions. The sucrase subunit is the only enzyme in the intestine which hydrolyzes sucrose to glucose and fructose. The isomaltase subunit performs most of the hydrolysis of α-1,6 bonds between glucosyl residues in the isomaltose formed from starch.

Glucoamylase Complex

The glucoamylase complex also has two different enzyme subunits, but they have only small differences in substrate specificity. Both of these enzyme subunits are exoglucosidases (sometimes referred to as α-glucosidases), and their major function is the hydrolysis of the α-1,4 bonds between glucosyl units in oligosaccharides, start-

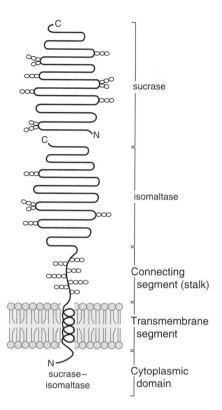

Fig. 25.14. Sucrase-isomaltase complex. This complex is attached to the cell membrane of the intestinal epithelial cell (the brush-border membrane). From Hunziker W, Spiess M, Semenza G, Lodish H. Cell 1986;46:231. Copyright by Cell Press.

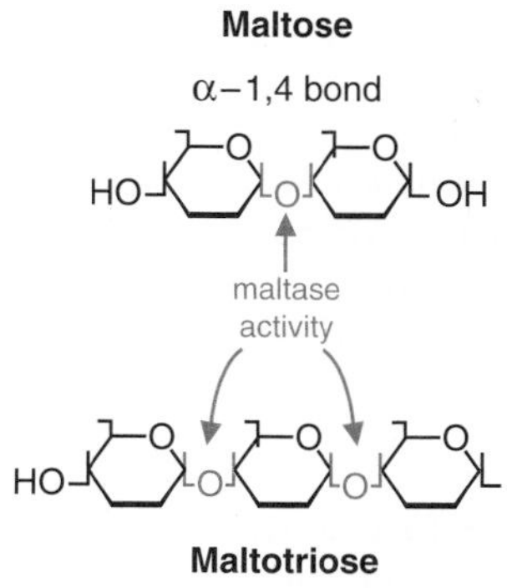

ing from the nonreducing end of the chains. They also cleave the $\alpha(1\rightarrow4)$ bond of maltose and, thus, act as maltases. Glucoamylase activity progressively increases along the length of the small intestine and is highest in the ileum.

β-Glycosidase Complex (Lactase)

Lactase activity (specific for the β-1,4 bond between galactose and glucose in lactose) is also part of a large glycoprotein found in the brush border, the β-glycosidase complex (Fig. 25.17). Its distribution along the gastrointestinal tract is similar to that of the sucrase-isomaltase complex and is highest in the jejunum. Unlike sucrase, maltase, isomaltase, and glucoamylase activities, which are present in excess, lactase activity is low and can be rate-limiting for lactose absorption. For most of the world's population, lactase activity increases during the late gestational period (27–32 weeks), and remains elevated until about 5–7 years of age. After this time, it falls to adult levels, which are less than 10% of that present in infants. In people who are derived mainly from Northern Europeans, the levels of lactase remain at, or only slightly below, infant levels throughout adulthood. Low adult levels of lactase are sometimes referred to as "late-onset lactase deficiency" (Table 25.1).

Diseases that injure the absorptive cells of the intestinal villi diminish lactase activity along the intestine, producing a condition known as secondary lactase deficiency. Kwashiorkor (protein malnutrition), colitis, gastroenteritis, tropical and nontropical sprue, and excessive alcohol consumption fall into this category. These diseases also affect other disaccharidases, but sucrase, maltase, isomaltase, and

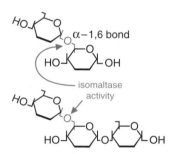

Fig. 25.15. Maltase activity (in the sucrase-isomaltase and glucoamylase complexes). Arrows indicate the α-1,4 bonds that are cleaved.

Fig. 25.16. Isomaltase activity. Arrows indicate the α-1,6 bonds that are cleaved.

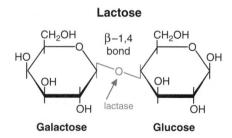

Fig. 25.17. Lactase activity. Lactase is a β-galactosidase. It cleaves the β-galactoside lactose, the major sugar in milk, forming galactose and glucose.

A 25.2: Bonds (1) and (3) would first be hydrolyzed by glucoamylase. Bond (2) would require isomaltase. Bonds (4) and (5) could then be hydrolyzed by the sucrase-isomaltase complex, or by the glucoamylase complex, all of which can convert maltotriose and maltose to glucose.

Q 25.3: Beans, peas, soybeans, and other leguminous plants contain oligosaccharides with (1,6)-linked galactose residues that cannot be hydrolyzed for absorption, including sucrose with one, 2, or 3 galactose residues attached (see Fig. 25.19). What is the fate of these polysaccharides in the intestine?

Individuals with genetic deficiencies of the sucrase-isomaltase complex show symptoms of sucrose intolerance, but are able to digest normal amounts of starch in a meal, without problems. The maltase activity in the glucoamylase complex, and residual activity in the sucrase-isomaltase complex (which is normally present in excess of need) is apparently sufficient to digest normal amounts of dietary starch.

Trehalose

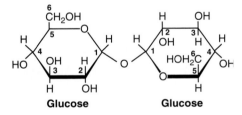

Fig. 25.18. Trehalose. This disaccharide contains 2 glucose moieties linked by an unusual bond that joins their anomeric carbons. It is cleaved by trehalase.

Carrageenan is a type of fiber derived from seaweed. It is composed of sulfated galactose and galacturonic acid derivatives (see Fig. 25.19). The negatively charged sulfate groups form hydrogen bonds with water and convert the polysaccharide into a gel-like substance. It is added to many foods such as ice cream and McDonald's McLean burger.

The dietician explained to **Ann Sulin** the rationale for adding a variety of fibers to her diet. The gel-forming, water-retaining pectins and gums delay gastric emptying and retard the rate of absorption of di- and monosaccharides.

Table 25.1. Prevalence of Late Onset Lactase Deficiency

Group	Prevalence (%)
U.S. population	
Asians	100
American Indians (Oklahoma)	95
Black Americans	81
Mexican Americans	56
White Americans	24
Others	
Ibo, Yoruba (Nigeria)	89
Italians	71
Aborigines (Australia)	67
Greeks	53
Danes	3
Dutch	0

Reproduced, with permission, from Annu Rev Med 1990;41:145. © 1990 by Annual Reviews, Inc.

glucoamylase activities are usually present at such excessive levels that there are no pathological effects. Lactase is usually the first activity lost and the last to recover.

Trehalase

The fourth glycosidase complex, trehalase, hydrolyzes the glycosidic bond in trehalose, a sugar found in insects, algae, mushrooms, and other fungi (Fig. 25.18). Although trehalose is not currently a major dietary component in the United States, a deficiency can have adverse consequences. Trehalase deficiency was discovered when a person became very sick after eating mushrooms and was initially thought to have mushroom poisoning.

The glycosidic bonds of other dietary sugars, including the sugar residues attached to lipids and proteins, are all hydrolyzed by digestive enzymes, and the sugars are released for absorption into the intestinal mucosal cell. For example, β-glycosidase is capable of hydrolyzing the glycosidic bond of the lipid glycosylceramide.

DIETARY FIBER

Dietary fiber is the portion of the diet that is not enzymatically digested by human digestive enzymes and thus does not directly serve as a source of nourishment (Fig. 25.19). Its five major categories include cellulose, hemicellulose, pectins, mucilages and gums, and lignins (which are not carbohydrates, but polymers of phenylpropane). Although human enzymes cannot digest fiber, the bacterial flora in the normal human gut may degrade the more soluble dietary fibers, releasing the products into the lumen of the gut. The endproducts of bacterial metabolism are CO_2, H_2O, H_2, methane, and short chain fatty acids (acetate, propionate, and butyrate). Some of these fatty acids may be absorbed and utilized by the epithelial cells of the gut and some may travel to the liver via the hepatic portal vein. We may obtain as much as 10% of our total calories from compounds produced by bacterial digestion of substances in our digestive tract.

The National Research Council has recommended that Americans increase the fiber content of their diet. One beneficial effect of fiber is seen in diverticular disease, where sacs or pouches may develop in the colon due to a weakening of the muscle and submucosal structures. Fiber is thought to "soften" the stool, thereby reducing pressure on the colonic wall and enhancing expulsion of feces. Epidemiological and other types of studies suggest that the low consumption of fiber by Americans may be related to an increased incidence of colon cancer.

Certain types of fiber (e.g., pectins) may be able to lower blood cholesterol levels by binding bile acids. Pectins may also have a beneficial effect in the diet of individuals with diabetes mellitus by slowing the rate of absorption of simple sugars and preventing high blood glucose levels following meals. However, each of the beneficial effects which have been related to "fiber" are relatively specific for the type of fiber, and the physical form of food which contains the fiber. This factor, along with many others, has made it difficult to obtain conclusive results from studies of the effects of fiber on human health.

A 25.3: These sugars are not digested well by the human intestine, but form good sources of energy for the bacteria of the gut. These bacteria convert the sugars to H_2, lactic acid, and short chain fatty acids. The amount of gas released after a meal containing beans is especially notorious.

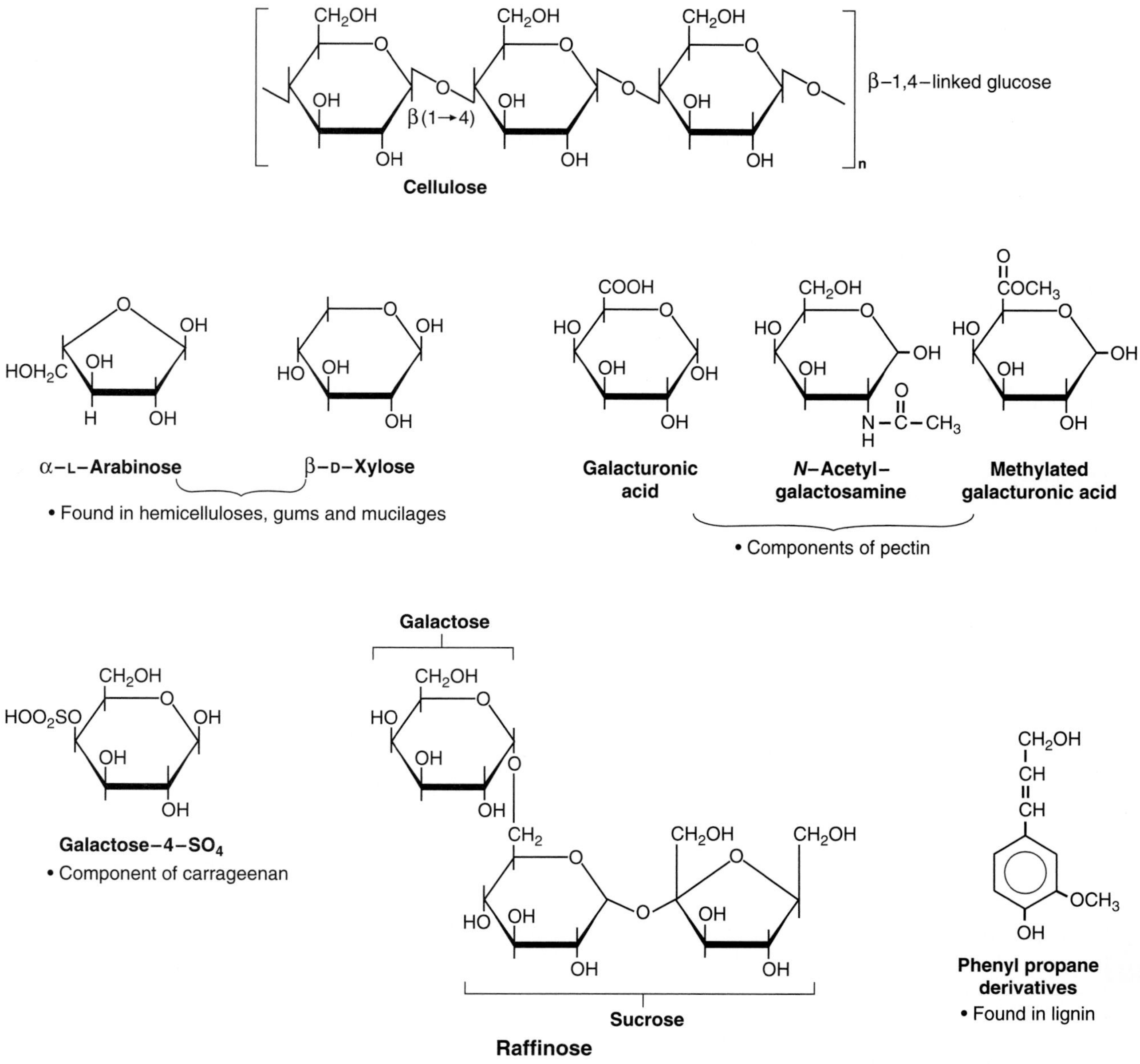

Fig. 25.19. Some indigestible carbohydrates. These compounds are components of dietary fiber.

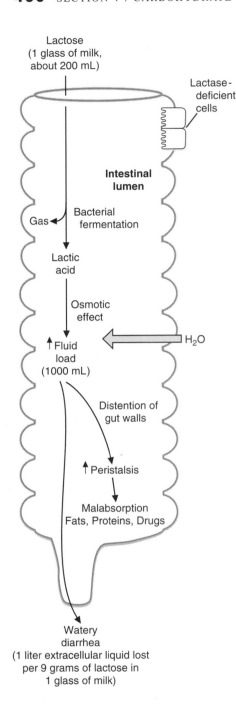

Lactose
(1 glass of milk,
about 200 mL)

Lactase-
deficient
cells

Intestinal
lumen

Gas ← Bacterial
fermentation

Lactic
acid

Osmotic
effect

↑ Fluid
load
(1000 mL)   ← H₂O

Distention of
gut walls

↑ Peristalsis

Malabsorption
Fats, Proteins, Drugs

Watery
diarrhea
(1 liter extracellular liquid lost
per 9 grams of lactose in
1 glass of milk)

Nona Melos's stool sample had a pH of 5 and gave a positive test for sugar. Her urine produced a negative reducing sugar test. The possibility of carbohydrate malabsorption was considered and a hydrogen breath test was recommended.

Lactose intolerance can either be the result of a primary deficiency of lactase production in the small bowel (as is the case for **Deria Voider**) or it can be secondary to an injury to the intestinal mucosa where lactase is normally produced. The lactose that is not absorbed is converted by colonic bacteria to lactic acid, methane gas (CH_4), and H_2 gas (see figure on left). The osmotic effect of the lactose and lactic acid in the bowel lumen is responsible for the diarrhea often seen as part of this syndrome. Similar symptoms can result from a sensitivity to milk proteins (milk intolerance) or from the malabsorption of other dietary sugars.

In adults suspected of having a lactase deficiency, the diagnosis is usually made inferentially when avoidance of all dairy products results in relief of symptoms and a rechallenge with these foods reproduces the characteristic syndrome. If the results of these measures are equivocal, however, the malabsorption of lactose can be more specifically determined by measuring the H_2 content of the patient's breath after a test dose of lactose has been consumed.

Deria Voider's symptoms did not appear if she took tablets containing lactase when she ate dairy products.

ABSORPTION OF SUGARS

Glucose is transported through the absorptive cells of the intestine by facilitated diffusion and by Na^+-dependent facilitated transport. (See Chapter 10 for a description of transport mechanisms.) The glucose molecule is extremely polar and cannot diffuse through the hydrophobic phospholipid bilayer of the cell membrane. Each –OH of the glucose molecule forms at least two hydrogen bonds with water molecules, and random movement would require energy to dislodge the polar OH groups from their hydrogen bonds and to disrupt the Van der Waals' forces between the hydrocarbon tails of the fatty acids in the membrane phospholipid. Glucose, therefore, enters the absorptive cells by binding to transport proteins, membrane-spanning proteins which bind the glucose molecule on one side of the membrane and release it on the opposite side (Fig. 25.20). Two types of glucose transport proteins are present in the intestinal absorptive cells: the Na^+-dependent glucose transporters and the facilitative glucose transporters (Fig. 25.21).

Na^+-dependent glucose transporters, which are located on the luminal side of the absorptive cells, enable these cells to concentrate glucose from the intestinal lumen. A low intracellular Na^+ concentration is maintained by a Na^+,K^+-ATPase on the serosal (blood) side of the cell that utilizes the energy from ATP cleavage to pump Na^+ out of the cell into the blood. Thus, the transport of glucose from a low concentration in the lumen to a high concentration in the cell is promoted by the cotransport of Na^+ from a high concentration in the lumen to a low concentration in the cell (secondary active transport) (see Chapter 10). Facilitative glucose transporters, which do not bind Na^+, are located on the serosal side of the cells. Glucose moves via the facilitative transporters from the high concentration inside the cell to the lower concentration in the blood without the expenditure of energy. In addition to the Na^+-dependent glucose transporters, facilitative transporters for glucose also exist on the luminal side of the absorptive cells.

Facilitative glucose transporters exist in different cells as a family of similar proteins (isoforms) with a 50–76% similarity in amino acid sequence. The protein isoforms are products of different genes on different chromosomes. The different isoforms have different tissue distributions and properties, and some cell types have more than one isoform. The properties and tissue distribution of five of these isoforms found in the plasma membranes of cells (referred to as GLUT 1–GLUT 5), are shown in Table 25.2.

Galactose is absorbed via the same mechanisms as glucose. It enters the absorptive cells on the luminal side via the Na^+-dependent glucose transporters and facili-

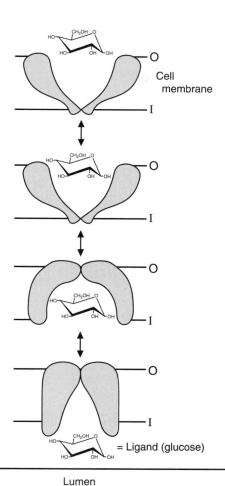

Fig. 25.20 (left). Facilitative transport. Transport of glucose occurs without rotation of the glucose molecule. Multiple groups on the protein bind the –OH groups of glucose and close behind it as it is released into the cell (i.e., the transporter acts like a "gated pore"). O = outside; I = inside.

The association of **Nona Melos's** symptoms with her ingestion of fruit juices suggests that she might have a problem with fructose or sucrose malabsorption resulting from a deficiency of sucrase activity or an inability to absorb fructose. Her ability to thrive and her adequate weight gain suggest that any deficiencies of the sucrase-isomaltase complex must be partial and do not result in a functionally important reduction in maltase activity (maltase activity is also present in the glucoamylase complex). Therefore, a hydrogen breath test after Nona ingested test meals containing fructose, lactose, and sucrose was performed. The basis for this test is that if a sugar is not absorbed, it is metabolized in the intestinal lumen by bacteria that produce various gases, including hydrogen.

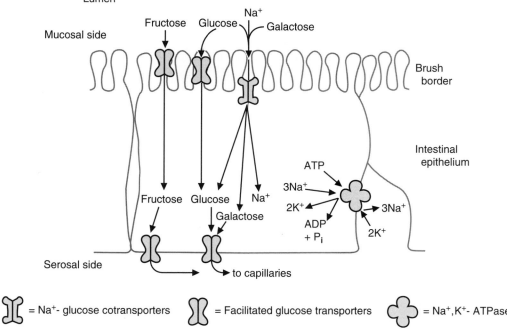

Fig. 25.21. Na^+-dependent and facilitative transporters in the intestinal epithelial cells. Both glucose and fructose are transported by the facilitated glucose transporters on the luminal and serosal sides of the absorptive cells. Glucose and galactose are transported by the Na^+-glucose cotransporters on the luminal (mucosal) side of the absorptive cells.

The epithelial cells of the kidney, which reabsorb glucose into the blood, have Na+-dependent glucose transporters similar to those of intestinal epithelial cells. They are thus also able to transport glucose against its concentration gradient. Other types of cells use mainly facilitative glucose transporters that carry glucose down its concentration gradient.

Table 25.2. Properties of GLUT 1–GLUT 5, Isoforms of the Glucose Transport Proteins

Transporter	Tissue Distribution	Special Properties
GLUT 1	• Red blood cells, brain microvessels (blood-brain barrier), kidney, colon and other cells	• May limit glucose transport into brain
GLUT 2	• Liver, pancreatic β cells, basolateral surface of small intestine	• High capacity, low affinity. K_m of 15 mM or higher
GLUT 3	• Neurons, placenta, testes	• Low K_m, possibly 1 mM
GLUT 4	• Fat, skeletal muscle, heart	• Mediates insulin-stimulated glucose uptake
GLUT 5	• Small intestine, testes and sperm. Lower levels in kidney, skeletal muscle, adipose tissue, and brain	• Fructose transporter

tative glucose transporters and is transported through the serosal side on the facilitative glucose transporters.

Fructose both enters and leaves absorptive epithelial cells via facilitated diffusion, apparently via transport proteins that are part of the GLUT family. The transporter on the luminal side has been identified as GLUT 5. Although this transporter can transport glucose, it has a much higher activity with fructose (see Fig. 25.21). Other fructose transport proteins may also be present. For reasons as yet unknown, fructose is absorbed at a much more rapid rate when it is ingested as sucrose than when it is ingested alone.

TRANSPORT OF MONOSACCHARIDES INTO TISSUES

The properties of the GLUT transport proteins differ between tissues, reflecting the function of glucose metabolism in each tissue. In most cell types, the rate of glucose transport across the cell membrane is not rate-limiting for glucose metabolism. The isoform of transporter present has a relatively low K_m for glucose and/or is present in relatively high concentration in the cell membrane so that the intracellular glucose concentration reflects that in the blood. Since the hexokinase isozyme present in these cells has an even lower K_m for glucose (0.05–0.10 mM), variations in blood glucose levels do not affect the intracellular rate of glucose phosphorylation. However, in several tissues, the rate of transport becomes rate-limiting when the serum level of glucose is low or when low levels of insulin signal the absence of dietary glucose.

In the liver, the K_m for the glucose transporter is relatively high compared to that of other tissues, probably 15 mM or above. The properties of the transporter are related to those of glucokinase, the liver enzyme that converts glucose to glucose 6-phosphate. Glucokinase also has a high $S_{0.5}$ ($\cong K_m$) for glucose and exhibits little inhibition by glucose 6-phosphate. These properties favor a net flux of glucose into the liver as the blood glucose concentration rises after a high carbohydrate meal and a net efflux as the blood glucose concentration decreases. The net flux of glucose into liver cells is also accelerated by the utilization of "excess" glucose for glycogen and fatty acid synthesis.

In muscle and adipose tissue, the transport of glucose is greatly stimulated by insulin. The mechanism involves the recruitment of glucose transporters from intracellular vesicles into the plasma membrane (Fig. 25.22). In adipose tissue, the stimulation of glucose transport across the plasma membrane by insulin increases its availability for the synthesis of fatty acids and glycerol from the glycolytic pathway. In skeletal muscle, the stimulation of glucose transport by insulin increases its availability for glycolysis and glycogen synthesis.

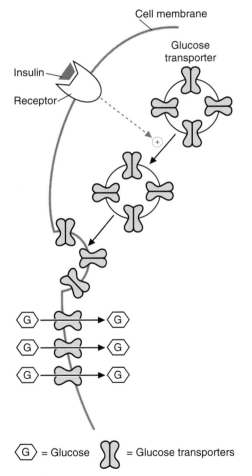

Fig. 25.22. Stimulation by insulin of glucose transport into muscle and adipose cells. Binding of insulin to its cell membrane receptor causes vesicles containing glucose transport proteins to move from inside the cell to the cell membrane.

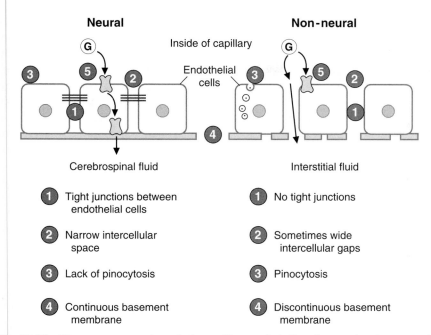

Fig. 25.23. Glucose transport through the capillary endothelium in neural and nonneural tissues. Characteristics of transport in each type of tissue are listed by numbers that refer to the numbers in the drawing. G = glucose.

GLUCOSE TRANSPORT THROUGH THE BLOOD-BRAIN BARRIER AND INTO NEURONS

A hypoglycemic response is elicited by a decrease of blood glucose concentration to some point between 18 and 54 mg/dL (1 and 3 mM). The hypoglycemic response is a result of a decreased supply of glucose to the brain and starts with lightheadedness and dizziness and may progress to coma. The slow rate of transport of glucose through the blood-brain barrier (from the blood into the cerebrospinal fluid) at low levels of glucose is thought to be responsible for this hypoglycemic response. Glucose transport from the cerebrospinal fluid across the plasma membranes of neurons is exceedingly fast and is not rate limiting for ATP generation from glycolysis.

In the brain, the endothelial cells of the capillaries have extremely tight junctions, and glucose must pass from the blood into the extracellular cerebrospinal fluid by transporters in the endothelial cell membranes (Fig. 25.23), and then through the basement membrane. Measurements of the overall process of glucose transport from the blood into the neural cells show a $K_{m,app}$ of 7–11 mM, and a maximal velocity not much greater than the rate of glucose utilization by the brain. Thus, decreases of blood glucose below the fasting level of 80–90 mg/dL (about 5 mM) are likely to significantly affect the rate of glucose metabolism in the brain.

The erythrocyte (red blood cell) is an example of a tissue in which glucose transport is not rate-limiting. Although the glucose transporter (GLUT 1) has a K_m of 1–7 mM, it is present in extremely high concentrations, comprising about 5% of all membrane proteins. Consequently, as the blood glucose levels fall from a postprandial level of 160 mg/dL (10 mM) to the normal fasting level of 80 mg/dL (5 mM), or even the hypoglycemic level of 40 mg/dL (2.5 mM), the supply of glucose is still adequate for the rates at which glycolysis and the pentose phosphate pathway operate.

CLINICAL COMMENTS. One out of five Americans experiences some form of gastrointestinal discomfort from 30 minutes to 12 hours after ingesting lactose-rich foods. Most become symptomatic when they consume more than 25 g (e.g., 1 pint of milk or its equivalent). **Deria Voider's** symptoms were caused by her "new" diet in this country, which included a glass of milk in addition to the milk she used on her cereal with breakfast each morning.

Management of lactose intolerance includes a reduction or avoidance of lactose-containing foods depending upon the severity of the deficiency of intestinal lactase. Hard cheeses (cheddar, Swiss, Jarlsberg) are low in lactose and may be tolerated by patients with only moderate lactase deficiency. Yogurt with "live and active cultures" printed on the package contain bacteria that release free lactases when the bacteria are lysed by gastric acid and proteolytic enzymes. The free lactases then digest the lactose. Commercially available milk products that have been hydrolyzed with a lactase enzyme provide a 70% reduction in total lactose content which may be adequate to prevent digestive symptoms in mildly affected patients. Tablets and capsules containing lactase are also available and should be taken one-half hour before meals.

Many adults who have a lactase deficiency develop the ability to ingest small amounts of lactose in dairy products without experiencing symptoms. This adaptation probably involves an increase in the population of colonic bacteria that can cleave lactose and not a recovery or induction of human lactase synthesis. For many individuals, dairy products are the major dietary source of calcium, and their complete elimination from the diet can lead to osteoporosis.

It is important to note that lactose is used as a "filler" or carrying agent in more than 1,000 prescription and over-the-counter drugs in this country. People with lactose intolerance often unwittingly ingest lactose with their medications.

Poorly controlled diabetic patients like **Ann Sulin** frequently have elevations in serum total and low density lipoprotein (LDL) cholesterol levels. The pectins and gums as well as the lignins bind bile acids and cholesterol and remove them from micelles in the proximal small bowel. This action tends to decrease the absorption of these substances into the blood, which may chronically lower serum total and LDL cholesterol levels in patients with diabetes mellitus.

The large amount of H_2 produced with fructose suggested that **Nona Melos's** problem was one of a deficiency in fructose transport into the absorptive cells of the intestinal villi. To confirm the diagnosis, a jejunal biopsy was taken; lactase, sucrase, maltase and trehalase activities were normal in the jejunal cells. The tissue was also tested for the enzymes of fructose metabolism; these were in the normal range as well. Although Nona had no sugar in her urine, malabsorption of disaccharides can result in their appearance in the urine if damage to the intestinal mucosal cells allows their passage into the interstitial fluid. When Nona was placed on a diet free of fruit juices and other foods containing fructose, she did well and could tolerate small amounts of pure sucrose.

It is estimated that over 50% of the adult population cannot absorb fructose in high doses (50 g) and over 10% cannot completely absorb 25 g of fructose. These individuals, like those with other disorders of fructose metabolism, must avoid fruits and other foods containing high concentrations of fructose.

BIOCHEMICAL COMMENTS. Cholera is an acute watery diarrheal disorder caused by the water-borne, Gram-negative bacterium *Vibrio cholerae*. It is a disease of antiquity; descriptions of epidemics of the disease date before 500 BC. During epidemics, the infection is spread by large numbers of vibrio that enter water sources from the voluminous liquid stools and contaminate the environment, particularly in areas of extreme poverty where plumbing and modern waste-disposal systems are primitive or nonexistent.

After being ingested, the *V. cholerae* organisms attach to the brush border of the intestinal epithelium and secrete an exotoxin which binds irreversibly to a specific chemical receptor (G_{M1} ganglioside) on the cell surface. This exotoxin catalyses an

ADP-ribosylation reaction that increases adenylate cyclase activity and thus cAMP levels in the enterocyte. As a result, the normal absorption of sodium, anions, and water from the gut lumen into the intestinal cell is markedly diminished. The exotoxin also stimulates the crypt cells to secrete chloride, accompanied by cations and water, from the bloodstream into the lumen of the gut. The resulting loss of solute-rich diarrheal fluid may, in severe cases, exceed 1 liter/hour, leading to rapid dehydration and even death.

The therapeutic approach to cholera takes advantage of the fact that the Na^+-dependent transporters for glucose and amino acids are not affected by the cholera exotoxin. As a result, coadministration of glucose and Na^+ by mouth results in the uptake of glucose and Na^+, accompanied by chloride and water, thereby partially correcting the ion deficits and fluid loss. Amino acids and small peptides are also adsorbed by Na^+-dependent cotransport involving transport proteins distinct from the Na^+-dependent glucose transporters. Therefore, addition of protein to the glucose-sodium replacement solution enhances its effectiveness and markedly decreases the severity of the diarrhea. Adjunctive antibiotic therapy also shortens the diarrheal phase of cholera, but does not decrease the need for the oral replacement therapy outlined earlier.

Suggested Readings

Bell GJ, Burant CF, Takeda J, Gould GW. Structure and function of mammalian facilitative sugar transporters. J Biol Chem 1993;268:19161–19164.

Buller HA, Grand RJ. Lactose intolerance. Annu Rev Med 1990;41:141–148.

Linder MC (ed). Nutrition and metabolism of carbohydrates. In: Nutritional biochemistry and metabolism with clinical applications. 2nd ed. New York: Elsevier, 1991:21–50.

Semenza G, Auricchio S. Small-intestinal disaccharidases. In: Scriver CR, Beaudet AL, Sly WS, Valle D, eds. The metabolic and molecular bases of inherited disease. New York: McGraw-Hill, 1995:4451–4480.

PROBLEMS

1. An alcoholic patient developed a pancreatitis which affected his exocrine pancreatic function. He exhibited discomfort after eating a high carbohydrate meal. The patient probably had an abnormally low ability to digest

   A. starch

   B. lactose

   C. fiber

   D. sucrose

   E. maltose

2. If a person with insulin-dependent diabetes mellitus neglects to take his insulin injections while on a weekend vacation, what will happen to the transport of glucose into his cells? Which cells would be most severely affected?

ANSWERS

1. **A.** The pancreas produces an α-amylase that digests starch. If pancreatic α-amylase is not entering the intestine, some digestion of starch could still occur in this patient by the action of salivary α-amylase, but his overall ability to digest starch would be much lower than normal. In the human, salivary amylase accounts for very

little of the total amount of starch digested. Its principal function may be the removal of bits of crackers and other food debris that get stuck between the teeth. Lactose, sucrose, and maltose are digested by enzymes produced by intestinal epithelial cells and located on their brush border. However, these enzymes protrude into the lumen and their effectiveness is highest when the acidic chyme from the stomach is neutralized by HCO_3^- from the pancreas. Fiber is not digestible even in a normal individual.

2. Insulin stimulates the recruitment to the cell membrane of glucose transporters located in membranes of vesicles within the cell. An increased number of glucose transporters on the cell membrane permits more glucose to be transported into the cells. The greatest effect of this action of insulin occurs in muscle and adipose cells. If a diabetic patient neglects to take insulin, the number of transporters on his muscle and adipose cell membranes will be markedly reduced. The result is a decreased transport of glucose into these cells, which contributes to the elevation of blood glucose levels that the patient experiences.

26 Formation and Degradation of Glycogen

Glycogen is the storage form of glucose found in most types of cells. It is composed of glucosyl units linked by α-1,4 glycosidic bonds, with α-1,6 branches occurring about every 8–10 glucosyl units. The liver and skeletal muscle contain the largest glycogen stores (Fig. 26.1).

The formation of glycogen from glucose is an energy-requiring pathway which begins, like most of glucose metabolism, with the phosphorylation of glucose to glucose 6-phosphate. Glycogen synthesis from glucose 6-phosphate involves the formation of UDP-glucose and the transfer of glucosyl units from UDP-glucose to the ends of the glycogen chains by the enzyme glycogen synthase. Once the chains reach approximately 11 glucosyl units, a branching enzyme moves 6–8 units to form an α(1→6) branch.

Glycogenolysis, the pathway for glycogen degradation, is not the reverse of the biosynthetic pathway. The degradative enzyme glycogen phosphorylase removes glucosyl units one at a time from the ends of the glycogen chains, converting them to glucose 1-phosphate without resynthesizing UDP-glucose or UTP. A debranching enzyme removes the glucosyl residues near each branchpoint.

Liver glycogen serves as a source of blood glucose. To generate glucose, the glucose 1-phosphate produced from glycogen degradation is converted to glucose 6-phosphate. Glucose 6-phosphatase, an enzyme found only in liver and kidney, converts glucose 6-phosphate to free glucose, which then enters the blood.

Glycogen synthesis and degradation are regulated in liver by hormonal changes which signal the need for blood glucose. The body maintains blood glucose levels at about 80 mg/dL to ensure that the brain and other tissues which are dependent on glucose for the generation of ATP have a continuous supply. The lack of dietary glucose, signaled by a decrease of the insulin/glucagon ratio, activates liver glycogenolysis and inhibits glycogen synthesis. Epinephrine, which signals an increased utilization of blood glucose and other fuels for exercise or emergency situations, also activates liver glycogenolysis. The hormones which regulate liver glycogen metabolism work principally through changes in the phosphorylation state of glycogen synthase in the biosynthetic pathway and glycogen phosphorylase in the degradative pathway.

In skeletal muscle, glycogen supplies glucose 6-phosphate for ATP synthesis in the glycolytic pathway. Muscle glycogen phosphorylase is stimulated during exercise by the increase of AMP, an allosteric activator of the enzyme, and also by phosphorylation. The phosphorylation is stimulated by calcium released during contraction, and by the "fight-or-flight" hormone epinephrine. Glycogen synthesis is activated in resting muscles by the elevation of insulin following carbohydrate ingestion.

The neonate must rapidly adapt to an intermittent fuel supply after birth. Once the umbilical cord is clamped, the supply of glucose from the maternal circulation is interrupted. The combined effect of epinephrine and glucagon on the liver glycogen stores of the neonate rapidly restore glucose levels to normal.

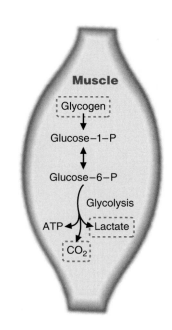

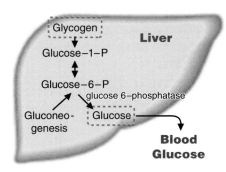

Fig. 26.1. Glycogenolysis in skeletal muscle and liver. Glycogen stores serve different functions in muscle cells and liver. In the muscle and most other cell types, glycogen stores serve as a fuel source for the generation of ATP. In the liver, glycogen stores serve as a source of blood glucose.

A newborn baby girl, **Getta Carbo**, was born after a 38-week gestation. Her mother, a 36-year-old woman, had moderate hypertension during the last trimester related to a recurrent urinary tract infection that resulted in a severe loss of appetite and recurrent vomiting in the month preceding delivery. Fetal bradycardia (slower than normal fetal heart rate) was detected with each uterine contraction of labor, a sign of possible fetal distress.

At birth Getta was cyanotic (a bluish discoloration caused by a lack of adequate oxygenation of tissues) and limp. She responded to several minutes of assisted ventilation. Her Apgar score of 3 was low at 1 minute after birth, but improved to a score of 7 at 5 minutes.

Physical examination in the nursery at 10 minutes showed a thin, malnourished female newborn. Her body temperature was slightly low, her heart rate was rapid, and her respiratory rate of 35/minute was elevated. Getta's birth weight was only 2,100 g, compared to a normal value of 3,300 g. Her length was 47 cm and her head circumference was 33 cm (low normal). The laboratory reported that Getta's serum glucose level when she was unresponsive was 14 mg/dL. A glucose value below 40 mg/dL (2.5 mM) is considered to be abnormal in newborn infants.

At 5 hours of age, she was apneic (not breathing) and unresponsive. Ventilatory resuscitation was initiated and a cannula placed in the umbilical vein. Blood for a glucose level was drawn through this cannula, and 5 mL of a 20% glucose solution was injected. Getta slowly responded to this therapy.

The Apgar score is an objective estimate of the overall condition of the newborn. The best score is 10 (normal in all respects).

Jim Bodie, a 19-year-old body builder, was rushed to the hospital emergency room in a coma. One-half hour earlier, his mother had heard a loud crashing sound in the basement where Jim had been lifting weights and completing his daily workout on the treadmill. She found her son on the floor having severe jerking movements of all muscles (a grand mal seizure).

In the emergency room, the doctors learned that despite the objections of his family and friends, Jim regularly used androgens and other anabolic steroids in an effort to bulk up his muscle mass.

On initial physical examination, he was comatose with occasional involuntary jerking movements of his extremities. A foamy saliva dripped from his mouth. He had bitten his tongue and had lost bowel and bladder control at the height of the seizure.

The laboratory reported a serum glucose level of 18 mg/dL (extremely low). The intravenous infusion of 5% glucose (5 g of glucose per 100 mL of solution), which had been started earlier, was increased to 10%. In addition, 50 g of glucose was given over 30 seconds through the intravenous tubing.

Jim Bodie's treadmill exercise and most other types of moderate exercise involving whole body movement (running, skiing, dancing, tennis) increase the utilization of blood glucose and other fuels by skeletal muscles. This glucose is normally supplied by the stimulation of liver glycogenolysis and gluconeogenesis.

STRUCTURE OF GLYCOGEN

Glycogen, the storage form of glucose, is a branched glucose polysaccharide composed of chains of glucosyl units linked by α-1,4 bonds with α-1,6 branches every 8–10 residues (Fig. 26.2). In a molecule of this highly branched structure, only one glucosyl residue has an anomeric carbon that is not linked to another glucose residue. This anomeric carbon at the beginning of the chain is attached to the protein glycogenin. The other ends of the chains are called nonreducing ends (see Chapter 6). The branched structure permits rapid degradation and rapid synthesis of glycogen because enzymes can work on several chains simultaneously from the multiple nonreducing ends.

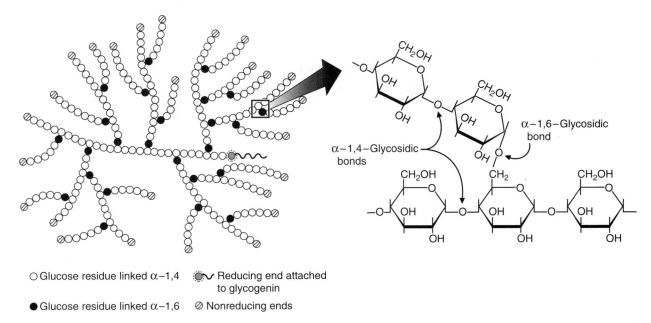

Fig. 26.2. Glycogen structure. Glycogen is composed of glucosyl units linked by α-1,4-glycosidic bonds and α-1,6-glycosidic bonds. The branches occur more frequently in the center of the molecule, and less frequently in the periphery. The anomeric carbon that is not attached to another glucosyl residue (the reducing end) is attached to the protein glycogenin by a glycosidic bond.

Glycogen is present in tissues as polymers of very high molecular weight (10^7–10^8) collected together in glycogen particles. The enzymes involved in glycogen synthesis and degradation, and some of the regulatory enzymes, are bound to the surface of the glycogen particles.

FUNCTION OF GLYCOGEN IN SKELETAL MUSCLE AND LIVER

Glycogen is found in all cell types, where it serves as a reservoir of glucosyl units for ATP generation from glycolysis.

Glycogen is degraded mainly to glucose 1-phosphate, which is converted to glucose 6-phosphate. In skeletal muscle and other cell types, the glucose 6-phosphate enters the glycolytic pathway (see Fig. 26.1). Glycogen is an extremely important fuel source for skeletal muscle when ATP demands are high and when glucose 6-phosphate is used rapidly in anaerobic glycolysis. In many other cell types, the small glycogen reservoir serves a similar purpose; it is an emergency fuel source which supplies glucose for the generation of ATP in the absence of oxygen or during restricted blood flow. In general, glycogenolysis and glycolysis are activated together in these cells.

Glycogen serves a very different purpose in liver than in skeletal muscle and other tissues (see Fig. 26.1). Liver glycogen is the first and immediate source of glucose for the maintenance of blood glucose levels. In the liver, the glucose 6-phosphate which is generated from glycogen degradation is hydrolyzed to glucose by glucose 6-phosphatase, an enzyme present only in the liver and kidneys. Glycogen degradation thus provides a readily mobilized source of blood glucose as dietary glucose decreases, or as exercise increases the utilization of blood glucose by muscles.

The pathways of glycogenolysis and gluconeogenesis in the liver both supply blood glucose, and, consequently, these two pathways are activated together. Gluconeogenesis, the synthesis of glucose from amino acids and other nongluconeogenic precursors, also forms glucose 6-phosphate, so that glucose 6-phosphatase serves as a "gateway" to the blood for both pathways (see Fig. 26.1).

SYNTHESIS AND DEGRADATION OF GLYCOGEN

Glycogen synthesis, like almost all the pathways of glucose metabolism, begins with the phosphorylation of glucose to glucose 6-phosphate by hexokinase or, in the liver,

Regulation of glycogen synthesis serves to prevent futile cycling and waste of ATP. Futile cycling refers to a situation in which a substrate is converted to a product through one pathway, and the product converted back to the substrate through another pathway. Since the biosynthetic pathway is energy-requiring, futile cycling results in a waste of high energy phosphate bonds. Thus, glycogen synthesis is activated when glycogen degradation is inhibited, and vice versa.

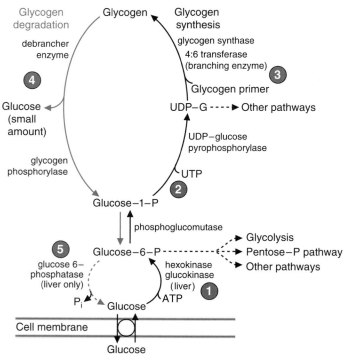

Fig. 26.3. Scheme of glycogen synthesis and degradation. **1.** Glucose 6-phosphate is formed from glucose by hexokinase in most cells, and glucokinase in the liver. It is a metabolic branch-point for the pathways of glycolysis, the pentose phosphate pathway, and glycogen synthesis. **2.** UDP-Glucose (UDP-G) is synthesized from glucose 1-phosphate. UDP-Glucose is the branchpoint for glycogen synthesis and other pathways requiring the addition of carbohydrate units. **3.** Glycogen synthesis is catalyzed by glycogen synthase and the branching enzyme. **4.** Glycogen degradation is catalyzed by glycogen phosphorylase and a debrancher enzyme. **5.** Glucose 6-phosphatase in the liver generates free glucose from glucose 6-phosphate.

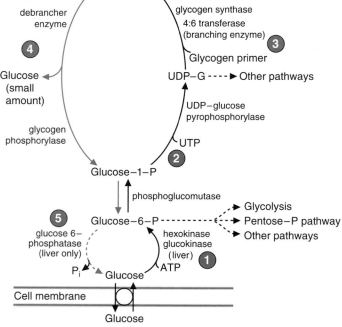

Fig. 26.4. Formation of UDP-glucose. The high energy phosphate bond of UTP provides the energy for the formation of a high energy bond in UDP-glucose. Pyrophosphate (PP_i), released by the reaction, is cleaved to 2 P_i.

glucokinase (Fig. 26.3). Glucose 6-phosphate is the precursor of glycolysis, the pentose phosphate pathway, and of pathways for the synthesis of other sugars. In the pathway for glycogen synthesis, glucose 6-phosphate is converted to glucose 1-phosphate by phosphoglucomutase, a reversible reaction.

Glycogen is both formed from—and degraded to—glucose 1-phosphate, but the biosynthetic and degradative pathways are separate and involve different enzymes (see Fig. 26.3). The biosynthetic pathway is an energy-requiring pathway; high energy phosphate from UTP is utilized to activate the glucosyl residues to UDP-glucose (Fig. 26.4). In the degradative pathway, the glycosidic bonds between the glucosyl residues in glycogen are simply cleaved by the addition of phosphate to produce glucose 1-phosphate (or water to produce free glucose), and UDP-glucose is not resynthesized. The existence of separate pathways for the formation and degradation of important compounds is a common theme in metabolism. Because the synthesis and degradation pathways utilize different enzymes, one can be activated while the other is inhibited.

Glycogen Synthesis

Glycogen synthesis requires the formation of α-1,4-glycosidic bonds to link glucosyl residues in long chains and the formation of an α-1,6 branch every 8–10 residues (Fig. 26.5). Most of glycogen synthesis occurs through the lengthening of the polysaccharide chains of a preexisting glycogen molecule (a glycogen primer) in which the reducing end of the glycogen is attached to the protein glycogenin. To lengthen the glycogen chains, glucosyl residues are added from UDP-glucose to the nonreducing ends of the chain by glycogen synthase. The anomeric carbon of each glucosyl residue is attached in an α-1,4 bond to the hydroxyl on carbon 4 of the terminal glucosyl residue. When the chain reaches 11 residues in length, a 6–8 residue piece is cleaved by amylo-4:6-transferase and reattached to a glucosyl unit by an α-1,6 bond. Both chains continue to lengthen until they are long enough to produce two new branches. This process continues, producing highly branched molecules. Glycogen synthase, the enzyme which attaches the glucosyl residues in 1,4- bonds, is the regulated step in the pathway.

The synthesis of new glycogen primer molecules also occurs. Glycogenin, the protein to which glycogen is attached, glycosylates itself (autoglycosylation) by attaching a glucosyl residue to the OH of a tyrosine residue. The addition of glucosyl residues continues until the glucosyl chain is long enough to serve as a substrate for glycogen synthase.

Degradation of Glycogen

Glycogen is degraded by two enzymes, glycogen phosphorylase and the debrancher enzyme (Fig. 26.6). The enzyme glycogen phosphorylase starts at the end of a chain and successively cleaves glucosyl residues by adding phosphate to the terminal glycosidic bond, thereby releasing glucose 1-phosphate. However, glycogen phosphorylase cannot act on the glycosidic bonds of the 4 glucosyl residues closest to a branchpoint because the branching chain sterically hinders a proper fit into the catalytic site of the enzyme. The debrancher enzyme, which catalyzes the removal of the 4 residues closest to the branchpoint, has two catalytic activities: it acts as a 4:4 transferase and a 1,6-glucosidase. As a 4:4 transferase, the debrancher first removes a unit containing 3 glucose residues, and adds it to the end of a longer chain by an α-1,4 bond. The one glucosyl residue remaining at the 1,6-branch is hydrolyzed by the amylo-1,6-glucosidase of the debrancher, resulting in the release of free glucose. Thus, one glucose and about 7–9 glucose 1-phosphate residues are released for every branchpoint.

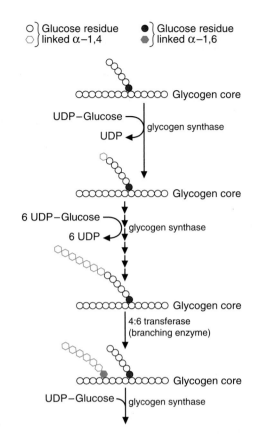

Fig. 26.5. Glycogen synthesis. See text for details.

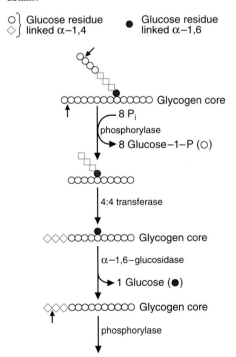

Fig. 26.6. Glycogen degradation. See text for details.

A genetic defect of lysosomal glucosidase, called type II glycogen storage disease, leads to the accumulation of glycogen particles in large, membrane-enclosed residual bodies, which disrupt the function of liver and muscle cells. Children with this disease usually die of heart failure at a few months of age.

Some degradation of glycogen also occurs within lysosomes when glycogen particles become surrounded by membranes which then fuse with the lysosomal membranes. A lysosomal glucosidase hydrolyzes this glycogen to glucose.

REGULATION OF GLYCOGEN SYNTHESIS AND DEGRADATION

The regulation of glycogen synthesis in different tissues matches the function of glycogen in each tissue. Liver glycogen serves principally for the support of blood glucose during fasting or during extreme need (e.g., exercise), and the degradative and biosynthetic pathways are regulated principally by changes in the insulin/glucagon ratio and by blood glucose levels, which reflect the availability of dietary glucose (Table 26.2). Degradation of liver glycogen is also activated by epinephrine, which is released in response to exercise, hypoglycemia, or another stress situation in which there is an immediate demand for blood glucose. In contrast, in skeletal muscles, glycogen is a reservoir of glucosyl units for the generation of ATP from glycolysis and glucose oxidation. As a consequence, muscle glycogenolysis is regulated principally by AMP, which signals a lack of ATP, and by Ca^{2+} released during contraction. Epinephrine, which is released in response to exercise and other stress situations, also activates skeletal muscle glycogenolysis. The glycogen stores of resting muscle decrease very little during fasting.

26.1: A series of inborn errors of metabolism, the glycogen storage diseases, result from deficiencies in the enzymes of glycogenolysis (see Table 26.1). Muscle glycogen phosphorylase, the key regulatory enzyme of glycogen degradation, is genetically different from liver glycogen phosphorylase, and thus a person may have a defect in one and not the other. Why do you think that a genetic deficiency in muscle glycogen phosphorylase (McArdle's disease) is a mere inconvenience, while a deficiency of liver glycogen phosphorylase (Hers' disease) can be lethal?

Table 26.1. Glycogen Storage Diseases

Type	Enzyme Affected	Primary Organ Involved	Manifestations[a]
O	Glycogen synthase	Liver	Hypoglycemia, hyperketonemia, FTT[b], early death
I[c]	Glucose 6-phosphatase (Von Gierke's disease)	Liver	Enlarged liver and kidney, growth failure, fasting hypoglycemia, acidosis, lipemia, thrombocyte dysfunction. Hypoglycemia is the most severe.
II	Lysosomal α-glucosidase	All organs with lysosomes	Infantile form: early-onset progressive muscle hypotonia, cardiac failure, death before 2 years; juvenile form: later-onset myopathy with variable cardiac involvement: adult form: limb-girdle muscular dystrophy-like features. Glycogen deposits accumulate in lysosomes.
III	Amylo-1,6-glucosidase (debrancher)	Liver, skeletal muscle, heart	Fasting hypoglycemia; hepatomegaly in infancy in some, myopathic features. Glycogen deposits have short outer branches.
IV	Amylo-4,6-glucosidase (branching enzyme)	Liver	Hepatosplenomegaly; symptoms may arise from a hepatic reaction to the presence of a foreign body (glycogen with long outer branches). Usually fatal.
V	Muscle glycogen phosphorylase (McArdle's disease)	Skeletal muscle	Exercise-included muscular pain, cramps, and progressive weakness, sometimes with myoglobinuria.
VI	Liver glycogen phosphorylase	Liver	Hepatomegaly, mild hypoglycemia, good prognosis
VII	Phosphofructokinase	Muscle, RBC	As in V, in addition, enzymopathic hemolysis
IX[d]	Phosphorylase kinase	Liver	As in VI. Hepatomegaly
X	Protein kinase A (cAMP dependent)	Liver	Hepatomegaly

Reproduced with permission, from Annu Rev Nutr 1993;13:85. © 1993 by Annual Reviews, Inc.

[a]All of these diseases but Type O are characterized by increased glycogen deposits.

[b]FTT = failure to thrive

[c]Glucose 6-phosphatase is comprised of several subunits which also transport glucose, glucose 6-phosphate, phosphate, and pyrophosphate across the endoplasmic reticulum membranes. Therefore there are several subtypes of this disease, corresponding to defects in the different subunits.

[d]There are several subtypes of this disease, corresponding to different mutations and patterns of inheritance.

Regulation of Glycogen Metabolism in Liver

Liver glycogen is synthesized during a carbohydrate meal when blood glucose levels are elevated, and degraded as blood glucose levels decrease. When an individual eats a carbohydrate-containing meal, blood glucose levels immediately increase, insulin levels increase, and glucagon levels decrease (see Fig. 24.8). The increase of blood glucose levels and the rise of the insulin/glucagon ratio inhibit glycogen degradation and stimulate glycogen synthesis. The immediate storage of blood glucose as glycogen helps to bring circulating blood glucose levels back to the normal 80–100 mg/dL range. As the length of time after a carbohydrate-containing meal increases, insulin levels decrease and glucagon levels increase. The fall of the insulin/glucagon ratio results in inhibition of the biosynthetic pathway and activation of the degradative pathway. As a result, liver glycogen is rapidly degraded to glucose, which is released into the blood.

Although glycogenolysis and gluconeogenesis are activated together by the same regulatory mechanisms, glycogenolysis responds more rapidly, with a greater outpouring of glucose. A substantial proportion of liver glycogen is degraded within the first few hours after eating (Table 26.3). Liver glycogen stores are, therefore, a rapidly rebuilt and degraded store of glucose—ever responsive to small and rapid changes of blood glucose levels.

REGULATION OF LIVER GLYCOGEN METABOLISM BY INSULIN AND GLUCAGON

Insulin and glucagon regulate liver glycogen metabolism by changing the phosphorylation state of glycogen phosphorylase in the degradative pathway and glycogen synthase in the biosynthetic pathway. An increase of glucagon and decrease of insulin during the fasting state initiates a cAMP-directed phosphorylation cascade, which results in the phosphorylation of glycogen phosphorylase to an active enzyme, and

Table 26.2. Regulation of Liver and Muscle Glycogen Stores[a]

State	Regulators	Response of Tissue
	Liver	
Fasting	Blood: Glucagon ↑; insulin ↓ Tissue: cAMP ↑	Glycogen degradation ↑; glycogen synthesis ↓
Carbohydrate meal	Blood: Glucagon ↓, insulin ↑, glucose ↑ Tissue: cAMP ↓, glucose ↑	Glycogen degradation ↓; glycogen synthesis ↑
Exercise and stress	Blood: epinephrine ↑ Tissue: cAMP ↑ Ca^{2+}-calmodulin ↑	Glycogen degradation ↑; glycogen synthesis ↓
	Muscle	
Fasting (rest)	Blood: Insulin ↓	Glycogen synthesis ↓; glucose transport ↓
Carbohydrate meal (rest)	Blood: Insulin ↑	Glycogen synthesis ↑; glucose transport ↑
Exercise	Blood: Epinephrine ↑ Tissue: AMP ↑ Ca^{2+}-calmodulin ↑	Glycogen synthesis ↓ Glycogen degradation ↑ Glycolysis ↑

↑ = increased compared to other physiological states; ↓ = decreased compared to other physiological states.

Table 26.3. Effect of Fasting on Liver Glycogen Content in the Human

Length of Fast (hrs)	Glycogen Content (μmol/g liver)
0	300
2	260
4	216
24	42
64	16

A 26.1: Muscle glycogen is utilized within the muscle to support exercise. Thus, an individual with McArdle's disease (type V glycogen storage disease) experiences no other symptoms but unusual fatigue and muscle cramps during exercise. These symptoms may be accompanied by myoglobinuria and release of muscle creatine kinase into the blood.

Liver glycogen is the first reservoir for the support of blood glucose levels, and a deficiency in glycogen phosphorylase or any of the other enzymes of liver glycogen degradation can result in fasting hypoglycemia. The hypoglycemia is usually mild because patients can still synthesize glucose from gluconeogenesis (see Table 26.1).

Q 26.2: A patient was diagnosed as an infant with type III glycogen storage disease, a deficiency of debrancher enzyme (Table 26.1). The patient had hepatomegaly (an enlarged liver) and experienced bouts of mild hypoglycemia. To diagnose the disease, glycogen was obtained from the patient's liver by biopsy after the patient had fasted overnight and compared to normal glycogen. The glycogen samples were treated with a preparation of commercial glycogen phosphorylase and commercial debrancher enzyme. The amounts of glucose 1-phosphate and glucose produced in the assay were then measured. The ratio of glucose 1-phosphate to glucose for the normal glycogen sample was 9:1, and the ratio for the patient was 3:1. Can you explain these results?

Maternal blood glucose readily crosses the placenta to enter the fetal circulation. During the last 9 or 10 weeks of gestation, glycogen formed from maternal glucose is deposited in the fetal liver under the influence of the insulin-dominated hormonal milieu of that period. At birth, maternal glucose supplies cease, causing a temporary physiological drop in glucose levels in the newborn's blood, even in normal healthy infants. This drop serves as one of the signals for glucagon release from the newborn's pancreas, which, in turn, stimulates glycogenolysis. As a result, the glucose levels in the newborn return to normal.

Healthy full-term babies have adequate stores of liver glycogen to survive short (12 hours) periods of caloric deprivation provided other aspects of fuel metabolism are normal. Because **Getta Carbo's** mother was markedly anorexic during the critical period when the fetal liver is normally synthesizing glycogen from glucose supplied in the maternal blood, and since fetal glycogen is the major source of fuel for the newborn in the early hours of life, Getta became profoundly hypoglycemic within 5 hours of birth.

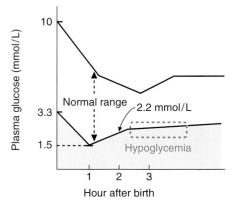

Fig. 26.A. Plasma glucose levels in the neonate. The normal range of blood glucose levels in the neonate lies between the two black lines. The stippled blue area represents the range of hypoglycemia in the neonate which should be treated. Treatment of neonates with blood glucose levels that fall within the dashed blue box, the zone of clinical uncertainty, is controversial. The units of plasma glucose are given in millimoles/L. Both milligrams/dL (milligrams/100 mL) and millimoles/L are used clinically for the values of blood glucose. 80 mg/dL glucose is equivalent to 5 mmol/L (5 mM). From Mehta A. Arch Dis Child 1994;70:F54.

A 26.2: With a deficiency of debrancher enzyme, but normal levels of glycogen phosphorylase, the glycogen chains of the patient could be degraded in vivo only to within 4 residues of the branchpoint. When the glycogen samples were treated with the commercial preparation containing normal enzymes, one glucose residue was released for each α-1,6 branch. In the patient's glycogen sample, with the short outer branches, three glucose 1-phosphates and one glucose residue were obtained for each α-1,6 branch. Normal glycogen has 8–10 glucosyl residues per branch, and thus gives a ratio of about 9 moles of glucose 1-phosphate to one mole of glucose.

the phosphorylation of glycogen synthase to an inactive enzyme (Fig. 26.7). As a consequence, glycogen degradation is stimulated and glycogen synthesis is inhibited.

Glucagon Activates a Phosphorylation Cascade That Converts Glycogen Phosphorylase b to Glycogen Phosphorylase a

Glucagon regulates glycogen metabolism through its intracellular second messenger cAMP and protein kinase A (see Chapter 24). Glucagon, by binding to its cell membrane receptor, transmits a signal through G proteins which activates adenylate cyclase, causing cAMP levels to increase (see Fig. 26.7). cAMP binds to the regulatory subunits of protein kinase A, which dissociate from the catalytic subunits. The catalytic subunits of protein kinase A are activated by the dissociation, and phosphorylate the enzyme phosphorylase kinase. Phosphorylase kinase is also a protein kinase which converts the inactive liver glycogen phosphorylase b conformer to the active glycogen phosphorylase a conformer by transferring a phosphate from ATP to specific serine residues on the phosphorylase subunits. As a result of the activation of glycogen phosphorylase, glycogenolysis is stimulated.

Inhibition of Glycogen Synthase by Glucagon-Directed Phosphorylation

When glycogen degradation is activated by the cAMP-stimulated phosphorylation cascade, glycogen synthesis is simultaneously inhibited. The enzyme glycogen synthase is also phosphorylated by protein kinase A, but this phosphorylation results in a less active form, glycogen synthase b.

Glycogen synthase is far more complex than glycogen phosphorylase. It has multiple phosphorylation sites and is acted upon by many different protein kinases. Phosphorylation by protein kinase A does not, by itself, inactivate glycogen synthase. Instead, phosphorylation by protein kinase A facilitates the subsequent addition of phosphate groups by other kinases, and these inactivate the enzyme. A term which has been applied to changes of activity resulting from multiple phosphorylation is hierarchical or synergistic phosphorylation—the phosphorylation of one site makes another site more reactive and easier to phosphorylate by a different protein kinase.

 To remember whether a particular enzyme has been activated or inhibited by cAMP-dependent phosphorylation, consider whether it makes sense for the enzyme to be active or inhibited under fasting conditions (In a **PHast, PHosphorylate**).

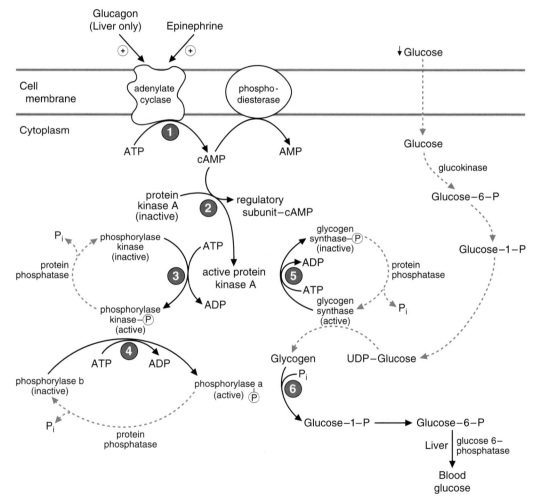

Fig. 26.7. Regulation of glycogen synthesis and degradation in the liver. **1.** Glucagon binding to the glucagon receptor or epinephrine binding to a β receptor in the liver activates adenylate cyclase, which synthesizes cAMP from ATP. **2.** cAMP binds to protein kinase A (cAMP-dependent protein kinase), thereby activating the catalytic subunits. **3.** Protein kinase A activates phosphorylase kinase by phosphorylation. **4.** Phosphorylase kinase adds a phosphate to specific serine residues on phosphorylase b, thereby converting it to the active phosphorylase a. **5.** Protein kinase A also phosphorylates glycogen synthase, thereby decreasing its activity. **6.** As a result of the inhibition of glycogen synthase and the activation of glycogen phosphorylase, glycogen is degraded to glucose 1-phosphate. The blue dashed lines denote reactions which are decreased in the livers of fasting individuals.

Most of the enzymes which are regulated by phosphorylation have multiple phosphorylation sites. Glycogen phosphorylase, which has only one serine per subunit, and can be phosphorylated only by phosphorylase kinase, is the exception. For some enzymes, the phosphorylation sites are antagonistic and phosphorylation initiated by one hormone counteracts the effects of other hormones. For other enzymes, the phosphorylation sites are synergistic, and phosphorylation at one site stimulated by one hormone can act synergistically with phosphorylation at another site.

Most of the enzymes which are regulated by phosphorylation can also be converted to the active conformation by allosteric effectors. Glycogen synthase b, the less active form of glycogen synthase, can be activated by the accumulation of glucose 6-phosphate above physiological levels. The activation of glycogen synthase by glucose 6-phosphate may be important in individuals with glucose 6-phosphatase deficiency, a disorder known as type I or von Gierke's glycogen storage disease. When glucose 6-phosphate produced from gluconeogenesis accumulates in the liver, it activates glycogen synthesis even though the individual may be hypoglycemic and have low insulin levels. Glucose 1-phosphate is also elevated, resulting in the inhibition of glycogen phosphorylase. As a consequence, large glycogen deposits accumulate and hepatomegaly occurs.

Regulation of Protein Phosphatases

At the same time that protein kinase A and phosphorylase kinase are adding phosphate groups to enzymes, the protein phosphatases which remove this phosphate are inhibited. Protein phosphatases remove the phosphate groups, bound to serine or other residues of enzymes, by hydrolysis. Hepatic protein phosphatase-1 (hepatic PP-1), one of the major protein phosphatases involved in glycogen metabolism, removes phosphate groups from phosphorylase kinase, glycogen phosphorylase, and glycogen synthase. During fasting, hepatic PP-1 is inactivated by glucagon-directed phosphorylation, dissociation from the glycogen particle, and the binding of inhibitor proteins, such as the protein called inhibitor-1. Insulin indirectly activates hepatic PP-1 through its own phosphorylation cascade initiated at the insulin receptor tyrosine kinase.

Insulin in Liver Glycogen Metabolism

Insulin is antagonistic to glucagon in the degradation and synthesis of glycogen. The glucose level in the blood is the signal controlling the secretion of insulin and glucagon. Glucose stimulates insulin release and suppresses glucagon release; one increases while the other decreases after a high carbohydrate meal. However, insulin levels in the blood change much more with the fasting-feeding cycle than the glucagon levels, and thus insulin is considered the principal regulator of glycogen synthesis and degradation. The role of insulin in glycogen metabolism is often overlooked because the mechanisms by which insulin reverses all of the effects of glucagon on individual metabolic enzymes is unknown. In addition to the activation of hepatic PP-1 through the insulin receptor tyrosine kinase phosphorylation cascade, insulin may activate the phosphodiesterase which converts cAMP to AMP, thereby decreasing cAMP levels. Regardless of the mechanisms involved, insulin is able to reverse all of the effects of glucagon and is the most important hormonal regulator of blood glucose levels.

Blood Glucose Levels and Glycogen Synthesis and Degradation

When an individual eats a high carbohydrate meal, glycogen degradation immediately stops. Although the changes in insulin and glucagon levels are relatively rapid (10–15 minutes), the direct inhibitory effect of rising glucose levels on glycogen degradation is even more rapid. Glucose inhibits liver glycogen phosphorylase a by stimulating dephosphorylation of this enzyme. As insulin levels rise and glucagon levels fall, cAMP levels decrease and protein kinase A reassociates with its inhibitory subunits and becomes inactive. The protein phosphatases are activated, and phosphorylase a and glycogen synthase are dephosphorylated. The collective result of these effects is rapid inhibition of glycogen degradation, and rapid activation of glycogen synthesis.

EPINEPHRINE AND CALCIUM IN THE REGULATION OF LIVER GLYCOGEN

Epinephrine, the "fight-or-flight" hormone, is released from the adrenal medulla in response to neural signals reflecting an increased demand for glucose. To flee from a dangerous situation, skeletal muscles utilize increased amounts of blood glucose to generate ATP. As a result, liver glycogenolysis must be stimulated. In the liver, epinephrine stimulates glycogenolysis through two different types of receptors, the α- and β-agonist receptors.

Epinephrine Acting at the β-Receptors

Epinephrine, acting at the β-receptors, transmits a signal through G proteins to adenylate cyclase, which increases cAMP and activates protein kinase A. Hence, regulation of glycogen degradation and synthesis in liver by epinephrine and glucagon are similar (see Fig. 26.7).

Epinephrine Acting at α-Receptors

Epinephrine also binds to α-receptors in the liver. This binding activates glycogenolysis and inhibits glycogen synthesis principally by increasing the Ca^{2+} levels in the liver. The effects of epinephrine at the α-agonist receptor are mediated by the phosphatidylinositol bisphosphate (PIP_2)-Ca^{2+} signal transduction system, one of the principal intracellular second messenger systems employed by many hormones (Fig. 26.8) (see Chapter 43).

In the PIP_2-Ca^{2+} signal transduction system, the signal is transferred from the epinephrine receptor to membrane-bound phospholipase C by G proteins. Phospholipase C hydrolyzes PIP_2 to form diacylglycerol (DAG) and inositol triphosphate (IP_3). IP_3 stimulates the release of Ca^{2+} from the endoplasmic reticulum. Ca^{2+} and DAG activate protein kinase C. The amount of calcium bound to one of the calcium binding proteins, calmodulin, is also increased.

Calcium-calmodulin associates as a subunit with a number of enzymes and modifies their activities. It binds to inactive phosphorylase kinase, thereby partially activating this enzyme. (The fully activated enzyme is both bound to the calcium-calmodulin subunit and phosphorylated.) Phosphorylase kinase then phosphorylates glycogen phosphorylase b, thereby activating glycogen degradation. Calcium-calmodulin is also a modifier protein which activates one of the glycogen synthase

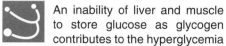

An inability of liver and muscle to store glucose as glycogen contributes to the hyperglycemia in patients, like **Di Beatty**, with insulin-dependent diabetes mellitus (IDDM) and in patients, like **Ann Sulin**, with non-insulin-dependent diabetes mellitus (NIDDM). The absence of insulin in IDDM patients and the high levels of glucagon result in decreased activity of glycogen synthase. Glycogen synthesis in skeletal muscles of IDDM patients is also limited by the lack of insulin-stimulated glucose transport. Insulin resistance in NIDDM patients has the same effect.

An injection of insulin suppresses glucagon release and alters the insulin/glucagon ratio. The result is rapid uptake of glucose into skeletal muscle and rapid conversion of glucose to glycogen in skeletal muscle and liver.

In the neonate, the release of epinephrine during labor and birth normally contributes to restoring blood glucose levels. Unfortunately, **Getta Carbo** did not have adequate liver glycogen stores to support her blood glucose levels.

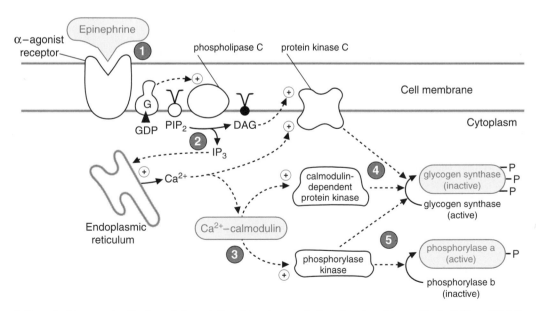

Fig. 26.8. Regulation of glycogen synthesis and degradation by epinephrine and Ca^{2+}. The effect of epinephrine binding to α-agonist receptors in liver transmits a signal via G proteins to phospholipase C, which hydrolyzes PIP_2 to DAG and IP_3. IP_3 stimulates the release of Ca^{2+} from the endoplasmic reticulum. Ca^{2+} binds to the modifier protein calmodulin which activates calmodulin-dependent protein kinase and phosphorylase kinase. Both Ca^{2+} and DAG activate protein kinase C. These three kinases phosphorylate glycogen synthase at different sites and decrease its activity. Phosphorylase kinase phosphorylates glycogen phosphorylase b to the active form. It therefore activates glycogenolysis as well as inhibiting glycogen synthesis.

kinases (calcium-calmodulin synthase kinase). Protein kinase C, calcium-calmodulin protein kinase, and phosphorylase kinase all phosphorylate glycogen synthase at different serine residues on the enzyme, thereby inhibiting glycogen synthase, and thus glycogen synthesis.

The effect of epinephrine in the liver, therefore, enhances or is synergistic with the effects of glucagon. Epinephrine release during bouts of hypoglycemia or during exercise can stimulate hepatic glycogenolysis and inhibit glycogen synthesis very rapidly.

Regulation of Glycogen Synthesis and Degradation in Skeletal Muscle

The regulation of glycogenolysis in skeletal muscle is related to the availability of ATP for muscular contraction. Skeletal muscle glycogen produces glucose 1-phosphate and a small amount of free glucose. Glucose 1-phosphate is converted to glucose 6-phosphate, which is committed to the glycolytic pathway; the absence of glucose 6-phosphatase in skeletal muscle prevents conversion of the glucosyl units from glycogen to blood glucose. Skeletal muscle glycogen is therefore degraded only when the demand for ATP generation from glycolysis is high. The highest demands occur during anaerobic glycolysis, which requires more moles of glucose for each ATP produced than oxidation of glucose to CO_2 (see Chapter 22). Anaerobic glycolysis occurs in tissues that have fewer mitochondria, a higher content of glycolytic enzymes, and higher levels of glycogen, i.e., fast twitch glycolytic fibers. It occurs most frequently at the onset of exercise—before vasodilation occurs to bring in blood-borne fuels. The regulation of skeletal muscle glycogen degradation must therefore respond very rapidly to the need for ATP, indicated by the rise of AMP.

The regulation of skeletal muscle glycogen synthesis and degradation differs from that in liver in several important respects: (*a*) glucagon has no effect on muscle, and thus glycogen levels in muscle do not vary with the fasting/feeding state; (*b*) AMP is an allosteric activator of the muscle isozyme of glycogen phosphorylase, but not liver glycogen phosphorylase (Fig. 26.9); (*c*) the effects of Ca^{2+} in muscle result principally from the release of Ca^{2+} from the sarcoplasmic reticulum after neural stimulation, and not from epinephrine-stimulated uptake; (*d*) glucose is not a physiological activator of glycogen synthase in muscle; (*e*) glycogen is a stronger feedback inhibitor of muscle glycogen synthase than of liver glycogen synthase, resulting in a smaller amount of stored glycogen per gram weight of muscle tissue. However, the effects of epinephrine-stimulated phosphorylation by protein kinase A on skeletal muscle glycogen degradation and glycogen synthesis are similar to those occurring in liver (see Fig. 26.7).

Muscle glycogen phosphorylase is a genetically distinct isozyme of liver glycogen phosphorylase, and contains an amino acid segment which has a purine nucleotide binding site. When AMP binds to this site, it changes the conformation at the catalytic site to a structure very similar to that in the phosphorylated enzyme (see Fig. 9.31). Thus hydrolysis of ATP to ADP and the consequent increase of AMP generated by adenylate kinase during muscular contraction can directly stimulate glycogenolysis to provide fuel for the glycolytic pathway. AMP also stimulates glycolysis by activating phosphofructokinase-1, so this one effector activates both glycogenolysis and glycolysis. The activation of the calcium-calmodulin subunit of phosphorylase kinase by the Ca^{2+} released from the sarcoplasmic reticulum during muscle contraction also provides a direct and rapid means of stimulating glycogen degradation. These differences accomplish the coordination of muscle glycogenolysis with the demand for ATP, the activation of glycolysis by AMP, and the activation of pyruvate dehydrogenase and the tricarboxylic acid cycle enzymes by ADP and Ca^{2+}.

Jim Bodie gradually regained consciousness with continued infusions of high concentration glucose titrated to keep his serum glucose level between 120 and 160 mg/dL. Although he remained somnolent and moderately confused over the next 12 hours, he was eventually able to tell his physicians that he had self-injected about 80 units of regular (short-acting) insulin every 6 hours while eating a high carbohydrate diet for the last 2 days preceding his seizure. Normal subjects under basal conditions secrete an average of 40 units of insulin daily. He had last injected insulin just before exercising. An article in a body-building magazine that he had recently read cited the anabolic effects of insulin on increasing muscle mass. He had purchased the insulin and necessary syringes from the same underground drug source from whom he regularly bought his anabolic steroids.

Normally, muscle glycogenolysis supplies the glucose required for the kinds of high intensity exercise which require anaerobic glycolysis, such as weight-lifting. Jim's treadmill exercise also utilizes blood glucose, which is supplied by liver glycogenolysis. The high serum insulin levels, resulting from the injection he gave himself just prior to his workout, activated both glucose transport into skeletal muscle and glycogen synthesis, while inhibiting glycogen degradation. His exercise, which would continue to utilize blood glucose, could normally be supported by breakdown of liver glycogen. However, glycogen synthesis in his liver was activated, and glycogen degradation was inhibited by the insulin injection.

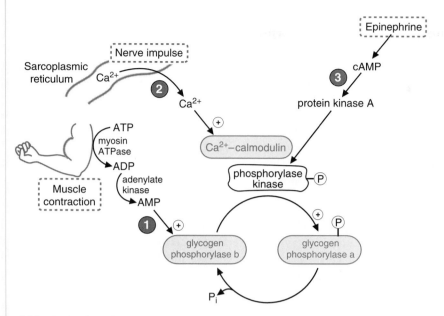

Fig. 26.9. Activation of muscle glycogen phosphorylase during exercise. Glycogenolysis in skeletal muscle is initiated by muscle contraction, neural impulses, and epinephrine. **1.** AMP produced from the degradation of ATP during muscular contraction allosterically activates glycogen phosphorylase b. **2.** The neural impulses which initiate contraction release Ca^{2+} from the sarcoplasmic reticulum. The Ca^{2+} binds to calmodulin, which is a modifier protein that activates phosphorylase kinase. **3.** Phosphorylase kinase is also activated through phosphorylation by protein kinase A. The formation of cAMP and the resultant activation of protein kinase A are initiated by the binding of epinephrine to plasma membrane receptors.

CLINICAL COMMENTS. **Getta Carbo's** hypoglycemia illustrates the importance of glycogen stores in the neonate. At birth, the fetus must make two major adjustments in the way fuels are utilized: it must adapt to using a greater variety of fuels than were available in utero and must adjust to intermittent feeding. In utero, the fetus receives a relatively constant supply of glucose from the maternal circulation via the placenta, producing a level of glucose in the fetus which approximates 75% of maternal blood levels. With regard to the hormonal regulation of fuel utilization in utero, fetal tissues function in an environment dominated by insulin, which promotes growth. During the last 10 weeks of gestation, this hormonal milieu leads to glycogen formation and storage. At birth, the infant's diet changes to one containing greater amounts of fat and lactose (galactose and glucose in equal ratio), presented at intervals rather than in a constant fashion. At the same time, the neonate's need for glucose will be relatively larger than that of the adult because her ratio of brain to liver weight is greater. Thus, the infant has even greater difficulty in maintaining glucose homeostasis than the adult.

At the moment that the umbilical cord is clamped, the normal neonate is faced with a metabolic problem: the high insulin levels of late fetal existence must be quickly reversed to prevent hypoglycemia. This reversal is accomplished through the secretion of the counterregulatory hormones epinephrine and glucagon. Glucagon release is triggered by the normal decline of blood glucose after birth. The neural response which stimulates the release of both glucagon and epinephrine is activated by the anoxia, cord clamping, and tactile stimulation which are part of a normal delivery. These responses have been referred to as the "normal sensor function" of the neonate.

Within 3–4 hours of birth, these counterregulatory hormones reestablish normal serum glucose levels in the newborn's blood through their glycogenolytic and gluconeogenic actions. The failure of Getta's normal "sensor function" was partly the result of maternal malnutrition, which resulted in an inadequate deposition of glycogen in Getta's liver prior to birth. The consequence was a serious degree of postnatal hypoglycemia.

The ability to maintain glucose homeostasis during the first few days of life also depends on the activation of gluconeogenesis and the mobilization of fatty acids. Fatty acid oxidation in the liver not only promotes gluconeogenesis (see Chapter 27), but generates ketone bodies. The neonatal brain has an enhanced capacity to utilize ketone bodies relative to that of infants (4-fold) and adults (40-fold). This ability is consistent with the relatively high fat content of breast milk.

Jim Bodie attempted to build up his muscle mass with androgens and with insulin. The anabolic (nitrogen-retaining) effects of androgens on skeletal muscle cells enhance muscle mass by increasing amino acid flux into muscle and by stimulating protein synthesis. Exogenous insulin has the potential to increase muscle mass by similar actions and also by increasing the content of muscle glycogen.

The most serious side effect of exogenous insulin administration is the development of severe hypoglycemia, such as occurred in Jim Bodie. The immediate adverse effect relates to an inadequate flow of fuel (glucose) to the metabolizing brain. When hypoglycemia is extreme, the patient may suffer a seizure and, if the hypoglycemia worsens, may lapse into a coma. If untreated, irreversible brain damage occurs in those who survive.

BIOCHEMICAL COMMENTS. The regulatory effect of insulin is frequently described as one of activating protein phosphatases. The effect of insulin on the regulation of hepatic PP-1 is exerted through the insulin receptor tyrosine kinase phosphorylation cascade, which ultimately activates a serine protein kinase which can act on PP-1.

PP-1 is the protein phosphatase which dephosphorylates glycogen phosphorylase, one of the phosphorylation sites on phosphorylase kinase, and one or more of the phosphorylation sites on glycogen synthase. These enzymes are all bound to the glycogen particle. PP-1 is composed of two subunits, the catalytic subunit (PP-1$_c$) and a regulatory subunit (the G subunit). The G subunit binds to the glycogen particle, thereby localizing the catalytic subunit near the regulatory phosphate groups on its substrate enzymes (Fig. 26.10). Dissociation of the catalytic subunit from the bound G subunit renders the enzyme inactive.

PP-1 is inhibited by the binding of inhibitor-1, a modifier protein, to the catalytic subunit. This inhibitor binds best when it is phosphorylated by protein kinase A. In some way, insulin decreases this phosphorylation, thus indirectly activating PP-1.

Another regulatory phosphorylation occurs at the G subunit. The G subunit has two phosphorylation sites. When protein kinase A phosphorylates one of these sites, the catalytic subunit dissociates, thereby becoming less effective. When the insulin-stimulated protein kinase (ISPK) phosphorylates the other regulatory site on the G subunit, it decreases the ability of protein kinase A to act at its phosphorylation site. Thus, insulin again indirectly activates the protein phosphatase.

Suggested Readings

Chen VT, Burchell A. Glycogen storage diseases. In: Scriver CR, Beaudet AL, Sly WS, Valle D, eds. The metabolic and molecular bases of inherited disease. 7th ed, vol I. New York: McGraw-Hill, 1995:935–965.

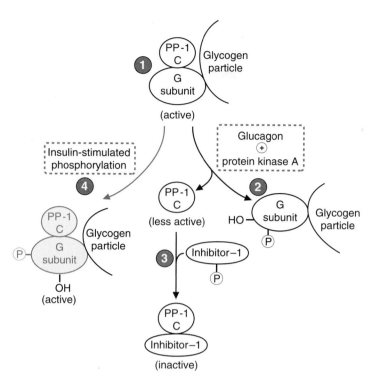

Fig. 26.10. Regulation of hepatic protein phosphatase-1. PP-1$_c$= the catalytic subunit of PP-1. G = the glycogen-binding subunit of PP-1. Inhibitor-1 = an inhibitory protein, best character-ized in skeletal muscle. **1.** Active PP-1 is bound to the glycogen particle through the G subunit. The G subunit has two different phosphorylation sites, one for glucagon-stimulated phospho-rylation, and one for insulin-stimulated phosphorylation. **2.** Protein kinase A, which is stimu-lated by glucagon binding to its receptor, phosphorylates the G subunit, resulting in the disso-ciation of a less active catalytic subunit (PP-1$_c$). **3.** Inhibitor-1 binds to PP-1c, decreasing its activity even more. cAMP-directed phosphorylation of inhibitor-1 protein increases its binding affinity for PP-1$_c$. **4.** The G subunit can also be phosphorylated through the insulin receptor tyrosine kinase phosphorylation cascade. Phosphorylation at the insulin-directed site prevents the phosphorylation by protein kinase A, thereby maintaining the activity of PP-1 and antago-nizing the effects of glucagon.

Cohen P. The structure and regulation of protein phosphatases. Annu Rev Biochem 1989;58:453–508.

Johnson LN, Barford D. Glycogen phosphorylase. J Biol Chem 1990;265:2409–2412.

Parker PH, Ballew M, Greene HL. Nutritional management of glycogen storage disease. Annu Rev Nutr 1993;13:83–109.

PROBLEM

An infant had recurring bouts of hypoglycemia from the time of birth. In a test to determine the cause of the hypoglycemia, the infant was given an injection of glucagon approximately 1 hour after a high carbohydrate meal. The blood glucose level of the infant rose from 70 mg/dL to 110 mg/dL. Approximately 3 hours after the meal, the infants' blood glucose level was 45 mg/dL. Another injection of glucagon was given, but no increase in the blood glucose level was detected. The infant was immediately fed.

From these results you conclude that the infant could have (Select all the answers that apply):

A. A deficiency of liver glycogen phosphorylase or the glycogen debrancher enzyme
B. A deficiency of glucose 6-phosphatase
C. A defect in the glucagon receptor
D. An inability to secrete adequate amounts of glucagon
E. A problem in gluconeogenesis

ANSWER

E. Only a problem in gluconeogenesis. You know from the patient's rapid response to glucagon 1 hour after her meal that she was able to rapidly degrade glycogen in response to injected glucagon. She was able, therefore, to synthesize glycogen and had adequate levels of glycogenolytic enzymes and glucose 6-phosphatase. Her proteins and enzymes necessary for the response (such as the glucagon receptor and protein kinase A) must also be functional. However, her blood glucose levels rapidly fell. The infant's glycogen stores were clearly unable to maintain blood glucose levels for very long. Once the glycogen stores were depleted, there was no response to glucagon. The alternate pathway for support of blood glucose is gluconeogenesis, which is also stimulated by the change in glucagon and insulin levels during fasting. To find out how gluconeogenesis is activated, go on to the next chapter. For a brief summary of the role of glucagon and its multitude of effects in regulating blood glucose, consult the "Ode to Glucagon."

ODE TO GLUCAGON

Canto I: Glucagon and Glycogen
After the meal is over,
    and blood glucose levels fall,
Brain and red blood cells panic,
    but the pancreas hears the call.
Alpha cells release glucagon,
    to find its binding site
On liver and adipose receptors,
    where it begins its fight.

In liver, active adenylate cyclase,
    increases cyclic AMP,
Which activates protein kinase
    phos. kinase, and phos. b.
Phosphorylated phosphorylase b,
    now called phosphorylase a,
Degrades liver glycogen
    in time to save the day.

Glycogen synthase is inhibited
    by phosphorylation, too.
Recycling is prevented
    (this is fortunately true).
Falling insulin levels
    enhance glucagon's effect.
Phosphatases stay inhibited
    to give glucagon due respect.

Canto II: Glucagon and Gluconeogenesis
But glucose must be synthesized
    (glycogen won't last too long),
From glycerol, lactate and amino acids,
    all of the precursor throng.

For essential gluconeogenic enzymes,
    transcription is induced,
And an increased supply of glycerol,
    gives the path a boost.

Canto III: Glucagon and Metabolic Homeostasis
But to conserve that glucose
    glucagon restricts its use,
Thereby decreasing the amount,
    the liver must produce.
Glucose to fatty acids
    is an inhibited pathway,
Due to enzyme phosphorylation
    by protein kinase A.

Glucagon in adipose tissue,
    activates adenylate cyclase.
And protein kinase A activates
    hormone-sensitive lipase.
Adipose tissue triglycerides,
    are rapidly hydrolyzed.
Skeletal muscles get fatty acids,
    which are then oxidized.

And when all is done,
    glucagon sighs relief
A glucose meal approaches;
    its reign has not been brief.
Insulin will take over,
    as blood glucose rises,
And dephosphorylate those enzymes
    with no compromises.

-C.M. Smith

27 Glucose Metabolism in the Liver: Glycolysis and Gluconeogenesis

Although glycolysis serves mainly to generate ATP in most tissues, this pathway has additional functions in the liver that change with the physiological state. After a meal, glycolysis provides carbon for the synthesis of fatty acids in the liver and for the production of glycerol 3-phosphate, which combines with fatty acids to form the triacylglycerols that are secreted in VLDL. During fasting, many of the reactions of glycolysis are reversed as the liver produces glucose to maintain blood glucose levels. This process of glucose production is called gluconeogenesis.

Gluconeogenesis, which occurs primarily in the liver, is the pathway for the synthesis of glucose from compounds other than carbohydrates. In humans, the major precursors of glucose are lactate, glycerol, and amino acids, particularly alanine. Except for three key sequences, the reactions of gluconeogenesis are reversals of the steps of glycolysis (Fig. 27.1). The sequences of gluconeogenesis that do not use enzymes of glycolysis involve the conversion of (a) pyruvate to phosphoenolpyruvate, (b) fructose 1,6-bisphosphate to fructose 6-phosphate, and (c) glucose 6-phosphate to glucose. These steps involve regulatory enzymes.

Al Martini, a known alcoholic, was brought to the emergency room by his landlady, who stated that he had been drinking heavily for the past week. During this time his appetite had gradually diminished, and he had not eaten any food for the past 3 days. He was confused, combative, tremulous, and sweating profusely. His speech was slurred. His heart rate was rapid (110 beats per minute). As his blood pressure was being determined, he had a grand mal seizure. His blood glucose, drawn just prior to the onset of the seizure, was 28 mg/dL or 1.6 mM (reference range for overnight fasting blood glucose = 80–100 mg/dL or 4.4–5.6 mM). His blood ethanol level drawn at the same time was 295 mg/dL (intoxication level, i.e., "confused" stage = 150–300 mg/dL).

Emma Wheezer presented to the emergency room 3 days after discharge from the hospital following a 10-day admission for severe refractory bronchial asthma. She required high dose intravenous dexamethasone (an antiinflammatory synthetic glucocorticoid) for the first 8 days of her stay. After 2 additional days on oral dexamethasone, she was discharged on substantial pharmacological doses of this steroid and instructed to return to her physician's office in 5 days. She presented now with marked polyuria (increased urination), polydipsia (increased thirst), and muscle weakness. Her blood glucose was 275 mg/dL or 15 mM (reference range = 80–100 mg/dL or 4.4–5.6 mM).

GLUCOSE METABOLISM IN THE LIVER

Glucose serves as a fuel for most tissues of the body. It is the major fuel for certain tissues such as the brain and red blood cells. After a meal, food is the source of blood

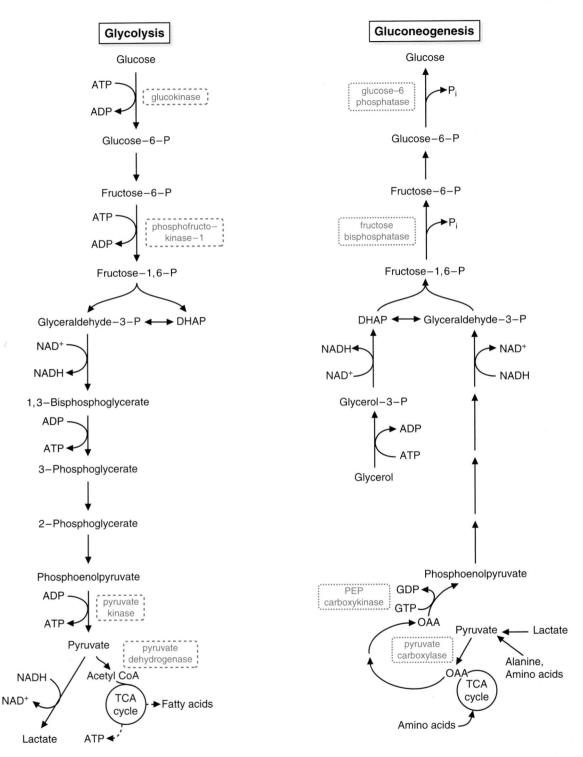

Fig. 27.1. Glycolysis and gluconeogenesis in the liver. The gluco-neogenic pathway is almost the reverse of the glycolytic pathway, except for three reaction sequences. At these three steps, the reactions are catalyzed by different enzymes. The energy requirements of these reactions differ, and one pathway can be activated while the other is inhibited.

glucose. The liver oxidizes glucose and stores the excess as glycogen. The liver also uses the pathway of glycolysis to convert glucose to pyruvate, which provides carbon for the synthesis of fatty acids. Glycerol 3-phosphate, produced from glycolytic intermediates, combines with fatty acids to form triacylglycerols, which are secreted into the blood in very low density lipoproteins (VLDL). During fasting, the liver releases glucose into the blood, so that glucose-dependent tissues do not suffer from a lack of energy. Two mechanisms are involved in this process: glycogenolysis and gluconeogenesis. Hormones, particularly insulin and glucagon, dictate whether glucose flows through glycolysis or whether the reactions are reversed and glucose is produced via gluconeogenesis.

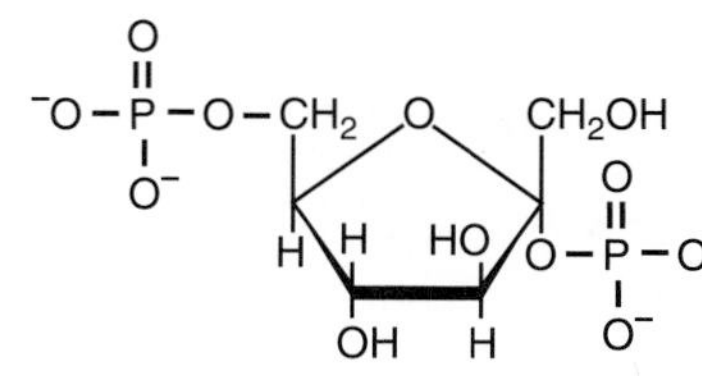

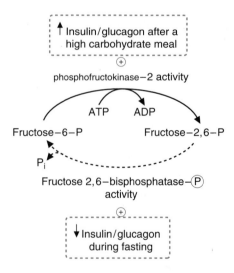

Fructose 2,6–bisphosphate

Fig. 27.2. Structure of fructose 2,6-bisphosphate.

GLYCOLYSIS

In the liver, the glycolytic pathway generates pyruvate to serve as a precursor for fatty acid synthesis as well as a source of ATP (Fig. 27.1). The major regulation of glycolysis occurs through the actions of insulin and glucagon, as well as ATP and related metabolites.

Regulation of Glucokinase

Glucokinase, the liver enzymes that phosphorylates glucose, has a high K_m for glucose. Therefore, it is most active after a meal, when glucose levels in the hepatic portal vein are high. This enzyme is induced by insulin.

Activation of Glycolysis by Fructose 2,6-Bisphosphate

An increase of the blood levels of insulin and a decrease of the blood levels of glucagon (i.e., an elevation of the blood insulin/glucagon ratio) after a high carbohydrate meal increases the concentration of fructose 2,6-bisphosphate (Fig. 27.2). This compound is not an intermediate of the glycolytic pathway, but a special allosteric activator of phosphofructokinase-1 (PFK-1) which acts like AMP (see Chapter 22). Its concentration is elevated in cells when levels of insulin increase and glucagon decrease, i.e., after a high carbohydrate meal.

Fructose 2,6-bisphosphate is produced in tissues by the enzyme phosphofructokinase-2/fructose 2,6-bisphosphatase. The unusually long name of the enzyme implies that it has dual functions (i.e., it is bifunctional). When the insulin/glucagon ratio is high (after a meal), the enzyme is dephosphorylated, its phosphofructokinase-2 activity is enhanced, and it synthesizes fructose 2,6-bisphosphate from fructose 6-phosphate and ATP (Fig. 27.3). When the insulin/glucagon ratio is low (during fasting), the enzyme is phosphorylated by protein kinase A (see Chapter 24). Phosphorylation enhances the phosphatase activity and inhibits the kinase activity of the bifunctional enzyme, and fructose 2,6-bisphosphate is converted back to fructose 6-phosphate. Note that this reaction is not a simple reversal of the reaction by which fructose 2,6-bisphosphate is synthesized. Synthesis utilizes ATP, but the conversion of fructose 2,6-bisphosphate to fructose 6-phosphate produces inorganic phosphate (P_i) rather than ATP.

Although fructose 2,6-bisphosphate has been found in a number of tissues, its function is understood only in liver (where it regulates both glycolysis and gluconeogenesis) and adipose tissue (where it regulates glycolysis). After a high carbohydrate meal, phosphofructokinase-2/fructose 2,6-bisphosphatase is dephosphorylated. As a result, the levels of fructose 2,6-bisphosphate are elevated, PFK-1 is activated, and glycolysis is stimulated, allowing glucose to be converted to fatty acids in the liver. During fasting, the levels of fructose 2,6-bisphosphate decrease because the

Fig. 27.3. Reactions catalyzed by phosphofructokinase-2/fructose 2,6-bisphosphatase. This is a bifunctional enzyme. It acts as a kinase after a meal when the insulin/glucagon ratio is elevated and as a phosphatase during fasting when the insulin/glucagon ratio is low. The activity of the enzyme is altered by phosphorylation and dephosphorylation. It is phosphorylated by protein kinase A in the fasting state (when it acts as a phosphatase) and dephosphorylated in the fed state (when it acts as a kinase).

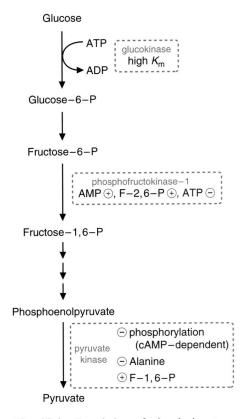

Fig. 27.4. Regulation of glycolysis. ⊖ = inhibited by; ⊕ = activated by.

bifunctional enzyme phosphofructokinase-2/fructose 2,6-bisphosphatase is phosphorylated and acts mainly as a phosphatase. When fructose 2,6-bisphosphate levels are low, the rate of glycolysis is decreased because PFK-1 is not activated. Activation of PFK-1 by fructose 2,6-bisphosphate and AMP is synergistic (Fig. 27.4). Glycolysis must not only provide carbon for fatty acid synthesis (and for other biosynthetic pathways), but it must also produce ATP to drive the process.

Regulation of Glycolysis by Pyruvate Kinase

Glycolysis in the liver is also regulated by the action of insulin and glucagon at the step catalyzed by pyruvate kinase (Fig. 27.5). During fasting, glucagon causes the activation of protein kinase A. In addition to phosphorylating enzymes involved in glycogen metabolism, this kinase also phosphorylates pyruvate kinase, converting it to a less active form. After a high carbohydrate meal, the high levels of insulin and low levels of glucagon decrease protein kinase A activity and stimulate a phosphatase which dephosphorylates pyruvate kinase. Dephosphorylation causes pyruvate kinase to become more active. The principal function of this regulatory mechanism is to inhibit glycolysis during a fast when the reverse pathway, gluconeogenesis, is activated.

Pyruvate kinase is also activated by fructose 1,6-bisphosphate. This mechanism is called the "feed forward" mechanism, i.e., the product of an earlier step in the pathway "feeds forward" and activates an enzyme that catalyzes a later step. Allosteric inhibitors ATP and alanine decrease the activity of pyruvate kinase, when the reverse pathway, gluconeogenesis, is activated (see Fig. 27.4).

GLUCONEOGENESIS

Gluconeogenesis, the process by which glucose is synthesized from noncarbohydrate precursors, occurs mainly in the liver under fasting conditions. Under the more extreme conditions of starvation, the kidney cortex may also produce glucose. For the most part, the glucose produced by the kidney cortex is used by the kidney medulla, but some may enter the bloodstream.

Starting with pyruvate, most of the steps of gluconeogenesis are simply reversals of those of glycolysis (Fig. 27.6). In fact, these pathways differ at only three points.

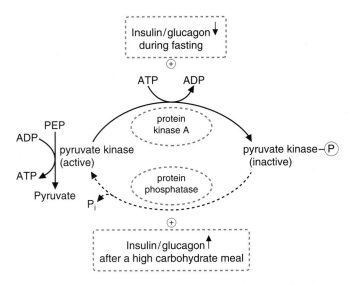

Fig. 27.5. Regulation of pyruvate kinase in liver by changes in the insulin/glucagon ratio.

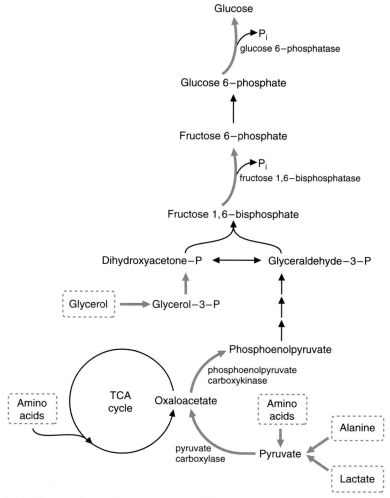

Fig. 27.6. Key reactions of gluconeogenesis. The precursors are amino acids (particularly alanine), lactate, and glycerol. Heavy arrows indicate steps that differ from those of glycolysis.

Enzymes involved in catalyzing these steps are regulated so that either glycolysis or gluconeogenesis predominates, depending on physiological conditions.

Most of the steps of gluconeogenesis use the same enzymes that catalyze the process of glycolysis. The flow of carbon, of course, is in the reverse direction. Three reaction sequences of gluconeogenesis differ from the corresponding steps of glycolysis. They involve the conversion of pyruvate to phosphoenolpyruvate (PEP) and the reactions that remove phosphate from fructose 1,6-bisphosphate to form fructose 6-phosphate and from glucose 6-phosphate to form glucose (see Fig. 27.6). The conversion of pyruvate to PEP is catalyzed during gluconeogenesis by a series of enzymes instead of the single enzyme used for glycolysis. The reactions that remove phosphate from fructose 1,6-bisphosphate and from glucose 6-phosphate each use single enzymes that differ from the corresponding enzymes of glycolysis. Although phosphate is added during glycolysis by kinases, which use ATP, it is removed during gluconeogenesis by phosphatases that release P_i. Thus, these gluconeogenic steps are more energetically favorable than they would be if ATP were produced.

Glucocorticoids are naturally occurring steroid hormones. In humans, the major glucocorticoid is cortisol. Glucocorticoids are produced in response to various types of stress (see Chapter 45). One of their actions is to stimulate the degradation of muscle protein. Thus, increased amounts of amino acids become available as substrates for gluconeogenesis. **Emma Wheezer** noted muscle weakness, a result of the muscle-degrading action of the synthetic glucocorticoid dexamethasone, which she was taking for its antiinflammatory effects.

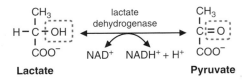

Fig. 27.7. Conversion of lactate to pyruvate.

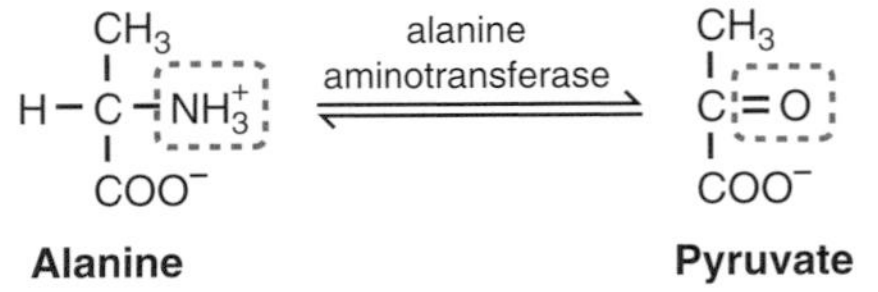

Fig. 27.8. Conversion of alanine to pyruvate. In this reaction, alanine aminotransferase transfers the amino group of alanine to α-ketoglutarate to form glutamate. The coenzyme for this reaction, pyridoxal phosphate, accepts and donates the amino group.

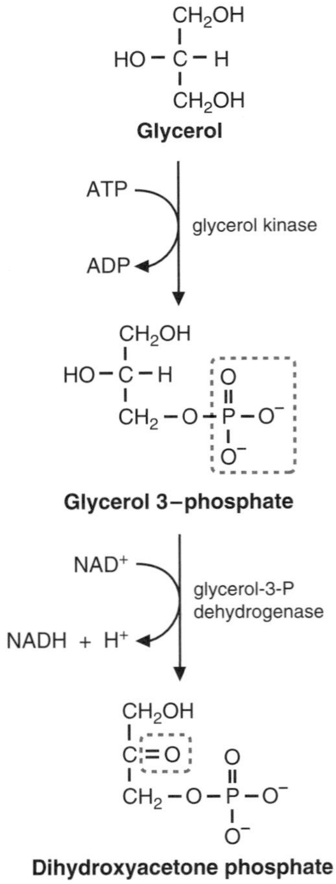

Fig. 27.9. Conversion of glycerol to dihydroxyacetone phosphate.

Precursors for Gluconeogenesis

The three major carbon sources for gluconeogenesis in humans are lactate, glycerol, and amino acids, particularly alanine. Lactate is produced by anaerobic glycolysis in tissues such as exercising muscle or red blood cells, glycerol is released from adipose stores of triacylglycerol, and amino acids come mainly from amino acid pools in muscle where they may be obtained by degradation of muscle protein. Alanine, the major gluconeogenic amino acid, is produced in muscle from other amino acids and from glucose (see Chapter 42).

Formation of Gluconeogenic Intermediates from Carbon Sources

The carbon sources for gluconeogenesis form pyruvate, intermediates of the tricarboxylic acid (TCA) cycle, or intermediates common both to glycolysis and gluconeogenesis.

LACTATE, AMINO ACIDS, AND GLYCEROL

Pyruvate is produced in the liver from the gluconeogenic precursors lactate and alanine. Lactate dehydrogenase oxidizes lactate to pyruvate, generating NADH (Fig. 27.7) and alanine aminotransferase converts alanine to pyruvate (Fig. 27.8).

Although alanine is the major gluconeogenic amino acid, other amino acids, such as serine, serve as carbon sources for the synthesis of glucose because they also form pyruvate, the substrate for the initial step in the process. Some amino acids form intermediates of the TCA cycle (see Chapter 19) which can enter the gluconeogenic pathway.

The carbons of glycerol are gluconeogenic because they form dihydroxyacetone phosphate (DHAP), a glycolytic intermediate (Fig. 27.9).

PROPIONATE

Fatty acids with an odd number of carbon atoms, which are obtained mainly from vegetables in the diet, produce propionyl CoA from the 3 carbons at the ω-end of the chain (see Chapter 23). These carbons are relatively minor precursors of glucose in humans. Propionyl CoA is converted to methylmalonyl CoA, which is rearranged to form succinyl CoA, a 4-carbon intermediate of the TCA cycle that can be used for gluconeogenesis. The remaining carbons of an odd chain fatty acid form acetyl CoA, from which no net synthesis of glucose occurs.

β-Oxidation of fatty acids produces acetyl CoA. Because the pyruvate dehydrogenase reaction is thermodynamically and kinetically irreversible, acetyl CoA does not form pyruvate for gluconeogenesis. Therefore, if acetyl CoA is to produce glucose, it must enter the TCA cycle and be converted to malate. For every 2 carbons of acetyl CoA that are converted to malate, 2 carbons are released as CO_2: one in the reaction catalyzed by isocitrate dehydrogenase and the other in the reaction catalyzed by α-ketoglutarate dehydrogenase. Therefore, there is no *net* synthesis of glucose from acetyl CoA.

Pathway of Gluconeogenesis

Gluconeogenesis occurs by a pathway that reverses many, but not all, of the steps of glycolysis.

CONVERSION OF PYRUVATE TO PHOSPHOENOLPYRUVATE

In glycolysis, PEP is converted to pyruvate by pyruvate kinase. In gluconeogenesis, a series of steps are required to accomplish the reversal of this reaction (Fig. 27.10).

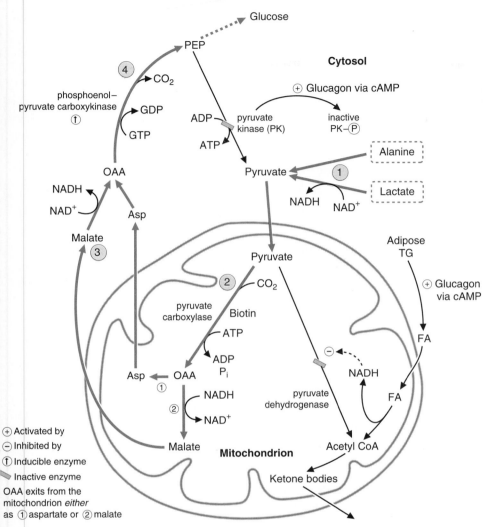

Fig. 27.10. Conversion of pyruvate to phosphoenolpyruvate (PEP). Follow the shaded circled numbers on the diagram starting with the precursors alanine and lactate. OAA = oxaloacetate; FA = fatty acid; TG = triacylglycerol. The white circled numbers are alternate routes for exit of carbon from the mitochondrion.

Pyruvate is carboxylated by pyruvate carboxylase to form oxaloacetate. This enzyme, which requires biotin, is the catalyst of an anaplerotic reaction of the TCA cycle (see Chapter 19). In gluconeogenesis, this reaction replenishes the oxaloacetate that is used for the synthesis of glucose (Fig. 27.11).

The CO_2 that was added to pyruvate to form oxaloacetate is released by phosphoenolpyruvate carboxykinase (PEPCK), and PEP is generated. For this reaction, GTP provides a source of energy as well as the phosphate group of PEP. The enzymes that catalyze these two steps are located in two different subcellular compartments. Pyruvate carboxylase is found in mitochondria. In various species, PEPCK is located either in the cytosol or in mitochondria, or it is distributed between these two compartments. In humans, the enzyme is distributed about equally in each compartment.

Oxaloacetate, generated from pyruvate by pyruvate carboxylase or from amino acids that form intermediates of the TCA cycle, does not readily cross the mitochondrial membrane. It is either decarboxylated to form PEP by the mitochondrial PEPCK, or it is converted to malate or aspartate (Fig. 27.10). The conversion of

 The metabolism of ethanol produces NADH from NAD^+.

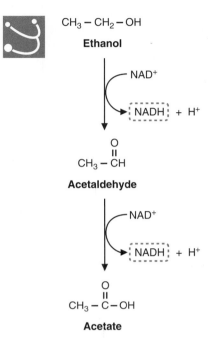

Cells have limited amounts of NAD, which exist either as NAD^+ or as NADH. As the levels of NADH rise, those of NAD^+ fall, and the ratio of the concentrations of NADH and NAD^+ ([NADH]/[NAD^+]) increases. In the presence of ethanol, which is very rapidly oxidized in the liver, the [NADH]/[NAD^+] ratio is much higher than it is in the normal fasting liver. High levels of NADH drive the lactate dehydrogenase reaction toward lactate. Therefore, lactate cannot enter the gluconeogenic pathway, and pyruvate that is generated from alanine is converted to lactate. The conversion of glycerol to glucose is also decreased by high levels of NADH. Consequently, the major precursors lactate, alanine, and glycerol are not used for gluconeogenesis.

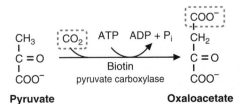

Fig. 27.11. Conversion of pyruvate to oxaloacetate.

Q 27.1: In a fatty acid with 19 carbons, how many carbons (and which ones) form glucose?

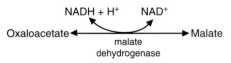

Fig. 27.12. Interconversion of oxaloacetate and malate.

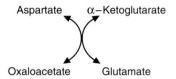

Fig. 27.13. Transamination of aspartate to form oxaloacetate. Note that the cytosolic reaction is the reverse of the mitochondrial reaction as shown in Figure 27.10.

Because glycerol is oxidized by NAD$^+$ during its conversion to DHAP, the conversion of glycerol to glucose is inhibited when NADH levels are elevated. Therefore, ethanol ingestion prevents all the major precursors—lactate, glycerol, and the gluconeogenic amino acids (especially alanine)—from being converted to glucose.

Amino acids that form intermediates of the TCA cycle are converted to malate, which enters the cytosol and is converted to oxaloacetate, which proceeds through gluconeogenesis to form glucose. When excessive amounts of ethanol are ingested, elevated NADH levels inhibit the conversion of malate to oxaloacetate in the cytosol. Therefore, carbons from amino acids that form intermediates of the TCA cycle cannot be converted to glucose as readily.

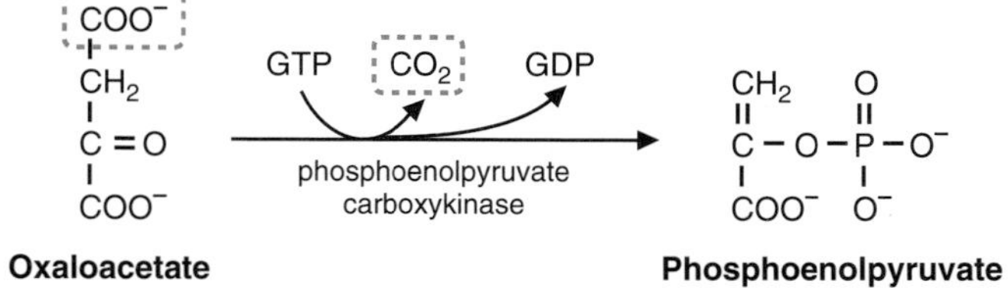

oxaloacetate to malate requires NADH. PEP, malate, and aspartate can be transported into the cytosol.

After malate and aspartate traverse the mitochondrial membrane and enter the cytosol, they are reconverted to oxaloacetate by reversal of the reactions given above (Figs. 26.12 and 26.13). The conversion of malate to oxaloacetate generates NADH. Whether oxaloacetate is transported across the mitochondrial membrane as malate or aspartate depends on the need for reducing equivalents in the cytosol. NADH is required to reduce 1,3-bisphosphoglycerate to glyceraldehyde 3-phosphate during gluconeogenesis.

Oxaloacetate, produced from malate or aspartate in the cytosol, is converted to PEP by the cytosolic PEPCK (Fig. 27.14).

CONVERSION OF PHOSPHOENOLPYRUVATE TO FRUCTOSE 1,6-BISPHOSPHATE

The remaining steps of gluconeogenesis occur in the cytosol (Fig. 27.15). PEP reverses the steps of glycolysis to form glyceraldehyde 3-phosphate. For every 2 molecules of glyceraldehyde 3-phosphate that are formed, 1 is converted to dihydroxyacetone phosphate (DHAP). These two triose phosphates, DHAP and glyceraldehyde 3-phosphate, condense to form fructose 1,6-bisphosphate by a reversal of the aldolase reaction.

Because glycerol forms DHAP, it enters the gluconeogenic pathway at this level.

CONVERSION OF FRUCTOSE 1,6-BISPHOSPHATE TO FRUCTOSE 6-PHOSPHATE

The enzyme fructose 1,6-bisphosphatase releases inorganic phosphate from fructose 1,6-bisphosphate to form fructose 6-phosphate. The glycolytic enzyme, PFK-1, does not catalyze this reaction but rather a reaction that involves ATP. In the next reaction of gluconeogenesis, fructose 6-phosphate is converted to glucose 6-phosphate by the same isomerase used in glycolysis.

CONVERSION OF GLUCOSE 6-PHOSPHATE TO GLUCOSE

Glucose 6-phosphatase cleaves P_i from glucose 6-phosphate, and free glucose is released into the blood. The glycolytic enzyme glucokinase, which catalyzes the reverse reaction, requires ATP.

Glucose 6-phosphatase is located in the membrane of the endoplasmic reticulum. It is used not only in gluconeogenesis, but also to produce blood glucose from the breakdown of liver glycogen.

REGULATION OF GLUCONEOGENESIS

Although gluconeogenesis occurs during fasting, it is also stimulated during prolonged exercise, by a high protein diet, and under conditions of stress. The factors that promote the overall flow of carbon from pyruvate to glucose include the availability of substrate and changes in the activity or amount of certain key enzymes of glycolysis and gluconeogenesis.

Fig. 27.14. Conversion of oxaloacetate to phosphoenolpyruvate.

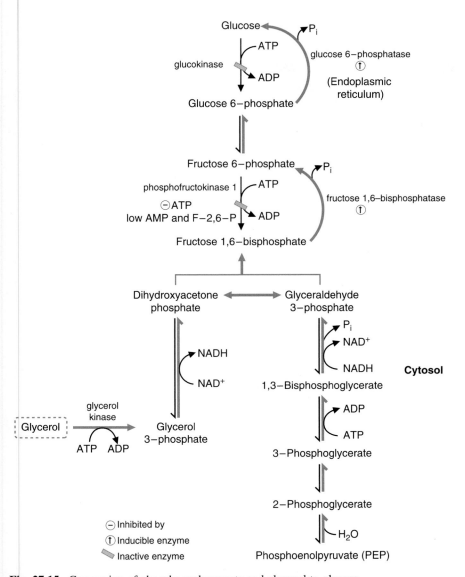

Al Martini had not eaten for 3 days, so he had no dietary source of glucose and his liver glycogen stores were essentially depleted. He was solely dependent on gluconeogenesis to maintain his blood glucose levels. One of the consequences of ethanol ingestion and the rise of NADH is that the major carbon sources for gluconeogenesis cannot readily be converted to glucose. After his alcoholic binges, Mr. Martini became hypoglycemic. His blood glucose was 28 mg/dL.

27.1: Only the 3 carbons at the ω-end of an odd chain fatty acid that form propionyl CoA are converted to glucose. The remaining 16 carbons of a fatty acid with 19 carbons form acetyl CoA, which does not form any net glucose.

Fig. 27.15. Conversion of phosphoenolpyruvate and glycerol to glucose.

Availability of Substrate

Gluconeogenesis is stimulated by the flow of its major substrates from peripheral tissues to the liver. Glycerol is released from adipose tissue whenever the levels of insulin are low and the levels of glucagon or the "stress" hormones, epinephrine and cortisol (a glucocorticoid), are elevated in the blood (see Chapter 24). Lactate is produced by muscle during exercise and by red blood cells. Amino acids are released from muscle whenever insulin is low or when cortisol is elevated. Amino acids are also available for gluconeogenesis when the dietary intake of protein is high and intake of carbohydrate is low.

Activity or Amount of Key Enzymes

Three steps in the pathway of gluconeogenesis are regulated:

1. pyruvate → phosphoenolpyruvate

In some species, propionate is a major source of carbon for gluconeogenesis. Ruminants can produce massive amounts of glucose from propionate. In cows, the cellulose in grass is converted to propionate by bacteria in the rumen. This substrate is then used to generate more than 5 lb of glucose each day by the process of gluconeogenesis.

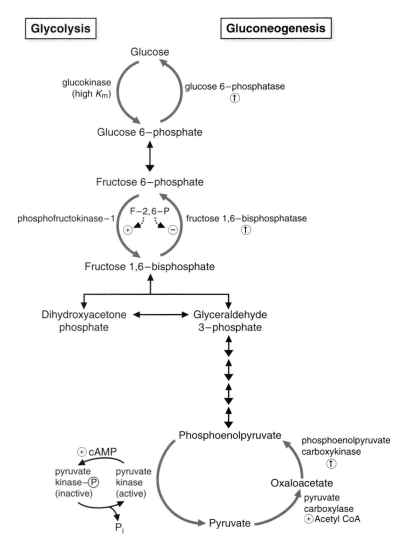

Fig. 27.16. Enzymes involved in regulating the substrate cycles of glycolysis and gluconeogenesis. Heavy arrows indicate the three substrate cycles. F-2,6-P, fructose 2,6-bisphosphate; ⊕, activated by; ⊖, inhibited by; ⊤, inducible enzyme.

2. fructose 1,6-bisphosphate → fructose 6-phosphate
3. glucose 6-phosphate → glucose.

These steps correspond to those in glycolysis that are catalyzed by regulatory enzymes. The enzymes involved in these steps of gluconeogenesis differ from those that catalyze the reverse reactions in glycolysis. The net flow of carbon, whether from glucose to pyruvate (glycolysis) or from pyruvate to glucose (gluconeogenesis), depends on the relative activity or amount of these glycolytic or gluconeogenic enzymes (Fig. 27.16 and Table 27.1).

CONVERSION OF PYRUVATE TO PHOSPHOENOLPYRUVATE

Pyruvate, a key substrate for gluconeogenesis, is derived from lactate and amino acids, particularly alanine. Pyruvate is not converted to acetyl CoA under conditions

Table 27.1. Regulation of Enzymes of Glycolysis and Gluconeogenesis in Liver

A. Glycolytic Enzymes	Mechanism
Pyruvate kinase	⊕ by F-1, 6-P
	⊖ by ATP, alanine
	⊖ by phosphorylation
	(glucagon and epinephrine
	→ cAMP ↑ which ⊕
	protein kinase A)
Phosphofructokinase-1	⊕ by F-2,6-P, AMP
Glucokinase	high K_m for glucose
	⇑ by insulin

B. Gluconeogenic Enzymes	Mechanism
Pyruvate carboxylase	⊕ by acetyl CoA
Phosphoenolpyruvate	
carboxykinase	⇑ by glucagon, epinephrine,
	glucocorticoids
	⇓ by insulin
Fructose 1,6-bisphosphatase	⊖ by F-2,6-P, AMP
	⇑ during fasting
Glucose 6-phosphatase	⇑ during fasting

⊕ = activated; ⊖ = inhibited; ↑ increased concentration; ⇑ = induced; ⇓ = repressed.

favoring gluconeogenesis because pyruvate dehydrogenase is relatively inactive. Instead, pyruvate is converted to oxaloacetate by pyruvate carboxylase. Subsequently, oxaloacetate is converted to PEP by PEPCK. Because pyruvate kinase is inactivated by phosphorylation and by alanine, PEP is not reconverted to pyruvate, a situation that would lead to a nonproductive substrate cycle (a futile cycle); rather, PEP reverses the steps of glycolysis, ultimately forming glucose.

Pyruvate dehydrogenase is inactive. Under conditions of fasting, insulin levels are low and glucagon levels are elevated. Consequently, fatty acids and glycerol are released from the triacylglycerol stores of adipose tissue. Fatty acids travel to the liver where they undergo β-oxidation, producing acetyl CoA, NADH, and ATP. As a consequence, the concentration of ADP decreases. These changes result in the phosphorylation of pyruvate dehydrogenase to the inactive form. Therefore, pyruvate is not converted to acetyl CoA.

Pyruvate carboxylase is active. Acetyl CoA, which is produced by oxidation of fatty acids, activates pyruvate carboxylase. Therefore, pyruvate, derived from lactate or alanine, is converted to oxaloacetate.

Phosphoenolpyruvate carboxykinase is induced. Oxaloacetate produces PEP in a reaction catalyzed by PEPCK. Cytosolic PEPCK is an inducible enzyme, which means that the quantity of the enzyme in the cell increases because of increased transcription of its gene and increased translation of its mRNA. The major inducer is cAMP, which is increased by hormones that activate adenylate cyclase. Adenylate cyclase produces cAMP from ATP. Glucagon is the hormone that causes cAMP to rise during fasting, while epinephrine acts during exercise or stress. cAMP activates protein kinase A which phosphorylates proteins that stimulate transcription of the

The mechanism of action of steroid hormones differs from that of glucagon or epinephrine (see Chapters 24 and 43). Glucocorticoids are steroid hormones that stimulate gluconeogenesis, in part because they induce the synthesis of PEPCK. **Emma Wheezer** had elevated levels of blood glucose because she was being treated with large pharmacological doses of dexamethasone, a potent synthetic glucocorticoid.

PEPCK gene. Increased synthesis of mRNA for PEPCK results in increased synthesis of the enzyme. Cortisol, the major human glucocorticoid, also induces PEPCK.

Pyruvate kinase is inactive. When glucagon is elevated, pyruvate kinase is phosphorylated and inactivated by a mechanism involving cAMP and protein kinase A. Therefore, PEP is not reconverted to pyruvate. Rather, it continues along the pathway of gluconeogenesis. If PEP were reconverted to pyruvate, these substrates would simply cycle, causing a net loss of energy with no net generation of useful products. The inactivation of pyruvate kinase prevents such futile cycling and promotes the net synthesis of glucose.

CONVERSION OF FRUCTOSE 1,6-BISPHOSPHATE TO FRUCTOSE 6-PHOSPHATE

The carbons of PEP reverse the steps of glycolysis, forming fructose 1,6-bisphosphate. Fructose 1,6-bisphosphatase acts on this bisphosphate to release inorganic phosphate and produce fructose 6-phosphate. A futile substrate cycle is prevented at this step because, under conditions that favor gluconeogenesis, the concentrations of the compounds that activate the glycolytic enzyme PFK-1 are low. These same compounds, fructose 2,6-bisphosphate and AMP, are allosteric inhibitors of fructose 1,6-bisphosphatase. When the concentrations of these allosteric effectors are low, PFK-1 is less active, fructose 1,6-bisphosphatase is more active, and the net flow of carbon is toward fructose 6-phosphate and, thus, toward glucose. Fructose 1,6-bisphosphatase is also induced during fasting.

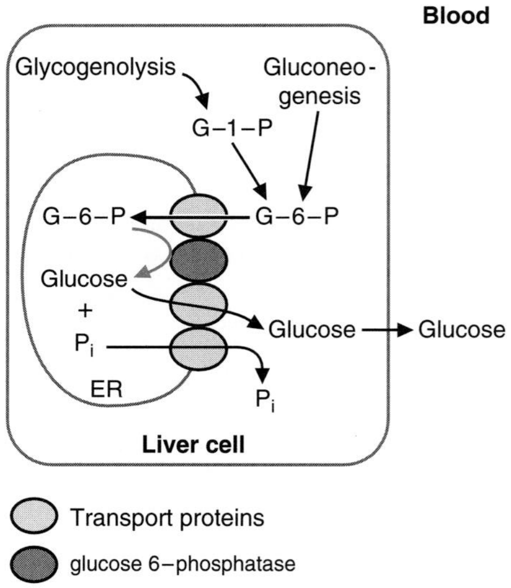

CONVERSION OF GLUCOSE 6-PHOSPHATE TO GLUCOSE

Glucose 6-phosphatase catalyzes the conversion of glucose 6-phosphate to glucose, which is released from the liver cell (Fig. 27.17). The glycolytic enzyme glucokinase, which catalyzes the reverse reaction, is relatively inactive during gluconeogenesis. Glucokinase, which has a high $S_{0.5}$ (K_m) for glucose (see Fig. 9.24), is not very active during fasting because the blood glucose level is low (about 5 mM).

Glucokinase is also an inducible enzyme. The concentration of the enzyme increases in the fed state when blood glucose and insulin levels are elevated and decreases in the fasting state when glucose and insulin are low.

ENERGY IS REQUIRED FOR THE SYNTHESIS OF GLUCOSE

During the gluconeogenic reactions, 6 moles of high energy phosphate bonds are cleaved. Two moles of pyruvate are required for the synthesis of 1 mole of glucose. As 2 moles of pyruvate are carboxylated by pyruvate carboxylase, 2 moles of ATP are hydrolyzed. PEPCK requires 2 moles of GTP (the equivalent of 2 moles of ATP) to convert 2 moles of oxaloacetate to 2 moles of PEP. An additional 2 moles of ATP are used when 2 moles of 3-phosphoglycerate are phosphorylated, forming 2 moles of 1,3-bisphosphoglycerate. Energy in the form of reducing equivalents (NADH) is also required for the conversion of 1,3-bisphosphoglycerate to glyceraldehyde 3-phosphate. Under fasting conditions, the energy required for gluconeogenesis is obtained from β-oxidation of fatty acids.

 Glucose 6-phosphatase is used both in glycogenolysis and gluconeogenesis.

 CLINICAL COMMENTS. The chronic excessive ingestion of ethanol concurrent with a recent reduction in nutrient intake caused **Al Martini's** blood glucose level to fall to 28 mg/dL. This degree of hypoglycemia caused the release of a number of "counterregulatory" hormones into the blood, including glucagon, growth hormone, cortisol, and epinephrine (adrenaline).

Fig. 27.17. Location and function of glucose 6-phosphatase. Glucose 6-phosphate travels on a transporter (shaded oval) into the endoplasmic reticulum (ER) where it is hydrolyzed by glucose 6-phosphatase (black oval) to glucose and P_i. These products travel back to the cytosol on transporters (shaded ovals).

Some of the patient's signs and symptoms are primarily the result of an increase in adrenergic nervous system activity following a rapid fall in blood glucose. The subsequent rise in epinephrine levels in the blood leads to tremulousness, excessive sweating, and rapid heart rate. Other manifestations arise when the brain has insufficient glucose, hence the term "neuroglycopenic symptoms." Mr. Martini was confused, combative, had slurred speech, and eventually had a grand mal seizure. If not treated quickly by intravenous glucose administration, Mr. Martini may have lapsed into a coma. Permanent neurological deficits and even death may result if severe hypoglycemia is not corrected in 6–10 hours.

The elevation in blood glucose which occurred in **Emma Wheezer's** case was primarily a consequence of the large pharmacological doses of a glucocorticoid which she received in an effort to reduce the intrabronchial inflammatory reaction characteristic of asthmatic bronchospasm. Although the development of hyperglycemia in this case could be classified as a "secondary" form of diabetes mellitus, the majority of patients treated with glucocorticoids do not develop glucose intolerance. Ms. Wheezer, therefore, may have a predisposition to the eventual development of "primary" diabetes mellitus.

In hyperglycemia, increased amounts of glucose enter the urine causing large amounts of water to be excreted. This "osmotic diuresis" is responsible for the increased volume of urine (polyuria) noted by the patient. Because of increased urinary water loss, the effective circulating blood volume is reduced. Therefore, less blood reaches volume-sensitive receptors in the central nervous system, which then trigger the sensation of thirst, causing increased drinking activity (polydipsia).

A diabetic diet and the tapering of her steroid dose over a period of several weeks gradually returned Mrs. Wheezer's blood glucose level into the normal range.

BIOCHEMICAL COMMENTS. Changes in activity that result from the binding of activators or inhibitors to enzymes occur rapidly and cause changes in the flux of metabolites within seconds. Changes in activity that result from phosphorylation or dephosphorylation of enzymes are also very rapid. However, induction of enzymes is a slower process that occurs over periods of hours or days (see Chapter 15).

PEPCK is an example of an inducible enzyme. The gene for the cytosolic form of the enzyme contains regulatory sequences in its 5'-flanking region. cAMP, which is produced as a result of the binding of hormones such as glucagon or epinephrine to receptors on the cell surface, causes one of these sequences to be activated. Glucocorticoids affect a different regulatory sequence. cAMP or glucocorticoids independently cause increased transcription of the PEPCK gene. The mRNA produced during transcription travels to the cytosol combines with ribosomes and is translated, producing increased amounts of the enzyme PEPCK.

Although less thoroughly studied, other enzymes of glycolysis and gluconeogenesis also appear to be regulated by induction and its reverse counterpart, repression (the decreased transcription of a gene). cAMP induces synthesis of gluconeogenic enzymes (PEPCK and fructose bisphosphatase) while repressing synthesis of certain glycolytic enzymes (glucokinase, PFK-1, and pyruvate kinase). Insulin has the opposite effect.

Suggested Readings

For more information on the regulation of gluconeogenesis see:

Granner D, Pilkis S. The genes of hepatic glucose metabolism. J Biol Chem 1990;265:10173–10176.

Gurney AL, Park EA, Liu J, et al. Metabolic regulation of gene transcription. J Nutr 1994;124: 15335–15395.

Pilkis S, Granner D. Molecular physiology of the regulation of hepatic gluconeogenesis and glycolysis. Annu Rev Physiol 1992;54:885–909.

PROBLEMS

1. **Al Martini's** blood lactate level was 7.2 mM or 65 mg/dL (reference range = 0.6–2.2 mM or 5.4–19.8). His blood pH of 7.14 (reference range = 7.36–7.45) was indicative of a lactic acidosis.

    Why did Mr. Martini have a lactic acidosis?

2. Individuals with a glucose 6-phosphatase deficiency (Type I glycogen storage disease, von Gierke's disease) often develop a lactic acidosis during fasting. Explain why.

ANSWERS

1. Lactate is one of the major carbon sources for gluconeogenesis. When NADH levels are elevated due to ethanol ingestion, the lactate dehydrogenase reaction favors lactate.

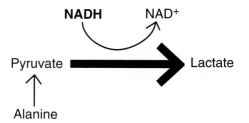

Alanine, another major substrate for gluconeogenesis, is converted to pyruvate by transamination. This pyruvate is also reduced to lactate because of the high NADH levels.

Because, under these conditions, lactate cannot be further metabolized in the liver, it passes into the blood and causes elevated lactate levels. Lactate (lactic acid) causes hydrogen ions (H⁺) to increase in the blood, and an acidosis develops (see Chapter 22).

2. During fasting, liver glycogenolysis forms glucose 6-phosphate which cannot be converted to blood glucose. Glucose 6-phosphate accumulates and floods the glycolytic pathway, increasing lactate production. Gluconeogenic precursors also accumulate and are shunted toward lactate.

28 Pentose Phosphate Pathway

The pentose phosphate pathway oxidizes glucose 6-phosphate to intermediates of the glycolytic pathway, generating NADPH and ribose 5-phosphate for nucleotide synthesis in the process (Fig. 28.1). The NADPH is utilized for reductive pathways, such as fatty acid biosynthesis, detoxification of drugs by monooxygenases, and the glutathione defense system against injury by reactive oxygen species (ROS).

The pentose phosphate pathway can be divided into two phases, an oxidative and a nonoxidative phase. In the oxidative phase of the pentose phosphate pathway, NADPH is generated by the irreversible oxidation of glucose 6-phosphate to a pentose, ribulose 5-phosphate. In the nonoxidative phase of the pathway, ribulose 5-phosphate is converted to ribose 5-phosphate and to intermediates of the glycolytic pathway. Ribose 5-phosphate provides the sugar for nucleotide synthesis. This portion of the pathway is reversible; therefore, ribose 5-phosphate can also be formed

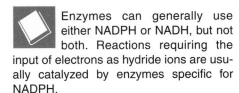
Enzymes can generally use either NADPH or NADH, but not both. Reactions requiring the input of electrons as hydride ions are usually catalyzed by enzymes specific for NADPH.

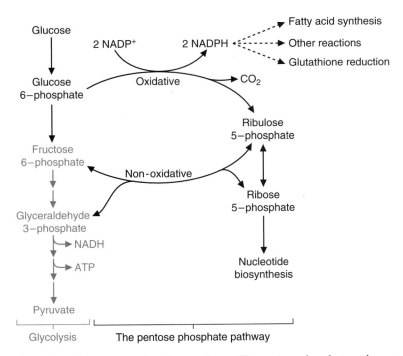

The pentose phosphate pathway is also called the hexose monophosphate shunt. It shunts hexoses from glycolysis, forming pentoses, which may be reconverted to glycolytic intermediates.

Fig. 28.1. Overview of the pentose phosphate pathway. The pentose phosphate pathway generates NADPH for reactions requiring reducing equivalents (electrons) or ribose 5-phosphate for nucleotide biosynthesis. Glucose 6-phosphate is a substrate for both the pentose phosphate pathway and glycolysis. The 5-carbon sugar intermediates of the pentose phosphate pathway are reversibly interconverted to intermediates of glycolysis. The portion of glycolysis which is not part of the pentose phosphate pathway is shown in blue.

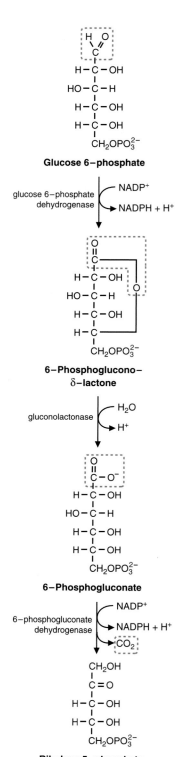

Fig. 28.2. Oxidative portion of the pentose phosphate pathway. Carbon 1 of glucose 6-phosphate is oxidized to an acid, and then released as CO_2 in an oxidative decarboxylation reaction. The two oxidation steps each generate NADPH.

from intermediates of glycolysis. One of the enzymes involved in these sugar interconversions, transketolase, uses thiamine pyrophosphate as a coenzyme.

The sugars produced by the pentose phosphate pathway enter glycolysis as fructose 6-phosphate and glyceraldehyde 3-phosphate, and their further metabolism in the glycolytic pathway generates NADH, ATP, and pyruvate. The overall equation for the pentose phosphate pathway is:

$$3 \text{ glucose-6-P} + 6 \text{ NADP}^+ \rightarrow 3 \text{ CO}_2 + 6 \text{ NADPH} + 6 \text{ H}^+ + 2 \text{ fructose-6-P} + \text{glyceraldehyde-3-P}.$$

Al Martini developed a fever of 101.5°F on the second day of his hospitalization for acute alcoholism. He had a cough productive of gray sputum. A chest x-ray revealed a right lower lobe pneumonia. A stain of his sputum revealed many small pleomorphic Gram-negative bacilli. Sputum was sent for culture and a determination of which antibiotics would be effective in treating the causative organism (sensitivity testing). Because his landlady stated that he had an allergy to penicillin, he was started on a course of the antibiotic combination of trimethoprim and sulfamethoxazole (TMP/sulfa). To his landlady's knowledge, he had never been treated with a sulfa drug previously.

On the third day of therapy with TMP/sulfa for his pneumonia, Al Martini was slightly jaundiced. His hemoglobin level had fallen by 3.5 g/dL from the value on admission and his urine was red-brown in color due to the presence of free hemoglobin. Mr. Martini had apparently suffered acute hemolysis (lysis or destruction of some of his red blood cells) induced by his infection and exposure to the sulfa drug.

REACTIONS OF THE PENTOSE PHOSPHATE PATHWAY

The pentose phosphate pathway is essentially a detour to the pathway of glycolysis which generates NADPH en route. Glucose 6-phosphate (the common precursor to both pathways) is oxidatively decarboxylated in the oxidative first phase of the pathway, and the products reconverted to intermediates of glycolysis in the nonoxidative second phase of the pathway (see Fig. 28.1). The enzymes of the pentose phosphate pathway, like the enzymes of glycolysis, are located solely in the cytosol.

Oxidative Phase of the Pentose Phosphate Pathway

In the oxidative first phase of the pentose phosphate pathway, glucose 6-phosphate is oxidatively decarboxylated to a pentose sugar, ribulose 5-phosphate (Fig. 28.2). The first enzyme of this pathway, glucose 6-phosphate dehydrogenase, oxidizes the aldehyde at C1 and reduces NADP$^+$ to NADPH. The gluconolactone which is formed is rapidly hydrolyzed to 6-phosphogluconate, a sugar acid with a carboxyl group instead of an aldehyde at C1. The next oxidation step releases this carboxyl group as CO_2, again transferring the electrons to NADP$^+$. Two moles of NADPH per mole of glucose 6-phosphate are formed from this portion of the pathway.

Nonoxidative Phase of the Pentose Phosphate Pathway

The nonoxidative portion of the pentose phosphate pathway consists of a series of rearrangement and transfer reactions which convert ribulose 5-phosphate to ribose 5-phosphate and xylulose 5-phosphate, and then to intermediates of the glycolytic pathway. To form a balanced equation for the entire pathway, the conversion of 3 moles of ribulose 5-phosphate to 2 moles of fructose 6-phosphate plus 1 mole of glyceraldehyde 3-phosphate needs to be considered (Fig. 28.3). The enzymes involved are an epimerase, an isomerase, transketolase, and transaldolase.

The epimerase and isomerase convert ribulose 5-phosphate to two other 5-carbon sugars (Fig. 28.4). The isomerase converts ribulose 5-phosphate to ribose 5-phosphate. The epimerase changes the stereochemical position of one –OH group, converting ribulose 5-phosphate to xylulose 5-phosphate.

Transketolase and transaldolase transfer 2- and 3-carbon fragments, respectively, of sugars to other sugars. Transketolase picks up a 2-carbon fragment from xylulose 5-phosphate by cleaving the carbon-carbon bond between the keto group and the adjacent carbon, thereby releasing glyceraldehyde 3-phosphate (Fig. 28.5). The 2-carbon fragment is covalently bound to thiamine pyrophosphate, which plays essentially the same role in this reaction as it does in the decarboxylation of α-keto acids. However, instead of releasing CO_2, transketolase releases the remaining 3 carbons of the compound as an aldehyde. The enzyme then transfers the 2-carbon fragment to the aldehyde carbon of another sugar, forming a new ketose. Two reactions in the pentose phosphate pathway utilize transketolase; in the first, the 2-carbon keto fragment from xylulose 5-phosphate is transferred to ribose 5-phosphate to form sedoheptulose 7-phosphate, and in the other, it is transferred to erythrose 4-phosphate to form fructose 6-phosphate (see Fig. 28.3).

Transaldolase transfers a 3-carbon keto fragment from sedoheptulose 7-phosphate to glyceraldehyde 3-phosphate to form erythrose 4-phosphate and fructose 6-phosphate. The aldol cleavage occurs between the 2 carbons adjacent to the keto group. This reaction is similar to the aldolase reaction in glycolysis, except that here the 3-carbon fragment containing the keto group is transferred to another sugar aldehyde instead of being released (the keto fragment is released as dihydroxyacetone phosphate in glycolysis) (Fig. 28.6).

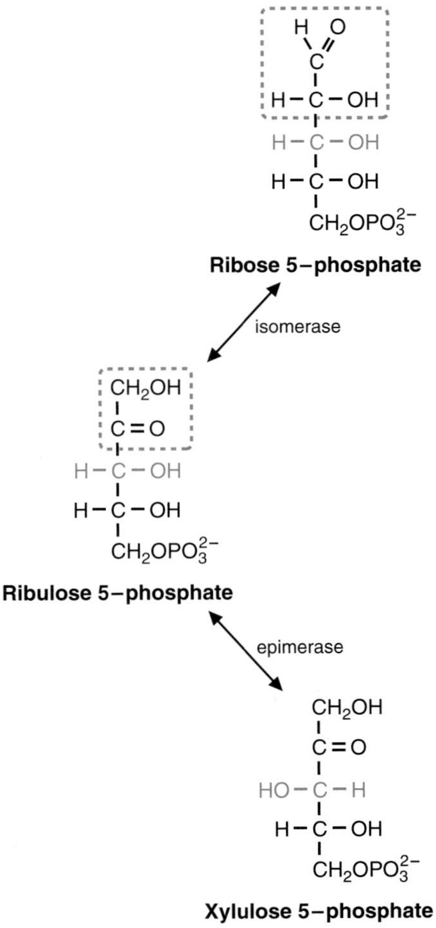

Fig. 28.4. Ribulose 5-phosphate is epimerized and isomerized.

Doctors suspected that the underlying factor in the destruction of **Al Martini's** red blood cells was an X-linked defect in the gene which codes for glucose 6-phosphate dehydrogenase. The red blood cell is dependent on this enzyme for a source of NADPH to maintain reduced levels of glutathione, one of its major defenses against oxidative stress (see Chapter 21). Glucose 6-phosphate dehydrogenase deficiency is the most common known enzymopathy, and affects about 7% of the world's population and about 2% of the U.S. population. Most glucose 6-phosphate dehydrogenase-deficient individuals are asymptomatic but can undergo an episode of hemolytic anemia if exposed to certain drugs, to certain types of infections, or if they ingest fava beans. When questioned, Al Martini replied that he did not know what a fava bean was, and had no idea whether or not he was sensitive to them.

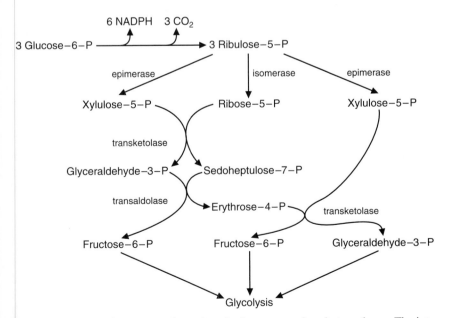

Fig. 28.3. A balanced sequence of reactions in the pentose phosphate pathway. The interconversion of sugars in the pentose phosphate pathway results in conversion of 3 glucose 6-phosphate to 6 NADPH, 3 CO_2, 2 fructose 6-phosphate, and one glyceraldehyde 3-phosphate.

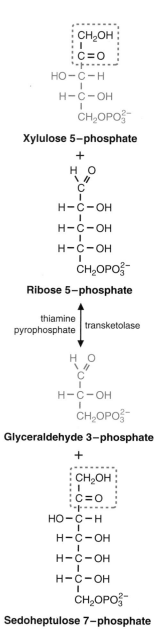

The transketolase activity of red blood cells is used to measure thiamine nutritional status and diagnose the presence of thiamine deficiency. The activity of transketolase is measured in the presence and absence of added thiamine pyrophosphate. If the thiamine intake of a patient is adequate, the addition of thiamine pyrophosphate does not increase the activity of transketolase because it already contains bound thiamine pyrophosphate. If the patient is thiamine deficient, transketolase activity will be low, and adding thiamine pyrophosphate will greatly stimulate the reaction. **Al Martini** was diagnosed in Chapter 19 as having beriberi heart disease resulting from thiamine deficiency. The diagnosis was based on laboratory tests confirming the thiamine deficiency.

Fig. 28.5. Two-carbon unit transferred by transketolase. Transketolase cleaves the bond next to the keto group and transfers the 2-carbon keto fragment to an aldehyde. Thiamine pyrophosphate carries the 2-carbon fragment, forming a covalent bond with the carbon of the keto group.

The net result of the metabolism of 3 moles of ribulose 5-phosphate in the pentose phosphate pathway is the formation of 2 moles of fructose 6-phosphate and 1 mole of glyceraldehyde 3-phosphate, which then continue through the glycolytic pathway with the production of NADH, ATP, and pyruvate. Because the pentose phosphate pathway begins with glucose 6-phosphate, and feeds back into the glycolytic pathway, it is sometimes called the hexose monophosphate shunt (a shunt or a pathway for glucose 6-phosphate).

Routes for Generation of Ribose 5-Phosphate

The reactions in the nonoxidative portion of the pentose phosphate pathway are all reversible under physiological conditions. Thus, ribose 5-phosphate for purine and pyrimidine synthesis can be generated from intermediates of the glycolytic pathway, as well as from the oxidative phase of the pentose phosphate pathway. The sequence of reactions which generate ribose 5-phosphate from intermediates of glycolysis is:

$$\text{2 fructose-6-P + glyceraldehyde-3-P} \rightarrow \text{2 xylulose-5-P + ribose-5-P}$$

$$\text{2 xylulose-5-P} \rightarrow \text{2 ribulose-5-P}$$

$$\text{2 ribulose-5-P} \rightarrow \text{2 ribose-5-P}$$

To generate ribose 5-phosphate from the oxidative pathway:

$$\text{glucose-6-P} \rightarrow \text{ribulose-5-P} \rightarrow \text{ribose-5-P.}$$

The ribose 5-phosphate then enters the pathway for nucleotide synthesis instead of forming intermediates of glycolysis.

The oxidative portion of the pathway can only proceed if NADPH is oxidized back to NADP$^+$ by NADPH-requiring enzymes. If conditions are not favorable for reoxidation of NADPH, ribose 5-phosphate can still be formed by reversal of the nonoxidative steps of the pathway, using glycolytic intermediates as precursors.

ROLE OF THE PENTOSE PHOSPHATE PATHWAY IN THE GENERATION OF NADPH

In general, the oxidative phase of the pentose phosphate pathway is the major source of NADPH in cells. NADPH provides the reducing equivalents for biosynthetic reactions, and for oxidation-reduction reactions involved in protection against toxicity of ROS (Fig. 28.7). The glutathione-mediated defense against oxidative stress is common to all cell types (including the red blood cell), and the requirement for NADPH to maintain levels of reduced glutathione probably accounts for the universal distribution of the pentose phosphate pathway among different types of cells. NADPH is also used for anabolic pathways, such as fatty acid synthesis, cholesterol synthesis, and fatty acid chain elongation (Table 28.1). It is the source of reducing equivalents for cytochrome P450 hydroxylation of aromatic compounds, steroids, alcohols, and drugs. The highest concentrations of glucose 6-phosphate dehydrogenase are found in phagocytic cells, where NADPH oxidase uses NADPH to form superoxide from molecular oxygen. The superoxide then generates the ROS which kills the microorganisms taken up by the phagocytic cells (see Chapter 21).

The entry of glucose 6-phosphate into the pentose phosphate pathway is controlled by the cellular concentration of NADPH. NADPH is a strong product inhibitor of glucose 6-phosphate dehydrogenase, the first enzyme of the pathway. As NADPH is oxidized in other pathways, the product inhibition of glucose 6-phosphate dehydrogenase is relieved and the rate of the enzyme is accelerated to produce more NADPH.

In the liver, the synthesis of fatty acids from glucose is a major route of NADPH reoxidation. The synthesis of liver glucose 6-phosphate dehydrogenase, like the key enzymes of glycolysis and fatty acid synthesis, is induced by the increased insulin/glucagon ratio after a high carbohydrate meal.

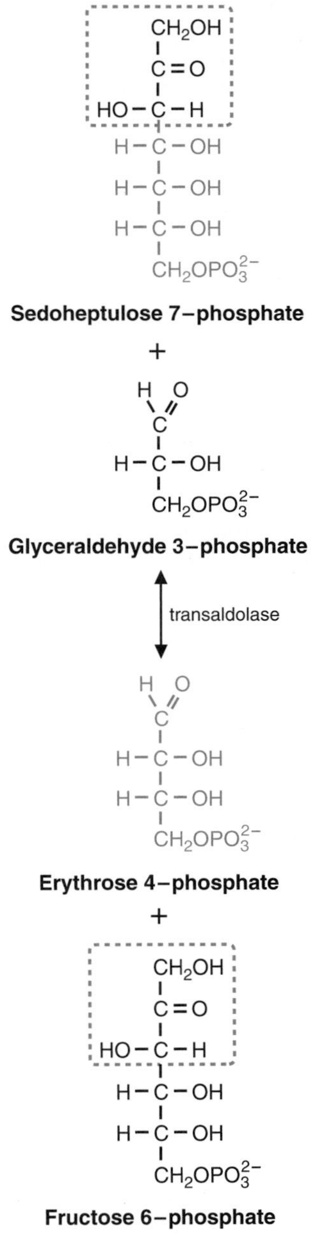

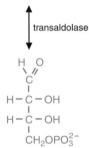

Sedoheptulose 7–phosphate

Glyceraldehyde 3–phosphate

transaldolase

Erythrose 4–phosphate

Fructose 6–phosphate

Fig. 28.6. Transaldolase transfers a 3-carbon fragment that contains an alcohol group next to a keto group.

CLINICAL COMMENTS. **Al Martini's** sputum culture sent on the second day of his admission for acute alcoholism and pneumonia grew out *Haemophilus influenzae*. This organism is sensitive to a variety of antibi-

Q 28.1: How does the net energy yield from the metabolism of 3 moles of glucose 6-phosphate through the pentose phosphate pathway to pyruvate compare to the yield of 3 moles of glucose 6-phosphate through glycolysis?

A 28.1: The net energy yield from 3 moles of glucose 6-phosphate metabolized through the pentose phosphate pathway and then the last portion of the glycolytic pathway is 6 moles of NADPH, 3 moles of CO_2, 5 moles of NADH, 8 moles of ATP, and 5 moles of pyruvate. In contrast, the metabolism of 3 moles of glucose 6-phosphate through glycolysis is 6 moles of NADH, 9 moles of ATP, and 6 moles of pyruvate.

otics, including TMP/sulfa. Unfortunately, it appeared that Mr. Martini had suffered an acute hemolysis (lysis or destruction of some of his red blood cells), probably induced by exposure to the sulfa drug and his infection with *H. influenzae*. The hemoglobin that escaped from the lysed red blood cells was filtered by his kidneys and appeared in his urine.

By mechanisms which are not fully delineated, certain drugs (such as sulfa drugs and antimalarials), a variety of infectious agents, and exposure to fava beans can cause red blood cell destruction in individuals with a genetic deficiency of glucose 6-phosphate dehydrogenase. Presumably, these patients cannot generate enough reduced NADPH to defend against the ROS. Although erythrocytes lack most of the other enzymatic sources of NADPH for the glutathione antioxidant system, they do have the defense mechanisms provided by the antioxidant vitamins E and C, and catalase. Thus, individuals who are not totally deficient in glucose 6-phosphate dehydrogenase

Table 28.1. Pathways That Require NADPH

Detoxification
- Reduction of oxidized glutathione
- Cytochrome P450 monooxygenases

Reductive synthesis
- Fatty acid synthesis
- Fatty acid chain elongation
- Cholesterol synthesis
- Neurotransmitter synthesis
- Nucleotide synthesis

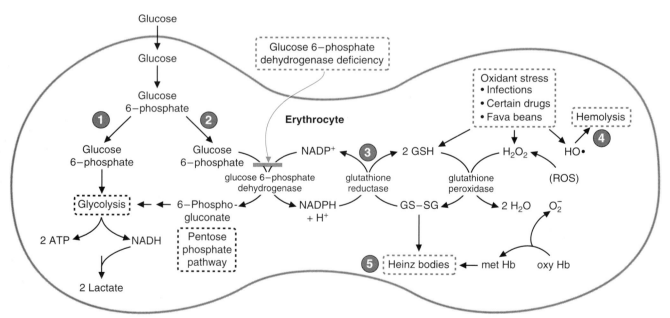

Fig. 28.7. Hemolysis caused by reactive oxygen species. **1.** Maintenance of the integrity of the erythrocyte membrane depends on its ability to generate ATP and NADH from glycolysis. **2.** NADPH is generated by the pentose phosphate pathway. **3.** NADPH is utilized for the reduction of oxidized glutathione to reduced glutathione. Glutathione is necessary for the removal of H_2O_2 and lipid peroxides generated by reactive oxygen species (ROS). **4.** In the erythrocytes of healthy individuals, the continuous generation of superoxide ion from the nonenzymatic oxidation of hemoglobin provides a source of reactive oxygen species. The glutathione defense system is compromised by glucose 6-phosphate dehydrogenase deficiency, infections, certain drugs, and the purine glycosides of fava beans. **5.** As a consequence, Heinz bodies, aggregates of cross-linked hemoglobin, form on the cell membranes and subject the cell to mechanical stress as it tries to go through small capillaries. The action of the ROS on the cell membrane as well as mechanical stress from the lack of deformability result in hemolysis.

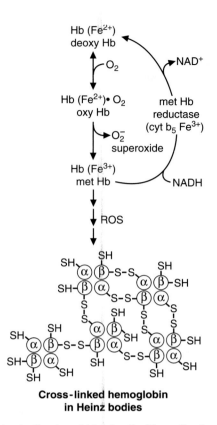

**Cross-linked hemoglobin
in Heinz bodies**

Fig. 28.8. Formation of Heinz bodies in red blood cells. Normally, the erythrocyte removes superoxide with superoxide dismutase, which converts superoxide to hydrogen peroxide. Glutathione peroxidase reduces the hydrogen peroxide to H_2O while oxidizing glutathione to the disulfide form. In individuals such as **Al Martini**, a deficiency of glucose 6-phosphate dehydrogenase prevents the production of a sufficient amount of NADPH. As a result, Heinz bodies are formed, and hemolysis occurs.

Red blood cells generate superoxide and ROS during the nonenzymatic oxidation of hemoglobin to methemoglobin, and depend on glucose 6-phosphate dehydrogenase to provide NADPH to protect against oxidative stress. Red blood cells do not have the mitochondrial metabolic pathways which normally account for most of the production of ROS in other tissues. However, methemoglobin is slowly and continuously produced by spontaneous transfer of an electron from the Fe^{2+} in hemoglobin to its bound oxygen by a reaction that generates superoxide. See Figure 28.8.

remain asymptomatic unless an additional oxidative stress, such as an infection, generates additional oxygen radicals.

Some drugs, such as the antimalarial primaquine and the sulfonamide which Al Martini is taking, affect the ability of red blood cells to defend against oxidative stress. Fava beans, which look like fat string beans and are sometimes called broad beans, contain the purine glycosides vicine and isouramil. These compounds react with glutathione. It has been suggested that cellular levels of reduced glutathione (GSH) fall to such an extent that critical sulfhydryl groups in some key proteins cannot be maintained in reduced form. Hemoglobin becomes cross-linked by disulfide bonds which result in the formation of bridges that are further oxidized, and the structures form aggregates on red blood cell membranes called Heinz bodies (see Fig. 28.8). Normally the red blood cells must deform to travel through the microvasculature. In the presence of Heinz bodies the membrane cannot deform and is predisposed to destruction or lysis, particularly if the cell membrane has suffered oxidative damage.

The highest prevalence rates for glucose 6-phosphate dehydrogenase deficiency are found in tropical Africa and Asia, in some areas of the Middle East and the Mediterranean, and in Papua New Guinea. The geographic distribution of this deficiency is similar to that of sickle cell trait, and is probably also related to the relative resistance it confers against the malaria parasite.

As red blood cells age during storage in a blood bank, hexokinase activity is lost and the cells are unable to generate ATP from glucose metabolism in the glycolytic pathway. However, they can generate ATP from inosine using the pentose phosphate pathway. Inosine (a nucleoside composed of the base hypoxanthine and the sugar ribose) is normally taken up by red blood cells and other cells for the synthesis of purines. When added to stored blood, it is converted to hypoxanthine and ribose 5-phosphate using inorganic phosphate. The ribose 5-phosphate is metabolized via the pentose phosphate pathway to fructose 6-phosphate and glyceraldehyde 3-phosphate. These metabolites are then converted to lactate via anaerobic glycolysis with the generation of 8 moles of ATP per 3 moles of ribose 5-phosphate.

Because the individuals with this deficiency are asymptomatic unless exposed to an "oxidant challenge," the clinical course of the hemolytic anemia is usually self-limited if the causative agent is removed. However, genetic polymorphism accounts for a substantial variability in the severity of the disease. Severely affected patients may have a chronic hemolytic anemia and other sequelae even without known exposure to drugs, infection, and other causative factors. In such patients, neonatal jaundice is also common and can be severe enough to cause death.

BIOCHEMICAL COMMENTS. NADPH, rather than NADH, is generally utilized in the cell for pathways which require the input of electrons for reductive reactions because the ratio of NADPH/NADP$^+$ is much greater than the NADH/NAD$^+$ ratio. The NADH which is generated from fuel oxidation is rapidly oxidized back to NAD$^+$ by NADH dehydrogenase in the electron transport chain, so the level of NADH is very low in the cell.

NADPH can be generated from a number of reactions in the liver and other tissues, but not the red blood cell. For example, in tissues with mitochondria, an energy-requiring transhydrogenase located near the complexes of the electron transport chain can transfer reducing equivalents from NADH to NADP$^+$ to generate NADPH.

NADPH, on the other hand, cannot be directly oxidized by the electron transport chain, and the ratio of NADPH to NADP$^+$ in cells is greater than one. The reduction potential of NADPH can therefore contribute to the energy needed for biosynthetic processes and provide a constant source of reducing power for detoxification reactions.

Suggested Readings

Hasler J, Lee S. Acute hemolytic anemia after ingestion of fava beans [letter]. Am J Emerg Med 1993;11:560–561.

Luzatto L, Mehta A. Glucose 6-phosphate dehydrogenase deficiency. In: Scriver CR, Beaudet AL, Sly WS, Valle D, eds. The metabolic and molecular bases of inherited disease. 7th ed, vol III. New York: McGraw-Hill, 1995:3367–3397.

PROBLEM

Vitamin E deficiency occasionally arises in individuals who have problems with fat absorption. The test for vitamin E deficiency involves treating the patient's red blood cells with H_2O_2 at a concentration of hydrogen peroxide that will not lyse red blood cells from normal, healthy individuals. Explain the rationale for this test in terms of your knowledge of erythrocyte metabolism.

ANSWER

Vitamin E is an antioxidant which can react with ROS (see Chapter 21). In healthy individuals, both vitamin E and the glutathione defense systems protect against H_2O_2. In the red blood cells of healthy individuals in vivo, these two systems provide a defense capacity which is more than adequate to deal with normal rates of H_2O_2 generation in vivo. However, when H_2O_2 is added to red blood cells in the test tube, the glutathione defense system alone is not sufficient in the absence of vitamin E. Membrane lipid peroxidation results in cell lysis.

29 Pathways for the Interconversion of Sugars

Glucose is at the center of carbohydrate metabolism and is the major dietary sugar. Other sugars in the diet are converted to intermediates of glucose metabolism, and their fates parallel that of glucose. When carbohydrates other than glucose are required for the synthesis of proteoglycans, gangliosides, or other carbohydrate-containing compounds, they are synthesized from glucose.

Fructose, the second most common sugar in the adult diet, is ingested principally as the monosaccharide or as part of sucrose (Fig. 29.1). It is metabolized principally in the liver (and to a lesser extent in the small intestine and kidney) by phosphorylation at the one-position and conversion to intermediates of the glycolytic pathway. The major products of its metabolism in liver include pyruvate, lactate, glucose, and glycogen. Essential fructosuria (fructokinase deficiency) and hereditary fructose intolerance (a deficiency of the fructose 1-phosphate aldolase activity of aldolase B) are inherited disorders of fructose metabolism.

Sugars are converted to their alcohol form by aldose reductase in the polyol pathway. Fructose can be synthesized from sorbitol, the sugar alcohol of glucose, in the seminal vesicles and other tissues. In the lens of the eye, elevated levels of sorbitol in diabetes mellitus and galactitol (the sugar alcohol of galactose) in galactosemia contribute to cataract formation.

Many of the pathways for interconversion of sugars or the formation of sugar derivatives utilize activated sugars attached to nucleotides. UDP-glucose, for example, can be epimerized to UDP-galactose, and the galactose then transferred to glucose to synthesize lactose in the mammary gland. UDP-glucose can also be oxidized to UDP-glucuronate, and the glucuronate transferred to bilirubin or a xenobiotic compound to make it more water-soluble and more readily excreted. Nucleotide sugars also donate sugar residues for the formation of glycosidic bonds with proteins and to extend the carbohydrate chains of glycoproteins and proteoglycans.

Galactose is ingested principally as lactose. It is converted to glucose 1-phosphate via phosphorylation and activation to the UDP-sugar. Classical galactosemia, a deficiency of galactosyl uridylyltransferase, results in the accumulation of galactose 1-phosphate and inhibition of glycogen metabolism and pathways which require UDP sugars.

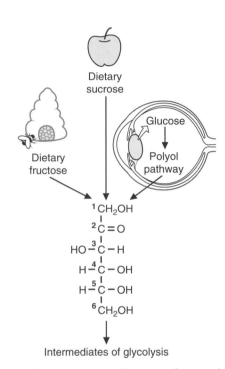

Fig. 29.1. Fructose. The sugar fructose is found in the diet as the free sugar in foods such as honey or as a component of the disaccharide sucrose in fruits and sweets. It can also be synthesized from glucose via the polyol pathway. In the lens of the eye, the polyol pathway contributes to the formation of cataracts. Fructose is metabolized by conversion to intermediates of glycolysis.

Candice Sucher is an 18-year-old female who presented to her physician for a precollege physical examination. While taking her medical history, the doctor learned that she carefully avoided eating all fruits and any foods that contained table sugar. She related that, from a very early age, she had learned that these foods caused severe weakness and symptoms suggestive of low blood sugar, such as tremulousness and sweating. Her past medical history also revealed that her mother had described her as having been a very irritable baby who often cried incessantly, especially after meals, and vomited frequently. At these times, Candice's abdomen had become distended, and she became drowsy and apathetic. Her mother had intuitively eliminated certain foods from Candice's diet, after which the severity and frequency of these symptoms diminished.

 Erin Galway is a 3-week-old female infant who began vomiting 3 days after birth, usually within 30 minutes after breastfeeding. Her abdomen became distended at these times and she became irritable and cried frequently. When her mother noted that the whites of Erin's eyes were yellow, she took her to a pediatrician. The doctor agreed that Erin was slightly jaundiced. He also noted an enlargement of her liver and questioned the possibility of early cataract formation in the lenses of Erin's eyes. He ordered liver and kidney function tests and did two separate dipstick urine tests in his office, one designed to measure only glucose in the urine and the other capable of detecting any of the reducing sugars.

FRUCTOSE

Fructose is found in the diet as a component of sucrose in fruit, as a free sugar in honey, and in high fructose corn syrup (see Fig. 29.1). Fructose enters epithelial cells and other types of cells by facilitated diffusion. Problems with fructose absorption and metabolism are relatively more common than with other sugars.

Fructose Metabolism

Fructose is metabolized by conversion to intermediates of glycolysis (Fig. 29.2). The first step in the metabolism of fructose, as with glucose, is phosphorylation. Fructokinase, the major kinase involved, phosphorylates fructose in the 1-position.

When individuals with defects of aldolase B ingest fructose, the extremely high levels of fructose 1-phosphate which accumulate in the liver and kidney cause a number of adverse effects. Hypoglycemia results from inhibition of glycogenolysis and gluconeogenesis. Glycogen phosphorylase (and possibly phosphoglucomutase and other enzymes of glycogen metabolism) are inhibited by the accumulated fructose 1-phosphate. Aldolase B is required for glucose synthesis from glyceraldehyde 3-phosphate and dihydroxyacetone phosphate, and its low activity in aldolase B-deficient individuals is further decreased by the accumulated fructose 1-phosphate. The inhibition of gluconeogenesis results in lactic acidosis. The accumulation of fructose 1-phosphate also substantially depletes the phosphate pools. The low levels of phosphate activate adenosine deaminase, which then converts AMP to inosine monophosphate (IMP). The nitrogenous base of IMP (hypoxanthine) is degraded to uric acid. The lack of phosphate and depletion of adenine nucleotides lead to a loss of ATP, further contributing to the inhibition of biosynthetic pathways.

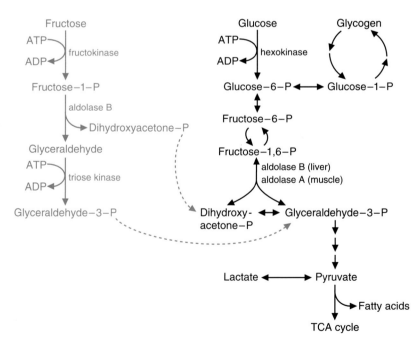

Fig. 29.2. Fructose metabolism. The pathway for the conversion of fructose to dihydroxyacetone phosphate and glyceraldehyde 3-phosphate is shown in blue. These two compounds are intermediates of glycolysis and are converted in the liver principally to glucose, glycogen, or fatty acids. Aldolase B cleaves both fructose 1-phosphate in the pathway for fructose metabolism, and fructose 1,6-bisphosphate in the pathway for glycolysis.

Since the only fructose-containing intermediates of glycolysis are fructose 6-phosphate and fructose 1,6-bisphosphate, the fructose 1-phosphate formed by fructokinase must be further metabolized before it can enter the glycolytic and gluconeogenic pathways. Fructose 1-phosphate is cleaved by aldolase B to dihydroxyacetone phosphate and glyceraldehyde, and the glyceraldehyde is phosphorylated by a triose kinase. Both dihydroxyacetone phosphate and glyceraldehyde 3-phosphate are intermediates of the glycolytic pathway and can proceed through it to pyruvate and lactate. In the liver, these intermediates are also converted to glucose 6-phosphate by reversal of the glycolytic pathway (i.e., by gluconeogenesis), and released into the blood as glucose or converted to glycogen. The pyruvate is either oxidized to CO_2 or converted to fatty acids. In other words, the fate of fructose parallels that of glucose.

The metabolism of fructose occurs principally in the liver and to a lesser extent in the small intestinal mucosa and proximal epithelium of the renal tubule because these tissues have both fructokinase and aldolase B. The aldolase which cleaves fructose 1,6-bisphosphate in the glycolytic pathway exists as several isoforms: aldolases A, B, C, and fetal aldolase. Only aldolase B can cleave both fructose 1-phosphate and fructose 1,6-bisphosphate. Aldolase A, present in muscle and most other tissues, and aldolase C, present in brain, have almost no ability to cleave fructose 1-phosphate. Fetal aldolase, present in the liver prior to birth, is similar to aldolase C.

Aldolase B is the rate-limiting enzyme of fructose metabolism, although it is not a rate-limiting enzyme of glycolysis. It has a much lower affinity for fructose 1-phosphate than fructose 1,6-bisphosphate (although the k_{cat} is the same) and is very slow at physiological levels of fructose 1-phosphate. As a consequence, after ingesting a high dose of fructose, normal individuals accumulate fructose 1-phosphate in the liver while it is slowly converted to glycolytic intermediates. Individuals with hereditary fructose intolerance (a deficiency of aldolase B) accumulate much higher amounts of fructose 1-phosphate in their livers.

Other tissues also have the capacity to metabolize fructose, but do so much more slowly. The hexokinase isoforms present in muscle, adipose tissue, and other tissues can convert fructose to fructose 6-phosphate, but react so much more efficiently with glucose that fructose phosphorylation is very slow in the presence of physiological levels of intracellular glucose and glucose 6-phosphate.

Polyol Pathway

The polyol pathway is named for the first step of the pathway in which sugars are reduced to the sugar alcohol by the enzyme aldose reductase (Fig. 29.3) One of the functions of the polyol pathway is the synthesis of fructose from glucose. Glucose is reduced to the sugar alcohol sorbitol, and sorbitol is then oxidized to fructose. This pathway is present in seminal vesicles, which synthesize fructose for the seminal fluid. Spermatozoa utilize fructose as a major fuel source while in the seminal fluid, and then switch to glucose once in the female reproductive tract. Utilization of fructose is thought to prevent acrosomal breakdown of the plasma membrane (and consequent activation) while the spermatozoa are still in the seminal fluid.

The polyol pathway is present in many tissues, but its function in all tissues is not understood. Aldose reductase is relatively nonspecific, and its major function may be the metabolism of an aldehyde sugar other than glucose. The enzyme causes major problems in the lens of the eye, where it is responsible for the production of sorbitol from glucose and galactitol from galactose. When glucose or galactose is elevated in the blood, their respective sugar alcohols are synthesized in the lens more rapidly than they are removed.

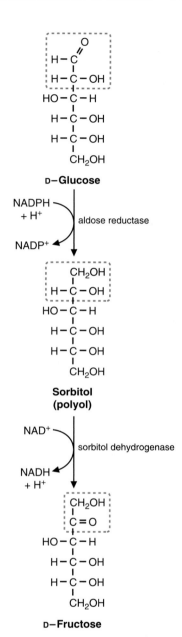

Fig. 29.3. The polyol pathway converts glucose to fructose.

The accumulation of sorbitol in muscle and nerve tissues may contribute to the peripheral neuropathy characteristic of patients with poorly controlled diabetes mellitus. This is one of the reasons it is so important for **Di Beatty** (who has IDDM) and **Ann Sulin** (who has NIDDM) to achieve good glycemic control.

Q 29.1: Essential fructosuria is a rare and benign genetic disorder caused by a deficiency of the enzyme fructokinase. Why is this disease benign, when a deficiency of aldolase B (hereditary fructose intolerance) can be fatal? Could **Candice Sucher** have essential fructosuria?

The accumulation of sugars and sugar alcohols in the lens of patients with hyperglycemia (e.g., diabetes mellitus) results in the formation of cataracts. Glucose levels are elevated and increase the synthesis of sorbitol and fructose. As a consequence, a high osmotic pressure is created in the lens. The high glucose and fructose levels also result in nonenzymatic glycosylation of lens proteins. The result of the increased osmotic pressure and the glycosylation of the lens protein is an opaque cloudiness of the lens known as a cataract. **Erin Galway** seemed to have an early cataract, probably caused by the accumulation of galactose and its sugar alcohol galactitol.

A 29.1: In essential fructosuria, fructose cannot be converted to fructose 1-phosphate. This condition is benign because no toxic metabolites of fructose accumulate in the liver and the patient remains nearly asymptomatic. Some of the ingested fructose is slowly phosphorylated by hexokinase in nonhepatic tissues and metabolized via glycolysis, and some appears in the urine. There is no renal threshold for fructose, so that the appearance of fructose in the urine (fructosuria) does not require a high fructose concentration in the blood.

Hereditary fructose intolerance, on the other hand, results in the accumulation of fructose 1-phosphate and fructose. By inhibiting glycogenolysis and gluconeogenesis, the high levels of fructose 1-phosphate caused the hypoglycemia which **Candice Sucher** experienced as an infant when she became apathetic and drowsy, and as an adult when she experienced sweating and tremulousness.

INTERCONVERSIONS INVOLVING UDP-SUGARS

Activated sugars attached to nucleotides are converted to other sugars, oxidized to sugar acids, and joined to proteins, lipids, or other sugars through glycosidic bonds.

Reactions of UDP-Glucose

UDP-glucose is an activated sugar nucleotide which is a precursor of glycogen and lactose, UDP-glucuronate and glucuronides, and the carbohydrate chains in proteoglycans, glycoproteins, and glycolipids (Fig. 29.4). In the synthesis of many of the carbohydrate portions of these compounds, a sugar is transferred from the nucleotide sugar to an alcohol or other nucleophilic group to form a glycosidic bond (Fig. 29.5). The high energy bond between UDP and the sugar provides the energy for formation of the new bond. The enzymes which form glycosidic bonds are sugar transferases (for instance, glycogen synthetase is a glucosyltransferase). Transferases are also involved in the formation of the glycosidic bonds in bilirubin glucuronides, proteoglycans, and lactose.

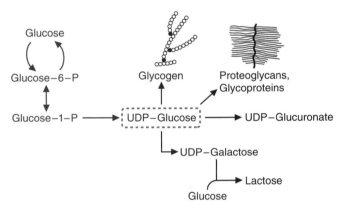

Fig. 29.4. Metabolism of UDP-glucose. The activated glucose moiety of UDP-glucose can be attached via a glycosidic bond to other sugars, as in glycogen or the sugar oligo- and polysaccharide side chains of proteoglycans and glycoproteins. UDP-glucose can also be oxidized to UDP-glucuronate, or epimerized to UDP-galactose, a precursor of lactose.

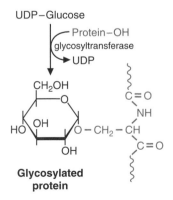

Fig. 29.5. Glycosyltransferases. These enzymes transfer sugars from nucleotide sugars to nucleophilic amino acid residues on proteins, such as the OH group of serine or the amide group of asparagine. Other transferases transfer specific sugars from a nucleotide sugar to the OH group of other sugars. The bond formed between the anomeric carbon of the sugar and the nucleophilic group of another compound is a glycosidic bond.

UDP-Glucuronate: A Source of Negative Charges

One of the major routes of UDP-glucose metabolism is the formation of UDP-glucuronate, which serves as a precursor of other sugars and of glucuronides (Fig. 29.6). Glucuronate is formed by the oxidation of the alcohol on C6 of glucose to an acid (through two oxidation states) by an NAD^+-dependent dehydrogenase (Fig. 29.7). Glucuronate is also present in the diet, and is formed from the degradation of inositol (the sugar alcohol which forms inositol trisphosphate (IP_3), an intracellular second messenger for many hormones).

GLUCURONATE IS INCORPORATED INTO GLYCOSAMINOGLYCANS

The acidic group of glucuronate carries a negative charge at physiological pH and increases the water solubility of the compounds to which it is attached. Once glucuronate is incorporated into glycosaminoglycans, some of the glucuronate residues are converted to the sugar acid iduronate. These two acids contribute to the strongly negative nature of the glycosaminoglycans. UDP-glucuronate is also the precursor of UDP-xylose, another sugar precursor of glycosaminoglycans.

FORMATION OF GLUCURONIDES

The function of glucuronate in the excretion of bilirubin, drugs, and xenobiotics and other compounds containing an OH group is to add negative charges and increase their solubility. Bilirubin is a degradation product of heme which is formed in the reticuloendothelial system, and is only slightly soluble in plasma. It is transported to the liver bound to albumin. In the liver, glucuronate residues are transferred from UDP-glucuronate to two carboxyl groups on bilirubin, sequentially forming bilirubin monoglucuronide and bilirubin diglucuronide, the "conjugated" forms of bilirubin (Fig. 29.8). The more soluble bilirubin diglucuronide is then actively transported into the bile for excretion.

Many xenobiotics, drugs, steroids, and other compounds with OH groups and a low solubility in water are converted to glucuronides in a similar fashion by glucuronyltransferases present in the endoplasmic reticulum and cytoplasm of the liver and kidney (Table 29.1). This is one of the major conjugation pathways for excretion of these compounds.

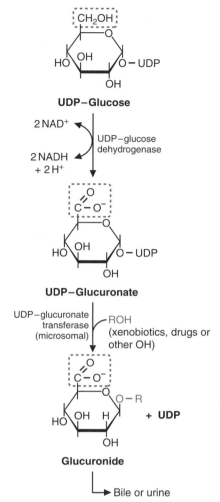

Fig. 29.7. Formation of glucuronate and glucuronides. A glycosidic bond is formed between the anomeric OH of glucuronate and an OH of a nonpolar compound. The negatively charged carboxyl group of the glucuronate increases the water solubility and allows otherwise nonpolar compounds to be excreted in the urine or bile.

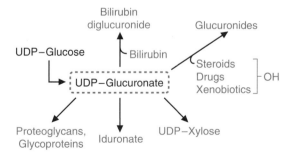

Fig. 29.6. Metabolic routes of UDP-glucuronate. UDP-glucuronate is formed from UDP-glucose (shown in black). Glucuronate from UDP-glucuronate is incorporated into glycosaminoglycans, where certain of the glucuronate residues are converted to iduronate. UDP-glucuronate is a precursor of UDP-xylose, another sugar residue incorporated into glycosaminoglycans. Glucuronate is also transferred to the carboxyl groups of bilirubin or the alcohol groups of steroids, drugs, and xenobiotics to form glucuronides. The "ide" in the name glucuronide denotes that these compounds are glycosides.

A failure of the liver to transport, store, or conjugate bilirubin results in the accumulation of unconjugated bilirubin in the blood. Jaundice, the yellowish tinge to the skin and the whites of the eyes (sclera) experienced by **Erin Galway**, occurs when plasma becomes supersaturated with bilirubin (>2–2.5 mg/dL) and the excess diffuses into tissues.

Q 29.2: A pregnant woman who was extremely lactose intolerant asked her physician if she would still be able to breastfeed her infant since she could not drink milk or dairy products. What advice should she be given?

Table 29.1. Some Compounds Degraded and Excreted as Urinary Glucuronides

Estrogen (female sex hormone)
Progesterone (steroid hormone)
Triiodothyronine (thyroid hormone)
Acetylaminofluorene (xenobiotic carcinogen)
Meprobamate (drug for sleep)
Morphine (painkiller)

Glucuronate, once formed, can reenter the pathways of glucose metabolism through reactions which eventually convert it to D-xylulose 5-phosphate, an intermediate of the pentose phosphate pathway. In most mammals other than humans, an intermediate of this pathway is the precursor of ascorbic acid (vitamin C). Humans cannot synthesize vitamin C.

Synthesis of UDP-Galactose and Lactose from Glucose

Lactose is synthesized from UDP-galactose and glucose (Fig. 29.9). However, galactose is not required in the diet for lactose synthesis because galactose can be synthesized from glucose.

CONVERSION OF GLUCOSE TO GALACTOSE

Galactose and glucose are epimers; they differ only in the stereochemical position of one OH group. Thus, the formation of UDP-galactose from UDP-glucose is an epimerization (Fig. 29.10). The epimerase does not actually transfer the OH group; it oxidizes the OH to a ketone by transferring electrons to NAD^+, and then donates electrons back to re-form the alcohol group on the other side of the carbon.

LACTOSE SYNTHESIS

Lactose is unique in that it is synthesized only in the mammary gland of the adult for short periods of time during lactation. Lactose synthase, an endoplasmic reticulum enzyme present in the lactating mammary gland, catalyzes the last step in lactose biosynthesis—the transfer of galactose from UDP-galactose to glucose (see Fig. 29.9). Lactose synthase has two protein subunits, a galactosyltransferase and α-lactalbumin. α-Lactalbumin is a modifier protein synthesized after parturition (child-

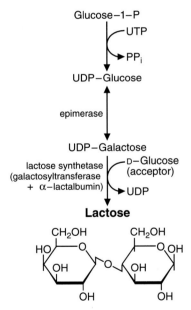

Fig. 29.9. Lactose synthesis. Lactose is a disaccharide composed of galactose and glucose. UDP-galactose for the synthesis of lactose in the mammary gland is usually formed from the epimerization of UDP-glucose. Lactose synthase attaches the anomeric carbon of the galactose to the C4 alcohol group of glucose to form a glycosidic bond. Lactose synthetase is composed of galactosyltransferase and α-lactalbumin.

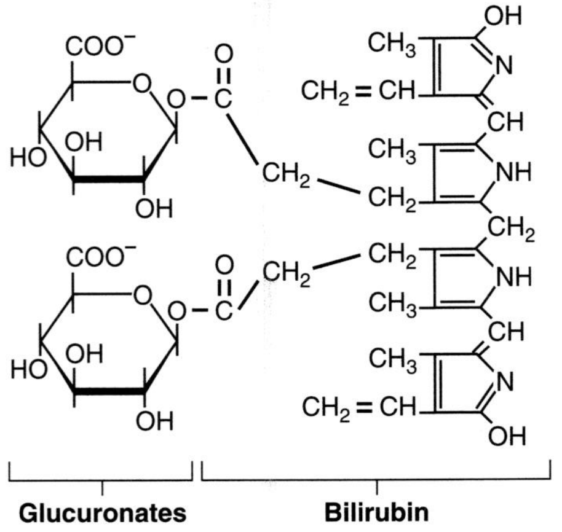

Fig. 29.8. Bilirubin diglucuronide. In bilirubin diglucuronide, the glycosidic bonds are between the anomeric carbon of the glucuronate residues and the carboxyl groups of bilirubin.

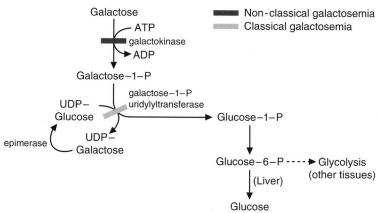

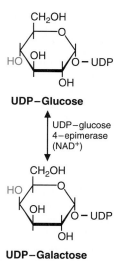

Fig. 29.11. Metabolism of galactose. Galactose is phosphorylated to galactose 1-phosphate by galactokinase. Galactose 1-phosphate reacts with UDP-glucose to release glucose 1-phosphate. Galactose can thus be converted to blood glucose, enter glycolysis, or enter any of the metabolic routes of glucose. In classical galactosemia, a deficiency of galactose 1-phosphate uridylyltransferase (shown in blue) results in the accumulation of galactose 1-phosphate in tissues and the appearance of galactose in the blood and urine. In nonclassical galactosemia, a deficiency of galactokinase results in the accumulation of galactose.

Fig. 29.10. Epimerization of UDP-glucose to UDP-galactose. The epimerization of glucose to galactose occurs on UDP-sugars. The epimerase utilizes NAD^+ to oxidize the alcohol to a ketone, and then reduce the ketone back to an alcohol. The reaction is reversible; glucose → galactose forms galactose for lactose synthesis, and galactose → glucose is part of the pathway for the metabolism of dietary galactose.

birth) in response to the hormone prolactin. This enzyme subunit lowers the K_m of the galactosyltransferase for glucose from 1,200 to 1 mM, thereby increasing the rate of lactose synthesis. In the absence of α-lactalbumin, galactosyltransferase transfers galactosyl units to glycoproteins.

GALACTOSE METABOLISM

Dietary galactose is metabolized principally by phosphorylation to galactose 1-phosphate, and then conversion to UDP-galactose and glucose 1-phosphate (Fig. 29.11). The route is circuitous. The phosphorylation of galactose, again an important first step in the pathway, is carried out by a specific kinase, galactokinase. The formation of UDP-galactose is accomplished by exchanging the galactose in galactose 1-phosphate for the glucose on UDP-glucose. The enzyme that catalyzes this reaction is called galactose 1-phosphate uridylyltransferase. The UDP-galactose is then converted to UDP-glucose by the reversible UDP-glucose epimerase. The net result of this sequence of reactions is that galactose is converted to glucose 1-phosphate.

(1) Galactose + ATP $\xrightarrow{\text{galactokinase}}$ Galactose -1-P + ADP

(2) Galactose-1-P + UDP-glucose $\xrightarrow[\text{uridylyltransferase}]{\text{galactose-1-P}}$ UDP-galactose + glucose -1-P

(3) UDP-galactose $\xrightarrow{\text{UDP-glucose epimerase}}$ UDP-glucose

Net equation:

Galactose + ATP $\xrightarrow{\hspace{4cm}}$ glucose-1-P + ADP

A 29.2: Although the lactose in dairy products is a major source of galactose, the ingestion of lactose is not required for lactation. UDP-galactose in the mammary gland is derived principally from the epimerization of glucose. Dairy products are, however, a major dietary source of Ca^{2+}, so breast-feeding mothers need increased Ca^{2+} from another source.

Q 29.3: High concentrations of galactose 1-phosphate inhibit phosphoglucomutase, the enzyme which converts glucose 6-phosphate to glucose 1-phosphate. How can this inhibition account for the hypoglycemia and jaundice which accompany galactose 1-phosphate uridylyltransferase deficiency?

Erin Galway's urine was negative for glucose using the glucose oxidase strip but was positive for the presence of a reducing sugar. The reducing sugar was identified as galactose. Her liver function tests showed an increase in serum bilirubin and in several liver enzymes. Albumin was present in her urine. These findings and the clinical history increased her physician's suspicion that Erin had classical galactosemia.

Classical galactosemia is caused by a deficiency of galactose 1-phosphate uridylyltransferase. In this disease, galactose 1-phosphate accumulates in tissues, and galactose is elevated in the blood and urine. This condition differs from the rarer deficiency of galactokinase (nonclassical galactosemia), in which galactosemia and galactosuria occur, but galactose 1-phosphate is not formed. Both enzyme defects result in cataracts from galactitol formation by aldose reductase in the polyol pathway. Aldose reductase has a relatively high K_m for galactose, about 12–20 mM, so that galactitol is formed only in galactosemic patients who have eaten galactose. Galactitol is not further metabolized, and diffuses out of the lens very slowly. Thus hypergalactosemia is even more likely to cause cataracts than hyperglycemia. **Erin Galway**, although only 3 weeks old, appeared to have early cataracts forming in the lens of her eyes.

One of the most serious problems of classical galactosemia is an irreversible mental retardation. Realizing this problem, Erin Galway's physician wanted to begin immediate dietary therapy. A test which measures galactose 1-phosphate uridylyltransferase in erythrocytes was ordered. The enzyme activity was virtually absent, confirming the diagnosis of classical galactosemia.

The enzymes for galactose conversion to glucose 1-phosphate are present in many tissues, including the adult erythrocyte, fibroblasts, and fetal tissues. The liver has a high activity of these enzymes, and can convert dietary galactose to blood glucose and glycogen. The fate of dietary galactose, like that of fructose, therefore parallels that of glucose. The ability to metabolize galactose is even higher in infants than in adults. Newborn infants ingest up to 1 g of galactose per kg per feeding (as lactose). Yet the rate of metabolism is so high that the blood level in the systemic circulation is less than 3 mg/dL, and none of the galactose is lost in the urine.

Formation of Sugars for Proteoglycan and Glycolipid Synthesis

The transferases which produce the oligo- and polysaccharide side chains of glycosaminoglycans and glycolipids and attach sugar residues to proteins are specific for the sugar moiety and for the donating nucleotide (e.g., UDP, CMP, or GDP). Some of the sugar-nucleotides utilized for proteoglycan and glycolipid formation are listed in Table 29.2. They include the derivatives of glucose and galactose which we have already discussed, as well as acetylated amino sugars and derivatives of mannose. The reason for the large variety of sugars attached to proteins and lipids is that they have relatively specific and different functions, such as targeting a protein toward a membrane; providing recognition sites on the cell surface for other cells, hormones, or viruses; or acting as lubricants or molecular sieves (see Chapter 30).

The pathways for utilization and formation of many of these sugars are summarized in Figure 29.12. Note that many of the steps are reversible, so that glucose and other dietary sugars enter a common pool from which the diverse sugars can be formed.

The amino sugars are all derived from glucosamine 6-phosphate. To synthesize glucosamine 6-phosphate, an amino group is transferred from the amide of glutamine to fructose 6-phosphate (Fig. 29.13). Amino sugars, such as glucosamine, can then be *N*-acetylated by an acetyltransferase.

Mannose is found in the diet in small amounts. Like galactose, it is an epimer of glucose, and mannose and glucose are interconverted by epimerization reactions. The interconversion can take place either at the level of fructose 6-phosphate to mannose 5-phosphate, or at the level of the derivatized sugars (see Fig. 29.12). *N*-Acetylmannosamine is the precursor of *N*-acetylneuraminic acid (NANA, a sialic acid) and GDP-mannose is the precursor of GDP-fucose (see Fig. 29.12). The negative charge on NANA is obtained by the addition of a 3-carbon carboxyl moiety from PEP.

 CLINICAL COMMENTS. Hereditary fructose intolerance (HFI) is caused by a low level of fructose 1-phosphate aldolase activity in aldolase B, an isozyme of fructose 1,6-bisphosphate aldolase which is also capable of cleaving fructose 1-phosphate. In patients of European descent, the most common defect is a single missense mutation in exon 5 (G → C), resulting in an amino acid

Table 29.2. Some Sugar Nucleotides Which Are Precursors for Transferase Reactions

UDP-glucose
UDP-galactose
UDP-glucuronic acid
UDP-xylose
UDP-*N*-acetylglucosamine
UDP-*N*-acetylgalactosamine
CMP-*N*-acetylneuraminic acid
GDP-fucose
GDP-mannose

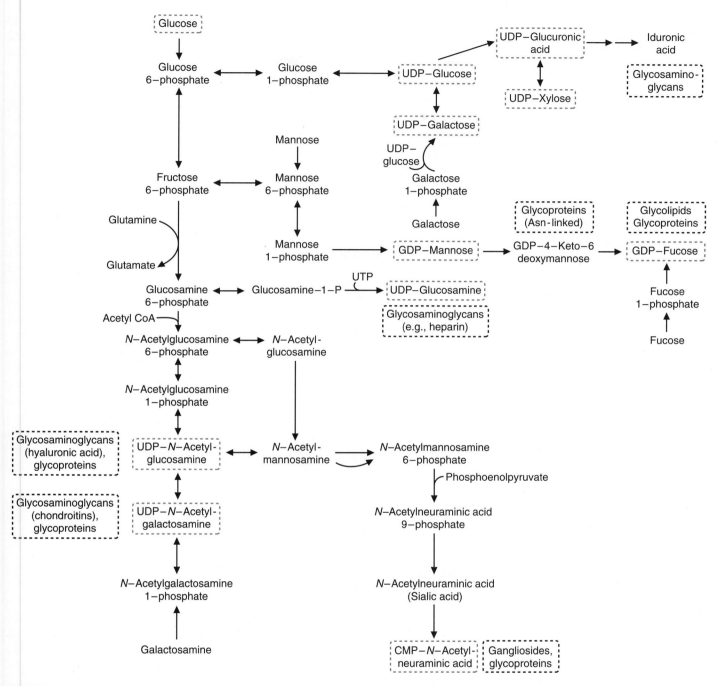

Fig. 29.12. Pathways for the interconversion of sugars. All of the different sugars found in glycosaminoglycans, gangliosides, and other compounds in the body can be synthesized from glucose. Dietary glucose, fructose, galactose, mannose, and other sugars enter a common pool from which other sugars are derived. The activated sugar is transferred from the nucleotide sugar, shown in blue boxes, to form a glycosidic bond with another sugar or amino acid residue. The box next to each nucleotide sugar lists some of the compounds which contain the sugar. Iduronic acid, in the upper right hand corner of the diagram, is formed only after glucuronic acid is incorporated into a glycosaminoglycan.

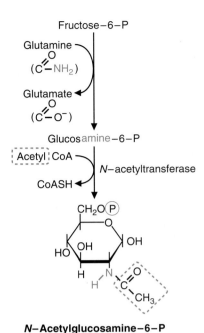

Fig. 29.13. The formation of *N*-acetylglucosamine 6-phosphate. The amino sugar is formed by a transfer of the amino group from the amide of glutamine to a carbon of the sugar. The amino group is acetylated by the transfer of an acetyl group from acetyl CoA.

substitution (Ala → Pro). As a result of this substitution, a catalytically impaired aldolase B is synthesized in abundance. The exact prevalence of HFI in the United States is not established but is approximately 1 per 15,000 to 25,000 population. The disease is autosomal recessive.

When affected patients like **Candice Sucher** ingest fructose, fructose is converted to fructose 1-phosphate. Because of the deficiency of aldolase B, fructose 1-phosphate cannot be further metabolized to dihydroxyacetone phosphate and glyceraldehyde, and accumulates in those tissues which have fructokinase (liver, kidney, and small intestine). Fructose is detected in the urine with the reducing sugar test (see Chapter 6). The new DNA screening tests provide a safe method to confirm a diagnosis of hereditary fructose intolerance (see Problems, below).

In the infant and small child, the major symptoms include poor feeding, vomiting, intestinal discomfort, and failure to thrive. The higher the intake of dietary fructose, the more severe the clinical reaction. The result of prolonged ingestion of fructose is ultrastructural changes in the liver and kidney resulting in hepatic and renal failure. Hereditary fructose intolerance is usually a disease of infancy, since adults with fructose intolerance who have survived avoid the ingestion of fruits, table sugar, and other sweets.

Erin Galway has galactosemia, which is caused by a deficiency of galactose 1-phosphate uridylyltransferase; it is one of the most common genetic diseases. Galactosemia is an autosomal recessive disorder of galactose metabolism which occurs in about 1 in 60,000 newborns. Approximately two-thirds of the states in the U.S. screen newborns for this disease because failure to begin immediate treatment results in mental retardation. Failure to thrive is the most common initial clinical symptom. Vomiting or diarrhea is found in most patients, usually starting within a few days of milk ingestion. Signs of deranged liver function, either jaundice or hepatomegaly, are present almost as frequently after the first week of life. The jaundice of intrinsic liver disease may be accentuated by the severe hemolysis in some patients. Cataracts have been observed within a few days of birth.

Management of patients requires elimination of galactose from the diet. Failure to eliminate this sugar results in progressive liver failure and death. In infants, an artificial milk made from casein or soybean hydrolysate is used.

BIOCHEMICAL COMMENTS. Before the metabolic toxicity of fructose was appreciated, substitution of fructose for glucose in intravenous solutions, and of fructose for sucrose in enteral tube feeding, or diabetic diets was frequently recommended. (Enteral tube feeding refers to tubes placed into the gut; parenteral tube feeding refers to tubes placed into the vein, feeding intravenously.) Administration of intravenous fructose to patients with diabetes mellitus or other forms of insulin resistance avoided the hyperglycemia found with intravenous glucose, possibly because fructose metabolism in the liver bypasses the insulin-regulated step at phosphofructokinase-1. However, because of the unregulated flow of fructose through glycolysis, intravenous fructose feeding frequently resulted in lactic acidosis (see Fig. 29.2). Moreover, many individuals with hereditary fructose intolerance died. Fructose is less toxic in the diet or in enteral feeding due to the relatively slow rate of fructose absorption.

N-Acetyltransferases are present in the endoplasmic reticulum and cytosol and provide another means of chemically modifying sugars, metabolites, drugs, and xenobiotic compounds. Individuals may vary greatly in their capacity for acetylation reactions.

Suggested Readings

Cox TM. Aldolase B and fructose intolerance. FASEB J 1994;8:62–71.

Kador PF, Robison WG Jr, Kinoshita JH. The pharmacology of aldose reductase inhibitors. Annu Rev Pharmacol Toxicol 1985;25:691–714.

Segal S, Berry GT. Disorders of galactose metabolism. In: Scriver CR, Beaudet AL, Sly WS, Valle D, eds. The metabolic and molecular basis of inherited disease. 7th ed, vol. I. New York: McGraw-Hill, 1995:967–1000.

Van den Berghe G. Inborn errors of fructose metabolism. Annu Rev Nutr 1994;14:41–58.

PROBLEMS

Hereditary fructose intolerance is a rare recessive genetic disease that is most commonly caused by a mutation in exon 5 of the aldolase B gene. The mutation fortuitously creates a new *Aha*II recognition sequence. To test for the mutation, DNA was extracted from a wife, husband, and their two children, Jack and Jill. The DNA for exon 5 of the aldolase B gene was amplified by polymerase chain reaction (PCR), treated with *Aha*II, subjected to electrophoresis on an agarose gel, and stained with a dye that binds to DNA.

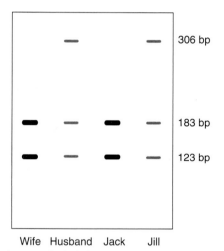

				306 bp
				183 bp
				123 bp

Wife Husband Jack Jill

1. From these data, it can be concluded that
   A. Both of the children have the disease.
   B. Neither of the children has the disease.
   C. Jill has the disease, Jack does not.
   D. Jack has the disease, Jill does not.

2. Upon examining the gel himself, the husband became concerned that he might not be the biological father of one or both of the children. From the pattern on the gel, you can reasonably conclude that
   A. He is probably not Jill's father.
   B. He is probably not Jack's father.
   C. He could be the father of both children.
   D. He is probably not the father of either child.

ANSWERS

1. The answer is **D**. The aldolase B gene has two alleles. One or both may have mutations. Because HFI is recessive, both alleles must be mutated for the disease to be expressed. Examination of the gel shows that the normal gene is cleaved by *Aha*II to produce a 306 bp restriction fragment. When a mutation creates a new *Aha*II site within the gene, this 306 bp fragment is cleaved into two fragments of 183 and 123 bp (which together contain 306 bp).

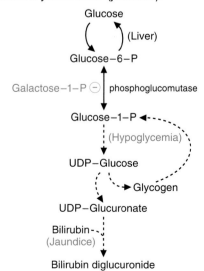

A 29.3: The inhibition of phosphoglucomutase can result in hypoglycemia by interfering with the formation of UDP-glucose (the glycogen precursor) and the degradation of glycogen back to glucose 6-phosphate. The lack of UDP-glucose prevents the formation of UDP-glucuronate, which is necessary to convert bilirubin to the diglucuronide form for transport into the bile. Bilirubin accumulates in tissues, giving them a yellow color (jaundice).

Glucose

(Liver)

Glucose–6–P

Galactose–1–P ⊖ | phosphoglucomutase

Glucose–1–P

(Hypoglycemia)

UDP–Glucose

Glycogen

UDP–Glucuronate

Bilirubin
(Jaundice)

Bilirubin diglucuronide

The husband and Jill, thus, are carriers. They have one normal allele that produces the 306 bp fragment and one that has an additional *Aha*II site, which is cleaved to yield the two fragments of 183 and 123 bp. The wife and Jack have the disease. Both of their alleles have the additional *Aha*II site and produce only 183 and 123 bp fragments.

2. The answer is **C**. This man could be the father of both children. He could provide either a normal gene (which produces a 306 bp *Aha*II fragment) or a mutant gene (which produces 183 and 123 bp *Aha*II fragments) to his offspring. This mother could provide only the mutant gene (of which she has two copies). Jill is a carrier. She received the mutant gene from her mother and could have received the normal gene from this man. Jack has the disease. He received one mutant gene from his mother and another from his father.

30 Proteoglycans, Glycoproteins, and Glycolipids

In addition to serving as fuel, carbohydrates are often found attached to proteins or lipids of the proteoglycans, glycoproteins, and glycolipids. These carbohydrate groups have many different types of functions.

Proteoglycans consist of a core protein covalently attached to many long, linear chains of glycosaminoglycans, which contain repeating disaccharide units. The repeating disaccharides usually contain a hexosamine and a uronic acid, and these sugars are frequently sulfated. Synthesis of the proteoglycans starts with the attachment of a sugar to a serine or threonine residue of the protein. Additional sugars add sequentially to the nonreducing end, with UDP-sugars serving as the precursors. The proteoglycans are secreted from cells and form the extracellular matrix (Fig. 30.1).

Glycoproteins contain short chains of carbohydrates (oligosaccharides) that are usually branched. These oligosaccharides are generally composed of glucose, galactose, and their amino derivatives. In addition, mannose, L-fucose, and N-acetylneuraminic acid (NANA) are frequently present. The carbohydrate chains grow by the sequential addition of sugars to a serine or threonine residue of the protein. UDP-sugars are the precursors. Branched carbohydrate chains may also be attached to the amide nitrogen of asparagine in the protein. In this case, the chains are synthesized on dolichol phosphate and subsequently transferred to the protein. Glycoproteins are found in mucus, in the blood, in compartments within the cell (such as lysosomes), in the extracellular matrix, and embedded in the cell membrane with the carbohydrate portion extending into the extracellular space.

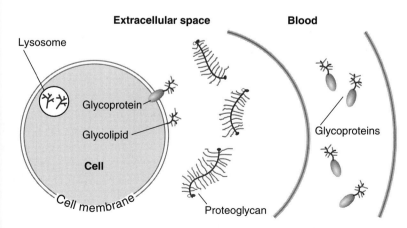

Fig. 30.1. Location of proteoglycans, glycoproteins, and glycolipids. Proteins containing carbohydrates are usually found outside the cell, in membrane-enclosed vesicles within the cell, or in the cell membrane. Glycolipids are located in the cell membrane.

Glycolipids belong to the class of sphingolipids. They are synthesized from UDP-sugars that add monosaccharides sequentially to the hydroxymethyl group of the lipid ceramide (related to sphingosine). They often contain branches of N-acetylneuraminic acid produced from CMP-NANA. They are found in the cell membrane with the carbohydrate portion extruding from the cell surface. These carbohydrates, as well as some of the carbohydrates of glycoproteins, serve as cell recognition factors.

Proteoglycans, glycoproteins, and glycolipids are synthesized in the endoplasmic reticulum (ER) and the Golgi complex. They are degraded by lysosomal enzymes that cleave one sugar at a time from the nonreducing end.

Sellie D'Souder noted a moderate reduction in pain and swelling in the joints of her fingers when she was taking a 6-week course of high dose prednisone, an antiinflammatory steroid. As the dose of this drug was tapered to minimize its long term side effects, however, the pain in the joints of her fingers returned, and, for the first time, her left knee became painful, swollen, and warm to the touch. Her rheumatologist described to her the underlying tissue changes that her systemic lupus erythematosus (SLE) was causing in the joint tissues.

Jay Sakz's psychomotor development has become progressively more abnormal. At 2 years of age, he is obviously mentally retarded and nearly blind. His muscle weakness has progressed to the point that he cannot sit up or even crawl. As the result of a weak cough reflex, he is unable to clear his normal respiratory secretions and has had recurrent respiratory infections.

To help support herself through medical school, **Erna Nemdy** works evenings in a hospital blood bank. She is responsible for assuring that compatible donor blood is available to patients requiring blood transfusions. As part of her training, Erna has learned that the external surfaces of all blood cells contain large numbers of antigenic determinants. These determinants are often glycoproteins or glycolipids that differ from one individual to another. As a result, all blood transfusions expose the recipient to many foreign immunogens. Most of these, fortunately, do not induce antibodies or they induce antibodies that elicit little or no immunological response. For routine blood transfusions, therefore, tests are performed only for the presence of antigens that determine whether the patient's blood type is A, B, AB, or O.

The extracellular matrix is not simply a glue that holds cells together; it also serves to keep cells from moving to other locations and to prevent large molecules and other particles, such as microorganisms, from reaching cells. Consequently, this matrix is medically important. Changes in the matrix are caused by agents that infect cells. Cancer cells that metastasize (migrate to other tissues) can do so only by altering the matrix. Diseases such as rheumatoid arthritis (an autoimmune destruction of joints) and osteoarthritis (degenerative joint disease often associated with aging) involve damage to molecules of the matrix. Destruction of the matrix of the renal glomerulus may allow proteins to be excreted into the urine. Genetic defects may cause components of the matrix to be abnormal, resulting in diseases such as the Ehlers-Danlos syndrome (a defect in the protein collagen) and Marfan's syndrome (a defect in the protein fibrillin). Deficiencies of lysosomal enzymes involved in normal degradation of molecules of the matrix result in diseases such as the mucopolysaccharidoses and the sphingolipidoses or gangliosidoses.

PROTEOGLYCANS

Structure and Function

Proteoglycans are found in the synovial fluid of joints, the vitreous humor of the eye, arterial walls, and bone and cartilage. They are major components of the extracellular matrix or ground substance, a gelatinous material that forms a meshwork between cells. The proteoglycans interact with proteins in the matrix, such as collagen and elastin (which play structural roles), fibronectin (which is involved in cell adhesion and migration), and laminin (which is found in basal laminae, such as the renal glomerulus).

Proteoglycans are proteins that contain many chains of glycosaminoglycans (formerly called mucopolysaccharides). Glycosaminoglycans are long, unbranched polysaccharides composed of repeating disaccharide units (Fig. 30.2). The repeating disaccharides usually contain a uronic acid and a hexosamine, and are frequently sulfated.

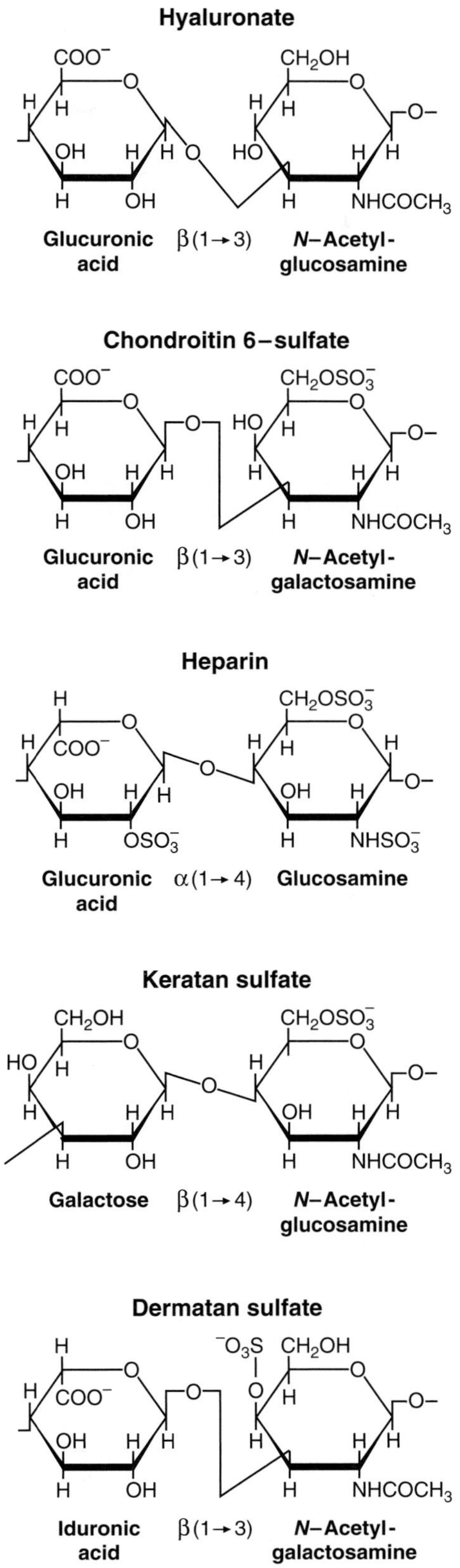

Fig. 30.2. Repeating disaccharides of some glycosaminoglycans. These repeating disaccharides usually contain an *N*-acetylated sugar and a uronic acid, which usually is glucuronic acid or iduronic acid. Sulfate groups are often present, but are not included in the sugar names in this figure.

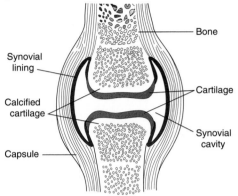

The functional properties of a normal joint depend, in part, on the presence of a soft, well-lubricated, deformable, and compressible layer of cartilaginous tissue covering the ends of the long bones that comprise the joint.

Bone

Synovial lining

Cartilage

Calcified cartilage

Synovial cavity

Capsule

In **Sellie D'Souder's** case, the pathological process which characterizes SLE disrupts the structural and functional integrity of her articular (joint) cartilage.

Consequently, they carry a negative charge, are hydrated, and act as lubricants. After synthesis, proteoglycans are secreted from cells; thus, they function extracellularly. Because the long, negatively charged glycosaminoglycan chains repel each other, the proteoglycans occupy a very large space and act as "molecular sieves," determining which substances approach and leave cells (Table 30.1). Their properties also give resilience to substances such as cartilage, permitting compression and reexpansion.

There are at least seven types of glycosaminoglycans, which differ in the monosaccharides present in their repeating disaccharide units—chondroitin sulfate, dermatan sulfate, heparin, heparan sulfate, hyaluronic acid, and keratan sulfate I and II. Except fo hyaluronic acid, the glycosaminoglycans are linked to proteins, usually attached covalently to serine or threonine residues (Fig. 30.3). Keratan sulfate I is attached to asparagine.

Synthesis

The protein component of the proteoglycans is synthesized on the ER. It enters the lumen of this organelle, where the initial glycosylations occur. UDP-sugars serve as the precursors that add sugar units, one at a time, first to the protein and then to the nonreducing end of the growing carbohydrate chain (Fig. 30.4). Glycosylation occurs

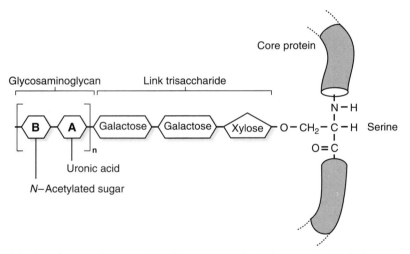

Fig. 30.3. Attachment of glycosaminoglycans to proteins. The sugars are linked to a serine or threonine residue of the protein. A and B represent the sugars of the repeating disaccharide.

Table 30.1. Some Specific Functions of the Glycosaminoglycans

Glycosaminoglycan	Function
Hyaluronic acid	Cell migration in: Embryogenesis Morphogenesis Wound healing
Chondroitin sulfate	Formation of bone, cartilage, cornea
Keratan sulfate	Transparency of cornea
Dermatan sulfate	Transparency of cornea Binds LDL to plasma walls
Heparin	Anticoagulant (binds antithrombin III) Causes release of lipoprotein lipase from capillary walls
Heparan sulfate	Component of skin fibroblasts and aortic wall; commonly found on cell surfaces

CHAPTER 30 / PROTEOGLYCANS, GLYCOPROTEINS, AND GLYCOLIPIDS **461**

initially in the lumen of the ER and subsequently in the Golgi complex. Glycosyltransferases, the enzymes that add sugars to the chain, are specific for the sugar being added, the type of linkage that is formed, and the sugars already present in the chain. Once the initial sugars are attached to the protein, the alternating action of two glycosyltransferases adds the sugars of the repeating disaccharide to the growing glycosaminoglycan chain. Sulfation occurs after addition of the sugar. 3'-Phosphoadenosine 5'-phosphosulfate (PAPS), also called active sulfate, provides the sulfate groups (Fig. 30.5). An epimerase converts glucuronic acid residues to iduronic acid residues.

After synthesis, the proteoglycan is secreted from the cell. Its structure resembles a bottle brush, with many glycosaminoglycan chains extending from the core protein (Fig. 30.6). The proteoglycans may form large aggregates, noncovalently attached by a "link" protein to hyaluronic acid (Fig. 30.7). The proteoglycans interact with the protein fibronectin, which is attached to the cell membrane protein integrin. Cross-linked fibers of collagen also associate with this complex, forming the extracellular matrix (Fig. 30.8).

3'−Phosphoadenosine 5'−phosphosulfate (PAPS−"active sulfate")

Fig. 30.5. 3′-Phosphoadenosine 5′-phosphosulfate (PAPS). PAPS transfers sulfate groups to the glycosaminoglycan. Ad = adenine.

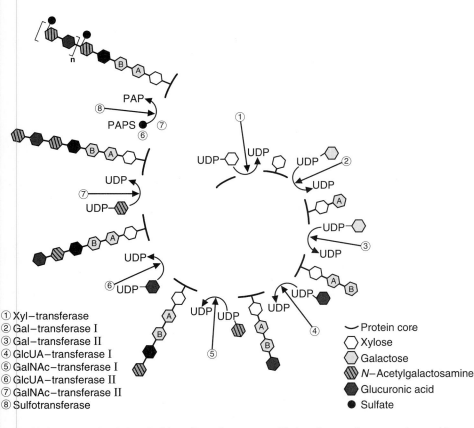

① Xyl−transferase
② Gal−transferase I
③ Gal−transferase II
④ GlcUA−transferase I
⑤ GalNAc−transferase I
⑥ GlcUA−transferase II
⑦ GalNAc−transferase II
⑧ Sulfotransferase

Protein core
Xylose
Galactose
N−Acetylgalactosamine
Glucuronic acid
Sulfate

Fig. 30.4. Synthesis of chondroitin sulfate. Sugars are added to the protein on at a time, with UDP-sugars serving as the precursors. Initially a xylose residue is added to a serine in the protein. Then 2 galactose residues are added, followed by a glucuronic acid (GlcUA) and an N-acetylgalactosamine (GalNAc). Subsequent additions occur by the alternating action of two enzymes that produce the repeating disaccharide units. One enzyme (**6**) adds GlcUA residues and the the other (**7**) adds GalNAc. As the chain grows, sulfate groups are added by phosphoadenosine phosphosulfate (PAPS). Modified from Roden L. In: Fishman WH, ed. Metabolic conjugation and metabolic hydrolysis, vol. II. Orlando, FL: Academic Press, 2970:401.

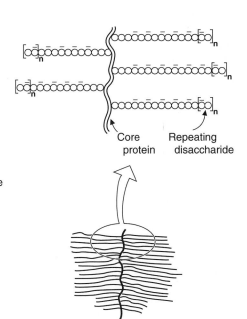

Fig. 30.6. "Bottle-brush" structure of a proteoglycan, with a magnified segment.

The principal components of the matrix of cartilage are collagen and proteoglycans, both of which are produced and degraded by the chondrocytes which are embedded in this matrix. Abnormalities in these processes are causing **Sellie D'Souder's** problem.

The collagen component forms a network of fine fibrils that give shape to the cartilage. The proteoglycans embedded in the cartilage are responsible for its compressible and deformable properties.

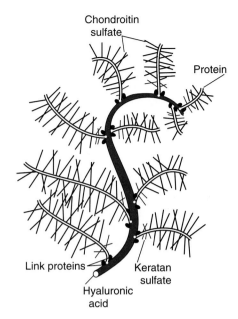

Fig. 30.7. Proteoglycan aggregate.

The long polysaccharide side chains of the proteoglycans in cartilage contain many anionic groups. This high concentration of negative charges attracts cations which create a high osmotic pressure within cartilage, drawing water into this specialized connective tissue and placing the collagen network under tension. At equilibrium, the resulting tension balances the swelling pressure caused by the proteoglycans. The complementary roles of this macromolecular organization give cartilage its resilience. Cartilage can thus withstand the compressive load of weight-bearing and then reexpand to its previous dimensions when that load is relieved.

The inflammatory intraarticular process of SLE causes a breakdown in this critical balance. This breakdown leads to the joint pain and swelling that **Sellie D'Souder** is experiencing.

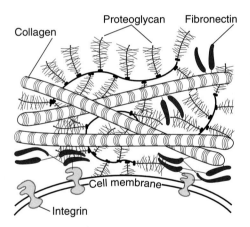

Fig. 30.8. Interactions between the cell membrane and the components of the extracellular matrix.

GLYCOPROTEINS

Structure and Function

Glycoproteins contain much shorter carbohydrate chains than proteoglycans. These oligosaccharide chains are often branched, and they do not contain repeating disaccharides (Fig. 30.9). Most proteins in the blood are glycoproteins. They serve as hormones, antibodies, enzymes (including those of the blood clotting cascade), and as structural components of the extracellular matrix. Collagen contains galactosyl units and disaccharides composed of galactosyl-glucose attached to hydroxylysine residues (see Chapter 8). The secretions of mucus-producing cells, such as salivary mucin, are glycoproteins (Fig. 30.10).

Although most glycoproteins are secreted from cells, some are segregated in lysosomes where they serve as the lysosomal enzymes that degrade various types of cellular and extracellular material. Other glycoproteins are produced like secretory proteins, but hydrophobic regions of the protein remain attached to the cell membrane and the carbohydrate portion extends into the extracellular space (Fig. 30.11). These glycoproteins serve as receptors for compounds such as hormones, as transport proteins, and as cell attachment and cell-cell recognition sites. Bacteria and viruses also bind to these sites.

Synthesis

The protein portion of glycoproteins is synthesized on the ER. The carbohydrate chains are attached to the protein in the lumen of the ER and the Golgi complex. In some cases, the initial sugar is added to a serine or a threonine residue in the protein, and the carbohydrate chain is extended by the sequential addition of sugar residues to the nonreducing end. UDP-sugars are the precursors for the addition of four of the seven sugars that are usually found in glycoproteins—glucose, galactose, N-acetylglucosamine, and N-acetylgalactosamine. GDP-sugars are the precursors for the addition of mannose and L-fucose, and CMP-NANA is the precursor for NANA. Dolichol phosphate is involved in transferring branched sugar chains to the amide nitrogen of asparagine residues (Fig. 30.12). Sugars are removed and added, as the glycoprotein moves from the ER through the Golgi complex (Fig. 30.13).

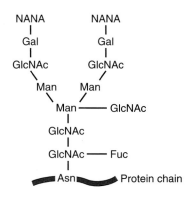

Fig. 30.9. Branched glycoprotein. NANA = N-acetylneuraminic acid; Gal= galactose; GlcNAc = N-acetylglucosamine; Man = mannose; Fuc = fucose.

I-cell (inclusion cell) disease is a rare condition in which lysosomal enzymes lack the mannose-phosphate marker that targets them to lysosomes. Consequently, lysosomal enzymes are secreted from the cells. Because lysosomes lack their normal complement of enzymes, undegraded molecules accumulate within membranes inside these cells, forming inclusion bodies.

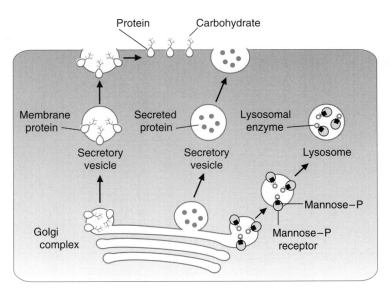

Fig. 30.11. Route from the Golgi complex to the final destination for lysosomal enzymes, cell membrane proteins, and secreted proteins, which include glycoproteins and proteoglycans.

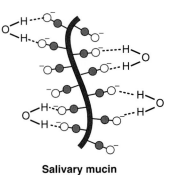

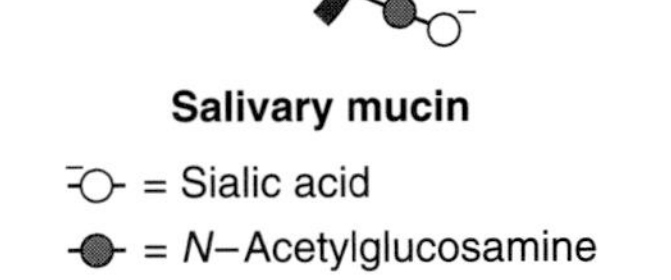

Salivary mucin

⊖ = Sialic acid
⬤ = N–Acetylglucosamine

Fig. 30.10. Structure of salivary mucin. The sugars form hydrogen bonds with water. Sialic acid provides a negatively charged carboxylate group. The protein is extremely large, and the negatively charged sialic acids extend the carbohydrate chains so the molecules occupy a large space. All of the salivary glycoproteins are O-linked. NANA is a sialic acid.

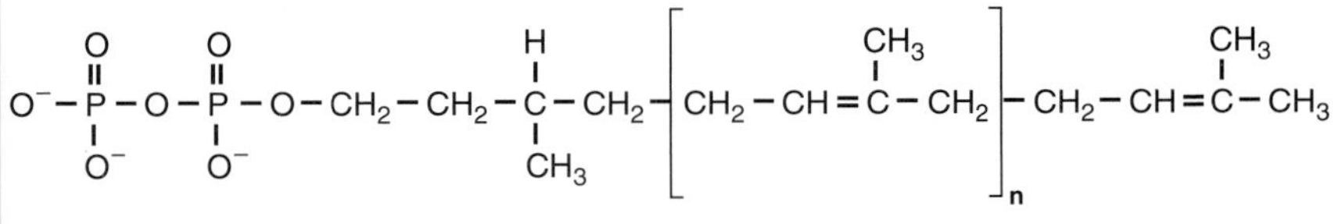

Fig. 30.12. Structure of dolichol phosphate. In humans the isoprene unit (in brackets) is repeated about 17 times (n = ~17).

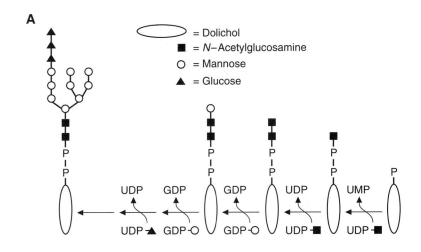

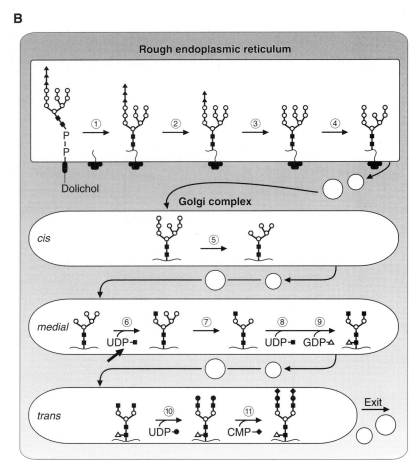

Fig. 30.13. Action of dolichol phosphate in transferring carbohydrate groups to proteins (**A**) and processing of these carbohydrate groups (**B**). Transfer of the branched oligosaccharide from dolichol phosphate to a protein in the lumen of the rough endoplasmic reticulum (RER) (step 1) and processing of the oligosaccharide (steps 2–11). Steps 1 through 4 occur in the RER. The glycoprotein is transferred in vesicles to the Golgi complex where further modifications of the oligosaccharides occur (steps 5–11). **B** modified with permission from Kornfeld R, Kornfeld S. Annu Rev Biochem 1985;54:640. © 1985 by Annual Reviews, Inc.

GLYCOLIPIDS

Function and Structure

Glycolipids are derivatives of the lipid sphingosine. These sphingolipids include the cerebrosides and the gangliosides (Fig. 30.14). They contain ceramide, with carbohydrate moieties attached to its hydroxymethyl group.

Glycolipids are involved in intercellular communication. Oligosaccharides of identical composition are present in both the glycolipids and glycoproteins associated with the cell membrane, where they serve as cell recognition factors. For example, carbohydrate residues in these oligosaccharides are the antigens of the ABO blood group substances (Fig. 30.15).

Synthesis

Cerebrosides are synthesized from ceramide and UDP-glucose or UDP-galactose. They contain a single sugar (a monosaccharide). Gangliosides contain oligosaccharides produced from UDP-sugars. CMP-NANA is the precursor for the *N*-acetylneuraminic acid residues that branch from the linear chain. (The synthesis of the sphingolipids is described in more detail in Chapter 33).

Sphingolipids are produced in the Golgi complex. Their lipid component becomes part of the membrane of the secretory vesicle that buds from the *trans* face of the Golgi. After the vesicle membrane fuses with the cell membrane, the lipid component of the glycolipid remains in the outer layer of the cell membrane and the carbohydrate component extends into the extracellular space.

By identifying the nature of antigenic determinants on the surface of the donor's red blood cells, **Erna Nemdy** is able to classify the donor's blood as belonging to certain specific blood groups. These antigenic determinants are located in the oligosaccharides of the glycoproteins and glycolipids of the cell membranes. The most important blood group in humans is the ABO group, which is comprised of two antigens, A and B. Individuals with the A antigen on their cells belong to blood group A. Those with B belong to group B, and those with both A and B belong to group AB. The absence of both the A and the B antigen results in blood type O (see Fig. 30.15).

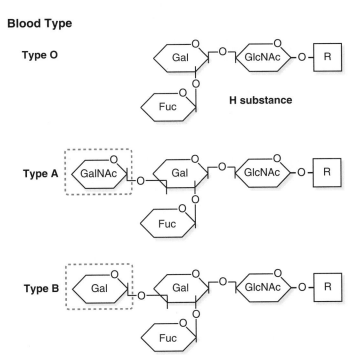

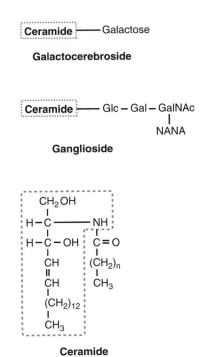

Fig. 30.14. Structures of cerebrosides and gangliosides. In these glycolipids, sugars are attached to ceramide (shown below the glycolipids). The boxed portion of ceramide is sphingosine, from which the name sphingolipids is derived.

Fig. 30.15. Structures of the blood group substances. Note that these structures are the same except that type A has *N*-acetylgalactosamine (GalNAc) at the nonreducing end, type B has galactose (Gal), and type O has neither. R is either a protein or the lipid ceramide. Each antigenic determinant is boxed. Fuc = fucose; GlcNAc = *N*-acetylglucosamine; Gal = galactose.

Deficiencies of lysosomal glycosidases cause partially degraded carbohydrates from proteoglycans, glycoproteins, and glycolipids to accumulate within membrane-enclosed vesicles inside cells. These "residual bodies" can cause marked enlargement of the organ with impairment of its function.

In the mucopolysaccharidoses (caused by accumulation of partially degraded glycosaminoglycans), deformities of the skeleton occur (Table 30.2). Mental retardation often accompanies these conditions.

Jay Sakz has Tay-Sachs disease, which belongs to a group of gangliosidoses that include Fabry's and Gaucher's diseases. They mainly affect the brain, the skin, and the reticuloendothelial system (e.g., liver and spleen). In these diseases, complex lipids accumulate. Each of these lipids contains a ceramide as part of its structure (Table 30.3). The rate at which the lipid is synthesized is normal. However, the lysosomal enzyme required to degrade it is not very active either because it is made in deficient quantities due to a mutation in a gene which specifically codes for the enzyme or because a critical protein required to activate the enzyme is deficient. Because the lipid cannot be degraded, it accumulates and causes degeneration of the affected tissues with progressive malfunction, e.g., the psychomotor deficits which occur as a result of the central nervous system involvement seen in most of these storage diseases.

DEGRADATION OF PROTEOGLYCANS, GLYCOPROTEINS, AND GLYCOLIPIDS

Lysosomal enzymes degrade proteoglycans, glycoproteins, and glycolipids, which are brought into the cell by the process of endocytosis. Lysosomes fuse with the endocytic vesicles, and lysosomal proteases digest the protein component. The carbohydrate component is degraded by lysosomal glycosidases.

Lysosomes contain both endoglycosidases and exoglycosidases. The endoglycosidases cleave the chains into shorter oligosaccharides. Then exoglycosidases specific for each type of linkage remove the sugar residues, one at a time, from the nonreducing ends.

CLINICAL COMMENTS. Articular cartilage is a living tissue with a turnover time determined by a balance between the rate of its synthesis and that of its degradation (Fig. 30.16). The chondrocytes embedded in the matrix of cartilage participate in both synthesis and enzymatic degradation. The latter occurs as a result of cleavage of proteoglycan aggregates by enzymes produced and secreted by the chondrocytes.

In SLE, the condition that affects **Sellie D'Souder**, this delicate balance is disrupted in favor of enzymatic degradation, leading to a dissolution of articular cartilage and, with it, the loss of its critical functions. The underlying mechanisms responsible for this process in SLE include the production of antibodies directed against specific normal cellular proteins in joint tissues. The cellular proteins thus serve as

Table 30.2. Defective Enzymes in the Mucopolysaccharidoses

Disease	Enzyme Deficiency	Accumulated Products
Hunter	Iduronate sulfatase	Heparan sulfate Dermatan sulfate
Hurler + Scheie	α-L-Iduronidase	Heparan sulfate Dermatan sulfate
Maroteaux-Lamy	N-Acetylgalactosamine sulfatase	Dermatan sulfate
Mucolipidosis VII	β-Glucuronidase	Heparan sulfate Dermatan sulfate
Sanfilippo A	Heparan sulfamidase	Heparan sulfate
Sanfilippo B	N-Acetylglucosaminidase	Heparan sulfate
Sanfilippo D	N-Acetylglucosamine 6-sulfatase	Heparin sulfate

Table 30.3. Defective Enzymes in the Gangliosidoses

Disease	Enzyme Deficiency	Accumulated Lipid
Fucosidosis	α-Fucosidase	Cer–Glc–Gal–GalNAc–Gal⋮Fuc H-isoantigen
Generalized gangliosidosis	G_{M1}-β-galactosidase	Cer–Glc–Gal(NeuAc)–GalNAc⋮Gal G_{M1} ganglioside
Tay-Sachs disease	Hexosaminidase A	Cer–Glc–Gal(NeuAc)⋮GalNAc G_{M2} ganglioside
Tay-Sachs variant or Sandhoff's disease	Hexosaminidase A and B	Cer–Glc–Gal–Gal⋮GalNAc Globoside plus G_{M2} ganglioside
Fabry's disease	α-Galactosidase	Cer–Glc–Gal⋮Gal Globotriaosylceramide
Ceramide lactoside lipidosis	Ceramide lactosidase (β-galactosidase)	Cer–Glc⋮Gal Ceramide lactoside
Metachromatic leukodystrophy	Arylsulfatase A	Cer–Gal⋮OSO₃ 3-Sulfogalactosylceramide
Krabbe's disease	β-Galactosidase	Cer⋮Gal Galactosylceramide
Gaucher's disease	β-Glucosidase	Cer⋮Glc Glucosylceramide
Niemann-Pick disease	Sphingomyelinase	Cer⋮P–choline Sphingomyelin
Farber's disease	Ceramidase	Acyl⋮sphingosine Ceramide

NeuAc, N-acetylneuraminic acid; Cer, ceramide; Glc, glucose; Gal, galactose; Fuc, fucose. ⋮, site of deficient enzyme reaction.

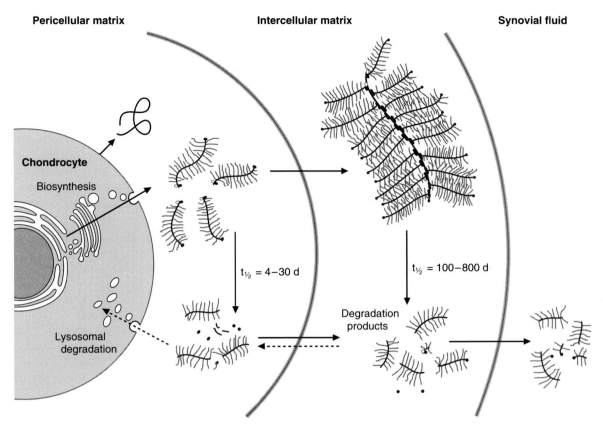

Fig. 30.16. Synthesis and degradation of proteoglycans by chondrocytes. From Cohen RD, et al. The metabolic basis of acquired disease, vol 2. London: Bailliere Tindall, 1990:1859.

the "antigens" to which these antibodies react. In this sense, SLE is an "autoimmune" disease because antibodies are produced by the host which attack "self" proteins. This process excites the local release of cytokines such as interleukin-1 (IL-1), which increases the proteolytic activity of the chondrocytes causing a loss of articular proteoglycans. The associated inflammatory cascade is responsible for Sellie D'Souder's joint pain.

During her stint in the hospital blood bank, **Erna Nemdy** learned that the importance of the ABO blood group system in transfusion therapy is based on two principles (see Table 30.4). (*a*) Antibodies to A and to B antigens occur naturally in the blood serum of persons whose red blood cell surfaces lack the corresponding antigen (i.e., individuals with A antigens on their red blood cells have B antibodies in their serum and vice versa). These antibodies may arise as a result of previous exposure to cross-reacting antigens in bacteria and foods or to blood transfusions. (*b*) Antibodies to A and B are usually present in high titers and are capable of activating the entire complement system. As a result, these antibodies may cause intravascular destruction of a large number of incompatible red blood cells given during a blood transfusion. Individuals with type AB blood have both A and B antigens and do not produce antibodies to either. Hence, they are "universal" recipients. They can safely receive red blood cells from individuals of A, B, AB, or O blood type. (However, they cannot safely receive serum from these individuals because it contains antibodies to A and/or B antigens.) Those with type O blood do not have either antigen. They are "universal" donors, i.e., their red cells can safely be infused into type A, B, O, or AB individuals. (However, their serum contains antibodies to both A and B antigens and cannot safely be used.)

Table 30.4. Characteristics of the ABO Blood Groups

Red cell type	O	A	B	AB
Possible genotypes	OO	AA or AO	BB or BO	AB
Antibodies in serum	Anti-A and B	Anti-B	Anti-A	None
Frequency (in Caucasians)	45%	40%	10%	5%

The second important red blood cell group is the Rh group. It is important because one of its antigenic determinants, the D antigen, is a very potent immunogen, stimulating the production of a large number of antibodies.

The unique carbohydrate composition of the glycoproteins which comprise the antigenic determinants on red blood cells in part contributes to the relative immunogenicity of the A, B, and Rh (D) red blood cell groups in human blood.

Tay-Sachs disease, the problem afflicting **Jay Sakz**, is an autosomal recessive disorder which is rare in the general population (1 in 300,000 births) but its prevalence in Jews of Eastern European extraction (who make up 90% of the Jewish population in the United States) is much higher (1 in 3,600 births). One in 28 Ashkenazi Jews carries this defective gene. Its presence can be discovered by measuring the tissue level of the protein produced by the gene (hexosaminidase A) or by recombinant DNA techniques. Skin fibroblasts of concerned couples planning a family are frequently used for these tests.

Carriers of the affected gene have a reduced but functional level of this enzyme which normally hydrolyzes a specific bond between an N-acetyl-D-galactosamine and a D-galactose residue in the polar head of the ganglioside.

No effective therapy is currently available. Enzyme replacement has met with little success although recent attempts to chemically modify the administered enzyme to enhance its binding to receptors in target cells have shown some promise.

 BIOCHEMICAL COMMENTS. The blood group substances are oligosaccharide components of glycolipids and glycoproteins found in most cell membranes. Those located on red blood cells have been studied extensively. A single genetic locus with two alleles determines an individual's blood type. These genes encode glycosyltransferases involved in the synthesis of the oligosaccharides of the blood group substances.

Most individuals can synthesize the H substance, an oligosaccharide which contains a fucose linked to a galactose at the nonreducing end of the blood group substance (see Fig. 30.15). Type A individuals produce an N-acetylgalactosamine transferase (encoded by the A gene) that attaches N-acetylgalactosamine to the galactose residue of the H substance. Type B individuals produce a galactosyltransferase (encoded by the B gene) that links galactose to the galactose residue of the H substance. Type AB individuals have two different alleles and produce both transferases. Thus, some of the oligosaccharides of their blood group substances contain N-acetylgalactosamine and some contain galactose. Type O individuals produce a defective transferase, and, therefore, they do not attach either N-acetylgalactosamine or galactose to the H substance. Thus, individuals of blood type O have only the H substance.

Suggested Readings

Gravel RA, Clarke JTR, Kaback MM, et al. The G_{M2} gangliosidoses. In: Scriver CR, Beaudet AL, Sly WS, Valle D, eds. The metabolic and molecular bases of inherited disease. 7th ed, vol I. New York: McGraw-Hill, 1995:2839–2879.

Neufeld EF, Muenzer J. The mucopolysaccharidoses. In: Scriver CR, Beaudet AL, Sly WS, Valle D, eds. The metabolic and molecular bases of inherited disease. 7th ed, vol I. New York: McGraw-Hill, 1995:2465–2494.

PROBLEMS

1. A child with coarse facial features, short stature, skeletal deformities, and mental retardation was found to have glycosaminoglycan fragments in the urine. What was the cause of these abnormalities?

2. **Erna Nemdy** determined that a patient's blood type was AB. The new surgical resident was eager to give this patient a blood transfusion and, because AB blood is rare and an adequate amount was not available in the blood bank, he requested type A blood. Should Erna give him type A blood for his patient?

ANSWERS

1. An inability to degrade the glycosaminoglycans of proteoglycans results in the type of abnormalities exhibited by this child. The diseases, known as the mucopolysaccharidoses, are genetic and result from deficiencies of lysosomal enzymes. Skeletal abnormalities, mental retardation, and the other characteristics of the disease are the result of the accumulation of partially degraded glycosaminogly-cans (formerly called mucopolysaccharides) in lysosomes. These residual bodies pack the cells and interfere with their function. Less specific enzymes partially cleave the glycosaminoglycans into fragments, which may appear in the urine.

2. The patient could safely receive type A blood **cells** from another person because he has both A and B antigens on his own cells and does not have antibodies in his serum to either type A or B cells. However, he should not be given type A serum (or type A whole blood) because type A serum contains antibodies to type B antigens, which are present on his cells.

31 Maintenance of Blood Glucose Levels

Some tissues of the body, such as the brain and red blood cells, depend on glucose for energy. On a long term basis, most tissues also require glucose for other functions such as the synthesis of the ribose moiety of nucleotides or the carbohydrate portion of glycoproteins. Therefore, in order to survive, humans must have mechanisms for maintaining blood glucose levels.

After a meal containing carbohydrates, blood glucose levels rise (Fig. 31.1). Some of the glucose from the diet is stored in the liver as glycogen. After 2 or 3 hours of fasting, this glycogen begins to be degraded by the process of glycogenolysis, and glucose is released into the blood. As glycogen stores decrease, adipose triacylglycerols are also degraded, providing fatty acids as an alternative fuel and glycerol for the synthesis of glucose by gluconeogenesis. Amino acids are also released from muscle to serve as gluconeogenic precursors.

During an overnight fast, blood glucose levels are maintained by both glycogenolysis and gluconeogenesis. However, after about 30 hours of fasting, liver glycogen stores are depleted. Subsequently, gluconeogenesis is the only source of blood glucose.

Changes in the metabolism of glucose that occur during the switch from the fed to the fasting state are regulated by the hormones insulin and glucagon. Insulin is elevated in the fed state, and glucagon is elevated during fasting. Insulin stimulates the transport of glucose into certain cells such as those in muscle and adipose tissue. Insulin also alters the activity of key enzymes that regulate metabolism, stimulating the storage of fuels. Glucagon counters the effects of insulin, stimulating the release of stored fuels and the conversion of lactate, amino acids, and glycerol to glucose.

Blood glucose levels are maintained not only during fasting, but also during exercise when muscle cells take up glucose from the blood and oxidize it for energy. During exercise, the liver supplies glucose to the blood by the processes of glycogenolysis and gluconeogenesis.

Fed

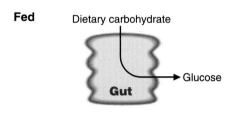

Fasting

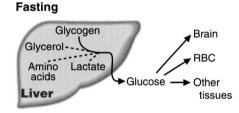

Starved

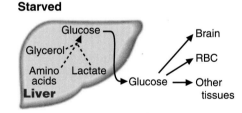

Fig. 31.1. Sources of blood glucose in the fed, fasting, and starved states. RBC = red blood cells.

Di Beatty could not remember whether she had taken her 6 PM insulin dose when, in fact, she had done so. Unfortunately, she decided to give herself the evening dose (for the second time). When she did not respond to her alarm clock at 6 AM the following morning, her roommate tried unsuccessfully to awaken her. The roommate called an ambulance and Di was rushed to the hospital emergency room in a coma. Her pulse and blood pressure at admission were normal. Her skin was flushed and slightly moist. Her respirations were slightly slow.

Priscilla Twigg continues to resist efforts on the part of her psychiatrist and family physician to convince her to increase her caloric intake. Her body weight varies between 97 and 99 lb, far below the desirable weight for a woman who is 5 feet 7 inches tall. In spite of her severe diet, her fasting blood glucose levels range from 55 to 70 mg/dL. She denies having any hypoglycemic symptoms.

Q 31.1: What clinical signs and symptoms help to distinguish a coma caused by an excess of blood glucose and ketone bodies due to a deficiency of insulin (diabetic ketoacidosis (DKA)) from a coma caused by a sudden lowering of blood glucose (hypoglycemic coma) induced by the inadvertent injection of excessive insulin—the current problem experienced by **Di Beatty**?

Ron Templeton has complied with his calorie-restricted diet and aerobic exercise program. He has lost another 7 lb and is closing in on his goal of weighing 154 lb. He notes increasing energy during the day, and remains alert during lectures and assimilates the lecture material noticeably better than he did prior to starting his weight loss and exercise program. He jogs for 45 minutes each morning before breakfast.

CHANGES IN BLOOD GLUCOSE LEVELS AFTER A MEAL

The metabolic transitions that occur as a person eats a meal and progresses through the various stages of fasting are described in detail in Chapters 24 through 27. This chapter summarizes the concepts presented in these previous chapters. Because a thorough understanding of these concepts is so critical to medicine, a summary is not only warranted but essential.

After a high carbohydrate meal, blood glucose rises from a fasting level of about 80–100 mg/dL (~5 mM) to a level of about 120–140 mg/dL (8 mM) within a period of 30 minutes to 1 hour (Fig. 31.2). The concentration of glucose in the blood then begins to decrease, returning to the fasting range by about 2 hours after the meal (see also Chapter 24).

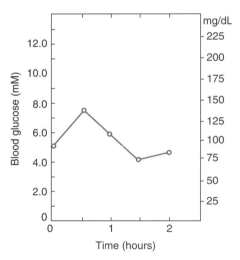

Fig. 31.2. Blood glucose concentrations at various times after a meal.

Diabetes mellitus (DM) should be suspected if a venous plasma glucose level drawn irrespective of when food was last eaten (a "random" sample of blood glucose) is "unequivocally elevated" (i.e., ≥ 200 mg/dL), particularly in a patient who manifests the classic signs and symptoms of chronic hyperglycemia (polydipsia, polyuria, blurred vision, headaches, rapid weight loss, sometimes accompanied by nausea and vomiting). To confirm the diagnosis, the patient should fast overnight (10–16 hours), and the blood glucose measurement should be repeated. Values of less than 115 mg/dL are considered normal. Values greater than 140 mg/dL are indicative of DM. Glycosylated hemoglobin should be measured to determine the extent of hyperglycemia over the past 4–8 weeks. Values of blood glucose between 115 and 140 mg/dL are borderline, and further testing should be performed to determine whether these individuals have impaired glucose tolerance (IGT) or diabetes mellitus.

Although the oral glucose tolerance test (OGTT) is contraindicated for patients who clearly have diabetes mellitus, it is used for patients with fasting blood glucose in the IGT range (between 115 and 140 mg/dL). In this test, a nonpregnant patient who has fasted overnight drinks 75 g of glucose in an aqueous solution of glucose. Blood samples are drawn before the oral glucose load and at 30, 60, 90, and 120 minutes thereafter. If any one of the 30, 60, and 90 minute samples and the 120 minute sample are greater than 200 mg/dL, DM is indicated.

The diagnosis of IGT and the more severe form of glucose intolerance (DM) is based on blood glucose levels because no more specific characteristic for the disorder exists. The distinction between IGT and DM is clouded by the fact that a patient's blood glucose level may vary significantly with serial testing over time under the same conditions of diet and activity.

The renal tubular transport maximum in the average healthy subject is such that glucose will not appear in the urine until the blood glucose level exceeds 180 mg/dL. As a result, reagent tapes (TesTape or Dextrostix) designed to detect the presence of glucose in the urine are not sensitive enough to establish a diagnosis of DM.

Blood glucose levels increase as dietary glucose is digested and absorbed. The values go no higher than about 140 mg/dL in a normal, healthy person because tissues take up glucose from the blood, storing it for subsequent use and oxidizing it for energy. After the meal is digested and absorbed, blood glucose levels decline because cells continue to metabolize glucose.

If blood glucose levels continued to rise after a meal, the high concentration of glucose would cause the release of water from tissues as a result of the osmotic effect of glucose. Tissues would become dehydrated and their function would be affected. A hyperosmolar coma could result from dehydration of the brain.

On the other hand, if blood glucose levels continued to drop after a meal, tissues that depend on glucose would suffer from a lack of energy. If blood glucose levels dropped abruptly, the brain would not be able to produce an adequate amount of ATP. Light-headedness and dizziness would result, followed by drowsiness and, eventually, coma. Red blood cells would not be able to produce enough ATP to maintain the integrity of their membranes. Hemolysis of these cells would decrease the transport of oxygen to the tissues of the body. Eventually, all tissues that rely on oxygen for energy production would fail to perform their normal functions. If the problem were severe enough, death could result.

Devastating consequences of glucose excess or insufficiency are normally avoided because the body is able to regulate its blood glucose levels. As the concentration of blood glucose approaches the normal fasting range of 80–100 mg/dL about 2 hours after a meal, the process of glycogenolysis is activated in the liver. Liver glycogen is the primary source of blood glucose during the first few hours of fasting. Subsequently, gluconeogenesis begins to play a role as an additional source of blood glucose. The carbon for gluconeogenesis, a process that occurs in the liver, is supplied by other tissues. Exercising muscle and red blood cells provide lactate via glycolysis; muscle also provides amino acids by degradation of protein; and glycerol is released from adipose tissue as triacylglycerol stores are mobilized.

Even during a prolonged fast, blood glucose levels do not fall dramatically. After 5–6 weeks of starvation, blood glucose levels decrease only to about 65 mg/dL (Table 31.1).

BLOOD GLUCOSE LEVELS IN THE FED STATE

The major factors involved in regulating blood glucose levels are the blood glucose concentration itself and hormones, particularly insulin and glucagon.

As blood glucose levels rise after a meal, the increased glucose concentration stimulates the B (or β) cells of the pancreas to release insulin (Fig. 31.3). Certain amino acids, particularly arginine and leucine, also stimulate insulin release from the pancreas.

Blood levels of glucagon, which is secreted by the A (or α) cells of the pancreas, may increase or decrease, depending on the content of the meal. Glucagon levels decrease in response to a high carbohydrate meal, but they increase in response to a high protein meal. After a typical mixed meal containing carbohydrate, protein, and fat, glucagon levels remain relatively constant, while insulin levels increase (Fig. 31.4).

Table 31.1. Blood Glucose Levels at Various Stages of Fasting

	Glucose (mg/dL)
Glucose, 700 g/day i.v.	100
Fasting, 12 hr	80
Starvation, 3 days	70
Starvation, 5–6 wk	65

Source of data: Ruderman NB, Aoki TT, Cahill GF, Jr. Gluconeogenesis and its disorders in man. In: Hanson RW, Mehlman MA, eds. Gluconeogenesis: its regulation in mammalian species. New York, John Wiley. 1976:517.

A 31.1: Comatose patients in diabetic ketoacidosis have the smell of acetone (a derivative of the ketone body acetoacetate) on their breath. In addition DKA patients have deep, relatively rapid respirations typical of acidotic patients (Kussmaul respirations). These respirations result from an acidosis-induced stimulation of the respiratory center in the brain. More CO_2 is exhaled in an attempt to reduce the amount of acid in the body: $H^+ + HCO_3^- \rightarrow H_2CO_3 \rightarrow H_2O + CO_2$ (exhaled).

The severe hyperglycemia of DKA also causes an osmotic diuresis (i.e., glucose entering the urine carries water with it) which, in turn, causes a contraction of blood volume. Volume depletion may be aggravated by vomiting, which is common in patients with DKA. DKA may cause dehydration (dry skin), a low blood pressure, and a rapid heart beat. Respiratory and hemodynamic alterations are not seen in patients with hypoglycemic coma. The flushed, wet skin of hypoglycemic coma is in contrast to the dry skin observed in DKA.

When **Di Beatty** inadvertently injected an excessive amount of insulin, she caused an acute reduction in her blood glucose levels 4–5 hours later while she was asleep. Had she been awake, she would have first experienced symptoms caused by a hypoglycemia-induced hyperactivity of her sympathetic nervous system (e.g., sweating, tremulousness, palpitations). Eventually, as her hypoglycemia became more profound, she would have experienced symptoms of "neuroglycopenia" (inadequate glucose supply to the brain) such as confusion, speech disturbances, emotional instability, possible seizure activity, and, finally, coma. While sleeping, she had reached this neuroglycopenic stage of hypoglycemia and could not be aroused at 6 am.

Priscilla Twigg, whose intake of glucose and of glucose precursors has been severely restricted, has not developed any of these manifestations. Her lack of hypoglycemic symptoms can be explained by the very gradual reduction of her blood glucose levels as a consequence of near starvation and her ability to maintain blood glucose levels within an acceptable fasting range through hepatic gluconeogenesis. In addition, lipolysis of adipose triacylglycerols produces fatty acids, which are used as fuel and converted to ketone bodies by the liver. The oxidation of fatty acids and ketone bodies spares blood glucose.

In **Di Beatty's** case, the excessive dose of insulin inhibited lipolysis and ketone body synthesis, so these alternative fuels were not available to spare blood glucose. The rapidity with which hypoglycemia was induced could not be compensated for quickly enough by hepatic gluconeogenesis, which was inhibited by the insulin, and hypoglycemia ensued.

A stat finger stick revealed that Di's capillary blood glucose level was less than 20 mg/dL. An intravenous infusion of a 50% solution of glucose was started, and her blood glucose level was determined frequently. When Di regained consciousness, the intravenous solution was eventually changed to 10% glucose. After 6 hours, her blood glucose levels stayed in the upper normal range, and she was able to tolerate oral feedings. She was transferred to the metabolic unit for overnight monitoring. By the next morning, her previous diabetes treatment regimen was reestablished. The reasons that she had developed hypoglycemic coma were explained to Di, and she was discharged to the care of her family doctor.

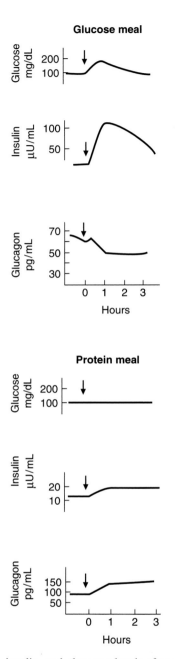

Fig. 31.3. Blood glucose, insulin, and glucagon levels after a high carbohydrate and a high protein meal.

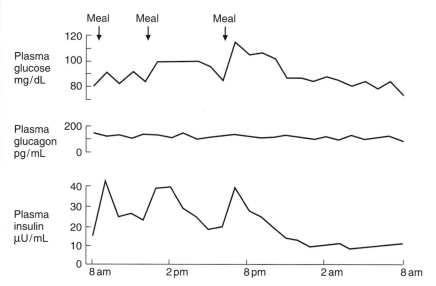

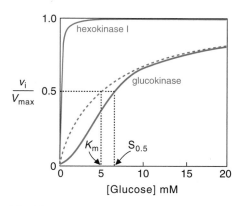

Fig. 31.5. Velocity of the glucokinase reaction.

Fig. 31.4. Blood glucose, insulin, and glucagon levels over a 24-hour period in a normal person eating mixed meals. Reprinted with permission from Tasaka Y, Sekine M, Wakatsuki M, et al. Horm Metab Res 1975;7:206. Copyright © Thieme Medical Publishers, Inc.

Fate of Dietary Glucose in the Liver

After a meal, the liver oxidizes glucose to meet its immediate energy needs. Any excess glucose is converted to stored fuels. Glycogen is synthesized and stored in the liver, and glucose is converted to fatty acids and to the glycerol moiety that reacts with the fatty acids to produce triacylglycerols. These triacylglycerols are packaged in very low density lipoproteins (VLDL) and transported to adipose tissue, where the fatty acids are stored in adipose triacylglycerols.

Regulatory mechanisms control the conversion of glucose to stored fuels. As the concentration of glucose increases in the hepatic portal vein, the concentration of glucose in the liver may increase from the fasting level of 80–100 mg/dL (~5 mM) to a concentration of 180–360 mg/dL (10–20 mM). Consequently, the velocity of the glucokinase reaction increases because this enzyme has a high $S_{0.5}$ (K_m) for glucose (Fig. 31.5). Glucokinase is also induced by a high carbohydrate diet; the quantity of the enzyme increases in response to elevated insulin levels.

Insulin promotes the storage of glucose as glycogen by countering the effects of glucagon-stimulated phosphorylation. It activates the phosphatases that dephosphorylate glycogen synthase (which is stimulated) and the enzymes of glycogen degradation (which are inhibited) (Fig. 31.6).

Insulin also promotes the synthesis of the triacylglycerols that are released from the liver into the blood as VLDL. The regulatory mechanisms for this process are described in Chapter 33.

Fate of Dietary Glucose in Peripheral Tissues

Almost every cell in the body oxidizes glucose for energy. Certain critical tissues, particularly the brain, other nervous tissue, and red blood cells, especially depend on glucose for their energy supply. In addition, all tissues require glucose for the pentose phosphate pathway, and many tissues use glucose for synthesis of glycoproteins and other carbohydrate-containing compounds.

Insulin stimulates the transport of glucose into adipose and muscle cells by promoting the recruitment of glucose transporters to the cell membrane. Other tissues,

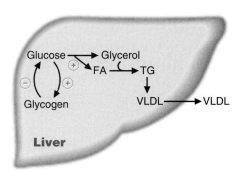

Fig. 31.6. Effect of insulin on glycogen synthesis and degradation and on VLDL synthesis in the liver. FA = fatty acids; TG = triacylglycerols; ⊕ = stimulated by insulin; ⊖ = inhibited by insulin.

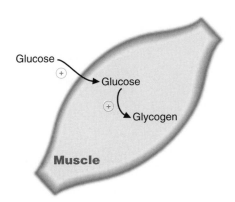

Fig. 31.7. Glucose metabolism in resting muscle in the fed state. The transport of glucose into cells and the synthesis of glycogen are stimulated (⊕) by insulin.

such as the liver, brain, and red blood cells, have a different type of glucose transporter that is not as significantly affected by insulin.

In muscle, glycogen is synthesized after a meal by a process similar to that in the liver (Fig. 31.7). Metabolic differences exist between these tissues (see Chapter 26), but, in essence, insulin stimulates glycogen synthesis in resting muscle as it does in the liver. A key difference between muscle and liver is that insulin greatly stimulates the transport of glucose into muscle cells but only slightly stimulates its transport into liver cells.

In adipose tissue, insulin stimulates the transport of glucose into cells (Fig. 31.8). This glucose produces energy for the cells and also provides the glycerol moiety for the synthesis of triacylglycerols. Glucose also may be converted to fatty acids in adipose tissue.

The brain, other nervous tissue, and red blood cells need a constant supply of blood glucose, both in the fed and the fasting states. The brain requires about 150 g of glucose per day. In addition, approximately 40 g are required by other glucose-dependent tissues. The brain and other nervous tissue oxidize glucose to CO_2 and H_2O. Because red blood cells lack mitochondria, they convert glucose to lactate.

Return of Blood Glucose to Fasting Levels

After a meal has been digested and absorbed, blood glucose levels reach a peak and then begin to decline. The uptake of dietary glucose by cells, particularly those in the liver, muscle, and adipose tissue, lowers blood glucose levels. By 2 hours after a meal, blood glucose levels return to the normal fasting level of about 80–100 mg/dL (~5 mM).

BLOOD GLUCOSE LEVELS IN THE FASTING STATE

Changes in Insulin and Glucagon Levels

During fasting, as blood glucose levels decrease, insulin levels decrease, and glucagon levels rise. These hormonal changes cause the liver to degrade glycogen by the process of glycogenolysis and to produce glucose by the process of gluconeogenesis so that blood glucose levels are maintained.

Stimulation of Glycogenolysis

Within a few hours after a high carbohydrate meal, glucagon levels begin to rise. Glucagon binds to cell surface receptors and activates adenylate cyclase, causing cAMP levels in liver cells to rise (Fig. 31.9). cAMP activates protein kinase A, which phosphorylates and inactivates glycogen synthase. Therefore, glycogen synthesis decreases.

At the same time, protein kinase A stimulates glycogen degradation by a two-step mechanism. Protein kinase A phosphorylates and activates phosphorylase kinase. This enzyme, in turn, phosphorylates and activates glycogen phosphorylase.

Phosphorylase catalyzes the phosphorolysis of glycogen, producing glucose 1-phosphate, which is converted to glucose 6-phosphate. Dephosphorylation of glucose 6-phosphate by glucose 6-phosphatase produces free glucose, which then enters the blood.

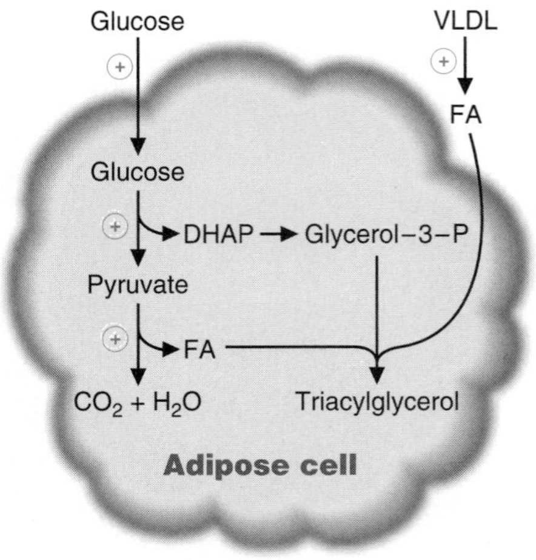

Stimulation of Gluconeogenesis

By 4 hours after a meal, the liver is supplying glucose to the blood not only by the process of glycogenolysis but also by the process of gluconeogenesis. Hormonal

Fig. 31.8. Glucose metabolism in adipose tissue in the fed state. ⊕ = stimulated by insulin. FA = fatty acids; DHAP = dihydroxyacetone phosphate.

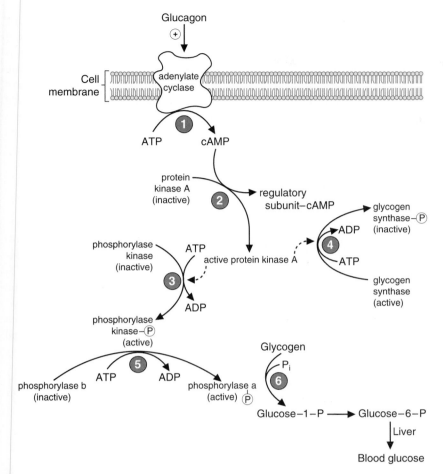

Fig. 31.9. Regulation of glycogenolysis in the liver.

The pathophysiology leading to an elevation of blood glucose after a meal differs between patients with insulin-dependent diabetes mellitus (IDDM) and those with non-insulin-dependent diabetes mellitus (NIDDM). **Di Beatty** who has IDDM, cannot secrete insulin adequately in response to a meal because of a defect in the B (or β) cells of her pancreas.

Ann Sulin, on the other hand, has NIDDM. In this form of the disorder, the etiology of glucose intolerance is more complex, involving at least a delay in the release of relatively appropriate amounts of insulin after a meal combined with a degree of resistance to the actions of insulin in skeletal muscle and adipocytes. Excessive hepatic gluconeogenesis occurs even though blood glucose levels are elevated.

changes cause peripheral tissues to release precursors that provide carbon for gluconeogenesis, specifically lactate, amino acids, and glycerol.

Regulatory mechanisms promote the conversion of gluconeogenic precursors to glucose (Fig. 31.10). These mechanisms prevent the occurrence of potential futile cycles, which would continuously convert substrates to products, while consuming energy but producing no useful result.

These regulatory mechanisms inactivate the glycolytic enzymes pyruvate kinase, phosphofructokinase-1 (PFK-1), and glucokinase during fasting and promote the flow of carbon to glucose via gluconeogenesis. These mechanisms operate at the three steps where glycolysis and gluconeogenesis differ:

1. Pyruvate (derived from lactate and alanine) is converted by the gluconeogenic pathway to phosphoenolpyruvate (PEP). PEP is not reconverted to pyruvate (a potential futile cycle) because glucagon-stimulated phosphorylation inactivates pyruvate kinase. Therefore, PEP reverses the steps of glycolysis and forms fructose 1,6-bisphosphate.

2. Fructose 1,6-bisphosphate is converted to fructose 6-phosphate by a bisphosphatase. Because the glycolytic enzyme PFK-1 is relatively inactive mainly as a result of low fructose 2,6-bisphosphate levels, fructose 6-phosphate is not converted back to fructose 1,6-bisphosphate, and a second potential futile cycle is avoided. Fructose 6-phosphate is converted to glucose 6-phosphate.

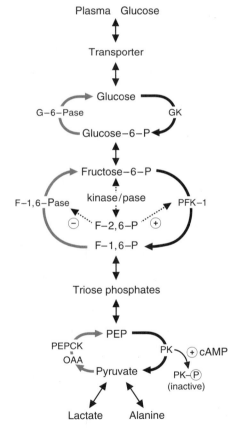

Fig. 31.10. Regulation of gluconeogenesis. GK = glucokinase; G-6-Pase = glucose 6-phosphatase; PK = pyruvate kinase; OAA = oxaloacetate; PEPCK = phosphoenolpyruvate carboxykinase; F-1,6-Pase = fructose 1,6-bisphosphatase; F-2,6-P = fructose 2,6-bisphosphate; PFK-1 = phosphofructokinase-1.

3. Glucose 6-phosphate is dephosphorylated by glucose 6-phosphatase, forming free glucose. Because glucokinase has a high $S_{0.5}$ (K_m) for glucose, and glucose concentrations are relatively low in liver cells during fasting, glucose is released into the blood. Therefore, the third potential futile cycle does not occur.

Enzymes that participate in gluconeogenesis, but not in glycolysis, are active under fasting conditions. Pyruvate carboxylase is activated by acetyl CoA, derived from oxidation of fatty acids. Phosphoenolpyruvate carboxykinase, fructose 1,6-bisphosphatase, and glucose 6-phosphatase are induced, that is the quantity of the enzymes increases. Fructose 1,6-bisphosphatase is also active because levels of fructose 2,6-bisphosphate, an inhibitor of the enzyme, are low.

Stimulation of Lipolysis

The hormonal changes that occur during fasting stimulate the breakdown of adipose triacylglycerols (see Chapters 3, 33, and 36). Consequently, fatty acids and glycerol are released into the blood (Fig. 31.11). Glycerol serves as a source of carbon for gluconeogenesis. Fatty acids become the major fuel of the body and are oxidized to CO_2 and H_2O by various tissues, which enables these tissues to decrease their utilization of glucose. Fatty acids are also oxidized to acetyl CoA in the liver. In this case, however, most of the acetyl CoA does not enter the tricarboxylic acid (TCA) cycle, but rather is converted to ketone bodies, which enter the blood and serve as an additional

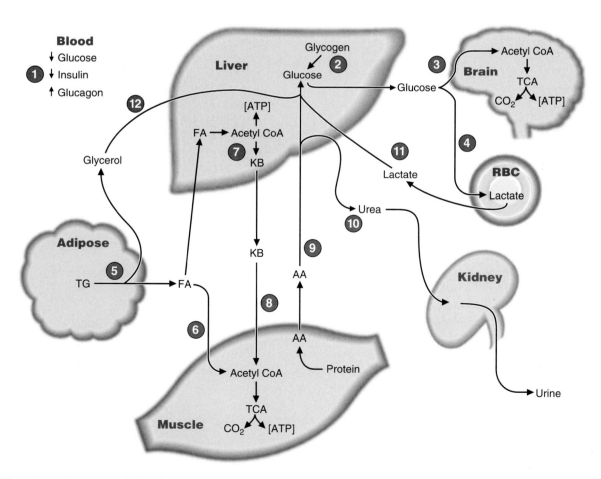

Fig. 31.11. Tissue interrelationships during fasting. KB = ketone bodies; FA = fatty acids; AA = amino acids; TG = triacylglycerols.

fuel source. β-Oxidation of fatty acids in the liver generates the ATP required to drive gluconeogenesis.

BLOOD GLUCOSE LEVELS DURING PROLONGED FASTING (STARVATION)

During prolonged fasting, a number of changes in fuel utilization occur. These changes cause tissues to use less glucose than they use during a brief fast and to use predominantly fuels derived from adipose triacylglycerols (i.e., fatty acids and their derivatives, the ketone bodies). Therefore, blood glucose levels do not decrease drastically. In fact, even after 5–6 weeks of starvation, blood glucose levels are still in the range of 65 mg/dL (Fig. 31.12).

The major change that occurs in starvation is a dramatic elevation of blood ketone body levels after 3–5 days of fasting (see Fig. 31.12). At these levels, the brain and other nervous tissues begin to use ketone bodies and, consequently, they oxidize less glucose, requiring about one-third as much glucose (about 40 g/day) as under normal dietary conditions. As a result of reduced glucose utilization, the rate of gluconeogenesis in the liver decreases, as does the production of urea (see Fig. 31.12). Protein from muscle and other tissues is, therefore, spared because there is less need for amino acids for gluconeogenesis.

Body protein, particularly muscle protein, is not primarily a storage form of fuel in the same sense as glycogen or triacylglycerol; proteins have many functions beside fuel storage. For example, proteins function as enzymes and in muscle contraction. If tissue protein is degraded to too great an extent, body function can be severely compromised. If starvation continues and no other problems, such as infections, occur, a starving individual usually dies because of severe protein loss that causes malfunction of major organs, such as the heart. Therefore, the increase in ketone body levels

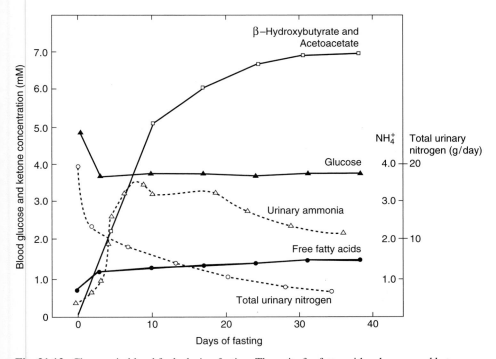

Fig. 31.12. Changes in blood fuels during fasting. The units for fatty acids, glucose, and ketone bodies are millimolar (on left) and for urinary nitrogen and ammonia are grams/day (on right). Modified from Linder MC. Nutritional biochemistry and metabolism, 2nd ed. Stamford CT: Appleton & Lange, 1991:103. © 1991 Appleton & Lange.

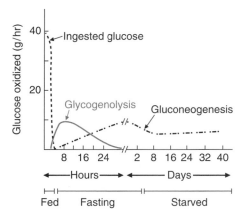

Fig. 31.13. Sources of blood glucose in fed, fasting, and starved states. Note that the scale changes from hours to days. From Ruderman NB, et al. In: Hanson RW, Mehlman MA, eds. Gluconeogenesis: its regulation in mammalian species. 1976:518. © 1976 John Wiley & Sons.

 Epidemiological studies have correlated the results of the OGTT with the current and subsequent development of the microvascular complications of DM in the eye (diabetic retinopathy) and in the kidney (diabetic nephropathy). Their development is usually limited to those patients whose fasting blood glucose level exceeded 140 mg/dL (7.8 mM) and/or whose 2-hour postprandial blood glucose level exceeded 200 mg/dL (11.1 mM).

As a consequence, the success of therapy with diet alone or with diet plus oral hypoglycemic agents is often determined by measuring blood glucose levels during fasting, prior to breakfast, and 2 hours after a meal. For patients taking an intermediate-acting insulin, blood glucose may also be measured at other times, such as when insulin action is expected to peak following its injection (e.g., around 5 PM when intermediate-acting insulin is given at 7 AM the same day).

 Remember that muscle glycogen is not used to maintain blood glucose levels.

that results in the sparing of body protein allows individuals to survive for long periods of time without ingesting food.

SUMMARY OF SOURCES OF BLOOD GLUCOSE

Immediately after a meal, dietary carbohydrates serve as the major source of blood glucose (Fig. 31.13). As blood glucose levels return to the fasting range within 2 hours after a meal, glycogenolysis is stimulated and begins to supply glucose to the blood. Subsequently, glucose is also produced by gluconeogenesis.

During a 12-hour fast, glycogenolysis is the major source of blood glucose. Thus, it is the major pathway by which glucose is produced in the basal state (after a 12-hour fast). However, by about 16 hours of fasting, glycogenolysis and gluconeogenesis contribute equally to the maintenance of blood glucose.

By 30 hours after a meal, liver glycogen stores are depleted. Subsequently, gluconeogenesis is the only source of blood glucose.

The mechanisms that cause fats to be used as the major fuel and that allow blood glucose levels to be maintained during periods of food deprivation result in the conservation of body protein and, consequently, permit survival during prolonged fasting for periods, often exceeding one or more months.

BLOOD GLUCOSE LEVELS DURING EXERCISE

During exercise, mechanisms very similar to those that are used during fasting operate to maintain blood glucose levels.

Use of Endogenous Fuels

Initially, exercising muscle uses endogenous fuels, fuels from its own stores. As the muscle contracts, ATP is hydrolyzed. Muscle cells avoid significant decreases in ATP levels initially by regenerating ATP from creatine phosphate. However, the amount of creatine phosphate in muscle cells could sustain exercise for only a few milliseconds. Therefore, muscle glycogen stores also begin to break down, supplying glucose which is oxidized within the muscle to produce ATP.

As ATP is converted to ADP during muscle contraction, the adenylate kinase reaction regenerates ATP, producing AMP in the process. AMP activates glycolysis by stimulating PFK-1. AMP also activates phosphorylase b, which then can break down muscle glycogen (Fig. 31.14). Phosphorylase b can also be activated by phosphorylation which produces phosphorylase a. Phosphorylation of phosphorylase b is also stimulated by calcium, released from the sarcoplasmic reticulum during exercise.

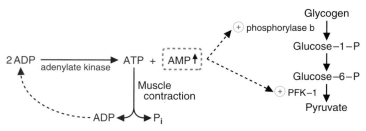

Fig. 31.14. Activation of muscle glycogenolysis and glycolysis by AMP. As muscle contracts, ATP is converted to ADP and P_i. In the adenylate kinase reaction, 2 ADP react to form ATP and AMP. The ATP is used for contraction. As AMP accumulates, it activates glycogenolysis and glycolysis.

Ca^{2+} binds to calmodulin, and this complex activates phosphorylase kinase, which phosphorylates and activates phosphorylase.

Glycogen stores in muscle are adequate to support an exercise such as push-ups or weight-lifting for only a short period of time (approximately 2 minutes in an average person). During intense exercise, the hormone epinephrine is released into the blood. It binds to receptors on the muscle cell membrane, activating adenylate cyclase (Fig. 31.15). As cAMP levels rise, protein kinase A is activated and phosphorylates phosphorylase kinase, causing it to phosphorylate glycogen phosphorylase. Phosphorylase b is converted to its more active, phosphorylated form, phosphorylase a. Phosphorylase a catalyzes the conversion of glycogen to glucose 1-phosphate, which via the phosphoglucomutase reaction, is converted to glucose 6-phosphate, which enters glycolysis. In muscles that contain many fast twitch, glycolytic fibers, such as the pectoral muscles in the chest, ATP is produced mainly by glycolysis, with lactate as the major product.

Use of Fuels from the Blood

In contrast to intense exercise, moderate to mild exercise can be sustained for very long periods of time. A trained individual, for example, can run for many hours. The leg muscles that are used contain many slow twitch oxidative fibers. Muscles containing slow twitch fibers tend to oxidize fuels to CO_2 and H_2O because they contain

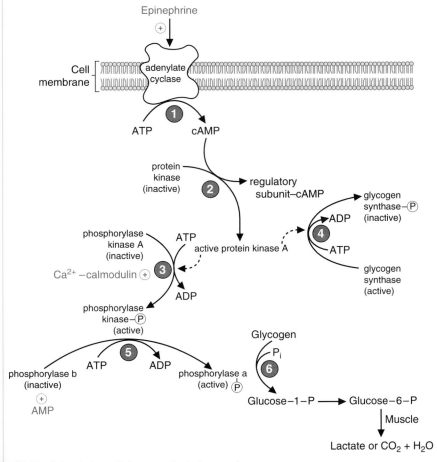

Fig. 31.15. Stimulation of glycogenolysis in muscle.

31.1: If **Ron Templeton** runs at a pace at which his muscles require about 500 Calories per hour, how long could he run on the amount of glucose that is present in circulating blood?

more mitochondria than muscles composed predominately of fast twitch glycolytic fibers.

Initially, when exercise of mild to moderate intensity begins, creatine phosphate and glycogen are used to regenerate ATP. However, as blood flow to the exercising muscle increases, a process that takes about 5–10 minutes, fuels travel to the muscle through the blood. The muscle takes up these fuels, mainly glucose and fatty acids, and oxidizes them to obtain ATP (Fig. 31.16).

At any given time during fasting, the blood contains only about 20 g of glucose, enough to support a person running at a moderate pace for a few minutes. Therefore, the blood glucose supply must be replenished. The liver performs this function by processes similar to those used during fasting. The liver produces glucose by breaking down its own glycogen stores and by gluconeogenesis. The major source of carbon for gluconeogenesis during exercise is, of course, lactate, produced by the exercising muscle, but amino acids and glycerol are also utilized (Fig. 31.17). Epinephrine released during exercise stimulates liver glycogenolysis and gluconeogenesis by causing cAMP levels to increase.

Obviously, fatty acids and a small amount of ketone bodies are present in the blood, and the muscle oxidizes these fuels in addition to glucose (see Fig. 31.16). They are produced as a consequence of lipolysis of the triacylglycerols of adipose tissue. During prolonged exercise, fatty acids become the major fuel for the exercising muscle.

CLINICAL COMMENTS. Chronically elevated levels of glucose in the blood may contribute to the development of the microvascular complications of diabetes mellitus, e.g., diabetic retinal damage, kidney damage, and nerve damage, as well as macrovascular complications such as cerebrovascular, peripheral vascular, and coronary vascular insufficiency. The precise mechanisms by which long term hyperglycemia induces these vascular changes is not fully established.

One postulated mechanism proposes that nonenzymatic glycation (glycosylation) of proteins in vascular tissue alters the structure and functions of these proteins. A protein exposed to chronically increased levels of glucose will covalently bind glucose, a process called glycation or glycosylation. This process is not regulated by enzymes (see Chapter 8). These nonenzymatically glycated proteins slowly form cross-linked protein adducts (often called advanced glycosylation products) within the micro- and macrovasculature.

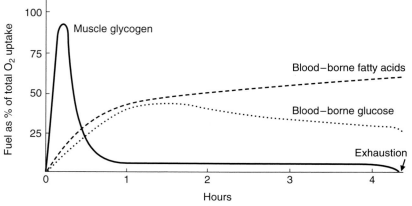

Fig. 31.16. Fuels used during exercise. The pattern of fuel utilization changes with the duration of the exercise. From Felig P, et al. Endocrinology & metabolism. New York: McGraw-Hill, 1981:796.

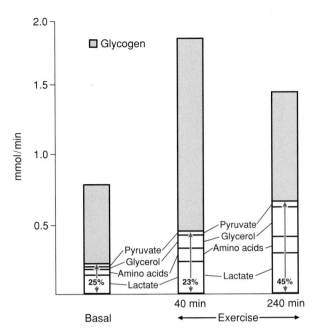

Fig. 31.17. Production of blood glucose by the liver from various precursors during rest and during prolonged exercise. The shaded area represents the contribution of liver glycogen to blood glucose, and the open area represents the contribution of gluconeogenesis. From Wahren J, et al. In: Howald H, Poortmans JR, eds. Metabolic adaptation to prolonged physical exercise. Cambridge, MA: Birkhauser, 1973:148.

By cross-linking vascular matrix proteins and plasma proteins, chronic hyperglycemia may cause narrowing of the luminal diameter of the microvessels in the retina (causing diabetic retinopathy), the renal glomeruli (causing diabetic nephropathy), and the microvessels supplying peripheral and autonomic nerve fibers (causing diabetic neuropathy). The same process has been postulated to accelerate atherosclerotic change in the macrovasculature, particularly in the brain (causing strokes), the coronary arteries (causing heart attacks), and the peripheral arteries (causing peripheral arterial insufficiency and gangrene). The abnormal lipid metabolism associated with poorly controlled diabetes mellitus may also contribute to the accelerated atherosclerosis associated with this metabolic disorder (see Chapters 33 and 34).

Until recently, it was argued that meticulous control of blood glucose levels in a diabetic patient would not necessarily prevent or even slow these complications of chronic hyperglycemia. The publication of the Diabetes Control and Complications Trial, however, suggests that maintaining long term euglycemia (normal blood glucose levels) in diabetic patients slows the progress of unregulated glycation of proteins as well as corrects their dyslipidemia. In this way, careful control may favorably affect the course of the micro- and macrovascular complications of diabetes mellitus in patients such as **Di Beatty** and **Ann Sulin**.

BIOCHEMICAL COMMENTS. Plants are the ultimate source of the earth's supply of glucose. Plants produce glucose from atmospheric CO_2 by the process of photosynthesis (see Fig. 31.18A). In contrast to plants, humans cannot synthesize glucose by the fixation of CO_2. Although we have a process called gluconeogenesis, the term may really be a misnomer. Glucose is not generated anew by gluconeogenesis; compounds produced from glucose are simply

Ron Templeton is able to jog for 45 minutes prior to eating breakfast without developing symptoms of hypoglycemia in spite of enhanced glucose utilization by skeletal muscle during exercise. He maintains his blood glucose level in an adequate range through hepatic glycogenolysis and gluconeogenesis.

31.1:
At 500 Calories per hour, Ron requires:

$$\frac{500 \text{ Calories}}{hr} \times \frac{1 \text{ g glucose}}{4 \text{ kcal}} \times \frac{1 \text{ hr}}{60 \text{ min}} = 2 \text{ g/min}$$

Blood contains only 20 g of glucose, so he could run for 10 minutes at this pace on the glucose present in his blood.

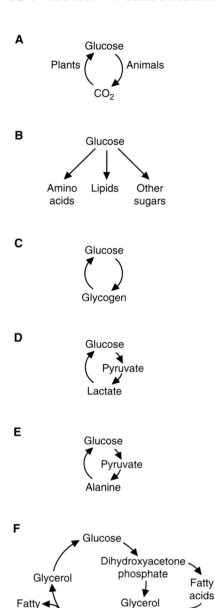

Fig. 31.18. Recycling of glucose.

recycled to glucose. We obtain glucose from the plants, including bacteria, that we eat and, to some extent, from animals in our food supply. We use this glucose both as a fuel and as a source of carbon for the synthesis of fatty acids, amino acids, and other sugars (see Fig. 31.18B). We store glucose as glycogen, which, along with gluconeogenesis, provides glucose when needed for energy (see Fig. 31.18C).

Lactate, one of the carbon sources for gluconeogenesis, is actually produced from glucose by tissues that obtain energy by oxidizing glucose to pyruvate via glycolysis. The pyruvate is then reduced to lactate, released into the bloodstream, and reconverted to glucose by the process of gluconeogenesis in the liver. This process is known as the Cori cycle (Fig. 31.18D).

Carbons of alanine, another carbon source for gluconeogenesis, may be produced from glucose. In muscle, glucose is converted via glycolysis to pyruvate and transaminated to alanine. Alanine from muscle is recycled to glucose in the liver. This process is known as the glucose-alanine cycle (Fig. 31.18E). Glucose may also be used to produce nonessential amino acids other than alanine which are subsequently reconverted to glucose in the liver via gluconeogenesis. Even the essential amino acids that we obtain from dietary proteins are synthesized in plants, particularly bacteria, using glucose as the major source of carbon. Therefore, all amino acids that are converted to glucose in humans, including the essential amino acids, were originally synthesized from glucose.

The production of glucose from glycerol, the third major source of carbon for gluconeogenesis, is also a recycling process. Glycerol is derived from glucose via the dihydroxyacetone phosphate intermediate of glycolysis. Fatty acids are then esterified to the glycerol and stored as triacylglycerol. When these fatty acids are released from the triacylglycerol, the glycerol moiety can travel to the liver and be reconverted to glucose (see Fig. 31.18F).

Suggested Readings

See the Suggested Readings for Chapters 26 and 27.

The Diabetes Control and Complications Trial Research Group. The effect of intensive treatment of diabetes on the development and progression of long-term complications in insulin-dependent diabetes mellitus. N Engl J Med 1993;329:977–986.

PROBLEMS

1. Patients with McArdle's disease (a muscle phosphorylase deficiency) and with PFK-1 deficiency have difficulty performing strenuous exercise. However, they can perform mild to moderate exercise for prolonged periods of time.
   A. Explain these observations in terms of the fuels that are used for each type of exercise and the pathways affected by the enzymatic defects.
   B. An oral glucose feeding improves the exercise tolerance of a person with McArdle's disease but causes a person with PFK-1 deficiency to become fatigued even more readily than usual. Explain these effects of glucose on exercise tolerance in these two enzyme deficiency diseases.

2. Why would a glucose 6-phosphatase deficiency be more devastating than a fructose 1,6-bisphosphatase deficiency?

3. **Ron Templeton** decided to enter a 10 km run to benefit the University Hospital. Because he wanted to do well, he decided to investigate the concept of glycogen loading and learned that if he exercised to exhaustion and then ate a high carbohydrate diet for 2 days before the race, his performance should improve. Explain in bio-

chemical terms how glycogen loading (i.e., eating large amount of starch on the days preceding a race) improves exercise performance.

4. Phosphofructokinase-2/fructose 2,6-bisphosphatase is a bifunctional enzyme involved in regulating glycolysis. Different promoters are used for expression of the gene in muscle and in liver. Transcription in muscle begins at exon 1 and in liver at exon 1′ (about 5 kb downstream from exon 1). Alternative splicing of the primary transcript produces an mRNA that contains exon 1 and exons 2 to 14 in muscle and exon 1′ and exons 2 to 14 in liver.

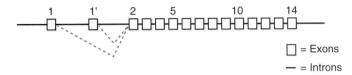

$\square$ = Exons

— = Introns

The base sequences at the splice junctions between the first exon and the first intron and between the first intron and exon 2 are as follows:

```
                        Intron
     Exon 1 (or 1′)                 Exon 2
Muscle  - - C A G g t a g g t - - - - c c a g C C T - - -
Liver  - - - - G C T g t a a g t - - c c a g C C T - - -
```

Bases in exons are capital letters and bases in introns are lowercase letters. The three underlined bases produce a critical codon.

A. What amino acid is specified by the codon produced by splicing at these exon-intron boundaries in muscle and in liver?

B. This amino acid is critical in terms of the regulation of the enzyme in these two tissues. Based on what you know about the regulation of this enzyme in liver, explain why the liver enzyme responds to changes in the insulin/glucagon ratio while the muscle enzyme does not.

ANSWERS

1A. In McArdle's disease, the isozyme of glycogen phosphorylase found in muscle is defective, and these individuals cannot readily degrade glycogen. Although individuals with a PFK-1 deficiency can break down glycogen, the rate of ATP production via glycolysis is low because the key glycolytic enzyme PFK-1 is defective. Therefore, individuals with either of these diseases become fatigued rapidly when attempting to perform strenuous exercise, such as weight lifting, that relies on muscle glycogen as the major fuel source.

Both types of individuals, however, can use blood-borne fatty acids, the major fuel for mild to moderate exercise of long duration. Individuals with McArdle's disease can also use blood-borne glucose.

1B. Glucose given orally can be used as fuel for mild to moderate exercise by individuals with McArdle's disease. However, individuals with PFK-1 deficiency cannot use blood glucose to support exercise. In fact, because glucose increases insulin levels and thus inhibits lipolysis in adipose tissue, the exercise tolerance of these individuals is adversely affected by a glucose feeding because they have less fatty acid in the blood to serve as fuel. The result has been called the "out of wind effect" (in contrast to the "second wind" experienced by normal individuals as lipolysis begins to supply additional fuel to their exercising muscles).

2. Fructose 1,6-bisphosphatase is a gluconeogenic enzyme. Individuals with a deficiency of this enzyme cannot maintain blood glucose by gluconeogenesis. However, they can produce blood glucose by glycogenolysis. Thus, they can tolerate short, but not lengthy, periods of fasting.

Glucose 6-phosphatase is involved in producing blood glucose both from glycogenolysis and gluconeogenesis. Individuals with a deficiency of this enzyme (von Gierke's disease, glycogen storage disease type I) cannot tolerate either long or short periods of fasting and must eat at very frequent intervals to obtain blood glucose.

3. Glycogen loading increases glycogen stores in muscle and also in the liver. Therefore, more fuel is stored in muscle to be used to support exercise and more glycogen is stored in the liver to supply glucose to the exercising muscle. Since Ron is not a well-trained athlete, but rather a medical student, the mitochondrial content of his muscle cells is not optimal. Therefore, he must rely to a greater extent on muscle glycolysis to meet his ATP needs than a well-trained athlete.

4A. In muscle, splicing produces a codon for alanine, (GCC). In liver, a codon for serine (TCC or UCC in the mRNA) is produced.

4B. Phosphorylation occurs at the serine residue produced by splicing of exon 1′ to exon 2 in liver, where the activity of the bifunctional enzyme phosphofructokinase 2 is regulated by fasting and feeding (i.e., by changes in the insulin/glucagon ratio). The enzyme is phosphorylated during fasting when the insulin/glucagon ratio is low (promoting gluconeogenesis) and dephosphorylated after a meal when the insulin/glucagon ratio is high (promoting glycolysis, which is used in the conversion of glucose to fatty acids). In muscle, the use of an alternative promoter, exon 1, and an alternative splice site results in the loss of this serine residue. Thus, in muscle, glycolysis is not regulated by phosphorylation and dephosphorylation of this enzyme in response to fasting and feeding. The role of fructose 2,6-bisphosphate in muscle is not well-defined.

Lipid Metabolism

Most of the lipids found in the body fall into the categories of fatty acids and triacylglycerols; glycerophospholipids and sphingolipids; eicosanoids; cholesterol, bile salts, and steroid hormones; and fat-soluble vitamins. These lipids have very diverse chemical structures and functions. However, they are related by a common property: their relative insolublity in water.

Fatty acids, which are stored as triacylglycerols, serve as fuels, providing the body with its major source of energy (Fig. 32.1). Glycerophospholipids and sphingolipids, which contain esterified fatty acids, are found in membranes and in blood lipoproteins at the interfaces between the lipid components of these structures and the surrounding water. These membrane lipids form hydrophobic barriers between subcellular compartments and between cellular constituents and the extracellular milieu. Polyunsaturated fatty acids containing 20 carbons form the eicosanoids, which regulate many cellular processes (Fig. 32.2).

Cholesterol adds stability to the phospholipid bilayer of membranes. It serves as the precursor of the bile salts, detergent-like compounds that function in the process of lipid digestion and absorption (Fig. 32.3). Cholesterol also serves as the precursor of the steroid hormones, which have many actions, including the regulation of metabolism, growth, and reproduction.

The fat-soluble vitamins are lipids that are involved in such varied functions as vision, growth, and differentiation (vitamin A), blood clotting (vitamin K), prevention of oxidative damage to cells (vitamin E), and calcium metabolism (vitamin D).

Triacylglycerols, the major dietary lipids, are digested in the lumen of the intestine (Fig. 32.4). The digestive products are reconverted to triacylglycerols in intestinal epithelial cells, packaged in lipoproteins known as chylomicrons, and secreted into the lymph. Ultimately, chylomicrons enter the blood, serving as one of the major blood lipoproteins.

Very low density lipoprotein (VLDL) is produced in the liver, mainly from dietary carbohydrate. Lipogenesis is the process by which glucose is converted to fatty acids, which are subsequently esterified to glycerol to form the triacylglycerols that are packaged in VLDL and secreted from the liver.

The triacylglycerols of chylomicrons and VLDL are digested by lipoprotein lipase (LPL), an enzyme found attached to capillary endothelial cells. The fatty acids that are released are taken up by muscle and many other tissues and oxidized to CO_2 and water to produce energy. After a meal, these fatty acids are taken up by adipose tissue and stored as triacylglycerols.

LPL converts chylomicrons to chylomicron remnants and VLDL to intermediate density lipoprotein (IDL). These products, which have a relatively low triacylglycerol content, are taken up by the liver by the process of endocytosis and degraded by lysosomal action. IDL may also be converted to low density lipoprotein (LDL) by further digestion of triacylglycerol. Endocytosis of LDL occurs in peripheral tissues as well as the liver (Table 32.1).

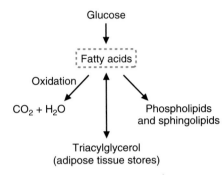

Fig. 32.1. Summary of fatty acid metabolism.

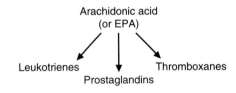

Fig. 32.2. Summary of eicosanoid synthesis.

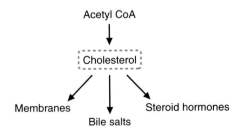

Fig. 32.3. Summary of cholesterol metabolism.

487

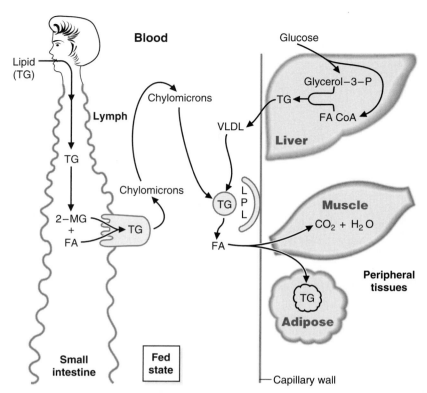

Fig. 32.4. Overview of triacylglycerol metabolism in the fed state. TG = triacylglycerol; 2-MG = 2-monoacylglycerol; FA = fatty acid; circled TG = triacylglycerols of VLDL and chylomicrons.

Table 32.1. Blood Lipoproteins

Chylomicrons
- produced in intestinal epithelial cells from dietary fat
- carries triacylglycerol in blood

VLDL (very low density lipoprotein)
- produced in liver mainly from dietary carbohydrate
- carries triacylglycerol in blood

IDL (intermediate density lipoprotein)
- produced in blood (remnant of VLDL after triacylglycerol digestion)
- endocytosed by liver or converted to LDL

LDL (low density lipoprotein)
- produced in blood (remnant of IDL after triacylglycerol digestion—endproduct of VLDL)
- contains high concentration of cholesterol and cholesterol esters
- endocytosed by liver and peripheral tissues

HDL (high density lipoprotein)
- produced in liver and intestine
- exchanges proteins and lipids with other lipoproteins
- functions in the return of cholesterol from peripheral tissues to the liver

The principal function of high density lipoprotein (HDL) is to transport cholesterol obtained from peripheral tissues to the liver and to exchange proteins and lipids with chylomicrons and VLDL.

During fasting, fatty acids and glycerol are released from adipose triacylglycerol stores (Fig. 32.5). The glycerol travels to the liver and is used for gluconeogenesis. The fatty acids form complexes with albumin in the blood and are taken up by muscle, kidney, and other tissues, where ATP is generated by their oxidation to CO_2 and water. Liver also converts some of the carbon to ketone bodies, which are released into the blood. Ketone bodies are oxidized for energy in muscle, kidney, and other tissues during fasting, and in the brain during prolonged starvation.

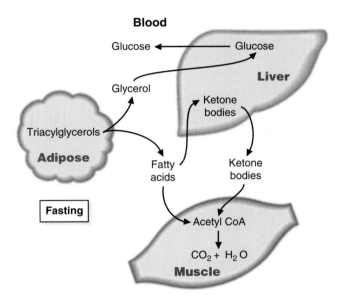

Fig. 32.5. Overview of triacylglycerol metabolism during fasting.

32   Digestion and Transport of Dietary Lipids

Triacylglycerols are the major fat in the human diet. These water-insoluble lipids are emulsified in the small intestine by bile salts and digested by a lipase secreted by the pancreas. The fatty acids and 2-monoacylglycerols that are produced by digestion are absorbed by intestinal epithelial cells and reconverted to triacylglycerols. Intestinal epithelial cells package the triacylglycerols derived from dietary fat into chylomicrons and secrete them via the lymph into the blood.

LPL on blood capillary endothelial cells digests the triacylglycerols of the chylomicrons to fatty acids and glycerol. After a normal mixed meal, the major fate of the fatty acids is storage as triacylglycerols in adipose tissue. Some of the fatty acids are also taken up by other tissues, such as muscle, and oxidized for energy.

Michael Sichel had several episodes of mild back and lower extremity pain over the last year, probably caused by minor sickle cell crises. He then developed severe right upper abdominal pain radiating to his lower right chest and his right flank 36 hours before admission to the emergency room. He states that the pain is not like his usual crisis pain. Intractable vomiting began 12 hours after the onset of these new symptoms. He reports that his urine is the color of iced tea and his stool now has a light clay color.

On physical examination, his body temperature is slightly elevated and his heart rate is rapid. The whites of his eyes (the sclerae) are obviously jaundiced (discolored by bilirubin pigment). He is exquisitely tender to pressure over his right upper abdomen.

The emergency room physician suspects that Michael is not in sickle cell crisis but instead has either acute cholecystitis (gallbladder inflammation) and/or a gallstone lodged in his common bile duct, causing cholestasis (the inability of the bile from the liver to reach his small intestine). His hemoglobin level was low at 7.6 g/dL (reference range = 12–16), but unchanged from his baseline 3 months earlier. His serum total bilirubin level was 3.2 mg/dL (reference range = 0.2–1.0), and his direct (conjugated) bilirubin level was 0.9 mg/dL (reference range = 0–0.2).

Intravenous fluids were started, a nasogastric tube was passed and placed on constant suction, and symptomatic therapy was started for pain and nausea. When his condition had stabilized, Michael was sent for an ultrasonographic (ultrasound) study of his upper abdomen.

Al Martini has continued to abuse alcohol and to eat poorly. After a particularly heavy intake of vodka, a steady severe pain began in his upper mid-abdomen, then spread to the left upper quadrant, and eventually radiated to his mid-back. He began vomiting nonbloody material and was brought to the hospital emergency room with fever, a rapid heart beat, and a mild reduction in blood pressure. On physical examination he was dehydrated and tender to pressure over the upper abdomen. His vomitus and stool were both negative for occult blood.

Blood samples were sent to the laboratory for a variety of hematological and chemical tests including a measurement of serum amylase and lipase, digestive

491

Currently, 38% of the calories (kcal) in the typical American diet come from fat. The content of fat in the diet increased from the early 1900s until the 1960s, and then decreased as we became aware of the unhealthy effects of a high fat diet. According to current recommendations, fat should provide no more than 30% of the total calories of a healthy diet.

In patients like **Michael Sichel** who have severe and recurrent episodes of increased red blood cell destruction (hemolytic anemia), greater than normal amounts of the red cell pigment, heme, must be processed by the liver and spleen. In these organs, heme (derived from hemoglobin) is degraded to bilirubin, which is excreted by the liver via the bile.

Large quantities of bilirubin can overwhelm the capacity of the liver to conjugate it, i.e., convert it to the water-soluble bilirubin diglucuronide. As a result, a greater percentage of the bilirubin entering the hepatic biliary ducts in patients with hemolysis is in the less water-soluble forms. In the gallbladder, they tend to precipitate as gallstones rich in calcium bilirubinate. In some patients, one or more stones may leave the gallbladder through the cystic duct and enter the common bile duct. The majority pass harmlessly into the small intestine and are later excreted in the stool. Larger stones, however, may become entrapped in the common bile duct where they cause varying degrees of obstruction to bile flow (cholestasis) with associated ductal spasm, producing pain. If adequate amounts of bile salts do not enter the intestinal lumen, dietary fats cannot readily be emulsified and digested.

enzymes normally secreted from the exocrine pancreas through the pancreatic ducts into the lumen of the small intestine.

DIGESTION OF TRIACYLGLYCEROLS

Triacylglycerols are the major fat in the human diet because they are the major storage lipid in the plants and animals that comprise our food supply. Triacylglycerols contain a glycerol backbone to which 3 fatty acids are esterified (Fig. 32.6). The main route for digestion of triacylglycerols involves hydrolysis to fatty acids and 2-monoacylglycerols in the lumen of the intestine. However, the route depends to some extent on the chain length of the fatty acids. Lingual and gastric lipases are produced by cells at the back of the tongue and in the stomach, respectively. These lipases preferentially hydrolyze short and medium chain fatty acids (containing 12 or fewer carbon atoms) from dietary triacylglycerols. Therefore, they are most active in infants and young children who drink relatively large quantities of cow's milk, which contains triacylglycerols with a high percentage of short and medium chain fatty acids.

Action of Bile Salts

Dietary fat leaves the stomach and enters the small intestine, where it is emulsified (suspended in small particles in the aqueous environment) by bile salts (Fig. 32.7). The bile salts are amphipathic compounds (containing both hydrophobic and hydrophilic components), synthesized in the liver and secreted via the gallbladder into the intestinal lumen. The contraction of the gallbladder and secretion of pancreatic enzymes is stimulated by the gut hormone cholecystokinin. Bile salts act as detergents, binding to the globules of dietary fat as they are broken up by peristaltic action. This emulsified fat is attacked by digestive enzymes from the pancreas (Fig. 32.8).

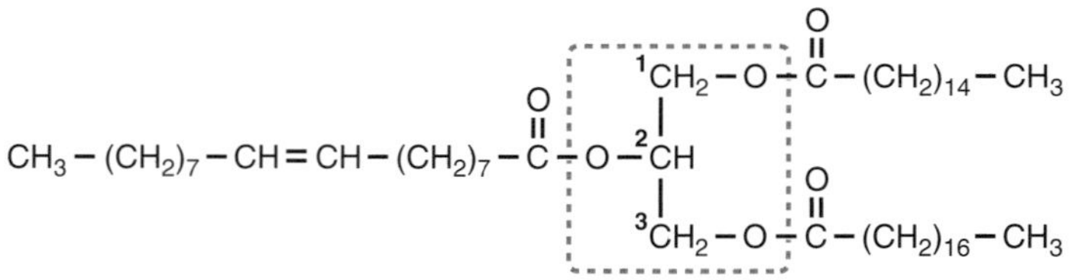

$$CH_3-(CH_2)_7-CH=CH-(CH_2)_7-C-O-\!^2CH$$

Fig. 32.6. Structure of a triacylglycerol. The glycerol moiety is highlighted and its carbons are numbered

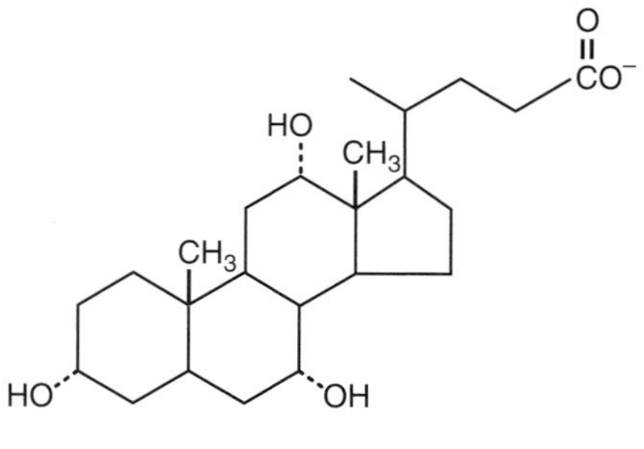

Cholate

Fig. 32.7. Structure of a bile salt. The bile salts are derived from cholesterol and retain the cholesterol ring structure. They differ from cholesterol in that the rings contain more hydroxyl groups and a polar side chain and lack a 5-6 double bond.

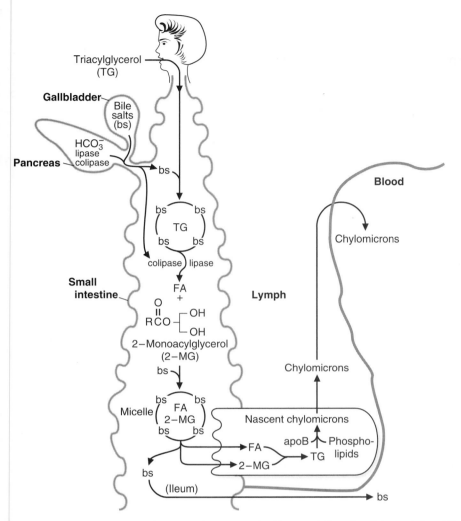

Fig. 32.8. Digestion of triacylglycerols in the intestinal lumen. TG = triacylglycerol; bs = bile salts; FA = fatty acid; 2-MG = 2-monoacylglycerol.

Al Martini's serum levels of pancreatic amylase (which digests dietary starch) and pancreatic lipase were elevated, a finding consistent with a diagnosis of acute and possibly chronic pancreatitis. The elevated levels of these enzymes in the blood are the result of their escape from the inflamed exocrine cells of the pancreas into the surrounding pancreatic veins. The cause of this inflammatory pancreatic process in this case was related to the toxic effect of acute and chronic excessive alcohol ingestion.

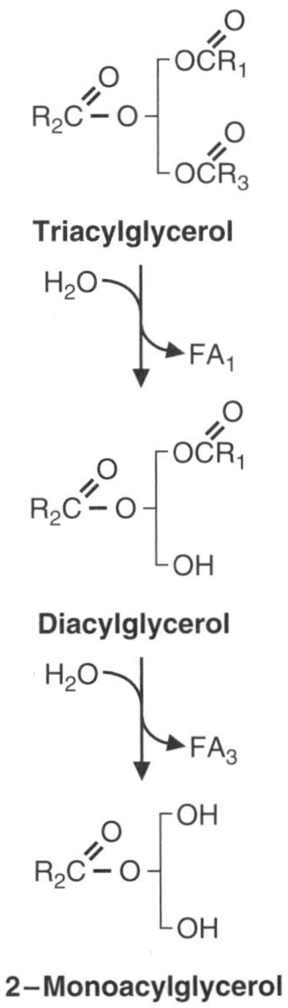

Action of Pancreatic Lipase

The major enzyme that digests dietary triacylglycerols is a lipase produced in the pancreas. Pancreatic lipase is secreted along with another protein, colipase. The pancreas also secretes bicarbonate, which neutralizes the acid that enters the intestine with partially digested food from the stomach. Bicarbonate raises the pH of the contents of the intestinal lumen into a range (pH ~ 6) that is optimal for the action of all of the digestive enzymes of the intestine.

The colipase binds to the dietary fat and to the lipase, causing it to be more active. Pancreatic lipase hydrolyzes fatty acids of all chain lengths from positions 1 and 3 of the glycerol moiety of the triacylglycerol, producing free fatty acids and 2-monoacylglycerol, i.e., glycerol with a fatty acid esterified at position 2 (Fig. 32.9). The pancreas also produces esterases that remove fatty acids from compounds (such as cholesterol esters) and phospholipases that digest phospholipids to their component parts.

Triacylglycerol

Diacylglycerol

2–Monoacylglycerol

Fig. 32.9. Action of pancreatic lipase. Fatty acids (FA) are cleaved from positions 1 and 3 of the triacylglycerol, and a monoacylglycerol with a fatty acid at position 2 is produced.

Q 32.1: When he was finally able to tolerate a full diet, **Al Martini's** stools became bulky, glistening, yellow-brown, and foul smelling. They floated on the surface of the toilet water. What caused this problem?

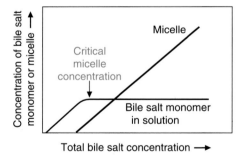

For bile salt micelles to form, the concentration of bile salts in the contents of the intestinal lumen must reach 5–15 µmol/mL. This critical concentration of bile salts is, therefore, required for optimal lipid absorption.

ABSORPTION OF DIETARY LIPIDS

The fatty acids and 2-monoacylglycerols produced by digestion are packaged into micelles, tiny microdroplets emulsified by bile salts (see Fig. 32.8). Other dietary lipids, such as cholesterol and fat-soluble vitamins, are also packaged in these micelles. The micelles travel through a layer of water (the unstirred water layer) to the microvilli on the surface of the intestinal epithelial cells where the fatty acids, 2-monoacylglycerols, and other dietary lipids are absorbed.

The bile salts, which remain in the gut, are extensively resorbed when they reach the ileum. Greater than 95% of the bile salts are recirculated, traveling via the enterohepatic circulation to the liver, which secretes them into the bile for storage in the gallbladder and ejection into the intestinal lumen during another digestive cycle (Fig. 32.10).

Short and medium chain fatty acids (C4 to C12) do not require bile salts for their absorption. They are absorbed directly into intestinal epithelial cells. Because they do not need to be packaged into chylomicrons, they enter the portal blood (rather than the lymph), and are transported to the liver bound to serum albumin.

SYNTHESIS OF CHYLOMICRONS

Within the intestinal epithelial cells, the fatty acids and 2-monoacylglycerols recombine by enzymatic reactions in the smooth endoplasmic reticulum to form triacylglycerols. The fatty acids are activated to fatty acyl CoA by the same process used for activation of fatty acids prior to β-oxidation (see Chapter 23). A fatty acyl CoA then reacts with a 2-monoacylglycerol to form a diacylglycerol, which reacts with another fatty acyl CoA to form a triacylglycerol (Fig. 32.11). The reactions for tri-

Because the fat-soluble vitamins (A, D, E, and K) are absorbed from micelles along with the long chain fatty acids and 2-monoacylglycerols, prolonged obstruction of the duct that carries secretions from the pancreas and the gallbladder into the intestine (the common duct) could lead to a deficiency of these metabolically important substances. If the obstruction of **Michael Sichel's** common duct continues, he will eventually suffer from a fat-soluble vitamin deficiency. (Graph from Devlin T. Textbook of biochemistry, 3rd ed. 1992:1084. Copyright © John Wiley & Sons, Inc.)

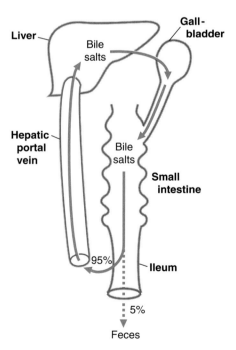

Fig. 32.10. Recycling of bile salts. Bile salts are synthesized in the liver, stored in the gallbladder, secreted into the small intestine, resorbed in the ileum, and returned to the liver. Only 5% are excreted.

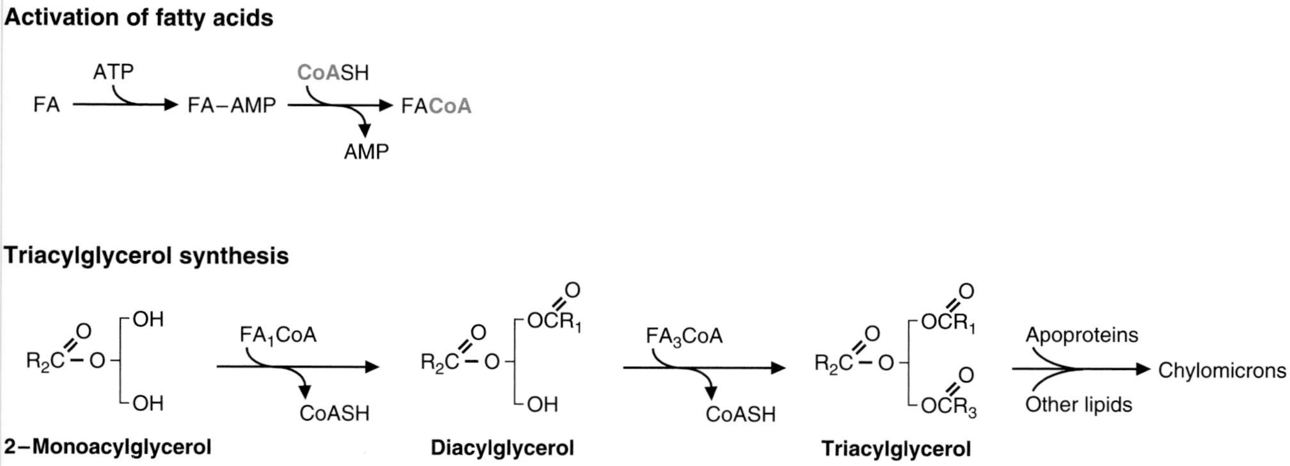

Activation of fatty acids

$$FA \xrightarrow{\text{ATP}} FA\text{--}AMP \xrightarrow[\displaystyle AMP]{\text{CoASH}} FACoA$$

Triacylglycerol synthesis

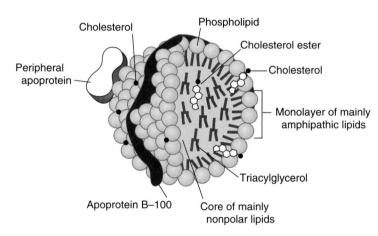

2–Monoacylglycerol   Diacylglycerol   Triacylglycerol

Fig. 32.11. Resynthesis of triacylglycerols in intestinal epithelial cells. Fatty acids (FA), produced by digestion, are activated in intestinal epithelial cells and then esterified to the 2-monoacylglycerol produced by digestion. The triacylglycerols are packaged in chylomicrons and secreted into the lymph.

Fig. 32.12. Example of the structure of a blood lipoprotein. VLDL is depicted. Lipoproteins contain phospholipids and proteins on the surface with their hydrophilic regions interacting with water. Hydrophobic molecules are in the interior. The hydroxyl group of cholesterol is near the surface. In cholesterol esters, the hydroxyl group is esterified to a fatty acid. Cholesterol esters are found in the interior of lipoproteins.

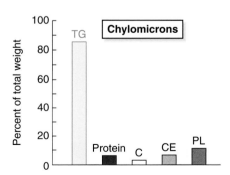

Fig. 32.13. Composition of a typical chylomicron. Although the composition varies to some extent, the major component is triacylglycerol (TG). C = cholesterol; CE = cholesterol ester; PL = phospholipid.

acylglycerol synthesis in intestinal cells differ from those in liver and adipose cells in that 2-monoacylglycerol is an intermediate in intestinal cells and phosphatidic acid is not.

Triacylglycerols are transported in lipoprotein particles because they are insoluble in water. If triacylglycerols directly entered the blood, they would coalesce, impeding blood flow. Intestinal cells package triacylglycerols together with proteins and phospholipids in chylomicrons, which are lipoprotein particles that do not readily coalesce in aqueous solutions (Figs. 32.12 and 32.13). Chylomicrons also contain cholesterol and fat soluble vitamins. The proteins constituents of the lipoproteins are known as apoproteins.

Because of their high triacylglycerol content, chylomicrons are the least dense of the blood lipoproteins. When blood collected from patients with certain types of hyperlipoproteinemias (high concentrations of lipoproteins in the blood) in which chylomicron levels are elevated is allowed to stand in the refrigerator overnight, the chylomicrons float to the top of the liquid and coalesce, forming a creamy layer.

The major apoprotein associated with chylomicrons as they leave the intestinal cells is B-48 (Fig. 32.14). The B-48 apoprotein is structurally and genetically related to the B-100 apoprotein synthesized in the liver that serves as a major protein of VLDL. These two apoproteins are encoded by the same gene. In the intestine, the primary transcript of this gene undergoes RNA editing (see Chapter 15). A stop codon is generated that causes a protein to be produced in the intestine that is 48% of the size of the protein produced in the liver, hence the designations B-48 and B-100.

The protein component of the lipoproteins is synthesized on the rough endoplasmic reticulum. Lipids, which are synthesized in the smooth endoplasmic reticulum, are complexed with the proteins to form the chylomicrons (Fig. 32.14).

TRANSPORT OF DIETARY LIPIDS IN THE BLOOD

By the process of exocytosis, chylomicrons are secreted by the intestinal epithelial cells into the chyle of the lymphatic system and enter the blood via the thoracic duct. Chylomicrons begin to enter the blood within 1–2 hours after the start of a meal, and as the meal is digested and absorbed, they continue to enter the blood for many hours. Initially, the particles are called nascent (newborn) chylomicrons. As they accept proteins from HDL within the lymph and the blood, they become "mature" chylomicrons.

HDL transfers proteins to the nascent chylomicrons, particularly apoprotein E (apoE) and apoprotein C_{II} (apoC_{II}) (Fig. 32.15). ApoE is recognized by membrane receptors, particularly those on the surface of liver cells, allowing ApoE-bearing lipoproteins to enter these cells by endocytosis for subsequent digestion by lysosomes. ApoC_{II} acts as an activator of LPL, the enzyme on capillary endothelial cells that digests the triacylglycerols of the chylomicrons and VLDL in the blood.

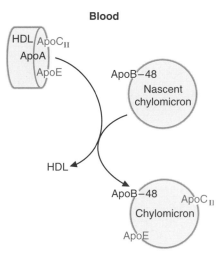

Fig. 32.15. Transfer of proteins from HDL to chylomicrons. Newly synthesized chylomicrons (nascent chylomicrons) mature as they receive apoproteins C_{II} and E from HDL. HDL functions in the transfer of these apoproteins and also in transfer of cholesterol from peripheral tissues to the liver (see Table 32.1).

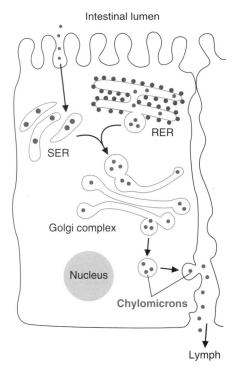

Fig. 32.14. Formation and secretion of chylomicrons. The triacylglycerol is produced in the smooth endoplasmic reticulum (SER) of intestinal epithelial cells from the digestive products, fatty acids and 2-monoacylglycerols. The protein is synthesized in the rough endoplasmic reticulum (RER). The major protein is B-48. Assembly of the lipoproteins occurs in the Golgi complex.

FATE OF CHYLOMICRONS

The triacylglycerols of the chylomicrons are digested by LPL attached to the proteoglycans in the basement membranes of endothelial cells that line the capillary walls (Fig. 32.16). LPL is produced by adipose cells, muscle cells (particularly cardiac muscle), and cells of the lactating mammary gland. The isozyme synthesized in adipose cells has a higher K_m than the isozyme synthesized in muscle cells. Therefore, adipose LPL is more active after a meal when chylomicrons levels are elevated in the blood. Insulin stimulates the synthesis and secretion of adipose LPL.

The fatty acids released from triacylglycerols by LPL are not very soluble in water. They become soluble in blood by forming complexes with the protein albumin. The major fate of the fatty acids is storage as triacylglycerol in adipose tissue. However, these fatty acids also may be oxidized for energy in muscle and other tissues (see Fig. 32.16). The LPL in the capillaries of muscle cells has a lower K_m than adipose LPL. Thus muscle cells can obtain fatty acids from blood lipoproteins whenever they are needed for energy even if the concentration of the lipoproteins is low.

The glycerol released from triacylglycerols by LPL may be used for triacylglycerol synthesis in the liver in the fed state.

The portion of a chylomicron that remains in the blood after LPL action is known as a chylomicron remnant. This remnant binds to receptors on hepatocytes (the major cells of the liver) and is taken up by the process of endocytosis. Lysosomes fuse with the endocytic vesicles, and the chylomicron remnants are degraded by lysosomal enzymes. The products of lysosomal digestion (e.g., fatty acids, amino acids, glycerol, cholesterol, phosphate) can be reutilized by the cell.

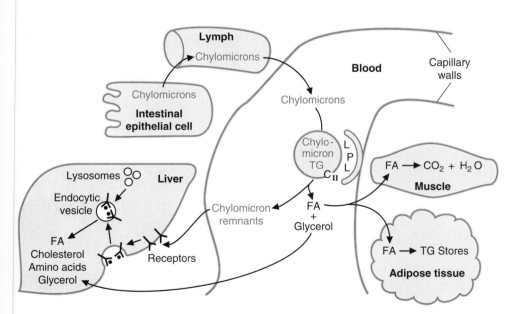

Fig. 32.16. Fate of chylomicrons. Chylomicrons are synthesized in intestinal epithelial cells, secreted into the lymph, pass into the blood, and become mature chylomicrons (see Fig. 32.15). On capillary walls, lipoprotein lipase (LPL) activated by apoC$_{II}$ digests the triacylglycerols (TG) of chylomicrons to fatty acids and glycerol. Fatty acids (FA) are oxidized or stored in cells as triacylglycerols. The remnants of the chylomicrons are taken up by the liver by receptor-mediated endocytosis. Lysosomal enzymes digest the remnants, releasing the products into the cytosol.

CLINICAL COMMENTS. The upper abdominal ultrasound study demonstrated a large gallstone lodged in **Michael Sichel's** common duct with dilatation of this duct proximal to the stone. Michael was scheduled for endoscopic retrograde cholangiopancreatography (ERCP). (An ERCP involves cannulation of the common bile duct—and, if necessary, the pancreatic duct—via a tube placed through the mouth and stomach and into the upper small intestine.) With this technique, a stone can be snared in the common duct and removed to relieve an obstruction.

If common duct obstruction is severe enough, bilirubin flows back into the venous blood draining from the liver. As a consequence, serum bilirubin levels, particularly the indirect (unconjugated) fraction, increase. Tissues such as the sclerae of the eye take up this pigment, which causes them to become yellow (jaundiced). Michael Sichel's condition was severe enough to cause jaundice by this mechanism.

Alcohol excess may produce proteinaceous plugs in the small pancreatic ducts, causing back pressure injury and autodigestion of the pancreatic acini drained by these obstructed channels. This process causes one form of pancreatitis. **Al Martini** had an acute episode of alcohol-induced pancreatitis superimposed on a more chronic alcohol-related inflammatory process in the pancreas, i.e., a chronic pancreatitis. As a result of decreased secretion of pancreatic lipase through the pancreatic ducts and into the lumen of the small intestine, dietary fat was not absorbed at a normal rate and steatorrhea occurred. If abstinence from alcohol does not allow adequate recovery of the enzymatic secretory function of the pancreas, Mr. Martini will have to take a commercial preparation of pancreatic enzymes with meals that contain even minimal amounts of fat.

 BIOCHEMICAL COMMENTS. The mammary gland produces milk, which is the major source of nutrients for the breast-fed human infant. The fatty acid composition of human milk varies, depending on the diet of the mother. However, long chain fatty acids predominate, particularly palmitic, oleic, and linoleic acids. Although the amount of fat contained in human milk and cow's milk is similar, cow's milk contains more short and medium chain fatty acids and does not contain the long chain, polyunsaturated fatty acids found in human milk which are important in brain development.

Although pancreatic lipase and bile salts are low in the newborn infant, the fat of human milk is readily absorbed. Lingual and gastric lipases produced by the infant partially compensate for the lower levels of pancreatic lipase. The human mammary gland also produces lipases that enter the milk. One of these lipases, which requires lower levels of bile salts than pancreatic lipase, is not inactivated by stomach acid and functions in the intestine for a number of hours.

Suggested Readings

Linder MC (ed). Nutrition and metabolism of fats. In: Nutritional biochemistry and metabolism with clinical applications. New York: Elsevier, 1991:51–85.

Zlotkin SH. Neonatal nutrition. In: Linder MC, ed. Nutritional biochemistry and metabolism with clinical applications. New York: Elsevier, 1991:357–360.

PROBLEMS

1. Abetalipoproteinemias are rare inherited disorders in which the B-apoproteins

(formerly called beta- or β-apoproteins) are not produced. What problems would you expect patients with these disorders to have?

2. In cystic fibrosis, mucous secretions block the pancreatic duct and prevent the excretion of exocrine enzymes. How would fat absorption be affected?

ANSWERS

1. Individuals with abetalipoproteinemia cannot form chylomicrons in the intestine or VLDL in the liver because both of these lipoproteins contain B-apoproteins. Triacylglycerols will accumulate in intestinal and liver cells, and blood lipoprotein levels will be low. Dietary fat, particularly long chain fatty acids, are a major source of fuel, which will not be available to these individuals. Short and medium chain fatty acids, however, will still be absorbed because they enter the intestinal cells directly and are transported to the liver complexed with albumin.

Because fat-soluble vitamins and essential fatty acids are absorbed from the diet and transported in the blood in chylomicrons, a deficiency of these nutrients will also occur.

2. The blockage caused by mucous secretions in cystic fibrosis prevents pancreatic secretions, including pancreatic lipase, colipase, and HCO_3^- from entering the intestine. Therefore, normal quantities of enzymes for the digestion of fats would not be available. This condition can lead to steatorrhea and also to fat-soluble vitamin deficiencies.

33 Synthesis of Fatty Acids, Triacylglycerols, and the Major Membrane Lipids

Fatty acids are synthesized mainly in the liver in humans, with dietary glucose serving as the major source of carbon. Glucose is converted via glycolysis to pyruvate, which enters the mitochondrion and forms both acetyl CoA and oxaloacetate (Fig. 33.1). These two compounds condense, forming citrate. Citrate is transported to the cytosol, where it is cleaved to form acetyl CoA, the source of carbon for the reactions that occur on the fatty acid synthase complex. The key regulatory enzyme for the process, acetyl CoA carboxylase, produces malonyl CoA from acetyl CoA.

The growing fatty acid chain, attached to the fatty acid synthase complex in the cytosol, is elongated by the sequential addition of 2-carbon units provided by malonyl CoA. NADPH, produced by the pentose phosphate pathway and the malic enzyme, provides reducing equivalents. When the growing fatty acid chain is 16 carbons in length, it is released as palmitate. After activation, palmitate can be elongated and desaturated to produce a series of fatty acids.

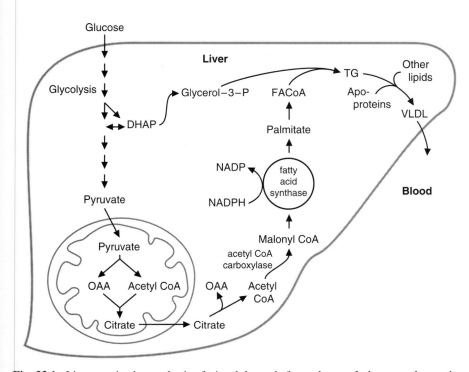

Fig. 33.1. Lipogenesis, the synthesis of triacylglycerols from glucose. In humans, the synthesis of fatty acids from glucose occurs mainly in the liver. Fatty acids (FA) are converted to triacylglycerols (TG), packaged in VLDL, and secreted into the blood. OAA = oxaloacetate.

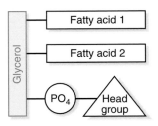

Fig. 33.3. General structure of a glycerophospholipid. The fatty acids are joined by ester bonds to the glycerol moiety. Various combinations of fatty acids may be present. The fatty acid at carbon 2 of the glycerol is usually unsaturated. The head group is the group attached to the phosphate on position 3 of the glycerol moiety. The most common head group is choline, but ethanolamine, serine, inositol, or phosphatidylglycerol may also be present. The phosphate group is negatively charged, and the head group may carry a positive charge (choline and ethanolamine), or both a positive and a negative charge (serine). The inositol may be phosphorylated and, thus, negatively charged.

Fatty acids, produced in cells or obtained from the diet, are used by various tissues for the synthesis of triacylglycerols (the major storage form of fuel) and the glycerophospholipids and sphingolipids (the major components of cell membranes).

In the liver, triacylglycerols are produced from fatty acyl CoA and glycerol 3-phosphate. Phosphatidic acid serves as an intermediate in this pathway. The triacylglycerols are not stored in the liver, but rather packaged with apoproteins and other lipids in very low density lipoprotein (VLDL) and secreted into the blood (see Fig. 33.1).

In the capillaries of various tissues (particularly adipose tissue, muscle, and the lactating mammary gland), lipoprotein lipase (LPL) digests the triacylglycerols of VLDL, forming fatty acids and glycerol (Fig. 33.2). The glycerol travels to the liver and other tissues where it is utilized. Some of the fatty acids are oxidized by muscle and other tissues. After a meal, however, most of the fatty acids are converted to triacylglycerols in adipose cells, where they are stored. These fatty acids are released during fasting and serve as the predominant fuel for the body.

Glycerophospholipids are also synthesized from fatty acyl CoA, which forms esters with glycerol 3-phosphate, producing phosphatidic acid. Various groups are added to carbon 3 of the glycerol 3-phosphate moiety of phosphatidic acid, generating amphipathic compounds such as phosphatidylcholine, phosphatidylinositol, and cardiolipin (Fig. 33.3). In the formation of plasmalogens and platelet-activating factor (PAF), a long chain fatty alcohol forms an ether with carbon 1, replacing the fatty acyl ester (Fig. 33.4). Cleavage of phospholipids is catalyzed by phospholipases found in cell membranes, lysosomes, and pancreatic juice.

Sphingolipids, which are prevalent in membranes and the myelin sheath of the central nervous system, are built on serine rather than glycerol. In the synthesis of sphingolipids, serine and palmitoyl CoA condense, forming a compound which is related to sphingosine. Reduction of this compound, followed by addition of a second fatty acid in amide linkage, produces ceramide. Carbohydrate groups attach to ceramide, forming glycolipids such as the cerebrosides, globosides, and gangliosides (Fig. 33.5). The addition of phosphocholine to ceramide produces sphingomyelin. These sphingolipids are degraded by lysosomal enzymes.

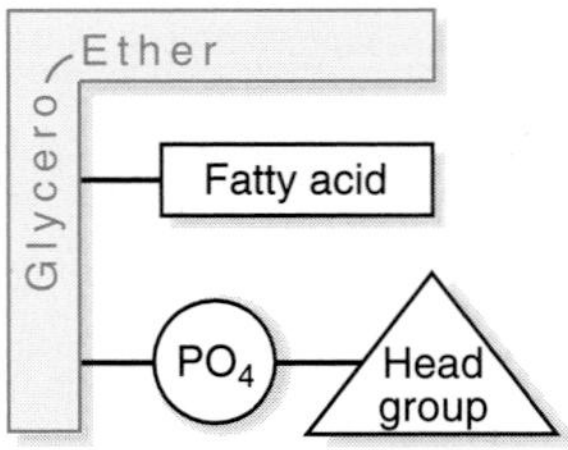

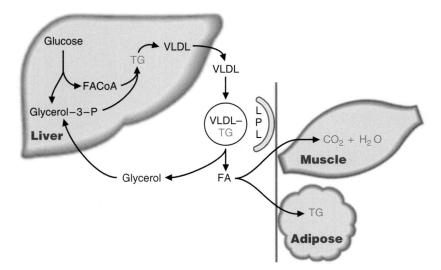

Fig. 33.2. Fate of VLDL triacylglycerol (TG). The TG of VLDL, produced in the liver, is digested by lipoprotein lipase (LPL) on capillary walls. Fatty acids are released and either oxidized or stored in tissues as TG. Glycerol is used by the liver and other tissues that contain glycerol kinase. FA = fatty acid (or fatty acyl group).

Fig. 33.4. General structure of a plasmalogen. Carbon 1 of glycerol is joined to a long chain fatty alcohol by an ether linkage. The fatty alcohol group has a double bond between carbons 1 and 2. The head group is usually ethanolamine or choline.

Teresa Livermore's mental depression slowly responded to antidepressant medication, to the therapy sessions with her psychiatrist, and to frequent visits from an old high school beau whose wife had died several years earlier. While hospitalized for malnutrition, Mrs. Livermore's appetite returned. By the time of discharge, she had gained back 18 of the 41 lb she had lost and weighed 108 lb.

During the next few months, Mrs. Livermore developed a craving for "sweet foods" to which her friend gladly responded by bringing her boxes of candy. After 6 months of this high carbohydrate courtship, Teresa had gained another 22 lb and now weighed 130 lb, just 3 lb less than she weighed when her depression began. She became concerned about the possibility that she would soon be overweight and consulted her dietician, explaining that she had faithfully followed her low fat diet, but had "gone overboard" with carbohydrates. She asked if it was possible to become fat without eating fat.

 Cora Nari's hypertension and heart failure have been well-controlled on medication, and she has lost 10 lb since she had her recent heart attack. Her fasting serum lipid profile on discharge from the hospital revealed a slightly elevated serum low density lipoprotein (LDL) cholesterol level of 175 mg/dL (recommended level for a patient with known coronary artery disease = 100 mg/dL or less), a serum triacylglycerol level of 280 mg/dL (reference range = 60–160), and a serum high density lipoprotein (HDL) cholesterol level of 34 mg/dL (reference range > 45 for healthy women). While still in the hospital, she was asked for the most recent serum lipid profiles of her older brother and her younger sister, both of whom were experiencing chest pain. Her brother's profile revealed normal triacylglycerols, moderately elevated LDL cholesterol, and significantly suppressed HDL cholesterol levels. Her sister's profile showed only hypertriglyceridemia (high blood triacylglycerols).

 Colleen Lakker was born 6 weeks prematurely. She appeared normal until about 30 minutes after delivery, when her respirations became rapid at 64 per minute with audible respiratory grunting. The spaces between her ribs (intercostal spaces) retracted inward with each inspiration and her lips and fingers became cyanotic from a lack of oxygen in her arterial blood. An arterial blood sample revealed a low partial pressure of oxygen (pO_2) and a slightly elevated partial pressure of carbon dioxide (pCO_2). The arterial pH was somewhat suppressed, in part from an accumulation of lactic acid secondary to the hypoxemia. A chest x-ray revealed a fine reticular granularity of the lung tissue especially in the left lower lobe area. From this clinical data, a diagnosis of respiratory distress syndrome (RDS), also known as hyaline membrane disease, was made.

Colleen was immediately transferred to the neonatal intensive care unit, where, with intensive respiration therapy, she slowly improved.

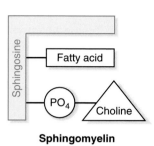

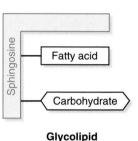

Fig. 33.5. General structures of the sphingolipids. The "backbone" is sphingosine rather than glycerol. Ceramide is sphingosine with a fatty acid joined to its amino group by an amide linkage. Sphingomyelin contains phosphocholine, whereas glycolipids contain carbohydrate groups.

FATTY ACID SYNTHESIS

Fatty acids are synthesized whenever there is a caloric excess in the diet. The major source of carbon for the synthesis of fatty acids is dietary carbohydrate. A caloric excess of dietary protein can also result in fatty acid synthesis. In this case, the carbon source is amino acids that can be converted to acetyl CoA or tricarboxylic acid (TCA) cycle intermediates (see Chapter 39). Fatty acid synthesis occurs mainly in the liver in humans, although the process also occurs in adipose tissue.

When an excess of dietary carbohydrate is consumed, glucose is converted to acetyl CoA, which provides the 2-carbon units that condense in a series of reactions

The dietician did a careful analysis of **Teresa Livermore's** diet, which was indeed low in fat, adequate in protein, but excessive in carbohydrates, especially in refined sugars. Teresa's total caloric intake averaged about 430 kilocalories (kcal) a day in excess of her isocaloric requirements. This excess carbohydrate was being converted to fats, accounting for Teresa's weight gain. A new diet with a total caloric content that would prevent further gain in weight was prescribed.

on the fatty acid synthase complex, producing palmitate (see Fig. 33.1). Palmitate is then converted to other fatty acids. The fatty acid synthase complex is located in the cytosol, and therefore it uses cytosolic acetyl CoA.

Conversion of Glucose to Cytosolic Acetyl CoA

The pathway for the synthesis of cytosolic acetyl CoA from glucose begins with glycolysis, which converts glucose to pyruvate in the cytosol (Fig. 33.6). Pyruvate enters mitochondria, where it is converted to acetyl CoA by pyruvate dehydrogenase and to oxaloacetate by pyruvate carboxylase. Acetyl CoA and oxaloacetate condense to form citrate, which is transported across the inner mitochondrial membrane. In the cytosol, citrate is cleaved by citrate lyase to reform acetyl CoA and oxaloacetate. This circuitous route is required because pyruvate dehydrogenase, the enzyme that converts pyruvate to acetyl CoA, is found only in mitochondria and because acetyl CoA cannot directly cross the mitochondrial membrane.

The NADPH required for fatty acid synthesis is generated by the pentose phosphate pathway and from recycling of the oxaloacetate produced by citrate lyase (Fig. 33.7). Oxaloacetate is converted back to pyruvate in two steps: the reduction of oxaloacetate to malate by NAD-dependent malate dehydrogenase and the oxidative decarboxylation of malate to pyruvate by an NADP-dependent malate dehydrogenase (malic enzyme) (Fig. 33.8). The pyruvate formed by malic enzyme is reconverted to citrate. The NADPH that is generated by malic enzyme, along with the NADPH generated by glucose 6-phosphate dehydrogenase in the pentose phosphate pathway, is used for the reduction reactions that occur on the fatty acid synthase complex (Fig. 33.9).

The generation of cytosolic acetyl CoA from pyruvate is stimulated by elevation of the insulin/glucagon ratio after a carbohydrate meal. Insulin activates pyruvate dehydrogenase by stimulating the phosphatase that dephosphorylates the enzyme to an active form (see Chapter 19). The synthesis of malic enzyme, glucose 6-phosphate dehydrogenase, and citrate lyase is induced by the high insulin/glucagon ratio. The concerted regulation of glycolysis and fatty acid synthesis is described in Chapter 36.

Conversion of Acetyl CoA to Malonyl CoA

Cytosolic acetyl CoA is converted to malonyl CoA, which serves as the immediate donor of the 2-carbon units that are added to the growing fatty acid chain on the fatty

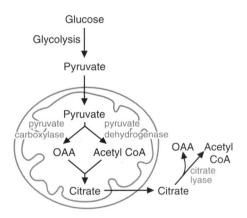

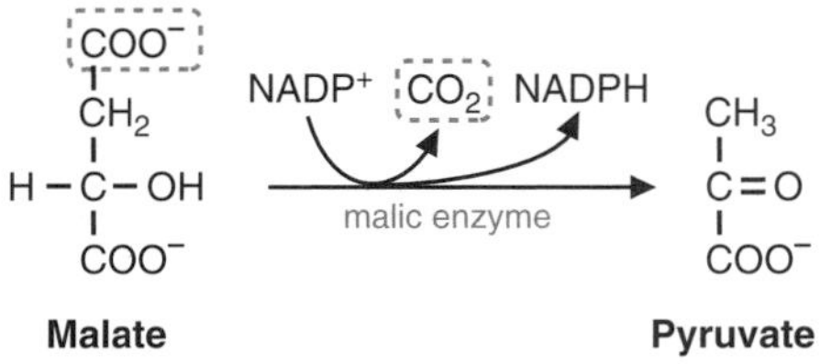

Fig. 33.6. Conversion of glucose to cytosolic acetyl CoA. OAA = oxaloacetate.

Fig. 33.8. Reaction catalyzed by malic enzyme. This enzyme is also called the decarboxylating or NADP-dependent malate dehydrogenase.

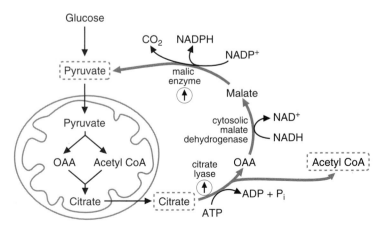

Fig. 33.7. Fate of citrate in the cytosol. Citrate lyase is also called citrate cleavage enzyme. OAA = oxaloacetate; circled ↑ = inducible enzyme.

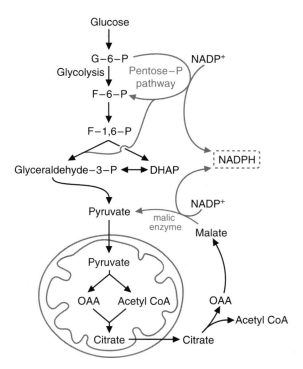

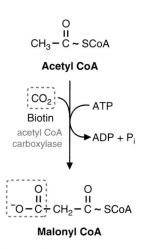

Fig. 33.10. Reaction catalyzed by acetyl CoA carboxylase. CO_2 is covalently attached to biotin which is linked by an amide bond to the ε-amino group of a lysine residue of the enzyme. Hydrolysis of ATP is required for the attachment of CO_2 to biotin.

Fig. 33.9. Sources of NADPH for fatty acid synthesis. NADPH is produced by the pentose phosphate pathway and by malic enzyme. OAA = oxaloacetate.

acid synthase complex. To synthesize malonyl CoA, acetyl CoA carboxylase adds a carboxyl group to acetyl CoA in a reaction requiring biotin and ATP (Fig. 33.10).

Acetyl CoA carboxylase is the rate-limiting enzyme of fatty acid synthesis. Its activity is regulated by hormonally directed phosphorylation, allosteric modification, and induction/repression of its synthesis (Fig. 33.11). Citrate allosterically activates acetyl CoA carboxylase by causing the individual enzyme protomers (each composed of 4 subunits) to polymerize. Palmitoyl CoA, produced from palmitate (the endproduct of fatty acid synthase), inhibits acetyl CoA carboxylase. Phosphorylation by cAMP-dependent protein kinase A inhibits the enzyme in the fasting state when glucagon levels are elevated. The enzyme is activated by dephosphorylation in the fed state when insulin levels are high. A high insulin/glucagon ratio also results in induction of the synthesis of both acetyl CoA carboxylase and the next enzyme in the pathway, fatty acid synthase.

Fatty Acid Synthase Complex

Fatty acid synthase sequentially adds 2-carbon units from malonyl CoA to the growing fatty acyl chain to form palmitate. After the addition of each 2-carbon unit, the growing chain undergoes two reduction reactions that require NADPH.

Fatty acid synthase is a large enzyme composed of two identical dimers, which each have seven catalytic activities and an acyl carrier protein (ACP) segment in a continuous polypeptide chain. The ACP segment contains a phosphopantetheine residue that is derived from the cleavage of coenzyme A (Fig. 33.12). The two dimers associate in a head-to-tail arrangement, so that the phosphopantetheinyl sulfhydryl group on one subunit and a cysteinyl sulfhydryl group on another subunit are closely aligned.

Q 33.1: Where does the methyl group of the first acetyl CoA that binds to fatty acid synthase appear in palmitate, the final product?

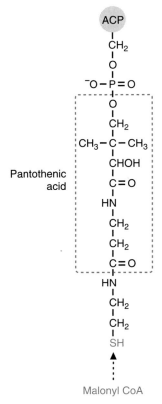

Fig. 33.12. Phosphopantetheinyl residue of the fatty acid synthase complex. The portion derived from the vitamin, pantothenic acid, is indicated. Phosphopantetheine is covalently linked to a serine residue of the acyl carrier protein (ACP) segment of the enzyme. The sulfhydryl group reacts with malonyl CoA to form a thioester.

 The phosphopantetheinyl group of the fatty acid synthase complex is also found in coenzyme A.

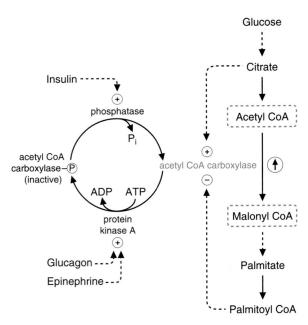

Fig. 33.11. Regulation of acetyl CoA carboxylase. This enzyme is regulated by activation ⊕ and inhibition ⊖, by phosphorylation (circled P) and dephosphorylation, and by induction (circled ↑). It is active in the dephosphorylated state when citrate causes it to polymerize. Dephosphorylation is catalyzed by an insulin-stimulated phosphatase. Glucagon and epinephrine cause the enzyme to be phosphorylated and inactivated via protein kinase A. The ultimate product of fatty acid synthesis, palmitate, is converted to its CoA derivative palmitoyl CoA, which inhibits the enzyme.

In the initial step of fatty acid synthesis, an acetyl moiety is transferred from acetyl CoA to the ACP phosphopantetheinyl sulfhydryl group of one subunit, and then to the cysteinyl sulfhydryl group of the other subunit. The malonyl moiety from malonyl CoA then attaches to the ACP phosphopantetheinyl sulfhydryl group of the first subunit. The acetyl and malonyl moieties condense, with the release of the malonyl carboxyl group as CO_2. A 4-carbon α-keto acyl chain is now attached to the ACP phosphopantetheinyl sulfhydryl group (Fig. 33.13).

A series of three reactions reduces the 4-carbon keto group to an alcohol, removes water to form a double bond, and reduces the double bond (Fig. 33.14). NADPH provides the reducing equivalents for these reactions. The net result is that the original acetyl group is elongated by 2 carbons.

The 4-carbon fatty acyl chain is then transferred to the cysteinyl sulfhydryl group and subsequently condenses with a malonyl group. This sequence of reactions is repeated until the chain is 16 carbons in length. At this point, hydrolysis occurs and palmitate is released (Fig. 33.15).

Palmitate is elongated and desaturated to produce a series of fatty acids. In the liver, palmitate and other newly synthesized fatty acids are converted to triacylglycerols that are packaged into VLDL for secretion.

In the liver, the oxidation of newly synthesized fatty acids back to acetyl CoA via the mitochondrial β-oxidation pathway is prevented by malonyl CoA. Carnitine:palmitoyltransferase I, the enzyme involved in the transport of long chain fatty acids into mitochondria (see Fig. 23.4), is inhibited by malonyl CoA (Fig. 33.16). Malonyl CoA levels are elevated when acetyl CoA carboxylase is activated, and, thus, fatty acid oxidation is inhibited while fatty acid synthesis is proceeding. This inhibition prevents the occurrence of a futile cycle.

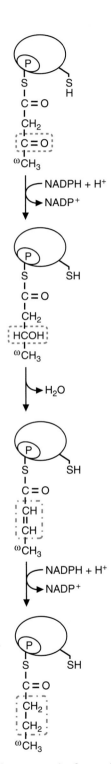

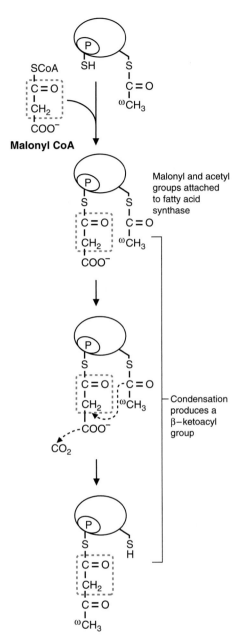

Fig. 33.13. Addition of a 2-carbon unit to an acetyl group on fatty acid synthase. The malonyl group attaches to the phosphopantetheinyl residue (P) of the ACP of the fatty acid synthase. The acetyl group, which is attached to a cysteinyl sulfhydryl group, condenses with the malonyl group. CO_2 is released, and a 3-ketoacyl group is formed.

A 33.1: The methyl group of acetyl CoA becomes the ω-carbon (the terminal methyl group) of palmitate. Each new 2-carbon unit is added to the carboxyl end of the growing fatty acyl chain (see Fig. 33.13).

Fig. 33.14. Reduction of a β-ketoacyl group on the fatty acid synthase complex. NADPH is the reducing agent. The carbon that eventually forms the ω-methyl group of palmitate is labeled ω.

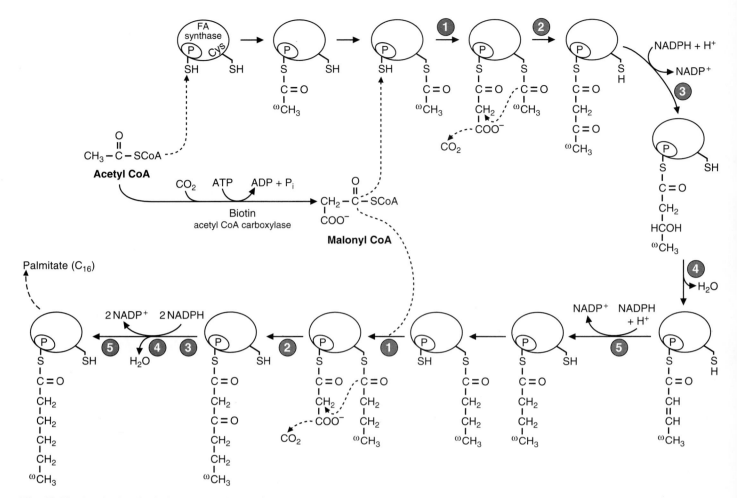

Fig. 33.15. Synthesis of palmitate on the fatty acid synthase complex. Initially, acetyl CoA adds to the synthase. It provides the ω-methyl group of palmitate. Malonyl CoA provides the 2-carbon units that are added to the growing fatty acyl chain. The addition and reduction steps are repeated until palmitate is produced. **1.** Transfer of the malonyl group to the phosphopantetheinyl residue. **2.** Condensation of the malonyl and fatty acyl groups. **3.** Reduction of the β-ketoacyl group. **4.** Dehydration. **5.** Reduction of the double bond. P = a phosphopantetheinyl group attached to the fatty acid synthase complex; Cys-SH = a cysteinyl residue.

ELONGATION OF FATTY ACIDS

After synthesis on the fatty acid synthase complex, palmitate is activated, forming palmitoyl CoA. Palmitoyl CoA and other activated long chain fatty acids can be elongated, 2 carbons at a time, by a series of reactions that occur in the endoplasmic reticulum (Fig. 33.17). Malonyl CoA serves as the donor of the 2-carbon units, and NADPH provides the reducing equivalents. The series of elongation reactions resemble those of fatty acid synthesis except that the fatty acyl chain is attached to coenzyme A rather than to the phosphopantetheinyl residue of an ACP. The major elongation reaction that occurs in the body involves the conversion of palmitoyl CoA (C16) to stearoyl CoA (C18). Very long chain fatty acids (C22 to C24) are also produced, particularly in the brain.

Fatty acids can also be elongated in mitochondria. In this case, the source of the 2-carbon units is acetyl CoA and the substrates are usually fatty acids containing less than 16 carbons, i.e., mainly short and medium chain fatty acids.

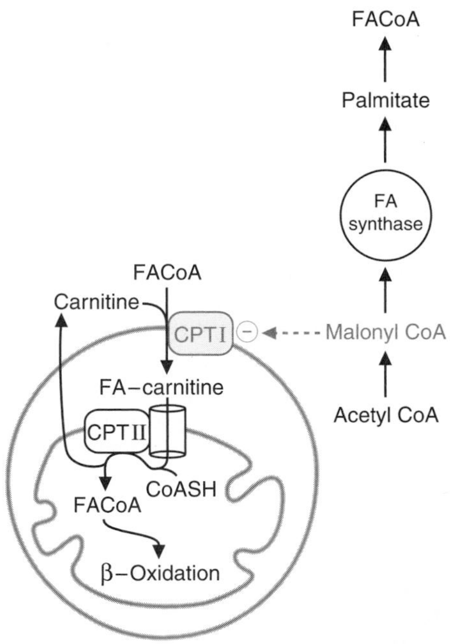

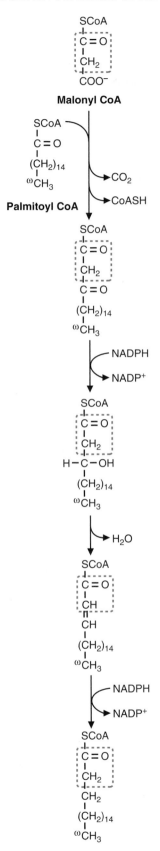

Malonyl CoA

Palmitoyl CoA

CO_2

$CoASH$

$NADPH$

$NADP^+$

H_2O

$NADPH$

$NADP^+$

Stearoyl CoA

Fig. 33.16. Inhibition of carnitine:palmitoyl-transferase (CPTI, also called carnitine:acyl-transferase I) by malonyl CoA. During fatty acid synthesis, malonyl CoA levels are high. This compound inhibits CPTI, which is involved in the transport of long chain fatty acids into mitochondria for β-oxidation. This mechanism prevents newly synthesized fatty acids from undergoing immediate oxidation.

Fig. 33.17. Elongation of long chain fatty acids in the endoplasmic reticulum. The reactions are similar to those of fatty acid synthesis expect that a fatty acyl CoA is the substrate which condenses with malonyl CoA.

Plants are able to introduce double bonds into fatty acids in the region between C10 and the ω-end and, therefore, can synthesize ω3 and ω6 polyunsaturated fatty acids. Fish oils also contain ω3 and ω6 fatty acids, particularly EPA (ω3,20:5,$\Delta^{5,8,11,14,17}$) and docosahexaenoic acid (DHA; ω3,22:6, $\Delta^{4,7,10,13,16,19}$). The fish obtain these fatty acids by eating phytoplankton (plants that float in water).

Arachidonic acid is listed in some textbooks as an essential fatty acid. Although it is an ω6 fatty acid, it is not essential in the diet if linoleic acid is present because arachidonic acid can be synthesized from dietary linoleic acid (see Fig. 33.19).

The essential fatty acid, linoleic acid is required in the diet for at least two reasons. (a) It serves as a precursor of arachidonic acid from which eicosanoids are produced. (b) It covalently binds another fatty acid attached to cerebrosides in the skin, forming an unusual lipid (acylglucosylceramide) that helps to make the skin impermeable to water. This function of linoleic acid may help to explain the red, scaly dermatitis and other skin problems associated with a dietary deficiency of essential fatty acids.

The other essential fatty acid, α-linolenic acid (18:3,$\Delta^{9,12,15}$), also forms eicosanoids. Note that it differs from the γ-linolenoyl derivative that we can synthesize (see Fig. 33.19).

Desaturation of Fatty Acids

Desaturation of fatty acids involves a process that requires molecular oxygen (O_2), NADH, and cytochrome b_5. The reaction, which occurs in the endoplasmic reticulum, results in the oxidation of both the fatty acid and NADH (Fig. 33.18). Human desaturase enzymes can place double bonds only between carbon 10 and the carboxyl group. They cannot place double bonds between carbon 10 and the ω-carbon. The most common desaturation reactions involve the placement of a double bond between carbons 9 and 10 in the conversion of palmitic acid to palmitoleic acid (16:1,Δ^9) and the conversion of stearic acid to oleic acid (18:1,Δ^9).

Polyunsaturated fatty acids with double bonds 3 carbons from the methyl end (ω3 fatty acids) and 6 carbons from the methyl end (ω6 fatty acids) are required for the synthesis of eicosanoids (see Chapter 35). Because humans cannot synthesize these fatty acids de novo (i.e., from glucose via palmitate), they must be present in the diet or the diet must contain other fatty acids that can be converted to these fatty acids. We obtain ω6 and ω3 polyunsaturated fatty acids mainly from dietary plant oils which contain the ω6 fatty acid linoleic acid (18:2,$\Delta^{9,12}$) and the ω3 fatty acid α-linolenic acid (18:3,$\Delta^{9,12,15}$). In the body, linoleic acid can be converted by elongation and desaturation reactions to arachidonic acid (20:4,$\Delta^{5,8,11,14}$), which is used for the synthesis of the major class of human prostaglandins and other eicosanoids (Fig. 33.19). Elongation and desaturation of α-linolenic acid produces eicosapentaenoic acid (EPA; 20:5,$\Delta^{5,8,11,14,17}$), which is the precursor of a different class of eicosanoids (see Chapter 35).

Synthesis of Triacylglycerols

In liver and adipose tissue, triacylglycerols are produced by a pathway containing a phosphatidic acid intermediate (Fig. 33.20). Phosphatidic acid is also the precursor of the glycerolipids found in cell membranes and the blood lipoproteins.

The sources of glycerol 3-phosphate, which provides the glycerol moiety for triacylglycerol synthesis, differ in liver and adipose tissue. In liver, glycerol 3-phosphate is produced from the phosphorylation of glycerol by glycerol kinase or from the reduction of dihydroxyacetone phosphate derived from glycolysis. Adipose tissue lacks glycerol kinase and can produce glycerol 3-phosphate only from glucose via dihydroxyacetone phosphate. Thus, adipose tissue can store fatty acids only when glycolysis is activated, i.e., in the fed state.

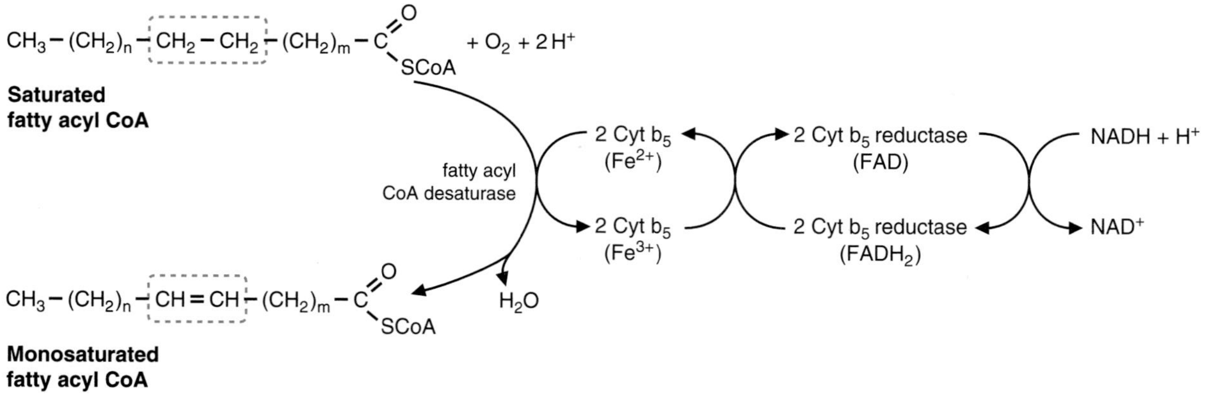

Fig. 33.18. Desaturation of fatty acids. The process occurs in the endoplasmic reticulum and uses molecular oxygen. Both the fatty acid and NADH are oxidized. Human desaturases cannot introduce double bonds between carbon 9 and the methyl end. Therefore, m ≤ 7.

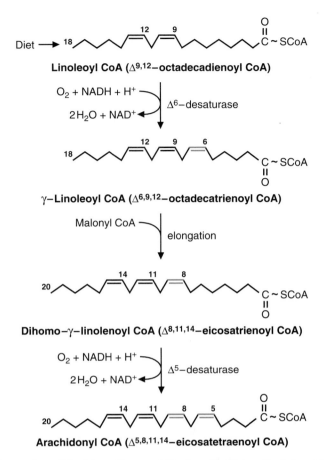

Fig. 33.19. Conversion of linoleic acid to arachidonic acid. Dietary linoleic acid (as linoleoyl CoA) is desaturated at carbon 6, elongated by 2 carbons, and then desaturated at carbon 5 to produce arachidonyl CoA.

In both adipose tissue and liver, triacylglycerols are produced by a pathway in which glycerol 3-phosphate reacts with fatty acyl CoA to form phosphatidic acid. Dephosphorylation of phosphatidic acid produces diacylglycerol. Another fatty acyl CoA reacts with the diacylglycerol to form a triacylglycerol (see Fig. 33.20).

The triacylglycerol, which is produced in the smooth endoplasmic reticulum of the liver, is packaged with cholesterol, phospholipids, and proteins (synthesized in the rough endoplasmic reticulum) to form VLDL (Fig. 33.21). The major protein of VLDL is apoB-100. There is one long apoB-100 molecule wound through the surface of each VLDL particle. ApoB-100 is encoded by the same gene as the apoB-48 of chylomicrons, but is a longer protein (Fig. 33.22). In intestinal cells, RNA editing produces a smaller mRNA and, thus, a shorter protein, apoB-48.

VLDL is processed in the Golgi complex and secreted into the blood by the liver (Figs. 33.23 and 33.24). The fatty acid residues of the triacylglycerols ultimately are stored in the triacylglycerols of adipose cells.

FATE OF VLDL TRIACYLGLYCEROL

LPL, which is attached to the basement membrane proteoglycans of capillary endothelial cells, cleaves the triacylglycerols in both VLDL and chylomicrons, forming fatty acids and glycerol. The C_{II} apoprotein, which these lipoproteins obtain from

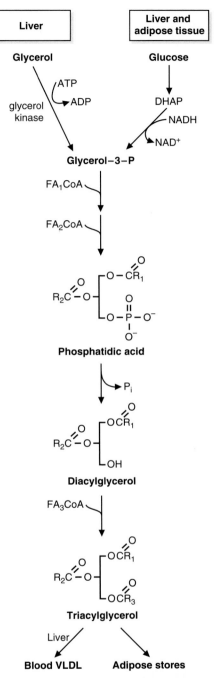

Fig. 33.20. Synthesis of triacylglycerol in liver and adipose tissue. Glycerol 3-phosphate is produced from glucose in both tissues. It is also produced from glycerol in liver, but not in adipose tissue, which lacks glycerol kinase. The steps from glycerol 3-phosphate are the same in the two tissues. FA = fatty acyl group.

Q 33.2: Why do some alcoholics have high VLDL levels?

Fatty acids for VLDL synthesis in the liver may be obtained from the blood or they may be synthesized from glucose. In a healthy individual, the major source of the fatty acids of VLDL triacylglycerol is excess dietary glucose. In individuals with diabetes mellitus, fatty acids mobilized from adipose triacylglycerols in excess of the oxidative capacity of tissues are a major source of the fatty acids re-esterified in liver to VLDL triacylglycerol. These individuals frequently have elevated levels of blood triacylglycerols.

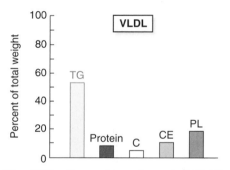

Fig. 33.21. Composition of a typical VLDL particle. The major component is triacylglycerol (TG). C = cholesterol; CE = cholesterol ester; PL = phospholipid.

A 33.2: In alcoholism, NADH levels in the liver are elevated (see Chapter 27). High levels of NADH inhibit the oxidation of fatty acids. Therefore, fatty acids, mobilized from adipose tissue, are re-esterified to glycerol in the liver, forming triacylglycerols, which are packaged into VLDL and secreted into the blood. Elevated VLDL is frequently associated with chronic alcoholism. As alcoholic liver disease progresses, the ability to secrete the triacylglycerols is diminished, resulting in a fatty liver.

HDL, activates LPL. The low K_m of the muscle LPL isozyme permits muscle to use the fatty acids of chylomicrons and VLDL as a source of fuel even when the blood concentration of these lipoproteins is very low. The isozyme in adipose tissue has a high K_m and is most active following a meal when blood levels of chylomicrons and VLDL are elevated.

STORAGE OF TRIACYLGLYCEROLS IN ADIPOSE TISSUE

After a meal, the triacylglycerol stores of adipose tissue increase (Fig. 33.25). Adipose cells synthesize LPL and secrete it into the capillaries of adipose tissue when the insulin/glucagon ratio is elevated. This enzyme digests the triacylglycerols of both chylomicrons and VLDL. The fatty acids enter adipose cells and are activated, forming fatty acyl CoA, which reacts with glycerol 3-phosphate to form triacylglycerol by the same pathway used in the liver (see Fig. 33.20). Because adipose tissue lacks glycerol kinase and cannot use the glycerol produced by LPL, the glycerol travels through the blood to the liver, which uses it for the synthesis of triacylglycerol. In adipose cells, glycerol 3-phosphate is derived from glucose.

In addition to stimulating the synthesis and release of LPL, insulin stimulates glucose metabolism in adipose cells. Insulin activates the glycolytic enzyme phosphofructokinase-1 by increasing fructose 2,6-bisphosphate levels. It also stimulates the dephosphorylation of pyruvate dehydrogenase, so that the pyruvate produced by glycolysis can be oxidized in the TCA cycle. Furthermore, insulin stimulates the conversion of glucose to fatty acids in adipose cells, although the liver is the major site of fatty acid synthesis in humans.

RELEASE OF FATTY ACIDS FROM ADIPOSE TRIACYLGLYCEROLS

During fasting, the decrease of insulin and the increase of glucagon cause cAMP levels to rise in adipose cells, stimulating lipolysis (Fig. 33.26). Protein kinase A phosphorylates hormone-sensitive lipase to produce a more active form of the enzyme. Hormone-sensitive lipase, also known as adipose triacylglycerol lipase, cleaves a fatty acid from a triacylglycerol. Subsequently, other lipases complete the process of lipolysis, and fatty acids and glycerol are released into the blood.

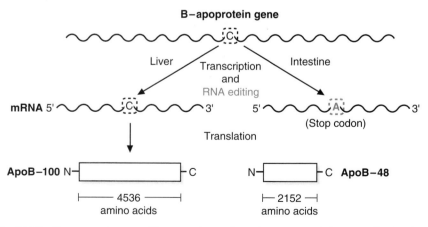

Fig. 33.22. B-apoprotein gene. The gene, located on chromosome 2, is transcribed and translated in liver to produce apoB-100, which is 4,536 amino acids in length (one of the longest single polypeptide chains). In intestinal cells, RNA editing converts a cytosine (C) to an adenine (A), producing a stop codon. Consequently, the B-apoprotein of intestinal cells (apoB-48) contains only 2,152 amino acids. ApoB-48 is 48% of the size of apoB-100.

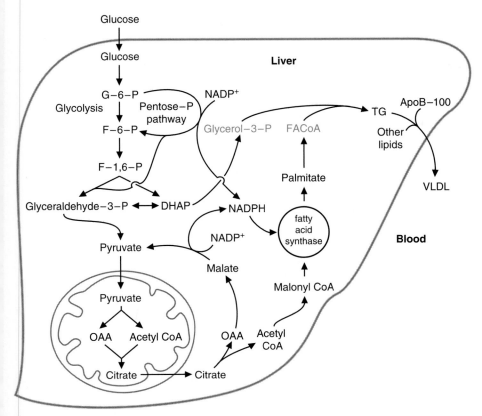

Fig. 33.23. Synthesis of VLDL from glucose in the liver. G-6-P = glucose 6-phosphate; F-6-P = fructose 6-phosphate; F-1,6-P = fructose 1,6-bisphosphate; FA = fatty acyl group; TG = triacylglycerol.

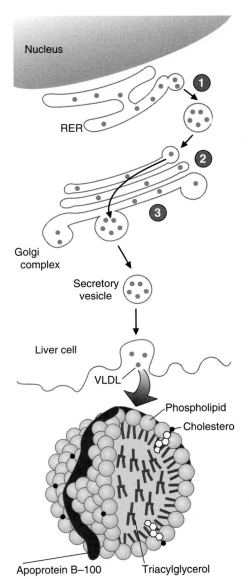

Fig. 33.24. Synthesis, processing, and secretion of VLDL. Proteins synthesized on the rough endoplasmic reticulum (RER) are packaged with triacylglycerols in the Golgi complex to form VLDL. VLDL are transported to the cell membrane in secretory vesicles and secreted by endocytosis. Blue dots represent VLDL particles. An enlarged VLDL particle is depicted at the bottom of the figure.

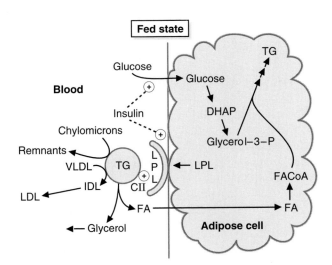

Fig. 33.25. Conversion of the fatty acid (FA) from the triacylglycerols (TG) of chylomicrons and VLDL to the triacylglycerols stored in adipose cells. Note that insulin stimulates (⊕) the transport of glucose into adipose cells. Glucose provides the glycerol 3-phosphate for TG synthesis. Insulin also stimulates the synthesis and secretion of lipoprotein lipase (LPL). Apoprotein C$_{II}$ activates LPL.

Q 33.3: In some cases of hyper-lipidemia, LPL is defective. If a blood lipid profile is performed on patients with an LPL deficiency, which lipids would be elevated?

The fact that a number of different abnormal lipoprotein profiles were found in **Cora Nari** and her siblings and that each had evidence of coronary artery disease, suggests that Cora has familial combined hyperlipidemia (FCH). This diagnostic impression is further supported by the finding that Cora's profile of lipid abnormalities appeared to change somewhat from one determination to the next, a characteristic of FCH. This hereditary disorder of lipid metabolism is believed to be quite common with an estimated prevalence of about 1 per 100 population.

The mechanisms for FCH are incompletely understood but may involve a genetically determined increase in the production of apoprotein B-100. As a result, packaging of VLDL is increased, and blood VLDL levels may be elevated. Depending on the efficiency of lipolysis of VLDL by LPL, VLDL levels may be normal and LDL levels may be elevated, or both VLDL and LDL levels may be high. In addition, the phenotypic expression of FCH in any given family member may be determined by the degree of associated obesity, the diet, the use of specific drugs, or other factors which change over time.

Because the fatty acids of adipose triacylglycerols come both from chylomicrons and VLDL, we produce our major fat stores both from dietary fat (which produces chylomicrons) and dietary sugar (which produces VLDL). An excess of dietary protein can also be used to produce the fatty acids for VLDL synthesis.

The dietician carefully explained to **Teresa Livermore** that we can get fat from eating excess fat, excess sugar, or excess protein.

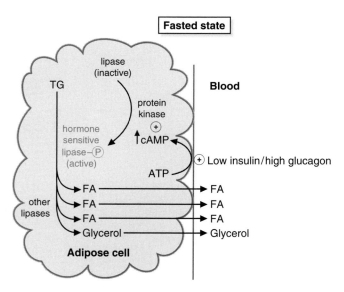

Fig. 33.26. Mobilization of adipose triacylglycerol (TG). In the fed state, when insulin levels are low and glucagon is elevated, cAMP increases and activates (⊕) protein kinase A, which phosphorylates hormone-sensitive lipase (HSL). Phosphorylated HSL is active and initiates the breakdown of adipose TG. HSL is also called triacylglycerol lipase. FA = fatty acid.

The fatty acids, which travel in the blood complexed with albumin, enter cells of muscle and other tissues, where they are oxidized to CO_2 and water to produce energy. During fasting, acetyl CoA produced by β-oxidation of fatty acids in the liver is converted to ketone bodies, which are released into the blood. The glycerol derived from lipolysis in adipose cells is used by the liver during fasting as a source of carbon for gluconeogenesis.

METABOLISM OF GLYCEROPHOSPHOLIPIDS AND SPHINGOLIPIDS

Fatty acids, obtained from the diet or synthesized from glucose, are the precursors of glycerophospholipids and of sphingolipids (Fig. 33.27). These lipids are major components of cellular membranes. Glycerophospholipids are also components of blood lipoproteins, bile, and lung surfactant. They are the source of the polyunsaturated fatty acids, particularly arachidonic acid, that serve as precursors of the eicosanoids (e.g., prostaglandins, thromboxanes, leukotrienes). Ether glycerophospholipids differ from other glycerophospholipids in that the alkyl or alkenyl chain (an alkyl chain with a double bond) is joined to carbon 1 of the glycerol moiety by an ether rather than an ester bond. Examples of ether lipids are the plasmalogens and platelet activating factor. Sphingolipids are particularly important in forming the myelin sheath surrounding nerves in the central nervous system.

In glycerolipids and ether glycerolipids, glycerol serves as the backbone to which fatty acids and other substituents are attached. Sphingosine, derived from serine, provides the backbone for sphingolipids.

Synthesis of Phospholipids Containing Glycerol

GLYCEROPHOSPHOLIPIDS

The initial steps in the synthesis of glycerophospholipids are similar to those of triacylglycerol synthesis. Glycerol 3-phosphate reacts with fatty acyl CoA to form

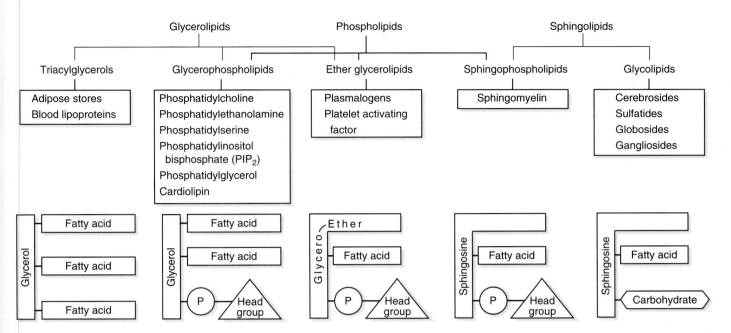

Fig. 33.27. Types of glycerolipids and sphingolipids. Glycerolipids contain glycerol, and sphingolipids contain sphingosine. The category of phospholipids overlaps both glycero- and sphingolipids. The head groups include choline, ethanolamine, serine, inositol, glycerol, and phosphatidylglycerol. The carbohydrates are monosaccharides (which may be sulfated), oligosaccharides, and oligosaccharides with branches of N-acetylneuraminic acid. P = phosphate.

phosphatidic acid. Two different mechanisms are then used to add a head group to the molecule (Fig. 33.28). A head group is a chemical group, such as choline or serine, attached to carbon 3 of a glycerol moiety that contains hydrophobic groups, usually fatty acids, at positions 1 and 2. Head groups are hydrophilic, either charged or polar.

In the first mechanism, phosphatidic acid is cleaved by a phosphatase to form diacylglycerol (DAG). DAG then reacts with an activated head group. In the synthesis of phosphatidylcholine, the head group choline is activated by combining with CTP to form CDP-choline (Fig. 33.29). Phosphocholine is then transferred to carbon 3 of DAG, and CMP is released. Phosphatidylethanolamine is produced by a similar reaction involving CDP-ethanolamine.

Various types of interconversions occur among these phospholipids (see Fig. 33.29). Phosphatidylserine is produced by a reaction in which the ethanolamine moiety of phosphatidylethanolamine is exchanged for serine. Phosphatidylserine can be converted back to phosphatidylethanolamine by a decarboxylation reaction. Phosphatidylethanolamine can be methylated to form phosphatidylcholine (see Chapter 40).

In the second mechanism for the synthesis of glycerolipids, phosphatidic acid reacts with CTP to form CDP-diacylglycerol (Fig. 33.30). This compound can react with phosphatidylglycerol to produce cardiolipin or with inositol to produce phosphatidylinositol. Cardiolipin is a component of the inner mitochondrial membrane. Phosphatidylinositol can be phosphorylated to form phosphatidylinositol 4,5-bisphosphate (PIP_2), which is a component of cell membranes. In response to signals such as the binding of hormones to membrane receptors, PIP_2 can be cleaved to form the second messengers diacylglycerol and inositol trisphosphate (see Chapter 43).

A 33.3: Individuals with a defective LPL have high blood triacylglycerol levels. Their levels of chylomicrons and VLDL (which contain large amounts of triacylglycerols) are elevated because they are not digested at the normal rate by LPL.

LPL can be dissociated from capillary walls by treatment with heparin (a glycosaminoglycan). Measurements can be made on blood after heparin treatment to determine if LPL levels are abnormal.

Phosphatidylcholine (lecithin) is not required in the diet because it can be synthesized in the body. The components of phosphatidylcholine (including choline) can all be produced as shown in Figure 33.29 and can be synthesized from glucose.

Because choline is widely distributed in the food supply, primarily in phosphatidylcholine (lecithin), deficiencies have not been observed in humans on a normal diet. Deficiencies may occur, however, in patients on total parental nutrition (TPN), i.e., supported solely by intravenous feeding. The fatty livers which have been observed in these patients probably result from a decreased ability to synthesize phospholipids for VLDL formation.

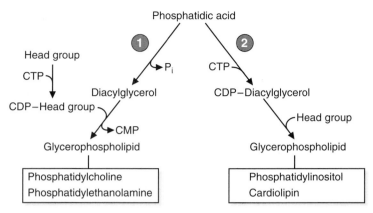

Fig. 33.28. Strategies for addition of the head group to form glycerophospholipids. In both cases, CTP is used to drive the reaction.

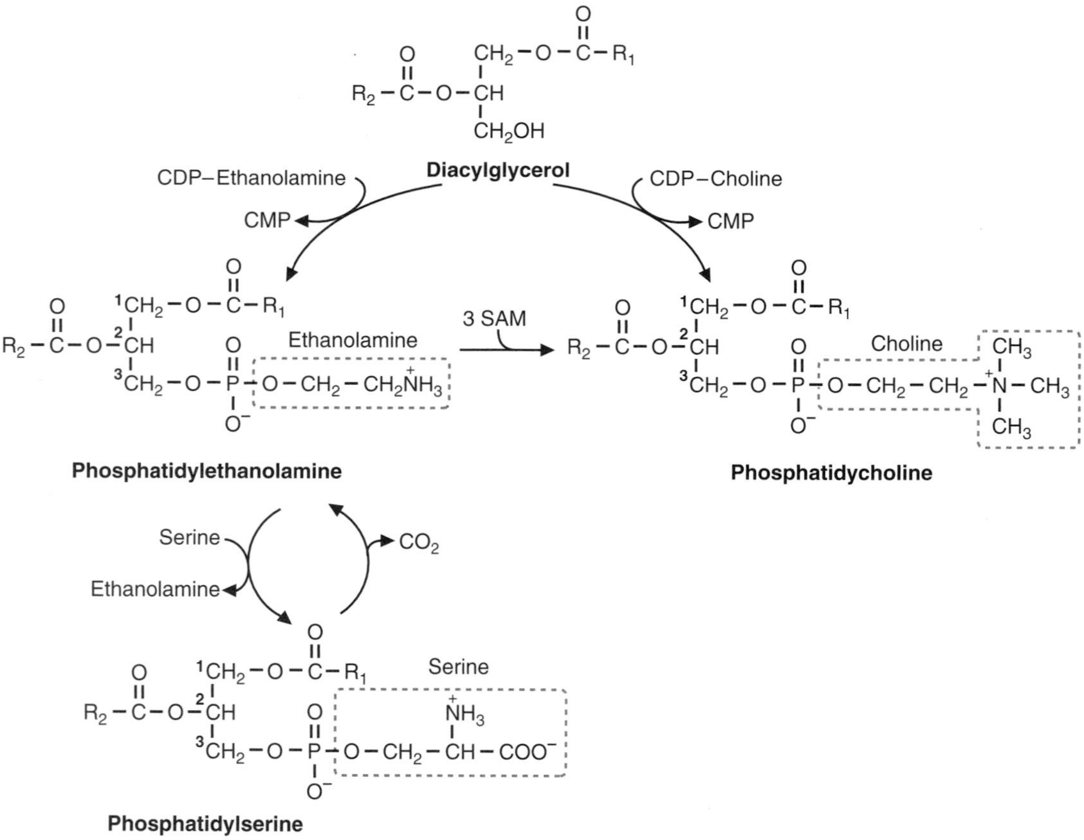

Fig. 33.29. Synthesis of phosphatidylcholine, phosphatidylethanolamine, and phosphatidylserine. The multiple pathways reflect the importance of phospholipids in membrane structure. For example, phosphatidylcholine (PC) can be synthesized from dietary choline when it is available. If choline is not available, PC can be made from dietary carbohydrate. SAM is *S*-adenosylmethionine, a methyl group donor for many biochemical reactions (see Chapter 40).

The respiratory distress syndrome (RDS) of a premature infant like **Colleen Lakker** is, in part, related to a deficiency in the synthesis of a substance known as lung surfactant. The major constituents of surfactant are dipalmitoylphosphatidylcholine, phosphatidylglycerol, apoproteins (surfactant proteins: Sp-A,B,C), and cholesterol.

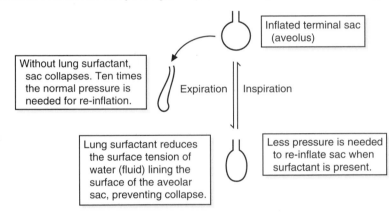

**Dipalmitoylphosphatidycholine,
the major component of
lung surfactant**

These components of lung surfactant normally contribute to a reduction in the surface tension within the air spaces (alveoli) of the lung, preventing their collapse. The premature infant has not yet begun to produce adequate amounts of lung surfactant.

Inflated terminal sac (aveolus)

Without lung surfactant, sac collapses. Ten times the normal pressure is needed for re-inflation.

Expiration | Inspiration

Lung surfactant reduces the surface tension of water (fluid) lining the surface of the aveolar sac, preventing collapse.

Less pressure is needed to re-inflate sac when surfactant is present.

The effect of lung surfactant

ETHER GLYCEROLIPIDS

The ether glycerolipids are synthesized from the glycolytic intermediate dihydroxyacetone phosphate (DHAP). A fatty acyl CoA reacts with carbon 1 of DHAP, forming an ester (Fig. 33.31). This fatty acyl group is exchanged for a fatty alcohol, produced by reduction of a fatty acid. Thus the ether linkage is formed. Then the keto group on carbon 2 of the DHAP moiety is reduced and esterified to a fatty acid. Addition of the head group proceeds by a series of reactions analogous to those for synthesis of phosphatidylcholine. Formation of a double bond between carbons 1 and 2 of the alkyl group produces a plasmalogen. Ethanolamine plasmalogen is found in myelin and choline plasmalogen in heart muscle. Platelet activating factor (PAF) is similar to choline plasmalogen except that an acetyl group replaces the fatty acyl group at carbon 2 of the glycerol moiety and the alkyl group on carbon 1 is saturated. PAF is released from phagocytic blood cells in response to various stimuli. It causes platelet aggregation, edema, and hypotension, and is involved in the allergic response.

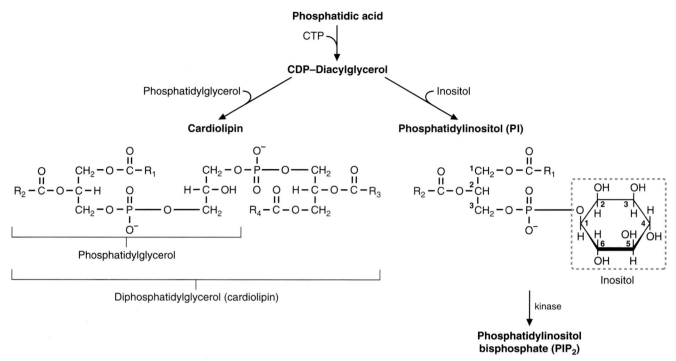

Fig. 33.30. Synthesis of cardiolipin and phosphatidylinositol.

Degradation of Glycerophospholipids

Phospholipases located in cell membranes or in lysosomes degrade glycerophospholipids. Phospholipase A_1 removes the fatty acyl group on carbon 1 of the glycerol moiety, and phospholipase A_2 removes the fatty acid on carbon 2 (Fig. 33.32). The C2 fatty acid in cell membrane phospholipids is frequently arachidonic acid. It is removed in response to signals for the synthesis of eicosanoids. The bond joining carbon 3 of the glycerol moiety to phosphate is cleaved by phospholipase C. Hormonal stimuli activate phospholipase C, which hydrolyzes PIP_2 to produce the second messengers DAG and inositol trisphosphate (IP_3) (see Chapter 43). The bond between the phosphate and the head group is cleaved by phospholipase D.

Sphingolipids

Sphingolipids serve in intercellular communication and as the antigenic determinants of the ABO blood group. Some are used as receptors by viruses and bacterial toxins, although it is unlikely that this was the purpose for which they originally evolved. Before the functions of the sphingolipids were elucidated, these compounds appeared to be inscrutable riddles. They were, therefore, named for the Sphinx of Thebes, who killed passersby that could not solve her riddle.

The synthesis of sphingolipids begins with the formation of ceramide (Fig. 33.33). Serine and palmitoyl CoA condense to form a product that is reduced. A very long chain fatty acid (usually containing 22 carbons) forms an amide with the amino group, a double bond is generated, and ceramide is formed.

Ceramide reacts with phosphatidylcholine to form sphingomyelin, a component of the myelin sheath (Fig. 33.34). Ceramide also reacts with UDP-sugars to form cerebrosides (which contain a single monosaccharide, usually galactose or glucose). Galactocerebroside may react with 3′-phosphoadenosine 5′-phosphosulfate (PAPS) to form sulfatides, the major sulfolipids of brain.

Phospholipase A_2 provides the major repair mechanism for membrane lipids damaged by oxidative free radical reactions. Arachidonic acid, which is a polyunsaturated fatty acid, can be peroxidatively cleaved in free radical reactions to malondialdehyde and other products. Phospholipase A_2 recognizes the distortion of membrane structure caused by the partially degraded fatty acid, and removes it. Acyltransferases then add back a new arachidonic acid molecule.

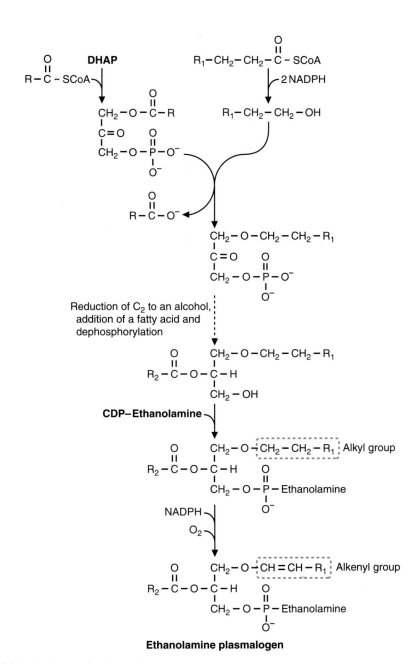

Fig. 33.31. Synthesis of a plasmalogen.

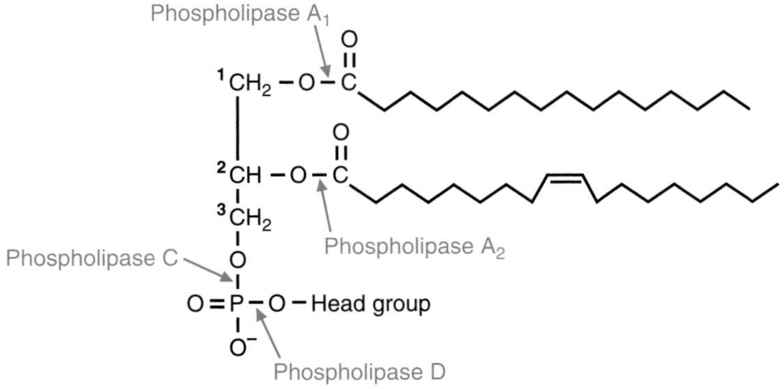

Fig. 33.32. Bonds cleaved by phospholipases.

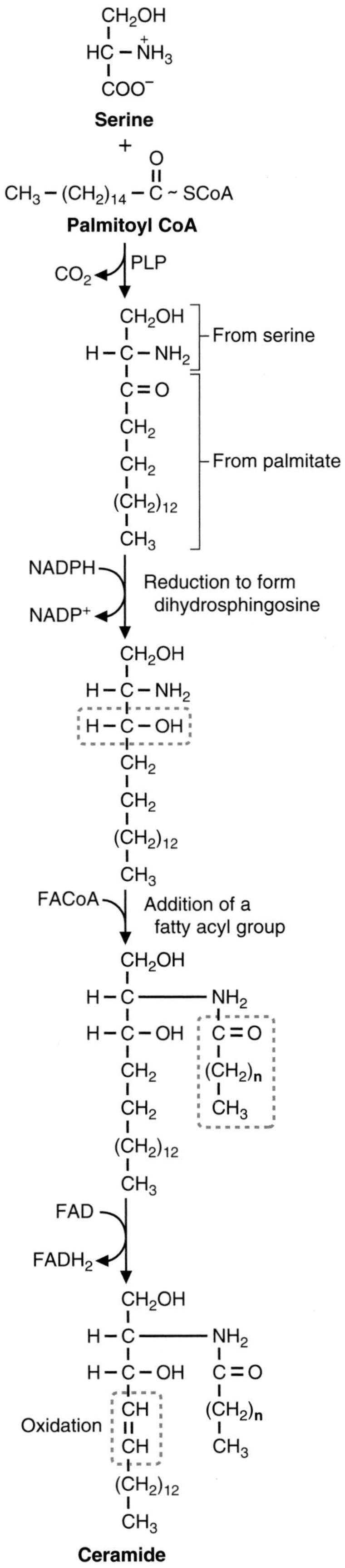

Fig. 33.33. Synthesis of ceramide. The changes that occur in each reaction are highlighted.

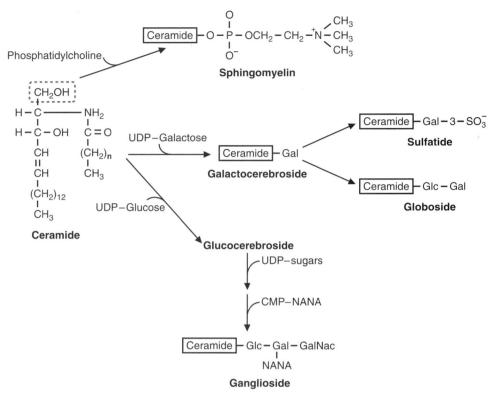

Fig. 33.34. Synthesis of sphingolipids from ceramide. Phosphocholine or sugars add to the hydroxymethyl group of ceramide (in blue) to form sphingomyelins, cerebrosides, sulfatides, globosides, and gangliosides.

Gal = galactose; Glc = gucose; GalNAc = *N*-acetylgalactosamine; NANA = *N*-acetylneuraminic acid.

Additional sugars may be added to ceramide to form globosides, and gangliosides are produced by the addition of *N*-acetylneuraminic acid (NANA) as branches from the oligosaccharide chains (see Fig. 33.34 and Chapter 30).

Sphingolipids are degraded by lysosomal enzymes (see Chapter 30). Deficiencies of these enzymes result in a group of lysosomal storage diseases known as the sphingolipidoses.

CLINICAL COMMENTS. If **Teresa Livermore** had continued to eat a hypercaloric diet rich in carbohydrates, she would have become obese. In an effort to define obesity, it has been agreed internationally that the ratio of the patient's body weight in kilograms and their height in meters squared (W/H^2) is the most useful and reproducible measure. This ratio is referred to as the body mass index or BMI. Normal men and women fall into the range of 20–25. Teresa's current value is 23.4 and rising.

It is estimated that approximately 36 million people in the United States have a BMI greater than 27.8 (for men) or 27.3 (for women). At this level of obesity, which is quite close to a 20% weight increase above the "ideal" or desirable weight, an attempt at weight loss should be strongly advised. The idea that obesity is a benign condition unless accompanied by other risk factors for cardiovascular disease is disputed by several long term properly controlled prospective studies. These studies show that obesity is an independent risk factor not only for heart attacks and strokes, but for the development of insulin resistance, diabetes mellitus (NIDDM), hypertension, and gallbladder disease.

Cholera toxin, produced by the bacterium *Vibrio cholerae*, binds to the G_{M1} ganglioside on intestinal mucosal cells. The B subunit of the toxin contains the binding site, and the A subunit enters the cell and activates adenylate cyclase. cAMP levels rise and stimulate the transport of chloride ions into the lumen of the gut, causing severe diarrhea that, if untreated, is often fatal.

Teresa did not want to become overweight and decided to follow her new diet faithfully.

Because **Cora Nari's** lipid profile revealed an elevation in both serum triacylglycerols and LDL cholesterol, she was classified as having a combined hyperlipidemia. The dissimilarities in the lipid profiles of Cora and her two siblings, both of whom were experiencing anginal chest pain, is characteristic of the multigenic syndrome referred to as familial combined hyperlipidemia (FCH).

Approximately 1% of the North American population has FCH. It is the most common cause of coronary artery disease in the United States. In contrast to patients with familial hypercholesterolemia (FH), patients with FCH do not have fatty deposits within the skin or tendons (xanthomas) (see Chapter 34). In FCH, coronary artery disease usually appears by the fifth decade of life.

Treatment of FCH includes restriction of dietary fat. Patients who do not respond adequately to dietary therapy are treated with antilipidemic drugs. Selection of the appropriate antilipidemic drugs depends upon the specific phenotypic expression of the patient's multigenic disease as manifest by their particular serum lipid profile. In Cora's case, a decrease in both serum triacylglycerols and LDL cholesterol must be achieved. If possible, her serum HDL cholesterol level should also be raised to a level above 45 mg/dL.

To accomplish these therapeutic goals, her physician initially prescribed fast-release nicotinic acid (niacin) because this agent has the potential to lower serum triacylglycerol levels and cause a reciprocal rise in serum HDL cholesterol levels, as well as to lower serum total and LDL cholesterol levels. The mechanisms suggested for niacin's triacylglycerol-lowering action include enhancement of the action of LPL, inhibition of lipolysis in adipose tissue, and a decrease in esterification of triacylglycerols in the liver. The mechanism by which niacin lowers the serum total and LDL cholesterol levels is related to the decrease in hepatic production of VLDL. When the level of VLDL in the circulation falls, the production of its daughter particles, IDL and LDL, also falls. Cora found niacin's side effects of flushing and itching to be intolerable and the drug was discontinued.

Pravastatin was given instead. Pravastatin inhibits cholesterol synthesis by inhibiting hydroxymethylglutaryl CoA (HMG-CoA) reductase, the rate limiting enzyme in the pathway (see Chapter 34). After 3 months of therapy, pravastatin decreased Cora's LDL cholesterol from a pretreatment level of 175 to 122 mg/dL (still higher than the recommended treatment goal of 100 mg/dL or less in a patient with established coronary artery disease). Her fasting serum triacylglycerol concentration was decreased from a pretreatment level of 280 to 178 mg/dL (a treatment goal for serum triacylglycerol when the pretreatment level is less than 500 mg/dL has not been established).

Colleen Lakker suffered from respiratory distress syndrome (RDS), which is a major cause of death in the newborn. RDS is preventable if prematurity can be avoided by appropriate management of high risk pregnancy and labor. Prior to delivery, the obstetrician must attempt to predict and possibly treat pulmonary prematurity in utero. For example, estimation of fetal head circumference by ultrasonography, monitoring for fetal asphyxia, and determination of the ratio of the concentrations of phosphatidylcholine (lecithin) and that of sphingomyelin in the amniotic fluid may help to identify premature infants who are predisposed to RDS (Fig. 33.35).

The administration of synthetic corticosteroids 48–72 hours prior to delivery of a fetus of less than 33 weeks of gestation in women who have toxemia of pregnancy, diabetes mellitus, or chronic renal disease may reduce the incidence and/or mortality of RDS by stimulating fetal synthesis of lung surfactant.

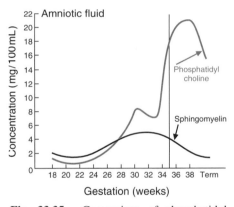

Fig. 33.35. Comparison of phosphatidylcholine and sphingomyelin in amniotic fluid. Phosphatidylcholine is the major lipid in lung surfactant. The concentration of phosphatidylcholine relative to sphingomyelin rises at 35 weeks of gestation, indicating pulmonary maturity.

The administration of one dose of surfactant into the trachea of the premature infant immediately after birth may transiently improve respiratory function but does not improve overall mortality. In Colleen's case, intensive therapy allowed her to survive this acute respiratory complication of prematurity.

 BIOCHEMICAL COMMENTS. Biochemically, what makes people become obese? Obviously, the amount of fat an individual can store depends on the number of fat cells in the body and the amount of triacylglycerol each cell can accommodate. In obese individuals, both the number of fat cells and the size of the cells (i.e., the total storage capacity) is greater than in individuals with no history of obesity. In order to fill these stores, however, an individual must eat more than required to support the basal metabolic rate and physical activity.

Fat cells begin to proliferate early in life, starting in the third trimester of gestation. Proliferation essentially ceases before puberty, and thereafter fat cells change mainly in size. However, some increase in the number of fat cells can occur in adulthood if preadipocytes are induced to proliferate by growth factors and changes in the nutritional state. Weight reduction results in a decrease in the size of fat cells rather than a decrease in number. After weight loss, the amount of LPL, an enzyme involved in the transfer of fatty acids from blood triacylglycerols to the triacylglycerol stores of adipocytes, increases. In addition, the amount of mRNA for LPL also increases. All of these factors suggest that individuals who become obese, particularly those who do so early in life, will have difficulty losing weight and maintaining a lower body mass.

Signals that initiate or inhibit feeding are extremely complex and include psychological and hormonal factors as well as neurotransmitter activity. These signals are integrated and relayed through the hypothalamus. Destruction of specific regions of the hypothalamus can lead to overeating and obesity or to anorexia and weight loss. Overeating and obesity are associated with damage to the ventromedial or the paraventricular nucleus, whereas weight loss and anorexia are related to damage to more lateral hypothalamic regions. Recently, two new compounds that act as satiety signals have been identified in brain tissue. They are leptin and glucagon-like peptide-1 (GLP-1). Appetite suppressors developed from compounds such as these may be used in the future for the treatment of obesity.

Although an increase in food intake beyond the daily requirements results in an increase in body weight and in fat stores, there is a large variation among individuals in the amount of weight gained for a given number of excess calories consumed. Both genetic and environmental factors influence the development of obesity. Studies of identical twins who were purposely overfed showed that the amount of weight gained was more similar within sets than between sets. Other studies of identical and fraternal twins, where the members of a set were reared apart, support the conclusion that heredity plays a major role in determining body weight.

Suggested Readings

Bouchard C, Tremblay A, Despres J-P, et al. The response to long-term overfeeding in identical twins. N Engl J Med 1990;322:1477–1482.

Girard J, Perderbeau D, Foufelle F, Prip-Buus C, Ferre P. Regulation of lipogenic enzyme gene expression by nutrients and hormones. FASEB J 1994;8:36–42.

Kern PA, Ong JM, Bahman S, Carty J. The effects of weight loss on the activity and expression of adipose-tissue lipoprotein lipase in very obese humans. N Engl J Med 1990;322:1053–1059.

Stunkard A, Harris J, Pedersen N, McClearn G. The body-mass index of twins who have been reared apart. N Engl J Med 1990;322:1483–1487.

PROBLEM

Under which conditions do we get fatter: (*a*) if we eat excess calories in the form of dietary fat, or (*b*) if we eat the same number of excess calories in the form of dietary carbohydrate?

ANSWER

We use more energy to produce fat stores from dietary glucose than from dietary fat. Therefore, if the same number of excess calories are consumed, we should get fatter by eating fat than by eating sugar.

The conversion of dietary triacylglycerols to the triacylglycerols of chylomicrons and then to the triacylglycerols of adipose tissue does not require as much energy as the conversion of dietary glucose to fatty acids, then to the triacylglycerols secreted as VLDL from the liver, followed by storage as adipose triacylglycerol.

For storage of dietary fat, energy is consumed in the intestinal epithelial cell and the adipocyte during the activation of the fatty acids. Energy is also required to convert glucose to glycerol 3-phosphate in the adipocyte. In addition, to store dietary glucose as fat, ATP is also required to convert glucose to palmitate. The ATP produced by phosphoglycerate kinase and pyruvate kinase is more than offset by the ATP required by glucokinase, phosphofructokinase-1, pyruvate carboxylase, citrate lyase, and acetyl CoA carboxylase. Although energy in the form of the reducing equivalents of NADH is generated by glyceraldehyde 3-phosphate dehydrogenase and pyruvate dehydrogenase, it is consumed in the form of NADPH by the reactions of the fatty acid synthase complex.

Try this exercise: Calculate the amount of ATP required to produce tripalmitin in adipose tissue from dietary tripalmitin or from dietary glucose. (Remember that tripalmitin has 51 carbon atoms.)

34 Cholesterol Metabolism and the Blood Lipoproteins

Cholesterol, which is transported in the blood in lipoproteins, serves as a stabilizing component of cell membranes and as a precursor of the bile salts and steroid hormones (Fig. 34.1). Precursors of cholesterol are converted to ubiquinone, dolichol, and, in the skin, to cholecalciferol, the active form of vitamin D (see Chapter 46).

Cholesterol is obtained from the diet or synthesized by a pathway that occurs in most cells of the body, but to a greater extent in cells of the liver and intestine. The precursor for cholesterol synthesis is acetyl CoA, which can be produced from glucose, fatty acids, or amino acids. Two molecules of acetyl CoA form acetoacetyl CoA, which condenses with another molecule of acetyl CoA to form hydroxymethylglutaryl CoA (HMG-CoA). Reduction of HMG-CoA produces mevalonate. This reaction, catalyzed by HMG-CoA reductase, is the major rate-limiting step of cholesterol synthesis. Mevalonate produces isoprene units that condense, eventually forming squalene. Cyclization of squalene produces the steroid ring system, and a number of subsequent reactions generates cholesterol (Fig. 34.2).

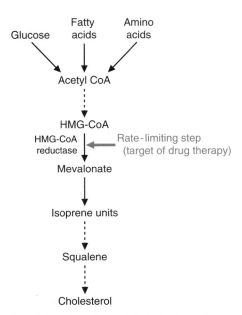

Fig. 34.2. Overview of cholesterol synthesis.

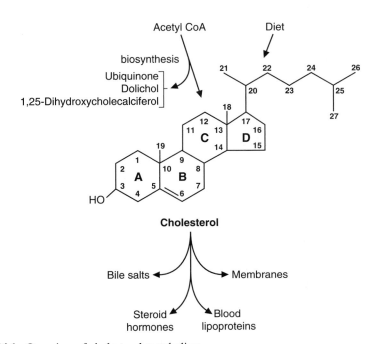

Fig. 34.1. Overview of cholesterol metabolism.

Cholesterol is packaged in chylomicrons in the intestine and in very low density lipoprotein (VLDL) in the liver (Table 34.1). It is transported in the blood in these lipoprotein particles, which also transport triacylglycerols. As the triacylglycerols of the blood lipoproteins are digested by lipoprotein lipase, chylomicrons are converted to chylomicron remnants and VLDL is converted to intermediate density lipoprotein (IDL) and subsequently to low density lipoprotein (LDL). These products return to the liver, where they bind to receptors in cell membranes and are taken up by endocytosis and digested by lysosomal enzymes. LDL is also endocytosed by nonhepatic (peripheral) tissues. Cholesterol and other products of lysosomal digestion are released into the cellular pools. The liver uses this recycled cholesterol, and the cholesterol that is synthesized from acetyl CoA, to produce VLDL and to synthesize bile salts.

Intracellular cholesterol obtained from blood lipoproteins decreases the synthesis of cholesterol within cells, stimulates the storage of cholesterol as cholesterol esters, and decreases the synthesis of LDL receptors. LDL receptors are found on the surface of the cells and bind various classes of lipoproteins prior to endocytosis.

Although high density lipoprotein (HDL) contains triacylglycerols and cholesterol, its function is very different from that of the chylomicrons and VLDL, which transport triacylglycerols (Table 34.2). HDL exchanges proteins and lipids with the other lipoproteins in the blood. HDL transfers apolipoprotein E (apoE) and apoC$_{II}$ to chylomicrons and VLDL. Following digestion of the VLDL triacylglycerols, apoE and apoC$_{II}$ are transferred back to HDL. In addition, HDL obtains cholesterol from other lipoproteins and from cell membranes and converts it to cholesterol esters by the lecithin:cholesterol acyltransferase (LCAT) reaction. Then HDL either directly transports cholesterol and cholesterol esters to the liver or transfers cholesterol esters to other lipoproteins via the cholesterol ester transfer protein (CETP). Ultimately, lipoprotein particles carry the cholesterol and cholesterol esters to the liver, where endocytosis and lysosomal digestion occur. Thus, "reverse cholesterol transport" (i.e., the return of cholesterol to the liver) is a major function of HDL (see Table 34.2).

Elevated levels of cholesterol in the blood are associated with the formation of atherosclerotic plaques that can occlude blood vessels, causing heart attacks and strokes. Although high levels of LDL cholesterol are especially atherogenic, high levels of HDL cholesterol are protective because HDL particles are involved in the process of removing cholesterol from tissues and returning it to the liver.

Table 34.1. Blood Lipoproteins[a]

Chylomicrons
  Chylomicron remnants

VLDL
  IDL
    LDL

HDL

[a]The major blood lipoproteins are listed. Indented lipoproteins are derivatives of the lipoprotein listed above.

Table 34.2. Functions of HDL

• Transfers proteins to other lipoproteins
• Picks up lipids from other lipoproteins
• Picks up cholesterol from cell membranes
• Converts cholesterol to cholesterol esters via the LCAT reaction
• Transfers cholesterol esters to other lipoproteins, which transport them to the liver

Bile salts, which are produced in the liver from cholesterol obtained from the blood lipoproteins or synthesized from acetyl CoA, are secreted into the bile. They are stored in the gallbladder and released into the intestine during a meal. The bile salts emulsify dietary triacylglycerols, thus aiding in digestion. The digestive products are absorbed by intestinal epithelial cells from bile salt micelles, tiny micro-droplets that contain bile salts at their water interface. After the contents of the micelles are absorbed, most of the bile salts travel to the ileum, where they are resorbed and recycled by the liver. Less than 5% of the bile salts that enter the lumen of the small intestine are eventually excreted in the feces.

Although the fecal excretion of bile salts is relatively low, it is a major means by which the body disposes of the steroid nucleus of cholesterol. Because the ring structure of cholesterol cannot be degraded in the body, it is excreted mainly in the bile as free cholesterol and bile salts.

At his current office visit, **Thomas Appleman's** case was reviewed by his physician. Mr. Appleman has several of the major risk factors for coronary heart disease (CHD) (Table 34.3). These include a sedentary lifestyle, marked obesity, hypertension, hyperlipidemia, and early non-insulin-dependent diabetes mellitus (NIDDM). Unfortunately, he has not followed his doctor's advice with regard to a diabetic diet designed to effect a significant loss of weight nor has he followed an aerobic exercise program. As a consequence, his weight has gone from 270 to 281 lb. After a 14-hour fast, his serum glucose is now 214 mg/dL (normal < 115) and his serum total cholesterol level is 314 mg/dL (desired level is 200 or less). His serum triacylglycerol level is 295 mg/dL (desired level is 160 or less), and his serum HDL cholesterol level is 24 mg/dL (desired level is 35 or more for a male). His calculated serum LDL cholesterol level is 231 mg/dL (desired level for a person with two or more risk factors for CHD is 130 or less). (See Table 34.4 for a list of the desirable levels of serum cholesterol and triacylglycerols in adults.)

Table 34.3. Some Risk Factors for Coronary Heart Disease (CHD)

- Increasing age
- Family history of premature CHD
- Current cigarette smoking
- Hypertension
- Marked obesity
- Sedentary lifestyle
- Diabetes mellitus
- High serum LDL cholesterol level
- Low serum HDL cholesterol level

Table 34.4. Desirable Levels of Serum Cholesterol and Triacylglycerols in Adults

Total cholesterol	≤200 mg/dL
LDL cholesterol	
Without CHD and with fewer than 2 risk factors	≤160 mg/dL
Without CHD and with 2 or more risk factors	≤130 mg/dL
With established CHD	<100 mg/dL
HDL cholesterol	
Female	≥45 mg/dL
Male	≥35 mg/dL
Triacylglycerols	60–160 mg/dL[a] ("normal" range)
	<500 mg/dL to prevent pancreatitis

Based on: NCEP, Second Report of the Adult Treatment Panel, JAMA 1993;269:3015–3023.

[a]Although epidemiological evidence suggests that chronic hypertriglyceridemia represents a risk for coronary heart disease (CHD), an elevation in serum triacylglycerols has not yet been proven to be a definite risk factor in atherogenesis.

Until recently, the concentration of LDL cholesterol could only be directly determined by sophisticated laboratory techniques not available for routine clinical use. As a consequence, the LDL cholesterol concentration in the blood was derived indirectly using the Friedewald formula: the sum of the HDL cholesterol level and the triacylglycerol (TG) level divided by 5 (which gives an estimate of the VLDL cholesterol level) subtracted from the total cholesterol level.

LDL cholesterol = Total cholesterol −
[HDL cholesterol + (TG/5)]

This equation yields inaccurate LDL cholesterol levels 15–20% of the time and fails completely when serum triacylglycerol levels exceed 400 mg/dL.

A new test called "LDL direct" isolates LDL cholesterol by using a special immunoseparation reagent. Not only is this direct assay for LDL cholesterol more accurate than the indirect Friedewald calculation, it also is not affected by high serum triacylglycerol levels and can be used for a patient who has not fasted. It does not require the expense of determining serum total cholesterol, HDL cholesterol, and triacylglycerol levels.

William Hartman was carefully followed by his physician after he survived his heart attack. Prior to discharge from the hospital, after a 14-hour fast, his serum triacylglycerol level was 158 mg/dL (in the upper range of normal) and his HDL cholesterol level was slightly low at 32 mg/dL (normal for men is ≥35) (see Table 34.4). His serum total cholesterol level was elevated at 420 mg/dL (reference range ≤ 200 for a male with known CHD). From these values, his LDL cholesterol level was calculated to be 356 mg/dL (desirable level for a person with established heart disease is < 100).

Both of Mr. Hartman's younger brothers had "very high" serum cholesterol levels and both had suffered heart attacks in their mid-forties. With this information, a tentative diagnosis of familial hypercholesterolemia, type IIA was made, and the patient was started on a Step I diet as recommended by the National Cholesterol Education Program (NCEP) Adult Treatment Panel II. This panel recommends that decisions with regard to when dietary and drug therapy are initiated be based on the serum LDL cholesterol level as depicted in Table 34.5.

Since a Step I diet usually lowers serum total and LDL cholesterol levels by no more than 15%, it is likely that Mr. Hartman's diet will eventually have to be further restricted in cholesterol and fat and that one or more lipid-lowering drugs will have to be added to his treatment plan.

SOURCES OF CHOLESTEROL

Cholesterol can be synthesized by most cells of the body and it is obtained from the diet in foods of animal origin. The major sources of dietary cholesterol are egg yolks and meats, particularly red meats and liver. Because cholesterol is not synthesized in plants, vegetables and fruits play a major role in low cholesterol diets. The Step I and Step II low cholesterol diets recommended by the NCEP are shown in Table 34.6. Although most animal tissues can synthesize the amount of cholesterol they require beyond that obtained from dietary sources, the liver and intestine are the major sites of cholesterol synthesis.

Table 34.5. Treatment Decisions Based on LDL Cholesterol Level

Patient Category	Initiation Level	LDL Goal
Dietary Therapy		
Without CHD and with fewer than two risk factors	≥160 mg/dL (4.1 mmol/L)	<160 mg/dL (4.1 mmol/L)
Without CHD and with two or more risk factors	≥130 mg/dL (3.4 mmol/L)	<130 mg/dL (3.4 mmol/L)
With CHD	>100 mg/dL (2.6 mmol/L)	≤100 mg/dL (2.6 mmol/L)
Drug Treatment		
Without CHD and with fewer than two risk factors	≥190 mg/dL (4.9 mmol/L)	<160 mg/dL (4.1 mmol/L)
Without CHD and with two or more risk factors	≥160 mg/dL (4.1 mmol/L)	<130 mg/dL (3.4 mmol/L)
With CHD	≥130 mg/dL (3.4 mmol/L)	≤100 mg/dL (2.6 mmol/L)

From NCEP, Second Report of the Adult Treatment Panel, JAMA, 1993; 269(23):3015–3023.

CHD = coronary heart disease.

Table 34.6. Dietary Therapy of Elevated Blood Cholesterol

Nutrient	Step I Diet	Step II Diet[a]
Cholesterol[b]	<300 mg/day	<200 mg/day
Total fat	≤30%[b]	≤30%
Saturated fat	8–10%	<7%
Polyunsaturated fat	≤10%	≤10%
Monounsaturated fat	≤15%	≤15%
Carbohydrates	≥55%	≥55%
Protein	~15%	~15%
Calories	To achieve and maintain desirable body weight	

Based on: NCEP, Second Report of the Adult Treatment Panel, JAMA, 1993;269(23):3015–3023.

[a]The Step II diet is applied if 3 months on the Step I diet has failed to reduce blood cholesterol to the desired level (see Table 34.4).

[b]Except for the values given in mg/day, all the values are percentage of total calories eaten daily.

William Hartman's serum total and LDL cholesterol levels improved only modestly after 3 months on a Step I diet. Three additional months on a more stringent low fat diet (Step II diet) brought little further improvement.

SYNTHESIS OF CHOLESTEROL

Precursors for Cholesterol Synthesis

The precursor for cholesterol synthesis is cytosolic acetyl CoA. Acetyl CoA is produced from its major precursors, glucose and fatty acids, principally in mitochondria. It is also produced from catabolism of amino acids. Acetyl CoA generated in mitochondria is carried to the cytosol by citrate, as it is for fatty acid synthesis (see Chapter 33). In the cytosol, citrate is cleaved, forming oxaloacetate and acetyl CoA.

Pathway for Cholesterol Synthesis

The pathway for the synthesis of cholesterol occurs in three phases (Fig. 34.3). In the first phase, acetyl CoA units condense to form mevalonate. In the second phase, mevalonate is converted to 5-carbon isoprene units, which are phosphorylated and

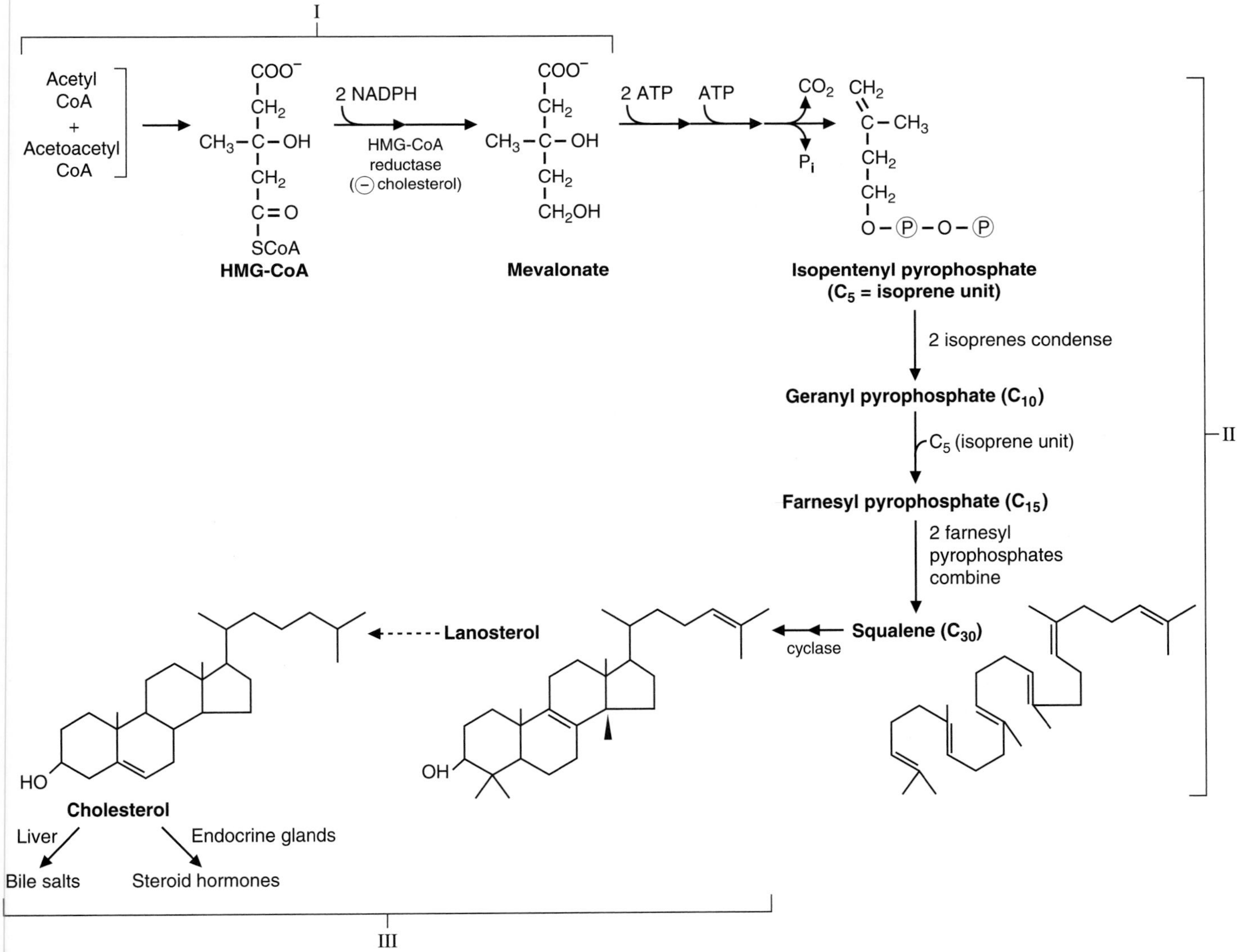

In plants, isoprene units condense to form vitamins A, E, and K, as well as many other compounds including rubber, plastoquinone (an electron carrier), the phytol chain of chlorophyll, and the carotenoid pigments.

Fig. 34.3. Synthesis of cholesterol. All the carbons of cholesterol are derived from acetyl CoA. Squalene is cyclized to produce the ring structure. Many steps are required to convert lanosterol to cholesterol. I, II, and III are the phases referred to in the text.

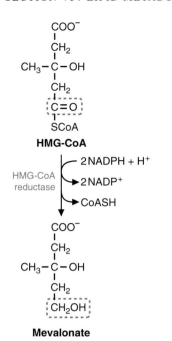

Fig. 34.4. Reduction of HMG-CoA to mevalonate.

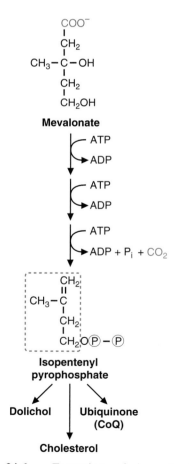

Fig. 34.6. Formation of isopentenyl pyrophosphate. The isoprene unit is highlighted. Isoprene units are precursors for dolichol, ubiquinone, and cholesterol synthesis in humans. CoQ = coenzyme Q.

condensed to form a 30-carbon compound, squalene. In the third phase, squalene cyclizes, forming lanosterol, which contains the rings of the steroid nucleus. Lanosterol is modified in a series of steps to form cholesterol.

In the initial phase of cholesterol synthesis, two molecules of cytosolic acetyl CoA condense to form acetoacetyl CoA. Another molecule of acetyl CoA combines with acetoacetyl CoA to form HMG-CoA. This sequence of reactions is similar to those involved in the synthesis of ketone bodies except that ketone body synthesis occurs in mitochondria (Fig. 23.15).

The next reaction in cholesterol biosynthesis is catalyzed by HMG-CoA reductase. This enzyme converts HMG-CoA to mevalonate, using reducing equivalents provided by NADPH (Fig. 34.4), and it is located in the endoplasmic reticulum with its active site extending into the cytosol. Although other enzymes are regulated, the reductase is the major rate-limiting and regulated enzyme for the pathway.

Cholesterol synthesis is controlled in most tissues by a type of feedback regulation in which cholesterol, the endproduct of the pathway, represses the synthesis of HMG-CoA reductase. In the liver, the rate of cholesterol synthesis is much higher than in other tissues because cholesterol serves as a precursor of bile salts. Thus, the synthesis of HMG-CoA reductase is also repressed by bile salts (Fig. 34.5). In addition to induction and repression, the liver enzyme is regulated by phosphorylation and dephosphorylation. When glucagon levels are elevated, HMG-CoA reductase is phosphorylated and inactive. When insulin levels are elevated, it is dephosphorylated and active. Thyroid hormone increases the activity of the reductase, while glucocorticoids decrease the activity.

Mevalonate is phosphorylated by ATP and subsequently decarboxylated to produce isopentenyl pyrophosphate (Fig. 34.6). These isoprene units may condense to form cholesterol. They may also form dolichol (a compound used to transfer branched oligosaccharides during glycoprotein synthesis) or ubiquinone (a component of the electron transport chain).

In cholesterol biosynthesis, 2 isoprene units condense to form geranyl pyrophosphate (see Fig. 34.3). An additional isoprene unit is added to produce farnesyl pyrophosphate. The condensation of 2 farnesyl pyrophosphates generates squalene, a compound containing 30 carbon atoms. After oxidation at carbon 3, squalene is cyclized to produce lanosterol, which contains the four rings that form the steroid

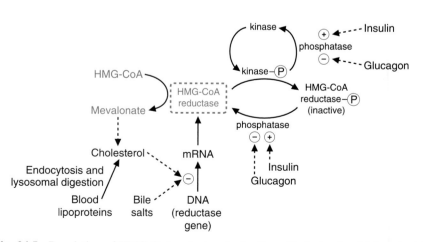

Fig. 34.5. Regulation of HMG-CoA reductase in the liver. Cholesterol and bile salts inhibit synthesis of the enzyme. Phosphorylation inactivates the enzyme. Glucagon probably acts by stimulating the phosphorylation of an inhibitor of the phosphatase, which causes the inhibitor to become active. The process may be similar to that for regulation of glycogen synthase (see Chapter 26).

nucleus of cholesterol. In a series of steps, 3 carbons are released from lanosterol as it is converted to cholesterol.

Esterification of Cholesterol

Cholesterol contains 27 carbon atoms. It has 8 carbons in its branched aliphatic side chain, and its steroid nucleus contains a double bond between carbons 5 and 6 and a hydroxyl group at position 3 (see Fig. 34.1). This hydroxyl group can be esterified to fatty acids, producing cholesterol esters. The esterification of cholesterol causes the molecule to become more hydrophobic, and, thus, it can more readily be packaged in lipoprotein particles or in lipid droplets in the cytosol of cells.

The enzymes that esterify cholesterol are (a) lecithin:cholesterol acyltransferase (LCAT), which is located in the blood and esterifies cholesterol associated with HDL particles, and (b) acyl:cholesterol acyltransferase (ACAT), which is located in cells, particularly those that need to store cholesterol for the synthesis of steroid hormones.

Transport of Cholesterol by Blood Lipoproteins

Cholesterol is very insoluble in water. Therefore, it is transported in the blood as a component of the blood lipoproteins.

CHYLOMICRON CHOLESTEROL

Dietary cholesterol is absorbed from bile salt micelles into intestinal epithelial cells. This cholesterol, along with that synthesized by the cells, is packaged in chylomicrons, which enter the blood via the lymph. The major protein of the nascent chylomicrons is apoB-48. In the lymph and the blood, chylomicrons obtain apoC$_{II}$ and

Farnesyl and geranyl groups covalently bind to proteins, particularly the G proteins and certain protooncogene products involved in signal transduction. These hydrophobic groups anchor the proteins in the cell membrane.

Because **William Hartman** continued to experience intermittent chest pain in spite of good control of his hypertension and a 20-lb weight loss, his physician decided that a two-drug regimen to lower his blood LDL cholesterol level must be added to the dietary changes already made. Consequently, treatment with a bile acid sequestrant, cholestyramine, and with an HMG-CoA reductase inhibitor, pravastatin, was initiated.

Pravastatin and other HMG-CoA reductase inhibitors, such as lovastatin, simvastatin, and fluvastatin, are structural analogs of intermediates in the conversion of HMG-CoA to mevalonate.

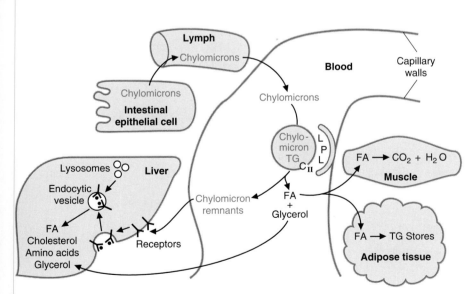

Fig. 34.7. Fate of chylomicron remnants. Chylomicrons, produced from dietary lipid, enter the blood by way of the lymphatic system. Chylomicron triacylglycerols (TG) are digested by LPL on capillary walls. The remnants of this digestion are much smaller and higher in density than the original chylomicrons. They are recognized by receptors on liver cells. Endocytosis followed by lysosomal action converts the remnants to their component parts. Cholesterol, obtained by the liver from the remnants, inhibits cholesterol synthesis. FA = fatty acids.

34.1: If a patient has high VLDL levels in the blood, what dietary change might help to lower them?

apoE from HDL. After digestion of the chylomicron triacylglycerols by lipoprotein lipase in the blood, the chylomicron remnants bind to receptors on liver cells and are internalized via endocytosis. Lysosomal digestion occurs, and the proteins and lipids are degraded, fatty acids are cleaved from cholesterol esters, and cholesterol and the other products of digestion of the chylomicron remnants enter the pools of liver cells (Fig. 34.7). The resultant increase of the free cholesterol pool inhibits cholesterol synthesis and down-regulates LDL receptor synthesis by the hepatocyte, i.e., synthesis of the receptors is inhibited. Consequently, as receptors are taken up by endocytosis, their number in the cell membrane decreases.

VLDL CHOLESTEROL

As the liver produces triacylglycerols, they are packaged along with cholesterol from the cholesterol pools, phospholipids, and apoB-100 into VLDL, which is secreted into the blood. The cholesterol pools of the liver are derived by endocytosis and lysosomal digestion of blood lipoproteins or by synthesis from acetyl CoA. In the blood, HDL transfers $apoC_{II}$ and apoE, as well as cholesterol esters, to VLDL.

VLDL is converted to IDL in the blood by digestion of its triacylglycerols by lipoprotein lipase (Fig. 34.8). The triacylglycerols of IDL may be degraded to produce LDL, or IDL may return to the liver, where it binds to cell surface receptors, is taken up by endocytosis, and is degraded by lysosomal enzymes. Fatty acids, amino acids, and cholesterol are returned to the pools in the liver.

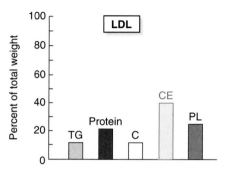

Fig. 34.9. Composition of a typical LDL particle. Cholesterol (C) and cholesterol esters (CE) are the major components of LDL. TG = triacylglycerol; PL = phospholipid.

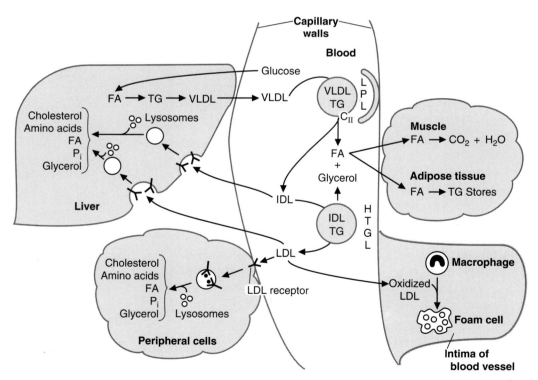

Fig. 34.8. Fate of VLDL. VLDL triacylglycerol (TG) is degraded by LPL, forming IDL. IDL can either be endocytosed by the liver via a receptor-mediated process or further digested, mainly by hepatic triacylglycerol lipase (HTGL) to form LDL. LDL may be endocytosed by receptor-mediated processes in the liver or in peripheral cells. LDL may also be oxidized and taken up by "scavenger" receptors on macrophages. The scavenger pathway plays a role in atherosclerosis (see Figs. 34.12 and 34.13). FA = fatty acids; P_i = inorganic phosphate.

LDL CHOLESTEROL

If the triacylglycerols of IDL are digested further, either by lipoprotein lipase (LPL) in various tissues or by hepatic triacylglycerol lipase in the liver sinusoids, LDL is produced. Its composition is shown in Figure 34.9. LDL is taken up by the liver where receptor-mediated endocytosis and lysosomal digestion return LDL cholesterol to the hepatic cholesterol pools. Endocytosis and lysosomal digestion of LDL also occur in extrahepatic tissues which contain LDL receptors (Fig. 34.10). In addition, uptake of LDL occurs via nonspecific "scavenger" receptors on cells such as macrophages.

Lipoprotein Receptors

The best-characterized lipoprotein receptor, the LDL receptor, recognizes apoE and apoB-100. Therefore, it binds VLDL, IDL, and chylomicron remnants in addition to LDL. The LDL receptor binds its ligands with high affinity, and it has a narrow range of specificity. Other receptors, such as the LDL receptor related protein (LRP) and the macrophage scavenger receptor, have broad specificity and bind many other ligands in addition to the blood lipoproteins.

LDL Receptor

The LDL receptor, located in the cell membrane, binds LDL and brings it into the cell by the process of endocytosis. Normal cells contain many copies of the LDL receptor. For example, fibroblasts contain 20,000 to 50,000 copies per cell. These receptors are synthesized in the endoplasmic reticulum and the Golgi complex and travel to the cell surface, where they cluster in coated pits lined with the protein clathrin. These pits invaginate, and the clathrin coat dissociates, producing endosomes (membrane enclosed vesicles generated by endocytosis). The internal pH of the endosomes decreases due to the action of ATP-driven proton pumps in the endosome membrane. The decrease in pH causes lipoproteins to dissociate from their receptors in the endosome, and many of the receptors are recycled to the cell surface by vesicles. The endosomes fuse with lysosomes, which contain hydrolytic enzymes that digest the lipoprotein particles and remaining receptors.

The uptake and lysosomal digestion of LDL by extrahepatic cells results in the release of cholesterol within these cells, which has a number of consequences (Fig. 34.11).

1. The cells may use this cholesterol to maintain their cell membranes.
2. When intracellular levels of cholesterol are elevated, synthesis of cholesterol from acetyl CoA in the cells decreases because an expansion of the intracellular free cholesterol pool reduces the synthesis of HMG-CoA reductase.
3. The increase in intracellular free cholesterol levels stimulates the activity of acyl CoA:cholesterol acyltransferase (ACAT), the enzyme that converts cholesterol to cholesterol esters for storage within the cell.
4. An increase in intracellular free cholesterol levels decreases the synthesis of LDL receptors by acting at the level of gene expression. As the concentration of these receptors on the cell membrane decreases, less LDL is taken up from the blood, and cellular cholesterol levels decline. This mechanism is known as down-regulation of receptor synthesis.

When intracellular levels of cholesterol decrease, these processes are reversed and cells act to increase their cholesterol levels. Both synthesis of cholesterol from acetyl CoA and synthesis of LDL receptors are stimulated. An increased number of receptors results in an increased uptake of LDL cholesterol from the blood.

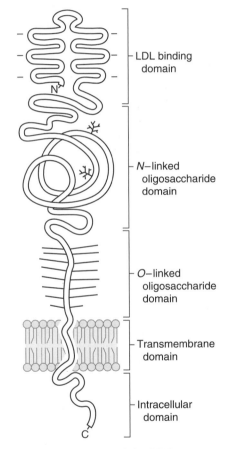

Fig. 34.10. Structure of the LDL receptor. The protein has five major domains.

A 34.1: Low carbohydrate diets may decrease triacylglycerol and cholesterol levels in patients who have high concentrations of VLDL. The triacylglycerols of VLDL are synthesized in the liver mainly from dietary carbohydrate (see Chapter 33). As VLDL are secreted from the liver, they carry cholesterol into the blood.

William Hartman's blood lipid levels (in mg/dL) were:

Triacylglycerol	158
Total cholesterol	420
HDL cholesterol	32
LDL cholesterol	356

He was diagnosed as having familial hypercholesterolemia (FH) type IIA, which is caused by genetic defects in the gene that encodes the LDL receptor (see Biochemical Comments). As a result of the receptor defect, LDL cannot readily be taken up by cells, and its concentration in the blood is elevated.

LDL particles contain a high percentage, by weight, of cholesterol and cholesterol esters, more than the other blood lipoproteins. However, LDL triacylglycerol levels are low because LDL is produced by digestion of the triacylglycerols of VLDL and IDL. Therefore, individuals with a type IIA hyperlipoproteinemia have very high blood cholesterol levels but their levels of triacylglycerols may be in or near the normal range (see Table 34.4).

Thomas Appleman's blood lipid levels were:

Triacylglycerol	295
Total cholesterol	314
HDL cholesterol	24
LDL cholesterol	231

The elevated serum levels of LDL cholesterol found in patients such as Thomas Appleman who have NIDDM is multifactorial. One of the mechanisms responsible for this increase involves the presence of chronically elevated levels of glucose in the blood of poorly controlled diabetics. This prolonged hyperglycemia increases the rate of nonenzymatic attachment of glucose to various proteins in the body, a process referred to as glycation or glycosylation of proteins.

Glycation may adversely affect the structure and/or the function of the protein involved. For example, glycation of the LDL receptor and of proteins in the LDL particle may interfere with the normal "fit" of LDL particles with their specific receptors. As a result, less circulating LDL is internalized into cells and the serum LDL cholesterol level rises.

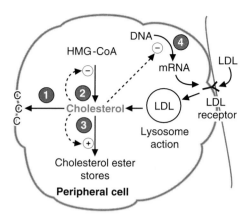

Fig. 34.11. Effect of uptake of cholesterol on intracellular cholesterol levels. LDL is taken up by receptor-mediated endocytosis. Lysosomes fuse with the endosomes, and the components of the LDL are digested. Free cholesterol from cholesterol esters is released into the cellular pools. This cholesterol is used to maintain cell membranes (**1**), to repress the synthesis of HMG-CoA reductase, which reduces the de novo synthesis of cholesterol (**2**), to stimulate the storage of cholesterol as cholesterol esters via the ACAT reaction (**3**), and to down-regulate LDL receptors (i.e., to repress synthesis of the receptor protein) (**4**).

LDL RECEPTOR-RELATED PROTEIN (LRP)

LRP is structurally related to the LDL receptor, but recognizes a broader spectrum of ligands. In addition to lipoproteins, it binds the blood proteins α_2-macroglobulin (a protein that inhibits blood proteases) and tissue plasminogen activator (TPA) and its inhibitors. The LRP receptor recognizes the apoE of lipoproteins and binds remnants produced by the digestion of the triacylglycerols of chylomicrons and VLDL by LPL. Thus, one of its functions is believed to be the clearance of these remnants from the blood. The LRP receptor is abundant in the cell membranes of the liver, brain, and placenta. In contrast to the LDL receptor, synthesis of the LRP receptor is not significantly affected by an increase in the intracellular concentration of cholesterol. However, insulin causes the number of these receptors on the cell surface to increase.

MACROPHAGE SCAVENGER RECEPTOR

Some cells, particularly the phagocytic macrophages, have nonspecific receptors known as "scavenger" receptors that bind various types of molecules, including modified LDL particles. Modification of LDL frequently involves oxidative damage, particularly of polyunsaturated fatty acyl groups (see Chapter 21). In contrast to the LDL receptors, the scavenger receptors are not subject to down-regulation. The continued presence of scavenger receptors in the cell membrane allows the cells to take up oxidatively modified LDL long after intracellular cholesterol levels are elevated. When the macrophages become engorged with lipid, they are called foam cells (Fig. 34.12). An accumulation of these foam cells in the subendothelial space of blood vessels forms the earliest gross evidence of a developing atherosclerotic plaque known as a fatty streak.

The processes that cause oxidation of LDL involve superoxide radicals, nitric oxide, hydrogen peroxide, and other oxidants (see Chapter 21). Antioxidants, such as vitamin E, ascorbic acid (vitamin C), and carotenoids, may be involved in protecting LDL from oxidation.

ATHEROSCLEROSIS

Atherosclerosis is a disease in which plaques form in the walls of the major arteries, constricting the lumen of the vessel (which impedes blood flow) and decreasing vessel elasticity. The plaques are composed of smooth muscle cells, connective tissue, lipids, and debris that accumulate in the intima of the arterial wall. Studies of humans of all age groups, as well as animals, suggest that the formation of these plaques progresses with age in the following sequence (Fig. 34.13):

The endothelial cells of the artery wall are injured, either mechanically or by cytotoxic agents (including oxidized LDL). The injured area is exposed to the blood and attracts monocytes, which are converted to macrophages that engulf material in the region (including oxidized LDL). As these phagocytic cells fill with lipid, they become foam cells, which accumulate causing a fatty streak to develop within the blood vessel wall.

Endothelial cells normally produce prostaglandin I_2 (PGI$_2$), a prostacyclin that inhibits platelet aggregation (see Chapter 35). When endothelial cells are damaged, platelets begin to aggregate and release thromboxane A_2 (TXA$_2$), a substance that further stimulates platelet aggregation. These cells also release platelet-derived growth factor (PDGF). Macrophages produce additional growth factors. The growth factors cause proliferation of smooth muscle cells, which migrate from the medial to the intimal layer of the arterial wall.

Cells within the intimal layer release lipids (triacylglycerols and cholesterol) which accumulate in the developing plaque. Blood lipoproteins, particularly LDL, continue to enter the area, contributing to the lipid buildup.

Cells in the lesion secrete collagen, elastin, and glycosaminoglycans, forming a fibrous cap, and cholesterol crystals appear in the core of the plaque. Cells are trapped in the plaque, where they die, adding to the debris. Calcification also occurs. Rupture and hemorrhage of the encapsulated plaque in a coronary vessel may cause the acute formation of a clot (thrombus), which further occludes the vessel, causing a myocardial infarction.

ROLE OF HDL

HDL, which helps to retard the atherosclerotic process, is synthesized in a nascent (immature) form in the liver and the gut. After HDL is secreted into the blood, it is altered by interacting with chylomicrons and VLDL, with which it exchanges lipids and proteins. It also picks up cholesterol from the surface of cells and from other lipoproteins and converts it to cholesterol esters. These cholesterol esters are ultimately returned to the liver, and thus HDL is said to participate in "reverse cholesterol transport."

HDL contains a much higher percentage of its weight as protein and a much lower percentage as triacylglycerol than the other blood lipoproteins (Fig. 34.14 and Table 34.7), and, therefore, it is the most dense.

HDL transfers the proteins apoC$_{II}$ and apoE to chylomicrons and VLDL, the triacylglycerol-rich lipoproteins (Fig. 34.15). ApoC$_{II}$ stimulates the degradation of the triacylglycerols of these particles by activating LPL. This degradation produces chylomicron remnants (from chylomicrons) and IDL (from VLDL). The apoE, which these particles contain, serves as a ligand for receptors on liver cell membranes that are involved in the uptake of chylomicron remnants and IDL.

When secreted into the blood, HDL particles are small and discoid in shape (see Fig. 34.15). These nascent HDL particles are nearly devoid of cholesterol ester and triacylglycerols. As they pick up cholesterol from other lipoproteins and from cell membranes, the cholesterol is converted to cholesterol esters by the LCAT reaction, which is stimulated by apoA$_I$, a component of the nascent HDL particle. As the particles fill with cholesterol ester and triacylglycerol, they become large and spherical in shape.

These large HDL particles (known as HDL$_2$ transfer cholesterol esters to VLDL in exchange for triacylglycerols (Fig. 34.16). Cholesterol ester transfer protein

In addition to dietary therapy, aimed at reducing his blood cholesterol levels, **William Hartman** was treated with pravastatin, an HMG-CoA reductase inhibitor. The HMG-CoA reductase inhibitors decrease the rate of synthesis of cholesterol in cells. As cellular cholesterol levels decrease, the synthesis of LDL receptors increases. As the number of receptors rises on the cell surface, the uptake of LDL is increased. Consequently, the blood level of LDL cholesterol decreases.

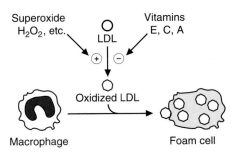

Fig. 34.12. Production of foam cells by phagocytosis of oxidized LDL. This process occurs in the subendothelial space of blood vessels. Vitamins E, C, and A inhibit oxidation of LDL. It has been claimed that diets that contain ample quantities of fruits and vegetables (five servings per day) prevent coronary heart disease, possibly because they contain vitamins E, C, and A.

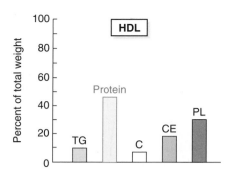

Fig. 34.14. Composition of a typical HDL particle. The composition of HDL is quite variable because these particles exchange proteins and lipids with other lipoproteins. However, their major component is protein. Therefore, HDL particles have a higher density than other lipoprotein particles.

HDL is considered to be the "good cholesterol," because it accepts free cholesterol from peripheral tissues, such as cells in the walls of blood vessels. This cholesterol is converted to cholesterol ester, part of which is transferred to VLDL by CETP, and returned to the liver by IDL and LDL. The liver reutilizes the cholesterol, converting it to bile salts, or excretes it directly into the bile. HDL, therefore, tends to lower blood cholesterol levels. Lower blood cholesterol levels correlate with a lower death rate. Figure from Arch Intern Med 1988;148:36–69.

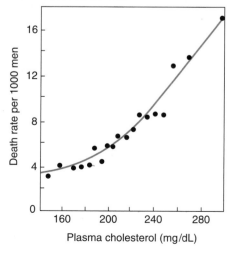

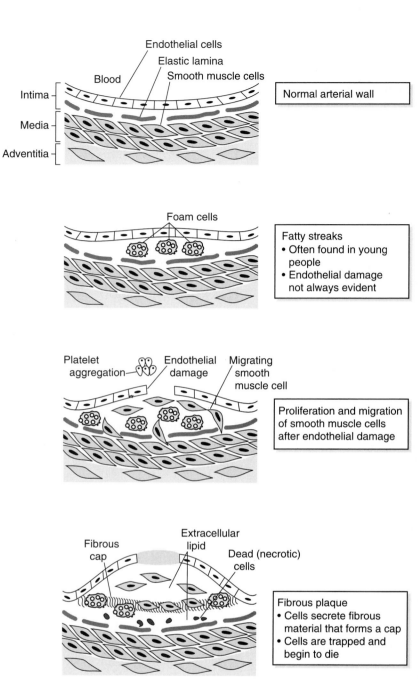

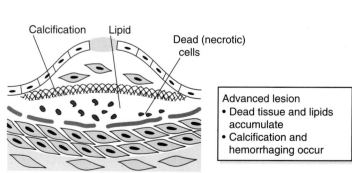

Fig. 34.13. Progression of atherosclerotic plaque formation in endothelial cells of blood vessels.

Table 34.7. Composition of the Blood Lipoproteins[a]

	Density (g/mL)	Diameter (nm)	Triacyl-glycerol (%)	Protein (%)	Type of Protein	Cholesterol (%)	Cholesterol Ester (%)	Phospholipid (%)
Chylomicrons	0.93	75–1,200	85	2	B,C,E	1	2	8
VLDL	0.930–1.006	30–80	55	9	B,C,E	7	10	20
IDL	1.006–1.019	25–35	26	11	B,E	8	30	23
LDL	1.019–1.063	18–25	10	20	B	10	35	20
HDL	1.063–1.210	5–12	8	45	A,C,E	5	15	25

[a]The composition is expressed as percent of the total weight. Because lipoprotein particles are constantly undergoing changes, these are not absolute values, only averages. Slightly different values may be listed in other texts. Chylomicrons are the least dense because of their high triacylglycerol and low protein content, and HDL (with low triacylglycerol and high protein content) is the most dense. The predominant proteins of chylomicrons and VLDL and its derivatives (IDL and LDL) are the B-apoproteins, while the A-apoproteins predominate in HDL.

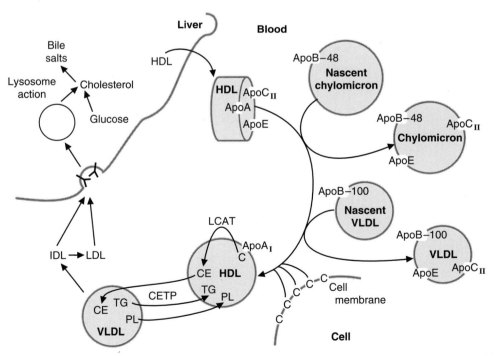

Fig. 34.15. Functions and fate of HDL. Nascent HDL is synthesized in liver and intestinal cells. It exchanges proteins with chylomicrons and VLDL. HDL picks up cholesterol (C) from cell membranes. This cholesterol is converted to cholesterol ester (CE) by the LCAT reaction. HDL transfers CE to VLDL in exchange for triacylglycerol (TG). The cholesterol ester transfer protein (CETP) mediates this exchange. PL = phospholipids.

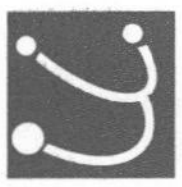

In patients such as **William Hartman** and **Thomas Appleman**, who have elevated levels of VLDL and/or LDL, HDL levels are often low. These patients are predisposed to atherosclerosis and suffer from a high incidence of heart attacks and strokes.

Exercise and estrogen increase HDL levels. This is one of the reasons exercise is often recommended to aid in the prevention or treatment of heart disease and estrogen replacement therapy is often prescribed for postmenopausal women. Prior to menopause, the incidence of heart attacks is low in women, but it rises following menopause and increases to the level found in men. Moderate consumption of ethanol (alcohol) has also been correlated with increased HDL levels. Recent studies suggest that the beneficial amount of ethanol may be quite low, about two small glasses of wine a day and that beneficial effects ascribed to ethanol may result from other components of wine and alcoholic beverages.

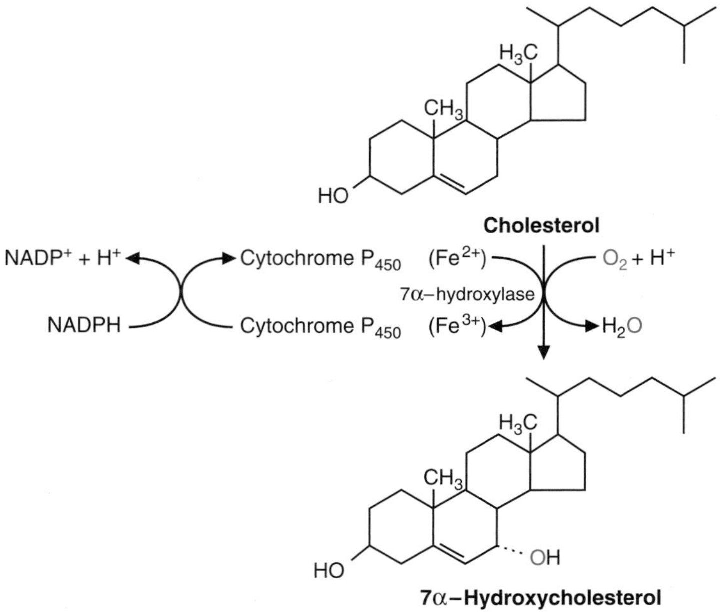

Fig. 34.17. Reaction catalyzed by 7α-hydroxylase. An α-hydroxyl group is formed at position 7 of cholesterol. This reaction, which is inhibited by bile salts, is the rate-limiting step in bile salt synthesis.

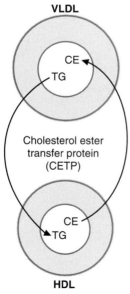

Fig. 34.16. Function of cholesterol ester transfer protein (CETP). CETP transfers cholesterol esters (CE) from HDL to VLDL in exchange for TG.

(CETP) mediates this exchange. As VLDL is degraded by LPL, it transfers the C_{II} apoprotein, originally obtained from HDL particles, back to these particles. As a result of these transfers of lipids and proteins to HDL and of triacylglycerol degradation, VLDL is converted to the smaller and more dense IDL (see Fig. 34.15). The triacylglycerols of someof the IDL particles are degraded, mainly by hepatic triglyceride lipase, apoE is transferred to HDL, and LDL is formed. LDL has a low content of triacylglycerols, a high content of cholesterol esters, and is lacking the C_{II} and E apoproteins. The altered HDL particles become much smaller in size and are now known as HDL_3. The fate of these particles is not clearly defined.

IDL and LDL particles are endocytosed by liver cells and their contents are released following lysosomal action. Thus cholesterol, collected by HDL, is returned to the liver. LDL is also endocytosed by peripheral cells, supplying them with cholesterol.

Synthesis of Bile Salts

CONVERSION OF CHOLESTEROL TO CHOLIC ACID AND CHENOCHOLIC ACID

Bile salts are synthesized in the liver from cholesterol by reactions that hydroxylate the steroid nucleus and cleave the side chain. In the first reaction, an α-hydroxyl group is added to carbon 7 (on the α side of the B ring). The activity of the 7α-hydroxylase that catalyzes this rate-limiting step is decreased by bile salts (Fig. 34.17).

In subsequent steps, the double bond is reduced and an additional hydroxylation may occur. Two different sets of compounds are produced. One set has α-hydroxyl groups at positions 3, 7, and 12, and produces the cholic acid series of bile salts. The other set has α-hydroxyl groups only at positions 3 and 7, and produces the chenocholic acid series (Fig. 34.18). Three carbons are removed from the side chain by an oxidation reaction. The remaining 5-carbon fragment attached to the ring structure contains a carboxyl group (see Fig. 34.18).

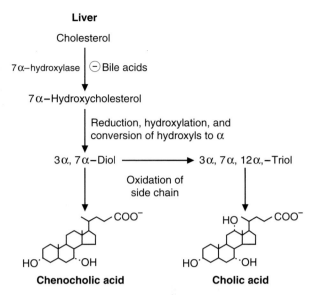

Fig. 34.18. Synthesis of bile salts. Bile salts are produced from cholesterol by hydroxylation, reduction of the 4,5 double bond, and oxidation of the side chain. Two sets of bile salts are generated: one with α-hydroxyl groups at positions 3 and 7, and the other with hydroxyls at positions 3, 7, and 12.

The pK of the bile acids is about 6. Therefore, in the contents of the intestinal lumen, which normally have a pH of 6, about half of the molecules are present in the protonated form and half are ionized, forming bile salts. (The terms bile acids and bile salts are often used interchangeably, but bile salts actually refers to the ionized form.)

CONJUGATION OF BILE SALTS

The carboxyl group at the end of the side chain of the bile salts is activated by a reaction that requires ATP and coenzyme A (CoA). The acyl CoA derivatives can react with either glycine or taurine, forming amides that are known as the conjugated bile salts. In glycocholic acid and glycochenocholic acid, the bile acids are conjugated with glycine. These compounds have a pK of about 4, so compared to their unconjugated forms, a higher percentage of the molecules is present in the ionized form at the pH of the intestine. The taurine conjugates, taurocholic and taurochenocholic acid, have a pK of about 2. Therefore, compared to the glycoconjugates, an even greater percentage of the molecules of these conjugates are ionized in the lumen of the gut (Fig. 34.19).

 Taurine is synthesized from the amino acid cysteine.

Fate of the Bile Salts

The bile salts are produced in the liver and secreted into the bile (Fig. 34.20). They are stored in the gallbladder and released into the intestine during a meal, where they serve as detergents that aid in the digestion of dietary lipids (see Chapter 32).

Intestinal bacteria deconjugate and dehydroxylate the bile salts, removing the glycine and taurine residues and the hydroxyl group at position 7. The bile salts that lack a hydroxyl group at position 7 are called secondary bile salts. The deconjugated and dehydroxylated bile salts are less soluble and, therefore, less readily resorbed from the intestinal lumen than the bile salts which have not been subjected to bacterial action (Fig. 34.21). Lithocholic acid, a secondary bile salt that has a hydroxyl group only at position 3, is the least soluble bile salt. Its major fate is excretion.

Lipoprotein(a) is essentially an LDL particle that is covalently bound to apoprotein(a). It is called "lipoprotein little a" to avoid confusion with the apoprotein A found in HDL. The structure of apoprotein(a) is very similar to plasminogen, a precursor of the protease plasmin that degrades fibrin, a major component of blood clots. Lipoprotein(a), however, cannot be converted to active plasmin. There are reports that high concentrations of lipoprotein(a) correlate with an increased risk of coronary artery disease, even in patients in whom the lipid profile is otherwise normal.

Greater than 95% of the bile salts are resorbed in the ileum and return to the liver via the enterohepatic circulation (see Fig. 34.20). The secondary bile salts may be reconjugated in the liver, but they are not rehydroxylated. The bile salts are recycled by the liver, which secretes them into the bile. This enterohepatic recirculation of bile salts is extremely efficient. Less than 5% of the bile salts entering the gut are excreted in the feces each day. Because the steroid nucleus cannot be degraded in the body, the excretion of bile salts serves as a major route for removal of the steroid nucleus and, thus, of cholesterol from the body.

CLINICAL COMMENTS. William Hartman is typical of patients with essentially normal serum triacylglycerol levels and elevated serum total cholesterol levels that are repeatedly in the upper 1% of the general population (e.g., 325–500 mg/dL). When similar lipid abnormalities are present in other

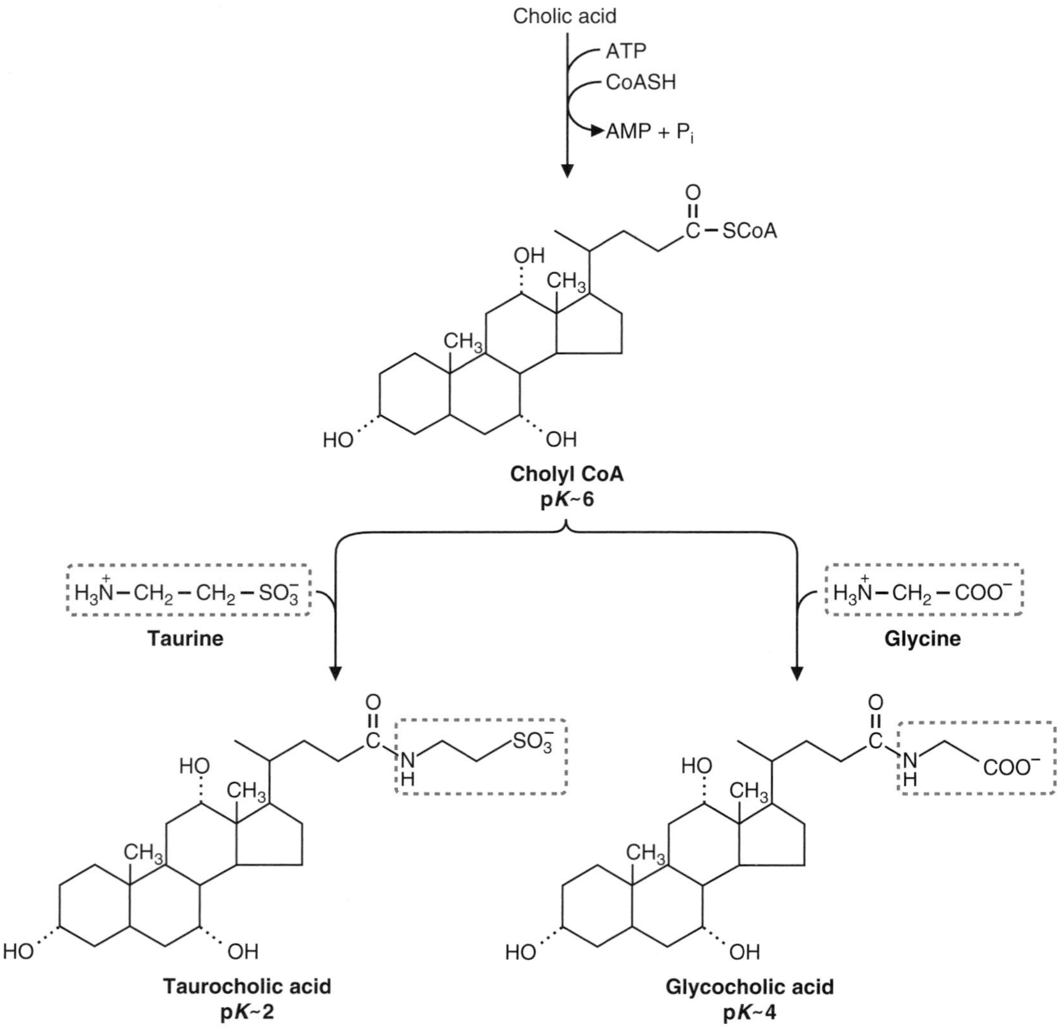

Fig. 34.19. Conjugation of bile salts. Conjugates form with taurine (derived from the amino acid cysteine) or glycine. Both cholic acid and chenocholic acid may be conjugated. Conjugation lowers the pK of the bile salts, making them better detergents, i.e., they are more ionized in the contents of the intestinal lumen (pH ~ 6) than are the unconjugated bile salts (pK ~ 6). Glycoconjugates have a pK of about 4, and tauroconjugates have a pK of about 2.

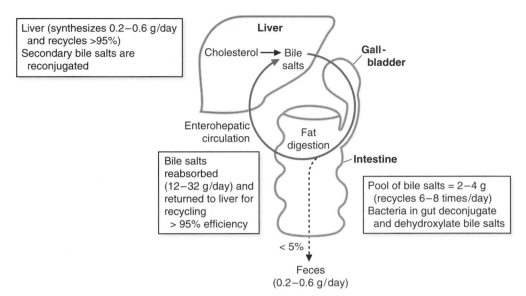

Fig. 34.20. Overview of bile salt metabolism.

family members in a pattern of autosomal dominant inheritance and no secondary causes for these lipid alterations (e.g., hypothyroidism) are present, the entity referred to as "familial hypercholesterolemia (FH), type IIA" is the most likely cause of this hereditary dyslipidemia.

FH is a genetic disorder caused by an abnormality in one or more alleles responsible for the formation and/or the functional integrity of high affinity LDL receptors on the plasma membrane of cells which normally initiate the internalization of circulating LDL and other blood lipoproteins. Heterozygotes for FH (1 in 500 of the population) have roughly one-half of the normal complement or functional capacity of such receptors while homozygotes (1 in 1 million of the population) have essentially no functional LDL receptors. The rare patient with the homozygous form of FH has a more extreme elevation of serum total and LDL cholesterol than does the heterozygote and, as a result, has a more profound predisposition to premature coronary artery disease.

Chronic hypercholesterolemia may cause the deposition of lipids within the skin and eye. When this occurs in the medial aspect of the upper and lower eyelids, it is referred to as xanthelasma. Similar deposits known as xanthomas may occur in the iris of the eye (arcus juvenilis) as well as the tendons of the hands and the Achilles tendons.

Although therapy aimed at inserting competent LDL receptor genes into the cells of patients with homozygous FH is undergoing clinical trials, the current pharmacological approach in the heterozygote is to attempt to increase the rate of synthesis of LDL receptors in cells.

William Hartman was treated with cholestyramine, a resin that binds some of the bile salts in the intestine, causing them to be excreted in the feces rather than recycled to the liver. The liver must now synthesize more bile salts, which lowers the intrahepatic free cholesterol pool. As a result, hepatic LDL receptor synthesis is induced and more circulating LDL is taken up by the liver.

HMG-CoA reductase inhibitors, such as pravastatin, also stimulate the synthesis of additional LDL receptors but do so by inhibiting HMG-CoA reductase, the rate-limiting enzyme for cholesterol synthesis. The subsequent decline in the intracellular free cholesterol pool also stimulates the synthesis of additional LDL receptors.

A combination of strict dietary and dual pharmacological therapy, aimed at decreasing the cholesterol levels of the body is usually quite effective in correcting

William Hartman was treated with cholestyramine. Bile salt sequestrants, such as cholestyramine, are positively charged resins capable of binding to the negatively charged bile salts in the lumen of the small intestine. This binding reduces the percentage of bile salts in the gut lumen which are resorbed and recirculated to the liver from the normal 95–98% to 90–92%. This relatively small reduction in the return of bile salts to the liver "signals" the liver cells that more bile salts must now be synthesized from the cholesterol located in the hepatic cholesterol pool. The consequent reduction in this pool size causes the liver cell to synthesize more LDL receptors which, in turn, will internalize more circulating LDL. The cholesterol component of this LDL is used to replenish the hepatic cell's pool of free cholesterol.

Primary bile salts

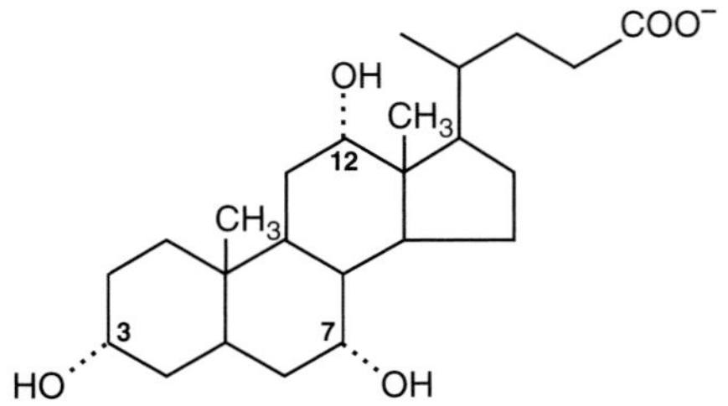

Cholic acid

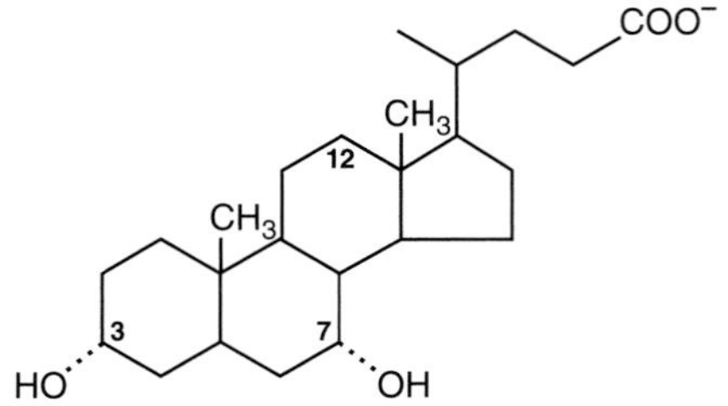

Chenocholic acid

Secondary bile salts

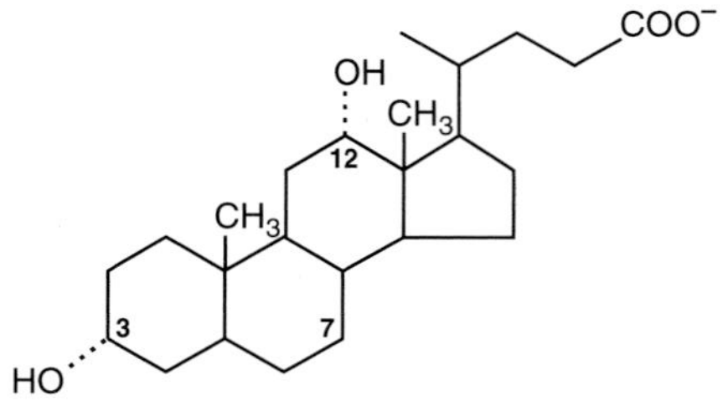

Deoxycholic acid

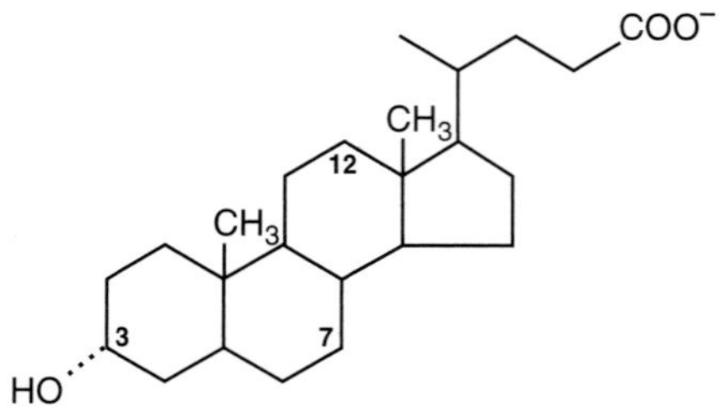

Lithocholic acid

Fig. 34.21. Structures of the primary and secondary bile salts. Primary bile salts form conjugates with taurine or glycine in the liver. After secretion into the intestine, they may be deconjugated and dehydroxylated by the bacterial flora, forming secondary bile salts. Note that dehydroxylation occurs at position 7. Primary and secondary bile salts are resorbed and returned to the liver. Lithocholic acid is very insoluble and is mainly excreted.

the lipid abnormality and, hopefully, the associated risk of atherosclerotic cardiovascular disease in patients with heterozygous familial hypercholesterolemia.

Low density lipoprotein cholesterol is the primary target of cholesterol lowering therapy because both epidemiological and experimental evidence strongly suggest a benefit of lowering serum LDL cholesterol in the prevention of atherosclerotic cardiovascular disease. Similar evidence for raising subnormal levels of serum HDL cholesterol is less conclusive but adequate to support such efforts particularly in high risk patients, such as **Thomas Appleman**, who have multiple cardiovascular risk factors.

The first-line therapy in this attempt is nonpharmacological and includes such measures as increasing aerobic exercise, weight loss in overweight patients, avoidance of excessive alcohol intake, and cessation of smoking. If these efforts fail, drug therapy to raise serum HDL cholesterol levels must be considered.

So far, Mr. Appleman has failed in his attempts to diet and exercise. His LDL cholesterol level is 231 mg/dL. According to Table 34.5, he is a candidate for more stringent dietary therapy and for drug treatment. He could be given an HMG-CoA reductase inhibitor such as pravastatin and, perhaps, a bile salt binding resin such as cholestyramine. Other lipid-lowering drugs such as the fibric acid derivatives, which decrease triacylglycerol levels and possibly increase HDL levels, should also be considered.

 BIOCHEMICAL COMMENTS. Defects in the LDL receptor gene are responsible for the elevated blood levels of LDL, and thus of cholesterol, in FH. At least 18 mutations have been found in the LDL receptor gene, affecting all stages in the production and functioning of the receptor.

The LDL receptor gene, which contains 18 exons and is 45 kilobases (kb) in length, is located on the short arm of chromosome 19. The exons share sequences with a number of other genes; the ligand-binding domain is homologous to the gene for the C9 component of complement (a blood protein involved in the immune response), and the N-linked oligosaccharide domain is homologous to the genes for the precursor of epidermal growth factor (EGF) and also for three proteases of the blood clotting system, Factors IX and X and protein C (see Chapter 9). The LDL receptor gene encodes a glycoprotein that contains 839 amino acids.

Heterozygotes for FH have one normal and one mutant allele. Their cells produce approximately one-half the normal amount of receptor and take up LDL at about one-half the normal rate. Homozygotes have two mutant alleles, which may either be identical or may differ. They produce very little functional receptor.

The genetic mutations are mainly deletions, but insertions or duplications also occur, as well as missense and nonsense point mutations (Fig. 34.22). Four classes of mutations have been identified. The first class involves "null" alleles that either direct the synthesis of no protein at all or a protein that cannot be precipitated by antibodies to the LDL receptor. In the second class, the alleles encode proteins, but they cannot be transported to the cell surface. The third class of mutant alleles encodes proteins that reach the cell surface but cannot bind LDL normally. Finally, the fourth class encodes proteins that reach the surface and bind LDL, but fail to cluster and internalize the LDL particles. The result of each of these mutations is that blood levels of LDL are elevated because cells cannot take up these particles at a normal rate.

Suggested Readings

Goldstein JL, Hobbs HH, Brown MS. Familial hypercholesterolemia. In: Scriver CR, Beaudet AL, Sly WS, Valle D, eds. The metabolic and molecular bases of inherited disease. 7th ed, vol II. New York: McGraw-Hill, 1995:1981–2030.

Havel RJ, Kane JP. Introduction: structure and metabolism of plasma lipoproteins. In: Scriver CR, Beaudet AL, Sly WS, Valle D, eds. The metabolic and molecular bases of inherited disease. 7th ed, vol II. New York: McGraw-Hill, 1995:1841–1851.

Krieger M, Herz J. Structures and functions of multiligand lipoprotein receptors: macrophage scavenger receptors and LDL receptor-related protein (LRP). Annu Rev Biochem 1994;63:601–637.

Summary of the Second Report of the National Cholesterol Education Program (NCEP) Expert Panel on Detection, Evaluation, and Treatment of High Blood Cholesterol in Adults (Adult Treatment Panel II). JAMA 1993;269:3015–3023.

Tall A. Plasma lipid transfer proteins. Annu Rev Biochem 1995;64:235–257.

PROBLEMS

1. A patient had very elevated plasma triacylglycerol levels, but her LDL levels were low. Administration of insulin did not significantly reduce her triacylglycerol levels; however, the levels decreased to the normal range after a blood transfusion. Suggest two possible causes for this patient's problem, and explain how you could distinguish between them.

2. Explain why a patient with a decreased production of bicarbonate by the pancreas but normal production of lipase and colipase could develop steatorrhea (fat in feces).

ANSWERS

1. This patient could have a deficiency of LPL or a deficiency of apoC$_{II}$, the activator of LPL. If either the enzyme or its activator is defective, chylomicrons and VLDL

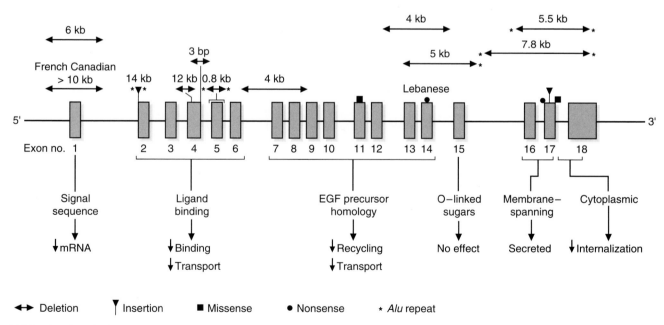

Fig. 34.22. Mutations in the LDL receptor gene. Exons, shown as shaded boxes, are separated by introns, which are drawn to approximate scale. Mutations that have been mapped or cloned are indicated above and below the gene. The mutations are: deletion of >10 kb (French-Canadian allele), deletion of 6 kb, 14 kb duplication (insertion in intron 1), 12 bp deletion in exon 4, 3 bp deletion in exon 4, missense mutation in exon 11, nonsense mutation in exon 14 (Lebanese allele), nonsense mutation in exon 17, 4 bp insertion in exon 17, missense mutation in exon 17, deletion of 0.8 kb, deletion of 4 kb involving exons 7 and 8, deletion of 4 kb involving exons 13 and 14, deletion of 5 kb, deletion of 7.8 kb, and deletion of 5.5 kb. From Goldstein JL, Brown MS. Familial hypercholesterolemia. In: Scriver CR, Beaudet AL, Sly WS, Valle D, eds. The metabolic and molecular bases of inherited disease. 6th ed, vol I. New York: McGraw-Hill, 1989:1232.

could not be normally degraded and triacylglycerols would accumulate in the blood within these lipoproteins. Because LDL is produced by degradation of the triacylglycerols of VLDL, LDL levels would be low. Normally, insulin stimulates the synthesis of LPL. In this case, no stimulation was observed. Therefore, the enzyme could be defective, or perhaps the enzyme is normal and insulin stimulated its production, but it could not be activated because of a deficiency in apoC$_{II}$. ApoC$_{II}$, a component of VLDL and chylomicrons, activates LPL.

The decreased triacylglycerol levels following a blood transfusion suggests that the problem is a lack of apoC$_{II}$. The blood transfusion supplied apoC$_{II}$, which activated the patient's LPL. LPL is attached to capillary walls and is not likely to be present in blood that is used for transfusions. Heparin treatment releases LPL from the capillary walls. Normal apoC$_{II}$ could be added to blood obtained after heparin treatment of the patient. If the lipolytic activity of the blood increases, the most likely defect is in apoC$_{II}$.

2. Digestion of dietary fats requires the action of bile salts. Although lipase and colipase are present in this case, if the bile salts are not functioning effectively as detergents, fats will not be digested and absorbed, and the result will be steatorrhea.

Bile salts must be ionized in order to function as detergents. If bicarbonate is not produced by the pancreas, stomach acid entering the intestine will not be neutralized. If the pH in the intestine is too low, the bile salts will not be adequately ionized and, therefore, they will not be very effective detergents. The pK of the unconjugated bile salts is about 6, the pK of the glycoconjugates is about 4, and the pK of the tauroconjugates is about 2. This is the order in which the bile salts will lose their detergent activity as the pH in the intestinal lumen decreases.

35 Metabolism of the Eicosanoids

The eicosanoids, which include the prostaglandins (PG), thromboxanes (TX), and leukotrienes (LT), are among the most potent regulators of cellular function in nature and are produced by almost every cell in the body. They act mainly as "local" hormones, affecting the cells that produce them or neighboring cells of a different type.

Eicosanoids participate in many processes in the body, particularly the inflammatory response that occurs following infection or injury. This response is the sum of the body's efforts to destroy invading organisms and to repair damage. It includes the control of bleeding through the formation of blood clots. In the process of protecting the body from a variety of insults, the inflammatory response can produce symptoms such as pain, swelling, and fever. An exaggerated or inappropriate expression of the normal inflammatory response may occur in individuals who have allergic or hypersensitivity reactions.

In addition to participating in the inflammatory response, eicosanoids also regulate smooth muscle contraction (particularly in the intestine and uterus). They increase water and sodium excretion by the kidney and are involved in regulating blood pressure. They frequently serve as modulators; some eicosanoids stimulate while others inhibit the same process. For example, some serve as constrictors and others as dilators of blood vessels. They are also involved in regulating bronchoconstriction and bronchodilation.

Eicosanoids are derived from polyunsaturated fatty acids containing 20 carbon atoms, which are found in cell membranes esterified to membrane phospholipids. Compounds that serve as signals for eicosanoid production bind to cell membrane receptors and activate phospholipases that cleave the polyunsaturated fatty acids from cell membrane phospholipids (Fig. 35.1). The major dietary sources of these eicosanoid precursors are the essential fatty acids, linoleate and α-linolenate, obtained from plant oils. Arachidonic acid, derived from the diet or synthesized from linoleate, is the compound from which most of the eicosanoids are produced in the body.

Arachidonic acid is metabolized by three pathways. The two pathways that have been most thoroughly studied are the cyclooxygenase pathway (which produces prostaglandins and thromboxanes) and the lipoxygenase pathway (which produces leukotrienes). The cytochrome P450 pathway generates eicosanoids with less well-defined functions.

Many eicosanoids have very short half-lives, in the range of a few minutes or less. They are rapidly inactivated and excreted.

 "Eicosa" is the Greek word for the number 20. Eicosanoids are synthesized from polyunsaturated fatty acids with 20 carbon atoms.

Since his admission to the hospital for an acute myocardial infarction, **William Hartman** has been taking the bile salt sequestrant cholestyramine and the HMG-CoA reductase inhibitor pravastatin to lower his blood cholesterol levels (see Chapter 34). He also takes 160 mg of acetylsalicylic acid (ASA;

Dietary deficiencies of essential fatty acids are rare. However, some cases have been reported in patients receiving total parenteral nutrition (TPN). Although the most obvious symptom is a red scaly dermatitis, deficiencies of essential fatty acids also result in a decreased availability of precursors for eicosanoid synthesis.

 The composition of the diet affects the fatty acid content of membrane phospholipids. Individuals with a high content of saturated fatty acids in their diets have a high content of saturated fatty acids in their membrane lipids. Likewise, individuals with a high content of polyunsaturated fatty acids in their diets have a high content of polyunsaturated fatty acids in their membrane lipids.

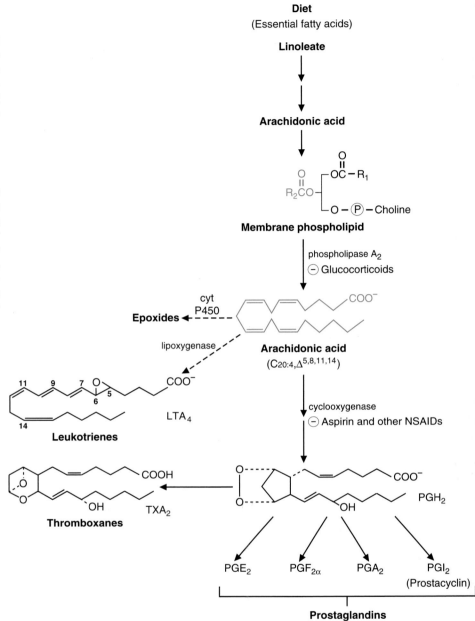

Fig. 35.1. Overview of eicosanoid metabolism. Eicosanoids are produced from fatty acids released from membrane phospholipids. In humans, arachidonic acid is the major precursor of the eicosanoids, which include the prostaglandins, leukotrienes, and thromboxanes. ⊖ = inhibits; cyt = cytochrome.

aspirin) each day. At his most recent visit to his cardiologist, he asked if he should continue to take aspirin because he no longer has any chest pain. He was told that the use of aspirin in his case was not to alleviate pain but to reduce the risk of a second heart attack and that he should continue to take this drug for the remainder of his life unless a complication, such as gastrointestinal bleeding, occurred as a result of its use.

Emma Wheezer has done well with regard to her respiratory function since her earlier hospitalization for an acute asthmatic attack. She has been maintained on two puffs of triamcinolone acetonide, a potent inhaled corticosteroid, three times a day and has not required systemic steroids for months. The glucose intolerance precipitated by high intravenous and oral doses of the synthetic glucocorticoid, dexamethasone, during her earlier hospitalization resolved after this drug was discontinued. She has come to her doctor now because she is concerned that the low grade fever and cough she has developed over the last 36 hours may trigger another acute asthma attack.

SOURCE OF THE EICOSANOIDS

The most abundant and, therefore, the most common precursor of the eicosanoids is arachidonic acid (eicosatetraenoic acid, $\omega 6,20{:}4,\Delta^{5,8,11,14}$), a polyunsaturated fatty acid with 20 carbons and 4 double bonds (see Fig. 35.1). It is esterified to phospholipids located in the lipid bilayer that comprises the plasma membrane of the cell. Because arachidonic acid cannot be synthesized de novo in the body, the diet must contain arachidonic acid or other fatty acids from which arachidonic acid can be produced. The major dietary precursor for arachidonic acid synthesis is the essential fatty acid linoleate, which is present in plant oils (see Chapter 33).

The arachidonic acid present in membrane phospholipids is released from the lipid bilayer as a consequence of the activation of membrane-bound phospholipase A_2 or C (see Fig. 33.32). This activation occurs when a variety of stimuli (agonists), such as histamine and the cytokines, interact with a specific plasma membrane receptor on the target cell surface (Fig. 35.2). Phospholipase A_2 is specific for the sn-2 position of phosphoacylglycerols, the site of attachment of arachidonic acid to the glycerol moiety. Phospholipase C hydrolyzes phosphorylated inositol from the inositol glycerophospholipids, generating a diacylglycerol containing arachidonic acid. This arachidonic acid is subsequently released by the action of other lipases.

Inflammation involving the mucosal and smooth muscle layers of the respiratory tract plays a major role in the development of acute asthmatic bronchospasm in patients such as **Emma Wheezer**. Dexamethasone and other potent glucocorticoids are capable of preventing or suppressing this inflammation.

In part, the glucocorticoids act by inhibiting the recruitment of leukocytes and monocytes-macrophages into affected areas. They also limit the ability of these cells to elaborate a variety of chemotactic factors and other substances, such as certain eicosanoids, which enhance the inflammatory process. Glucocorticoids, for example, induce the synthesis of a protein or family of proteins (lipocortins or macrocortins) that inhibit the activity of phospholipase A_2. As a result, the synthesis of prostaglandins and leukotrienes is decreased and the inflammatory response in bronchial tissues is reduced (see Figs. 35.1 and 35.2).

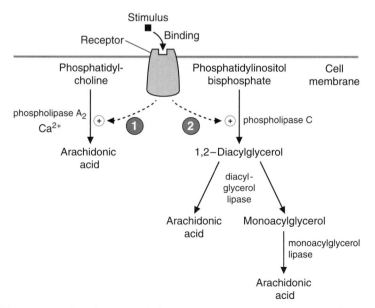

Fig. 35.2. Release of arachidonic acid from membrane lipids. The binding of a stimulus to its receptor activates pathway **1** or **2**.

PATHWAYS FOR EICOSANOID SYNTHESIS

After arachidonic acid is released into the cytosol, it is converted to eicosanoids by a variety of enzymes with activities that vary among tissues. This variation explains why some cells, such as those in the vascular endothelium, synthesize prostaglandins E$_2$ and I$_2$ (PGE$_2$ and PGI$_2$) whereas cells, such as platelets, synthesize primarily thromboxane A$_2$ (TXA$_2$) and 12-hydroxyeicosatetraenoic acid (12-HETE).

Three pathways for the metabolism of arachidonic acid occur in various tissues (Fig. 35.3). The first of these, the cyclooxygenase pathway, leads to the synthesis of prostaglandins and thromboxanes. The second, the lipoxygenase pathway, yields the leukotrienes, HETEs, and lipoxins. The third pathway, catalyzed by the cytochrome P450 system, is responsible for the synthesis of the epoxides, HETEs, and diHETEs.

Cyclooxygenase Pathway: Synthesis of the Prostaglandins and Thromboxanes

STRUCTURES OF THE PROSTAGLANDINS

Prostaglandins are fatty acids containing 20 carbon atoms, including an internal, saturated, 5-carbon ring. In addition to this ring, each of the biologically active prostaglandins has a hydroxyl group at carbon 15, a double bond between carbons 13 and 14, and various substituents on the ring (Fig. 35.4)

The nomenclature for the prostaglandins (PGs) involves the assignment of a capital letter (PGE), an Arabic numeral subscript (PGE$_1$), and, for the PGF family, a Greek letter subscript (e.g., PGF$_{2\alpha}$). The capital letter, in this case "F," refers to the ring substituents shown in Figure 35.5.

The subscript that follows the capital letter (PGF$_1$) refers to the PG series 1, 2, or 3, determined by the number of unsaturated bonds present in the linear portion of the hydrocarbon chain (Fig. 35.6). It does not include double bonds in the internal ring. Prostaglandins of the 1-series have one double bond (between carbons 13 and 14). The 2-series has two double bonds (between carbons 13 and 14, and 5 and 6), and the 3-series has three double bonds (between carbons 13 and 14, 5 and 6, and 17 and 18). The double bonds between carbons 13 and 14 are *trans*; the others are *cis*.

The Greek letter subscript, found only in the F series, refers to the position of the hydroxyl group at carbon 9. In nature, this hydroxyl group is found only in the α position; it lies below the plane of the ring as does the hydroxyl group at carbon 11 (see Figs. 35.4 and 35.5).

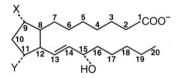

Fig. 35.4. Structural features common to the biologically active prostaglandins. These compounds have 20 carbons, with a carboxyl group at carbon 1. Carbons 8 through 12 form a 5-membered ring with substituents (usually a hydroxyl or keto group) at carbons 9 (X) and 11 (Y). Carbon 15 contains a hydroxyl group, and a *trans* double bond connects carbons 13 and 14. Double bonds also may be present between carbons 5 and 6 and between carbons 17 and 18 (see Fig. 35.6).

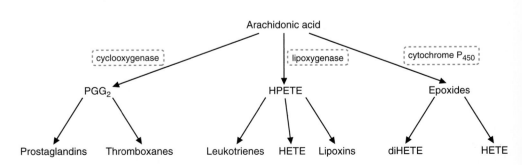

Fig. 35.3. Pathways for the metabolism of arachidonic acid.

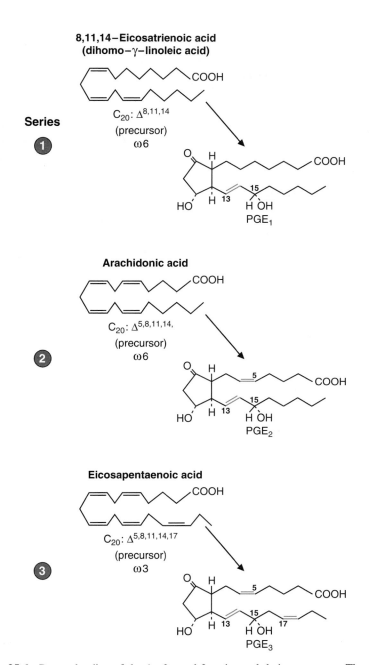

Fig. 35.6. Prostaglandins of the 1-, 2-, and 3-series and their precursors. The numeral (as a subscript in the name of the compound) refers to the number of double bonds in the non-ring portion of the prostaglandin. *Trans* double bonds are at position 13, and *cis* double bonds at positions 5 and 17. The hydroxyl group at carbon 15 is required for biological activity.

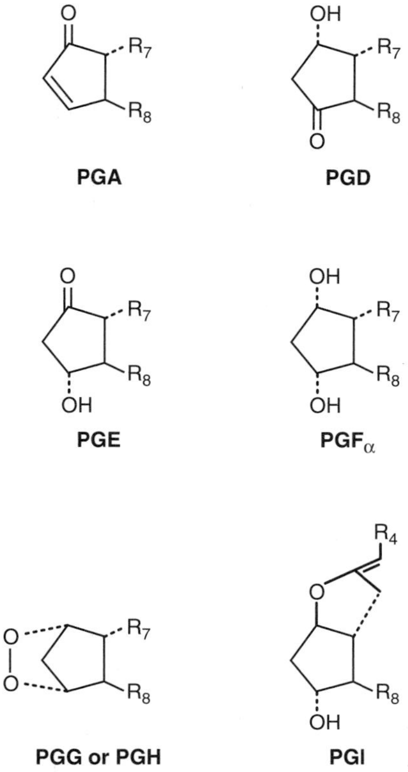

PGA

PGD

PGE

PGF$_\alpha$

PGG or PGH

PGI

Fig. 35.5. Ring substituents of the prostaglandins (PG). The letter after PG denotes the configuration of the ring and its substituents. R_4, R_7, and R_8 represent the non-ring portions of the molecule. R_4 contains 4 carbons (including the carboxyl group). R_7 and R_8 contain 7 and 8 carbons, respectively, and correspond to the 1-, 2-, or 3-series shown in Figure 35.6. Note that the prostacyclins (PGI) contain two rings.

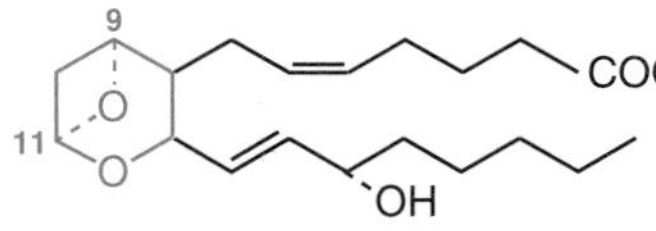

Thromboxane A$_2$
(TXA$_2$)

Fig. 35.7. The thromboxane ring. In contrast to the prostaglandins which have a 5-membered carbon ring, thromboxanes have a 6-membered ring (shown in blue) containing an oxygen atom. Substituents are attached to the ring at carbons 9 and 11. In the case of TXA$_2$ (shown above), an oxygen atom connects carbons 9 and 11.

STRUCTURE OF THE THROMBOXANES

The thromboxanes, derived from arachidonic acid via the cyclooxygenase pathway, closely resemble the prostaglandins in structure except that they contain a 6-membered ring that includes an oxygen atom (Fig. 35.7). The most common thromboxane, TXA$_2$, contains an additional oxygen atom attached both to carbon 9 and carbon 11 of the ring.

The prostaglandins were discovered in the 1930s when seminal vesicle fluid from animals and humans was found to decrease blood pressure and to produce contraction of uterine and intestinal smooth muscle. Because the prostate gland was believed (erroneously) to be the source of these acidic lipids, they were called "prostaglandins."

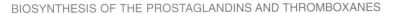

Only the biosynthesis of those prostaglandins derived from arachidonic acid (e.g., the 2-series such as PGE_2, PGI_2, TXA_2) will be described since those derived from eicosatrienoic acid (the 1-series) or from eicosapentaenoic acid (the 3-series) are present in very small amounts in humans on a normal diet (see Fig. 35.6).

The biochemical reactions that lead to the synthesis of prostaglandins and thromboxanes are illustrated in Figure 35.8. The initial step, which is catalyzed by a cyclooxygenase, forms the 5-membered ring and adds 4 atoms of oxygen (two between carbons 9 and 11, and two at carbon 15) to form the unstable endoperoxide, PGG_2. The hydroperoxy group at carbon 15 is quickly reduced to a hydroxyl group by a peroxidase to form another endoperoxide, PGH_2.

The next step is tissue specific (see Fig. 35.8). Depending upon the type of cell involved, PGH_2 may be reduced to PGE_2 or PGD_2 by specific isomerases (PGE synthase and PGD synthase). PGE_2 may be further reduced by PGE 9-ketoreductase to form $PGF_{2\alpha}$. Some of the major functions of the prostaglandins are listed in Table 35.1.

The thromboxanes were named for their action in producing blood clots (thrombi).

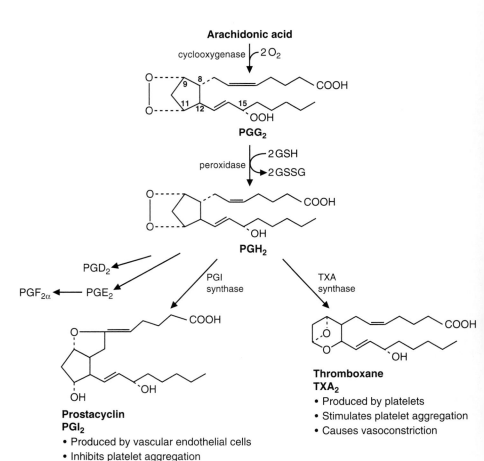

Fig. 35.8. Formation of prostaglandins (including the prostacyclin, PGI_2) and thromboxane TXA_2 from arachidonic acid. The conversion of arachidonic acid to PGH_2 is catalyzed by a membrane-bound enzyme, prostaglandin endoperoxide synthase, which has cyclooxygenase and peroxidase activities. The reducing agent is glutathione (GSH), which is oxidized to GSSG.

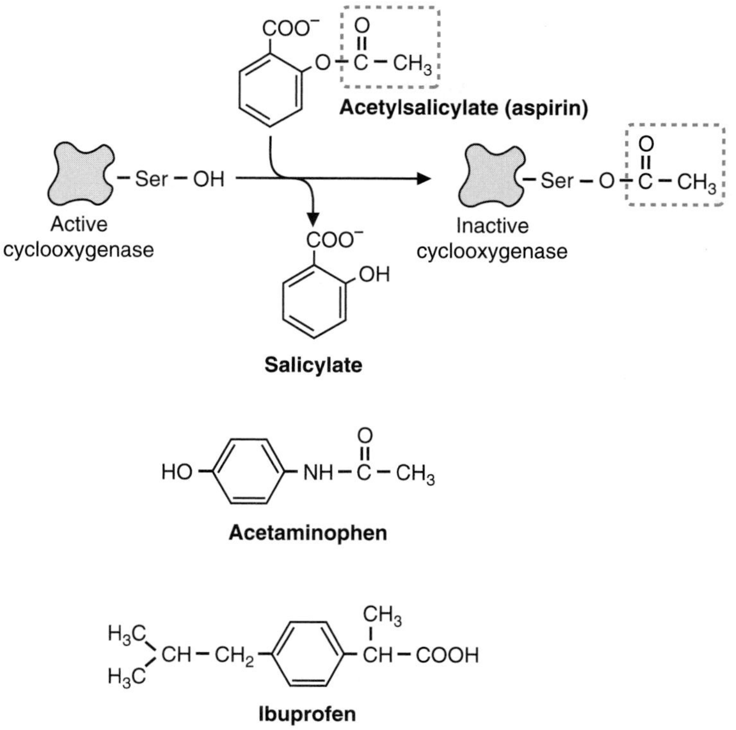

Fig. 35.9. Action of aspirin and other nonsteroidal antiinflammatory drugs.

The cyclooxygenase is inhibited by all nonsteroidal antiinflammatory drugs (NSAIDs) such as aspirin (acetylsalicylic acid). Aspirin transfers an acetyl group to the enzyme, irreversibly inactivating it. Other NSAIDs (e.g., acetaminophen, ibuprofen) act as reversible inhibitors of cyclooxygenase. Acetaminophen is the major ingredient in Tylenol, and ibuprofen is the major ingredient in other NSAIDs such as Motrin, Nuprin, and Advil (see Fig. 35.9).

Table 35.1. Some Functions of the Prostaglandins

PGI$_2$, PGE$_2$, PGD$_2$

Increase
- Vasodilation
- cAMP

Decrease
- Platelet aggregation
- Leukocyte aggregation
- IL-1[a] and IL-2
- T-cell proliferation
- Lymphocyte migration

PGF$_{2\alpha}$

Increases
- Vasoconstriction
- Bronchoconstriction
- Smooth muscle contraction

[a] IL = interleukin, a cytokine that augments the activity of many cells in the immune system.

PGH$_2$ may be converted to the thromboxane TXA$_2$, a reaction catalyzed by TXA synthase (see Fig. 35.8). This enzyme is present in high concentration in platelets. In the vascular endothelium, on the other hand, PGH$_2$ is converted to the prostaglandin PGI$_2$ (prostacyclin) by PGI synthase (see Fig. 35.8). TXA$_2$ and PGI$_2$ have important antagonistic biological effects on vasomotor and smooth muscle tone and on platelet aggregation. Some of the known functions of the thromboxanes are listed in Table 35.2.

The predominant eicosanoid in platelets is TXA$_2$, a potent vasoconstrictor and a stimulator of platelet aggregation. The latter action initiates thrombus formation at sites of vascular injury as well as in the vicinity of a ruptured atherosclerotic plaque in the lumen of vessels such as the coronary arteries. Such thrombi may cause sudden total occlusion of the vascular lumen causing acute ischemic damage to tissues distal to the block (i.e., acute myocardial infarction).

Aspirin, by covalently acetylating the active site of cyclooxygenase, blocks the production of TXA$_2$ from its major precursor, arachidonic acid. By causing this mild hemostatic defect, low dose aspirin has been shown to be effective in prevention of acute myocardial infarction (see Clinical Comments). For **Thomas Appleman** (who has symptoms of coronary heart disease), aspirin is used to prevent a first heart attack (primary prevention). For **William Hartman** and **Cora Nari** (who already have had heart attacks), aspirin is used to prevent a second heart attack (secondary prevention).

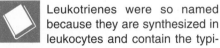

Diets that include cold water fish (e.g., salmon, mackerel, brook trout, herring) with a high content of the polyunsaturated fatty acids, eicosapentaenoic acid (EPA) and docosahexaenoic acid (DHA) (see Chapter 33), result in a high content of these fatty acids in membrane phospholipids. It has been suggested that such diets are effective in preventing heart disease, in part because they lead to formation of more TXA_3 relative to TXA_2. TXA_3 is less effective in stimulating platelet aggregation than its counterpart in the 2-series, TXA_2.

Leukotrienes were so named because they are synthesized in leukocytes and contain the typical triene structure, i.e., three double bonds in series (in this case, at positions 7, 9, and 11) (see Fig. 35.10).

Table 35.2. Some Functions of Thromboxane A$_2$

Increases
Vasoconstriction
Platelet aggregation
Lymphocyte proliferation
Bronchoconstriction

INACTIVATION OF THE PROSTAGLANDINS AND THROMBOXANES

Prostaglandins and thromboxanes are rapidly inactivated. Their half lives ($t_{1/2}$) range from seconds to minutes. The prostaglandins are inactivated by oxidation of the 15-hydroxy group, critical for their activity, to a ketone. The double bond at carbon 13 is reduced. Subsequently, both β- and ω-oxidation of the non-ring portions occur, producing dicarboxylic acids which are excreted in the urine. Active TXA_2 is rapidly metabolized to TXB_2 by cleavage of the oxygen bridge between carbons 9 and 11 to form two hydroxyl groups. TXB_2 has no biological activity.

Lipoxygenase Pathway: Synthesis of the Leukotrienes, HETE, and Lipoxins

In addition to serving as a substrate for the cyclooxygenase pathway, arachidonic acid also acts as a substrate for the lipoxygenase pathway. The lipoxygenase enzymes catalyze the incorporation of an oxygen molecule onto a carbon of one of several double bonds of arachidonic acid, forming a hydroperoxy (–OOH) group at these positions. With this oxygenation, the double bond isomerizes to a position one carbon removed from the hydroperoxy group and is transformed from the *cis* to the *trans* configuration (Fig. 35.10).

Lipoxygenases may act at carbon 5, 12, or 15. The type of lipoxygenase varies from tissue to tissue. For example, polymorphonuclear leukocytes contain primarily 5-lipoxygenase, platelets are rich in 12-lipoxygenase, and eosinophilic leukocytes contain primarily 15-lipoxygenase.

LEUKOTRIENE SYNTHESIS

As shown in Figure 35.11, the synthesis of the leukotrienes begins with the formation of hydroperoxyeicosatetraenoic acids (HPETEs). This product is either reduced to the corresponding hydroxy metabolites, HETEs (see Fig. 35.10), or it is metabolized to form leukotrienes or lipoxins (see Figs. 35.11 and 35.12). The major leukotrienes are produced by 5-lipoxygenase.

In leukocytes and mast cells, 5-HPETE is converted to an epoxide, leukotriene A$_4$ (LTA$_4$). The subscript number 4 refers to the presence of four double bonds in the leukotriene. Three of the double bonds (7, 9, 11) are conjugated, i.e., form a triene.

Other functional leukotrienes are formed from LTA$_4$ by one of two pathways. In the first, LTA$_4$ is converted to LTB$_4$, a 5,12-dihydroxy derivative. The second metabolic pathway involves the addition of reduced glutathione to carbon 6 to form LTC$_4$, a reaction catalyzed by glutathione *S*-transferase. Glutamate is removed from the glutathione moiety of LTC$_4$ through the action of γ-glutamyl transpeptidase to form LTD$_4$. A dipeptidase then cleaves the glycine residue from LTD$_4$ to form LTE$_4$ (see Fig. 35.11). The major functions of some of the leukotrienes are listed in Table 35.3.

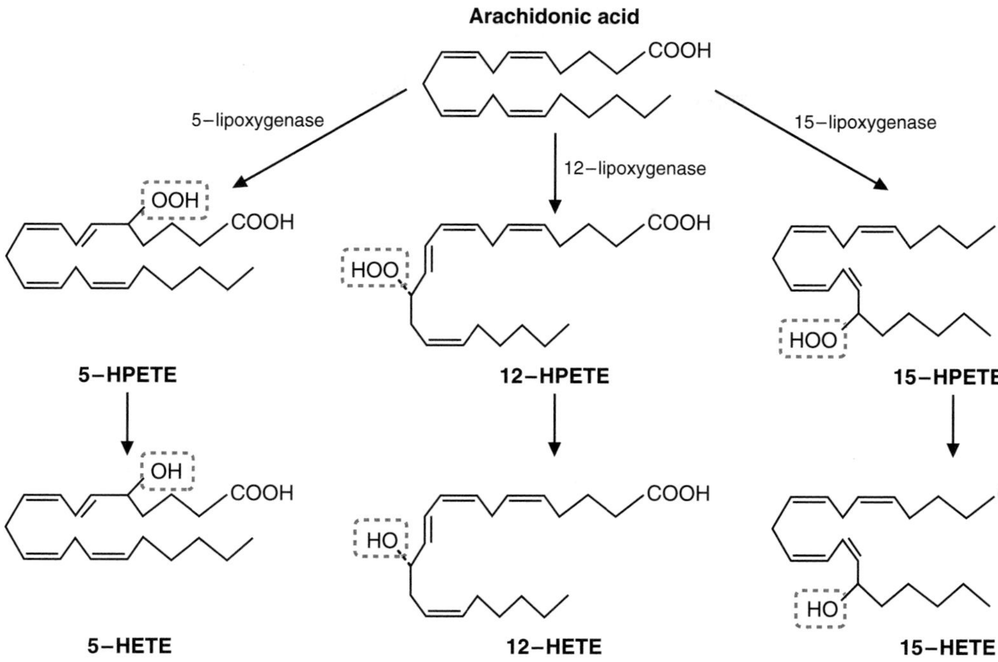

Fig. 35.10. Action of lipoxygenases in the formation of HPETEs and HETEs. Lipoxygenases add hydroperoxy groups at position 5, 12, or 15 with rearrangement of the double bond. HPETEs are unstable and are rapidly reduced to form HETEs or converted to leukotrienes and lipoxins (see Figs. 35.11 and 35.12).

LIPOXIN SYNTHESIS AND ACTIONS

The lipoxins are formed through the action of 15-lipoxygenase followed by the action of 5-lipoxygenase on arachidonic acid. A series of reductions of the resultant hydroperoxy groups leads to the formation of trihydroxy derivatives of arachidonic acid known as the lipoxins (Fig. 35.12). Lipoxins cause chemotaxis and stimulate superoxide anion production in leukocytes.

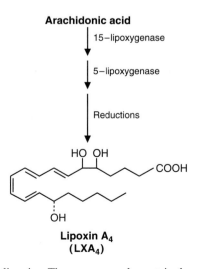

Fig. 35.12. Formation of the lipoxins. These compounds contain three hydroxyl groups.

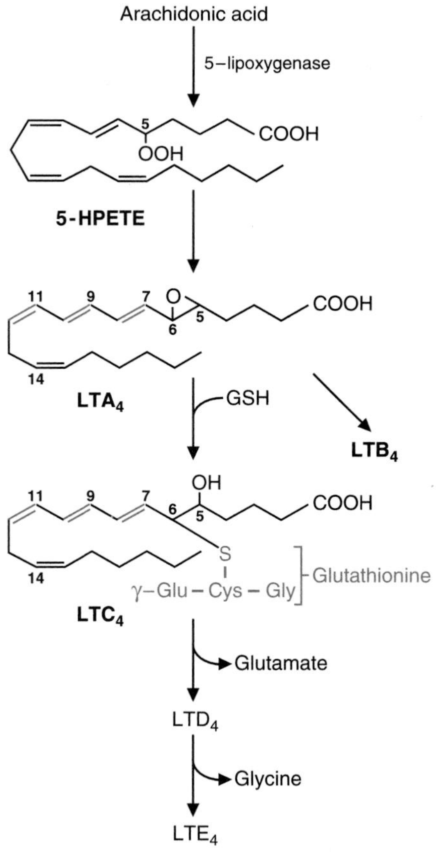

Fig. 35.11. Formation of leukotrienes and their glutathione (GSH) derivatives.

Table 35.3. Some Functions of Leukotrienes

LTB$_4$
Increases
    Vascular permeability
    T-cell proliferation
    Leukocyte aggregation
    INF-γ
    IL-1
    IL-2

LTC$_4$ and LTD$_4$
Increase
    Bronchoconstriction
    Vascular permeability
    INF-γ

INF = interferon; IL = interleukin.

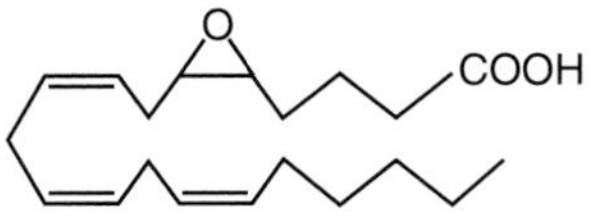

Epoxide
(5,6-EET)

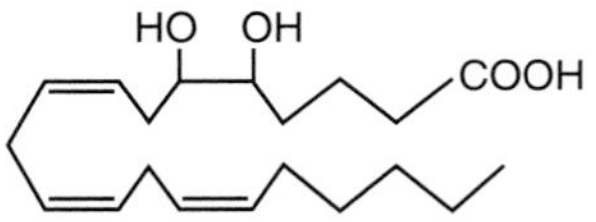

Dihydroxide
(5,6-diHETE)

Fig. 35.13. Examples of compounds produced from arachidonic acid by the cytochrome P450 pathway.

Paracrine action: A substance released from one type of cell alters the function of neighboring cells of a different type without entry into the bloodstream.

Autocrine action: A substance produced in one type of cell alters the activity of cells of that same type.

Cytochrome P450 Pathway: Synthesis and Actions of Epoxides, HETEs, and diHETES

A third mechanism for the oxygenation of arachidonic acid involves the cytochrome P450 pathway. The activity of the monoxygenases in this microsomal system yields epoxides, certain forms of HETEs (e.g., ω-hydroxy derivatives), and diol forms (diHETEs) (Fig. 35.13). The biological activity of these compounds has not been determined but some may alter the tone of vascular smooth muscle in part by inhibiting the Na$^+$,K$^+$-ATPase.

MECHANISM OF ACTION OF THE EICOSANOIDS

The eicosanoids have a wide variety of physiological effects, which are generally initiated through an interaction of the eicosanoid with a specific receptor on the plasma membrane of a target cell. This eicosanoid-receptor binding either activates the adenylate cyclase-cAMP-protein kinase A system (PGE, PGD, and PGI series) or causes an increase in the level of calcium in the cytosol of target cells (PGF$_{2\alpha}$, TXA$_2$, the endoperoxides, and the leukotrienes).

In some systems, the eicosanoids appear to modulate the degree of activation of adenylate cyclase in response to other stimuli. In these instances the eicosanoid may bind to a regulatory subunit of the GTP-binding proteins (G proteins) within the plasma membrane of the target cell (see Chapter 43). If the eicosanoid binds to the stimulatory subunit, the effect of the stimulus is amplified. On the other hand, if the eicosanoid binds to the inhibitory subunit, the cellular response to the stimulus is reduced. Through these influences on the activation of adenylate cyclase, eicosanoids contribute to the regulation of cell function.

Some of the biological effects of certain eicosanoids occur as a result of a paracrine or autocrine action. One paracrine action is the contraction of vascular smooth muscle cells caused by TXA$_2$ released from circulating platelets. An autocrine action of eicosanoids is exemplified by platelet aggregation induced by TXA$_2$ produced by the platelets themselves.

The eicosanoids influence the cellular function of almost every tissue of the body. Certain organ systems are affected to a greater degree than others.

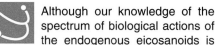

Although our knowledge of the spectrum of biological actions of the endogenous eicosanoids is incomplete, several actions are well-enough established to allow their application in a variety of clinical situations or diseases. For example, drugs that are analogs of PGE$_1$ and PGE$_2$ suppress the gastric secretion of hydrochloric acid through the blockade of type 2 histamine receptors in the mucosal cells of the stomach. These drugs, known as H$_2$ blockers, have improved the rate of healing of gastric and duodenal ulcers. Analogues of PGE$_1$ decrease the venous outflow of blood from the penis. Therefore, men with certain forms of sexual impotence can self-inject this agent into the corpus cavernosum of the penis to induce immediate but temporary penile tumescence. Finally, the stimulatory action of PGE$_2$ and PGF$_{2\alpha}$ on uterine muscle contraction has led to the use of these prostaglandins to induce labor and to control postpartum bleeding.

CLINICAL COMMENTS. In the presence of aspirin, cyclooxygenase is irreversibly inactivated by acetylation. New cyclooxygenase molecules are not produced in platelets because these cells have no nuclei and, therefore, cannot synthesize new mRNA. Thus the inhibition of cyclooxygenase by aspirin persists for the lifespan of the platelet (7–10 days). When aspirin is taken daily at doses between 80 and 320 mg, new platelets are affected as they are generated. Higher doses do not improve efficacy but do increase side effects, such as gastrointestinal bleeding and easy bruisability.

Patients with established or suspected atherosclerotic coronary disease, such as **William Hartman, Cora Nari,** and **Thomas Appleman,** benefit from the action of low-dose aspirin (approximately 160 mg/day), which produces a mild defect in hemostasis. This action of aspirin helps to prevent thrombus formation in the area of an atherosclerotic plaque at critical sites in the vascular tree.

Corticosteroids reduce inflammation, in part, through their inhibitory effect on phospholipase A$_2$. Despite the unquestionable value of glucocorticoid therapy in a variety of diseases associated with acute inflammation of tissues, the suppression of the inflammatory response with pharmacological doses of corticosteroids is potentially hazardous. The sudden appearance of temporary glucose intolerance when **Emma Wheezer** was treated with large doses of dexamethasone, a gluconeogenic steroid (glucocorticoid), is just one of the many potential adverse effects of this class of drugs when given systemically in pharmacological doses over an extended period (see Chapter 45). The inhaled steroids, on the other hand, have far fewer systemic side effects because their absorption across the bronchial mucosa into the circulation is very limited. This property allows them to be used over prolonged periods in the treatment of asthma. The fact that inhalation allows direct delivery of the agent to the primary site of inflammation, adds to their effectiveness in the treatment of these patients.

BIOCHEMICAL COMMENTS. Inflammation is the response of the body to infection or injury, directed at destroying the infectious agents and repairing the damaged areas. It involves an increase of the blood supply to the affected region by means of vasodilation. The capillaries become more permeable so that fluid, large molecules, and white blood cells can cross, leaving the blood and entering the tissue. White blood cells (particularly neutrophils and monocytes) move by chemotaxis to the injured site. Redness, heat, swelling, and pain are associated with the inflammatory process. Redness and heat are caused by the increased blood flow. Swelling is the result of the increased movement of fluid and white blood cells into the area of inflammation. Pain is caused by the release of chemical compounds and the compression of nerves in the vicinity of the inflammatory process.

The chemical mediators of inflammation usually are produced by activation of complement (a family of blood proteins that are cleaved to form active fragments) or of the blood clotting cascade (see Chapter 9). These processes cause the release of histamine from mast cells, and the production of kinins by cleavage of kininogens. Among their other effects, both histamine and kinins increase vascular permeability. They stimulate the synthesis of eicosanoids that act on the motility and metabolism of white blood cells and cause the aggregation of platelets to arrest bleeding. Some of the prostaglandins act on thermoregulatory centers of the brain, producing fever. Cytokines are also released that stimulate the proliferation of cells involved in the immune response.

Although uncomfortable, the pain, swelling, and fever that are part of the inflammatory response serve as an important warning sign that the host is threatened and that some specific counteractions must be taken against the offending agent or process. Although the use of antiinflammatory drugs may bring welcome symptomatic relief, their use may, in part, diminish the effectiveness of the host's response to the inciting agent.

PROBLEMS

1. Write a series of reactions by which α-linolenic acid ($\omega 3, 18{:}3, \Delta^{9,12,15}$) can be converted to eicosapentaenoic acid (EPA, $\omega 3, 20{:}5, \Delta^{5,8,11,14,17}$). Hints: (*a*) Humans have a Δ^6- and a Δ^5-desaturase. (*b*) See conversion of linoleic acid to arachidonic acid in Chapter 33.

2. Some patients with asthma have an exacerbation of their symptoms when they take NSAIDs. Develop a biochemical rationale for this problem.

ANSWERS

1. The original bonds in α-linolenate are indicated by solid lines. Changes as linolenate is converted to EPA are indicated by dashed lines. Note that the position of the original double bonds changes because the chain is elongated at the carboxyl end.

2. NSAIDs inhibit cyclooxygenase but do not inhibit lipoxygenase. Because arachidonic acid cannot proceed through the cyclooxygenase pathway at a normal rate in the presence of NSAIDs, more substrate is available for the lipoxygenase pathway that produces the leukotrienes which cause bronchoconstriction (see Fig. 35.1). (An alternative or additional reason is that synthesis of bronchodilator prostaglandins and thromboxanes may be more inhibited than synthesis of those that cause bronchoconstriction.)

36 Integration of Carbohydrate and Lipid Metabolism

The purpose of this chapter is to summarize and integrate the major pathways for the utilization of carbohydrates and fats as fuels. We will concentrate on reviewing the regulatory mechanisms that determine the flux of metabolites in the fed and fasting states, integrating the pathways that were described separately under carbohydrate and lipid metabolism. The next section of the book covers the mechanisms by which the pathways of nitrogen metabolism are coordinated with fat and carbohydrate metabolism.

In order for the species to survive, it is necessary for us to store excess food when we eat and to use these stores when we are fasting. Regulatory mechanisms direct compounds through the pathways of metabolism involved in the storage and utilization of fuels. These mechanisms are controlled by hormones, by the concentration of available fuels, and by the energy needs of the body.

Changes in hormone levels, in the concentration of fuels, and in energy requirements affect the activity of key enzymes in the major pathways of metabolism. Intracellular enzymes are generally regulated by activation and inhibition, by phosphorylation and dephosphorylation (or other covalent modifications), by induction and repression, and by degradation. Activation and inhibition of enzymes cause immediate changes in metabolism. Phosphorylation and dephosphorylation of enzymes affect metabolism slightly less rapidly. Induction and repression of enzyme synthesis are much slower processes, usually affecting metabolic flux over a period of hours. Degradation of enzymes decreases the amount available to catalyze reactions.

The pathways of metabolism have multiple control points and multiple regulators at each control point. The function of these complex mechanisms is to produce a graded response to a stimulus and to provide sensitivity to multiple stimuli so that an exact balance is maintained between flux through a given step (or series of steps) and the need or use for the product. Pyruvate dehydrogenase is an example of an enzyme that has multiple regulatory mechanisms. Regardless of insulin levels, the enzyme cannot become fully activated in the presence of products and absence of substrates.

The major hormones that regulate the pathways of fuel metabolism are insulin and glucagon. In liver, all effects of glucagon are reversed by insulin, and some of the pathways that insulin activates are inhibited by glucagon. Thus, the pathways of carbohydrate and lipid metabolism are generally regulated by changes in the insulin/glucagon ratio.

Although glycogen is a critical storage form of fuel because blood glucose levels must be carefully maintained, adipose triacylglycerols are quantitatively the major fuel store in the human. Following a meal, both dietary glucose and fat are stored in adipose tissue as triacylglycerol. This fuel is released during fasting, when it provides the main source of energy for the tissues of the body. The length of time we can survive without food depends mainly on the size of our bodies' fat stores.

557

Within 2 months of her surgery to remove a benign insulin-secreting B cell tumor of the pancreas, **Bea Selmass** was again jogging lightly. She had lost the 8 lb that she had gained in the 6 weeks prior to her surgery. Since her hypoglycemic episodes were no longer occurring, she had no need to eat frequent carbohydrate snacks to prevent the adrenergic and neuroglycopenic symptoms that she had experienced when her tumor was secreting excessive amounts of insulin.

A few months after her last hospitalization, **Di Beatty** was once again brought to the hospital emergency room in diabetic ketoacidosis (DKA). Blood samples for glucose and electrolytes were drawn repeatedly during the first 24 hours. The hospital laboratory reported that the serum in each of these specimens appeared opalescent rather than having its normal clear or transparent appearance. This opalescence results from light scattering caused by the presence of elevated levels of triacylglycerol-rich lipoproteins in the blood

When **Ann Sulin** initially presented with non-insulin-dependent diabetes mellitus (NIDDM) at age 39, she was approximately 30 lb above her ideal weight. Her high serum glucose levels were accompanied by abnormalities in her 14-hour fasting lipid profile. Her serum total cholesterol, low density lipoprotein (LDL) cholesterol, and triacylglycerol levels were elevated and her serum high density lipoprotein (HDL) cholesterol level was below the normal range.

REGULATION OF CARBOHYDRATE AND LIPID METABOLISM IN THE FED STATE

Mechanisms That Affect Glycogen and Triacylglycerol Synthesis in Liver

After a meal, the liver synthesizes glycogen and triacylglycerol. The level of glycogen stored in the liver can increase from about 80 g after an overnight fast to a limit of about 200–300 g. Although the liver synthesizes triacylglycerol, it does not store this fuel, but rather packages it in VLDL and secretes it into the blood. The fatty acids of the VLDL triacylglycerols are stored as adipose triacylglycerols. Adipose tissue has an almost infinite capacity to store fat, limited mainly by the ability of the heart to pump blood through the capillaries of the tissue. Although we store fat throughout our bodies, it tends to accumulate in places where it does not interfere too much with our mobility: in the abdomen, hips, thighs, and buttocks.

Both the synthesis of liver glycogen and the conversion by the liver of dietary glucose to triacylglycerol (lipogenesis) are regulated by mechanisms involving key enzymes in these pathways.

GLUCOKINASE

After a meal, glucose can be converted to glycogen or to triacylglycerol in the liver. For both processes, glucose is first converted to glucose 6-phosphate by glucokinase, a liver enzyme that has a high K_m for glucose (Fig. 36.1). This enzyme is most active in the fed state when the concentration of glucose is particularly high because the hepatic portal vein carries digestive products directly from the intestine to the liver. Synthesis of glucokinase is also induced by insulin (which is elevated after a meal) and repressed by glucagon (which is elevated during fasting).

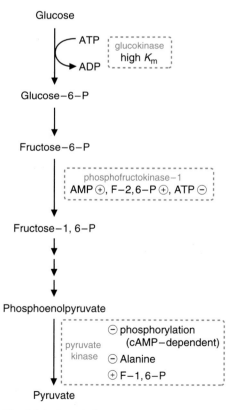

Fig. 36.1. Regulation of glucokinase, PFK-1, and pyruvate kinase in the liver.

GLYCOGEN SYNTHASE

In the conversion of glucose 6-phosphate to glycogen, the key regulatory enzyme is glycogen synthase. This enzyme is activated by the dephosphorylation which occurs when insulin is elevated and glucagon is decreased (Fig. 36.2) and by the increased level of glucose.

PHOSPHOFRUCTOKINASE-1 AND PYRUVATE KINASE

For lipogenesis, glucose 6-phosphate is converted via glycolysis to pyruvate. Key enzymes that regulate this pathway in the liver are phosphofructokinase-1 (PFK-1) and pyruvate kinase. PFK-1 is allosterically activated in the fed state by fructose 2,6-bisphosphate and AMP (see Fig. 36.1). Phosphofructokinase-2, the enzyme that produces this activator, is dephosphorylated and following a meal (see Chapter 27). Pyruvate kinase is also activated by dephosphorylation, which is stimulated by the increase of the insulin/glucagon ratio in the fed state (see Fig. 36.1).

PYRUVATE DEHYDROGENASE AND PYRUVATE CARBOXYLASE

The conversion of pyruvate to fatty acids requires a source of acetyl CoA in the cytosol. Pyruvate can only be converted to acetyl CoA in mitochondria, so it enters mitochondria and forms acetyl CoA via the pyruvate dehydrogenase (PDH) reaction. This enzyme is dephosphorylated and most active when its supply of substrates and ADP is high, its products are utilized, and insulin is present (Fig. 36.3).

Pyruvate is also converted to oxaloacetate. The enzyme that catalyzes this reaction, pyruvate carboxylase, is activated by acetyl CoA. Because acetyl CoA cannot directly cross the mitochondrial membrane to form fatty acids in the cytosol, it condenses with oxaloacetate, producing citrate. The citrate that is not required for tricarboxylic acid (TCA) cycle activity crosses the membrane and enters the cytosol.

CITRATE LYASE, MALIC ENZYME, AND GLUCOSE 6-PHOSPHATE DEHYDROGENASE

In the cytosol, citrate is cleaved by citrate lyase, an inducible enzyme, to form oxaloacetate and acetyl CoA (Fig. 36.4). The acetyl CoA is used for fatty acid biosynthesis and for cholesterol synthesis, which are also activated by insulin. Oxaloacetate is recycled to pyruvate via cytosolic malate dehydrogenase and malic enzyme, which is inducible. Malic enzyme generates NADPH for the reactions on the fatty acid synthase complex. NADPH is also produced by the two enzymes of the pentose phosphate pathway, glucose 6-phosphate dehydrogenase and 6-phosphogluconate dehydrogenase. Glucose 6-phosphate dehydrogenase is also induced by insulin.

ACETYL CoA CARBOXYLASE

Acetyl CoA is converted to malonyl CoA, which provides the 2-carbon units for elongation of the growing fatty acyl chain on the fatty acid synthase complex. Acetyl CoA carboxylase, the enzyme that catalyzes the conversion of acetyl CoA to malonyl CoA, is controlled by three of the major mechanisms that regulate enzyme activity (Fig. 36.5). It is activated by citrate, which causes the enzyme to polymerize, and inhibited by long chain fatty acyl CoA. A phosphatase stimulated by insulin activates the enzyme by dephosphorylation. The third means by which this enzyme is regulated is induction; the quantity of the enzyme increases in the fed state.

Malonyl CoA, the product of the acetyl CoA carboxylase reaction, provides the carbons for the synthesis of palmitate on the fatty acid synthase complex. Malonyl CoA also inhibits carnitine:palmitoyltransferase I (CPTI, also known as carnitine:acyltransferase I), the enzyme that prepares long chain fatty acyl CoA for

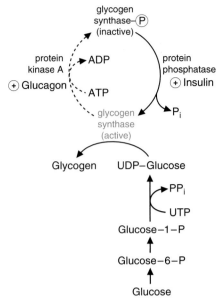

Fig. 36.2. Regulation of glycogen synthase. This enzyme is phosphorylated by a cAMP-mediated mechanism during fasting. It is dephosphorylated and active after a meal, and glycogen is stored. Circled P = phosphate; ⊕ = activated by; ⊖ = inhibited by.

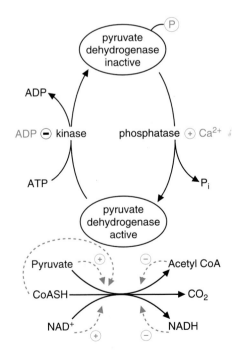

Fig. 36.3. Regulation of pyruvate dehydrogenase (PDH). A kinase associated with the PDH complex phosphorylates and inactivates the enzyme.

36.1: Why does **Ann Sulin** have a hypertriglyceridemia?

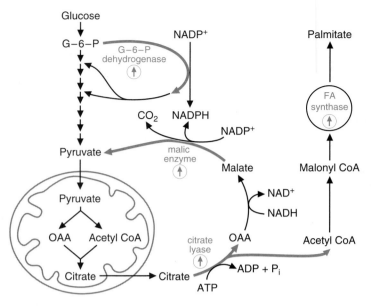

Fig. 36.4. Regulation of citrate lyase, malic enzyme, glucose 6-phosphate dehydrogenase, and fatty acid synthase. Citrate lyase, which provides acetyl CoA for fatty acid biosynthesis, the enzymes that provide NADPH (malic enzyme, glucose 6-phosphate dehydrogenase), as well as fatty acid synthase are inducible (circled ↑).

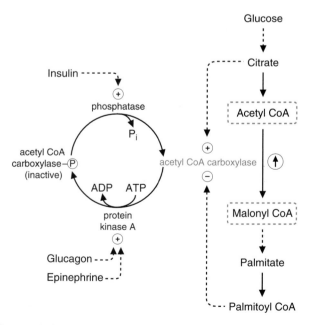

Fig. 36.5. Regulation of acetyl CoA carboxylase (AcC). AcC is regulated by activation and inhibition, by phosphorylation (mediated by cAMP) and dephosphorylation (via an insulin-stimulated phosphatase), and by induction and repression. It is active in the fed state.

transport into mitochondria (Fig. 36.6). In the fed state, when acetyl CoA carboxylase is active and malonyl CoA levels are elevated, newly synthesized fatty acids are converted to triacylglycerols for storage, rather than being transported into mitochondria for oxidation and ketone body formation.

FATTY ACID SYNTHASE COMPLEX

In a well-fed individual, the quantity of the fatty acid synthase complex is increased (see Fig. 36.4). The genes that produce this enzyme complex are induced by increases in the insulin/glucagon ratio. The amount of the complex increases slowly, after a few days of a high carbohydrate diet.

Glucose 6-phosphate dehydrogenase, which generates NADPH in the pentose phosphate pathway, and malic enzyme, which produces NADPH, are also induced by the increase of insulin.

The palmitate produced by the synthase complex is converted to palmitoyl CoA and elongated and desaturated to form other fatty acyl CoA molecules, which are converted to triacylglycerols. These triacylglycerols are packaged and secreted into the blood as VLDL.

Mechanisms That Affect the Fate of Chylomicrons and VLDL

The lipoprotein triacylglycerols in chylomicrons and VLDL are hydrolyzed to fatty acids and glycerol by lipoprotein lipase (LPL), an enzyme attached to endothelial cells of capillaries in muscle and adipose tissue. The enzyme found in muscle, particularly heart muscle, has a low K_m for these blood lipoproteins. Therefore, it acts even when these lipoproteins are present at very low concentrations in the blood. The fatty acids enter muscle cells and are oxidized for energy. The enzyme found in adipose tissue has a higher K_m and is most active after a meal when blood lipoprotein levels are elevated.

Mechanisms That Affect Triacylglycerol Storage in Adipose Tissue

Insulin stimulates adipose cells to synthesize and secrete LPL, which hydrolyzes the chylomicron and VLDL triacylglycerols. The C_{II} apoprotein, donated to chylomicrons and VLDL by HDL, activates LPL (Fig. 36.7).

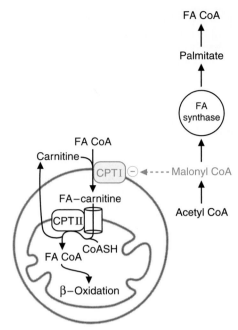

Fig. 36.6. Inhibition of transport of fatty acids (FA) into mitochondria by malonyl CoA. In the fed state, malonyl CoA (the substrate for fatty acid synthesis produced by acetyl CoA carboxylase) is elevated. It inhibits CPTI, preventing the transport of long chain fatty acids into mitochondria. Therefore, substrate is not available for β-oxidation and ketone body synthesis.

Di Beatty has insulin-dependent diabetes mellitus (IDDM), a disease associated with a severe deficiency or absence of insulin production by the B (β) cells of the pancreas. One of the effects of insulin is to stimulate production of LPL. Because of low insulin levels, Di Beatty tends to have low levels of this enzyme. Hydrolysis of the triacylglycerols in chylomicrons and in VLDL is decreased, and hypertriglyceridemia results.

A 36.1: **Ann Sulin** has NIDDM. She produces insulin but her adipose tissue is resistant to its actions. Therefore, her adipose tissue does not produce as much LPL as a normal person, which is one of the reasons why VLDL and chylomicrons remain elevated in her blood.

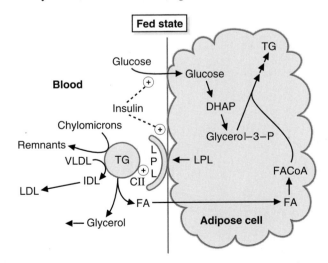

Fig. 36.7. Regulation of the storage of triacylglycerols (TG) in adipose tissue. Insulin stimulates the secretion of LPL from adipose cells and the transport of glucose into these cells. ApoC$_{II}$ activates LPL. FA= fatty acids.

Twenty to 30% of patients with an insulinoma gain weight as part of their syndrome. **Bea Selmass** gained 8 lb in the 6 weeks prior to her surgery. Although she was primed by her high insulin levels both to store and to utilize fuel more efficiently, she would not have gained weight if she had not consumed more calories than she required for her daily energy expenditure during her illness (see Chapter 1). Bea consumed extra carbohydrate calories, mostly as hard candies and table sugar, in order to avoid the symptoms of hypoglycemia.

Fatty acids released from chylomicrons and VLDL by LPL are stored as triacylglycerols in adipose cells. The glycerol released by LPL is not utilized by adipose cells because they lack glycerol kinase. Glycerol can be used by liver cells, however, because these cells do contain glycerol kinase. In the fed state, liver cells convert glycerol to the glycerol moiety of the triacylglycerols of VLDL.

Insulin causes the number of glucose transporters in adipose cell membranes to increase. Glucose enters these cells, producing energy and providing the glycerol moiety for triacylglycerol synthesis (via the dihydroxyacetone phosphate intermediate of glycolysis).

REGULATION OF CARBOHYDRATE AND LIPID METABOLISM DURING FASTING

Mechanisms in Liver that Serve to Maintain Blood Glucose Levels

During fasting, the insulin/glucagon ratio decreases. Liver glycogen is degraded to produce blood glucose because enzymes of glycogen degradation are activated by cAMP-directed phosphorylation (Fig. 36.8). Glucagon stimulates adenylate cyclase to produce

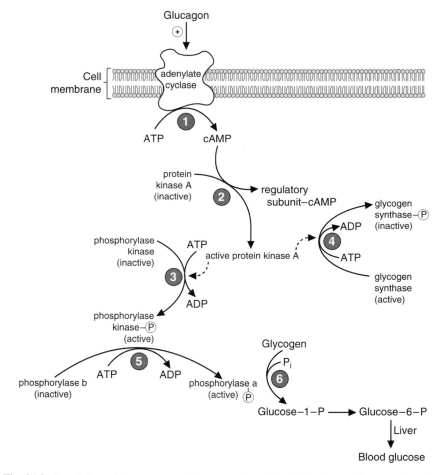

Fig. 36.8. Regulation of the enzymes of glycogen degradation in the liver. Glucagon (or epinephrine) binds to its cell membrane receptor, activating adenylate cyclase. As cAMP levels rise, inhibitory subunits are removed from protein kinase A, which now phosphorylates phosphorylase kinase. Phosphorylated phosphorylase kinase phosphorylates glycogen phosphorylase. Phosphorylated glycogen phosphorylase catalyzes the phosphorolysis of glycogen, producing glucose 1-phosphate. These events occur during fasting and produce glucose to maintain blood levels.

cAMP, which activates protein kinase A. Protein kinase A phosphorylates phosphorylase kinase, which then phosphorylates and activates glycogen phosphorylase. Protein kinase A also phosphorylates but, in this case, **in**activates glycogen synthase.

Gluconeogenesis is stimulated because the synthesis of phosphoenolpyruvate carboxykinase, fructose 1,6-bisphosphatase, and glucose 6-phosphatase is induced and because there is an increased availability of precursors. Fructose 1,6-bisphosphatase is also activated because the levels of its inhibitor, fructose 2,6-bisphosphate, are low (Fig. 36.9). During fasting, the activity of the corresponding enzymes of glycolysis is decreased.

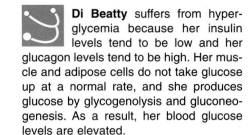

Di Beatty suffers from hyperglycemia because her insulin levels tend to be low and her glucagon levels tend to be high. Her muscle and adipose cells do not take glucose up at a normal rate, and she produces glucose by glycogenolysis and gluconeogenesis. As a result, her blood glucose levels are elevated.

Ann Sulin is in a similar metabolic state. However, in this case, she produces insulin, but her tissues are resistant to its actions.

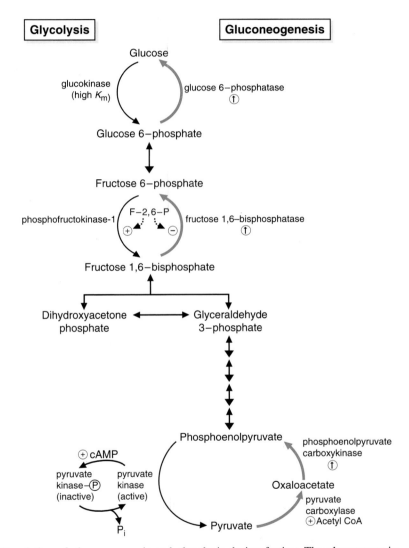

Fig. 36.9. Regulation of gluconeogenesis and glycolysis during fasting. The gluconeogenic enzymes phosphoenolpyruvate carboxykinase, fructose 1,6-bisphosphatase, and glucose 6-phosphatase are induced. Fructose 1,6-bisphosphatase is also active because, during fasting, the level of its inhibitor, fructose 2,6-bisphosphate, is low. The corresponding enzymes of glycolysis are not very active during fasting. The rate of glucokinase is low because it has a high K_m for glucose and the glucose concentration is low. Phosphofructokinase-1 is not very active because the concentration of its activator fructose 2,6-bisphosphate is low. Pyruvate kinase is inactivated by cAMP-mediated phosphorylation.

Q 36.2: Would **Ann Sulin's** serum triacylglycerol level be elevated?

Mechanisms That Affect Lipolysis in Adipose Tissue

During fasting, as blood insulin levels fall and glucagon levels rise, the level of cAMP rises in adipose cells. Consequently, protein kinase A is activated and causes phosphorylation of hormone-sensitive lipase (HSL). The phosphorylated form of this enzyme is active and cleaves fatty acids from triacylglycerols (Fig. 36.10). Other hormones (e.g., epinephrine, adrenocorticotropic hormone (ACTH), growth hormone) also activate this enzyme (see Chapter 45).

Mechanisms That Affect Ketone Body Production by the Liver

As fatty acids are released from adipose tissue during fasting, they travel in the blood complexed with albumin. These fatty acids are oxidized by various tissues, particularly muscle. In the liver, fatty acids are transported into mitochondria because acetyl CoA carboxylase is inactive, malonyl CoA levels are low, and CPTI (carnitine:acyltransferase I) is active (see Fig. 36.6). Acetyl CoA, produced by β-oxidation, is converted to ketone bodies.

Regulation of the Use of Glucose and Fatty Acids by Muscle

During exercise, the fuel that is used initially by muscle cells is muscle glycogen. As exercise continues and the blood supply to the tissue increases, glucose is taken up from the blood and oxidized. Liver glycogenolysis and gluconeogenesis replenish the blood glucose supply.

As fatty acids become available because of increased lipolysis of adipose triacylglycerols, the exercising muscle begins to oxidize fatty acids. β-Oxidation produces NADH and acetyl CoA, which slow the flow of carbon from glucose through the reaction catalyzed by pyruvate dehydrogenase (see Fig. 36.3). Thus, the oxidation of fatty acids provides a major portion of the increased demand for ATP generation and spares blood glucose.

Insulin normally inhibits lipolysis by decreasing the lipolytic activity of HSL in the adipocyte. Individuals, such as **Di Beatty**, who have a deficiency of insulin, have an increase in lipolysis and a subsequent increase in the concentration of free fatty acids in the blood. The liver, in turn, uses some of these fatty acids to synthesize triacylglycerols which are then used in the hepatic production of VLDL. VLDL is not stored in the liver but is secreted into the blood, raising its serum concentration. Di also has low levels of LPL because of decreased insulin levels. Her hypertriglyceridemia is the result, therefore, of both overproduction of VLDL by the liver and decreased breakdown of VLDL triacylglycerol for storage in adipose cells.

The serum begins to appear cloudy when the triacylglycerol level reaches 200 mg/dL. As the triacylglycerol level increases still further, the degree of serum opalescence increases proportionally.

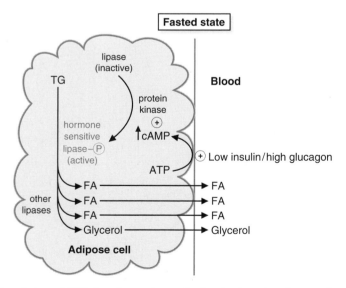

Fig. 36.10. Regulation of HSL in adipose tissue. During fasting, the glucagon/insulin ratio rises, causing cAMP levels to be elevated. Protein kinase A is activated and phosphorylates HSL, activating this enzyme. HSL-P initiates the mobilization of adipose triacylglycerol by removing a fatty acid (FA). Other lipases then act, producing fatty acids and glycerol. Insulin stimulates the phosphatase that inactivates HSL in the fed state.

CLINICAL COMMENTS. **Bea Selmass's** younger sister was very concerned that Bea's pancreatic tumor might be genetically determined and/or potentially malignant, so she accompanied Bea to her second postoperative visit to the endocrinologist. The doctor explained that insulinomas may be familial in up to 20% of cases and that in 10% of patients with insulinomas, additional secretory neoplasms may occur in the anterior pituitary and/or the parathyroid glands (a genetically determined syndrome known as multiple endocrine neoplasia, type I or, simply, MEN I). Bea's tumor showed no evidence of malignancy, and the histologic slides, although not always definitive, showed a benign-appearing process. The doctor was careful to explain, however, that close observation for recurrent hypoglycemia and for the signs and symptoms suggestive of other facets of MEN I would be necessary for Bea and her immediate family.

Diabetes mellitus is a well-accepted risk factor for the development of coronary artery disease; the risk is three to four times higher in the diabetic than in the nondiabetic population. Although chronically elevated serum levels of chylomicrons and VLDL may contribute to this atherogenic predisposition, the premature vascular disease seen in **Di Beatty** and other patients with IDDM, as well as **Ann Sulin** and other patients with NIDDM, is also related to other abnormalities in lipid metabolism. Among these are the increase in glycation (nonenzymatic attachment of glucose molecules to proteins) of LDL apoproteins as well as glycation of the proteins of the LDL receptor which occurs when serum glucose levels are chronically elevated. These glycations interfere with the normal interaction or "fit" of the circulating LDL particles with their specific receptors on cell membranes. As a consequence, the rate of uptake of circulating LDL by the normal target cells is diminished. The LDL particles, therefore, remain in the circulation and eventually bind nonspecifically to "scavenger" cells located on the endothelial surfaces of blood vessels, one of the early steps in the process of atherogenesis.

BIOCHEMICAL COMMENTS. All the material in this chapter was presented previously. However, because this information is so critical for understanding biochemistry in a way that will allow it to be used in interpreting clinical situations, it was summarized in this chapter. In addition, the information previously presented under carbohydrate metabolism was integrated with lipid metabolism. We have, for the most part, left out the role of allosteric modifiers and other regulatory mechanisms which finely coordinate these processes to an exquisite level. Because such details may be important for specific clinical situations, we hope this summary will serve as a framework to which the details can be fitted as students advance in their clinical studies.

Figure 36.11 is a comprehensive figure, and Table 36.1 provides a list of the major regulatory enzymes of carbohydrate and lipid metabolism in the liver and the mechanisms by which they are controlled. This figure and table should help students to integrate this mass of material.

Now that many of the details of the pathways have been presented, it would be worthwhile to re-read the first three chapters of this book. A student who understands biochemistry within the context of fuel metabolism is in a very good position to solve clinical problems that involve metabolic derangements.

Suggested Readings

Iritani N. Nutritional and hormonal regulation of lipogenic-enzyme gene expression in rat liver. Eur J Biochem 1992;205:433–442.

Because **Di Beatty** produces very little insulin, she is prone to developing ketoacidosis. When insulin levels are low, HSL of adipose tissue is very active, resulting in increased lipolysis. The fatty acids that are released travel to the liver where they are converted to the triacylglycerols of VLDL. They also undergo β-oxidation and conversion to ketone bodies. If Di does not take exogenous insulin or if her insulin levels decrease abruptly for some physiological reason, she may develop a ketoacidosis (DKA). In fact, she has had repeated bouts of DKA.

For reasons that are not well understood, individuals with NIDDM, such as **Ann Sulin**, do not tend to develop ketoacidosis.

36.2: Since the adipose tissue of individuals with NIDDM is relatively resistant to insulin's inhibition of HSL and its stimulation of LPL, **Ann Sulin's** serum triacylglycerol level would be elevated for the same reasons as those which caused the hypertriglyceridemia in **Di Beatty**.

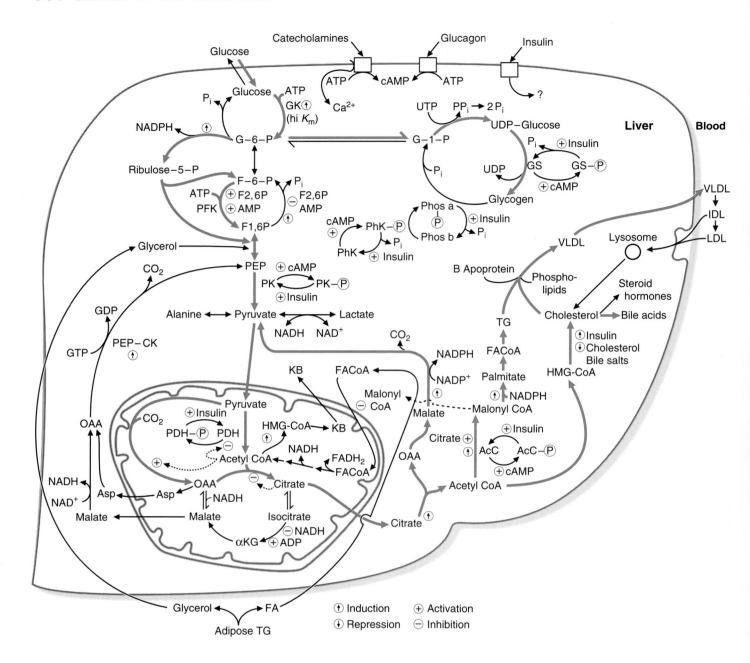

Fig. 36.11. Regulation of carbohydrate and lipid metabolism in the liver. Solid blue arrows indicate the flow of metabolites in the fed state. Solid black arrows indicate the flow during fasting. G = glucose; GK = glucokinase; F = fructose; PFK = phosphofructokinase-1; PEP = phospho-enolpyruvate; PK = pyruvate kinase; OAA = oxaloacetate; αKG = α-ketoglutarate; GS = glycogen synthase; Phos = glycogen phosphorylase; PhK = phosphorylase kinase; AcC = acetyl CoA carboxylase; FA = fatty acid or fatty acyl group; TG = triacylglycerol; circled P = phosphate group.

Table 36.1. Regulation of Liver Enzymes Involved in Glycogen, Blood Glucose, and Triacylglycerol Synthesis and Degradation

LIVER ENZYMES REGULATED BY ACTIVATION/INHIBITION		
Enzyme	Activated By	State in Which Active
Phosphofructokinase-1	Fructose-2,6-P, AMP	Fed
Pyruvate carboxylase	Acetyl CoA	Fed and fasting
Acetyl CoA carboxylase	Citrate	Fed
Carnitine:palmitoyltransferase I	↓ inhibitor (malonyl CoA)	Fasting
LIVER ENZYMES REGULATED BY PHOSPHORYLATION/DEPHOSPHORYLATION		
Enzyme	Active Form	State in Which Active
Glycogen synthase	Dephosphorylated	Fed
Phosphorylase kinase	Phosphorylated	Fasting
Glycogen phosphorylase	Phosphorylated	Fasting
Phosphofructokinase-2/F-2,6-bisphosphatase (acts as a kinase, increasing fructose-2,6-P levels)	Dephosphorylated	Fed
Phosphofructokinase-2/F-2,6-bisphosphatase (acts as a phosphatase, decreasing fructose-2,6-P levels)	Phosphorylated	Fasting
Pyruvate kinase	Dephosphorylated	Fed
Pyruvate dehydrogenase	Dephosphorylated	Fed
Acetyl CoA carboxylase	Dephosphorylated	Fed
LIVER ENZYMES REGULATED BY INDUCTION/REPRESSION		
Enzyme	State in Which Induced	Process Affected
Glucokinase	Fed	Glucose → TG
Citrate lyase	Fed	Glucose → TG
Acetyl CoA carboxylase	Fed	Glucose → TG
Fatty acid synthase	Fed	Glucose → TG
Malic enzyme	Fed	Production of NADPH
Glucose-6-P dehydrogenase	Fed	Production of NADPH
Glucose 6-phosphatase	Fasted	Production of blood glucose
Fructose 1,6-bisphosphatase	Fasted	Production of blood glucose
Phosphoenolpyruvate carboxykinase	Fasted	Production of blood glucose

Klip A, Tsakiridis T, Marette A, Ortiz PA. Regulation of expression of glucose transporters by glucose: a review of studies in vivo and in cell cultures. FASEB J 1994;8:43–53.

Pilkis SJ, Granner DK. Molecular physiology of the regulation of hepatic gluconeogenesis and glycolysis. Annu Rev Physiol 1992;54:885–909.

Sugden MC, Holness MJ. Interactive regulation of the pyruvate dehydrogenase complex and the carnitine palmitoyltransferase system. FASEB J 1994;8:54–61.

Vaulont S, Kahn A. Transcriptional control of metabolic regulation genes by carbohydrates. FASEB J 1994;8:28–35.

PROBLEM

Why is **Di Beatty** treated with insulin when she is in diabetic ketoacidosis (DKA)? Explain the biochemical mechanisms.

ANSWER

Insulin activates a phosphatase that causes HSL in adipose tissue to be inactivated by dephosphorylation. As a result, the release of fatty acids from adipose tissue is decreased. Less fatty acids reach the liver, so there is less substrate for β-oxidation and ketone body synthesis.

In addition, insulin stimulates fatty acid synthesis in liver. Acetyl CoA carboxylase is activated, producing malonyl CoA. This compound inhibits CPTI and thus the transport of fatty acids into mitochondria, where β-oxidation and ketone body synthesis occur.

Nitrogen Metabolism

Dietary proteins are the primary source of the nitrogen that is metabolized by the body (Fig. 37.1). Amino acids, produced by digestion of dietary proteins, are absorbed through intestinal epithelial cells and enter the blood. Various cells take up these amino acids, which enter the cellular pools. They are used for the synthesis of proteins and other nitrogen-containing compounds, or they are oxidized for energy.

Protein synthesis, the translation of mRNA on ribosomes (see Chapter 14), is a dynamic process. Within the body, proteins are constantly being synthesized and degraded, partially draining and then refilling the cellular amino acid pools.

Compounds derived from amino acids include cellular proteins, hormones (such as thyroxine, epinephrine, and insulin), neurotransmitters, creatine phosphate, the heme of hemoglobin and the cytochromes, the skin pigment melanin, and the purine and pyrimidine bases of nucleotides and nucleic acids. In fact, all of the nitrogen-containing compounds of the body are synthesized from amino acids. Many of these pathways are outlined in Chapters 41 and 42.

In addition to serving as the precursors for the nitrogen-containing compounds of the body and as the building blocks for protein synthesis, amino acids are also a source of energy. Amino acids are directly oxidized, or they are converted to glucose and then oxidized or stored as glycogen. They may also be converted to fatty acids and stored as adipose triacylglycerols. Glycogen and triacylglycerols are oxidized during periods of fasting. The liver is the major site of amino acid oxidation. However, most tissues can oxidize the branched chain amino acids (leucine, isoleucine, and valine).

Before the carbon skeletons of amino acids are oxidized, the nitrogen must be removed. Amino acid nitrogen forms ammonia, which is toxic to the body. In the liver, ammonia and the amino groups from amino acids are converted to urea, which is nontoxic, water-soluble, and readily excreted in the urine. The process by which urea is produced is known as the urea cycle.

Although urea is the major nitrogenous excretory product of the body, nitrogen is also excreted in other compounds (Table 37.1). Uric acid is the degradation product of the purine bases, creatinine is produced from creatine phosphate, and ammonia is released from glutamine, particularly by the kidney where it helps to buffer the urine by reacting with protons to form ammonium ions (NH_4^+). These compounds are excreted mainly in the urine, but substantial amounts are also lost in the feces and through the skin. Small amounts of nitrogen-containing metabolites are formed from the degradation of neurotransmitters, hormones, and other specialized amino acid products and excreted in the urine. Some of these degradation products, such as bilirubin (formed from the degradation of heme), are excreted mainly in the feces.

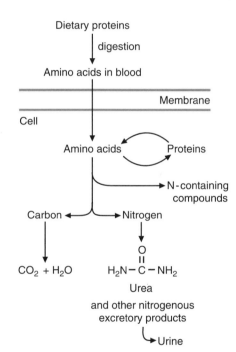

Fig. 37.1. Summary of amino acid metabolism. Dietary proteins are digested to amino acids, which are absorbed and taken up by cells. Amino acids are used to synthesize proteins and other nitrogen-containing compounds. The carbon skeletons of amino acids are also oxidized for energy, and the nitrogen is converted to urea and other nitrogenous excretory products.

Table 37.1. Major Nitrogenous Urinary Excretory Products

	Amount Excreted in urine/day[a]
Urea[b]	12–20 g urea nitrogen
NH_4^+	140–1,500 mg ammonia nitrogen
Creatinine	Males: 14–26 mg/kg
	Females 11–20 mg/kg
Uric acid	250–750 mg

[a]The amounts are expressed in units generally reported by clinical laboratories. Note that the amounts for creatinine and uric acid are for the whole compound, while those for urea and ammonia are for the nitrogen content.

[b]Under normal circumstances, about 90% of the nitrogen excreted in the urine is in the form of urea. The exact amounts of each component vary, however, depending on dietary protein intake and physiological state. For instance, NH_4^+ excretion increases during an acidosis because the kidney secretes ammonia to bind protons in the urine.

Table 37.2. Amino Acids Synthesized in the Body[a]

From Glucose	From an Essential Amino Acid
Serine	Tyrosine (from phenylalanine)
Glycine	
Cysteine[b]	
Alanine	
Aspartate	
Asparagine	
Glutamate	
Glutamine	
Proline	
Arginine	

[a]These amino acids are called "nonessential" or "dispensable," terms which refer to dietary requirements. Of course, within the body, they are necessary. We cannot survive without them.

[b]Although the carbons of cysteine can be derived from glucose, its sulfur is obtained from the essential amino acid methionine.

The healthy human adult is in nitrogen balance, i.e., the amount of nitrogen excreted each day (mainly in the urine) equals the amount consumed (mainly as dietary protein). Negative nitrogen balance occurs when the amount of nitrogen excreted is greater than the amount consumed, and positive nitrogen balance occurs when the amount excreted is less than that consumed (see Chapter 1).

Eleven of the twenty amino acids used to form proteins are synthesized in the body if an adequate amount is not present in the diet (Table 37.2). Ten of these amino acids can be produced from glucose; the eleventh, tyrosine, is synthesized from the essential amino acid phenylalanine. It should be noted that cysteine, one of the 10 amino acids produced from glucose, obtains its sulfur atom from the essential amino acid methionine.

Nine amino acids are essential in the human. "Essential" means that the carbon skeleton cannot be synthesized, and, therefore, these amino acids are required in the diet (Table 37.3). The essential amino acids are also called the indispensable amino acids.

After nitrogen is removed from amino acids, the carbon skeletons are oxidized (Fig. 37.2). Most of the carbons are converted to pyruvate, intermediates of the tricarboxylic acid (TCA) cycle, or to acetyl CoA. In the liver, particularly during fasting, these carbons may be converted to glucose or to ketone bodies and released into the blood. Other tissues then oxidize the glucose and ketone bodies. Ultimately, the carbons of the amino acids are converted to CO_2 and H_2O.

Table 37.3. Amino Acids Essential in the Diet[a]

Lysine
Isoleucine
Leucine
Threonine
Valine
Tryptophan
Phenylalanine
Methionine
Histidine
Arginine (not required by the adult, but required for growth)

[a]Mnemonic: Little TV Tonight (PM)—HA (LIL TV To PM—HA)

Another mnemonic often used by students is Pvt. Tim Hall.

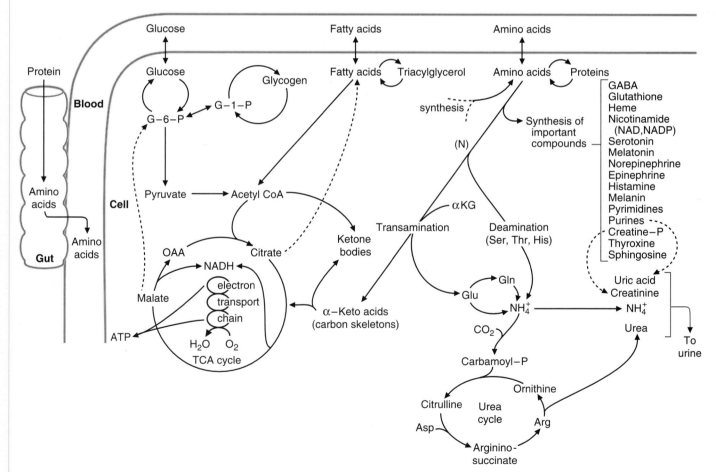

Fig. 37.2. Overview of nitrogen metabolism. The metabolism of nitrogen-containing compounds is shown on the right, and that of glucose and fatty acids is shown on the left. This figure shows a hypothetical, composite cell. No single cell type has all these pathways. αKG = α-ketoglutarate; OAA = oxaloacetate; G-6-P = glucose 6-phosphate; G-1-P = glucose 1-phosphate.

37 Protein Digestion and Amino Acid Absorption

Proteolytic enzymes (also called proteases) break down dietary proteins into their constituent amino acids in the stomach and the intestine. Many of these digestive proteases are synthesized as larger, inactive forms known as zymogens. After zymogens are secreted into the digestive tract, they are cleaved to produce the active proteases.

In the stomach, pepsin begins the digestion of proteins by hydrolyzing them to smaller polypeptides. The contents of the stomach pass into the small intestine, where enzymes produced by the exocrine pancreas act. The pancreatic proteases (trypsin, chymotrypsin, elastase, and the carboxypeptidases) cleave the polypeptides into oligopeptides and amino acids.

The cleavage of the oligopeptides to amino acids is accomplished by enzymes produced by the intestinal epithelial cells. These enzymes include aminopeptidases located on the brush border and other peptidases located within the cells. Ultimately, the amino acids produced by protein digestion are absorbed through the intestinal epithelial cells and enter the blood.

Sissy Fibrosa, a young child with cystic fibrosis, has had repeated bouts of bronchitis caused by *Pseudomonas aeruginosa*. With each of these infections, her response to aerosolized antibiotics has been good. However, her malabsorption of food continues, resulting in foul-smelling, glistening, bulky stools. Her growth records show a slow decline. She is now in the 24th percentile for height and the 20th percentile for weight. She is often listless and irritable, and she tires easily. When her pediatrician discovered that her levels of the serum proteins albumin, transferrin, and thyroid hormone binding prealbumin (transthyretin) were low to low-normal (indicating protein malnutrition), Sissy was given enteric coated microspheres of pancreatic enzymes. Almost immediately, the character of Sissy's stools became more normal and she began gaining weight. In the next 6 months, her growth curves showed improvement and she seemed brighter, more active, and less irritable.

For the first few months following a painful episode of renal colic, during which he passed a kidney stone, **Cal Kulis** had faithfully maintained a high daily fluid intake and had taken the medication required to increase the pH of his urine. Because he has cystinuria, these measures were necessary to increase the solubility of the large amounts of cystine present in his urine and, thereby, to prevent further formation of kidney stones (calculi). With time, however, he became increasingly complacent about his preventive program. After failing to take his medication for a month, he experienced another severe episode of renal colic with grossly bloody urine. Fortunately, he passed the stone spontaneously, after which he vowed to faithfully comply with therapy.

His mother heard that some dietary amino acids were not absorbed in patients with cystinuria and asked whether any dietary changes would reduce Cal's chances of developing additional renal stones.

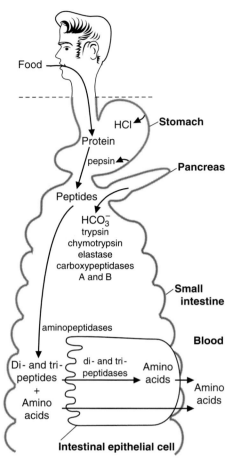

Fig. 37.3. Digestion of proteins. The proteolytic enzymes, pepsin, trypsin, chymotrypsin, elastase, and the carboxypeptidases, are produced as zymogens that are activated by cleavage after they enter the gastrointestinal lumen (see Fig. 37.4).

Kwashiorkor, a common problem of children in Third World countries, is caused by a deficiency of protein in a diet that is adequate in calories. Children with kwashiorkor suffer from muscle wasting and a decreased concentration of plasma proteins, particularly albumin. The result is an increase in interstitial fluid that causes edema and a distended abdomen that make the children appear "plump."

These problems may be compounded by a decreased ability to produce digestive enzymes and new intestinal epithelial cells because of a decreased availability of amino acids for the synthesis of new proteins.

PROTEIN DIGESTION

The digestion of proteins begins in the stomach and is completed in the intestine (Fig. 37.3). The enzymes that digest proteins are produced as inactive precursors (zymogens) that are larger than the active enzymes. The inactive zymogens are secreted from the cells in which they are synthesized and enter the lumen of the digestive tract, where they are cleaved to smaller forms that have proteolytic activity (Fig. 37.4). These active enzymes have different specificities; no single enzyme can completely digest a protein. However, by acting in concert, they can digest dietary proteins to amino acids and small peptides, which are cleaved by peptidases associated with intestinal epithelial cells.

Digestion of Proteins in the Stomach

Pepsinogen is secreted by the chief cells of the stomach. The parietal cells secrete HCl. The acid in the stomach lumen alters the conformation of pepsinogen so that it can cleave itself, producing the active protease pepsin. Thus, the activation of pepsinogen is autocatalytic.

Dietary proteins are denatured by the acid in the stomach. However, at this low pH, pepsin is not denatured, and it acts as an endopeptidase, cleaving peptide bonds at various points within the protein chain. Although pepsin has a fairly broad specificity, it tends to cleave peptide bonds in which the carboxyl group is provided by an aromatic or acidic amino acid (Fig. 37.5). Smaller peptides and some free amino acids are produced.

Digestion of Proteins by Enzymes from the Pancreas

As the gastric contents empty into the intestine, they encounter the secretions from the exocrine pancreas. In addition to bicarbonate, which neutralizes the stomach acid, these secretions contain a number of proteases in the inactive proenzyme form (zymogens). Because the active forms of these enzymes can digest each other, it is important for their zymogen forms all to be activated within a short span of time. This feat is accomplished by the cleavage of trypsinogen to the active enzyme trypsin,

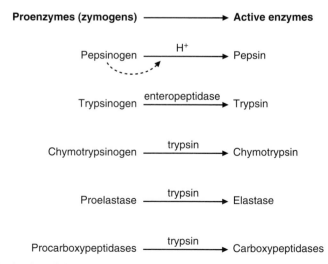

Fig. 37.4. Activation of the gastric and pancreatic zymogens. Pepsinogen catalyzes its own cleavage at the pH of the stomach. Trypsinogen is cleaved by enteropeptidase. The active form of the enzyme trypsin plays a key role by catalyzing the cleavage of the other pancreatic zymogens.

which then cleaves the other pancreatic zymogens, producing their active forms (see Fig. 37.4).

The zymogen trypsinogen is cleaved to form trypsin by enteropeptidase (a protease, formerly called enterokinase) secreted by the brush-border cells of the small intestine. Trypsin catalyzes the cleavages that convert chymotrypsinogen to the active enzyme chymotrypsin, proelastase to elastase, and the procarboxypeptidases to the carboxypeptidases. Thus, trypsin plays a central role in digestion because it both cleaves dietary proteins and activates other digestive proteases produced by the pancreas.

Trypsin, chymotrypsin, and elastase are serine proteases (see Chapter 9) that act as endopeptidases. Trypsin is the most specific of these enzymes, cleaving peptide bonds in which the carboxyl (carbonyl) group is provided by lysine or arginine (see Fig. 37.5). Chymotrypsin is less specific, but favors residues that contain hydrophobic or acidic amino acids. Elastase cleaves not only elastin (for which it was named) but also other proteins at bonds in which the carboxyl group is contributed by amino acid residues with small side chains (alanine, glycine, or serine). The actions of these pancreatic endopeptidases continue the digestion of dietary proteins begun by pepsin in the stomach.

The smaller peptides formed by the action of trypsin, chymotrypsin, and elastase are attacked by exopeptidases, which are proteases that cleave one amino acid at a time from the end of the chain. Procarboxypeptidases, zymogens produced by the pancreas, are converted by trypsin to the active carboxypeptidases. These exopeptidases remove amino acids from the carboxyl ends of peptide chains. Carboxypeptidase A preferentially releases hydrophobic amino acids, and carboxypeptidase B releases basic amino acids (arginine and lysine).

Digestion of Proteins by Enzymes from Intestinal Cells

Exopeptidases produced by intestinal epithelial cells act within the brush border and also within the cell. Aminopeptidases, located on the brush border, cleave one amino acid at a time from the amino end of peptides. Intracellular peptidases act on small peptides that are absorbed by the cells.

The concerted action of the proteolytic enzymes produced by cells of the stomach, pancreas, and intestine cleaves dietary proteins to amino acids. The digestive enzymes digest themselves as well as dietary protein. They also digest the intestinal cells that are regularly sloughed off into the lumen. These cells are replaced by cells that mature from precursor cells in the duodenal crypts. The amount of protein that is digested and absorbed each day from digestive juices and cells released into the intestinal lumen may be equal to, or greater than, the amount of protein consumed in the diet (50–100 g).

ABSORPTION OF AMINO ACIDS

Amino acids are absorbed from the intestinal lumen through secondary active Na^+-dependent transport, through facilitated diffusion, and through transport linked to the γ-glutamyl cycle.

Cotransport of Na⁺ and Amino Acids

Amino acids are absorbed from the lumen of the small intestine principally by semi-specific Na^+-dependent transport proteins in the luminal membrane of the intestinal cell brush border (Fig 37.6). The cotransport of Na^+ and the amino acid from the outside of the apical membrane to the inside of the cell is driven by the low intracellular Na^+ concentration. Low intracellular Na^+ results from the pumping of Na^+ out of

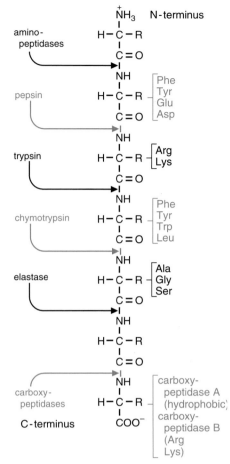

Fig. 37.5. Action of the digestive proteases. Pepsin, trypsin, chymotrypsin, and elastase are endopeptidases; they hydrolyze peptide bonds within chains. The others are exopeptidases; aminopeptidases remove the amino acid at the N-terminus, and the carboxypeptidases remove the amino acid at the C terminus. For each proteolytic enzyme, the amino acid residues involved in the peptide bond that is cleaved are listed beside the R group to the right of the enzyme name.

Patients with cystic fibrosis, such as **Sissy Fibrosa**, have a genetically determined defect in the function of the chloride channels present in the pancreatic secretory ducts, which carry pancreatic enzymes into the lumen of the small intestines. This defect causes inspissation (drying and thickening) of pancreatic exocrine secretions, eventually leading to obstruction of these ducts. One result of this problem is a lack of pancreatic enzymes in the intestinal lumen to digest dietary proteins.

Q 37.1: Why do patients with cystinuria and Hartnup disease have a hyperaminoaciduria without an associated hyperaminoacidemia?

Hartnup disease is another genetically determined and relatively rare autosomal recessive disorder. It involves a defect in the transport of neutral amino acids across both intestinal and renal epithelial cells. The signs and symptoms are, in part, caused by a deficiency of essential amino acids (see Clinical Comments). Cystinuria and Hartnup disease involve defects in two different transport proteins. In each case, the defect is present both in intestinal cells, causing malabsorption of the amino acids from the digestive products in the intestinal lumen, and in kidney tubular cells, causing a decreased resorption of these amino acids from the glomerular filtrate.

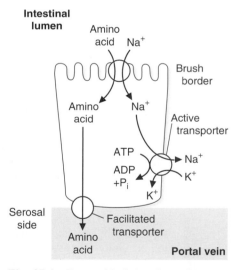

Fig. 37.6. Transepithelial amino acid transport. Na⁺-dependent carriers transport both Na⁺ and an amino acid into the intestinal epithelial cell from the intestinal lumen. Na⁺ is pumped out on the serosal side (across the basolateral membrane) in exchange for K⁺ by the Na⁺,K⁺-ATPase. On the serosal side, the amino acid is carried by a facilitated transporter down its concentration gradient into the blood. This process is an example of secondary active transport.

the cell by a Na⁺,K⁺-ATPase on the serosal membrane. This process allows the cells to concentrate amino acids from the intestinal lumen. The amino acids are then transported out of the cell into the interstitial fluid principally by facilitated transporters in the serosal membrane (see Fig. 37.6).

At least six different Na⁺-dependent amino acid carriers are located in the apical brush-border membrane of the epithelial cells. These carriers have an overlapping specificity for different amino acids. One carrier preferentially transports neutral amino acids, another transports proline and hydroxyproline, a third preferentially transports acidic amino acids, and a fourth transports basic amino acids (lysine, arginine, the urea cycle intermediate ornithine) and cystine. In addition to these Na⁺-dependent carriers, some amino acids are transported across the luminal membrane via facilitated transport carriers. Most amino acids are transported by more than one transport system.

As with glucose transport, the Na⁺-dependent carriers of the apical membrane of the intestinal epithelial cells are also present in the renal epithelium. However, different isozymes are present in the cell membranes of other tissues. On the other hand, the facilitated transport carriers in the serosal membrane of the intestinal epithelia are similar to those found in other cell types in the body. During starvation, the intestinal epithelia, like these other cells, take up amino acids from the blood. Thus amino acid transport across the serosal membrane is bidirectional.

γ-Glutamyl Cycle

The γ-glutamyl cycle is involved in the transport of amino acids into cells of the intestine and the kidney (Fig. 37.7). In this case, the extracellular amino acid reacts with glutathione (γ-glutamyl-cysteinyl-glycine) in a reaction catalyzed by a transpeptidase present in the cell membrane. A γ-glutamyl amino acid is formed, which travels across the cell membrane and releases the amino acid into the cell. The other products of these two reactions are reconverted to glutathione.

The reactions converting glutamate to glutathione in the γ-glutamyl cycle are the same reactions required for the synthesis of glutathione. The enzymes for glutathione synthesis, but not the transpeptidase, are found in most tissues. Glutathione is also involved in reducing compounds such as hydrogen peroxide (see Chapter 21).

Transport of Amino Acids into Cells

Amino acids that enter the blood are transported across cell membranes of the various tissues principally via Na⁺-dependent cotransporters and, to a lesser extent, by facilitated transporters. In this respect, amino acid transport differs from glucose transport, which is Na⁺-dependent transport in the intestinal and renal epithelium but facilitated transport in other cell types. The Na⁺ dependence of amino acid transport in liver, muscle, and other tissues allows these cells to concentrate amino acids from the blood. These transport proteins have a different genetic basis, amino acid composition, and somewhat different specificity than those in the luminal membrane of intestinal epithelia. They also differ somewhat between tissues. For instance, the N system for glutamine uptake is present in the liver, but either not present in other tissues or present as an isoform with different properties. There is also some overlap in specificity of the transport proteins, with most amino acids being transported by more than one carrier.

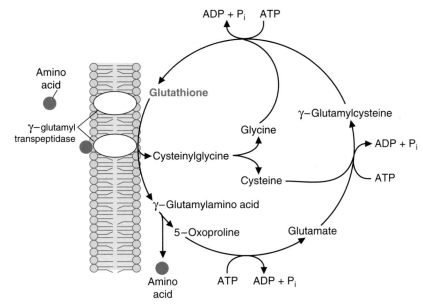

Fig. 37.7. γ-Glutamyl cycle. In cells of the intestine and kidney, amino acids are transported across the cell membrane by reacting with glutathione (γ-glutamyl-cysteinyl-glycine) to form a γ-glutamyl amino acid. The amino acid is released into the cell, and glutathione is resynthesized.

Trace amounts of polypeptides pass into the blood. They may be transported through intestinal epithelial cells, probably by pinocytosis, or they may slip between the cells that line the gut wall. This process is particularly troublesome for premature infants because it can lead to allergies caused by proteins in their food.

Cal Kulis and other patients with cystinuria have a genetically determined defect in the transport of cystine and the basic amino acids, lysine, arginine, and ornithine, across the brush-border membranes of cells in both their small intestine and renal tubules. However, they do not appear to have any symptoms of amino acid deficiency, in part because the amino acids cysteine (which is oxidized in blood and urine to form the disulfide cystine) and arginine can be synthesized in the body (i.e., they are "nonessential" amino acids). Ornithine (an amino acid that is not found in proteins but serves as an intermediate of the urea cycle) can also be synthesized. The most serious problem for these patients is the insolubility of cystine, which can form kidney stones that may lodge in the ureter causing bleeding and severe pain.

CLINICAL COMMENTS. **Sissy Fibrosa's** growth and weight curves were both subnormal until her pediatrician added pancreatic enzyme supplements to her treatment plan. These supplements digest dietary protein, releasing essential and other amino acids that are absorbed by the endothelial cells of Sissy's small intestine, through which they are transported into the blood. A discernable improvement in Sissy's body weight and growth curves was noted within months of the start of this therapy.

Apart from the proportions of essential amino acids present in various foods, the quality of a dietary protein is also determined by the rate at which it is digested and, in a more general way, by its capacity to contribute to the growth of the infant. In this regard, the proteins in foods of animal origin are more digestible than are those derived from plants. For example, the digestibility of proteins in eggs is approximately 97%, that for meats, poultry, and fish is 85–100%, while that from wheat, soybeans, and other legumes ranges from 75 to 90%.

The official dietary "protein requirement" accepted by the U.S. and Canadian governments is 0.8 g of protein per kilogram of desirable body weight for adults (about 56 g for an adult male and 44 g for an adult female). On an average weight basis, the requirement per kilogram is much greater for infants and children. This fact underscores the importance of improving Sissy Fibrosa's protein digestion to optimize her potential for normal growth and development.

In patients with cystinuria, like **Cal Kulis**, the inability to normally absorb cystine and basic amino acids from the gut and the increased loss of these amino acids in the urine would be expected to cause a deficiency of these compounds in the blood. However, because three of these amino acids can be synthesized in the body, (i.e., they are nonessential amino acids), their concentrations in the plasma remain normal and clinical manifestations of a deficiency state do not develop. It is not clear why symptoms related to a lysine deficiency have not been observed.

37.1: Patients with cystinuria and Hartnup disease have defective transport proteins both in the intestine and the kidney. These patients do not absorb the affected amino acids at a normal rate from the digestive products in the intestinal lumen. They also do not readily resorb these amino acids from the glomerular filtrate into the blood. Therefore, they do not have a hyper-aminoacidemia (a high concentration in the blood). Normally, only a few percent of the amino acids that enter the glomerular filtrate are excreted in the urine; most are resorbed. In these diseases, much larger amounts of the affected amino acids are excreted in the urine, resulting in a hyper-aminoaciduria.

The half-life of a compound (t½) is the time required for one-half of the compound to be degraded.

 Protein turnover is quite extensive. For example, red blood cells have a lifespan of 120 days. Every day 3×10^{11} (300,000 million) red blood cells die and are phagocytosed. The hemoglobin in these cells is degraded to amino acids by lysosomal proteases, and these amino acids are reutilized. About 6 lb of hemoglobin are recycled in this way every year.

As the aged cells are dying, newly generated reticulocytes are synthesizing hemoglobin in preparation for their conversion into new red blood cells, which replace the dying cells.

 Adults cannot increase the amount of muscle or other body proteins by eating an excess amount of protein. If dietary protein is consumed in excess of our needs, it is converted to glycogen and triacylglycerols, which are then stored.

In the disorder which was first observed in the Hartnup family and bears their name, the intestinal and renal transport defect involves the neutral amino acids (monoamine, monocarboxylic acids), including a number of the essential amino acids (isoleucine, leucine, phenylalanine, threonine, tryptophan, and valine) as well as certain nonessential amino acids (alanine, serine, and tyrosine). A reduction in the availability of these essential amino acids would be expected to cause a variety of clinical disorders. Yet children with the Hartnup disorder identified by routine newborn urine screening almost always remain clinically normal.

However, some patients with the Hartnup biochemical phenotype eventually develop pellagra-like manifestations, which usually include a photosensitivity rash, ataxia, and neuropsychiatric symptoms. Pellagra results from a dietary deficiency of the vitamin niacin and/or the essential amino acid tryptophan, which are both precursors for the nicotinamide moiety of NAD and NADP (see Chapter 41). In asymptomatic patients, the transport abnormality may be incomplete and so subtle as to allow no phenotypic expression of Hartnup disease. These patients may also be capable of absorbing some small peptides that contain the neutral amino acids.

The only rational treatment of patients having pellagra-like symptoms is the administration of niacin (nicotinic acid) in oral doses up to 300 mg/day. Although the rash, ataxia, and neuropsychiatric manifestations of niacin deficiency may disappear, the hyperaminoaciduria and intestinal transport defect do not respond to this therapy. In addition to niacin, a high protein diet may benefit some patients.

BIOCHEMICAL COMMENTS. Proteins are continuously being synthesized and degraded in the body. The half-life of proteins is quite variable, ranging from minutes to days. Proteins that contain regions rich in the amino acids proline (P), glutamate (E), serine (S), and threonine (T) have short half-lives. These regions are known as PEST sequences, based on the one-letter abbreviations used for these amino acids. Most of the amino acids produced by protein degradation are recycled and may be reutilized for protein synthesis.

Examples of proteins that undergo extensive synthesis and degradation are hemoglobin, muscle protein, digestive enzymes, and the proteins of cells sloughed off from the gastrointestinal tract. Hemoglobin is produced in reticulocytes and reconverted to amino acids by the phagocytic cells that remove mature red blood cells from the circulation on a daily basis. Muscle protein is degraded during periods of fasting, and the amino acids are used for gluconeogenesis. After ingestion of protein in the diet, muscle protein is resynthesized.

A large amount of protein is recycled daily in the form of digestive enzymes, which are themselves degraded by digestive proteases. In addition, about one-fourth of the cells lining the walls of the gastrointestinal tract are lost each day and replaced by newly synthesized cells. As cells leave the gastrointestinal wall, their proteins and other components are digested by enzymes in the lumen of the gut and the products are absorbed. Only about 6% (about 10 g) of the protein that enters the digestive tract (including dietary proteins, digestive enzymes, and the proteins in sloughed-off cells) is excreted in the feces each day. The remainder is recycled.

Proteins are also recycled within cells. The synthesis of many enzymes is induced in response to physiological demand (such as fasting or feeding). These enzymes are continuously being degraded. Intracellular proteins are also damaged by oxidation and other modifications that limit their function. Mechanisms for intracellular degradation of unnecessary or damaged proteins involve lysosomes or a protein known as ubiquitin. Lysosomes participate in the process of autophagy, in which intracellular components are surrounded by membranes that fuse with lysosomes. The digestive enzymes of the lysosomes, including cathepsins (lysosomal proteases), that degrade the membrane-enclosed material (see Chapter 10). Ubiquitin is a small protein (76 amino acids) that is highly conserved. Its amino acid sequence in yeast and humans differs by only 3 residues. Ubiquitin targets intracellular proteins for degradation by covalently binding to the ε-amino group of lysine residues. A protease degrades the targeted protein, releasing intact ubiquitin that can again mark other proteins for degradation.

The differences in amino acid composition of the various proteins of the body, the vast range in turnover times ($t_{1/2}$), and the recycling of amino acids are all important factors that help to determine the requirements for specific amino acids and total protein in the diet.

Suggested Readings

Argiles JF, Lopez-Soriano FJ. Intestinal amino acid transport: an overview. Int J Biochem 1990;22:931–939.

Christensen HN. Role of amino acid transport and countertransport in nutrition and metabolism. Physiol Rev 1990;70:43–77.

PROBLEMS

1. Explain why a deficiency of trypsin would be more detrimental than a deficiency of any of the other digestive proteases.

2. Children with kwashiorkor usually have a fatty liver. Propose a biochemical rationale for this observation.

ANSWERS

1. Trypsin not only serves as a digestive enzyme that cleaves dietary and other proteins in the lumen of the intestinal tract, but it also catalyzes the cleavages that activate the other digestive proteases produced by the pancreas (see Fig. 37.4). A deficiency of trypsin would cause chymotrypsin, elastase, and the carboxypeptidases to remain in their inactive forms. Although pepsin and the peptidases produced by intestinal cells would still be active, protein digestion would be incomplete because it requires the concerted action of all the digestive proteases.

2. Kwashiorkor is caused by a diet that is low in protein but contains an adequate amount of calories. It usually occurs when a child is weaned to accommodate a younger sibling. The child's diet, subsequently, is generally high in carbohydrate but low in protein. The dietary carbohydrate is converted to fatty acids and triacylglycerols by the liver. However, because of a deficiency of amino acids, liver protein synthesis is diminished. The B-apoprotein of VLDL is synthesized at a reduced rate, and triacylglycerols accumulate in the liver because of decreased VLDL production.

38 Fate of Amino Acid Nitrogen: Urea Cycle

In comparison to carbohydrate and lipid metabolism, the metabolism of amino acids is complex. We must be concerned not only with the fate of the carbon atoms of the amino acids but also with the fate of the nitrogen. During their metabolism, amino acids travel in the blood from one tissue to another. Ultimately, most of the nitrogen is converted to urea in the liver and the carbons are oxidized to CO_2 and H_2O by a number of tissues (Fig. 38.1).

After a meal that contains protein, amino acids released by digestion pass from the gut through the hepatic portal vein to the liver (see Fig. 38.2A). In a normal diet containing 60–100 g of protein, most of the amino acids are used for the synthesis of proteins in the liver and in other tissues. Excess amino acids may be converted to glucose.

During fasting, muscle protein is cleaved to amino acids. Some of the amino acids are partially oxidized to produce energy (see Fig. 38.2B). Portions of these amino acids are converted to alanine and glutamine, which, along with other amino acids, are released into the blood. Glutamine is oxidized by various tissues, including the gut and kidney, which convert some of the carbons and nitrogen to alanine. Alanine and other amino acids travel to the liver, where the carbons are converted to glucose and ketone bodies and the nitrogen is converted to urea, which is excreted by the kidneys. Glucose, produced by gluconeogenesis, is subsequently oxidized to CO_2 and H_2O by many tissues, and ketone bodies are oxidized by tissues such as muscle and kidney.

Several enzymes are important in the process of interconverting amino acids and in removing nitrogen so that the carbon skeletons can be oxidized. These include transaminases, glutamate dehydrogenase, and deaminases.

The conversion of amino acid nitrogen to urea occurs mainly in the liver. Urea is formed in the urea cycle from NH_4^+, CO_2, and the nitrogen of aspartate (see Fig. 38.1). Initially, NH_4^+, CO_2, and ATP react to produce carbamoyl phosphate, which reacts with ornithine to form citrulline. Aspartate then reacts with citrulline to form argininosuccinate, which releases fumarate, forming arginine. Finally, arginase cleaves arginine to release urea and regenerate ornithine.

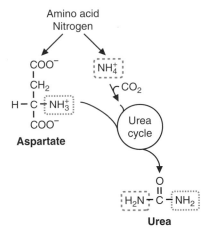

Fig. 38.1. Sources of nitrogen for urea synthesis. One nitrogen of urea comes from NH_4^+, the other from aspartate.

Teresa Livermore and her high school beau decided to take a Caribbean cruise, during which they sampled the cuisine of many of the islands on their itinerary. One month after their return to the United States, Teresa complained of severe malaise, loss of appetite, nausea, vomiting, and arthralgias (joint pains). She had a low grade fever and noted a constant increasing pain in the area of her liver. Her friend noted a yellow discoloration of the whites of her eyes and skin. Her urine turned the color of iced tea and her stool became a light-clay color. Her doctor found her liver to be enlarged and tender. Liver function tests were ordered.

Serological testing for viral hepatitis type B, C, and D were nonreactive but fecal studies showed "shedding" of hepatitis virus type A. Tests for antibodies to antigens of the hepatitis A virus (anti-HAV) in the serum were positive for the immunoglobulin M type.

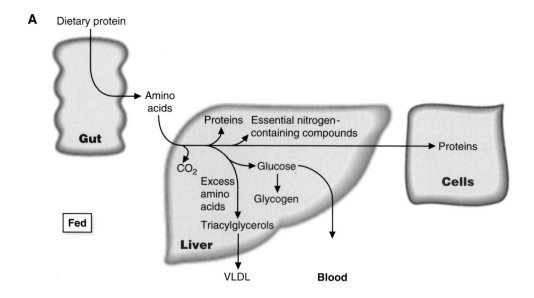

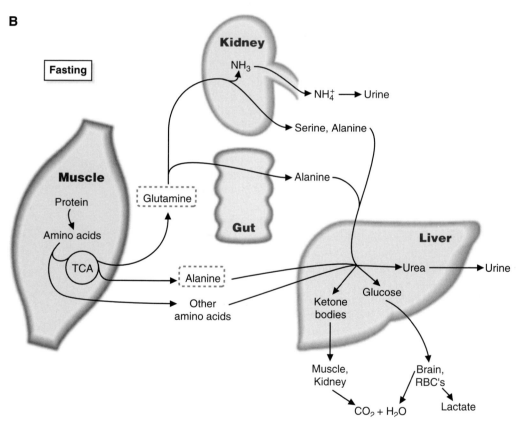

Fig. 38.2. Roles of various tissues in amino acid metabolism. **A.** In the fed state, amino acids released by digestion of dietary proteins travel through the hepatic portal vein to the liver where they are used for the synthesis of proteins, particularly the blood proteins, such as serum albumin. Excess amino acids are converted to glucose or to triacylglycerols which are packaged and secreted in VLDL. The glucose produced from amino acids in the fed state is stored as glycogen or released into the blood if blood glucose levels are low. Amino acids that pass through the liver are converted to proteins in cells of other tissues. **B.** During fasting, amino acids are released from muscle protein. Some enter the blood directly. Others are partially oxidized and converted to alanine and glutamine, which enter the blood. (Alanine is also produced from glucose.) In the kidney, glutamine releases ammonia into the urine and is converted to alanine and serine. In the cells of the gut, glutamine is converted to alanine. Alanine (the major gluconeogenic amino acid) and other amino acids enter the liver, where their nitrogen is converted to urea, which is excreted in the urine, and their carbons to glucose and ketone bodies, which are oxidized by various tissues for energy.

A diagnosis of acute viral hepatitis type A was made, probably contracted from virus-contaminated food Teresa had eaten while on her cruise. Her physician explained that there was no specific treatment for type A viral hepatitis but recommended symptomatic and supportive care and prevention of transmission to others by the fecal-oral route. Teresa took acetaminophen 3–4 times a day for fever and arthralgias throughout her illness.

 Jean Ann Tonich, a 46-year-old commercial artist, recently lost her job because of absenteeism. Her husband of 24 years had left her 10 months earlier. She complains of loss of appetite, fatigue, muscle weakness, and emotional depression. She has had occasional pain in the area of her liver, at times accompanied by nausea and vomiting.

On physical examination she appears somewhat disheveled and pale. The physician notes tenderness to light percussion over her liver and detects a small amount of ascites (fluid within the peritoneal cavity around the abdominal organs). The lower edge of her liver is palpable about 2 inches below the lower margin of her right rib cage, suggesting liver enlargement, and feels somewhat more firm and nodular than normal. Jean Ann's spleen is not palpably enlarged. There is a suggestion of mild jaundice (a yellow discoloration caused by the deposition of bilirubin) involving the sclerae (the "whites" of the eyes). No obvious neurological or cognitive abnormalities are present.

After detecting a hint of alcohol on Jean Ann's breath, the physician questions her about possible alcohol abuse, which the patient initially denies. With more intensive questioning, however, Jean Ann admits that for the last 5 or 6 years, while her marriage was faltering, she began drinking gin on a daily basis in quantities of about 50–70 g of ethanol while eating relatively poorly.

FATE OF AMINO ACID NITROGEN

Transamination Reactions

Transamination is the major process for removing nitrogen from amino acids. In most instances, the nitrogen is transferred as an amino group from the original amino acid to α-ketoglutarate, forming glutamate, while the original amino acid is converted to its corresponding α-keto acid (Fig. 38.3). For example, the amino acid aspartate can be transaminated to form its corresponding α-keto acid oxaloacetate. In the process, the amino group is transferred to α-ketoglutarate, which is converted to its corresponding amino acid glutamate.

All amino acids except lysine and threonine can undergo transamination reactions. The enzymes catalyzing these reactions are known as transaminases or aminotransferases. For most of these reactions, α-ketoglutarate and glutamate serve as one of the α-keto acid–amino acid pairs. Pyridoxal phosphate is the cofactor (Fig. 38.4).

Overall, in a transamination reaction, an amino group from one amino acid becomes the amino group of a second amino acid. Because these reactions are readily reversible, they can be used to remove nitrogen from amino acids or to transfer nitrogen to α-keto acids to form amino acids. Thus, they are involved both in amino acid degradation and in amino acid synthesis.

Removal of Amino Acid Nitrogen as Ammonia

Cells in the body and bacteria in the gut release the nitrogen of certain amino acids as ammonia or ammonium ion (NH_4^+) (Fig. 38.5). Because these two forms of nitro-

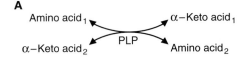

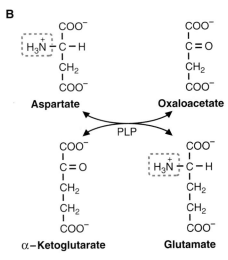

Fig. 38.3. Transamination. The amino group from one amino acid is transferred to another. Pairs of amino acids and their corresponding α-keto acids are involved in these reactions. α-Ketoglutarate and glutamate are usually one of the pairs. The reactions, which are readily reversible, use pyridoxal phosphate (PLP) as a cofactor. The enzymes are called transaminases or aminotransferases. **A.** A generalized reaction. **B.** The aspartate transaminase reaction.

Teresa Livermore's laboratory studies showed that her serum alanine transaminase (ALT) level was 294 units/L (reference range = 5–30) and her serum aspartate transaminase (AST) level was 268 units/L (reference range = 10–30). Her serum alkaline phosphatase level was 284 units/L (reference range for an adult female = 56–155), and her serum total bilirubin was 9.6 mg/dL (reference range = 0.2–1.0).

Cellular enzymes such as AST, ALT, and alkaline phosphatase leak into the blood through the membranes of cells that have been damaged as a result of the inflammatory process. In acute viral hepatitis, the serum ALT level is often elevated to a greater extent than the serum AST level. Alkaline phosphatase, which is present on membranes between liver cells and the bile duct, is also elevated in the blood in acute viral hepatitis.

The rise in serum total bilirubin occurs as a result of the inability of the infected liver to conjugate bilirubin and of a partial or complete occlusion of the hepatic biliary drainage ducts caused by inflammatory swelling within the liver. In fulminant hepatic failure, the serum bilirubin level may exceed 20 mg/dL, a poor prognostic sign.

Because of the possibility of mild alcoholic hepatitis and perhaps chronic alcoholic cirrhosis, the physician ordered liver function studies on **Jean Ann Tonich** which revealed an ALT level of 46 units/L (reference range = 5–30) and an AST level of 98 units/L (reference range = 10–30). The serum total bilirubin level was 2.4 mg/dL (reference range = 0.2–1.0). Her serum alkaline phosphatase level was 151 units/L (reference range = 56–155 for an adult female). Serological tests for viral hepatitis were nonreactive. Her blood hemoglobin and hematocrit levels were slightly below the normal range. Serum folate, vitamin B_{12}, and iron levels were also slightly suppressed. Her serum ethanol level on the initial office visit was 245 mg/dL (a level above 150 mg/dL is considered indicative of inebriation).

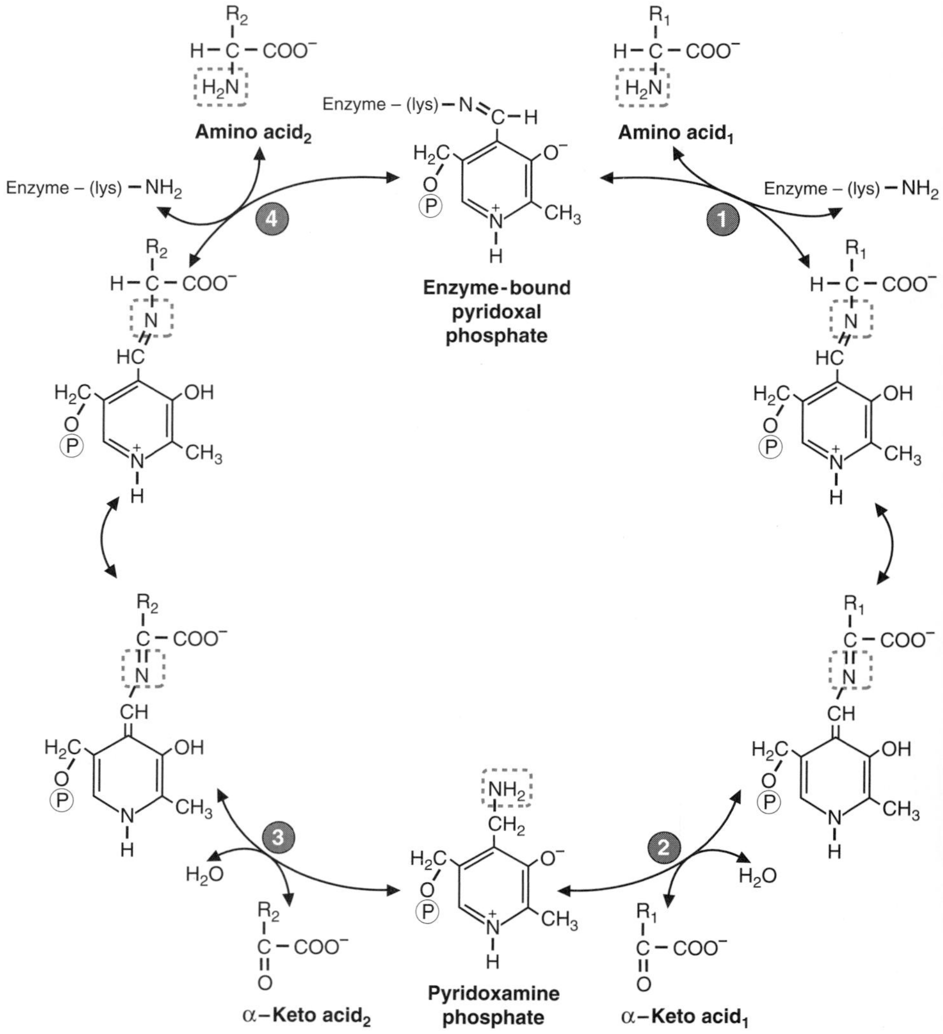

Fig. 38.4. Function of pyridoxal phosphate (PLP) in transamination reactions. The order in which the reactions occur is **1** to **4**. Pyridoxal phosphate (enzyme-bound) reacts with amino $acid_1$, forming a Schiff base. After a shift of the double bond, α-keto $acid_1$ is released and pyridoxamine phosphate is produced. Pyridoxamine phosphate then forms a Schiff base with α-keto $acid_2$. After the double bond shifts, amino $acid_2$ is released, and enzyme-bound pyridoxal phosphate is regenerated. The net result is that the amino group from amino $acid_1$ is transferred to amino $acid_2$. In all of the different kinds of reactions that require pyridoxal phosphate, the amino group of the substrate forms a Schiff base with pyridoxal phosphate. The reactions differ in which bond of the amino acid is cleaved in a subsequent step.

gen can be interconverted, the terms are sometimes used interchangeably. Ammonium ion releases a proton to form ammonia by a reaction with a pK of 9.3 (Fig. 38.6). Therefore, at physiological pH, the equilibrium favors NH_4^+ by a factor of about 100/1. However, it is important to note that NH_3 is also present in the body because this is the form that can cross cell membranes. For example, NH_3 passes into the urine from kidney tubule cells and decreases the acidity of the urine by binding protons, forming NH_4^+.

Glutamate can be oxidatively deaminated by a reaction catalyzed by glutamate dehydrogenase which produces ammonium ion and α-ketoglutarate (Fig. 38.7). Either NAD^+ or $NADP^+$ can serve as the cofactor. This reaction, which occurs in the

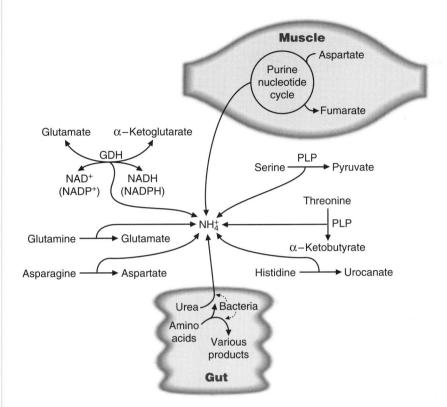

Fig. 38.5. Summary of the sources of NH₄⁺ for the urea cycle. All of the reactions are irreversible except glutamate dehydrogenase (GDH). Only the dehydratase reactions, which produce NH₄⁺ from serine and threonine, require pyridoxal phosphate as a cofactor. The reactions that are not shown occurring in the muscle or the gut can all occur in the liver, where the NH₄⁺ generated can be converted to urea.

mitochondria of most cells, is readily reversible; it can incorporate ammonia into glutamate or release ammonia from glutamate. Glutamate can collect nitrogen from other amino acids as a consequence of transamination reactions and then release ammonia via the glutamate dehydrogenase reaction. This process provides one source of the ammonia that enters the urea cycle.

In addition to glutamate, a number of amino acids release their nitrogen as NH₄⁺ (see Fig. 38.5). Histidine may be directly deaminated to form NH₄⁺ and urocanate. The deaminations of serine and threonine are dehydration reactions that require pyridoxal phosphate and are catalyzed by serine dehydratase. Serine forms pyruvate, and threonine forms α-ketobutyrate. In both cases, NH₄⁺ is released.

Glutamine and asparagine contain amide groups that may be released as NH₄⁺ by deamidation. Asparagine is deamidated by asparaginase, yielding aspartate and NH₄⁺. Glutaminase acts on glutamine, forming glutamate and NH₄⁺. The glutaminase reaction is particularly important in the kidney, where it produces the ammonia that buffers the urine, decreasing its acidity.

In muscle and brain but not in liver, the purine nucleotide cycle allows NH₄⁺ to be released from amino acids (see Fig. 38.5). Nitrogen is collected by glutamate from other amino acids by means of transamination reactions. Then, glutamate transfers its amino group to oxaloacetate to form aspartate, which supplies nitrogen to the purine nucleotide cycle (see Chapter 42). The reactions of the cycle release fumarate and NH₄⁺.

The more chronic inflammatory process associated with long term ethanol abuse in patients such as **Jean Ann Tonich** is accompanied by increases in the levels of serum ALT and AST which are significantly below those seen in acute viral hepatitis. In addition, the ratio of the absolute values for serum ALT and AST often differ in the two diseases, tending to be greater than one in acute viral hepatitis and less than one in chronic alcoholic cirrhosis. The reasons for these differences are not completely understood.

$$NH_4^+ \rightleftharpoons NH_3 + H^+$$
$$pK = 9.3$$

Fig. 38.6. Formation of ammonia from ammonium ion. Because the pK is 9.3, at physiological pH, the concentration of NH₄⁺ is almost 100 times that of NH₃.

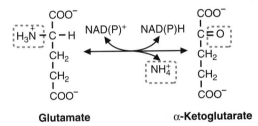

Glutamate   **α-Ketoglutarate**

Fig. 38.7. Reaction catalyzed by glutamate dehydrogenase. This reaction is readily reversible and can use either NAD or NADP as a cofactor. The oxygen on α-ketoglutarate is derived from H₂O.

Vitamin B₆ deficiency symptoms include dermatitis; a microcytic, hypochromic anemia; weakness; irritability; and, in some cases, convulsions. Xanthurenic acid (a degradation product of tryptophan) and other compounds appear in the urine because of an inability to completely metabolize amino acids. A decreased ability to synthesize heme from glycine may cause the microcytic anemia, and decreased decarboxylation of amino acids to form neurotransmitters may explain the convulsions.

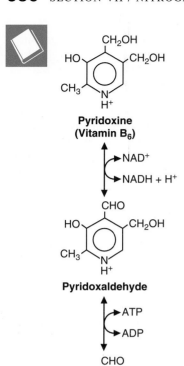

Pyridoxine (Vitamin B$_6$)

→ NAD$^+$
→ NADH + H$^+$

Pyridoxaldehyde

→ ATP
→ ADP

Pyridoxal phosphate (PLP)

Pyridoxal phosphate is derived from pyridoxine (vitamin B$_6$). Pyridoxal phosphate is the cofactor not only for transamination reactions, but also for decarboxylations and a number of other reactions involving amino acids.

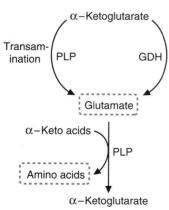

Fig. 38.8. Role of glutamate in amino acid synthesis. Glutamate transfers nitrogen by means of transamination reactions to α-keto acids to form amino acids. This nitrogen is either obtained by glutamate from transamination of other amino acids or from NH$_4^+$ by means of the glutamate dehydrogenase (GDH) reaction. PLP = pyridoxal phosphate.

Compounds that contain "glut" in their name have 5 carbons in a straight chain. At each end of the chain, the carbon is part of a carboxyl group. In glutamine, the carboxyl group has formed an amide, and in hydroxymethylglutaryl CoA (HMG-CoA), it has formed a thioester with coenzyme A.

Glutamine **Glutamate** **α–Ketoglutarate** **Hydroxymethyl-glutaryl CoA (HMG CoA)**

In summary, NH$_4^+$ that enters the urea cycle is produced in the body by deamination or deamidation of amino acids (see Fig. 38.5). A significant amount of NH$_4^+$ is also produced by bacteria that live in the lumen of the intestinal tract. This ammonia enters the hepatic portal vein and travels to the liver.

Role of Glutamate in the Metabolism of Amino Acid Nitrogen

Glutamate plays a pivotal role in the metabolism of amino acids. It is involved in both synthesis and degradation.

Glutamate provides nitrogen for amino acid synthesis (Fig. 38.8). In this process, glutamate obtains its nitrogen either from other amino acids by transamination reactions or from NH$_4^+$ by the glutamate dehydrogenase reaction. Transamination reactions then serve to transfer amino groups from glutamate to α-keto acids to produce their corresponding amino acids.

When amino acids are degraded and urea is formed, glutamate collects nitrogen from other amino acids by transamination reactions. Some of this nitrogen is released as ammonia by the glutamate dehydrogenase reaction, but much larger amounts of ammonia are produced from the other sources shown in Figure 38.5. NH$_4^+$ is one of the two forms in which nitrogen enters the urea cycle (Fig. 38.9).

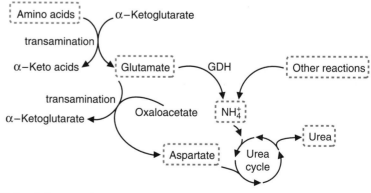

Fig. 38.9. Role of glutamate in urea production. Glutamate collects nitrogen from other amino acids by transamination reactions. This nitrogen can be released as NH$_4^+$ by glutamate dehydrogenase (GDH). NH$_4^+$ is also produced by other reactions (see Fig. 38.5). NH$_4^+$ provides one of the nitrogens for urea synthesis. The other nitrogen comes from aspartate and is obtained from glutamate by transamination of oxaloacetate.

The second form of nitrogen for urea synthesis is provided by aspartate (see Fig. 38.9). Glutamate is the source of the nitrogen. Glutamate transfers its amino group to oxaloacetate, and aspartate and α-ketoglutarate are formed.

UREA CYCLE

The normal human adult is in nitrogen balance, that is, the amount of nitrogen ingested each day, mainly in the form of dietary protein, is equal to the amount of nitrogen excreted. The major nitrogenous excretory product is urea, which exits from the body in the urine. This innocuous compound, produced mainly in the liver by the urea cycle, serves as the disposal form of ammonia, which is toxic, particularly to the brain and central nervous system. Normally, little ammonia (or NH_4^+) is present in the blood. The concentration ranges between 30 and 60 μM. Ammonia is rapidly removed from the blood and converted to urea by the liver. Nitrogen travels in the blood mainly in amino acids, particularly alanine and glutamine (see Fig. 38.1).

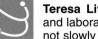

Teresa Livermore's symptoms and laboratory abnormalities did not slowly subside over the next 6 weeks as they usually do in uncomplicated viral hepatitis A infections. Instead, her serum total bilirubin, ALT, AST, and alkaline phosphatase levels increased further. Her vomiting became intractable and her friend noted jerking motions of her arms (asterixis), facial grimacing, restlessness, slowed mentation, and slight disorientation. She was admitted to the hospital with a diagnosis of hepatic failure with incipient hepatic encephalopathy (brain dysfunction caused by accumulation of various toxins in the blood), a rare complication of acute type A viral hepatitis alone. The possibility of a superimposed acute hepatic toxicity caused by the use of acetaminophen was considered.

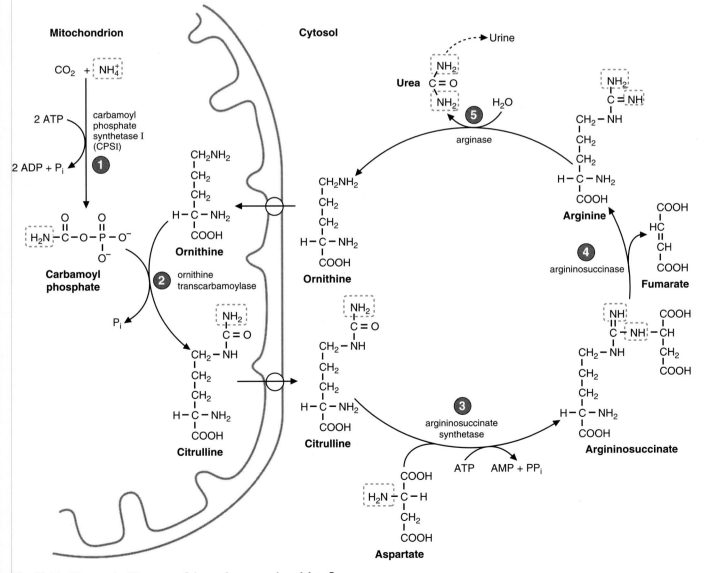

Fig. 38.10. Urea cycle. The steps of the cycle are numbered **1** to **5**.

The urea cycle was proposed in 1932 by Hans Krebs and a medical student, Kurt Henseleit, based on their laboratory observations. It was originally called the Krebs-Henseleit cycle. Subsequently, Krebs used this concept of metabolic cycling to explain a second process that also bears his name, the Krebs (or TCA) cycle.

When ornithine transcarbamoylase (OTC) is deficient, the carbamoyl phosphate that normally would enter the urea cycle accumulates and floods the pathway for pyrimidine biosynthesis. Under these conditions, excess orotic acid (orotate), an intermediate in pyrimidine biosynthesis, is excreted in the urine. It produces no ill effects, but is indicative of a problem in the urea cycle.

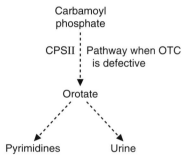

The precise pathogenesis of the central nervous system (CNS) signs and symptoms that accompany liver failure (hepatic encephalopathy) in patients such as **Teresa Livermore** are not completely understood. These changes are, however, attributable in part to toxic materials that are derived from the metabolism of nitrogenous substrates by bacteria in the gut which circulate to the liver in the portal vein. These materials "bypass" their normal metabolism by the liver cells, however, because the acute inflammatory process of viral hepatitis severely limits the ability of liver cells to degrade these compound to harmless metabolites. As a result, these toxins are "shunted" into the hepatic veins unaltered and eventually reach the brain through the systemic circulation ("portal-systemic encephalopathy").

Reactions of the Urea Cycle

Nitrogen enters the urea cycle as NH_4^+ and aspartate (Fig. 38.10). NH_4^+ forms carbamoyl phosphate, which reacts with ornithine, the compound that both initiates and is regenerated by the cycle. Aspartate reacts with citrulline, the compound produced from carbamoyl phosphate and ornithine. In two successive steps, arginine is formed. Cleavage of arginine by arginase releases urea and regenerates ornithine.

SYNTHESIS OF CARBAMOYL PHOSPHATE

In the first step of the urea cycle, NH_4^+, CO_2, and ATP react to form carbamoyl phosphate (see Fig. 38.10). The cleavage of 2 ATPs is required to form the high energy phosphate bond of carbamoyl phosphate. Carbamoyl phosphate synthetase I (CPSI), the enzyme that catalyzes this first step of the urea cycle, is found mainly in mitochondria of the liver. The Roman numeral suggests that another carbamoyl phosphate synthetase exists, and indeed, CPSII, located in the cytosol, produces carbamoyl phosphate for pyrimidine biosynthesis, using nitrogen from glutamine.

PRODUCTION OF ARGININE BY THE UREA CYCLE

Carbamoyl phosphate reacts with ornithine to form citrulline (see Fig. 38.10). The high energy phosphate bond of carbamoyl phosphate provides the energy required for this reaction, which occurs in mitochondria and is catalyzed by ornithine transcarbamoylase. The product citrulline is transported across the mitochondrial membranes and enters the cytosol.

Ornithine, which plays a role analogous to citrate in the TCA cycle, is an amino acid. However, it is not incorporated into proteins during the process of protein synthesis because no genetic codon exists for this amino acid.

In the cytosol, citrulline reacts with aspartate, the second source of nitrogen for urea synthesis, to produce argininosuccinate (see Fig. 38.10). This reaction, catalyzed by argininosuccinate synthetase, is driven by the hydrolysis of ATP to AMP and pyrophosphate. Aspartate is produced by transamination of oxaloacetate.

Argininosuccinate is cleaved by argininosuccinase to form fumarate and arginine (see Fig. 38.10). Fumarate is produced from the carbons of argininosuccinate provided by aspartate. Fumarate is converted to malate, which is used either for the synthesis of glucose by the gluconeogenic pathway or for the regeneration of oxaloacetate. Oxaloacetate is transaminated to form the aspartate that carries nitrogen into the urea cycle. Thus, the carbons of aspartate can be recycled to aspartate.

CLEAVAGE OF ARGININE TO PRODUCE UREA

Arginine, which contains nitrogens derived from NH_4^+ and aspartate, is cleaved by arginase, producing urea and regenerating ornithine (see Fig. 38.10). Urea is produced from the guanido group on the side chain of arginine. The portion of arginine originally derived from ornithine is reconverted to ornithine.

The reactions by which citrulline is converted to arginine and arginine is cleaved to produce urea occur in the cytosol. Ornithine, the other product of the arginase reaction, is transported into the mitochondrion, where it can react with carbamoyl phosphate, initiating another round of the cycle.

Regulation of the Urea Cycle

The human liver has a vast capacity to convert amino acid nitrogen to urea, thereby preventing toxic effects from ammonia, which would otherwise accumulate. In general, the urea cycle is regulated by substrate availability; the higher the rate of ammonia production, the higher the rate of urea formation. Regulation by substrate availability is a general characteristic of disposal pathways, like the urea cycle, which remove toxic compounds from the body. This is a type of "feed-forward" regulation, in contrast to the "feedback" regulation characteristic of pathways which produce functional endproducts.

Two other types of regulation control the urea cycle: allosteric activation of CPSI by N-acetylglutamate (NAG) and induction/repression of the synthesis of urea cycle enzymes. NAG is formed specifically to activate CPSI; it has no other known function. The synthesis of NAG from acetyl CoA and glutamate is stimulated by arginine (Fig. 38.11).

The induction of urea cycle enzymes occurs in response to conditions which require increased protein metabolism, such as a high protein diet or prolonged fasting. In both of these physiological states, as amino acid carbon is converted to glucose, amino acid nitrogen is converted to urea. The induction of the synthesis of urea cycle enzymes under these conditions occurs even though the uninduced enzyme levels are far in excess of the capacity required. The ability of a high protein diet to increase urea cycle enzyme levels is another type of "feed-forward" regulation.

Function of the Urea Cycle during Fasting

During fasting, the liver maintains blood glucose levels. Amino acids from muscle protein are a major carbon source for the production of glucose by the process of gluconeogenesis. As amino acid carbons are converted to glucose, the nitrogens are converted to urea. Thus, the urinary excretion of urea is high during fasting (Fig. 38.12). As fasting progresses, however, the brain begins to use ketone bodies, sparing blood glucose. Less muscle protein is cleaved to provide amino acids for gluconeogenesis, and decreased production of glucose from amino acids is accompanied by decreased production of urea (see Chapter 31).

The major amino acid substrate for gluconeogenesis is alanine, which is synthesized in peripheral tissues to act as a nitrogen carrier (see Fig. 38.1). Two molecules of alanine are required to generate one molecule of glucose. The nitrogen from the 2 molecules of alanine is converted to one molecule of urea (Fig. 38.13).

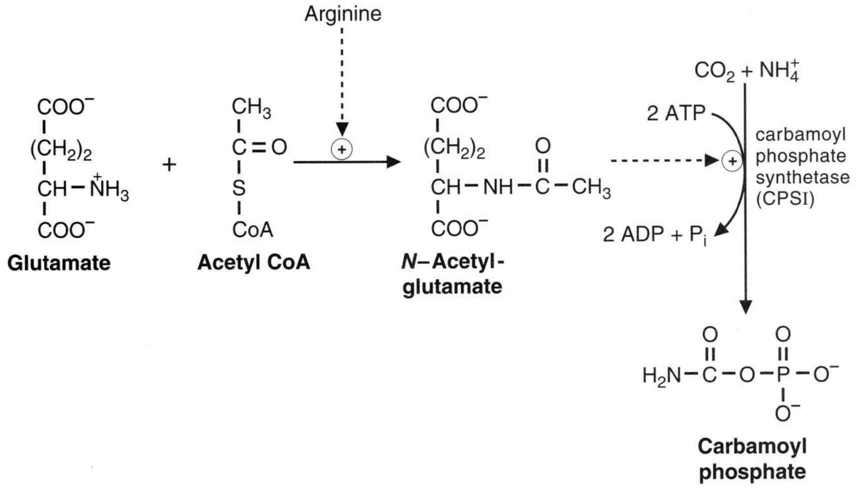

Fig. 38.11. Activation of carbamoyl phosphate synthetase I (CPSI). Arginine stimulates the synthesis of N-acetylglutamate, which activates CPSI.

Jean Ann Tonich's mild alcoholic hepatitis and associated early hepatic cirrhosis were not yet sufficiently severe or chronic to cause functional or anatomic shunting of metabolites of nitrogenous substrates formed in the gut into the systemic circulation. As a consequence, her brain was not exposed to elevated levels of ammonia and other potential neurotoxins believed to be involved in the pathogenesis of hepatic encephalopathy.

NH_4^+ is one of the toxins that results from the degradation of urea or proteins by intestinal bacteria and is not metabolized by the infected liver. The subsequent elevation of ammonia concentrations in the fluid bathing the brain causes depletion of tricarboxylic acid (TCA) cycle intermediates and ATP in the central nervous system. α-Ketoglutarate, a TCA cycle intermediate, combines with ammonia to form glutamate in a reaction catalyzed by glutamate dehydrogenase. Glutamate subsequently reacts with ammonia to form glutamine.

The absolute level of ammonia and its metabolites, such as glutamine, in the blood or cerebrospinal fluid in patients with hepatic encephalopathy correlates only roughly with the presence or severity of the neurological signs and symptoms. γ-Aminobutyric acid (GABA), an important inhibitory neurotransmitter in the brain, is also produced in the gut lumen and is shunted into the systemic circulation in increased amounts in patients with hepatic failure. In addition, other compounds (such as aromatic amino acids, false neurotransmitters, and certain short chain fatty acids) bypass liver metabolism and accumulate in the systemic circulation, eventually affecting the brain. Their relative importance in the pathogenesis of hepatic encephalopathy remains to be determined.

Although ornithine is normally regenerated by the urea cycle, it can be synthesized de novo if the need arises. It is produced from glutamate, which can be synthesized from glucose (see Chapter 39).

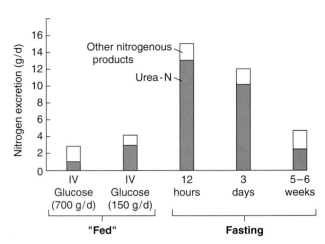

Fig. 38.12. Nitrogen excretion during fasting. Human subjects were initially given intravenous (IV) glucose as indicated, then fasted. Total nitrogen excretion was measured as well as the nitrogen in urea (dark area). Based on Ruderman NB, et al. Gluconeogenesis and its disorders in man. In: Hanson RW, Mehlman MA (eds). Gluconeogenesis: its regulation in mammalian species. New York: John Wiley, 1976:518.

 In addition to producing urea, the reactions of the urea cycle also serve as the pathway for the biosynthesis of arginine. Therefore, this amino acid is not required in the diet of the adult; however, it is required in the diet for growth.

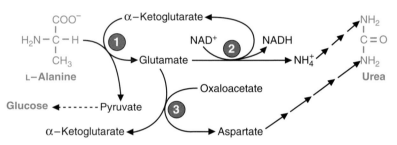

Fig. 38.13. Conversion of alanine to glucose and urea. **1.** Alanine, the key gluconeogenic amino acid, is transaminated to form pyruvate, which is converted to glucose. The nitrogen, now in glutamate, can be released as NH_4^+ (**2**) or transferred to oxaloacetate to form aspartate (**3**). NH_4^+ and aspartate enter the urea cycle, which produces urea. In summary, the carbons of alanine form glucose and the nitrogens form urea. Two molecules of alanine are required to produce one molecule of glucose and one molecule of urea.

 Urea is not cleaved by human enzymes. However, bacteria, including those in the human digestive tract, can cleave urea to ammonia and CO_2. (Urease, the enzyme that catalyzes this reaction, was the first enzyme to be crystallized.)

To some extent, humans excrete urea into the gut and saliva. Intestinal bacteria convert urea to ammonia. This ammonia, as well as ammonia produced by other bacterial reactions in the gut, is absorbed into the hepatic portal vein. It is normally extracted by the liver and converted to urea.

CLINICAL COMMENTS. The two most serious complications of acute viral hepatitis found in patients like **Teresa Livermore** are massive hepatic necrosis leading to fulminant liver failure and the eventual development of chronic hepatitis. Both complications are rare in acute viral hepatitis type A, however, suggesting that acetaminophen toxicity may have contributed to Teresa's otherwise unexpectedly severe hepatocellular dysfunction and early hepatic encephalopathy.

Fortunately, bed rest, rehydration, parenteral nutrition, and therapy directed at decreasing the production of toxins that result from bacterial degradation of nitrogenous substrates in the gut lumen (e.g., administration of lactulose which reduces gut ammonia levels by a variety of mechanisms, the use of enemas and antibiotics to decrease the intestinal flora, a low protein diet) prevented Teresa Livermore from progressing to the later stages of hepatic encephalopathy. As with most patients who survive an episode of fulminant hepatic failure, recovery to her previous state of health occurred over the next 3 months. Teresa's liver function studies returned to normal and a follow-up liver biopsy demonstrated no histological abnormalities.

Jean Ann Tonich's signs and symptoms as well as her laboratory profile were consistent with the presence of mild reversible alcohol-induced hepatocellular inflammation (alcoholic hepatitis) superimposed on a degree of irreversible scarring of liver tissues known as chronic alcoholic (Laënnec's) cirrhosis of the liver. She was cautioned strongly to abstain from alcohol immediately and to improve her nutritional status. In addition, Jean Ann was referred to the hospital drug and alcohol rehabilitation unit for appropriate psychological therapy and supportive social counseling. The physician also arranged for a follow-up office visit in 2 weeks.

Alcoholic liver disease, a common and sometimes fatal sequela of chronic ethanol abuse, may manifest in three forms: fatty liver, alcoholic hepatitis, and cirrhosis. Each may occur alone or they may be present in any combination in a given patient. Alcoholic cirrhosis is discovered in up to 9% of all autopsies performed in the United States, with a peak incidence in patients 40–55 years of age.

Alcohol is oxidized to acetaldehyde principally by cytosolic alcohol dehydrogenase (Fig. 38.14). Acetaldehyde is oxidized to acetate by mitochondrial and cytosolic acetaldehyde dehydrogenases. The acetate, for the most part, diffuses from the liver into the blood and is taken up by muscle and other tissues for oxidation in the TCA cycle. Alcohol is also oxidized to acetaldehyde by the microsomal ethanol oxidizing system (MEOS), part of the cytochrome P450 superfamily. MEOS has a much higher K_m for ethanol than alcohol dehydrogenase, and the synthesis of MEOS is induced by ethanol and by substrates for the other members of the cytochrome P450 family. MEOS, therefore, may account for as much as 30% of ethanol oxidation in individuals who chronically consume high doses of ethanol.

Much of the tissue damage in chronic alcoholism is believed to result from acetaldehyde, which accumulates in the liver and is released into the blood after heavy doses of alcohol. Acetaldehyde is highly reactive and binds covalently to amino groups, nucleotides, and phospholipids to form "adducts." Some of the proteins that are affected include hemoglobin, calmodulin, ribonuclease, and tubulin. Proteins in the heart and other tissues are affected as well as proteins in the liver.

One of the results of acetaldehyde-adduct formation is a diminished synthesis of proteins for hepatic lipoprotein particles, and a diminished tubulin-dependent secretion of proteins. As a consequence of the impaired secretory mechanisms, triacylglycerols and proteins accumulate in the liver. Although very low density lipoprotein (VLDL), formed in increased amounts from the inhibition of fatty acid oxidation, is increased in the blood, significant amounts of protein and triacylglycerols also accumulate in the liver. The accumulation of proteins results in an influx of water within the hepatocytes and a swelling of the liver that contributes to portal hypertension and a disruption of hepatic architecture.

Another consequence of acetaldehyde adduct formation is enhanced lipid peroxidation and the perpetuation of free radical damage. Acetaldehyde binds directly to glutathione and diminishes its ability to protect against H_2O_2, and enhances hydroxyl radical formation. The induction of MEOS also increases free radical formation.

Acetaldehyde damage is self-perpetuating because the protein and lipid damage diminish the capacity of mitochondria to oxidize NADH and acetaldehyde. As a consequence, even greater acetaldehyde levels accumulate. The higher $NADH/NAD^+$ ratio of chronic alcoholism can result in lactic acidosis, ketoacidosis, and hypoglycemia. Because lactate and ketone bodies interfere with uric acid excretion by the kidney, hyperuricemia can also occur.

The development of hepatic cirrhosis, or hepatic scarring, occurs in less than 20% of individuals who chronically consume ethanol, but a much greater percentage develop some of the biochemical changes found in alcoholic liver disease. The development of hepatic fibrosis after ethanol consumption is related to stimulation of the

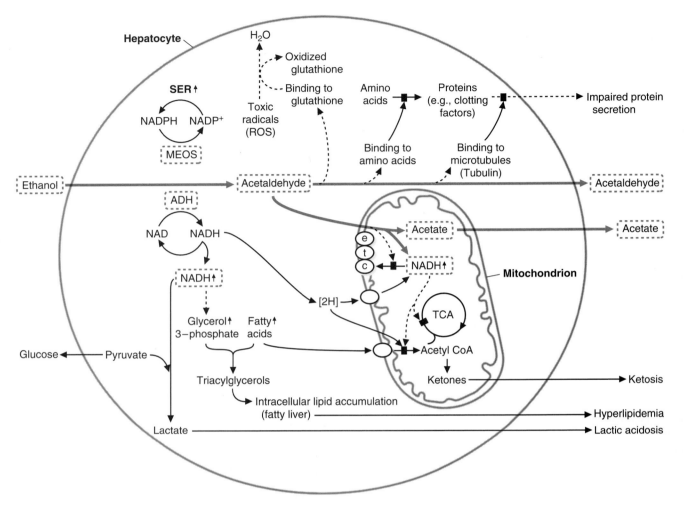

Fig. 38.14. Effects of ethanol on the liver. Ethanol is oxidized to acetaldehyde principally by alcohol dehydrogenase (ADH). Acetaldehyde is oxidized to acetate principally by mitochondrial acetaldehyde dehydrogenase. Ethanol at high concentrations can also be oxidized by MEOS in the endoplasmic reticulum (ER). ADH produces NADH, which inhibits gluconeogenesis by converting pyruvate to lactate. Accumulation of lactate results in a lacticacidosis. High NADH levels also slow the TCA cycle. Therefore, fatty acids are only partially oxidized and converted to ketone bodies, or diverted to triacylglycerol formation. Simultaneous induction of the enzymes of MEOS and other enzymes of the ER, such as the fatty acyl glycerol transferases, further enhances triacylglycerol formation. A fatty liver is produced by triacylglycerol accumulation. Acetaldehyde binds to molecules and prevents detoxification of toxic radicals. It also prevents the synthesis and secretion of proteins.

mitogenic development of Ito cells into fibroblasts, and stimulation of their production of collagen and fibronectin. Free radical damage also contributes to the fibrosis. There is also a genetic component, which may involve the collagen gene, the enzymes of ethanol metabolism, and/or the response of hepatic cells to inflammation or viral infection.

Once hepatic cirrhosis occurs, much of liver function is lost. The capacity for urea formation is altered, resulting in NH_4^+ accumulation and possibly hepatic encephalopathy. The liver decreases synthesis and secretion of serum albumin, the proteins of blood coagulation, and other serum proteins.

Because Jean Ann's case is mild, lifelong abstinence from ethanol and good nutrition should decrease the likelihood for progression to more serious liver dysfunction. In fact, because of the capacity of the liver to regenerate new and healthy cells, the prognosis for recovery of normal liver function is good.

BIOCHEMICAL COMMENTS. Because ammonia is toxic, it must be excreted rapidly. Animals that live in the sea excrete ammonia, which is diluted by the surrounding water. Land animals convert ammonia to urea, and the kidneys excrete it, dissolved in water. Birds, in order to fly, must have a lower body weight than land animals. Therefore, they excrete nitrogen as uric acid and other purine bases, in a solid white precipitate with little associated water.

The following verses from *The Biochemists' Songbook* by Harold Baum deal with these issues and the reactions of the urea cycle. Note that the British use oxoglutarate for α-ketoglutarate. GDH is glutamate dehydrogenase.

Those concerned about political issues should pay particular attention to the last verse and its definition of freedom.

WE'RE HERE BECAUSE UREA
(Tune: "The Bold Gendarmes," also known as "The Marine's Hymn")

The endogenous repletion of water in the sea
Lets nitrogenous excretion proceed quite easily
For ammonia though toxic is quickly washed away
So fish excrete (4 times) the ammonotelic way (repeat).

But new terrestrial creatures to survive where it was dry
Developed metabolic features in order to detoxify,
Since urea is quite soluble and it doesn't make you sick
We each excrete (4 times) as a ureotelic (repeat).

When protein breakdown is induced (to make new glucose, say)
Amino acids thus produced give nitrogen away,
Keto acids are acceptors; and oxaloacetate
Transaminates...giving rise to aspartate.

Glutamate too may be produced from oxoglutarate
And now that it's been introduced deamination is its fate
For inside each mitochondrion of every liver cell
Is GDH...(reducing NAD as well).

Ammonia that's thus set free combined with CO_2
Utilising ATP (and an extra squiggle too)
The effector of the synthetase is acetyl glutamate,
The product formed...carbamoylphosphate.

Two amino acid oddities now enter on the scene,
The essential commodities, ornithine and citrulline;
Ornithine starts in the cytosol, citrulline in mitos. free
Then they exchange...electrogenically.

Carbamoylphosphate carbamylates the ornithine
So we get a kind of steady state generating citrulline;
Citrulline now is exported, then combined with aspartate
And generates...argininosuccinate.

That Schiff base condensation utilises ATP
But there is now elimination and fumarate's set free;
Fumarate through citric cycle yields oxaloacetate
That then in turn...gives another aspartate.

That cleavage mentioned just before also yielded arginine
And what this pathway's called a cycle for can now readily be seen
For arginine is hydrolysed regenerating ornithine
Which can exchange...for another citrulline.

That arginase reaction then also yielded urea
(Aspartate gave one nitrogen, one from ammonia)
And we thus complete the cycle that let us leave the sea,
Sing urea...which set the people free.

– Harold Baum

From Baum H. The Biochemists' Songbook, 2nd ed. London: Taylor & Francis, 1995:51–52.

Suggested Readings

Brusilow S, Horwich A. Urea cycle enzymes. In: Scriver CR, Beaudet AL, Sly WS, Valle D, eds. The metabolic and molecular bases of inherited disease, 7th ed, vol I. New York: McGraw-Hill, 1995:629.

Goldin R. The pathogenesis of alcoholic liver disease. J Exp Path 1994;75:71–76.

PROBLEM

Deficiency diseases have been described which involve each of the five enzymes of the urea cycle. Clinical manifestations may appear in the neonatal period. Infants with defects in the first four enzymes usually appear normal at birth, but after 24 hours progressively develop lethargy, hypothermia, and apnea. They have high blood ammonia levels and the brain becomes swollen. One possible explanation for the swelling is the osmotic effect of the accumulation of glutamine in the brain produced by the reactions of ammonia with α-ketoglutarate and glutamate. Arginase deficiency is not as severe as deficiencies of the other urea cycle enzymes.

Given the following information about five newborn infants who appeared normal at birth but developed hyperammonemia after 24 hours, determine which urea cycle enzyme might be defective in each case. All infants had low levels of blood urea nitrogen (BUN). (Normal citrulline levels are 10–20 μM.)

Infant	Urine Orotate	Blood Citrulline	Blood Arginine	Blood Ammonia	Defective Enzyme
I	Low	Low	Low	High	
II	–*	High (>1,000 μM)	Low	High	
III	–	–	High	Moderately high	
IV	High	Low	Low	High	
V	–	High (200 μM)	Low	High	

* = value not determined; low = below normal; high = above normal.

ANSWER

Infant I has a defect in carbamoyl phosphate synthetase I (CPSI), and Infant IV has a defect in ornithine transcarbamoylase (OTC). Infants with high ammonia, low arginine, and low citrulline levels must have a defect in a urea cycle enzyme before the step that produces citrulline, i.e., CPSI or OTC. If CPSI is functional and carbamoyl phosphate is produced but cannot be further metabolized, more than the normal amount is diverted to the pathway for pyrimidine synthesis and the intermediate orotate appears in the urine. Therefore, Infant I has a defect in CPSI (citrulline is low and less than the normal amount of orotate is in the urine). Infant IV has an OTC defect; carbamoyl phosphate is produced, but it cannot be converted to citrulline, so citrulline is low and orotate is present in the urine.

Infants II and V have high levels of citrulline, but low levels of arginine. Therefore, they cannot produce arginine from citrulline. Argininosuccinate synthetase or argininosuccinase is defective. The very elevated citrulline levels in Infant II suggest that the block is in argininosuccinate synthetase. In Infant V, citrulline levels are more moderately elevated, suggesting that citrulline can be converted to argininosuccinate and that the defect is in argininosuccinase. Thus, the accumulated intermediates of the urea cycle are distributed between argininosuccinate and citrulline (which both can be excreted in the urine). The high levels of arginine and more moderate hyperammonemia in Infant III suggest that, in this case, the defect is in arginase.

39 Synthesis and Degradation of Amino Acids

Because each of the 20 common amino acids has a unique structure, their metabolic pathways differ. Many of these pathways are clinically relevant. Therefore, we will try to present most of the diverse pathways for the synthesis and degradation of the amino acids that occur in humans. However, to avoid burdening students with overwhelming details, we will be as succinct as possible.

Eleven of the twenty common amino acids can be synthesized in the body (Fig. 39.1). The other nine are required in the diet. Ten of these eleven "nonessential" amino acids can be produced from glucose plus, of course, a source of nitrogen. The eleventh nonessential amino acid, tyrosine, requires an essential amino acid, phenylalanine, for its synthesis.

The carbon skeletons of the 10 nonessential amino acids derived from glucose are produced from intermediates of glycolysis and the tricarboxylic acid (TCA) cycle. Four amino acids (serine, glycine, cysteine, and alanine) are produced from

 Genetic codons exist for 20 amino acids. Only these 20 common amino acids are incorporated into proteins during the process of protein synthesis.

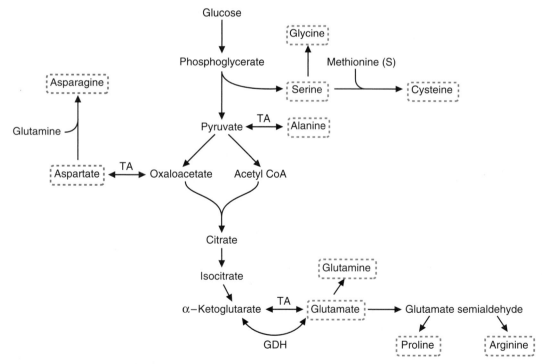

Fig. 39.1. Overview of the synthesis of the nonessential amino acids. Ten amino acids may be produced from glucose via intermediates of glycolysis or the TCA cycle. The eleventh nonessential amino acid, tyrosine, is synthesized by hydroxylation of the essential amino acid phenylalanine. Only the sulfur of cysteine comes from the essential amino acid methionine; its carbons and nitrogen come from serine. Transamination (TA) reactions involve pyridoxal phosphate (PLP) and another amino acid/α-keto acid pair.

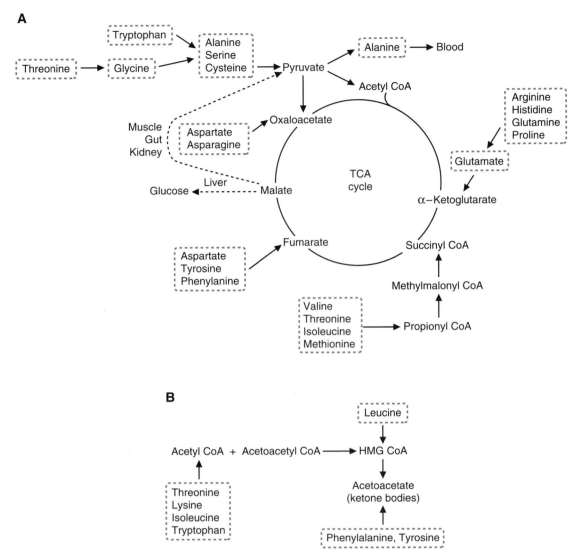

Fig. 39.2. Degradation of amino acids. **A.** Amino acids that produce pyruvate or intermediates of the TCA cycle. These amino acids are considered glucogenic because they can produce glucose in the liver. **B.** Amino acids that produce acetyl CoA or ketone bodies. These amino acids are considered ketogenic.

glucose via components of the glycolytic pathway. Intermediates of the TCA cycle (which are produced from glucose) provide carbon for synthesis of the six remaining nonessential amino acids. α-Ketoglutarate is the precursor for the synthesis of glutamate, glutamine, proline, and arginine. Oxaloacetate provides carbon for the synthesis of aspartate and asparagine.

The fate of the carbons of the amino acids depends on the physiological state of the individual and the tissue where the degradation occurs. For example, in the liver during fasting, the carbon skeletons of the amino acids produce glucose, ketone bodies, and CO_2. In the fed state, the liver can convert intermediates of amino acid metabolism to glycogen and triacylglycerols. Thus, the fate of the carbons of the amino acids parallels that of glucose and fatty acids. The liver is the only tissue which has all the pathways of amino acid synthesis and degradation.

As amino acids are degraded, their carbons are converted to (a) CO_2, (b) compounds that produce glucose in the liver (pyruvate and the TCA cycle intermediates α-ketoglutarate, succinyl CoA, fumarate, and oxaloacetate), and (c) ketone bodies or their precursors (acetoacetate and acetyl CoA) (Fig. 39.2). For simplicity, amino acids are considered to be glucogenic if their carbon skeletons can be converted to glucose, and ketogenic if their carbon skeletons can be converted to acetyl CoA or acetoacetate. Some amino acids contain carbons that produce glucose and other carbons that produce acetyl CoA or acetoacetate. These amino acids are both glucogenic and ketogenic. Amino acids that produce pyruvate are considered to be glucogenic because the liver converts pyruvate to glucose during fasting. Under fasting conditions in the liver, pyruvate does not produce acetyl CoA (and thus ketone bodies) because pyruvate dehydrogenase is inactive.

The amino acids that are synthesized from intermediates of glycolysis produce pyruvate when they are degraded (see Figs. 39.1 and 39.2A). The amino acids synthesized from TCA cycle intermediates are reconverted to these intermediates during degradation. Histidine, an essential amino acid, contains 5 carbons that are converted to glutamate and thence to the TCA cycle intermediate α-ketoglutarate.

Some essential amino acids (amino acids that cannot be synthesized) contain carbons that are converted to pyruvate or to TCA cycle intermediates. Tryptophan produces alanine, which is converted to pyruvate. Methionine, threonine, valine, and isoleucine form succinyl CoA, and phenylalanine (after conversion to tyrosine) forms fumarate. Because pyruvate and the TCA cycle intermediates produce glucose in the liver, these amino acids are glucogenic.

Some essential amino acids with carbons that produce glucose also contain other carbons that produce ketone bodies (see Fig. 39.2B). Tryptophan, isoleucine, and threonine produce acetyl CoA, and phenylalanine produces acetoacetate. These amino acids are both glucogenic and ketogenic.

Two of the essential amino acids (lysine and leucine) are strictly ketogenic. They do not produce glucose.

Piquet Yuria, a 4-month-old female infant, emigrated from the Soviet Union with her French mother and Russian father 1 month ago. She was normal at birth but in the last several weeks was noted to be less than normally attentive to her surroundings. Her psychomotor maturation seemed delayed and a tremor of her extremities had recently appeared. When her mother found her having gross twitching movements in her crib, she brought the infant to the hospital emergency room. A pediatrician examined Piquet and immediately noted a musty odor to the baby's wet diaper. A drop of her blood was obtained from a heel prick and used to perform a Guthrie bacterial inhibition assay using a special type of filter paper. This screening procedure was positive for the presence of an excess of phenylalanine in Piquet's blood.

Homer Sistine, a 14-year-old male, had a sudden grand mal seizure (with jerking movements of the torso and head) in his eighth grade classroom. The school physician noted mild weakness of the muscles of the left side of Homer's face and of his left arm and leg. Homer was hospitalized with a tentative diagnosis of a cerebrovascular accident involving the right cerebral hemisphere, which presumably triggered the seizure.

Homer's past medical history was normal, except for slight mental retardation requiring placement in a special education group. He also had a downward partial dislocation of the lenses of both eyes for which he had had a surgical procedure (a peripheral iridectomy).

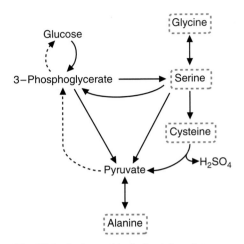

Fig. 39.3. Amino acids derived from intermediates of glycolysis. These amino acids can be synthesized from glucose. Their carbons can be reconverted to glucose in the liver.

Homer's left-sided neurological deficits cleared spontaneously within 3 days, but a computerized axial tomogram (CAT) showed changes consistent with a small infarction (damaged area caused by a temporary or permanent loss of adequate arterial blood flow) in the right cerebral hemisphere. A neurologist noted that Homer had a slight waddling gait, which his mother said began several years earlier and was progressing with time. Further studies confirmed the presence of decreased mineralization (decreased calcification) of the skeleton (osteopenia probably due to a process known as osteoporosis) and high methionine and homocysteine but low cystine levels in the blood.

All of this information, plus the increased length of the long bones of Homer's extremities and a slight curvature of his spine (scoliosis), caused his physician to suspect that Homer might have an inborn error of metabolism.

AMINO ACIDS DERIVED FROM INTERMEDIATES OF GLYCOLYSIS

Four amino acids are synthesized from intermediates of glycolysis. Serine, which produces glycine and cysteine, is synthesized from 3-phosphoglycerate, and alanine is formed by transamination of pyruvate, the product of glycolysis (Fig. 39.3). When these amino acids are degraded, they all are converted to pyruvate or to intermediates of the glycolytic/gluconeogenic pathway and, therefore, can produce glucose or be oxidized to CO_2.

Serine

In the biosynthesis of serine from glucose, 3-phosphoglycerate is first oxidized to a 2-keto compound (3-phosphohydroxypyruvate), which is then transaminated to form phosphoserine (Fig. 39.4). Phosphoserine phosphatase removes the phosphate, forming serine.

In many mammals, serine is degraded by serine dehydratase, an enzyme that requires pyridoxal phosphate (PLP) and produces NH_4^+ and pyruvate. This pathway appears to be a minor one in humans, and serine is generally degraded by transamination to hydroxypyruvate followed by reduction and phosphorylation to form 2-phosphoglycerate, an intermediate of gycolysis that forms PEP and, subsequently, pyruvate.

Regulatory mechanisms maintain serine levels in the body. When serine levels fall, serine synthesis is increased by induction of 3-phosphoglycerate dehydrogenase and by release of the feedback inhibition of phosphoserine phosphatase (caused by higher levels of serine). When serine levels rise, synthesis of serine decreases because the dehydrogenase is repressed and the phosphatase is inhibited (see Fig. 39.4).

Glycine

Glycine is metabolized by a number of different routes. Glycine is produced from serine by a reversible reaction that involves tetrahydrofolate (Fig. 39.5). Glycine also transfers a carbon atom (carbon 2) to tetrahydrofolate, forming CO_2, and NH_4^+. Tetrahydrofolate is a coenzyme that transfers one-carbon groups at different levels of oxidation. It is derived from the vitamin folate (see Chapter 40). Although threonine is not a major source of glycine, glycine can be produced by degradation of threonine.

Glycine is oxidized by D-amino acid oxidase (see Fig. 39.5). The product, glyoxalate, is converted back to glycine by transamination, further oxidized to oxalate, or oxidized to CO_2 and H_2O.

Oxalate, produced from glycine or obtained from the diet, forms precipitates with calcium. Kidney stones (renal calculi) are often composed of calcium oxalate.

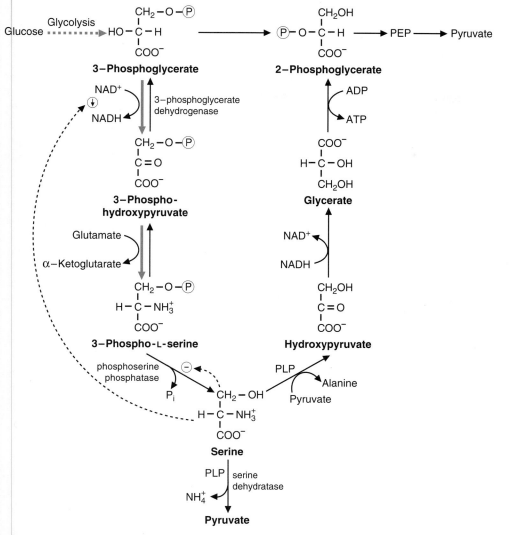

Fig. 39.4. Synthesis and degradation of serine. Serine levels are maintained because serine causes repression (circled ↓) of 3-phosphoglycerate dehydrogenase. Serine also inhibits (⊖) phosphoserine phosphatase.

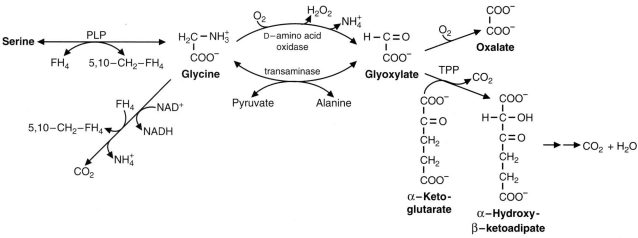

Fig. 39.5. Metabolism of glycine. Glycine forms serine or CO_2 and NH_4^+ by reactions that require tetrahydrofolate (FH_4). Glycine also forms glyoxylate, which is converted to oxalate or to CO_2 and H_2O.

39.1: Based on methionine, homocysteine, and cystine determinations, **Homer Sistine's** doctor concluded that he had homocystinuria due to an enzyme deficiency. What was the rationale for this conclusion?

Cystathionuria, the presence of cystathionine in the urine, is relatively common in premature infants. As they mature, cystathionase levels rise and the levels of cystathionine in the urine decrease.

In adults, a genetic deficiency of cystathionase causes cystathionuria. Individuals with a genetically normal cystathionase also develop cystathionuria if they have a dietary deficiency of pyridoxine (vitamin B$_6$). (Cystathionase requires the cofactor PLP, which is derived from vitamin B$_6$.) No characteristic clinical abnormalities have been observed in individuals with cystathionase deficiency. It is probably a benign disorder.

All transamination reactions involved in the synthesis or degradation of amino acids require PLP, derived from pyridoxine (vitamin B$_6$).

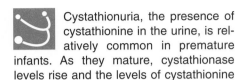

Cystinuria and cystinosis are disorders involving two different transport proteins for cystine, the disulfide formed from 2 molecules of cysteine. Cystinuria is caused by a defect in the transport protein that carries cystine, lysine, arginine, and ornithine into intestinal epithelial cells and that permits resorption of these amino acids by renal tubular cells. Cystine, which is not very soluble in the urine, forms renal calculi (stones). **Cal Kulis**, a patient with cystinuria, developed cystine stones (see Chapter 8).

Cystinosis is a rare disorder caused by a defective carrier that transports cystine across the lysosomal membrane from lysosomal vesicles to the cytosol. Cystine accumulates in the lysosomes in many tissues and forms crystals, impairing their function. Children with this disorder develop renal failure by 6–12 years of age.

Cysteine

The carbons and nitrogen for the synthesis of cysteine are provided by serine and the sulfur is provided by methionine (Fig. 39.6). Serine reacts with homocysteine (which is produced from methionine) to form cystathionine. This reaction is catalyzed by cystathionine synthase. Cleavage of cystathionine by cystathionase produces cysteine and α-ketobutyrate, which forms succinyl CoA via propionyl CoA. Both cystathionine synthase and cystathionase require PLP. This pathway serves as the major degradative route for methionine.

Cysteine inhibits cystathionine synthase and, therefore, regulates its own production. Because cysteine derives its sulfur from the essential amino acid methionine, cysteine becomes essential if it is low in the diet and the supply of methionine is inadequate for cysteine synthesis. On the other hand, an adequate dietary source of cysteine "spares" methionine, i.e., decreases the amount that must be degraded to produce cysteine.

When cysteine is degraded, the nitrogen is converted to urea, the carbons to pyruvate, and the sulfur to sulfate, which is excreted in the urine (see Fig. 39.6; see also Chapter 42).

Alanine

Alanine is produced from pyruvate by a transamination reaction catalyzed by alanine transaminase (ALT) and may be converted back to pyruvate by a reversal of the same reaction (see Fig. 39.3). Alanine is the major gluconeogenic amino acid because it is produced in many tissues for the transport of nitrogen to the liver.

AMINO ACIDS RELATED TO TCA CYCLE INTERMEDIATES

Two groups of amino acids are synthesized from TCA cycle intermediates, one group from α-ketoglutarate and one from oxaloacetate (see Fig. 39.1). During degradation, four groups of amino acids are converted to the TCA cycle intermediates α-ketoglutarate, oxaloacetate, succinyl CoA, and fumarate (see Fig. 39.2A).

Amino Acids Related through α-Ketoglutarate/Glutamate

GLUTAMATE

The 5 carbons of glutamate are derived from α-ketoglutarate either by transamination or by the glutamate dehydrogenase reaction. Because α-ketoglutarate can be synthesized from glucose, all of the carbons of glutamate can be obtained from glucose (see Fig. 39.1). When glutamate is degraded, it is converted back to α-ketoglutarate either by transamination or by glutamate dehydrogenase. In the liver, α-ketoglutarate forms malate, which via gluconeogenesis produces glucose. Thus, glutamate is derived from glucose and reconverted to glucose (Fig. 39.7).

A number of other amino acids (glutamine, proline, and arginine) are derived from glutamate (Fig. 39.7). Another function of glutamate is to provide the glutamyl moiety of glutathione (γ-glutamyl-cysteinyl-glycine), which is involved in transporting amino acids into cells of the kidney and intestine (see Chapter 37). Perhaps more importantly, glutathione reduces compounds such as hydrogen peroxide (H$_2$O$_2$) which cause severe free radical damage to cells (see Chapter 21).

GLUTAMINE

Glutamine is produced from glutamate by glutamine synthetase, which adds NH$_4^+$ to the carboxyl group of the side chain, forming an amide (Fig. 39.8). Glutamine is

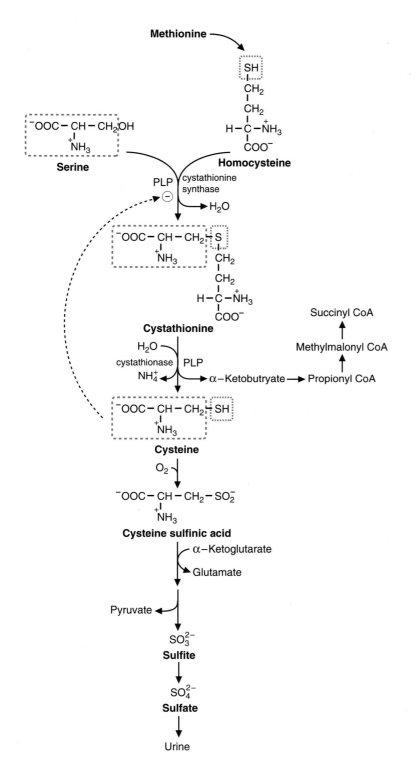

Fig. 39.6. Synthesis and degradation of cysteine. Cysteine is synthesized from the carbons and nitrogen of serine and the sulfur of homocysteine (which is derived from methionine). During the degradation of cysteine, the sulfur is converted to sulfate and excreted in the urine and the carbons are converted to pyruvate.

Homocysteine is oxidized to a disulfide, homocystine. To indicate that both forms are being considered, the term homocyst(e)ine is used.

Homocysteine

Homocysteine ⟷ Homocystine

Because a colorimetric screening test for urinary homocystine was positive, the doctor ordered several biochemical studies on **Homer Sistine's** serum which included tests for methionine, homocyst(e)ine (both free and protein-bound), cystine, vitamin B_{12}, and folate. The level of homocystine in a 24-hour urine collection was also measured.

The results were as follows: the serum methionine level was 980 μM (reference range < 30); serum homocyst(e)ine (both free and protein bound) was markedly elevated; cystine was not detected in the serum; the serum B_{12} and folate levels were normal. A 24-hour urine homocystine level was elevated.

A 39.1: If the blood levels of methionine and homocysteine are very elevated and cystine is low, cystathionine synthase could be defective, but a cystathionase deficiency is also a possibility. With a deficiency of either of these enzymes, cysteine could not be synthesized, and levels of homocysteine would rise. Homocysteine would be converted to methionine by reactions that require B_{12} and tetrahydrofolate (see Chapter 40), and it would be oxidized to homocystine, which would appear in the urine. The levels of cysteine (measured as its oxidation product cystine) would be low.

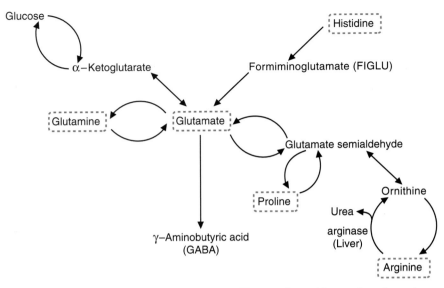

Fig. 39.7. Amino acids related through glutamate. These amino acids contain carbons that can be reconverted to glutamate, which can be converted to glucose in the liver. All of these amino acids except histidine can be synthesized from glucose.

reconverted to glutamate by a different enzyme, glutaminase, which is particularly important in the kidney. The ammonia it produces enters the urine and decreases its acidity ($NH_3 + H^+ \rightarrow NH_4^+$).

PROLINE

In the synthesis of proline, glutamate is first phosphorylated and then converted to glutamate 5-semialdehyde by reduction of the side chain carboxyl group to an aldehyde (Fig. 39.9). This semialdehyde spontaneously cyclizes, forming an internal Schiff base (between the aldehyde and the α-amino group). Reduction of this cyclic compound yields proline.

Proline is converted back to glutamate semialdehyde, which is reduced to form glutamate.

ARGININE

Arginine is synthesized from glutamate via the semialdehyde, which is transaminated to form ornithine, an intermediate of the urea cycle. The reactions of the cycle produce arginine (Fig. 39.10). However, the quantities of arginine that are generated are adequate only for the adult and are insufficient to support growth. Therefore, during periods of growth, arginine becomes an essential amino acid.

Arginine is cleaved by arginase to form urea and ornithine. If ornithine is present in amounts in excess of those required for the urea cycle, it is transaminated to glutamate semialdehyde, which is reduced to glutamate.

HISTIDINE

Although histidine cannot be synthesized in humans, five of its carbons form glutamate when it is degraded. In a series of steps, histidine is converted to formiminoglutamate (FIGLU). The subsequent reactions transfer one carbon of FIGLU to the tetrahydrofolate pool (see Chapter 40) and release NH_4^+ and glutamate (Fig. 39.11).

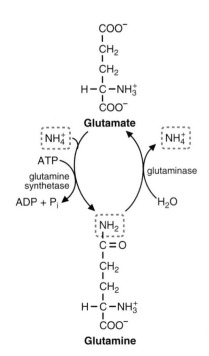

Fig. 39.8. Synthesis and degradation of glutamine. Different enzymes catalyze the addition and the removal of the amide nitrogen of glutamine.

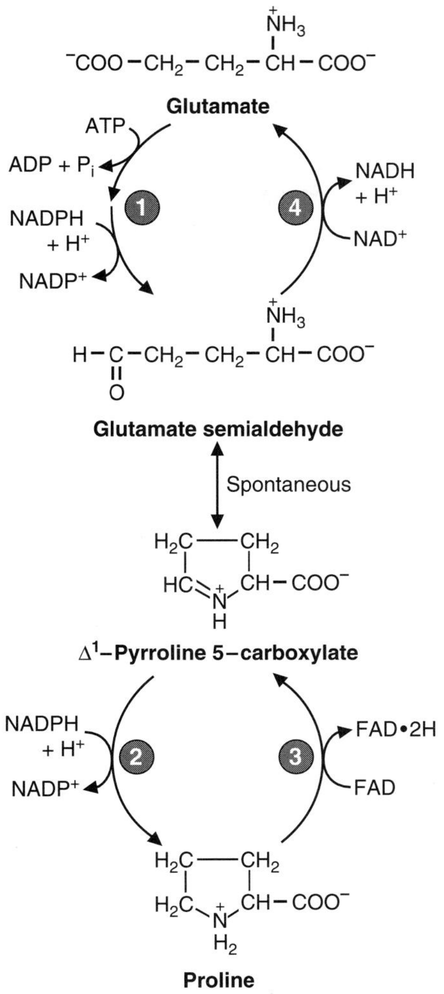

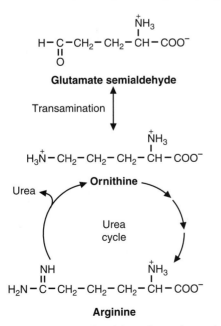

Fig. 39.9. Synthesis and degradation of proline. Reactions 1, 3, and 4 occur in mitochondria. Reaction 2 occurs in the cytosol. Synthesis and degradation involve different enzymes. The cyclization reaction (formation of a Schiff base) is nonenzymatic, i.e., spontaneous.

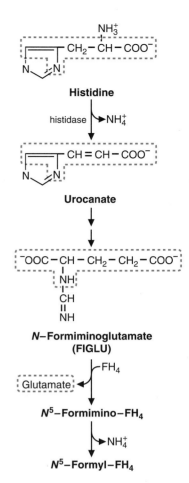

Fig. 39.11. Degradation of histidine. The highlighted portion of histidine forms glutamate. The remainder of the molecule provides one carbon for the tetrahydrofolate (FH_4) pool (see Chapter 40) and releases NH_4^+.

Fig. 39.10. Synthesis and degradation of arginine. The carbons of ornithine are derived from glutamate, which is converted to glutamate semialdehyde. Reactions of the urea cycle convert ornithine to arginine. Arginase converts arginine back to ornithine by releasing urea.

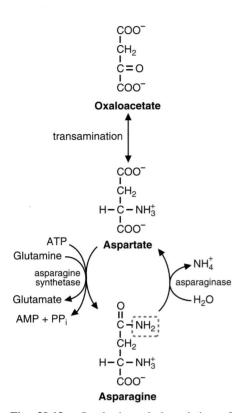

Fig. 39.12. Synthesis and degradation of aspartate and asparagine. Note that the amide nitrogen of asparagine is derived from glutamine. (The amide nitrogen of glutamine comes from NH_4^+. See Fig. 39.8.)

Certain types of tumor cells, particularly leukemic cells, require asparagine from the blood. Therefore, asparaginase has been used as an antitumor agent. It acts by converting asparagine to aspartate in the blood, decreasing the amount of asparagine available for tumor cell growth.

Amino Acids Related to Oxaloacetate (Aspartate and Asparagine)

Aspartate is produced by transamination of oxaloacetate. This reaction is readily reversible, so aspartate can be reconverted to oxaloacetate (Fig. 39.12).

Asparagine is formed from aspartate by a reaction in which glutamine provides the nitrogen for formation of the amide group. Thus, this reaction differs from the synthesis of glutamine from glutamate, in which NH_4^+ provides the nitrogen.

However, the reaction catalyzed by asparaginase, which hydrolyzes asparagine to NH_4^+ and aspartate, is analogous to the reaction catalyzed by glutaminase.

Amino Acids That Form Fumarate

ASPARTATE

Although the major route for aspartate disposal involves its conversion to oxaloacetate, carbons from aspartate can form fumarate. In the urea cycle, aspartate reacts with citrulline to form argininosuccinate, which is cleaved, forming arginine and fumarate. The carbons of the fumarate are derived from aspartate (see Fig. 38.10).

An analogous sequence of reactions occurs in the purine nucleotide cycle. Aspartate reacts with inosine monophosphate (IMP) to form an intermediate which is cleaved, forming AMP and fumarate (see Chapter 42).

PHENYLALANINE AND TYROSINE

Phenylalanine is converted to tyrosine by a hydroxylation reaction. Tyrosine, produced from phenylalanine or obtained from the diet, is oxidized, ultimately forming acetoacetate and fumarate. By forming malate, fumarate supplies carbons for gluconeogenesis. The conversion of phenylalanine to tyrosine and the production of acetoacetate will be considered further under the heading "Amino Acids That Form Acetyl CoA and Acetoacetate."

Amino Acids That Form Succinyl CoA

The amino acids that are degraded to form succinyl CoA cannot be synthesized in the human, so we only need to be concerned with their degradation. The reactions that convert propionyl CoA to succinyl CoA are common to the degradative pathways of methionine, valine, isoleucine, and threonine.

Propionyl CoA is carboxylated in a reaction that requires biotin and forms methylmalonyl CoA. Methylmalonyl CoA is then rearranged in a vitamin B_{12}-requiring reaction to produce succinyl CoA, a TCA cycle intermediate (see Fig. 23.8).

METHIONINE

Methionine is converted to *S*-adenosylmethionine (SAM), which donates its methyl group to other compounds by a sequence of reactions that produce homocysteine (Fig. 39.13). Methionine can be regenerated from homocysteine by a reaction that requires both tetrahydrofolate and vitamin B_{12} (a topic that will be considered in more detail in Chapter 40). Alternatively, by reactions that require PLP, homocysteine can provide the sulfur required for the synthesis of cysteine. Carbons of homocysteine are then converted to succinyl CoA. Thus, degradation of methionine produces succinyl CoA (see Fig, 39.13).

THREONINE

Threonine is degraded by two pathways. It is converted to acetyl CoA and glycine, or it is cleaved by a dehydratase to ammonia and α-ketobutyrate, which is decarboxylated to form propionyl CoA (see Fig. 39.13).

VALINE AND ISOLEUCINE

Two of the three branched chain amino acids contain carbons that form succinyl CoA. The initial step in the degradation of the branched chain amino acids is a transamination reaction. In the second step, the α-keto analogues of these amino acids are oxidatively decarboxylated by an α-keto acid dehydrogenase complex in a reaction similar in its mechanism and cofactor requirements to pyruvate dehydrogenase and α-ketoglutarate dehydrogenase (see Chapter 19). Subsequently, the pathways for degradation of these amino acids follow parallel routes (Fig. 39.14). The steps are analogous to those for β-oxidation of fatty acids and generate NADH and FAD(2H).

Valine and isoleucine are converted to succinyl CoA (see Fig. 39.13). Isoleucine also forms acetyl CoA. Leucine, the third branched chain amino acid, does not produce succinyl CoA. It forms acetoacetate and acetyl CoA.

AMINO ACIDS THAT FORM ACETYL COA AND ACETOACETATE

Seven amino acids produce acetyl CoA and/or acetoacetate, and are, therefore, categorized as ketogenic. Isoleucine, threonine, and the aromatic amino acids (phenyl-

39.2: What compounds form succinyl CoA via propionyl CoA and methylmalonyl CoA?

39.3: Homocystinuria is caused by deficiencies in the enzymes cystathionine synthase and cystathionase and also by deficiencies of methyltetrahydrofolate (CH_3-FH_4) or of methyl-B_{12}. The deficiencies of CH_3-FH_4 or of methyl-B_{12} are due either to an inadequate dietary intake of folate or B_{12} or to defective enzymes involved in joining methyl groups to tetrahydrofolate (FH_4), transferring methyl groups from FH_4 to B_{12}, or passing them from B_{12} to homocysteine to form methionine (see Chapter 40).

Is **Homer Sistine's** homocystinuria caused by any of these problems?

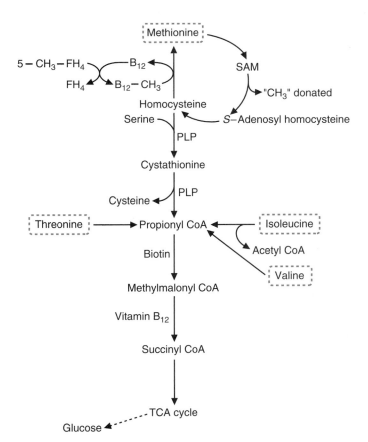

Fig. 39.13. Conversion of amino acids to succinyl CoA. The amino acids methionine, threonine, isoleucine, and valine, all of which form succinyl CoA via methylmalonyl CoA, are essential in the diet. The carbons of serine are converted to cysteine and do not form succinyl CoA by this pathway. SAM = S-adenosylmethionine.

39.2: In addition to methionine, threonine, isoleucine, and valine (see Fig. 39.13), the last 3 carbons at the ω-end of odd chain fatty acids form succinyl CoA by this route (see Chapter 23). In addition, the pyrimidine base thymine follows this route during its degradation (see Chapter 41).

39.3: **Homer Sistine's** methionine levels are elevated, and his B_{12} and folate levels are normal. Therefore, he does not have a deficiency of dietary folate or B_{12} or of the enzymes that transfer methyl groups from tetrahydrofolate to homocysteine to form methionine. In these cases, homocysteine levels are elevated, but methionine levels are low.

A biopsy specimen from Homer Sistine's liver was sent to the hospital's biochemistry research laboratory for enzyme assays. Cystathionine synthase activity was reported to be 7% of that found in normal liver.

In maple syrup urine disease, the α-keto acid dehydrogenase that oxidatively decarboxylates the branched chain amino acids is defective. As a result, the branched chain amino acids and their α-keto analogues (produced by transamination) accumulate. They appear in the urine, giving it the odor of maple syrup.

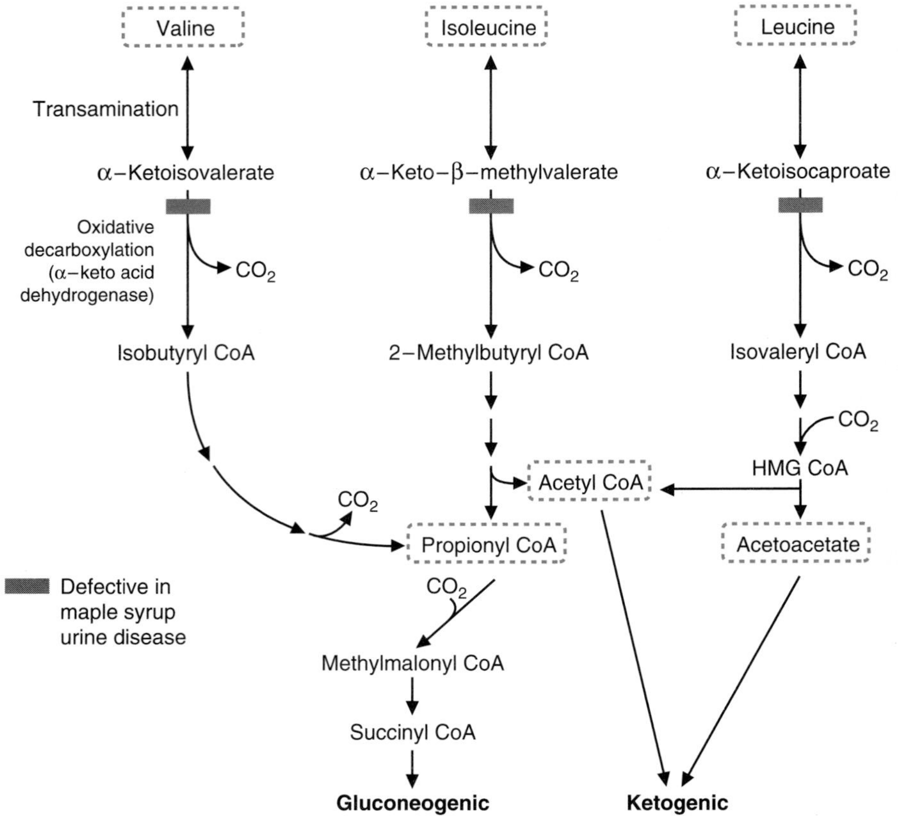

Fig. 39.14. Degradation of the branched chain amino acids. Valine forms propionyl CoA. Isoleucine forms propionyl CoA and acetyl CoA. Leucine forms acetoacetate and acetyl CoA.

A small subset of patients with hyperphenylalaninemia show an appropriate reduction in plasma phenylalanine levels with dietary restriction of this amino acid, yet develop progressive neurological symptoms and seizures and usually die within the first 2 years of life ("malignant" hyperphenylalaninemia). These infants exhibit normal phenylalanine hydroxylase (PAH) activity but have a deficiency in dihydropteridine reductase (DHPR), an enzyme required for the regeneration of tetrahydrobiopterin (BH$_4$), a cofactor of PAH (see Fig. 39.17). Less frequently, DHPR activity is normal but a defect in the biosynthesis of BH$_4$ exists. In either case, dietary therapy corrects the hyperphenylalaninemia. However, BH$_4$ is also a cofactor for two other hydroxylations required in the synthesis of neurotransmitters in the brain: the hydroxylation of tryptophan to 5-hydroxytryptophan and of tyrosine to L-dopa (see Chapter 41). It has been suggested that the resulting deficit in central nervous system neurotransmitter activity is, at least in part, responsible for the neurological manifestations and eventual death of these patients.

alanine, tyrosine, and tryptophan) are converted to compounds that produce both glucose and acetyl CoA or acetoacetate (Fig. 39.15). Leucine and lysine do not produce glucose; they produce acetyl CoA and acetoacetate.

Phenylalanine and Tyrosine

Phenylalanine is converted to tyrosine, which undergoes oxidative degradation (Fig. 39.16). The last step in the pathway produces both fumarate and the ketone body, acetoacetate. Deficiencies of different enzymes in the pathway result in phenylketonuria, tyrosinemia, and alcaptonuria.

Phenylalanine is hydroxylated to form tyrosine by a mixed function oxidase, phenylalanine hydroxylase (PAH), which requires molecular oxygen and tetrahydrobiopterin (Fig. 39.17). The cofactor, tetrahydrobiopterin is converted to dihydrobiopterin by this reaction. Tetrahydrobiopterin is not synthesized from a vitamin; it can be synthesized in the body from GTP. However, as is the case with other cofactors, the body contains limited amounts. Therefore, dihydrobiopterin must be reconverted to tetrahydrobiopterin in order for the reaction to continue to produce tyrosine.

Tryptophan

Tryptophan is oxidized to produce alanine (from the non-ring carbons), formate, and acetyl CoA. Tryptophan is, therefore, both glucogenic and ketogenic (Fig. 39.18).

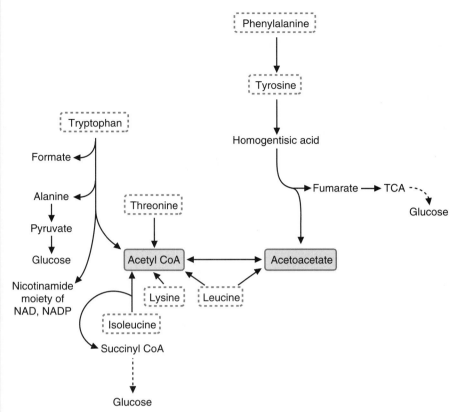

Fig. 39.15. Ketogenic amino acids. Some of these amino acids (tryptophan, phenylalanine, and tyrosine) also contain carbons that can form glucose. Leucine and lysine are strictly ketogenic; they do not form glucose.

NAD and NADP can be produced from the ring structure of tryptophan. Therefore, tryptophan "spares" the dietary requirement for niacin. The higher the dietary levels of tryptophan, the lower the levels of niacin required to prevent symptoms of deficiency.

Because the reactions converting tryptophan to NAD(P) require PLP, pyridoxine deficiency can result in pellagra-like symptoms.

Threonine

By one of its degradative pathways, threonine produces glycine and acetyl CoA in the liver. Acetyl CoA can be used by the liver for the synthesis of ketone bodies or oxidized to CO_2.

Isoleucine

Isoleucine produces both succinyl CoA and acetyl CoA. Therefore, it can produce both glucose and ketone bodies in the liver (see Figs. 39.13–39.15).

Leucine

Leucine produces hydroxymethylglutaryl CoA (HMG-CoA), which is cleaved to form acetyl CoA and the ketone body acetoacetate (see Figs. 39.14 and 39.15). It does not generate any compounds that can produce glucose. Most of the tissues where it is oxidized can utilize ketone bodies.

On more definitive testing of **Piquet Yuria's** blood, the plasma level of phenylalanine was found to be elevated at 18 mg/dL (reference range <1.2). Several phenyl ketones and other products of phenylalanine metabolism, which give the urine a characteristic odor, were found in significant quantities in the baby's urine.

A plasma sample was sent to the special chemistry research laboratory where it was determined that the level of activity of phenylalanine hydroxylase (PAH) in Piquet's blood was less than 1% of that found in normal infants. A diagnosis of "classic" phenylketonuria (PKU) was made.

Until gene therapy allows substitution of the defective PAH gene with its normal counterpart in vivo, the mainstay of therapy in classic PKU is to chronically maintain the levels of phenylalanine in the blood between 3 and 12 mg/dL through dietary restriction of this essential amino acid.

If the dietary levels of niacin and tryptophan are insufficient, the condition known as pellagra results. The symptoms of pellagra are dermatitis, diarrhea, dementia, and, finally, death.

Alcaptonuria occurs when homogentisate, an intermediate in tyrosine metabolism, cannot be further oxidized because the next enzyme in the pathway, homogentisate oxidase, is defective. Homogentisate accumulates and autooxidizes, forming a dark pigment, which discolors the urine and stains the diapers of affected infants. Later in life, the chronic accumulation of this pigment in cartilage may cause arthritic joint pain.

Tyrosinemia is frequently observed in newborn infants, especially those that are premature. For the most part, the condition appears to be benign, and dietary restriction of protein returns plasma tyrosine levels to normal. The biochemical defect has not been determined.

Other types of tyrosinemia are related to specific enzyme defects (see Fig. 39.16). Tyrosinemia II is caused by a genetic deficiency of tyrosine aminotransferase (TAT) and may involve eye and skin lesions as well as neurological problems. Patients are treated with a low tyrosine, low phenylalanine diet.

Tyrosinemia I (also called tyrosinosis) is caused by a genetic deficiency of fumarylacetoacetate hydrolase. The acute form is associated with liver failure, a cabbagelike odor, and death within the first year of life.

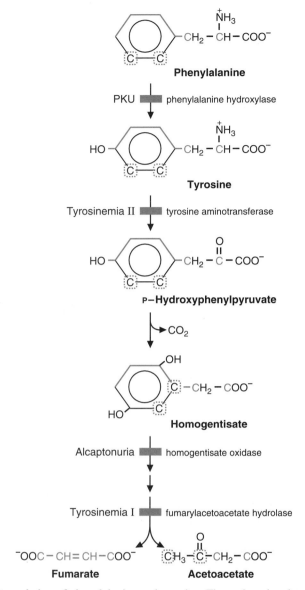

Fig. 39.16. Degradation of phenylalanine and tyrosine. The carboxyl carbon forms CO_2, and the other carbons form fumarate or acetoacetate as indicated. Deficiencies of enzymes (▓▓) result in the indicated diseases. PKU = phenylketonuria.

Lysine

Lysine cannot be directly transaminated at either of its two amino groups. Lysine is degraded by a complex pathway in which saccharopine, α-ketoadipate, and crotonyl CoA are intermediates. Ultimately, lysine generates acetyl CoA (see Fig. 39.15).

CLINICAL COMMENTS. The overall incidence of hyperphenylalaninemia is approximately 100 per million births with a wide geographic and ethnic variation. PKU occurs by autosomal recessive transmission of a defective PAH gene causing accumulation of phenylalanine in the blood well above the normal concentration in young children and adults (less than 1–2 mg/dL). In the new-

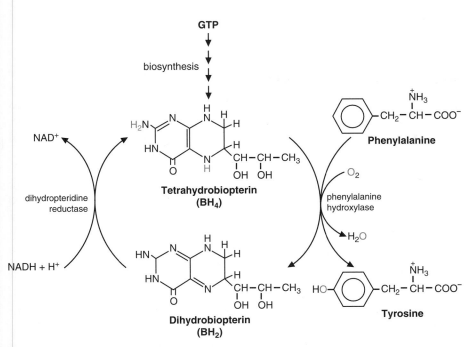

Fig. 39.17. Hydroxylation of phenylalanine. Phenylalanine hydroxylase (PAH) is a mixed function oxidase, i.e., molecular oxygen (O_2) donates one atom to water and one to the product, tyrosine. The cofactor, tetrahydrobiopterin (BH_4), is oxidized to dihydrobiopterin (BH_2), and must be reduced back to BH_4 in order for the phenylalanine to continue forming tyrosine. BH_4 is synthesized in the body from GTP. PKU results from deficiencies of PAH (the classic form), dihydrobiopterin reductase, or enzymes in the biosynthetic pathway for BH_4.

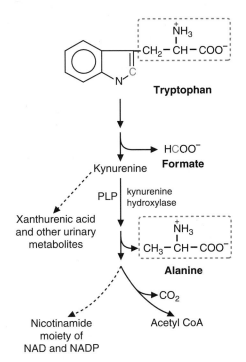

Fig. 39.18. Degradation of tryptophan. One of the ring carbons produces formate. The non-ring portion forms alanine. Kynurenine is an intermediate, which can be converted to a number of urinary excretion products (e.g., xanthurenate), degraded to CO_2 and acetyl CoA, or converted to the nicotinamide moiety of NAD and NADP, which can also be formed from the vitamin niacin.

born, the upper limit of normal is almost twice this value. Values above 16 mg/dL are usually found in patients, such as **Piquet Yuria**, with "classic" PKU.

Patients with classic PKU usually appear normal at birth. If the disease is not recognized and treated within the first month of life, the infant gradually develops varying degrees of irreversible mental retardation (IQ scores frequently under 50), delayed psychomotor maturation, tremors, seizures, eczema, and hyperactivity. It has been suggested that the neurological sequelae result in part from the competitive interaction of phenylalanine with brain amino acid transport systems and inhibition of neurotransmitter synthesis. These biochemical alterations lead to impaired myelin synthesis and delayed neuronal development which result in the clinical picture in patients like Piquet Yuria.

In order to restrict dietary levels of phenylalanine, special semisynthetic preparations such as Lofenalac or PKUaid are utilized in the United States. Use of these preparations reduces dietary intake of phenylalanine to 250–500 mg/day while maintaining normal intake of all other dietary nutrients. Although it is generally agreed that scrupulous adherence to this regimen is mandatory for the first decade of life, less consensus exists regarding its indefinite use. Evidence suggests, however, that without lifelong compliance with dietary restriction of phenylalanine, even adults will develop at least neurological sequelae of PKU. A pregnant woman with PKU must be particularly careful to maintain satisfactory plasma levels of phenylalanine throughout gestation to avoid the adverse effects of hyperphenylalaninemia on the fetus.

Piquet's parents were given thorough dietary instruction which they followed carefully. Although her pediatrician was not optimistic, it was hoped that the damage

Abnormal metabolism of tryptophan occurs in a vitamin B_6 deficiency. Kynurenine intermediates in tryptophan degradation cannot be cleaved because kynureninase requires PLP derived from vitamin B_6. Consequently, these intermediates enter a minor pathway for tryptophan metabolism that produces xanthurenic acid, which is excreted in the urine.

done to her nervous system prior to dietary therapy was minimal and that her subsequent psychomotor development would allow her to lead a relatively normal life.

The most characteristic biochemical features of the disorder affecting **Homer Sistine**, a cystathionine synthase deficiency, are the presence of an accumulation of both homocyst(e)ine and methionine in the blood. Because renal tubular reabsorption of methionine is highly efficient, this amino acid may not appear in the urine. Homocystine, the disulfide of homocysteine, is less efficiently reabsorbed, and amounts in excess of 1 mmol may be excreted in the urine each day.

In the type of homocystinuria in which the patient is deficient in cystathione synthase, the elevation in serum methionine levels is presumed to be the result of enhanced rates of conversion of homocysteine to methionine caused by increased availability of homocysteine (see Fig. 39.13). In type II and type III homocystinuria, in which there is a deficiency in the synthesis of methyl cobalamin and of N^5-methyltetrahydrofolate, respectively (both required for the methylation of homocysteine to form methionine), serum homocysteine levels are elevated but serum methionine levels are low (see Fig. 39.13).

The pathological findings which underlie the clinical features manifest by Homer Sistine are presumed (but not proven) to be the consequence of chronic elevations of homocysteine (and perhaps other compounds, e.g., methionine) in the blood and tissues. The zonular fibers which normally hold the lens of the eye in place become frayed and break, causing dislocation of the lens. The skeleton reveals a loss of bone ground substance (i.e., osteoporosis) which may explain the curvature of the spine. The elongation of the long bones beyond their normal genetically determined length leads to tall stature.

Animal experiments suggest that increased concentrations of homocysteine and methionine in the brain may trap adenosine as S-adenosylhomocysteine, diminishing adenosine levels. Since adenosine is normally depressant in cerebral actions, its deficiency may be associated with a lowering of the seizure threshold as well as a reduction in cognitive function.

Acute vascular events are common in these patients. Thrombi (blood clots) and emboli (clots that have broken off and traveled to a distant site in the vascular system) have been reported in almost every major artery and vein as well as in smaller vessels. These clots result in infarcts in vital organs such as the liver, the myocardium (heart muscle), the lungs, the kidneys, and many other tissues. Although increased serum levels of homocysteine have been implicated in enhanced platelet aggregation and damage to vascular endothelial cells (leading to clotting and accelerated atherosclerosis), no generally accepted mechanism for these vascular events has yet emerged.

Treatment is directed toward early reduction of the elevated levels of homocysteine and methionine in the blood. In addition to a diet low in methionine, very high oral doses of pyridoxine (vitamin B_6) have significantly decreased the plasma levels of homocysteine and methionine in some patients with cystathionine synthetase deficiency. (Genetically determined "responders" to pyridoxine treatment make up about 50% of type I homocystinurics.) PLP serves as a cofactor for cystathionine synthase; however, the molecular properties of the defective enzyme which confer the responsiveness to B_6 therapy are not known.

BIOCHEMICAL COMMENTS. Many enzyme deficiency diseases have been discovered that affect the pathways of amino acid metabolism. These deficiency diseases have helped researchers to elucidate the pathways in humans, where experimental manipulation is, at best, unethical. These spontaneous mutations ("experiments" of nature), although devastating to patients, have resulted in an understanding of these diseases that now permit treatment of inborn errors of metabolism that were once considered to be untreatable.

Classic PKU is caused by mutations in the gene located on chromosome 12 which encodes the enzyme phenylalanine hydroxylase (PAH). This enzyme normally catalyzes the hydroxylation of phenylalanine to tyrosine, the rate-limiting step in the major pathway by which phenylalanine is catabolized.

In early experiments, sequence analysis of mutant clones demonstrated a single base substitution in the gene with a G to A transition at the canonical 5′ donor splice site of intron 12 and expression of a truncated unstable protein product. This protein lacked the C-terminal region, a structural change which yielded less than 1% of the normal activity of PAH.

Since these initial studies, DNA analysis has demonstrated over 100 mutations (missense, nonsense, insertions, and deletions) in the PAH gene, associated with PKU and non-PKU hyperphenylalaninemia. That PKU is a heterogeneous phenotype is supported by studies measuring PAH activity in needle biopsy samples taken from the livers of a large group of patients with varying degrees of hyperphenylalaninemia. PAH activity varied from below 1% of normal in patients with classic PKU to up to 35% of normal in those with a non-PKU form of hyperphenylalaninemia.

The terms hypermethioninemia, homocystinuria (or -emia), and cystathioninuria (or -emia) designate biochemical abnormalities and are not specific clinical diseases. Each may be caused by more than one specific genetic defect. For example, at least seven distinct genetic alterations can cause increased excretion of homocystine in the urine. A deficiency of cystathionine synthase is the most common cause of homocystinuria; more than 600 such proven cases have been studied.

Suggested Readings

Mudd S, Levy H, Skovby F. Disorders of transsulfuration. In: Scriver CR, Beaudet AL, Sly WS, Valle D, eds. The metabolic and molecular bases of inherited disease. 7th ed, vol I. New York: McGraw-Hill, 1995:1279–1327.

Scriver C, Kaufman S, Eisensmith R, Woo S. The hyperphenylalaninemias. In: Scriver CR, Beaudet AL, Sly WS, Valle D, eds. The metabolic and molecular bases of inherited disease. 7th ed, vol I. New York: McGraw-Hill, 1995:1015–1075.

PROBLEMS

1. Why is PKU not treated by the complete elimination of phenylalanine from the diet?

2. How does the body produce tyrosine in patients with PKU?

3. Predict the blood levels of the compounds (listed at the top of the following chart) for a series of individuals, each of whom has a single dietary or enzyme deficiency (listed on the left). ($\uparrow$ = higher than normal; $\downarrow$ = lower than normal; N = normal)

Deficiency	Homocysteine	Methionine	Cystathionine
Dietary B_{12}			
Dietary folate			
Cystathionine synthase			
Cystathionase			
Methionine synthase (homocysteine $\rightarrow$ methionine)			

ANSWERS

1. Phenylalanine is an essential amino acid. Although it cannot be synthesized by the body, it is required for the synthesis of proteins. Therefore, at least a minimal amount must be present in the diet, even in the diet of patients with PKU.

2. Tyrosine can be synthesized in humans only from phenylalanine. When phenylalanine is restricted in the diet, tyrosine, in effect, becomes an essential amino acid. It must be supplied in the diet.

3.

Deficiency	Homocysteine	Methionine	Cystathionine
Dietary B_{12}	↑	↓	↑ (or N)
Dietary folate	↑	↓	↑ (or N)
Cystathionine synthase	↑	↑	↓
Cystathionase	↑	↑	↑ (or N)
Methionine synthase (homocysteine → methionine)	↑	↓	↑ (or N)

40 Tetrahydrofolate, Vitamin B$_{12}$, and S-Adenosylmethionine

Groups containing a single carbon atom can be transferred from one compound to another. This carbon atom may be in a number of different oxidation states. The most oxidized form, CO_2, is transferred by biotin. One-carbon groups at lower levels of oxidation than CO_2 are transferred by reactions involving tetrahydrofolate (FH_4), vitamin B_{12}, and S-adenosylmethionine (SAM).

Tetrahydrofolate, which is produced from the vitamin folate, obtains one-carbon units from serine, glycine, histidine, formaldehyde, and formate. While they are attached to FH_4, these one-carbon groups are oxidized and reduced. Once they are reduced to the methyl level, however, they cannot be re-oxidized. Collectively, these one-carbon groups attached to their carrier FH_4 are known as the one-carbon pool (Fig. 40.1).

The one-carbon groups carried by tetrahydrofolate are transferred to the pyrimidine base of deoxyuridine monophosphate (dUMP) to form deoxythymidine monophosphate (dTMP), to the amino acid glycine to form serine, to precursors of the purine bases to produce carbons C2 and C8 of the purine ring, and to vitamin B_{12}.

Vitamin B_{12} is involved in two reactions in the body. It participates in the rearrangement of the methyl group of methylmalonyl CoA to form succinyl CoA,

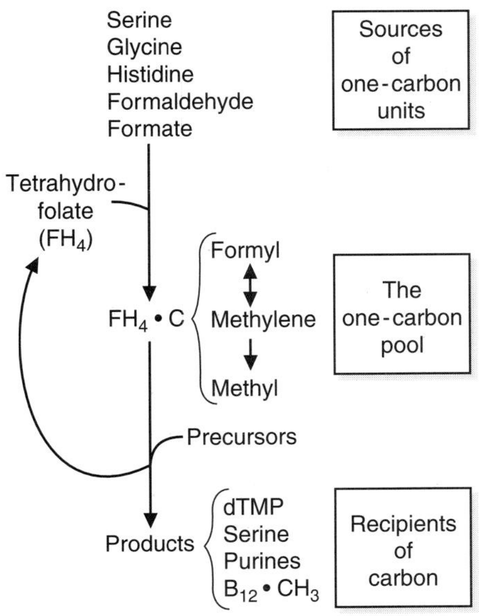

The recommended dietary allowance (RDA) for folate is approximately 200 μg in the adult male and in the nonpregnant, non-lactating adult female. A standard U.S. diet provides 50–500 μg of absorbable folate each day. If a folic acid deficiency is severe, supplements may be given in doses of 1–2 mg/day.

Virtually all foods contain significant amounts of folate, especially fresh green vegetables. In fact, the word "folate" is related to "foliage." Other good sources of this vitamin are liver, yeast, legumes, and some fruits. Protracted cooking of these foods, however, can destroy up to 90% of their folate content.

Folate deficiencies frequently occur, particularly in pregnant women and in alcoholics. Oral contraceptives and anticonvulsants interfere with folate absorption and metabolism. It is particularly important for women to have adequate levels of folate during the first few weeks of a pregnancy when the neural tube is developing in the fetus. Deficiencies can result in neural tube defects such as spina bifida.

Fig. 40.1. Overview of the one-carbon pool. FH$_4$•C indicates tetrahydrofolate (FH$_4$) containing a one-carbon unit that is at the formyl, methylene, or methyl level of oxidation (see Fig. 40.3).

Because of the possibility of a direct toxic effect of alcohol on hematopoietic tissues in **Jean Ann Tonich**, a bone marrow aspirate was performed. The aspirate contained a greater than normal number of red and white blood cell precursors, most of which were larger than normal (i.e., megaloblasts). Therefore, Jean Ann had a megaloblastic anemia, characteristic of a folate or B_{12} deficiency.

Jean Ann's serum folic acid level was 3.1 ng/mL (reference range = 6–15), and her serum B_{12} level was 154 pg/mL (reference range = 150–750). Her serum iron level was normal. It was clear, therefore, that Jean Ann's megaloblastic anemia was due to a folate deficiency (although her B_{12} levels were in the low range of normal). The management of a pure folate deficiency in an alcoholic patient includes cessation of alcohol intake and a diet rich in folate.

The abbreviation fL stands for *femtoliters*. One fL is 10^{-12} milliliters (mL).

Sulfa drugs, which are used to treat certain bacterial infections, are analogues of PABA. They prevent growth and cell division in bacteria by interfering with the synthesis of folate. Because we cannot synthesize folate, sulfa drugs do not affect human cells.

---

and it transfers a methyl group, obtained from tetrahydrofolate, to homocysteine, forming methionine. SAM, produced from methionine and ATP, transfers the methyl group to precursors that form compounds such as creatine, phosphatidylcholine, epinephrine, melatonin, and methylated nucleotides.

Following resection of the cancer in his large intestine and completion of a course of postoperative chemotherapy with 5-fluorouracil (5-FU), **Colin Tuma** returned to his gastroenterologist for routine follow-up colonoscopy. His colon was completely normal, with excellent healing at the site of the anastomosis. His physician expressed great optimism about a cure of Colin's previous malignancy but cautioned him about the need for regular colonoscopic examinations over the next few years.

Arlyn Foma's left ventricular function slowly improved after doxorubicin (adriamycin), an agent with known cardiotoxicity, was withdrawn from his multidrug chemotherapeutic regimen. Although the other drugs, including methotrexate, were continued, Arlyn's lymphoma continued its aggressive course.

The initial laboratory profile, determined when **Jean Ann Tonich** first presented to her physician with evidence of early alcoholic hepatitis, included a hematological analysis which showed that Jean Ann was anemic. Her hemoglobin was 11.0 g/dL (reference range = 12–16 for an adult female). The erythrocyte (red blood cell) count was 3.6 million cells/mm³ (reference range = 4.0–5.2 for an adult female). The average volume of her red blood cells (mean corpuscular volume, or MCV) was 108 fL (reference range = 80–100), and the hematology laboratory reported a striking variation in the size and shape of the red blood cells in a smear of her peripheral blood. The nuclei of the circulating granulocytic leukocytes had increased nuclear segmentation (polysegmented neutrophils). Because of these findings suggestive of a macrocytic anemia (in which blood cells are larger than normal), tests for serum folate and vitamin B_{12} (cobalamin) levels were ordered.

TETRAHYDROFOLATE (FH₄)

Tetrahydrofolate is produced in human cells by reduction of the vitamin folate (Fig. 40.2). Although FH_4 is related structurally to tetrahydrobiopterin (see Chapter 39), it differs functionally in that it is not involved in mixed-function oxidase reactions and it contains a vitamin. The vitamin folate is synthesized by bacteria and higher plants from the bicyclic pteridine ring, *p*-aminobenzoic acid (PABA), and glutamate. A number of additional glutamate residues can be joined to folate by amide linkages involving the carboxyl groups of the glutamate side chain.

Enzymes in the brush border of intestinal epithelial cells remove all but one of the glutamate residues from dietary folate before it is absorbed. Subsequently, folate is reduced, first to dihydrofolate and then to tetrahydrofolate (see Fig. 40.2). The enzyme catalyzing these reductions is dihydrofolate reductase, which uses NADPH as a cofactor. When tetrahydrofolate enters cells, 4 or 5 additional glutamate residues are added. The reduced polyglutamate derivative is the form that participates as a cofactor in biochemical reactions.

OXIDATION AND REDUCTION OF THE ONE-CARBON GROUPS OF TETRAHYDROFOLATE

One-carbon groups transferred by FH_4 are attached either to nitrogen N^5 or N^{10} or they form a bridge between N^5 and N^{10}. The collection of one-carbon groups attached to FH_4 is known as the one-carbon pool. While attached to FH_4, these one-carbon units are oxidized and reduced (Fig. 40.3). The most oxidized form, N^{10}-formyl-FH_4, releases H_2O to produce the N^5,N^{10}-methenyl (also called the methylidyne) derivative, without changing its oxidation state. Reduction of the methenyl derivative produces N^5,N^{10}-methylene-FH_4. A second reduction produces N^5-methyl-FH_4. This methyl derivative is not readily reoxidized. Further reduction to the methane level does not occur in humans. Bacteria, however, including those in the human intestinal tract, can produce methane gas (CH_4).

Sources of One-Carbon Groups Carried by FH_4

Carbon sources for the one-carbon pool include serine, glycine, formaldehyde, histidine, and formate (Fig. 40.4). Serine is the major carbon source. Its hydroxymethyl group is transferred to FH_4 by a reversible reaction that requires pyridoxal phosphate and produces N^5,N^{10}-methylene-FH_4 and glycine (Table 40.1). Because serine can be synthesized from glucose, dietary carbohydrate serves as a source of carbon for the one-carbon pool.

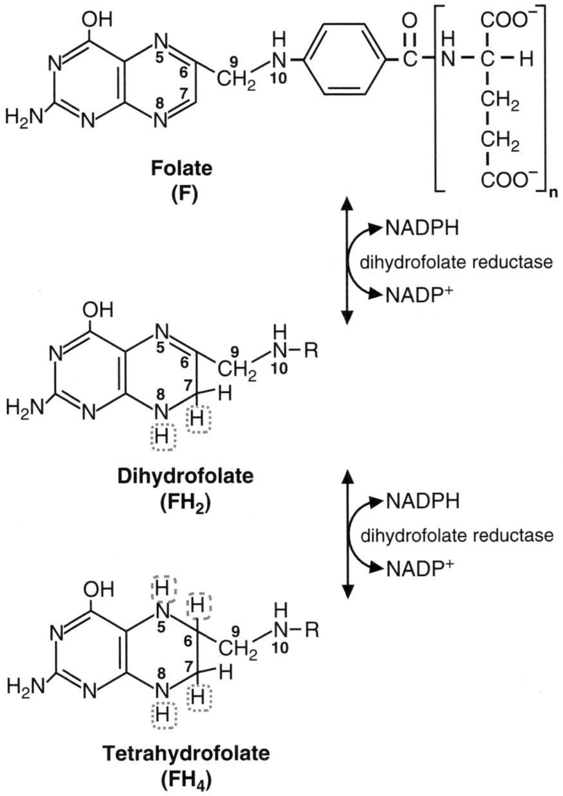

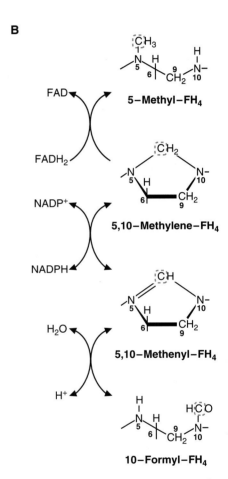

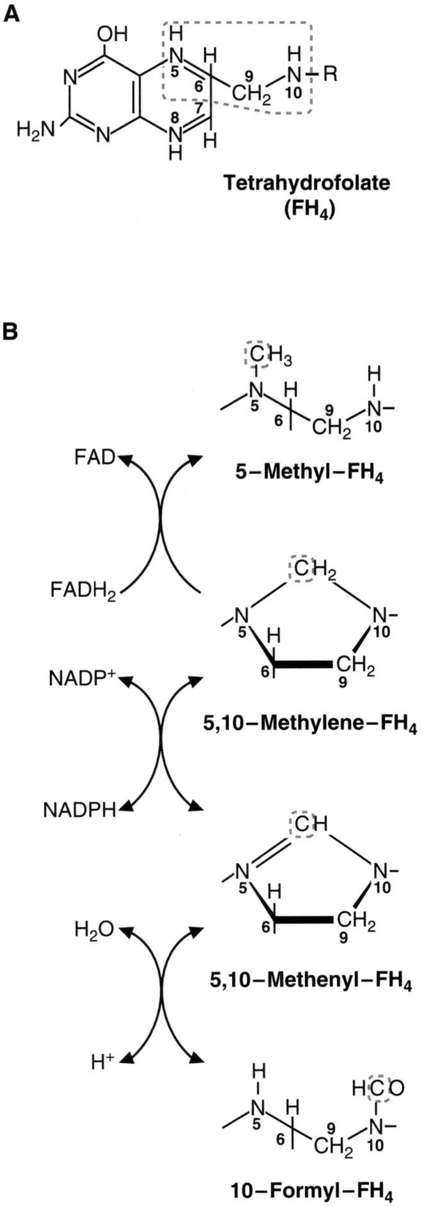

Fig. 40.3. One-carbon units attached to FH_4. **A.** The active form of FH_4. For definition of R, see Figure 40.2. **B.** Interconversions of one-carbon units of FH_4. Only the portion of FH_4 from N^5 to N^{10} is shown. After a formyl group forms a bridge between N^5 and N^{10}, two reductions can occur. Note that 5-methyl-FH_4 cannot be reoxidized.

Fig. 40.2. Reduction of folate to tetrahydrofolate (FH_4). The same enzyme, dihydrofolate reductase, catalyzes both reactions. Multiple glutamate residues are added within cells ($n \approx 5$). Plants can synthesize folate, but humans cannot. Therefore, folate is a dietary requirement. R is the portion of the folate molecule shown to the right of N^{10}.

Q 40.1: Because N^5-methyl-FH$_4$ is not readily reoxidized, it accumulates if the methyl group cannot be transferred to vitamin B$_{12}$. What effect would a B$_{12}$ deficiency have on folate metabolism?

Glycine reacts with FH$_4$ to produce NH$_4^+$, CO$_2$, and N^5,N^{10}-methylene-FH$_4$. NAD$^+$ serves as a cofactor for this reaction.

Formaldehyde, produced during the degradation of methyl groups of compounds such as choline or epinephrine, also reacts with FH$_4$ to form N^5,N^{10}-methylene-FH$_4$. Histidine, during its degradation, produces formiminoglutamate (FIGLU). FIGLU reacts with FH$_4$, forming glutamate and 5-formimino-FH$_4$, which releases NH$_4^+$ and generates N^5,N^{10}-methenyl-FH$_4$.

A deficiency of folate results in the accumulation of FIGLU, which is excreted in the urine. A histidine load test was formerly used for detecting folate deficiencies. Patients were given a test dose of histidine (a histidine load), and the amount of FIGLU that appeared in the urine was measured.

Table 40.1. One-Carbon Pool: Sources and Recipients of Carbon

Source[a]	Form of FH$_4$ Produced[b]	Recipient	Product
Formate →	N^{10}-Formyl	Purine precursor →	Purine (C2)
Histidine → (via formiminoglutamate)	N^5,N^{10}-Methenyl	Purine precursor →	Purine (C8)
Serine		dUMP →	dTMP
Glycine	N^5,N^{10}-Methylene	Glycine →	Serine
Formaldehyde			
Reduction of N^5,N^{10}-methylene-FH$_4$	N^5-Methyl	Vitamin B$_{12}$ →	Methyl-B$_{12}$

[a]The major source of carbon is serine.

[b]The carbon unit attached to FH$_4$ can be oxidized and reduced (see Fig. 40.3). At the methyl level, reoxidation does not occur.

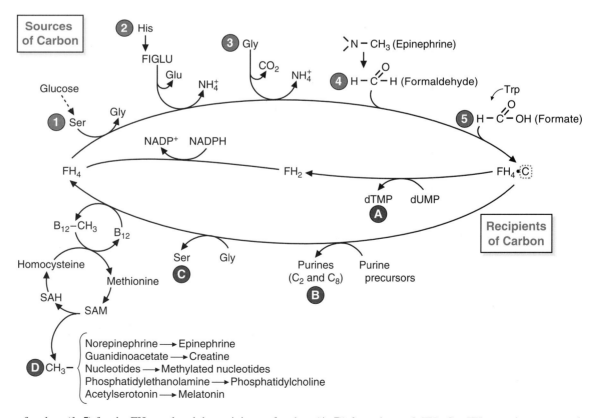

Fig. 40.4. Sources of carbon (**1–5**) for the FH$_4$ pool and the recipients of carbon (**A–D**) from the pool. FH$_4$•C = FH$_4$ carrying a one-carbon unit. The FH$_4$ derivatives involved in each reaction are listed in Table 40.1.

Formate also reacts with FH$_4$ to produce N^5,N^{10}-methenyl-FH$_4$. Formate is produced, for example, in the degradation of tryptophan (see Chapter 39). N^5-Methyl-FH$_4$ is produced by reduction of N^5,N^{10}-methylene-FH$_4$.

Recipients of One-Carbon Groups

The one-carbon groups on FH$_4$ may be oxidized or reduced and then transferred to other compounds (see Fig. 40.3 and Table 40.1). Transfers of this sort are involved in the synthesis of glycine from serine, the synthesis of the base thymine required for DNA synthesis, the purine bases required for both DNA and RNA synthesis, and the transfer of methyl groups to vitamin B$_{12}$ (see Fig. 40.4).

Because the conversion of serine to glycine is readily reversible, glycine can be converted to serine by drawing carbon from the one-carbon pool.

The base thymine is produced from uracil by a reaction in which dUMP is methylated to form dTMP (Fig. 40.5). The source of carbon is N^5,N^{10}-methylene-FH$_4$. Two hydrogen atoms from FH$_4$ are used to reduce the carbon to the methyl level. Consequently, FH$_2$ is produced. Reduction of FH$_2$ by NADPH in a reaction catalyzed by dihydrofolate reductase regenerates FH$_4$.

During the synthesis of the purine bases, carbon 2 and carbon 8 are obtained from the one-carbon pool (see Chapter 41). N^{10}-Formyl-FH$_4$ provides carbon 2, and N^5,N^{10}-methenyl-FH$_4$ provides carbon 8.

After the carbon group carried by FH$_4$ is reduced to the methyl level, it is transferred to vitamin B$_{12}$.

VITAMIN B$_{12}$

Structure of Vitamin B$_{12}$

The structure of vitamin B$_{12}$ (also known as cobalamin) is complex (Fig. 40.7). It contains a corrin ring, which is similar to the porphyrin ring found in heme. The corrin ring differs from heme, however, in that two of the four pyrrole rings are joined

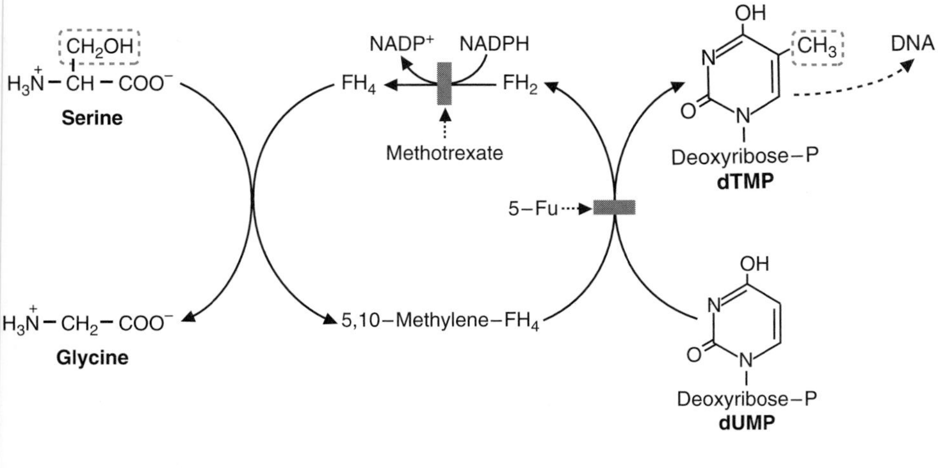

FH$_4$ is required for synthesis of thymine and the purine bases used to produce the precursors for DNA replication. Therefore, FH$_4$ is required for cell division. Blockage of the synthesis of thymine and the purine bases either by a dietary deficiency of folate or by drugs that interfere with folate metabolism results in a decreased rate of cell division and growth.

A better understanding of the structure and function of the purine and pyrimidine bases and of folate metabolism led to the development of compounds having antimetabolic and antifolate action useful for treatment of neoplastic disease. For example, **Colin Tuma** was successfully treated for colon cancer with 5-fluorouracil (5-FU) (see Chapter 17). 5-FU is a pyrimidine analogue, which is converted in cells to the nucleotide fluorodeoxyuridylate (FdUMP). FdUMP causes a "thymineless death," especially for tumor cells having a rapid turnover rate. It prevents the growth of cancer cells by blocking the thymidylate synthetase reaction, i.e., the conversion of dUMP to dTMP (see Fig. 40.5).

Fig. 40.5. Transfer of a one-carbon unit from serine to dUMP to form dTMP. FH$_4$ is oxidized to FH$_2$ (dihydrofolate) in this reaction. FH$_2$ is reduced to FH$_4$ by dihydrofolate reductase. Shaded bars indicate the steps at which the antimetabolites 5-FU and methotrexate act. 5-FU inhibits thymidylate synthetase. Methotrexate inhibits dihydrofolate reductase (see Fig. 40.6).

40.1: In a B$_{12}$ deficiency, most of the folate of the body is irreversibly "trapped" as its methyl derivative, and an adequate supply of free FH$_4$ is not available to carry out the reactions in which it normally participates. Thus, a B$_{12}$ deficiency can precipitate a folate deficiency via a mechanism known as the "methyl trap theory."

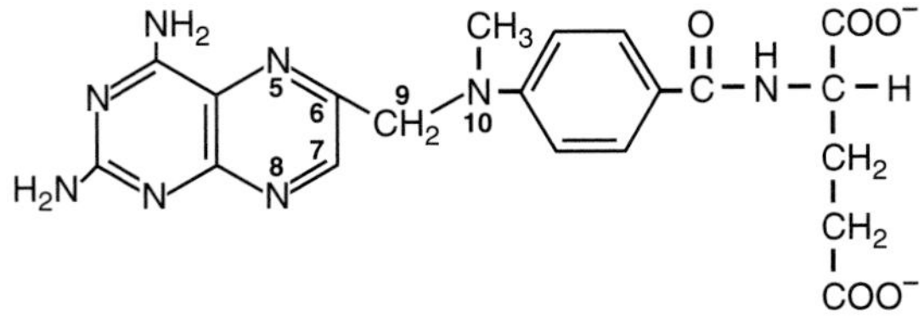

Methotrexate

Fig. 40.6. The structure of methotrexate.

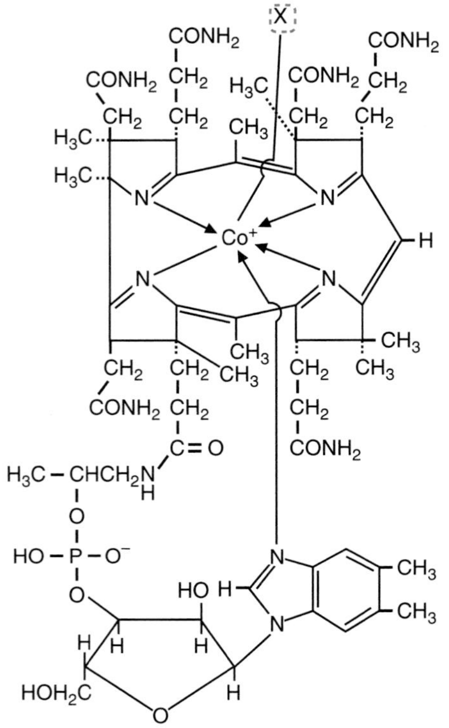

Fig. 40.7. Vitamin B_{12}. X = deoxyadenosine in deoxyadenosylcobalamin; X = CH_3 in methylcobalamin; X = CN in cyanocobalamin (the commercial form found in vitamin tablets).

40.2: **Arlyn Foma** received multidrug chemotherapy for treatment of non-Hodgkin's lymphoma. One of the drugs that he received was methotrexate (see Chapter 15). The structure of methotrexate is shown in Figure 40.6. What compound does methotrexate resemble?

Jean Ann Tonich's megaloblastic anemia was treated, in part, with folate supplements (see Clinical Comments). Within 48 hours of the initiation of folate therapy, megaloblastic erythropoiesis usually subsides and effective erythropoiesis begins.

A megaloblastic anemia is caused by a decrease in the synthesis of thymine and the purine bases. These deficiencies lead to an inability of hematopoietic (and other) cells to synthesize DNA and, therefore, to divide. Their persistently thwarted attempts at normal DNA replication, DNA repair, and cell division produce abnormally large cells (called megaloblasts) with abundant cytoplasm capable of RNA and protein synthesis, but with clumping and fragmentation of nuclear chromatin.

The average daily diet in Western countries contains 5–30 μg of vitamin B_{12}, of which 1–5 μg is absorbed into the blood. (The RDA is about 2 μg/day.) Total body content of this vitamin in an adult is approximately 2–5 mg, of which 1 mg is present in the liver. As a result, a dietary deficiency of B_{12} is uncommon.

In spite of **Jean Ann Tonich's** relatively malnourished state because of chronic alcoholism, her serum cobalamin level was still within the low-normal range. If her undernourished state had continued, a cobalamin deficiency would eventually have developed.

Pernicious anemia, a deficiency of intrinsic factor, is a relatively common problem caused by malabsorption of dietary cobalamin. It may result from an inherited defect that leads to a decreased ability of gastric parietal cells to synthesize intrinsic factor or from partial resection of the stomach or of the ileum. Production of intrinsic factor often declines with age and is low in elderly individuals.

directly rather than by a methylene bridge. Its most unusual feature is the presence of cobalt, coordinated with the corrin ring (similar to the iron coordinated with the porphyrin ring). This cobalt can form a bond with a carbon atom. In the body, it reacts with the carbon of a methyl group, forming methylcobalamin, or with the 5′-carbon of deoxyadenosine, forming 5′-deoxyadenosylcobalamin.

Although vitamin B_{12} is produced by bacteria, it cannot be synthesized by higher plants or animals. Humans obtain small amounts of vitamin B_{12} from their intestinal flora. However, the major source of vitamin B_{12} is dietary meat, eggs, dairy products, fish, poultry, and seafood. The animals that serve as the source of these foods obtain B_{12} mainly from the bacteria in their food supply.

Intrinsic factor, a glycoprotein produced by gastric parietal cells, is required for B_{12} absorption (Fig. 40.8). It complexes with B_{12} (the extrinsic factor) and facilitates the absorption of the vitamin by cells of the ileum, the distal segment of the small intestine. After absorption, the vitamin is stored in the liver in amounts such that 3–6 years are required for deficiency symptoms to develop after a shift from an adequate diet to one that contains little or no B_{12}.

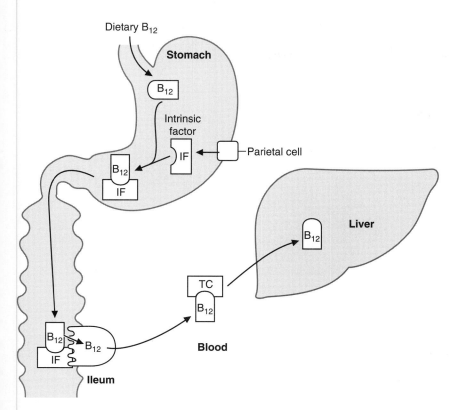

Fig. 40.8. Absorption, transport, and storage of vitamin B_{12}. Dietary B_{12} binds to intrinsic factor (IF), a glycoprotein secreted by gastric parietal cells. B_{12} is absorbed in the ileum and carried by blood proteins called transcobalamins (TC) to the liver, where B_{12} is stored.

Functions of Vitamin B_{12}

Vitamin B_{12} is involved in two reactions in the body: the transfer of a methyl group from FH_4 to homocysteine to form methionine and the rearrangement of the methyl group of methylmalonyl CoA to form succinyl CoA (Fig. 40.9).

Tetrahydrofolate receives a one-carbon group from serine or from other sources. This carbon is reduced to the methyl level. It is then transferred to vitamin B_{12}, forming methyl-B_{12} (or methylcobalamin). Vitamin B_{12} transfers the methyl group to homocysteine, which is converted to methionine. The methyl group of methionine is transferred to other compounds via SAM (Fig. 40.10).

Vitamin B_{12} also participates in the conversion of methylmalonyl CoA to succinyl CoA. In this case, the active form of the coenzyme is 5′-adenosylcobalamin. This reaction is part of the metabolic route for the conversion of carbons from valine, isoleucine, threonine, thymine, and the last 3 carbons of odd chain fatty acids, all of which form propionyl CoA, to the TCA cycle intermediate succinyl CoA (see Chapter 39).

S-Adenosylmethionine

S-Adenosylmethionine (SAM) participates in the synthesis of many compounds that contain methyl groups. SAM is required for the conversion of phosphatidylethanolamine to phosphatidylcholine, guanidinoacetate to creatine, norepinephrine to epinephrine, acetylserotonin to serotonin, and nucleotides to methylated

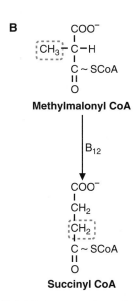

Fig. 40.9. The two reactions of vitamin B_{12} in humans.

A 40.2: Methotrexate has the same structure as folate except that it has an amino group on C4 and a methyl group on N10. Anticancer drugs such as methotrexate are folate analogues that act by inhibiting dihydrofolate reductase, preventing the conversion of FH_2 to FH_4 (see Fig. 40.5). Thus, the cellular pools of FH_4 are not replenished, and reactions requiring FH_4 cannot proceed.

40.3: How should vitamin B_{12} be administered to a patient with pernicious anemia?

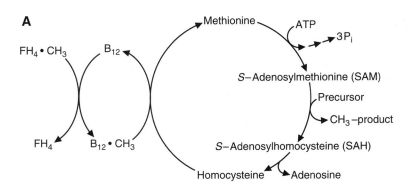

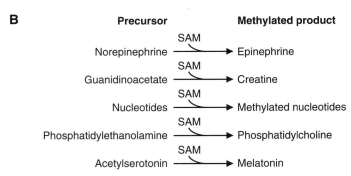

Fig. 40.10. Relationship between FH_4, B_{12}, and SAM. **A.** Overall scheme. **B.** Some specific reactions requiring SAM.

There are two major clinical manifestations of cobalamin (B_{12}) deficiency, hematopoietic (caused by the adverse effects of a B_{12} deficiency on folate metabolism) and neurological (caused by an inability to convert methylmalonyl CoA to succinyl CoA).

The hemopoietic problems caused by a B_{12} deficiency are identical to those observed in a folate deficiency, and, in fact, result from a folate deficiency secondary to (i.e., caused by) the B_{12} deficiency. In patients with a cobalamin deficiency, N^5-methyltetrahydrofolate cannot be converted to free FH_4 (see Fig. 40.9). Essentially all of the folate becomes "trapped" as the N^5-methyl derivative. As the FH_4 pool is exhausted, deficiencies of the tetrahydrofolate derivatives needed for purine and dTMP biosynthesis develop, leading to the characteristic megaloblastic anemia.

nucleotides (see Fig. 40.10). It is also required for the inactivation of catecholamines and serotonin (see Fig. 41.24).

SAM is synthesized from methionine and ATP. After transfer of its methyl group, SAM forms S-adenosylhomocysteine, which is cleaved to form homocysteine and adenosine.

Methionine, required for the synthesis of SAM, is obtained from the diet, or produced from homocysteine, which accepts a methyl group from vitamin B_{12} (see Fig. 40.10). Thus, the methyl group of methionine is regenerated. The portion of methionine that is essential in the diet is the homocysteine moiety. If we had an adequate dietary source of homocysteine, methionine would not be required in the diet. However, there is no good dietary source of homocysteine.

Homocysteine provides the sulfur atom for the synthesis of cysteine (see Figs. 39.6 and 39.13). In this case, homocysteine reacts with serine to form cystathionine, which is cleaved, yielding cysteine and α-ketobutyrate. The first reaction in this sequence is inhibited by cysteine. Thus, methionine, via homocysteine, is not utilized for cysteine synthesis unless the levels of cysteine in the body are lower than required for its metabolic functions. An adequate dietary supply of cysteine, therefore, can "spare" (or reduce) the dietary requirement for methionine.

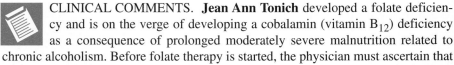

CLINICAL COMMENTS. Jean Ann Tonich developed a folate deficiency and is on the verge of developing a cobalamin (vitamin B_{12}) deficiency as a consequence of prolonged moderately severe malnutrition related to chronic alcoholism. Before folate therapy is started, the physician must ascertain that the megaloblastic anemia is not due to a pure B_{12} deficiency or a combined deficiency of folate and B_{12}.

If folate is given without cobalamin to a B$_{12}$-deficient patient, the drug only partially corrects the megaloblastic anemia because it will "bypass" the methyl-folate trap and provide adequate FH$_4$ coenzyme for the conversion of dUMP to dTMP and for a resurgence of purine synthesis. As a result, normal DNA synthesis, DNA repair, and cell division occur. However, the neurological syndrome, resulting from inhibition of methylmalonyl CoA mutase, may progress unless the physician realizes that B$_{12}$ supplementation is required. Jean Ann's case, in which the serum B$_{12}$ concentration was borderline low and in which the dietary history supported the possibility of a B$_{12}$ deficiency, requires a combination of folate and B$_{12}$ supplements to avoid this potential therapeutic trap.

Colin Tuma continued to do well and faithfully returned for his regular colonoscopic examinations. **Arlyn Foma's** course was not as positive. In spite of aggressive chemotherapy, his condition deteriorated. Interferon therapy was eventually tried, but, nevertheless, Mr. Foma succumbed to the progressive invasion of his tissues by colonies of cancer cells.

BIOCHEMICAL COMMENTS. Folate deficiencies result in decreased availability of the thymine and purine nucleotides that serve as precursors for DNA synthesis. The decreased concentrations of these precursors affect not only the DNA synthesis that occurs during replication prior to cell division, but also the DNA synthesis that occurs as a step in the processes that repair damaged DNA.

Decreased methylation of deoxyuridine monophosphate (dUMP) to form deoxythymidine monophosphate (dTMP), a reaction which requires $N^{5,10}$-methylene tetrahydrofolate as a coenzyme (see Fig. 40.5), leads to an increase in the intracellular dUTP/dTTP ratio. This change causes a significant increase in the incorporation of uracil into DNA. Although much of this uracil can be removed by DNA repair enzymes, the lack of available dTTP blocks the step of DNA repair catalyzed by DNA polymerase. The result is fragmentation of DNA as well as blockade of normal DNA replication.

These abnormal nuclear processes are responsible for the clumping and polysegmentation seen in the nuclei of leukocytes in the bone marrow and in the peripheral blood of patients with a megaloblastic anemia caused either by a primary folate deficiency or one that is secondary to a B$_{12}$ deficiency. The abnormalities in DNA synthesis and repair lead to an irreversible loss of the capacity for cell division and eventually to cell death.

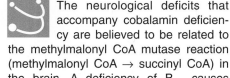

The neurological deficits that accompany cobalamin deficiency are believed to be related to the methylmalonyl CoA mutase reaction (methylmalonyl CoA → succinyl CoA) in the brain. A deficiency of B$_{12}$ causes methylmalonyl CoA to accumulate. Methylmalonic acid (methylmalonate) is produced and excreted in the urine.

Two mechanisms have been proposed for the pathogenesis of the neurological sequelae of cobalamin deficiency. When methylmalonyl CoA accumulates, (*a*) it may act as a competitive inhibitor of malonyl CoA in fatty acid synthesis (see Chapter 33) or (*b*) it may act as a substitute for malonyl CoA in the formation of fatty acids. The sphingolipids of the myelin sheaths turnover rapidly. Severe inhibition of fatty acid synthesis or incorporation of methylmalonyl CoA will eventually result in myelin degeneration with its subsequent adverse effects on neural function.

The classical clinical presentation of the neurological effects of a B$_{12}$ deficiency includes symmetric numbness and tingling of the hands and feet, diminishing vibratory and position sense, and progression to a spastic gait disturbance. The patient may become somnolent or may become extremely irritable ("megaloblastic madness"). Eventually, blind spots in the central portions of the visual fields develop accompanied by alterations in gustatory (taste) and olfactory (smell) function.

Suggested Readings

Allen RH. Megaloblastic anemias. In: Wyngaarden J, Smith L Jr, Bennett J, eds. Cecil textbook of medicine. Philadelphia: WB Saunders, 1992:846–854.

Linder MC, ed. Nutrition and metabolism of vitamins. In: Nutritional biochemistry and metabolism with clinical applications. New York: Elsevier, 1991:137–143.

PROBLEMS

1. What reactions or processes would be affected by a dietary deficiency of methionine?

2. Pregnant women frequently suffer from folate deficiencies. What reactions of folate are particularly important for the fetus?

3. What advice about folate and B$_{12}$ intake should a physician give to a patient who is a vegan (an individual who eats only vegetables)?

A 40.3: Because the problem in pernicious anemia is a lack of intrinsic factor which results in an inability to absorb vitamin B$_{12}$ from the gastrointestinal tract, B$_{12}$ cannot be administered orally to treat this condition. Therefore, it is usually given by injection.

4. A patient with a megaloblastic anemia has a serum methylmalonic acid level of 150 nM (reference range = 70–270) and a homocyst(e)ine level (homocysteine plus homocystine) of 200 µM (reference range = 5–16). Could this patient have a cobalamin or a folate deficiency?

ANSWERS

1. Methionine, an essential amino acid, is necessary for the formation of *S*-adenosylmethionine. SAM provides methyl groups for the synthesis of epinephrine from norepinephrine, of phosphatidylcholine from phosphatidylethanolamine, of creatine from guanidinoacetate, of methylated nucleotides from nucleotides, and of melatonin from serotonin. Methionine, of course, is also required for the synthesis of proteins. In fact, this amino acid is not only found within protein chains, but it is also the amino acid used for the initiation of protein synthesis on ribosomes (see Chapter 14).

2. Folate is required for growth and division of cells. It is required for the formation of thymine (dUMP to dTMP), which is used for DNA synthesis, and for the synthesis of purines, which are necessary for both DNA and RNA synthesis, and, therefore, for protein synthesis. FH_4 also transfers methyl groups to B_{12}, which, in turn, passes them to homocysteine to form methionine. Methionine, as SAM, provides methyl groups for many reactions required for normal bodily function.

3. Folate is plentiful in vegetables, and vegans should not have deficiencies of this vitamin. B_{12}, on the other hand, is synthesized by microorganisms, but not by higher plants. We obtain small amounts of B_{12} from the bacteria in our gut, but our major source is food prepared from the tissues of other animals, particularly liver where the vitamin is stored. Strict vegans eat only plants, and, therefore, do not obtain vitamin B_{12} from their diet. They may need to consider taking B_{12} supplements, particularly if they are women of childbearing age.

4. Measurement of serum homocyst(e)ine and methylmalonic acid is used to distinguish between folate and cobalamin deficiencies. This patient could have a folate deficiency. Homocysteine would be elevated in the blood because it could not be converted to methionine. A cobalamin deficiency would also result in elevated homocysteine, but, in this case, methylmalonic acid would be elevated as well because of decreased conversion of methylmalonyl CoA to succinyl CoA.

Folate therapy should restore the patient's homocyst(e)ine levels to normal within 5 to 10 days.

41   Special Products Derived from Amino Acids

All of the nitrogen-containing compounds synthesized in the body are derived from amino acids. In this chapter, we consider the synthesis and degradation of the most medically important of these compounds.

Glycine contributes both carbons and nitrogen for the synthesis of creatine, heme, and the purine bases. Creatine is synthesized from glycine, arginine, and S-adenosylmethionine (SAM). It reacts with ATP to form creatine phosphate, which stores and transports high energy phosphate within cells. Creatine phosphate spontaneously cyclizes to form creatinine, a nitrogenous waste product that is excreted in the urine. Serum creatinine is used as an indicator of the glomerular filtration rate of the kidney and urinary creatinine as a gauge in assessing the quantity of other compounds excreted in the urine.

Glycine reacts with a number of compounds, forming conjugates that are more readily excreted into the urine by virtue of their increased water solubility. Glycine forms glycoconjugates (e.g., glycocholate) with bile salts, as well as with other metabolites and drugs, such as benzoate and salicylate.

Heme is produced by a pathway initiated by the condensation of glycine and succinyl CoA to form δ-aminolevulinic acid (δ-ALA). Pyrroles, derived from δ-ALA, condense to form the porphyrin ring that complexes with iron (Fe^{2+}) to generate heme. Heme is found in the cytochromes, myoglobin, and hemoglobin. Iron, which serves as a component of heme and of certain metalloenzymes, is absorbed from the digestive tract, transported in the blood in transferrin, and stored in cells in ferritin.

Heme is degraded to form bilirubin, which is excreted by the liver into the bile as the diglucuronide (conjugated bilirubin) and converted by intestinal bacteria to other bile pigments, which are excreted in the feces. Jaundice, the result of the accumulation of bilirubin in tissues, is caused by excessive production of bilirubin (e.g., in hemolytic anemias), failure of the liver to conjugate bilirubin (e.g., in hepatitis), or interference with bilirubin excretion (e.g., in blockage of the bile ducts by a pancreatic cancer).

In purine biosynthesis, the entire glycine molecule is incorporated into the ring. Other nitrogens are provided by glutamine and aspartate, and the remaining carbons are derived from CO_2 and the tetrahydrofolate pool. Purines are degraded to uric acid, which is not very soluble. It can precipitate in the joints, causing gout.

The pyrimidine ring is formed from aspartate and carbamoyl phosphate. Degradation of the pyrimidines produces innocuous compounds such as urea, CO_2, and H_2O (Fig. 41.5).

A number of amino acids undergo decarboxylation reactions to produce amines that serve as neurotransmitters and/or hormones, such as γ-aminobutyric acid (GABA, an inhibitory neurotransmitter), histamine, serotonin, dopamine, norepinephrine, and epinephrine. (Other aspects of the metabolism of amino acids that produce neurotransmitters and hormones are described in Chapter 42 and in Section VIII.)

Putrescine is produced by decarboxylation of ornithine, a process associated with cell division. Decarboxylations of amino acids are also involved in the synthesis of sphingolipids and heme.

Compounds with a variety of functions are formed from the aromatic amino acids. Tryptophan, in addition to producing serotonin, forms melatonin and the nicotinamide moiety of NAD and NADP. Tyrosine forms the thyroid hormones triiodothyronine (T₃) and thyroxine (T₄), and the melanin pigments, as well as the catecholamines (dopamine, norepinephrine, and epinephrine).

Arginine produces nitric oxide (NO), which has neurotransmitter or paracrine actions that stimulate relaxation of smooth muscle cells, causing vasodilation and reduction of blood pressure. Macrophages release NO, which has cytotoxic effects on parasites and tumor cells.

Rena Felya, a 9-year-old girl, complained of a severe pain in her throat and difficulty in swallowing. She had chills, sweats, headache, and a fever of 102.4°F. When her symptoms persisted for several days, her mother took her to the pediatrician, who found diffuse erythema (redness) in her posterior pharynx (throat) with yellow exudates (patches) on her tonsils. Large, tender lymph nodes were present under her jaw on both sides of her neck. A throat culture was taken and therapy with penicillin was begun.

Although the sore throat and fever improved, 8 days after the onset of the original infection, Rena's eyes and legs became swollen, and her urine suddenly turned the color of "Coca-Cola." Her blood pressure was elevated. Protein and red blood cells were found in her urine. Her serum creatinine level was elevated at 1.8 mg/dL (reference range = 0.3–0.7 for a child). Because the throat culture grew out group A β-hemolytic streptococci, the doctor ordered a Streptozyme test. This test was positive for antibodies to streptolysin O and several other streptococcal antigens. As a result, a diagnosis of acute poststreptococcal glomerulonephritis was made. Supportive therapy, including bed rest and treatment for hypertension, was initiated.

Michael Sichel had not had a sickle cell crisis for 4 months when he experienced a severe steady ache in his right upper abdomen radiating to this right shoulder and scapular (shoulder blade) region. When he developed nausea and vomited a green bilious material, he realized that his current symptoms might be due to the presence of gallstones (cholelithiasis) discovered on x-ray f few years earlier. The physician in the sickle cell crisis center noted significant local tenderness to pressure over the right upper quadrant of Michael's abdomen. His bowel sounds were diminished and his sclerae (the whites of his eyes) were yellow. A urine specimen was the color of weak iced tea and Micheal's stool appeared lighter than normal in color. An ultrasound (sonogram) study of the abdomen revealed several gallstones within the lumen of the gallbaldder and another partially obstructing stone within the distal common bile duct. His serum bilirubin level was 6.7 mg/dL (reference range = 0.3–1.0) and the direct (or conjugated) bilirubin level was 5.0 mg/dL (reference range = 0.1–0.3). Michael's serum transaminase (ALT and AST) levels were only slightly elevated, whereas his serum alkaline phosphatase level was significantly increased at 465 units/L (reference range = 30–120). Serum levels of amylase and lipase (pancreatic enzymes) were normal. A diagnosis of extrahepatic obstructive jauntice caused by a common duct stone was made.

The initial acute inflammatory process which caused **Yves Topaigne** to experience a painful attack of gouty arthritis responded quickly to colchicine therapy (see Chapter 10). Several weeks after the inflammatory signs and symptoms in his right great toe subsided, Yves was placed on allopurinol. His serum uric acid level gradually fell from a pretreatment level of 9.2 mg/dL into the normal range (2.5–8.0 mg/dL). He remained free of gouty symptoms when he returned to his physician for a follow-up office visit.

Katie Colamin, a 34-year-old dress designer, developed alarming palpitations of her heart while bending forward to pick up her cat. She also developed a pounding headache and sweated profusely. After 5–10 minutes, these symptoms subsided. One week later, her aerobic exercise instructor, a registered nurse, noted that Katie grew very pale and was tremulous. The instructor took Katie's blood pressure, which was 220 mm Hg systolic (normal, up to 140 at rest) and diastolic 132 mm Hg (normal up to 90 at rest). Within 15 minutes, Katie recovered and her blood pressure returned to normal. The instructor told Katie to see her physician the next day.

The doctor told Katie that her symptom complex coupled with severe hypertension strongly suggested the presence of a tumor in the medulla of one of her adrenal glands (a pheochromocytoma) that was episodically secreting large amounts of catecholamines, such as norepinephrine (noradrenaline) and epinephrine (adrenaline). Her blood pressure was normal until moderate pressure to the left of her umbilicus caused Katie to suddenly develop a typical attack and her blood pressure rose rapidly. She was immediately scheduled for a magnetic resonance imaging (MRI) study of her adrenal glands. The MRI showed a 3.5 × 2.8 × 2.6 cm mass in the left adrenal gland, typical of a pheochromocytoma.

Each kidney normally contains approximately one million glomerular units. Each unit is supplied by arterial blood via the renal arteries and acts as a "filter." Metabolites such as creatinine leave the blood by passing through pores or channels in the glomerular capillaries and enter the fluid within the proximal kidney tubule for eventual excretion in the urine. When functionally intact, these glomerular tissues are impermeable to all but the smallest of proteins. When acutely inflamed, however, this barrier function is lost and albumin and other proteins may appear in the urine.

The marked inflammatory changes in the glomerular capillaries that accompany poststreptococcal glomerulonephritis significantly reduce the flow of blood to the filtering surfaces of these vessels. As a result, creatinine, urea, and other circulating metabolites which are filtered into the urine at a normal rate (the glomerular filtration rate or GFR) in the absence of kidney disease now fail to reach the filters, and, therefore, they accumulate in the plasma.

These changes explain **Rena Felya's** laboratory profile during her acute inflammatory glomerular disease.

CREATINE

Creatine synthesis begins in the kidney and is completed in the liver. In the first step of creatine synthesis, which occurs in the kidney, glycine combines with arginine to form guanidinoacetate. In this reaction, the guanidinium group of arginine (the group that also forms urea), is transferred to glycine, and the remainder of the arginine molecule is released as ornithine. Guanidinoacetate is then methylated in the liver by S-adenosylmethionine (SAM) to form creatine (Fig. 41.1).

Creatine travels through the bloodstream to other tissues, particularly muscle and brain, where it reacts with ATP to form the high energy compound creatine phosphate. This reaction, catalyzed by creatine phosphokinase (CK, also abbreviated as CPK), is reversible. Therefore, cells can use creatine phosphate to regenerate ATP.

Creatine phosphate, which serves as a small reservoir of high energy phosphate that can readily regenerate ATP from ADP, plays a particularly important role in muscle during exercise. It also carries high energy phosphate from mitochondria, where ATP is synthesized, to myosin filaments, where ATP is used for muscle contraction.

Creatine phosphate is an unstable compound. It spontaneously cyclizes, forming creatinine (see Fig. 41.1). Creatinine cannot be further metabolized. It is excreted in the urine. Particularly for individuals on a limited diet, the excretion of creatinine represents a significant loss of compounds that provide the methyl groups transferred by SAM.

The amount of creatinine excreted each day is constant and depends on body muscle mass. Therefore, it can be used as a gauge for determining the amounts of other compounds excreted in the urine. The volume of urine varies considerably with time and water intake. At any given moment, the concentration of a compound in a spec-

Muscle and brain cells contain large amounts of creatine phosphokinase (CK), and damage to these cells causes the enzyme to leak into the blood. Serum CK is measured to diagnose and evaluate patients who have had strokes and heart attacks. The presence of 5% or more of the CK in the blood as the MB isoform is indicative of a heart attack (see Chapters 8 and 9).

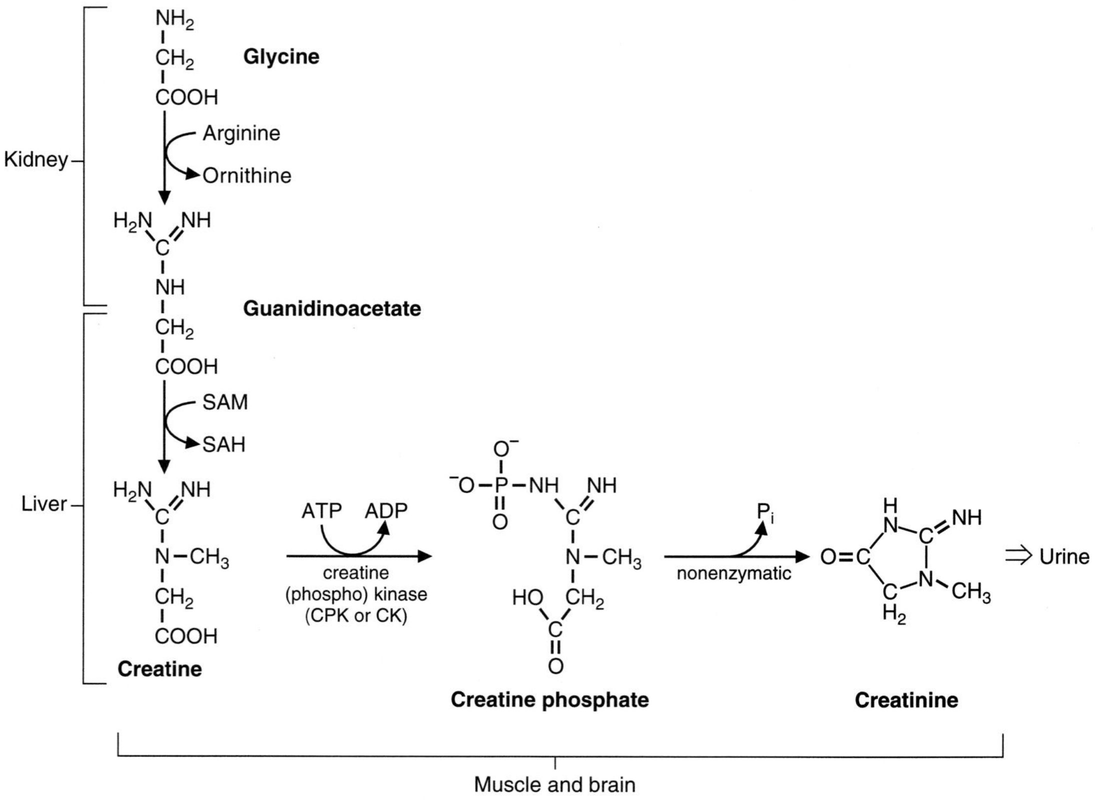

Fig. 41.1. Creatine metabolism. SAM = *S*-adenosylmethionine; SAH = *S*-adenosylhomocysteine.

In the liver, the food component and additive benzoate forms a conjugate with glycine known as hippuric acid (*N*-benzoylglycine). The ability of the liver to form hippuric acid formerly was used to evaluate liver function. Current tests measure specific enzymes such as AST that leak into the blood from damaged liver cells. The predominant urinary excretion product of aspirin is also a glycine conjugate, salicylglycine (also called salicylurate). Conjugation reactions of this type, in addition to the P450 system (see Chapter 21), serve as a means of ridding the body of foreign compounds.

Heme, which is red, is responsible for the color of red blood cells and of muscles that contain a large number of mitochondria.

Chlorophyll, the major porphyrin in plants, is similar to heme, except that it is coordinated with magnesium rather than iron, and it contains different substituents on the rings, including a long chain alcohol (phytol). As a result of these structural differences, chlorophyll is green.

imen of urine does not give a good indication of the total amount that is being excreted on a daily basis. However, if the concentration of the compound is divided by the concentration of creatinine, the result provides a better indication of the true excretion rate.

CONJUGATES FORMED BY GLYCINE

Glycine forms conjugates with a number of compounds. In Chapter 34, the reactions that produce conjugates of glycine and bile salts were described. These conjugated bile salts have a lower p*K* than the unconjugated bile salts, and therefore serve as better detergents in the process of lipid digestion in the intestinal lumen. Many lipid-soluble drugs also react with glycine to form more water-soluble derivatives.

HEME

Structure

Heme consists of a porphyrin ring coordinated with an atom of iron (Fig. 41.2). Four pyrrole rings are joined by methenyl bridges (—CH—) to form the porphyrin ring. Eight side chains serve as substituents on the porphyrin ring, two on each pyrrole. These side chains may be acetyl (A), propionyl (P), methyl (M), or vinyl (V) groups. In heme, the order of these groups (numbered 1 through 6) is M V M V M P P M. This order, in which the position of the methyl group is reversed on the fourth ring, is characteristic of the porphyrins of the type III series, the most abundant in nature.

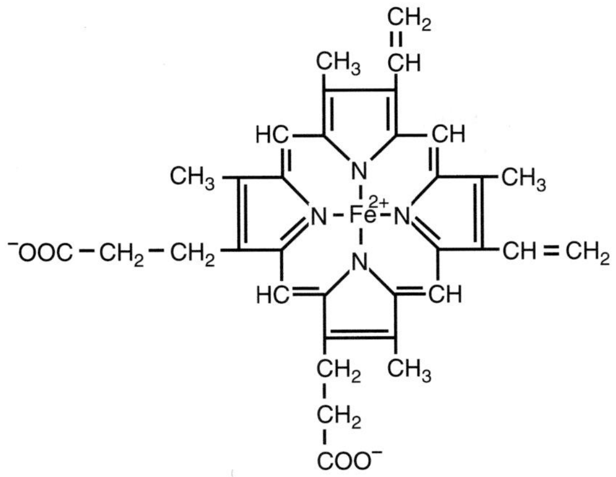

Fig. 41.2. Structure of heme. The side chains are MVMVMPPM. M = methyl (CH_3); V = vinyl (—CH=CH_2); P = propionyl (—CH_2—CH_2—COO^-).

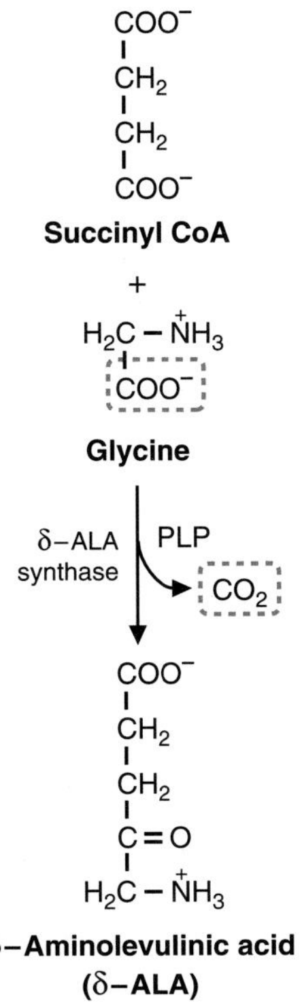

Heme is the most common porphyrin found in the body. It is complexed with proteins to form hemoglobin, myoglobin, and the cytochromes (see Chapters 9 and 20), including cytochrome P450 (see Chapter 21).

Synthesis of Heme

Heme is synthesized from glycine and succinyl CoA (Fig. 41.3), which condense in the initial reaction to form δ-aminolevulinic acid (δ-ALA). The enzyme that catalyzes this reaction, δ-ALA synthase, requires pyridoxal phosphate. In this reaction, glycine is decarboxylated.

In the second reaction of heme synthesis catalyzed by δ-ALA dehydratase, 2 molecules of δ-ALA condense to form the pyrrole porphobilinogen (Fig. 41.4). Four of these pyrrole rings condense to form a linear chain and then a series of porphyrinogens. The side chains of these porphyrinogens initially contain acetyl (A) and propionyl (P) groups. The acetyl groups are decarboxylated to form methyl groups. Then the first two propionyl side chains are decarboxylated and oxidized to vinyl groups, forming a protoporphyrinogen. The methylene bridges are subsequently oxidized to form protoporphyrin IX (see Fig. 41.5).

In the final step of the pathway, iron (as Fe^{2+}) is incorporated into protoporphyrin IX in a reaction catalyzed by ferrochelatase (also known as heme synthase).

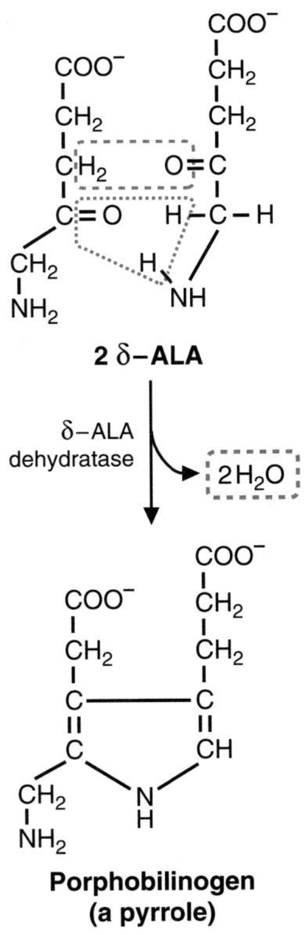

Source of Iron

Iron, which is obtained from the diet, has a Recommended Dietary Allowance (RDA) of 10 mg for adult males and postmenopausal females, and 15 mg for premenopausal females. The average American diet contains 10–50 mg of iron. However, only 10–15% is absorbed, and iron deficiencies are fairly common. The iron in meats is in the form of heme, which is readily absorbed. The non-heme iron in plants is not as readily absorbed, in part because plants often contain oxalates, phytates, tannins, and other phenolic compounds that chelate or form insoluble precipitates with iron, preventing its absorption. On the other hand, vitamin C (ascorbic acid) increases the uptake of non-heme iron from the digestive tract. The uptake of iron is also increased in times of need by mechanisms that are not yet understood. Iron is absorbed in the ferrous (Fe^{2+}) state (Fig. 41.6).

Fig. 41.3. Synthesis of δ-aminolevulinic acid (δ-ALA). PLP = pyridoxal phosphate.

Fig. 41.4. Two molecules of δ-ALA condense to form porphobilinogen.

41.1: Pyridoxine (vitamin B_6) deficiencies are often associated with a microcytic, hypochromic anemia. Why would a B_6 deficiency result in small (microcytic), pale (hypochromic) red blood cells?

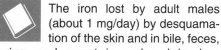

ALA dehydratase, which contains zinc, and ferrochelatase are inactivated by lead. Thus, in lead poisoning, γ-ALA and protoporphyrin IX accumulate, and the production of heme is decreased. Anemia results from a lack of hemoglobin, and energy production decreases due to lack of cytochromes for the electron transport chain.

Porphyrias are a group of rare inherited disorders resulting from deficiencies of enzymes in the pathway for heme biosynthesis (see Fig. 41.5). Intermediates of the pathway accumulate and may have toxic effects on the nervous system that cause neuropsychiatric symptoms. When porphyrinogens accumulate, they may be converted by light to porphyrins, which react with molecular oxygen to form oxygen radicals. These radicals may cause severe damage to the skin. Thus, individuals with excessive production of porphyrins are photosensitive.

The iron lost by adult males (about 1 mg/day) by desquamation of the skin and in bile, feces, urine, and sweat is replaced by iron absorbed from the diet. Men are not as likely to suffer from iron deficiencies as premenopausal adult women, who also lose iron during menstruation and who must supply iron to meet the needs of the growing fetus during a pregnancy.

Although spinach has been touted as a wonderful source of iron (mostly by the cartoon character Popeye), this iron is not readily absorbed because spinach has a high content of phytate (inositol with a phosphate group attached to each of its 6 hydroxyl groups).

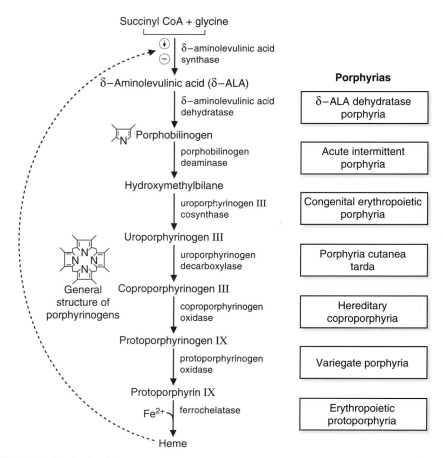

Fig. 41.5. Synthesis of heme. To produce one molecule of heme, 8 molecules each of glycine and succinyl CoA are required. A series of porphyrinogens are generated in sequence. Finally iron is added to produce heme. Heme regulates its own production by repressing the synthesis of δ-aminolevulinic acid (δ-ALA) synthase (circled ↓) and by directly inhibiting the activity of this enzyme (⊖). Deficiencies of enzymes in the pathway result in a series of diseases known as porphyrias (listed on the right, beside the deficient enzyme).

Because free iron is toxic, it is usually found in the body bound to proteins (see Fig. 41.6). Iron is carried in the blood (as Fe^{3+}) by the protein, apotransferrin, with which it forms a complex known as transferrin. Iron is oxidized from Fe^{2+} to Fe^{3+} by a ferroxidase known as ceruloplasmin (a copper-containing enzyme). Transferrin is usually only one-third saturated with iron. The total iron-binding capacity of blood, mainly due to its content of transferrin, is about 300 μg/dL.

Storage of iron occurs in most cells but especially those of the liver, spleen, and bone marrow. In these cells, the storage protein, apoferritin, forms a complex with iron (Fe^{3+}) known as ferritin. Normally, little ferritin is present in the blood. This amount increases, however, as iron stores increase. Therefore, the amount of ferritin in the blood is the most sensitive indicator of the amount of iron in the body's stores.

Iron can be drawn from ferritin stores, transported in the blood as transferrin, and taken up via receptor-mediated endocytosis by cells that require iron (e.g., by reticulocytes that are synthesizing hemoglobin). When excess iron is absorbed from the diet, it is stored as hemosiderin, a form of ferritin complexed with additional iron that cannot readily be mobilized.

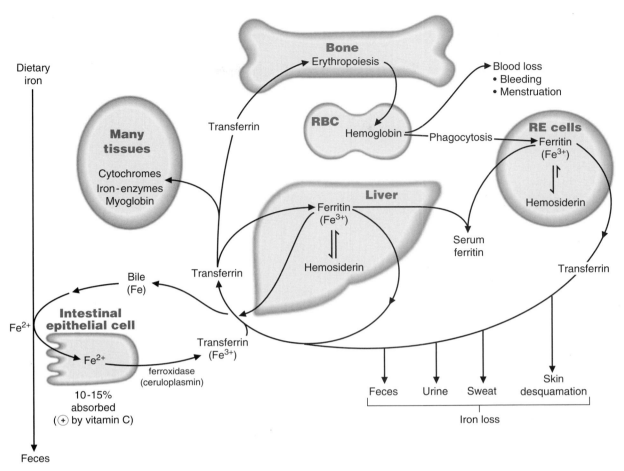

Fig. 41.6. Iron metabolism. Iron is absorbed from the diet, transported in the blood in transferrin, stored in ferritin, and utilized for the synthesis of cytochromes, iron-containing enzymes, hemoglobin, and myoglobin. It is lost from the body with bleeding and sloughed-off cells, sweat, urine, and feces. Hemosiderin is the protein in which excess iron is stored. Small amounts of ferritin enter the blood and can be used to measure the adequacy of iron stores. RE = reticuloendothelial.

Regulation of Heme Synthesis

Heme regulates its own synthesis by mechanisms that affect the first enzyme in the pathway, γ-ALA synthase (see Fig. 41.3). Heme represses the synthesis of this enzyme, and also directly inhibits it. Thus, heme is synthesized when heme levels fall. As heme levels rise, the rate of heme synthesis decreases.

Heme also regulates the synthesis of hemoglobin by stimulating synthesis of the protein globin. Heme maintains the ribosomal initiation complex in an active state (see Chapter 15).

Degradation of Heme

Heme is degraded to form bilirubin, which is conjugated with glucuronic acid and excreted in the bile (Fig. 41.7). Although heme from cytochromes and myoglobin also undergoes conversion to bilirubin, the major source of this bile pigment is hemoglobin. After red blood cells reach the end of their lifespan (about 120 days), they are phagocytosed by cells of the reticuloendothelial system. Globin is cleaved to its constituent amino acids, and iron is returned to the body's iron stores. Heme is oxidized and

Drugs, such as phenobarbital, induce enzymes of the drug-metabolizing systems of the endoplasmic reticulum that contain cytochrome P450. As heme is used for synthesis of cytochrome P450 and heme levels fall, γ-ALA synthase is induced and the rate of heme synthesis increases.

A 41.1: In a B_6 deficiency, the rate of heme production is slow because the first reaction in heme synthesis requires pyridoxal phosphate (see Fig. 41.3). Thus, less heme is synthesized, causing red blood cells to be small and pale. Iron stores are usually elevated.

41.2: In an iron deficiency, what characteristics would blood exhibit?

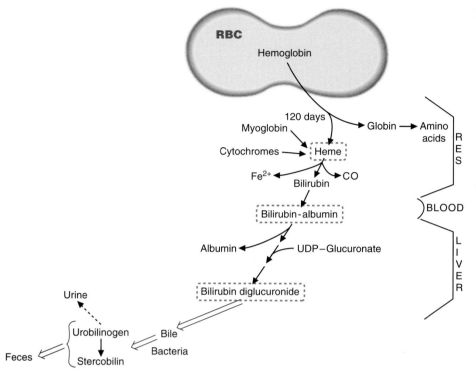

Fig. 41.7. Overview of heme degradation. Heme is degraded to bilirubin, carried in the blood by albumin, conjugated to form the diglucuronide in the liver, and excreted in the bile. The iron is returned to the body's iron stores. RES = reticuloendothelial system; RBC = red blood cells.

A sickle cell crisis accompanied by the intravascular destruction of red blood cells (hemolysis) experienced by patients with sickle cell disease, such as Michael Sichel, increase the amount of unconjugated bilirubin which is transported to the liver. If the concentration of this unconjugated bilirubin exceeds the capacity of the hepatocytes to conjugate it to the more soluble diglucuronide via interaction with hepatic UDP-glucuronate, both the total and the unconjugated bilirubin levels would rise in the blood. More unconjugated bilirubin would be secreted by the liver into the bile. The increase in unconjugated bilirubin (which is not very water soluble) results in its precipitation within the gallbladder lumen leading to the formation of pigmented (calcium bilirubinate) gallstones.

A bile duct obstruction can also result in increased bilirubin in the blood. If hemolysis is not occurring in a patient but a previously formed gallstone exits the gallbladder via the cystic duct, it may become lodged within the lumen of the common bile duct, causing extrahepatic obstruction to bile flow into the duodenum. Provided hepatocellular function is normal, conjugation of bilirubin could proceed, but the flow of this conjugated diglucuronide into the small intestine would be limited. As a consequence, "backflow" into the systemic circulation would increase the concentration of conjugated (and hence, total) bilirubin in the blood. In this case, the predominant subfraction of the total bilirubin in the blood would be the conjugated form of the pigment.

cleaved to produce carbon monoxide and biliverdin (Fig. 41.8). Biliverdin is reduced to bilirubin, which is transported to the liver complexed with serum albumin.

In the liver, bilirubin is converted to a more water-soluble compound by reacting with UDP-glucuronate to form bilirubin monoglucuronide, which is converted to the diglucuronide (see Fig. 29.8). This conjugated form of bilirubin is excreted into the bile.

In the intestine, bacteria deconjugate bilirubin diglucuronide and convert the bilirubin to urobilinogens (see Fig. 41.7). Some urobilinogen is absorbed into the blood and excreted in the urine. However, most of the urobilinogen is oxidized to urobilins, such as stercobilin, and excreted in the feces. These pigments give feces its brown color.

PURINES AND PYRIMIDINES

The purine and pyrimidine bases are found in nucleotides and in the nucleic acids. They are produced de novo by pathways that use amino acids as precursors and produce nucleotides. Most de novo synthesis occurs in the liver, and the nitrogenous bases and nucleosides are then transported to other tissues by red blood cells. The brain also synthesizes significant amounts of nucleotides.

Synthesis of the Purine Nucleotides

5-Phosphoribosyl-1-pyrophosphate (PRPP) is the source of the ribose moiety. It is synthesized from ATP and ribose 5′-phosphate (Fig. 41.9), which is produced from glucose via the pentose phosphate pathway (see Chapter 28). The purine bases are built on the ribose moiety (Fig. 41.10).

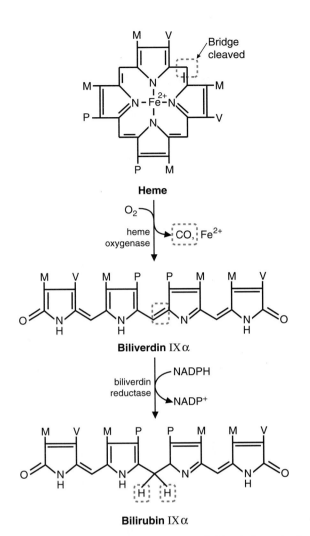

Fig. 41.8. Conversion of heme to bilirubin. A methylene bridge in heme is cleaved, releasing carbon monoxide (CO) and iron. Then, the center methylene bridge is reduced.

Neonatal jaundice occurs frequently because the system for conjugating and excreting bilirubin is not fully mature. This condition is treated by phototherapy of the infant, which converts bilirubin to other compounds that can be excreted in the urine as well as the bile.

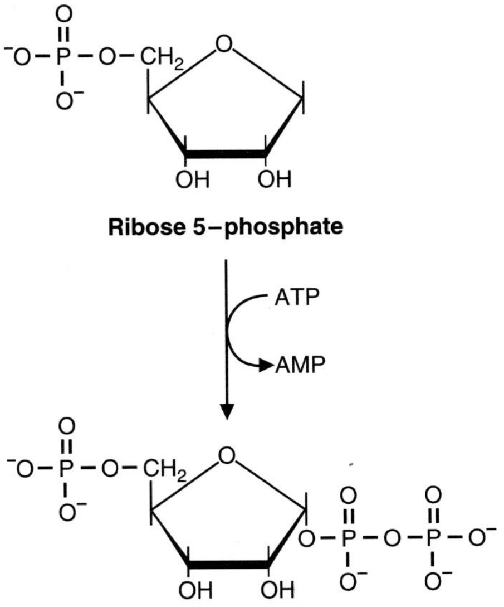

Fig. 41.9. Synthesis of PRPP. Ribose 5-phosphate is produced from glucose by the pentose phosphate pathway. The synthesis of PRPP is inhibited by purine and pyrimidine nucleotides.

41.2: Iron deficiency would result in a microcytic, hypochromic anemia. Red blood cells would be small and pale. In contrast to a vitamin B_6 deficiency, which also results in a microcytic, hypochromic anemia, iron stores are low in an iron deficiency anemia.

In the first step of the pathway, PRPP reacts with glutamine to form phosphoribosylamine (Fig. 41.11). This reaction, which produces nitrogen 9 of the purine ring, is catalyzed by PRPP glutamyl amidotransferase, an enzyme that is inhibited by three products of the pathway, IMP, AMP, and GMP. These three nucleotides also inhibit PRPP synthesis and thus slow purine nucleotide production by decreasing the levels of the substrate PRPP.

In the second step, the entire glycine molecule is added to the growing precursor. Glycine provides carbons 4 and 5 and nitrogen 7 of the purine ring (Fig. 41.12).

Subsequently, carbon 8 is provided by methenyl tetrahydrofolate, nitrogen 3 by glutamine, carbon 6 by CO_2, nitrogen 1 by aspartate, and carbon 2 by formyl tetrahydrofolate. Figure 41.10 shows the source of each of the atoms of the purine ring.

The first purine nucleotide formed by this pathway is inosine monophosphate (IMP). This nucleotide contains the base hypoxanthine joined by an *N*-glycosidic bond from nitrogen 9 of the purine ring to carbon 1 of the ribose (Fig. 41.13).

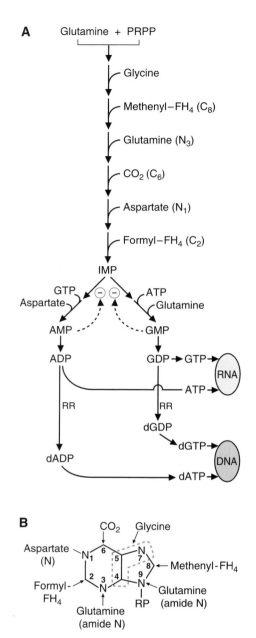

Fig. 41.10. Purine biosynthesis. **A.** Steps in the biosynthetic pathway. **B.** Origin of the atoms of the purine base. RR = ribonucleotide reductase; FH_4 = tetrahydrofolate.

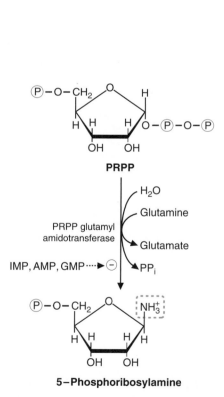

Fig. 41.11. The first step in purine biosynthesis. The purine base is built on the ribose moiety. The products of the pathway (IMP, AMP, and GMP) inhibit (⊖) the reaction. The availability of the substrate PRPP is a major determinant of the rate of this reaction (Fig. 41.10).

IMP serves as a branchpoint, and both adenine and guanine nucleotides are produced from IMP (see Fig. 41.10). Adenosine monophosphate (AMP) is derived from IMP by the addition of an amino group from aspartate to carbon 6 of the purine ring in a reaction that requires GTP. Guanosine monophosphate (GMP) is derived from IMP by the transfer of an amino group from the amide of glutamine to carbon 2 of the purine ring. In this case, the reaction requires ATP. AMP and GMP each inhibit their own production from IMP.

AMP and GMP can be phosphorylated to the di- and triphosphate levels and used for energy-requiring processes in the cell. The purine nucleoside triphosphates are also used as precursors for RNA synthesis (see Fig. 41.10).

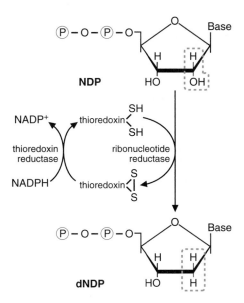

Fig. 41.14. Reduction of ribose to deoxyribose. Reduction occurs at the nucleoside diphosphate level. A ribonucleoside diphosphate (NDP) is converted to a deoxyribonucleoside diphosphate (dNDP). Thioredoxin is oxidized to a disulfide, which must be reduced for the reaction to continue producing dNDP. N = a nitrogenous base, usually adenine, guanine, or cytosine (see Figs. 41.9 and 41.16).

For DNA synthesis, the ribose moiety must be reduced to deoxyribose (Fig. 41.14). This reduction occurs at the dinucleotide level and is catalyzed by ribonucleotide reductase, which requires the protein thioredoxin. The deoxyribonucleoside diphosphates can be phosphorylated to the triphosphate level and used as precursors for DNA synthesis (see Fig. 41.10).

Degradation of the Purine Bases

The degradation of the purine nucleotides (AMP and GMP) occurs mainly in the liver (Fig. 41.15). AMP is first deaminated to produce IMP. Then IMP and GMP are dephosphorylated, and the ribose is cleaved from the base. Hypoxanthine, the base produced by cleavage of IMP, is converted by xanthine oxidase to xanthine, and guanine is deaminated to produce xanthine. The pathways for the degradation of adenine and guanine merge at this point. Xanthine is converted by xanthine oxidase to uric acid, which is excreted in the urine. Xanthine oxidase is a molybdenum-requiring enzyme that uses molecular oxygen and produces hydrogen peroxide (H_2O_2). Another form of xanthine oxidase exists that uses NAD^+ as the electron acceptor (see Chapter 21).

Uric acid has a pK of 5.4. It is ionized in the body to form urate. Urate is not very soluble in an aqueous environment. The quantity in normal human blood is very close to the solubility constant.

Synthesis of the Pyrimidine Nucleotides

In the synthesis of the pyrimidine nucleotides, the base is synthesized first, and then it is attached to the ribose 5′-phosphate moiety (Fig. 41.16). In the first reaction, glutamine reacts with CO_2 and ATP to form carbamoyl phosphate. This reaction is anal-

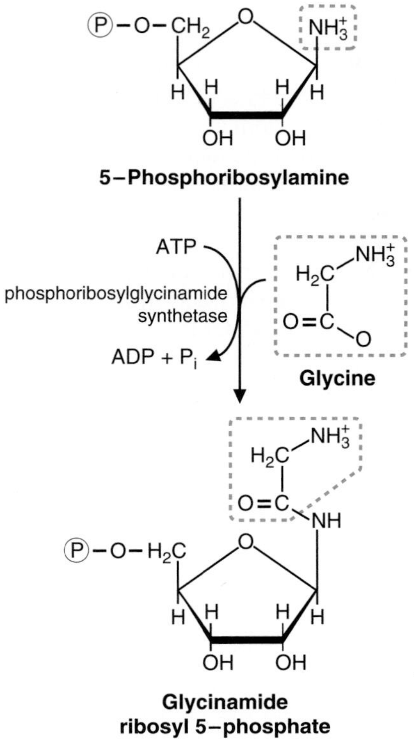

5-Phosphoribosylamine

ATP

phosphoribosylglycinamide synthetase

ADP + P_i

Glycine

Glycinamide ribosyl 5-phosphate

Fig. 41.12. Incorporation of glycine into the purine precursor.

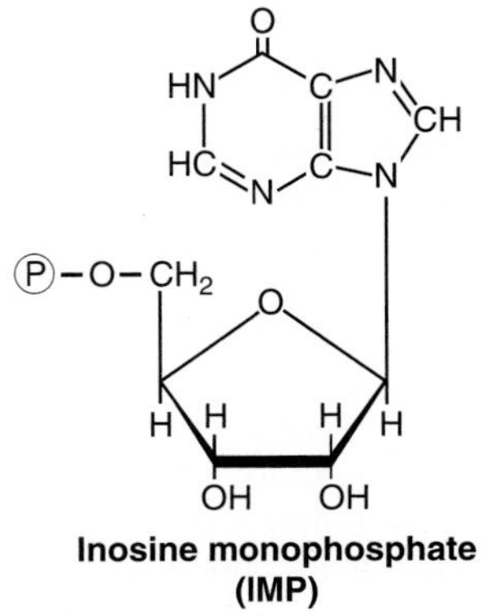

Inosine monophosphate (IMP)

Fig. 41.13. Structure of inosine monophosphate (IMP). The base is hypoxanthine.

Q 41.3: Gout is caused by excessive uric acid levels in the blood. To determine whether a person with gout has developed this problem because of overproduction of purine nucleotides or because of a decreased ability to excrete uric acid, an oral dose of an ^{15}N-labeled amino acid is sometimes used. Which amino acid would be most appropriate to use for this purpose?

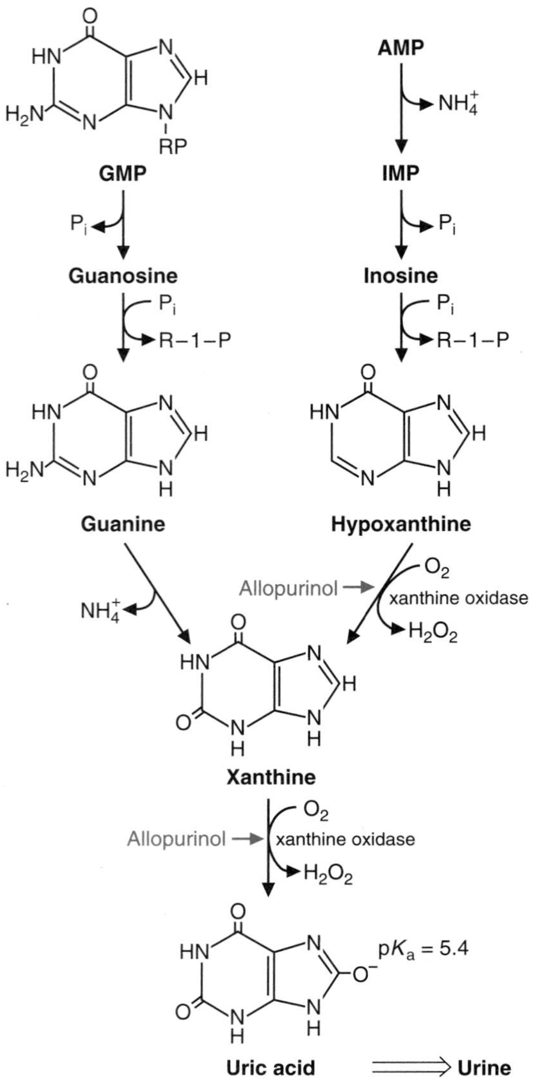

Fig. 41.15. Degradation of the purine bases. The reactions inhibited by allopurinol are indicated. A second form of xanthine oxidase exists that uses NAD^+ instead of O_2 as the electron acceptor.

Normally, as cells die, their purine nucleotides are degraded to hypoxanthine and xanthine which are converted to uric acid by xanthine oxidase (see Fig. 41.15). Allopurinol (a structural analogue of hypoxanthine) is a substrate for xanthine oxidase. It is converted to oxypurinol (also called alloxanthine) which remains tightly bound to the enzyme, preventing further catalytic activity (see Chapter 9). Thus, allopurinol is a suicide inhibitor. It reduces the production of uric acid and hence its concentration in the blood and tissues (e.g., the synovial lining of joints, such as that of **Yves Topaigne's** great toe). Xanthine and hypoxanthine accumulate and urate levels decrease. Overall, the amount of purine being degraded is spread over three products rather than appearing in only one. Therefore, none of the compounds exceeds its solubility constant, precipitation does not occur, and the symptoms of gout gradually subside.

ogous to the first reaction of the urea cycle, except that it uses glutamine as the source of the nitrogen (rather than ammonia) and it occurs in the cytosol (rather than in mitochondria). The reaction is catalyzed by carbamoyl phosphate synthetase II, which is inhibited by UTP, one of the products of the pathway. The analogous reaction in urea synthesis is catalyzed by carbamoyl phosphate synthetase I, which is activated by N-acetylglutamate (Table 41.1).

In the next step of pyrimidine biosynthesis, the entire aspartate molecule adds to carbamoyl phosphate. The molecule subsequently closes to produce a ring, which is oxidized to form orotic acid (or orotate). Orotate reacts with PRPP, producing orotidine 5'-phosphate, which is decarboxylated to form uridine monophosphate (UMP) (Fig. 41.17).

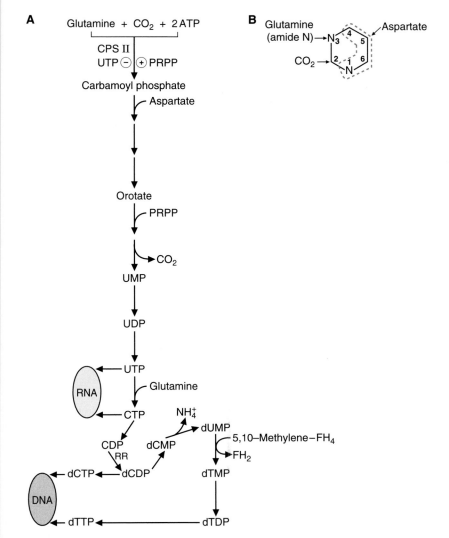

Fig. 41.16. Synthesis of the pyrimidine bases. **A.** Steps in the pathway. **B.** Source of the atoms of the pyrimidine base. CPSII = carbamoyl phosphate synthetase II. RR = ribonucleotide reductase; ⊕ = stimulated by; ⊖ = inhibited by; FH_2 and FH_4 = forms of folate.

In hereditary orotic aciduria, orotic acid is excreted in the urine because the enzymes that convert it to uridine monophosphate, orotate phosphoribosyltransferase and orotidine 5′-phosphate decarboxylase are defective (see Fig. 41.17). Pyrimidines cannot be synthesized, and, therefore, normal growth does not occur. Oral administration of uridine is used to treat this condition. Uridine, which is converted to UMP, bypasses the metabolic block and provides the body with a source of pyrimidines.

UMP is phosphorylated to UTP. An amino group, derived from the amide of glutamine, is added to carbon 4 to produce CTP. UTP and CTP are precursors for the synthesis of RNA (see Fig. 41.16).

CTP is dephosphorylated to form CDP, and at this diphosphate level the ribose moiety is reduced to deoxyribose by ribonucleotide reductase (see Fig. 41.14). dCDP is dephosphorylated and deaminated, forming dUMP. Methylene tetrahydrofolate transfers a methyl group to dUMP to form dTMP (see Chapter 40). Phosphorylation reactions produce dCTP and dTTP, precursors used for DNA synthesis.

Degradation of the Pyrimidine Bases

The pyrimidine nucleotides are dephosphorylated, and the nucleosides are cleaved to produce ribose 1-phosphate and the free pyrimidine bases cytosine, uracil, and

41.3: The entire glycine molecule is incorporated into the precursor of the purine nucleotides. The nitrogen of this glycine also appears in uric acid, the product of purine degradation. ^{15}N-labeled glycine could be used, therefore, to determine if purines are being overproduced.

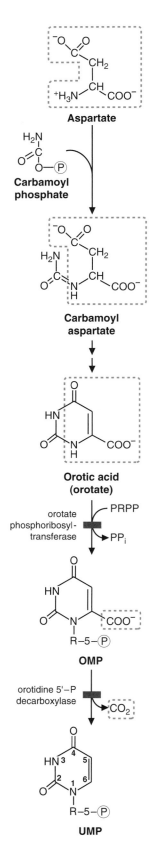

Aspartate

Carbamoyl phosphate

Carbamoyl aspartate

Orotic acid (orotate)

orotate phosphoribosyl-transferase

PRPP

PP_i

OMP

orotidine 5'–P decarboxylase

CO_2

UMP

▬ Block in hereditary orotic aciduria

Table 41.1. Comparison of Carbamoyl Phosphate Synthetases (CPSI and CPSII)

	CPSI	CPSII
Pathway	Urea cycle	Pyrimidine biosynthesis
Source of nitrogen	NH_4^+	Glutamine
Location	Mitochondria	Cytosol
Activator	N-Acetylglutamate	PRPP
Inhibitor	–	UTP

thymine. Cytosine is deaminated, forming uracil, which is converted to CO_2, NH_4^+, and β-alanine. Thymine is converted to CO_2, NH_4^+, and β-aminoisobutyrate. These products of pyrimidine degradation are excreted in the urine or converted to CO_2, H_2O, and NH_4^+ (which forms urea). They do not cause any problems for the body, in contrast to urate, which is produced from the purines and can precipitate, causing gout.

Salvage of Bases

Most of the de novo synthesis of the bases of nucleotides occurs in the liver, and to some extent in the brain neutrophils, and other cells of the immune system. In the liver, nucleotides are dephosphorylated to form nucleosides, which are frequently cleaved to form the free bases. The nucleosides and bases are transported to other tissues, where the nucleosides are rephosphorylated to nucleotides (Fig. 41.18), and the free bases are salvaged by reacting with PRPP to re-form nucleotides (Fig. 41.19). The salvage enzymes for the purine bases are hypoxanthine-guanine phosphoribosyltransferase (HGPRT) and adenine phosphoribosyltransferase (APRT). Analogous reactions occur with the pyrimidine bases.

DECARBOXYLATION OF AMINO ACIDS

Many amino acids are decarboxylated by reactions that require pyridoxal phosphate. These reactions produce amines that often serve as neurotransmitters and hormones (see Chapter 42 and Section VIII). They also serve as the initial steps in pathways that produce polyamines, heme, and sphingolipids.

Glutamate is decarboxylated at carbon 1 to form an amine, GABA, which serves as a neurotransmitter in inhibitory pathways (Fig. 41.20).

Histidine is decarboxylated to form histamine. Histamine causes dilation of blood vessels. In the lung, it causes bronchoconstriction, and in the stomach, it stimulates the secretion of HCl.

Ornithine, an amino acid found as a component of the urea cycle, is decarboxylated to form putrescine. The polyamines, spermine and spermidine, are produced from putrescine. The activity of ornithine decarboxylase, the enzyme that catalyzes the decarboxylation of ornithine, increases prior to cell division.

The initial step in sphingolipid synthesis involves the decarboxylation of serine as it condenses with palmitoyl CoA. The product is converted to ceramide, from which sphingomyelin, cerebrosides, and gangliosides are produced (see Chapter 33). Likewise, the initial step in the synthesis of heme involves the decarboxylation of glycine as it condenses with succinyl CoA to form δ-ALA (see Fig. 41.3).

Fig. 41.17. Conversion of carbamoyl phosphate and aspartate to UMP. The defective enzymes in hereditary orotic aciduria are indicated (▬).

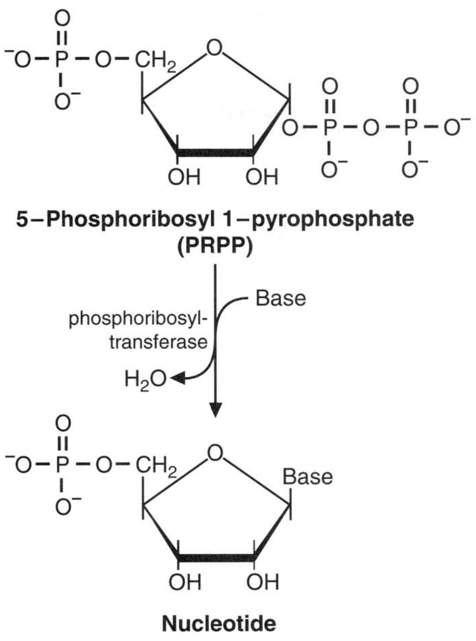

**5-Phosphoribosyl 1-pyrophosphate
(PRPP)**

phosphoribosyl-
transferase

H_2O

Nucleotide

Fig. 41.19. Salvage of bases. The purine bases hypoxanthine and guanine react with PRPP to form inosine and guanosine monophosphate, respectively. The enzyme is hypoxanthine-guanine phosphoribosyltransferase (HGPRT). Adenine forms AMP in a reaction catalyzed by adenine phosphoribosyltransferase. The pyrimidine bases also undergo salvage reactions.

The aromatic amino acids also undergo decarboxylations during their metabolism to produce compounds that serve as neurotransmitters and/or as hormones. Serotonin is formed from tryptophan, and the catecholamines, dopamine, norepinephrine, and epinephrine are produced from tyrosine.

PRODUCTS DERIVED FROM TRYPTOPHAN

Serotonin, melatonin, and the nicotinamide moiety of NAD and NADP are formed from tryptophan (Fig. 41.21). In the formation of serotonin, tryptophan is first hydroxylated in a tetrahydrobiopterin-requiring reaction (similar to the hydroxylation of phenylalanine to form tyrosine). The product, 5-hydroxytryptophan, is then decarboxylated to form serotonin.

Serotonin, in addition to serving as a neurotransmitter, is a potent vasoconstrictor and a stimulator of smooth muscle contraction. Serotonin undergoes acetylation by acetyl CoA, followed by methylation by *S*-adenosylmethionine to form melatonin. Melatonin is produced in the pineal gland in response to the light-dark cycle, and blood levels of melatonin rise at night. It is probably via melatonin that the pineal gland conveys information about light-dark cycles to the body, organizing seasonal and circadian rhythms. Melatonin may also be involved in regulating reproductive functions.

Tryptophan can be converted to the nicotinamide moiety of NAD and NADP, although the major precursor of nicotinamide is the vitamin niacin (nicotinic acid). Thus, the higher the amount of dietary tryptophan, the lower the dietary requirement for niacin, i.e., tryptophan spares the dietary requirement for niacin. Diets low in both tryptophan and niacin can result in pellagra (see Chapter 39).

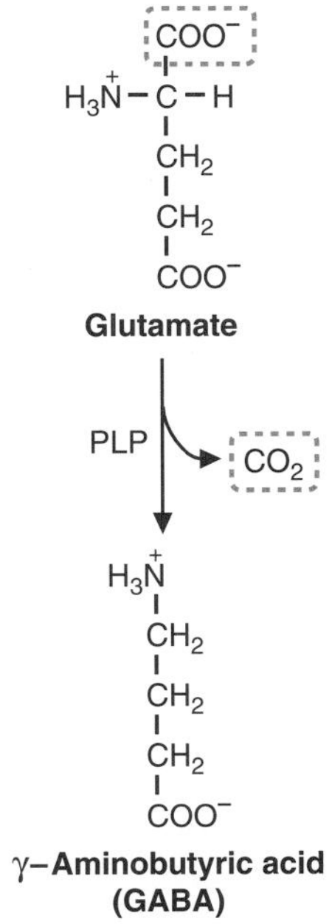

Nucleoside
monophosphate

ATP

kinase

ADP

Nucleoside
diphosphate

ATP

kinase

ADP

Nucleoside
triphosphate

Fig. 41.18. Phosphorylation of nucleosides.

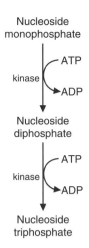 Lesch-Nyhan syndrome is caused by a defective hypoxanthine-guanine phosphoribosyltransferase (HGPRT) (see Fig. 41.19). In this condition, purine bases cannot be salvaged. Instead they are degraded, forming excessive amounts of uric acid. Individuals with this syndrome suffer from mental retardation. They are also prone to chewing off their fingers and performing other acts of self-mutilation.

COO⁻

$H_3\overset{+}{N}$ — C — H

CH_2

CH_2

COO⁻

Glutamate

PLP

CO_2

$H_3\overset{+}{N}$

CH_2

CH_2

CH_2

COO⁻

**γ-Aminobutyric acid
(GABA)**

Fig. 41.20. Synthesis of γ-aminobutyric acid (GABA).

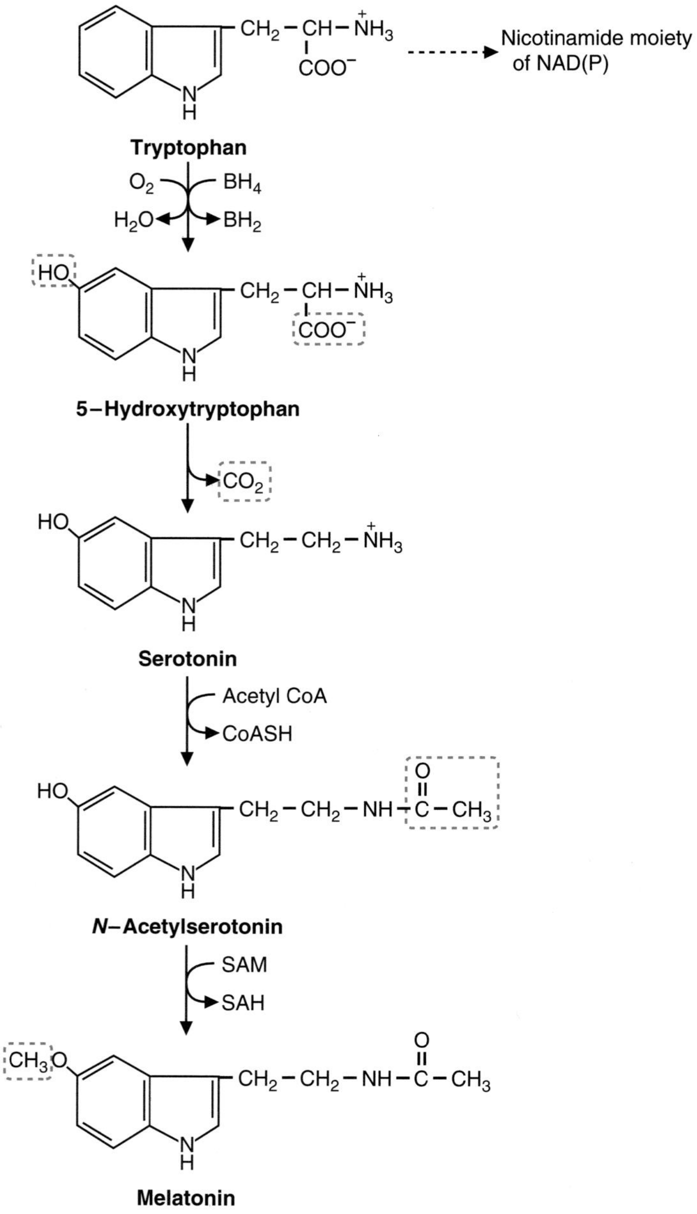

Fig. 41.21. Products derived from tryptophan. SAH = *S*-adenosylhomocysteine; SAM = *S*-adenosylmethionine; BH_4 and BH_2 = tetra- and dihydrobiopterin.

PRODUCTS DERIVED FROM PHENYLALANINE AND TYROSINE

The thyroid hormones T_3 and T_4 are produced in the thyroid gland from tyrosine residues in the protein thyroglobulin. This process is described in Chapter 44.

Phenylalanine is converted to tyrosine in a reaction catalyzed by phenylalanine hydroxylase (see Chapter 39), and tyrosine is hydroxylated to form 3,4-dihydroxyphenylalanine (dopa). Dopa can be converted to melanin pigments or to the catecholamines (Fig. 41.22).

In melanocytes of the skin, eye, and hair, dopa is oxidized to quinones that polymerize forming the melanin pigments. In these cells, the hydroxylation of tyrosine to form dopa is catalyzed by a copper-containing isozyme that differs from the one that converts tyrosine to catecholamines in other cell types.

The catecholamines are derived from tyrosine in neurons and in the adrenal medulla by a series of reactions. Tyrosine hydroxylase, the enzyme that converts tyrosine to dopa, is similar to phenylalanine hydroxylase and requires tetrahydrobiopterin as a cofactor. Decarboxylation of dopa produces the neurotransmitter dopamine. Dopamine can be hydroxylated on its aliphatic chain to form the neurotransmitter norepinephrine. Dopamine hydroxylase requires copper and vitamin C, rather than tetrahydrobiopterin.

In the adrenal medulla, norepinephrine is methylated to produce the hormone epinephrine. *S*-Adenosylmethionine provides the methyl group for this reaction.

NEUROTRANSMITTERS

General Mechanism of Action

Many amino acids serve as neurotransmitters (e.g., glutamate, glycine) or are converted to other compounds that serve as neurotransmitters (e.g., GABA from glutamate, the catecholamines from tyrosine, 5-hydroxytryptamine and serotonin from tryptophan).

In general, neurotransmitters are formed in the presynaptic terminals of axons. Many neurotransmitters are stored in vesicles until released by a transient change in electrical potential along the axon (Fig. 41.23). The neurotransmitter binds to a receptor on the postsynaptic terminal, initiating a nerve impulse in this neuron. It is then taken up by the postsynaptic terminal, or by an adjacent cell, such as the astroglial cell. Subsequent catabolism of the neurotransmitter often results in the formation of a urinary excretion product. The rapid catabolism of neurotransmitters requires a continuous supply of a precursor pool of amino acids to be available for their synthesis (see Chapter 42).

Inactivation and Excretion of Catecholamines

Catecholamines provide examples of neurotransmitters which are converted to urinary excretion products. Three basic types of reactions are involved in the inactivation and degradation of these neurotransmitters: oxidative deamination, oxidation, and *O*-methylation (Fig. 41.24). The oxidative deamination is catalyzed by monoamine oxidase (MAO), which is present in the cytosol of the presynaptic terminal, adjacent glial cells, erythrocytes, and other tissues. MAO oxidatively deaminates neurotransmitters, forming aldehydes. Further oxidation occurs through an aldehyde dehydrogenase. In addition, the hydroxyl group can be methylated by SAM in a reaction catalyzed by catecholamine *O*-methyltransferase (COMT). This reaction creates an $-O-CH_3$ (methoxy) group. These reactions can occur in almost any order and any combination, so that a wide range of urinary excretion products exists for these compounds. MAO also inactivates serotonin.

CONVERSION OF ARGININE TO NITRIC OXIDE

Nitric oxide (NO) is a biological messenger in a variety of physiological responses including vasodilation, neurotransmission, and the ability of the immune system to kill tumor cells and parasites. NO is synthesized from arginine in a reaction catalyzed by NO synthase (Fig. 41.25).

NO synthase exists as tissue-specific forms of two families of enzymes. The form present in macrophages is responsible for the overproduction of NO, leading to its

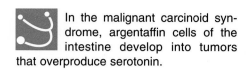
In the malignant carcinoid syndrome, argentaffin cells of the intestine develop into tumors that overproduce serotonin.

In albinism, either the copper-dependent tyrosine hydroxylase of melanocytes or other enzymes that convert tyrosine to melanins may be defective. Individuals with albinism suffer from a lack of pigment in the skin, hair, and eyes, and they are sensitive to sunlight.

In Parkinson's disease, dopamine levels in the central nervous system are decreased because of a deficiency of cells that produce dopamine (see Chapter 21).

Katie Colamin's doctor ordered plasma catecholamine (epinephrine, norepinephrine, and dopamine) levels and also had Katie collect a 24-hour urine specimen for the determination of catecholamines and their degradation products. All of these tests showed unequivocal elevations of these compounds in Katie's blood and urine. Katie was placed on phenoxybenzamine, an α_1- and α_2-adrenergic receptor antagonist which blocks the pharmacological effect of the elevated catecholamines on these receptors. After ruling out evidence to suggest metastatic disease to the liver or other organs (in case Katie's tumor was malignant), the doctor referred Katie to a surgeon with extensive experience in adrenal surgery.

The catecholamines exert their physiological and pharmacological effects by circulating in the bloodstream to target cells whose plasma membranes contain catecholamine receptors. This interaction initiates a biochemical cascade leading to responses that are specific for different types of cells. Patients like Katie Colamin experience palpitations, excessive sweating, hypertensive headaches, and a host of other symptoms when a catecholamine-producing tumor of the adrenal medulla suddenly secretes supraphysiological amounts of epinephrine and/or norepinephrine into the venous blood draining the neoplasm.

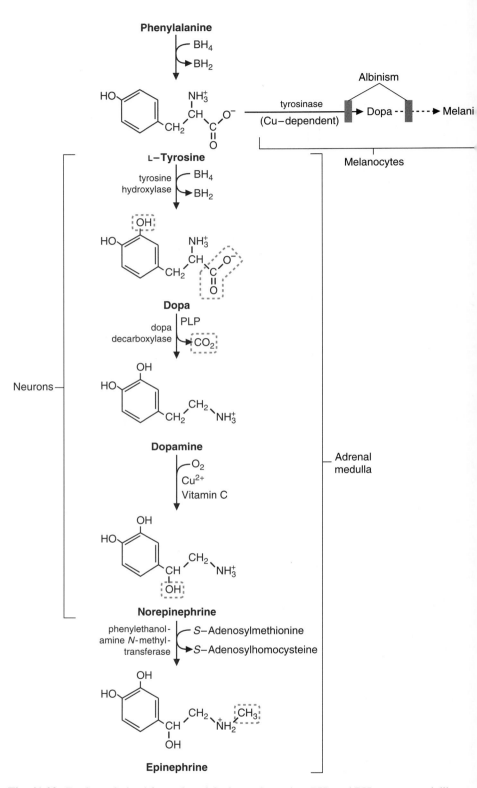

Fig. 41.22. Products derived from phenylalanine and tyrosine. BH_4 and BH_2 = tetra- and dihydrobiopterin; PLP = pyridoxal phosphate; ▓ = enzymes that are defective in albinism.

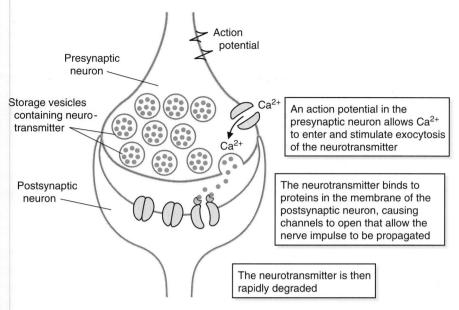

Fig. 41.23. Action of neurotransmitters.

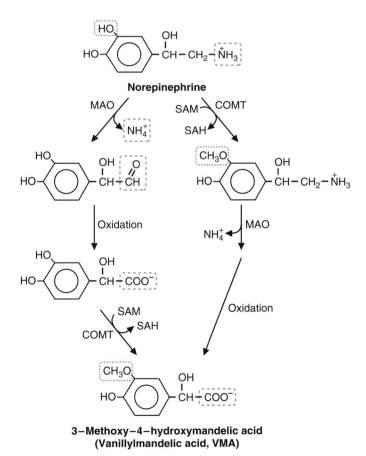

Fig. 41.24. Inactivation of catecholamines. Methylation and oxidation may occur in any order. Methylated and oxidized derivates of norepinephrine and epinephrine are produced, and 3-methoxy-4-hydroxymandelic acid is the final product. These compounds are excreted in the urine. MAO = monoamine oxidase; COMT = catechol *O*-methyltransferase; SAM = *S*-adenosylmethionine; SAH = *S*-adenosylhomocysteine.

The cytotoxic action of NO is related to its ability to react with iron. The activation of macrophages by an endotoxin induces NO synthase, which produces NO. NO interacts directly with Fe-S centers in the electron transport chain proteins of nearby parasites and tumor cells, inhibiting their respiration and ATP production.

cytotoxic actions on parasites and tumor cells. The enzyme present in nervous tissue, vascular endothelium, platelets, and other tissues is responsible for the physiological responses to NO in vasodilation and neural transmission. In these responses, NO activates a soluble guanylate cyclase which results in increased cellular levels of cGMP ($3',5'$-cyclic GMP) (see Fig. 41.26). In smooth muscle cells, cGMP, like cAMP, activates one or more protein kinases which are responsible for the relaxation of smooth muscle and the subsequent dilation of vessels. NO stimulates penile erection by acting as a neurotransmitter, stimulating smooth muscle relaxation that permits the corpus cavernosum to fill with blood.

NO lasts only about 100 msec in the blood, and only a few seconds in tissues because it combines with O_2 to form nitrite. Nitrite is converted to nitrate and excreted in the urine.

CLINICAL COMMENTS. Poststreptococcal glomerulonephritis (PSGN) may follow pharyngeal or cutaneous infection with one of a limited number of "nephritogenic" strains of group A β-hemolytic streptococci. The pathogenesis of PSGN involves a host immune (antibody) response to one or more of the enzymes secreted by the bacterial cells. The antigen-antibody complexes are deposited on the tissues of glomerular units, causing a local acute inflammatory response. Hypertension may occur as a consequence of sodium and water retention caused by an inability of the inflamed glomerular units to filter sodium and water into the urine. Proteinuria is usually mild if the immune response is self-limited.

Overall, one of the most useful clinical indicators of glomerular filtration rate in both health and disease is the serum creatinine concentration. The endogenous production of creatinine, which averages about 15 mg/kg of body weight per day, is correlated with muscle mass and, therefore, tends to be constant for a given individual if renal function is normal. Any rise in serum creatinine in patients like **Rena Felya**,

Arginine

NADPH
O_2
NO synthase
NADP$^+$

NO
Nitric oxide

Citrulline

Fig. 41.25. Synthesis of nitric oxide (NO).

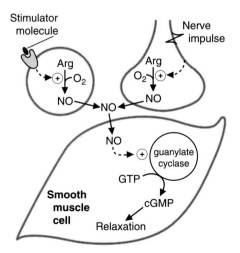

Fig. 41.26. Action of nitric oxide (NO) in vasodilation. The synthesis of NO occurs in response to a stimulator binding to a receptor on some cells or to a nerve impulse in neurons. NO enters smooth muscle cells, stimulating guanylate cyclase to produce cGMP, which causes smooth muscle relaxation. When the smooth muscle cells relax, blood vessels dilate.

therefore, can be assumed to result from decreased excretion of this metabolite into the urine. The extent of the rise in the blood is directly related to the severity of the pathological process involving the glomerular units within the kidneys.

The mechanism leading to jaundice in **Michael Sichel** was an obstruction of the common bile duct by a gallstone. Treatment included restricted oral intake, nasogastric suction, intravenous fluids, parenteral analgesics, and antibiotic therapy.

Michael's conservative therapy was gradually discontinued after a repeat ultrasound of his abdomen 2 days after admission revealed that he had spontaneously passed the obstructing stone. Because of the likelihood that future hemolytic crises would cause further gallstones to form, and because these, in turn, could later cause recurrence of bile duct obstruction, it was decided to do a laparoscopic cholecystectomy. In this procedure, a surgical laparoscope is passed through a small incision in the abdominal wall and the stone-containing gallbladder is removed. Michael tolerated the procedure well and was discharged just 2 days later, free of symptoms and with a rapid return of his serum bilirubin and liver enzyme levels to normal.

Hyperuricemia results from overproduction or underexcretion of uric acid. Overproduction is caused by enzymatic abnormalities in the de novo pathway for purine biosynthesis or by an increased rate of cell death (and hence nucleic acid degradation, such as that which follows radiation therapy for cancer). Underexcretion results from a variety of chronic renal disorders which reduce the ability of the kidneys to excrete uric acid into the urine.

Hyperuricemia in **Yves Topaigne's** case arose as a consequence of overproduction of uric acid. Treatment with allopurinol not only inhibits xanthine oxidase, lowering the formation of uric acid with an increase in the excretion of hypoxanthine and xanthine, but also decreases the overall synthesis of purine nucleotides. Hypoxanthine and xanthine produced by purine degradation are salvaged (i.e., converted to nucleotides) by a process that requires the consumption of PRPP. PRPP is both a substrate and an activator for the PRPP glutamyl amidotransferase reaction that initiates purine biosynthesis. Therefore, decreased levels of PRPP cause decreased synthesis of purine nucleotides.

Catecholamines affect nearly every tissue and organ in the body. Their integrated release from nerve endings of the sympathetic (adrenergic) nervous system plays a critical role in the reflex responses we make to sudden changes in our internal and external environment. For example, under stress, catecholamines appropriately increase heart rate, blood pressure, myocardial (heart muscle) contractility, and conduction velocity of the heart.

Episodic, inappropriate secretion of catecholamines in pharmacological amounts, such as occurs in patients with pheochromocytomas, like **Katie Colamin**, causes an often alarming array of symptoms and signs of a hyperadrenergic state.

Although the majority of the signs and symptoms related to catecholamine excess can be masked by phenoxybenzamine, a long-acting α_1- and α_2-adrenergic receptor antagonist, combined with a β_1- and β_2-adrenergic receptor blocker such as propranolol, pharmacological therapy alone is reserved for patients with inoperable pheochromocytomas (e.g., patients with malignant tumors with metastases and patients with severe heart disease). Because of the sudden, unpredictable, and sometimes life-threatening discharges of large amounts of catecholamines from these tumors, definitive therapy involves surgical resection of the neoplasms(s) after appropriate preoperative preparation of the patient with the agents mentioned above. Katie's tumor was resected without intra- or postoperative complications. Following surgery, she remained free of symptoms and her blood pressure fell to normal levels.

Nitroglycerin, a drug frequently used by patients with angina pectoris (heart pain caused by a narrowing of the coronary arteries), is converted to NO and causes dilation of blood vessels of the heart, increasing its blood flow and oxygen supply, thereby relieving pain. NO also causes vasodilation of other vessels in the body, reducing blood pressure and, therefore, the workload on the heart, which reduces its energy requirements.

In Chapter 20, **Cora Nari** was treated with nitroprusside, a drug that is converted to NO and, therefore, is used to treat high blood pressure.

Male sexual impotence can be treated by penile injection of drugs that inhibit cGMP phosphodiesterase, causing increased cGMP in cavernosal smooth muscle cells, the same effect produced by NO. However, in some patients, these drugs cause fibrotic nodules and priapism (unrelieved engorgement). For these reasons, prostaglandin E_1, which appears to have fewer side effects, is now being used for self-injection.

BIOCHEMICAL COMMENTS. Hyperbilirubinemia and jaundice (the deposition of bilirubin pigment in the tissues) can occur (*a*) as a result of the presentation of amounts of bilirubin to the liver in excess of the capacity of normal hepatocytes to conjugate the pigments (as in severe hemolysis); and/or (*b*) as a result of dysfunction of the hepatocytes per se (i.e., in alcoholic hepatitis or viral hepatitis) which limits the ability of the liver cells to metabolize bilirubin normally; and/or (*c*) as a result of intra- or extrahepatic obstruction of the drainage ducts leading from the liver to the small intestine.

Radiological studies may help to distinguish one mechanism for jaundice from the others. For example, an ultrasound study of the abdomen may reveal the presence of gallstones which obstruct the common bile duct, causing "backflow" of bilirubin into the blood.

An understanding of the biochemistry involved in the production and processing of bilirubin can also help to determine the cause of a hyperbilirubinemia. Laboratory studies may suggest that hemolysis is occurring, e.g., a falling hemoglobin level in association with an elevated reticulocyte count (an increase in the number of immature red blood cells) in the peripheral blood reflecting erythroid hyperplasia (increased production of new red cells in the bone marrow in response to hemolysis, the destruction of mature red blood cells). Tests that determine the functional capacity of the liver cells may indicate hepatocellular disease (e.g., elevated serum transaminase levels in acute alcoholic or viral hepatitis, positive tests for hepatitis antigens and antibodies in the peripheral blood).

Measurement of the total bilirubin as well as the proportion of unconjugated and conjugated bilirubin in the blood may indicate whether the patient's jaundice is due to acute hemolysis, hepatocellular dysfunction, or intra- or extrahepatic obstruction. Because alkaline phosphatase is produced in the cells lining the drainage ducts (biliary ducts) of the liver rather than in the hepatocytes themselves, an elevation of this enzyme in the blood suggests either an inflammatory or obstructive process in these drainage ducts. Either type of process may cause a discharge of alkaline phosphatase into the systemic circulation. A disproportionate increase in the serum concentration of this enzyme compared to that of the liver transaminases (e.g., alanine aminotransferase (ALT) and aspartate aminotransferase (AST)) would not be expected with acute hemolysis or with nonobstructive hepatocellular disease.

Suggested Reading

Cryer PE. The adrenal medullae. In: Wyngaarden JB, Smith LH Jr, Bennett JC, eds. Cecil textbook of medicine. Philadelphia: WB Saunders, 1988:1390–1393.

Moncada S, Higgs A. The L-arginine-nitric oxide pathway. N Engl J Med 1993;329:2002–2012.

Scharschmidt BR. Bilirubin metabolism and hyperbilirubinemia. In: Wyngaarden JB, Smith LH Jr, Bennett JC, eds. Cecil textbook of medicine. Philadelphia: WB Saunders, 1988:756–760.

Wyngaarden JB. Disorders of purine and pyrimidine metabolism. In: Wyngaarden JB, Smith LH Jr, Bennett JC, eds. Cecil textbook of medicine. Philadelphia: WB Saunders, 1988:1107–1115.

PROBLEMS

1. A professional body builder had an identical twin who was a very studious medical student with no time for exercise. Would the daily creatinine production of the twins be the same or different? Explain your answer.

2. When Teresa Livermore had acute viral hepatitis, she was noted to be jaundiced. Explain why serum bilirubin levels were elevated in this case.

3. An individual had a deficiency of an enzyme involved in the de novo synthesis of IMP. Why would feeding inosine be beneficial in this case?

ANSWERS

1. The body-building twin would produce more creatinine because the amount of creatinine produced per day depends on body muscle mass.

2. In viral hepatitis, the capacity of the infected liver to conjugate bilirubin is diminished. Therefore, unconjugated bilirubin builds up in the blood and accumulates in the tissues, causing jaundice.

3. Inosine (the nucleoside) or its base (hypoxanthine) can be used by tissues to form the purine nucleotides. Hypoxanthine via the salvage reaction catalyzed by HGPRT can form IMP. Inosine can also be phosphorylated to form IMP.

IMP can be converted to AMP and GMP which can be phosphorylated to the di- and triphosphate level, providing ATP and GTP for energy-requiring reactions and for RNA synthesis. At the diphosphate level (i.e., ADP and GDP), reduction of the ribose moiety to deoxyribose occurs. dADP and dGDP can be further phosphorylated to dATP and dGTP, which are precursors for DNA synthesis.

42 Intertissue Relationships in the Metabolism of Amino Acids

The body maintains a relatively large free amino acid pool in the blood, even during fasting. As a result, tissues have continuous access to individual amino acids for the synthesis of proteins and essential amino acid derivatives, such as neurotransmitters. The amino acid pool also provides the liver with amino acid substrates for gluconeogenesis, and provides several other cell types with a source of fuel. The free amino acid pool is derived from dietary amino acids and the turnover of proteins in the body. During an overnight fast and during hypercatabolic states, degradation of labile protein, particularly that in skeletal muscle, is the major source of free amino acids.

The liver is the major site of amino acid metabolism in the body and the major site of urea synthesis. The liver is also the major site of amino acid degradation, and partially oxidizes most amino acids, converting the carbon skeleton to glucose, ketone bodies, or CO_2. Because ammonia is toxic, the liver converts most of the nitrogen from amino acid degradation to urea, which is excreted in the urine. The nitrogen derived from amino acid catabolism in other tissues is transported to the liver as alanine or glutamine and converted to urea.

The branched chain amino acids (valine, isoleucine, and leucine) are oxidized principally in skeletal muscle and other tissues, and not in the liver. In skeletal muscle, the carbon skeletons and some of the nitrogen are converted to glutamine, which is released into the blood. The remainder of the nitrogen is incorporated into alanine, which is taken up by the liver and converted to urea and glucose.

The formation and release of glutamine from skeletal muscle and other tissues serves several functions. In the kidney, the NH_4^+ carried by glutamine is excreted into the urine. This process removes protons formed during fuel oxidation and helps to maintain the body's pH, especially during metabolic acidosis. Glutamine also provides a fuel for the kidney and gut. In rapidly dividing cells (e.g., lymphocytes and macrophages), glutamine is required as a fuel, as a nitrogen donor for biosynthetic reactions, and as a substrate for protein synthesis.

During conditions of sepsis, trauma, injury, or burns, the body enters a catabolic state characterized by a negative nitrogen balance (Fig. 42.1). An increased net protein degradation in skeletal muscle increases the availability of glutamine and other amino acids for cell division and protein synthesis in cells involved in the immune response and wound healing. In these conditions, an increased release of glucocorticoids from the adrenal cortex stimulates proteolysis.

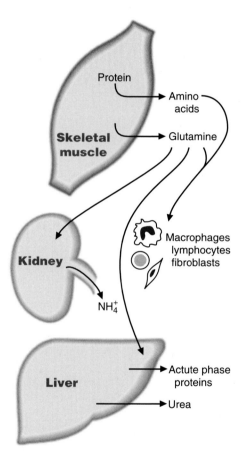

Fig. 42.1. Amino acid flux in sepsis and trauma. In sepsis and traumatic injury, glutamine and other amino acids are released from skeletal muscle for uptake by tissues involved in the immune response and tissue repair, such as macrophages, lymphocytes, fibroblasts, and the liver. Nitrogen excretion as urea and NH_4^+ results in negative nitrogen balance.

Rena Felya's daily urine output fell to an average of 320 mL (normal = 800–1,800) during the week after her poststreptococcal glomerulonephritis (PSGN) was diagnosed. When her oliguria (low urine output) persisted for an additional 2 weeks and her urinary sediment continued to show red and white

Q 42.1: What changes in hormone levels and fuel metabolism occur during an overnight fast?

blood cells, casts, and protein, she was referred to a nephrologist. The nephrologist admitted Rena to the hospital because her blood urea nitrogen (BUN) and serum creatinine levels were progressively rising. Her low arterial pH and her serum electrolytes indicated that Rena had developed a metabolic acidosis. A renal biopsy showed large cellular crescents (collections of granular deposits consisting of immunoglobulin, complement, fibrinogen, fibrin, and inflammatory cells surrounding and compressing the glomerular capillary tuft in Bowman's capsule) in approximately 65% of the visible glomeruli. A diagnosis of rapidly progressive glomerulonephritis complicating that caused by the streptococcal infection was made. Rena's ability to "clear" creatinine from her blood into her urine (the creatinine clearance) fell to 20 mL/min/1.73 m^2 (reference range = 88–128). Due to the compression of her glomeruli, her urine volume decreased, and she was unable to filter acids into the glomerular filtrate, and her metabolic acidosis worsened. The nephrologist decided to initiate "pulse" therapy (parenteral glucocorticoids in high doses for short periods) with methylprednisolone, as well as daily therapy with oral prednisone (another glucocorticoid) to relieve the inflammation and the compression of her glomeruli. Fortunately, after several such "pulses," Rena's urine volume began to increase, her creatinine clearance, BUN, and serum creatinine improved, and her metabolic acidosis slowly resolved. Within 4 months, she had regained her health and did not need steroids or antihypertensive medications.

Katta Bolic, a 62-year-old homeless woman, was found by a neighborhood child who heard Katta's moans coming from an abandoned building. The child's mother called the police, who took Katta to the hospital emergency room. The patient was semicomatose, incontinent of urine, and her clothes were stained with vomitus. She had a fever of 103°F, was trembling uncontrollably, appeared to be severely dehydrated, and had marked muscle wasting. Her heart rate was very rapid, and her blood pressure was low (85/46 mm Hg). Her abdomen was distended and without bowel sounds. She responded to moderate pressure on her abdomen with moaning and grimacing.

Blood was sent for a broad laboratory profile, and cultures of her urine, stool, throat, and blood were taken. Intravenous glucose, saline, and parenteral broad spectrum antibiotics were begun. X-rays performed after her vital signs were stabilized suggested a bowel perforation. These findings were compatible with a diagnosis of a ruptured viscus (e.g., an infected colonic diverticulum which perforated, allowing colonic bacteria to infect the tissues of the peritoneal cavity causing peritonitis). Further studies confirmed that a diverticulum had ruptured, and appropriate surgery was performed. All of the arterial blood cultures grew out *Escherichia coli*, indicating that Katta also had a Gram-negative infection of her blood (septicemia) which had been seeded by the proliferating organisms in her peritoneal cavity. Intensive fluid and electrolyte therapy and antibiotic coverage were continued. The medical team (surgeons, internists, and nutritionists) began developing a complex therapeutic plan to reverse Katta's severely catabolic state.

MAINTENANCE OF THE FREE AMINO ACID POOL IN BLOOD

The body maintains a relatively large free amino acid pool in the blood, even in the absence of an intake of dietary protein. The large free amino acid pool ensures the continuous availability of individual amino acids to tissues for the synthesis of proteins, neurotransmitters, and other nitrogen-containing compounds (Fig. 42.2). In a normal, well-fed, healthy individual, about 300–600 g of body protein is degraded

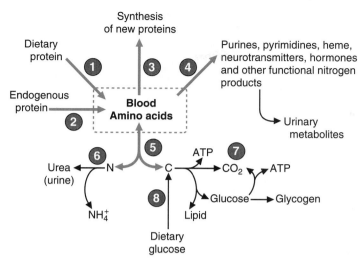

Fig. 42.2. Maintenance of the blood amino acid pool. Dietary protein (**1**) and degradation of endogenous protein (**2**) provide a source of indispensable amino acids (those which cannot be synthesized in the human). **3.** The synthesis of new protein is the major use of amino acids from the free amino acid pool. **4.** Compounds synthesized from amino acid precursors are essential for physiological functions. Many of these compounds are degraded to N-containing urinary metabolites and do not return to the free amino acid pool. **5.** In tissues, the nitrogen is removed from amino acids by transamination and deamination reactions. **6.** The nitrogen from amino acid degradation appears in the urine primarily as urea or NH_4^+, the ammonium ion. Ammonia excretion is necessary to maintain the pH of the blood. **7.** Amino acids are used as fuels either directly or after being converted to glucose by gluconeogenesis. **8.** Some amino acids can be synthesized in the human, provided that glucose and a nitrogen source are available.

per day. At the same time, about 100 g of protein is consumed in the diet per day, which adds additional amino acids. From this pool, tissues utilize amino acids for the continuous synthesis of new proteins (300–600 g) to replace those degraded. The continuous turnover of proteins in the body makes the complete complement of amino acids available for the synthesis of new and different proteins, such as antibodies. Protein turnover allows shifts in the quantities of different proteins produced in tissues in response to changes in physiological state, and continuously removes modified or damaged proteins. It also provides a complete pool of specific amino acids which can be utilized as oxidizable substrates: precursors for gluconeogenesis and for heme, creatine phosphate, purine, pyrimidine, and neurotransmitter synthesis; for ammoniagenesis to maintain blood pH levels; and for numerous other functions.

Interorgan Flux of Amino Acids in the Postabsorptive State

The fasting state provides an example of the interorgan flux of amino acids necessary to maintain the free amino acid pool in the blood and supply tissues with their required amino acids (Fig. 42.3). During an overnight fast, protein synthesis in the liver and other tissues continues, but at a diminished rate compared to the postprandial state. Net degradation of labile protein occurs in skeletal muscle (which contains the body's largest protein mass) and other tissues.

RELEASE OF AMINO ACIDS FROM SKELETAL MUSCLE DURING FASTING

The efflux of amino acids from skeletal muscle supports the essential amino acid pool

The concentration of free amino acids in the blood is not nearly as rigidly controlled as blood glucose levels. The free amino acid pool in the blood is only a small part (0.5%) of the total amino acid pool in whole body protein. Due to the large skeletal muscle mass, about 80% of the body's total protein is in skeletal muscle. Consequently, the concentration of individual amino acids in the blood is strongly affected by the rates of protein synthesis and degradation in skeletal muscle, as well as the rate of uptake and utilization of individual amino acids for metabolism in liver and other tissues. For the most part, changes in the rate of protein synthesis and degradation take place over a time span of hours.

 42.1: The hormonal changes that occur during an overnight fast include a decrease of blood insulin levels and an increase of glucagon relative to levels after a high carbohydrate meal. Glucocorticoid levels also increase in the blood. These hormones coordinate the changes of fat, carbohydrate, and amino acid metabolism. Fatty acids are released from adipose triacylglycerols and are utilized as the major fuel by heart, skeletal muscle, liver, and other tissues. The liver converts some of the fatty acids to ketone bodies. Liver glycogen stores are diminished, and gluconeogenesis becomes the major support of blood glucose levels for glucose-dependent tissues. The major precursors of gluconeogenesis include amino acids released from skeletal muscle, lactate, and glycerol.

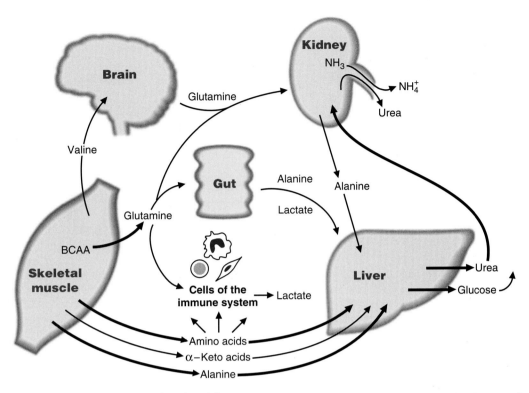

Fig. 42.3. Interorgan amino acid exchange after an overnight fast. After an overnight fast, (the postabsorptive state), the utilization of amino acids for protein synthesis, for fuels, and for the synthesis of essential functional compounds continues. The free amino acid pool is supported largely by net degradation of skeletal muscle protein. Glutamine and alanine serve as amino group carriers from skeletal muscle to other tissues. Glutamine brings NH_4^+ to the kidney for the excretion of protons, and serves as a fuel for the kidney, gut, and cells of the immune system. Alanine transfers amino groups from skeletal muscle, the kidney, and the gut to the liver, where they are converted to urea for excretion. The brain continues to use amino acids for neurotransmitter synthesis.

in the blood (see Fig. 42.3). Skeletal muscle oxidizes the branched chain amino acids (valine, leucine, isoleucine) to produce energy and glutamine. The amino groups of the branched chain amino acids (BCAA), and of aspartate and glutamate, are transferred out of skeletal muscle in alanine and glutamine. Alanine and glutamine account for about 50% of the total α-amino nitrogen released by skeletal muscle (Fig. 42.4).

The release of amino acids from skeletal muscle is stimulated during an overnight fast by the decrease of insulin and increase of glucocorticoid levels in the blood. Insulin promotes the uptake of amino acids and the general synthesis of proteins. The mechanisms for the stimulation of protein synthesis in human skeletal muscle are not all known, but probably include an activation of the A system for amino acid transport (a modest effect), a general effect on initiation of translation, and an inhibition of lysosomal proteolysis. The fall of blood insulin levels during an overnight fast results in net proteolysis and release of amino acids. As glucocorticoids increase, there is also an induction of ubiquitin synthesis and an increase of ubiquitin-dependent proteolysis.

AMINO ACID METABOLISM IN LIVER DURING FASTING

The major site of alanine uptake is the liver, which disposes of the amino nitrogen by incorporating it into urea (see Fig. 42.3). The liver also extracts free amino acids, α-keto acids, and some glutamine from the blood. Alanine and other amino acids are oxidized and their carbon skeletons converted principally to glucose. Glucagon and glucocorticoids stimulate the uptake of amino acids into liver and increase gluconeogenesis and ureagenesis (Fig. 42.5). Alanine transport into the liver, in particular, is enhanced by glucagon. The induction of the synthesis of gluconeogenic enzymes by glucagon and glucocorticoids during the overnight fast correlates with an induction of many of the enzymes of amino acid degradation (e.g., tyrosine aminotransferase), and an induction of urea cycle enzymes (see Chapter 38). Urea synthesis also increases because of the increased supply of NH_4^+ from amino acid degradation in the liver.

METABOLISM OF AMINO ACIDS IN OTHER TISSUES DURING FASTING

Glucose, produced by the liver, is utilized for energy by the brain and other glucose-dependent tissues, such as lymphocytes. The muscle also oxidizes some of this glucose to pyruvate, which is used for the carbon skeleton of alanine (see Fig. 42.12)

Glutamine is generated in skeletal muscle from the oxidation of BCAA, and by the lungs and brain for the removal of NH_4^+ formed from amino acid catabolism or entering from the blood. The kidney, the gut, and cells with rapid turnover rates such as those of the immune system are the major sites of glutamine uptake (see Fig. 42.3). Glutamine serves as a fuel for these tissues, as a nitrogen donor for purine synthesis, and as a substrate for ammoniagenesis in the kidney. Much of the unused nitrogen from glutamine is transferred to pyruvate to form alanine in these tissues, and alanine carries the unused nitrogen back to the liver.

The brain is glucose dependent, but like many cells in the body can utilize BCAA for energy. The BCAA also provide a source of nitrogen for neurotransmitter synthesis during fasting. Other amino acids released from skeletal muscle protein degradation also serve as precursors of neurotransmitters.

Principles Governing Amino Acid Flux between Tissues

The pattern of interorgan flux of amino acids is strongly affected by conditions which change the supply of fuels (for example the overnight fast, a mixed meal, a high protein meal), and by conditions which increase the demand for amino acids (metabolic

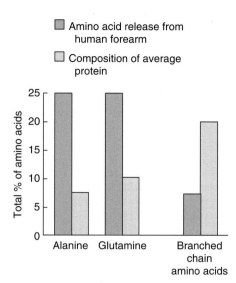

Fig. 42.4. Amino acid release from skeletal muscle. The arteriovenous difference (concentration in arterial blood minus the concentration in venous blood) across the human forearm has been measured for many amino acids. This graph compares the amount of alanine, glutamine, and BCAA released to their composition in the average protein. Alanine and glutamine represent a much higher percentage of total nitrogen released than originally present in the degraded protein, evidence that they are being synthesized in the skeletal muscle. The BCAA (leucine, valine, and isoleucine) are released in much lower amounts than are present in the degraded protein, evidence that they are being catabolized. Aspartate and glutamate also contribute nitrogen to the formation of alanine and glutamine.

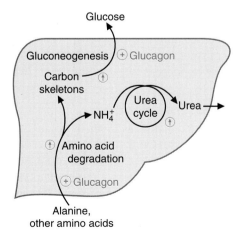

Fig. 42.5. Hormonal regulation of hepatic amino acid metabolism in the postabsorptive state. $\oplus$ = glucagon-mediated activation of enzymes or proteins; circled↑ = induction of enzyme synthesis mediated by glucagon and glucocorticoids. Induction of urea cycle enzymes occurs both during fasting and after a high protein meal. Since many individuals in the United States normally have a high protein diet, the levels of urea cycle enzymes may not fluctuate to any great extent.

Q 42.2: The body normally produces about 1 mmol of protons per kilogram of body weight per day. Nevertheless, the pH of the blood and extracellular fluid is normally maintained between 7.36 and 7.44. The narrow range is maintained principally by the bicarbonate (HCO_3^-) and phosphate (HPO_4^-) and hemoglobin buffering systems, and by the excretion of an amount of acid equal to that produced. The excretion of protons by the kidney regenerates bicarbonate, which can be reclaimed from the glomerular filtrate.

The acids are produced from normal fuel metabolism. The major acid is carbonic acid, which is formed from water and CO_2 produced in the TCA cycle and other oxidative pathways. The oxidation of sulfur-containing amino acids (methionine and cysteine) ultimately produces sulfuric acid (H_2SO_4), which dissociates into $2H^+ + SO_4^{2-}$, and the protons and sulfate are excreted. The hydrolysis of phosphate esters produces the equivalent of phosphoric acid. What other acids produced during metabolism appear in the blood?

Table 42.1. Functions of Glutamine

Protein synthesis
Ammoniagenesis for proton excretion
Nitrogen donor for synthesis of
    Purines
    Pyrimidines
    NAD^+
    Amino sugars
    Asparagine
    Other compounds
Glutamate donor for synthesis of
    Glutathione
    GABA
    Ornithine
    Arginine
    Proline
    Other compounds

acidosis, surgical stress, traumatic injury, burns, wound healing, and sepsis). The flux of amino acid carbon and nitrogen in these different conditions is dictated by several considerations:

1. Ammonia (NH_4^+) is toxic. Consequently, it is transported between tissues as alanine or glutamine. Alanine is the principal carrier of amino acid nitrogen from other tissues back to the liver, where the nitrogen is converted to urea and subsequently excreted into the urine by the kidneys. The amount of urea synthesized is proportional to the amount of amino acid carbon that is being oxidized as a fuel.

2. The pool of glutamine in the blood serves several essential metabolic functions (Table 42.1). It provides ammonia for excretion of protons in the urine as NH_4^+. It serves as a fuel for the gut, the kidney, and the cells of the immune system. Glutamine is also required by the cells of the immune system and other rapidly dividing cells in which its amide group serves as the source of nitrogen for biosynthetic reactions. In the brain, the formation of glutamine from glutamate and NH_4^+ provides a means of removing ammonia and of transporting glutamate between cells in the brain. The utilization of the blood glutamine pool is prioritized. During metabolic acidosis the kidney becomes the predominant site of glutamine uptake, at the expense of glutamine utilization in other tissues. On the other hand, during sepsis, cells involved in the immune response (macrophages, hepatocytes) become the preferential sites of glutamine uptake.

3. The BCAA (valine, leucine, and isoleucine) form a significant portion of the average protein, and can be converted to tricarboxylic acid (TCA) cycle intermediates and utilized as fuels by almost all tissues. They are also the major precursors of glutamine. Except for the BCAA and alanine, aspartate, and glutamate, the catabolism of amino acids occurs principally in the liver.

4. Amino acids are major gluconeogenic substrates, and most of the energy obtained from their oxidation is derived from oxidation of the glucose formed from their carbon skeletons. A much smaller percentage of amino acid carbon is converted to acetyl CoA or to ketone bodies and oxidized. The utilization of amino acids for glucose synthesis for the brain and other glucose-requiring tissues is subject to the hormonal regulatory mechanisms of glucose homeostasis.

5. The relative rates of protein synthesis and degradation (protein turnover) determine the size of the free amino acid pools available for the synthesis of new proteins and for other essential functions. For example, the synthesis of new proteins to mount an immune response is supported by the net degradation of other proteins in the body.

The pattern of amino acid flux between tissues is determined by the specific amino acid requirements of different tissues as their metabolic activities change and by metabolic changes in the tissues that serve as the source of these amino acids. As either need or dietary state changes, the pattern of amino acid flux changes. These changes are facilitated by the hormonal response to dietary intake (insulin and glucagon) and to physiological stress (glucocorticoids, epinephrine, and triiodothyronine). The levels of amino acids, fatty acids, glucose, and other compounds in the blood also influence amino acid utilization by individual tissues.

UTILIZATION OF AMINO ACIDS IN INDIVIDUAL TISSUES

Because tissues differ in their physiological functions, they have different amino acid requirements and contribute differently to whole body nitrogen metabolism.

However, all tissues share a common requirement for essential amino acids for protein synthesis, and protein turnover is an ongoing process in all cells.

Kidney

One of the primary roles of amino acid nitrogen is to provide ammonia in the kidney for the excretion of protons in the urine. NH_4^+ is released from glutamine by glutaminase and by glutamate dehydrogenase, resulting in the formation of α-ketoglutarate (Fig. 42.6). α-Ketoglutarate is used as a fuel by the kidney and is oxidized to CO_2, converted to glucose for use in cells in the renal medulla, or converted to alanine to return ammonia to the liver for urea synthesis.

USE OF GLUTAMINE NITROGEN TO BUFFER URINE

The rate of glutamine uptake from the blood and its utilization by the kidney depends principally on the amount of acid which must be excreted to maintain a normal pH in the blood. During a metabolic acidosis, the excretion of NH_4^+ by the kidney increases severalfold (Table 42.2). Because glutamine nitrogen provides about two-thirds of the NH_4^+ excreted by the kidney, glutamine uptake by the kidney also increases. Renal glutamine utilization for proton excretion takes precedence over the requirements of other tissues for glutamine.

Ammonia increases proton excretion by providing a buffer for protons which are transported into the renal tubular fluid (which is transformed into urine as it passes through the tubules of the kidney) (Fig. 42.7). Specific transporters in the membranes of the renal tubular cells transport protons from these cells into the tubular lumen in exchange for Na^+. The protons in the tubular fluid are buffered by phosphate, by bicarbonate, and by ammonia. Ammonia (NH_3), which is uncharged, enters the urine by free diffusion through the cell membrane. As it combines with a proton in the fluid, it forms ammonium ion (NH_4^+), which cannot be transported back into the cells and is excreted in the urine.

GLUTAMINE AS A FUEL FOR THE KIDNEY

Glutamine is used as a fuel by the kidney in the normal fed state, and to a greater extent during fasting and metabolic acidosis (Table 42.3). The carbon skeleton forms α-ketoglutarate, which is oxidized to CO_2, converted to glucose, or released as the carbon skeleton of serine or alanine (Fig. 42.8). α-Ketoglutarate can be converted to oxaloacetate by TCA cycle reactions, and oxaloacetate is converted to phosphoenolpyruvate (PEP) by PEP carboxykinase. PEP can then be converted to pyruvate and subsequently acetyl CoA, alanine, serine, or glucose. The glucose is utilized principally by the cells of the renal medulla, which have a relatively high dependence on anaerobic glycolysis due to their lower oxygen supply and mitochondrial capacity. The lactate released from anaerobic glycolysis in these cells is taken up and oxidized

The differences in amino acid metabolism between tissues are dictated by the types and amounts of different enzyme and transport proteins present in each tissue and the ability of each tissue to respond to different regulatory messages (hormones and neural signals).

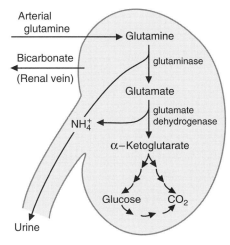

Fig. 42.6. Renal glutamine metabolism. Renal tubule cells preferentially oxidize glutamine. During metabolic acidosis, it is the major fuel for the kidney. Conversion of glutamine to α-ketoglutarate generates NH_4^+. Ammonium ion excretion helps to buffer systemic acidemia.

Table 42.3. Major Fuel Sources for the Kidney

Fuel	% of Total CO_2 Formed in Different Physiological States[a]		
	Normal	Acidosis	Fasted
Lactate	45	20	15
Glucose	25	20	0
Fatty acids	15	20	60
Glutamine	15	40	25

[a]Glucose utilized in the renal medulla is produced in the renal cortex.

42.2: Lactic acid is produced from glucose and amino acid metabolism, and the ketone bodies (acetoacetate and β-hydroxybutyrate) are acids. Many α-keto acids are also found in the blood.

Table 42.2. Excretion of Compounds in the Urine

Component	g/24 hrs	Nitrogen (mmol)
H_2O	1000	–
$SO_4^=$	2–5	–
$PO_4^=$	2–5	–
K^+	1–2	–
Urea	12–40	400–1300
Creatinine	1–1.8	25–50
Uric acid	0.5–1	10–20
NH_4^+	0.4–1 (up to 10 in acidosis)	22–55 (up to 550 in acidosis)

To maintain acid-base balance, the quantity of net acid excreted (the sum of H^+ bound to filtered buffers like phosphate and ammonia) must equal the quantity of acid entering the body fluids from all sources.

Rena Felya's metabolic acidosis developed as this delicate balance was upset by the inability of her kidneys to accomplish sufficient net acid excretion.

In the kidney, the rate of glutamine uptake from the blood is regulated by the pH of the blood and by glucocorticoid levels. Glutamine transport into kidney cells is principally Na^+ dependent and affected by the electrochemical potential of the plasma membrane. As the proton level of the blood increases (pH decreases), the membrane potential is altered and glutamine uptake increases. Increased blood glucocorticoid levels promote glutamine uptake by increasing mRNA levels for glutaminase. Glutaminase cleaves glutamine to NH_4^+ and glutamate, thereby decreasing the level of glutamine in the cell and increasing its rate of uptake.

During an overnight fast, the release of ketone bodies and other acids into the blood increases. This production of acids results in a mild metabolic acidosis during prolonged fasting (starvation). The acidosis and the elevation of glucocorticoid levels enhance glutamine uptake to compensate for the increased acidosis.

The acidosis experienced by **Rena Felya** is caused principally by her diminished glomerular filtration rate due to the PSGN. Protons and ammonia are not as rapidly entering the glomerular filtrate (which is transformed into urine). As a consequence, the type of compensatory response to metabolic acidosis which occurs in healthy individuals in the fasting state is unable to correct her metabolic acidosis.

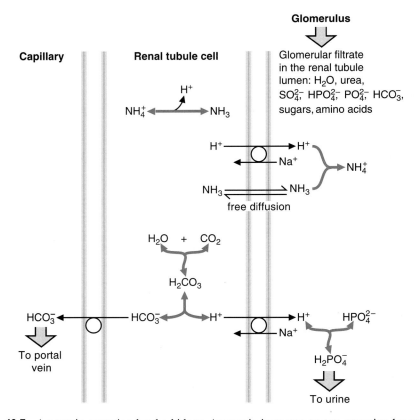

Fig. 42.7. Ammonia excretion by the kidney. Ammonia increases proton excretion by combining with a proton to form ammonium ion in the renal tubular fluid, which is transformed into urine as it passes through the tubules of the kidney. As blood is filtered in the capillary bed of the glomerulus, urea, sugars, amino acids, ions, and H_2O enter the renal tubular fluid (glomerular filtrate). As this fluid passes through a progression of tubules (the proximal convoluted tubule, the loop of Henle, the distal convoluted tubule, and the collecting duct) on its way to becoming urine, various components are reabsorbed or added to the filtrate by the epithelial cells lining the tubules. Specific transporters in the membranes of the renal tubule cells transport protons into the tubule lumen in exchange for Na^+ so that the glomerular filtrate becomes more acidic as it is transformed into urine. The protons in the tubule fluid are buffered by phosphate, by bicarbonate, and by NH_3. The ammonia, which is uncharged, is able to diffuse through the membrane of the renal tubule cells into the urine. As it combines with a proton in the urine, it forms NH_4^+, which cannot be transported back into the cells. The removal of protons as NH_4^+ decreases the requirement for bicarbonate excretion to buffer the urine.

in the renal cortical cells, which have a higher mitochondrial capacity and a greater blood supply.

Skeletal Muscle

Skeletal muscle, because of its large mass, is a major site of protein synthesis and degradation in the human. After a high protein meal, insulin promotes the uptake of certain amino acids and stimulates net protein synthesis. During fasting and other catabolic states, a net degradation of skeletal muscle protein and release of amino acids occur (see Fig. 42.3). The net degradation of protein affects functional proteins, like myosin, which are sacrificed to meet more urgent demands for amino acids in other tissues. During sepsis, degradation of skeletal muscle protein is stimulated by

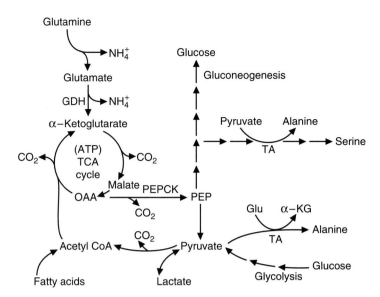

Fig. 42.8. Metabolism of glutamine and other fuels in the kidney. To completely oxidize glutamate carbon to CO_2, it must enter the TCA cycle as acetyl CoA. Carbon entering the TCA cycle as α-ketoglutarate (α-KG) exits as oxaloacetate, and is converted to phosphoenolpyruvate (PEP) by PEP carboxykinase. PEP is converted to pyruvate, which may be oxidized to acetyl CoA. PEP can also be converted to serine, glucose, or alanine. GDH = glutamate dehydrogenase; PEPCK = phosphoenolpyruvate carboxykinase; TA = transaminase; OAA = oxaloacetate.

Katta Bolic was in a severe stage of negative nitrogen balance on admission caused by both her malnourished state and her intraabdominal infection complicated by sepsis. The physiological response to her advanced catabolic status includes a degradation of muscle protein with the release of amino acids into the blood. This release is coupled with an increased uptake of amino acids for "acute phase" protein synthesis by the liver (systemic response) and other cells involved in the immune response to general and severe infection.

The ability to convert 4-carbon intermediates of the TCA cycle to pyruvate is required for oxidation of both BCAA and glutamine. This sequence of reactions requires PEP carboxykinase, or decarboxylating malate dehydrogenase (malic enzyme). Most tissues have one, or both, of these enzymes.

the glucocorticoid cortisol. The effect of cortisol is exerted through the activation of ubiquitin-dependent proteolysis. During fasting, the decrease of blood insulin levels and the increase of blood cortisol levels increase net protein degradation.

Skeletal muscle is a major site of glutamine synthesis, thereby satisfying the demand for glutamine during the postabsorptive state, during metabolic acidosis, and during septic stress and trauma. The carbon skeleton and nitrogen of glutamine are derived principally from the metabolism of BCAA. Amino acid degradation in skeletal muscle is also accompanied by the formation of alanine, which transfers amino groups from skeletal muscle to the liver in the glucose-alanine cycle.

OXIDATION OF BRANCHED CHAIN AMINO ACIDS IN SKELETAL MUSCLE

The BCAA play a special role in muscle and most other tissues because they are the major amino acids which can be oxidized in tissues other than the liver. (However, all tissues can interconvert amino acids and TCA cycle intermediates via transaminase reactions, i.e., alanine ↔ pyruvate, aspartate ↔ oxaloacetate, and α-ketoglutarate ↔ glutamate.) The first step of the pathway, transamination of the BCAA to α-keto acids, occurs principally in brain, heart, kidney, and skeletal muscles. These tissues have a high content of BCAA transaminase relative to the low levels in liver. The α-keto acids of the BCAA are then either released into the blood and taken up by liver, or oxidized to CO_2 or glutamine within the muscle or other tissue (Fig. 42.9). They can be oxidized by all tissues that contain mitochondria.

The oxidative pathways of the BCAA convert the carbon skeleton to either succinyl CoA or acetyl CoA (see Chapter 39 and Fig. 42.9). The pathways generate NADH and FAD(2H) for ATP synthesis prior to the conversion of carbon into intermediates of the TCA cycle, thus providing the muscle with energy. Leucine is "keto-

In an acidosis, such as that experienced by **Rena Felya**, the amount of glutamine which is formed from the degradation of BCAA depends on the free ammonia levels in the tissue, the pH of the blood, and the supply of BCAA. In an acidosis, the proportion of BCAA carbon released into the blood as glutamine increases, and the proportion released as the α-keto acids decreases.

The glucocorticoid cortisol contributes to the increase of glutamine formation by inducing the synthesis of glutamine synthetase, and by stimulating protein degradation, thereby increasing the availability of the BCAA and their α-keto acids formed via transamination reactions. The α-keto acid of one of the BCAA, leucine, is an activator of the branched chain amino acid dehydrogenase complex.

The branched chain α-keto acid dehydrogenase complex, the enzyme which catalyzes the oxidative decarboxylation of the BCAA, is the rate-limiting step in the oxidative pathway (see Chapter 39). Like the pyruvate dehydrogenase complex, which catalyzes a similar reaction, this enzyme is controlled through the actions of a bound kinase and a bound phosphatase which regulate its conversion to an inactive phosphorylated form. The BCAA α-keto acid dehydrogenase complex can be activated by increased levels of the α-keto acid of leucine, which inhibit the bound kinase.

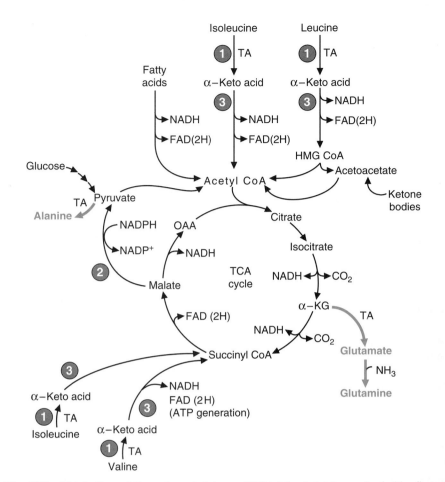

Fig. 42.9. Metabolism of the carbon skeletons of BCAA in skeletal muscle. **1.** The first step in the metabolism of BCAA is transamination (TA). **2.** Carbon from valine and isoleucine enters the TCA cycle as succinyl CoA and is converted to pyruvate by decarboxylating malate dehydrogenase. **3.** The oxidative pathways generate NADH and FAD(2H) even before the carbon skeleton enters the TCA cycle. The rate-limiting enzyme in the oxidative pathways is the α-keto acid dehydrogenase complex. The carbon skeleton can also be converted to glutamate and alanine, shown in blue.

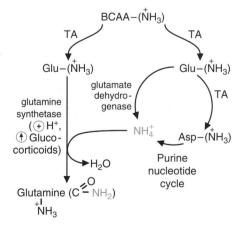

Fig. 42.10. Formation of glutamine from the amino groups of BCAA. TA = transamination.

genic" in that it is converted to acetyl CoA and acetoacetate. Skeletal muscle, adipocytes, and most other tissues are able to utilize these products and, therefore, directly oxidize leucine to CO_2. The portion of isoleucine converted to acetyl CoA is also oxidized directly to CO_2. For the portion of valine and isoleucine that enters the TCA cycle as succinyl CoA to be completely oxidized to CO_2, it must first be converted to acetyl CoA. To form acetyl CoA, succinyl CoA is oxidized to malate in the TCA cycle, and malate is then converted to pyruvate by decarboxylating malate dehydrogenase (malate + $NADP^+$ → pyruvate + NADPH + H^+) (see Fig. 42.9). Pyruvate can then be oxidized to acetyl CoA. Alternatively, pyruvate can form alanine or lactate.

CONVERSION OF BRANCHED CHAIN AMINO ACIDS TO GLUTAMINE

The major route of valine and isoleucine catabolism in skeletal muscle is to enter the TCA cycle as succinyl CoA and exit as α-ketoglutarate to provide the carbon skeleton for glutamine formation (see Fig. 42.9). Some of the glutamine and CO_2 which is formed from net protein degradation in skeletal muscle may also arise from the carbon skeletons of aspartate and glutamate. These amino acids are transaminated, and become part of the pool of 4-carbon intermediates of the TCA cycle.

Glutamine nitrogen is derived principally from the BCAA (Fig. 42.10). The α-amino group arises from transamination reactions which form glutamate from α-ketoglutarate, and the amide nitrogen is formed from the addition of free ammonia to glutamate by glutamine synthetase. Free ammonia in skeletal muscle arises principally from the deamination of glutamate by glutamate dehydrogenase, or from the purine nucleotide cycle.

In the purine nucleotide cycle (Fig. 42.11), the deamination of AMP to IMP releases NH_4^+. AMP is resynthesized with amino groups provided from aspartate. The aspartate amino groups can arise from the BCAA via transamination reactions.

GLUCOSE-ALANINE CYCLE

The nitrogen arising from the oxidation of BCAA in skeletal muscle can also be transferred back to the liver as alanine in the glucose-alanine cycle (Fig. 42.12). The amino group of the BCAA is first transferred to α-ketoglutarate to form glutamate, and then transferred to pyruvate to form alanine by sequential transamination reactions. The pyruvate arises principally from glucose via the glycolytic pathway. The alanine released from skeletal muscle is taken up principally by the liver, where the amino group is incorporated into urea and the carbon skeleton can be converted back to glucose via gluconeogenesis. Although the amount of alanine formed varies with dietary intake and physiological state, the transport of nitrogen from skeletal muscle to liver as alanine occurs almost continuously throughout our daily fasting-feeding cycle.

Gut

Amino acids are an important fuel for the intestinal mucosal cells following a protein-containing meal, and in catabolic states such as fasting or surgical trauma (Fig. 42.13). During fasting, glutamine is one of the major amino acids utilized by the gut. The principal fates of glutamine carbon in the gut are oxidation to CO_2 and conversion to the carbon skeletons of lactate, citrulline, and ornithine. The gut also oxidizes BCAA. Nitrogen derived from amino acid degradation is converted to citrulline, ala-

 The purine nucleotide cycle is found in skeletal muscle and brain, but is absent in liver and many other tissues. One of its functions in skeletal muscle is to respond to the rapid utilization of ATP during exercise. During exercise the rapid hydrolysis of ATP increases AMP levels, resulting in an activation of AMP deaminase (see Fig. 42.11). As a consequence, the cellular concentration of IMP increases, and ammonia is generated. IMP, like AMP, activates muscle glycogen phosphorylase during exercise (see Chapter 22). The ammonia which is generated may help to buffer the increased lactic acid production occurring in skeletal muscles during strenuous exercise.

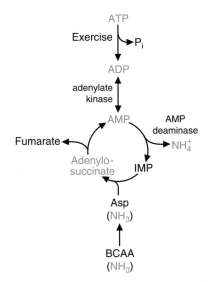

Fig. 42.11. Purine nucleotide cycle. In skeletal muscle, the purine nucleotide cycle can convert the amino groups of the BCAA to NH_4^+, which is incorporated into glutamine. The compounds containing the amino group released in the purine nucleotide cycle are shown in blue.

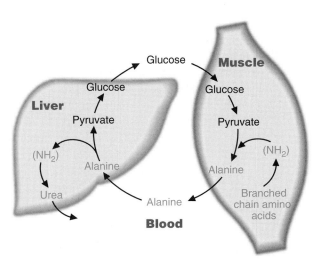

Fig. 42.12. Glucose-alanine cycle. The pathway for transfer of the amino groups from BCAA in skeletal muscle to urea in the liver is shown in blue.

Q 42.3: When the carbon skeleton of alanine is derived from glucose, the efflux of alanine from skeletal muscle and its uptake by liver provide no net transfer of amino acid carbon to the liver for gluconeogenesis. However, some of the alanine carbon is derived from sources other than glucose. Which amino acids can provide carbon for alanine formation? (Hint: See Fig. 42.9.)

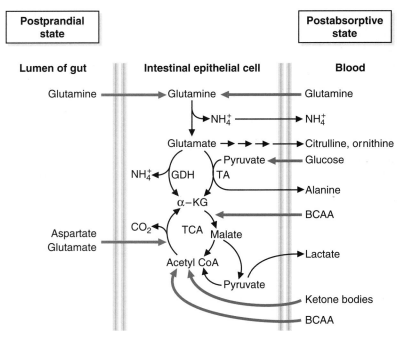

Fig. 42.13. Amino acid metabolism in the gut. The pathways of glutamine metabolism in the gut are the same whether it is supplied by the diet (postprandial state) or from the blood (postabsorptive state). Cells of the gut also metabolize aspartate, glutamate, and BCAA. Glucose is converted principally to the carbon skeleton of alanine. α-KG = α-ketoglutarate; GDH = glutamate dehydrogenase; TA = transaminase.

nine, NH_4^+, and other compounds which are released into the blood and taken up by the liver. Although most of the carbon in this alanine is derived from glucose, the oxidation of glucose to CO_2 is not a major fuel pathway for the gut. Fatty acids are also not a significant source of fuel for the intestinal mucosal cells, although they do utilize ketone bodies.

After a protein meal, dietary glutamine is a major fuel for the gut, and the products of glutamine metabolism are similar to those seen in the postabsorptive state. The gut also utilizes dietary aspartate and glutamate, which enter the TCA cycle. Colonocytes (the cells of the colon) also utilize short chain fatty acids, derived from bacterial action in the lumen.

The importance of the gut in whole body nitrogen metabolism arises from the high rate of division and death of intestinal mucosal cells, and the need to continuously provide these cells with amino acids to sustain the high rates of protein synthesis required for cellular division. Not only are these cells important for the uptake of nutrients, but they maintain a barrier against invading bacteria from the gut lumen and are, therefore, part of our passive defense system. As a result of these important functions, the intestinal mucosal cells are supplied with the amino acids required for protein synthesis and fuel oxidation at the expense of the more expendable skeletal muscle protein.

Liver

The liver is the major site of amino acid metabolism. It is the major site of amino acid catabolism, and converts most of the carbon in amino acids to intermediates of the TCA cycle or the glycolytic pathway (which can be converted to glucose or oxidized to CO_2), or to acetyl CoA and ketone bodies. The liver is also the major site for urea

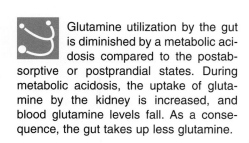

Glutamine utilization by the gut is diminished by a metabolic acidosis compared to the postabsorptive or postprandial states. During metabolic acidosis, the uptake of glutamine by the kidney is increased, and blood glutamine levels fall. As a consequence, the gut takes up less glutamine.

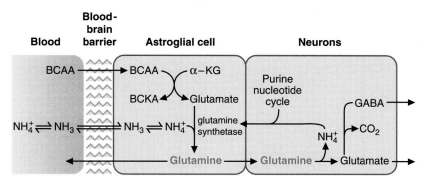

Fig. 42.14. Role of glutamine in the brain. Glutamine serves as a nitrogen transporter in the brain for the synthesis of many different neurotransmitters. Different neurons convert glutamine to γ-aminobutyric acid (GABA) or to glutamate. Glutamine also transports excess NH_4^+ from the brain into the blood. BCKA = branched chain keto acids; α-KG = α-ketoglutarate.

synthesis, and can take up both glutamine and alanine and convert the nitrogen to urea for disposal (see Chapter 38). Other pathways in the liver provide it with an unusually high amino acid requirement. The liver synthesizes plasma proteins, such as serum albumin, transferrin, and the proteins of the blood coagulation cascade. It is a major site for the synthesis of nonessential amino acids, the conjugation of xenobiotic compounds with glycine, the synthesis of heme and purine nucleotides, and the synthesis of glutathione.

Brain and Nervous Tissue

AMINO ACID POOL AND NEUROTRANSMITTER SYNTHESIS

A major function of amino acid metabolism in neural tissue is the synthesis of neurotransmitters. More than 40 compounds are believed to function as neurotransmitters, and all of these contain nitrogen derived from precursor amino acids. They include amino acids which are themselves neurotransmitters (e.g., glutamate, glycine), the catecholamines derived from tyrosine (dopamine and norepinephrine), serotonin (derived from tryptophan), GABA (derived from glutamate), acetylcholine (derived from choline synthesized in the liver and acetyl CoA), and many peptides. In general, neurotransmitters are formed in the presynaptic terminals of axons and stored in vesicles until released by a transient change in electrochemical potential along the axon. Subsequent catabolism of some of the neurotransmitter results in the formation of a urinary excretion product. The rapid metabolism of neurotransmitters requires the continuous availability of a precursor pool of amino acids for de novo neurotransmitter synthesis.

METABOLISM OF GLUTAMINE IN THE BRAIN

The brain is a net glutamine producer owing principally to the presence of glutamine synthetase in astroglial cells. Glutamate and aspartate are synthesized in these cells utilizing amino groups donated by the BCAA (principally valine) and TCA cycle intermediates formed from glucose and from the carbon skeletons of BCAA (Fig. 42.14) The glutamate is converted to glutamine by glutamine synthetase, which incorporates NH_4^+ released from deamination of amino acids and deamination of AMP in the purine nucleotide cycle in the brain. This glutamine may efflux from the brain, carrying excess NH_4^+ into the blood, or serve as a precursor of glutamate in neuronal cells.

The levels of serum albumin and transferrin in the blood may be used as indicators of the degree of protein malnutrition. In the absence of hepatic disease, decreased levels of these proteins in the blood indicate insufficient availability of amino acids to the liver for synthesis of serum proteins.

A 42.3: Some of the alanine released from skeletal muscle is derived directly from protein degradation. The carbon skeletons of valine, isoleucine, aspartate, and glutamate, which are converted to malate and oxaloacetate in the TCA cycle, can be converted to pyruvate and subsequently transaminated to alanine. The extent to which these amino acids contribute carbon to alanine efflux differs between different types of muscles in the human. These amino acids may also contribute to alanine efflux from the gut.

Q 42.4: In what ways does liver metabolism after a high protein meal resemble liver metabolism in the fasting state?

The rate of synthesis of neurotransmitters is usually independent of dietary supply of the precursor amino acid or the concentration of the precursor amino acid in the blood. The transport of amino acids across the blood-brain barrier is likewise not normally a rate-limiting factor in neurotransmitter synthesis, except in the presence of inhibitory drugs. The synthesis of serotonin from tryptophan may be an exception. The hydroxylase converting tryptophan to 5′-hydroxytryptophan has a high K_m for tryptophan, so that changes in tryptophan concentration could affect the rate of serotonin synthesis. For example, a reduction in the rate of tryptophan degradation in the liver in a patient with hepatic disease might increase blood tryptophan levels, resulting in higher serotonin levels in neural tissue.

Usually the rate of neurotransmitter synthesis within the neuron is regulated by a feedback mechanism which adjusts the supply of the neurotransmitter to the rate of firing of the nerve. Tyrosine hydroxylase, the rate-limiting enzyme in the synthesis of dopamine and norepinephrine, provides an example of an enzyme in neurotransmitter synthesis that is subject to feedback regulation. The enzyme has a very low K_m for tyrosine, and thus its rate is independent of tyrosine concentration in the physiological range present in neural tissue. However, depolarization of the neuronal membrane during firing of the neuron activates a kinase which phosphorylates the enzyme to an active form. Repetitive firing of the neuron also induces the synthesis of tyrosine hydroxylase.

During hyperammonemia, ammonia (NH_3) can diffuse into the brain from the blood. The ammonia is able to inhibit the neural isozyme of glutaminase, thereby decreasing additional ammonia formation in the brain and inhibiting the formation of glutamate and its subsequent metabolism to GABA. This effect of ammonia might contribute to the lethargy associated with the hyperammonemia found in patients with hepatic disease.

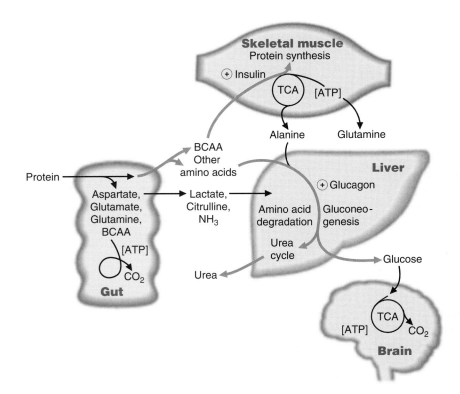

Fig. 42.15. Flux of amino acids after a high protein meal.

Glutamine synthesized in the astroglial cells is a precursor of glutamate (an excitatory neurotransmitter) and GABA (an inhibitory neurotransmitter) in the neuronal cells (see Fig. 42.14). It is converted to glutamate by a neuronal glutaminase isozyme. In GABAergic neurons, glutamate is then decarboxylated to GABA, which is released during excitation of the neuron. GABA is one of the neurotransmitters which is recycled; a transaminase converts it to succinaldehyde, which is then oxidized to succinate. Succinate enters the TCA cycle.

CHANGES IN AMINO ACID METABOLISM WITH DIETARY AND PHYSIOLOGICAL STATE

The rate and pattern of amino acid utilization by different tissues change with dietary and physiological state. Two such states, the postprandial period following a high protein meal and the hypercatabolic state produced by sepsis or surgical trauma, differ from the postabsorptive state with respect to the availability of amino acids and other fuels and the levels of different hormones in the blood. As a result, the pattern of amino acid utilization is somewhat different.

A High Protein Meal

Following the ingestion of a high protein meal, the gut and the liver utilize most of the absorbed amino acids (Fig. 42.15). Glutamate and aspartate are utilized as fuels by the gut, and very little enters the portal vein. The gut may also use some BCAA. The liver takes up 60–70% of the amino acids present in the portal vein. These amino acids, for the most part, are converted to glucose in the gluconeogenic pathway.

After a pure protein meal, the increased levels of dietary amino acids reaching the pancreas stimulate the release of glucagon above fasting levels, thereby increasing amino acid uptake into liver and stimulating gluconeogenesis. Insulin release is also stimulated, but not nearly to the levels found after a high carbohydrate meal. In general, the insulin released after a high protein meal is sufficiently high that the uptake of BCAA into skeletal muscle and net protein synthesis is stimulated, but gluconeogenesis in the liver is not inhibited. The higher the carbohydrate content of the meal, the higher the insulin/glucagon ratio and the greater the shift of amino acids away from gluconeogenesis into biosynthetic pathways in the liver such as the synthesis of plasma proteins.

Most of the amino acid nitrogen entering the peripheral circulation after a high protein meal or a mixed meal is present as the BCAA. Because the liver has low levels of transaminases for these amino acids, it cannot oxidize them to a significant extent and they enter the systemic circulation. The BCAA are slowly taken up by skeletal muscle and other tissues. These peripheral nonhepatic tissues utilize the amino acids derived from the diet principally for net protein synthesis.

Hypercatabolic States

Surgery, trauma, burns, and septic stress are examples of hypercatabolic states characterized by increased fuel utilization and a negative nitrogen balance (Fig. 42.16).

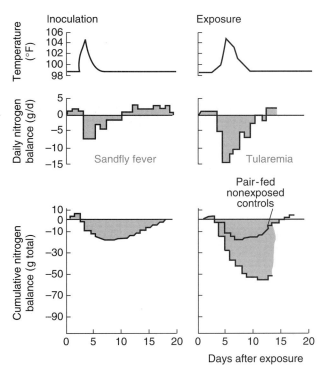

The degree of the body's hypercatabolic response depends upon the severity and duration of the trauma or stress. After an uncomplicated surgical procedure in an otherwise healthy patient, the net negative nitrogen balance may be limited to about 1 week. The mild nitrogen losses are usually reversed by dietary protein supplementation as the patient recovers. With more severe traumatic injury or septic stress, the body may catabolize body protein and adipose tissue lipids for a prolonged period and the negative nitrogen balance may not be corrected for weeks.

Fig. 42.16. Negative nitrogen balance during infection. The effects of experimentally induced infections on nitrogen balance were determined in human volunteers. After inoculation with sandfly fever, increased amino acid catabolism produced a negative nitrogen balance. A few days after exposure, the daily nitrogen balance became positive until the volunteers returned to their original state. Experiments with patients exposed to tularemia showed that the negative nitrogen balance was much larger than could be expected from a decreased appetite alone. Volunteers who ate the same amount of food as the infected individuals (pair-fed nonexposed controls) had a much smaller cumulative negative nitrogen balance than the infected volunteers. From Beisel WR. Am J Clin Nutr 1977;30:1236–1247. © 1977 American Society for Clinical Nutrition.

42.4: Both of these dietary states are characterized by an elevation of glucagon. Glucagon stimulates amino acid transport into the liver, stimulates gluconeogenesis through decreasing levels of fructose 2,6-bisphosphate, and induces the synthesis of enzymes in the urea cycle, the gluconeogenic pathway, and the pathways for degradation of some of the amino acids.

Katta Bolic's severe negative nitrogen balance was caused by both her malnourished state and her intraabdominal infection complicated by sepsis. The systemic and diverse responses the body makes to insults such as an acute febrile illness are termed the "acute phase response." An early event in this response is the stimulation of phagocytic activity (Fig. 42.17). Stimulated macrophages release cytokines, which are regulatory proteins that stimulate the release of cortisol, insulin, and growth hormone. Cytokines also directly mediate the acute phase response of the liver and skeletal muscle to sepsis.

The mobilization of body protein, fat, and carbohydrate stores serves to maintain normal tissue function in the presence of a limited dietary intake, as well as to support the energy and amino acid requirements for the immune response and wound healing. The negative nitrogen balance which occurs in these hypercatabolic states results from an accelerated protein turnover and an increased rate of net protein degradation, primarily in skeletal muscle.

The catabolic state of sepsis (acute, generalized, febrile infection) is one of enhanced mobilization of fuels and amino acids to provide the energy and precursors required by cells of the immune system, host defense mechanisms, and wound healing. The amino acids must provide the substrates for new protein synthesis and cell division. Glucose synthesis and release are enhanced to provide fuel for these cells and the patient may become mildly hyperglycemic.

In these hypercatabolic states, skeletal muscle protein synthesis decreases and protein degradation increases. Oxidation of BCAA is increased, and glutamine production enhanced. Amino acid uptake is diminished. Cortisol is the major hormonal mediator of these responses, although certain cytokines may also have direct effects on skeletal muscle metabolism. As occurs during fasting and metabolic acidosis, increased levels of cortisol stimulate ubiquitin-mediated proteolysis, induce the synthesis of glutamine synthetase, and enhance release of amino acids and glutamine from the muscle cells.

The amino acids released from skeletal muscle during periods of hypercatabolic stress are utilized in a prioritized manner, with the cellular components of the immune and antiinflammation systems receiving top priority. For example, the uptake of amino acids by the liver for the synthesis of acute phase proteins, which are part of the immune system, is greatly increased. On the other hand, during the early phase of the acute response, the synthesis of other plasma proteins (e.g., albumin) is decreased. The increased availability of amino acids and the increased cortisol levels also stimulate gluconeogenesis, thereby providing fuel for the glucose-dependent cells of the immune system (e.g., lymphocytes). An increase of urea synthesis accompanies the acceleration of amino acid degradation.

The increased efflux of glutamine from skeletal muscle during sepsis serves several functions (see Fig. 42.1). It provides the rapidly dividing cells of the immune system with an energy source. Glutamine is available as a nitrogen donor for purine synthesis, for NAD^+ synthesis, and for other biosynthetic functions essential to growth and division of the cells. An increased production of metabolic acids may accompany stress such as sepsis, so there is an increased utilization of glutamine by the kidney.

Under the influence of elevated levels of glucocorticoids, epinephrine, and glucagon, fatty acids are mobilized from adipose tissue to provide alternate fuels for other tissues and spare glucose. Under these conditions, fatty acids are the major energy source for skeletal muscle, and glucose uptake is decreased. These changes may lead to a mild hyperglycemia.

CLINICAL COMMENTS. In more than 90% of cases of poststreptococcal glomerulonephritis (PSGN), complete spontaneous recovery occurs with a diuresis (increase in urine output) occurring within 1 week. Fewer than 5% of patients have oliguria (reduced urine volume) lasting more than 8–10 days; in these patients the prognosis for full recovery of renal function is somewhat more guarded and their kidney biopsies frequently show the crescentic glomerular lesions. In spite of these ominous-appearing tissue changes, however, about half of these patients recover spontaneously with time. The remainder may show persistent proteinuria and progress to chronic renal insufficiency.

Rena Felya's nephrologist feared that she was entering a phase of rapid loss of renal function known as rapidly progressive glomerulonephritis (RPGN). Accurate prognosis and selection of appropriate therapy require that the underlying mechanism for RPGN be defined through kidney biopsy. About 40% of RPGN is caused by glomerular immune complex formation (usually in association with disorders like PSGN). The histological finding of glomerular crescent formation on Rena's kidney biopsy prompted the use of steroid therapy, a decision which contributed to the patient's full recovery.

The clinician can determine if a patient such as **Katta Bolic** is mounting an acute phase response to some insult, however subtle, by determining whether or not several unique acute phase proteins are being secreted by the liver. C-reactive protein, so named because of its ability to interact with the C-polysaccharide of pneumococci, and serum amyloid A protein, a precursor of the amyloid fibril found in secondary amyloidosis, are found only in patients undergoing the acute phase response and not in healthy individuals. Other proteins normally found in the blood of healthy individuals are present in increased concentrations in patients undergoing an acute phase response. These include haptoglobin, certain protease inhibitors, complement components, ceruloplasmin, and fibrinogen. The elevated concentration of these proteins in the blood increases the erythrocyte sedimentation rate (ESR), another laboratory measure of the presence of an acute phase response.

The weight loss often noted in septic patients is primarily due to a loss of appetite resulting from the effect of certain cytokines on the medullary appetite center. Other causes include an increased energy expenditure from fever, and enhanced muscle proteolysis.

BIOCHEMICAL COMMENTS. Following a catabolic insult such as injury, trauma, infection, or cancer, the interorgan flow of glutamine and fuels is dramatically altered. Teleologically, the changes in metabolism that occur give first priority to cells which are part of the immune system. Evidence suggests that the changes in glutamine and fuel metabolism are mediated by the insulin counterregulatory hormones, such as cortisol and epinephrine, and several different cytokines. Cytokines appear to play a more important role than hormones during sepsis, although they exert their effects, in part, via hormones (see Fig. 42.17). Although cytokines can be released from a variety of cells, macrophages are the principal source during trauma and sepsis.

Two cytokines that are important in sepsis are interleukin-1 (IL-1) and tumor necrosis factor (TNF). IL-1 and TNF affect amino acid metabolism both through regulation of the release of glucocorticoids, and through direct effects on tissues. Although cytokines are generally considered to be paracrine, with their effects being exerted over cells in the immediate vicinity, TNF and IL-1 increase in the blood during sepsis. Other cytokines, such as IL-6, may also be involved.

During sepsis, TNF, IL-1, and possibly other cytokines, bacterial products, or mediators act on the brain to stimulate the release of glucocorticoids from the adrenal cortex (a process mediated by adrenocorticotropic hormone (ACTH)), epinephrine from the adrenal medulla, and both insulin and glucagon from the pancreas. Although insulin is elevated during sepsis, the tissues exhibit an insulin resistance which is similar to that of the non-insulin-dependent diabetes mellitus patient, possibly resulting from the elevated levels of the insulin counterregulatory hormones (glucocorticoids, epinephrine, and glucagon). Changes in the rate of acute phase protein synthesis are mediated, at least in part, by effects of TNF, IL-1, and IL-6 on the synthesis of groups of proteins in the liver.

Hypercatabolic states may be accompanied by varying degrees of insulin resistance caused, in part, by the release of counterregulatory hormones into the blood. Thus, patients with diabetes mellitus may require higher levels of exogenous insulin during sepsis.

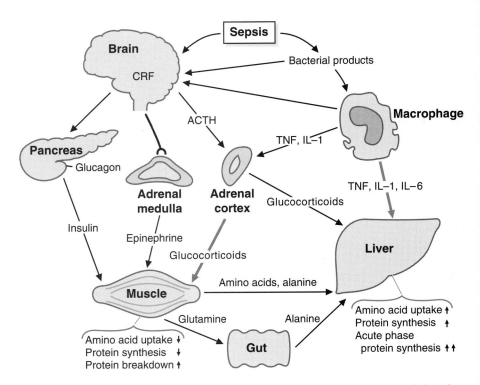

Fig. 42.17. Cytokines and hormones mediate amino acid flux during sepsis. Bacterial products act on macrophages to stimulate the release of cytokines and on the brain to stimulate the sympathoadrenal response. The result is a stimulation of the release of the insulin counterregulatory hormones, epinephrine, glucagon, and glucocorticoids. The glucocorticoid cortisol may be the principal mediator of net muscle protein degradation during sepsis. Hepatic protein synthesis, particularly that of acute phase proteins, is stimulated both by cortisol and cytokines. Amino acid metabolism in the gut is also probably affected by glucocorticoids and cytokines. Adapted with permission from Fisher J. Am J Surg 1991;161:270.

Suggested Readings

Abumrad NN, Williams P, Frexes-Steed M, et al. Inter-organ metabolism of amino acids in vivo. Diabetes/Metabol Rev 1989;5:213–226.

Beisel WR. Nutrition and infection. In: Linder MC, ed. Nutritional biochemistry and metabolism with clinical applications. 2nd ed. New York: Elsevier, 1991:507–542.

Fischer J, Hasselgren P-O. Cytokines and glucocorticoids in the regulation of the "hepato-skeletal muscle axis" in sepsis. Am J Surg 1991;161:266–271.

Skeie B, Kvetan V, Gil KM, et al. Branch-chain amino acids: their metabolism and clinical utility. Crit Care Med 1990;18:549–571.

PROBLEMS

1. The utilization of total parenteral solutions enriched in BCAA for nutritional support of septic patients and trauma patients has been suggested. What might be some of the benefits? Can you think of any disadvantages in increasing the content of BCAA above that found in normal protein?

2. What changes in amino acid metabolism would you expect to find in patients with untreated insulin-dependent diabetes mellitus?

ANSWERS

1. Some of the more obvious benefits are those associated with malnourishment. A patient depleted in the essential amino acids, which includes the BCAA, would have a diminished supply for the protein synthesis required for the immune response and wound healing. Leucine or its α-keto acid could inhibit muscle protein turnover and decrease muscle wasting. The metabolism of the BCAA to glutamine would provide glutamine for the cells of the immune system, intestine, and kidney. Metabolism of glutamine would also give these cells a source of energy. Many cells, in fact, could utilize BCAA directly as an energy source. However, BCAA supplied with other amino acids in a normal distribution, such as a high quality protein supplement, might still provide all these benefits. .

Some of the potential problems which could arise would be those related to an imbalance of amino acids. Too high levels of BCAA could stimulate insulin release and inhibit skeletal muscle proteolysis, thereby leading to a limited availability of other amino acids.

2. Although the mechanism of insulin action is not known, it is known that insulin stimulates the uptake of amino acids into skeletal muscle, increases general protein synthesis through stimulating translation and through other mechanisms, and inhibits protein degradation. A deficiency of insulin would increase net protein degradation, thereby increasing the release of glutamine, alanine, and other amino acids into the blood. The increased influx of gluconeogenic precursors into liver contributes to the hyperglycemia of diabetes mellitus. The presence of ketoacidosis in the patient with insulin-dependent diabetes mellitus would invoke the mechanisms for responding to an acidosis, resulting in an increased efflux of glutamine from muscle, enhanced glutamine uptake by the kidney, and enhanced excretion of NH_4^+. The result for the patient is pronounced muscle wasting.

Molecular Endocrinology

The ability of a variety of specialized tissues within the body to contribute in an integrated way to the normal function of the multicellular organism requires communication between cells. This communication is provided primarily by four distinct systems:

1. The nervous system, both central and peripheral, which operates via complex electrical and neurotransmitter signals and reflex arcs
2. The endocrine system, which, through a variety of glands, synthesizes and secretes hormones into the blood that have physiological effects on distal target tissues
3. The paracrine and autocrine systems, which synthesize and secrete substances into the intercellular space that modify cellular function without entering the bloodstream (Fig. 43.1), and
4. The immune system, which monitors and mediates the response to both external (e.g., infectious agents, foreign proteins) and internal (neoplastic) threats to the organism.

None of these systems operates independently of the others. For example, neurochemicals produced in the nervous system act as local neurosignals (neurotransmitters), and may also enter the circulation and act distally as true hormones. Several circulating hormones are also capable of having a regulatory effect in the central nervous system. Even the competence of the immune system depends upon endocrine and neural influences.

Although these interrelationships make it difficult to clearly delineate the limits of the discipline of endocrinology, the central theme of the endocrine system relates to hormones and their physiological actions as well as to the factors that control the synthesis of hormones, their secretion into the circulation, and their inactivation and degradation.

More than 100 hormones have been described in higher primates. Table 43.1 lists the abbreviations of many of the hormones and related compounds produced in humans. Major hormones that do not have standard abbreviations, such as cortisol and testosterone, are not listed in this table.

The normal sites of hormone synthesis include the hypothalamus, the anterior and posterior pituitary glands, the thyroid and parathyroid glands, the islet cells of the pancreas, the adrenal cortex and medulla, the gonads, the placenta, and certain cells of the gastrointestinal tract, the brain, and the myocardium. Hormones are also produced by nonendocrine neoplasms. This process is known as ectopic hormone production.

A. Endocrine

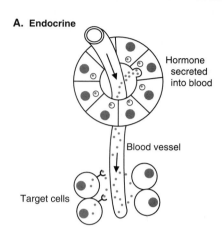

Hormone secreted into blood

Blood vessel

Target cells

B. Paracrine

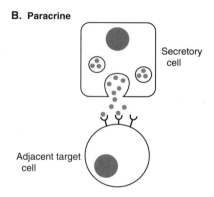

Secretory cell

Adjacent target cell

C. Autocrine

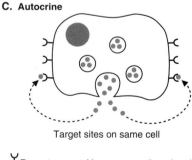

Target sites on same cell

Y Receptor   ● Hormone or other signal

Fig. 43.1. Endocrine, paracrine, and autocrine cell-to-cell communication. Hormones or other chemical compounds are secreted from cells. They act as signals that bind to cellular receptors, exerting an intracellular effect. **A.** Endocrine signals travel through the blood and affect cells in other tissues. **B.** Paracrine signals affect nearby cells without entering the blood. **C.** Autocrine signals affect the same cell (or cell type) from which they are secreted.

667

Those clinical disorders which result from primary or secondary deficiencies or excesses in the secretion of, or physiological response to, hormones make up the discipline of clinical endocrinology. This Section will present the biochemical basis for understanding the consequences of endocrine disease.

Table 43.1. Abbreviations for Some of the Hormones and Related Compounds Produced in Humans

ACTH	Adrenocorticotropic hormone
ABP	Androgen binding protein
ADH	Antidiuretic hormone (also known as AVP)
ANP	Atrionatriuretic peptide (or atriopeptin)
CCK	Cholecystokinin
CG	Chorionic gonadotropin (hCG, human CG)
CLIP	Corticotropin-like intermediate lobe peptide
CRH	Corticotropin releasing hormone
DHEA	Dehydroepiandrosterone
DHT	Dihydrotestosterone
$1,25\text{-}(OH)_2D_3$	1,25-Dihydroxycholecalciferol
E_2	Estradiol
FSH	Follicle stimulating hormone
GH	Growth hormone
GIP	Gastric inhibitory peptide
GnRH	Gonadotropin releasing hormone
GRH	Growth hormone releasing hormone (somatocrinin) (GHRH)
GRIH	Growth hormone release inhibiting hormone (somatostatin)
hCG	Human chorionic gonadotropin
IGF	Insulin-like growth factor
LH	Luteinizing hormone
LPH	Lipotropin
MSH	Melanocyte stimulating hormone
POMC	Proopiomelanocortin
PRH	Prolactin releasing hormone
PRIH	Prolactin release inhibiting hormone (PRIH)
PRL	Prolactin
PTH	Parathyroid hormone
T_3	Triidothyronine
T_4	Thyroxine (tetraidothyronine)
TRH	Thyrotropin releasing hormone
TSH	Thyroid stimulating hormone
VIP	Vasoactive intestinal polypeptide
VP	Vasopressin (ADH)

Hormones circulate in the plasma in very low concentrations (picomolar to micromolar range). Therefore, in order for hormones to exert their physiological effects on target tissues, the cells must contain receptors on their plasma membranes or within their interior which recognize and bind the circulating hormones with high affinity and specificity.

A distinguishing characteristic of the endocrine system is the homeostatic feedback mechanism which, in part, determines the rate of hormone production for virtually all endocrine organs. For example, the plasma concentration of a hormone produced by a peripheral endocrine gland in response to a hormone from the anterior pituitary acts as a feedback signal to the secretory cells of the hypothalamus and/or the anterior pituitary. The secretory activity of the hypothalamic or pituitary cells is stimulated if the peripheral hormone level is subnormal and inhibited if the peripheral level is greater than normal.

Finally, the duration of the physiological effect of a hormone is determined in part by the extent of its binding to transport proteins in the circulation (transport proteins exist for thyroid hormone and for adrenal and gonadal steroid hormones), by the rate of its inactivation caused by a variety of degradative processes occurring primarily in the liver, and by the rate of excretion of the hormone or of its metabolites into the feces or the urine. Polypeptide hormones, for example, are taken up by cells by the process of endocytosis. These internalized hormones are then degraded by lysosomal enzyme systems within the cell.

43 Structure, Synthesis, and Basic Actions of Hormones

According to the classic definition, a hormone is a substance produced in an endocrine gland, secreted into the blood, and delivered to a target cell in a separate tissue of the body where it has a specific physiological effect. However, this definition is now expanding to include compounds that have autocrine or paracrine actions (see Fig. 43.1). Table 43.2 lists the major human hormones and categorizes them into classes (i.e., peptide, steroid, or amino acid derivative).

Most hormones are either peptides or compounds derived from amino acids. Some of the peptide hormones are complex glycoproteins, such as thyroid-stimulating hormone (TSH), and the gonadotropins (luteinizing hormone (LH) and follicle-stimulating hormone (FSH)). Other peptide hormones are of intermediate size, such as growth hormone (GH) and prolactin. Others are very small peptides, for example, thyrotropin-releasing hormone (TRH) is a tripeptide. Hormones derived from a single amino acid include the catecholamines (e.g., epinephrine and norepinephrine) (Fig. 43.2) and the thyroid hormones (triiodothyronine (T_3) and thyroxine (T_4)).

Table 43.2. Major Hormones of the Body[a]

Polypeptides	Glycoproteins	Steroid-Related	Amines
Adrenocorticotropic hormone (ACTH)	Follicle stimulating hormone (FSH)	Aldosterone	Epinephrine
Angiotensins I and II	Human chorionic gonadotropin (hCG)	Cortisol	Norepinephrine
Calcitonin (CT)	Luteinizing hormone (LH)	1,25-Dihydroxychole-calciferol	Thyroxine (T_4)
Cholecystokinin	Thyroid stimulating hormone (TSH)	Estradiol	Triidothyronine (T_3)
Gastrin		Progesterone	
Glucagon		Retinoic acid	
Growth hormone (GH)		Testosterone	
Insulin			
Insulin-like growth factors (IGFs, somatomedins)			
Melanocyte stimulating hormone (MSH)			
Oxytocin (OT)			
Parathyroid hormone (PTH)			
Prolactin (PRL)			
Vasopressin (VP; antidiuretic hormone, ADH)			

[a]The releasing and release inhibiting hormones produced in the hypothalamus are not included in this table.

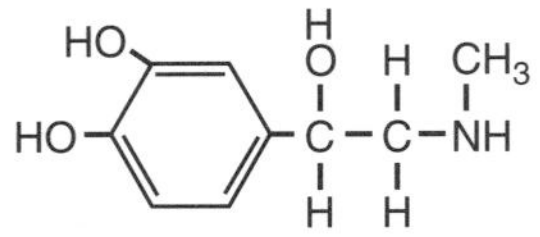

Epinephrine

Fig. 43.2. Epinephrine, an example of a hormone derived from an amino acid. Epinephrine is derived from tyrosine.

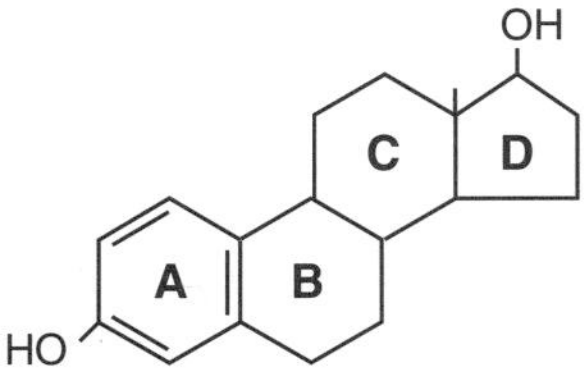

17−β−Estradiol

Fig. 43.3. 17β-Estradiol, an example of a hormone derived from cholesterol.

The remaining hormones are derivatives of cholesterol or one of its precursors (Fig. 43.3). The steroid hormones, derived from cholesterol, include the adrenal cortical hormones (e.g., cortisol, aldosterone, the adrenal sex steroids) and the gonadal hormones (e.g., the ovarian and testicular sex steroids). Vitamin D and its metabolites are derived from a precursor of cholesterol. Vitamin A and the carotenoids such as β-carotene are synthesized in plants (from the isoprene unit used in animals for the synthesis of cholesterol), and converted in the body to the hormone retinoic acid.

The initial step in the action of a hormone is its binding to a receptor. The receptors for some hormones are located on the cell surface, while those for other hormones are located within the cell. A variety of mechanisms increase the likelihood that hormones, which are present in very low concentrations in the blood, will interact with their specific receptors. These mechanisms include the local formation of a hormone within its target tissue (e.g., the conversion of testosterone to the more active dihydrotestosterone within the hair follicle). Hormones may also diffuse directly into adjacent cells, having a paracrine effect (e.g., testosterone produced in the Leydig cells of the testicle diffuses into the neighboring seminiferous tubules of the testes and, along with its more potent metabolite dihydrotestosterone, initiates spermatogenesis). Finally, hormones may be targeted to specific receptors by virtue of the presence of a portal vasculature (e.g., the entry of hypothalamic releasing hormones into the hypophyseal-portal vessels through which they are delivered to their receptors on cells of the anterior pituitary gland).

Some hormones require a mechanism of signal transduction. These hormones (the first messengers) bind to receptors located on the surface of cells of their target tissue. They trigger the transformation of this binding phenomenon into a signal that alters cellular functions and/or growth via the formation of an intracellular signal (the second messenger), such as cyclic AMP (cAMP) or inositol trisphosphate (IP$_3$). Hormones that bind to receptors on the surface of the cell membrane of target tissues include the catecholamines (such as epinephrine) and the peptide hormones (such as insulin and glucagon).

Other hormones exert their effects by binding to receptors located within the target cells (e.g., the steroid hormones, thyroid hormone, retinoic acid, and the active form of vitamin D$_3$). The intracellular hormone-receptor complexes then bind to hormone response elements of DNA, inducing the synthesis of specific mRNAs and the proteins for which they code. These proteins mediate the particular hormone-induced change in cellular function, growth, or differentiation.

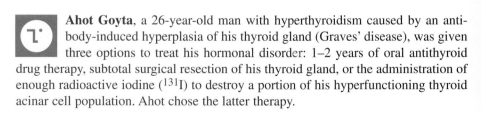

Ahot Goyta, a 26-year-old man with hyperthyroidism caused by an antibody-induced hyperplasia of his thyroid gland (Graves' disease), was given three options to treat his hormonal disorder: 1–2 years of oral antithyroid drug therapy, subtotal surgical resection of his thyroid gland, or the administration of enough radioactive iodine (^{131}I) to destroy a portion of his hyperfunctioning thyroid acinar cell population. Ahot chose the latter therapy.

Vera Leizd is a 34-year-old woman in whom pubertal changes began at age 12, leading to the development of normal secondary sexual characteristics and the onset of menses at age 13. Her menstrual periods occurred on a monthly basis over the next 7 years but the flow was scant. At age 20 she noted a gradual increase in the intermenstrual interval from her normal of 28 days to 32–38 days. The volume of her menstrual flow also gradually diminished. After 7 months, her menstrual periods ceased. She complained of increasing oiliness of her skin, the appearance of acnelike lesions on her face and upper back, and the appearance of short dark terminal hairs on the mustache and sideburn areas of her face. The amount of extremity hair also increased, and she noticed a disturbing loss of hair from her scalp.

SYNTHESIS OF HORMONES

Peptide Hormones

Polypeptide hormones are synthesized like other proteins from amino acids by a process that requires mRNA and occurs on ribosomes (see Chapter 14). During the synthesis of most of the polypeptide hormones, large, biologically inactive precursor molecules are first translated from mRNA and then cleaved to form smaller, biologically active peptides. For example, parathyroid hormone (PTH) is translated from a mRNA for preproPTH. This protein is synthesized on ribosomes attached to the rough endoplasmic reticulum (RER). As synthesis proceeds, the pre- or signal sequence is removed by the signal peptidase, and proPTH enters the lumen of the RER (see Fig. 14.13). Six additional residues are cleaved from the amino (NH_2) end of proPTH within the Golgi complex to form the active 84 amino acid PTH which is then stored in the secretory vesicles of the parathyroid cell awaiting secretion into the blood (Fig. 43.4). Similar cleavages of a precursor preprohormone within the secretory cell to form the final secretory product occur in the β cells of the pancreas during the synthesis of insulin (see Chapter 24) and in the α cells of the pancreas during the synthesis of glucagon.

Most polypeptide hormones are each encoded by a single gene. However, in some cases, a group of peptide hormones are encoded together on one gene which produces a single polyprotein. For example, proopiomelanocortin (POMC), a gene product of the anterior pituitary corticotrophic cells, is cleaved to form eight different peptides, at least some of which act as hormones (see Chapter 44).

Hormones Derived from Single Amino Acids

THYROID HORMONE

The secretory products of the thyroid acinar cells are tetraiodothyronine (thyroxine, T_4) and triiodothyronine (T_3). Their structures are shown in Figure 43.5. The basic steps in the synthesis of T_3 and T_4 in these cells involve the transport of iodide from the blood into the thyroid acinar cell against an electrochemical gradient; the oxidation of iodide to form an iodinating species; the iodination of tyrosyl residues on the protein, thyroglobulin, to form iodotyrosines; and the coupling of residues of monoiodo- and diiodotyrosine in thyroglobulin to form residues of T_3 and T_4 (Fig. 43.6). Proteolytic cleavage of thyroglobulin releases free T_3 and T_4. The steps in thyroid hormone synthesis are stimulated by TSH, a hormone produced by the anterior pituitary.

Iodide transport from the blood into the thyroid acinar cell is accomplished through an energy-requiring, iodide-trapping mechanism which is poorly defined but may involve the Na^+,K^+-ATPase coupled to a cotransporter for Na^+ and iodide in the plasma membrane of the acinar cell.

The rate of iodide transport is influenced by the absolute concentration of iodide within the thyroid cell. An internal autoregulatory mechanism decreases transport of iodide into the cell when the intracellular iodide concentration exceeds a certain threshold and increases transport when intracellular iodide is low.

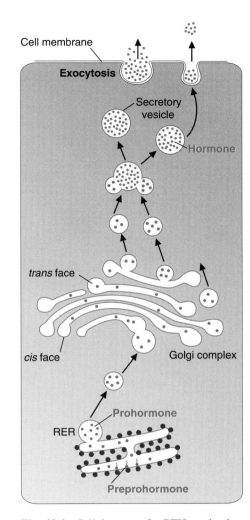

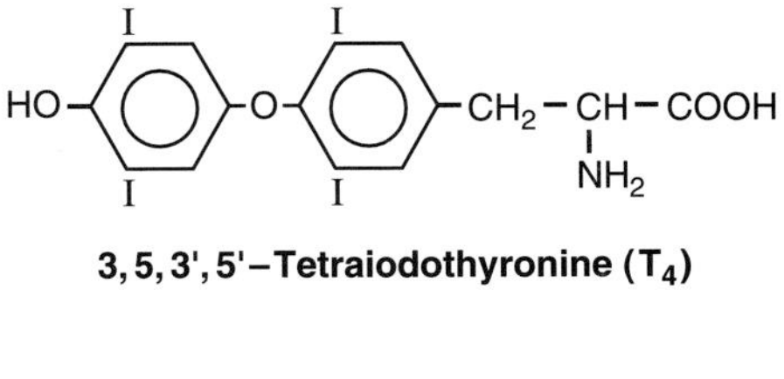

Fig. 43.4. Cellular route for PTH production and secretion. The hormone is synthesized on the RER, where the pre-sequence (signal sequence) is removed. The pro-sequence is removed in the Golgi complex, and the mature hormone is secreted by exocytosis.

3,5,3',5'–Tetraiodothyronine (T_4)

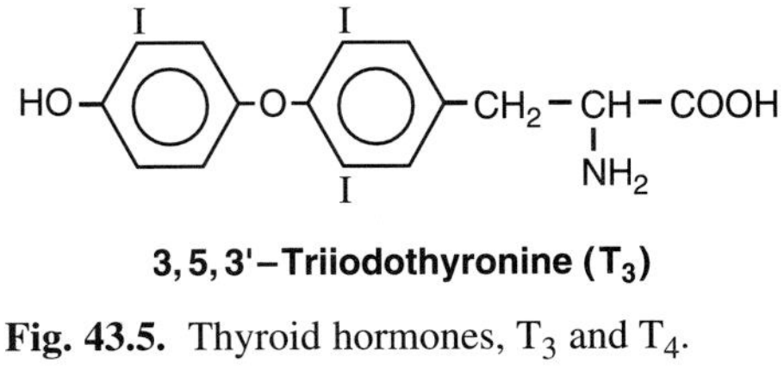

3,5,3'–Triiodothyronine (T_3)

Fig. 43.5. Thyroid hormones, T_3 and T_4.

The concentrating process for iodide creates iodide levels within the thyroid cell that are several hundred fold greater than those in the blood, depending upon the current size of the total body iodide pool and the present need for new hormone synthesis.

Radioactive iodine (^{131}I), used in the therapy of Graves' disease, is concentrated in the thyroid gland. It exerts its therapeutic effect within the acinar cells primarily via tissue-destroying β-particle emissions with an average acinar cell penetration of 2.2 mm.

Unfortunately, the dose of ^{131}I administered to **Ahot Goyta** had an unexpectedly potent effect. He was left with an insufficient number of undamaged acinar cells and slowly became hypothyroid. Ahot was started on thyroid hormone replacement therapy, treatment he would require for the rest of his life.

In areas of the world where the soil is deficient in iodide, hypothyroidism is prevalent. The thyroid gland enlarges (forms a goiter) in an attempt to produce more thyroid hormone. In the United States, table salt (NaCl) enriched with iodide (iodized salt) is used to prevent hypothyroidism caused by iodine deficiency.

The thyroid gland is unique in that it has the capacity to store large amounts of hormone as amino acid residues in thyroglobulin within its colloid space. This storage accounts for the low overall turnover rate of T_3 and T_4 in the body.

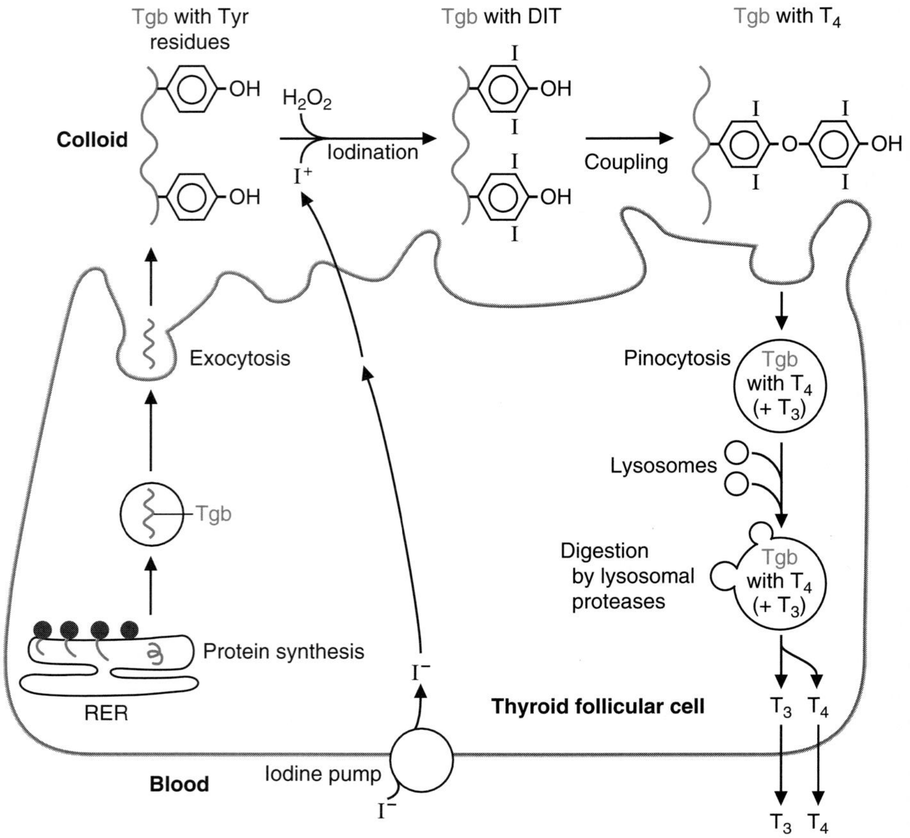

Fig. 43.6. Synthesis of the thyroid hormones (T_3 and T_4). The protein thyroglobulin (Tgb) is synthesized in thyroid follicular cells and secreted into the colloid. Iodination and coupling of tyrosine residues in Tgb produce T_3 and T_4 residues, which are released from Tgb by pinocytosis (endocytosis) and lysosomal action. The coupling of a monoiodotyrosine with a diiodotyrosine (DIT) to form triiodothyronine (T_3) is not depicted here.

The oxidation of intracellular iodide is catalyzed by thyroid peroxidase (located at the apical border of the thyroid acinar cell) in what may be a 2-electron oxidation step forming I^+ (iodinium ion). Iodinium ion may react with a tyrosine residue in the protein thyroglobulin to form a tyrosine quinoid and then a 3'-monoiodotyrosine (MIT) residue. It has been suggested that a second iodide is added to the ring by similar mechanisms to form a 3,5-diiodotyrosine (DIT) residue. Because iodide is added to these organic compounds, iodination is also referred to as the "organification of iodide."

The biosynthesis of thyroid hormone proceeds with the coupling of an MIT and a DIT residue to form a triiodothyronine (T_3) residue or of 2 DIT residues to form a tetraiodothyronine (T_4) residue. T_3 and T_4 are stored in the thyroid follicle as amino acid residues in thyroglobulin. Under most circumstances, the T_4/T_3 ratio in thyroglobulin is approximately 13:1.

The release of T_3 and T_4 from thyroglobulin is controlled by TSH from the anterior pituitary. TSH stimulates the endocytosis of thyroglobulin to form endocytic vesicles within the thyroid acinar cells (see Fig. 43.6). Lysosomes fuse with these vesicles, and lysosomal proteases hydrolyze thyroglobulin, releasing free T_4 and T_3 into the blood in a 10:1 ratio. In various tissues, T_4 is deiodinated, forming T_3, which is the most active form of the hormone.

CATECHOLAMINES

In humans, the catecholamines (epinephrine, norepinephrine, and dopamine) are synthesized primarily in the sympathetic neurons, the adrenal medulla, and specific locations in the central nervous system (CNS). Most of the epinephrine in the body is found in the adrenal medulla in concentrations of milligrams per gram of tissue. The concentration in brain and sympathetic neurons is relatively small. On the other hand, significant amounts of norepinephrine are found in the adrenal medulla as well as in peripheral sympathetic neurons, the CNS (hypothalamus and brain stem primarily), and in extraadrenal chromaffin tissues.

Dopamine (DA) is found in relatively high levels in the CNS especially in the basal ganglia and, to some extent, in the ventral hypothalamus, areas where it functions as a neurotransmitter. Some DA is present in the sympathetic ganglia and carotid body as well.

The major pathway for catecholamine synthesis was described in Chapter 41 and is summarized in Figure 43.7. In some tissues, no further biochemical modification of norepinephrine occurs. However, in the adrenal medulla, in the neurons of the CNS, and in peripheral sympathetic ganglia that use epinephrine as a neurotransmitter, norepinephrine is N-methylated to form epinephrine, a reaction which is catalyzed by the enzyme phenylethanolamine N-methyltransferase (PNMT).

The catecholamines in the adrenal medulla and sympathetic neural endings are stored in chromaffin granules. They are released from these granules following stimulation by acetylcholine (ACh) acting on nicotinic receptors in the granule membrane. Catecholamines are secreted via exocytosis through a calcium-dependent mechanism.

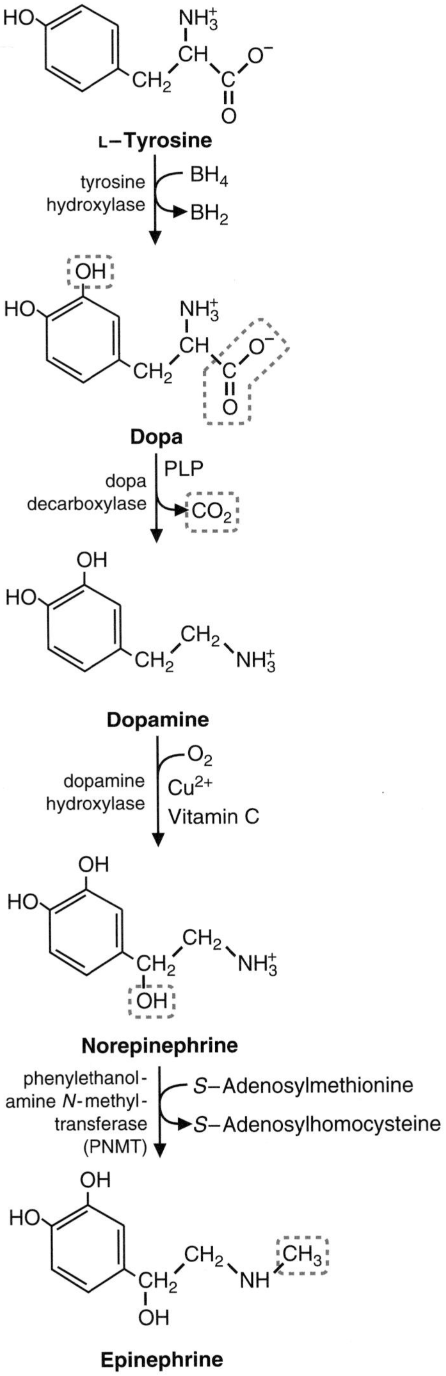

Steroid Hormones

Steroid hormones are derived from cholesterol (Fig. 43.8), which is either synthesized in the tissues from acetyl CoA, extracted from intracellular cholesterol ester pools, or taken up by the cell in the form of cholesterol-containing lipoproteins which are internalized by a plasma membrane receptor-mediated process. In general, glucocorticoids and progestins contain 21 carbons, androgens contain 19 carbons, and estrogens contain 18 carbons. The specific complement of enzymes present in the cells of an organ determines which hormones the organ can synthesize.

The biosynthesis of glucocorticoids and mineralocorticoids (in the adrenal cortex), and that of sex steroids (in the adrenal cortex and gonads), requires four cytochrome P450 enzymes (see Chapter 21). These monooxygenases are involved in the transfer of electrons from NADPH through electron transfer protein intermediates to molecular oxygen, which then oxidizes a variety of the ring carbons of cholesterol.

Cholesterol is converted to progesterone in the first two steps of synthesis of all steroid hormones. Cytochrome $P450_{SCC}$ side-chain cleavage enzyme, located in the mitochondrial inner membrane, removes 6 carbons from the side chain of cholesterol, forming pregnenolone, which has 21 carbons. The next step, the conversion of pregnenolone to progesterone, is catalyzed by 3β-hydroxysteroid dehydrogenase, an enzyme that is not a member of the cytochrome P450 family. Other steroid hormones are produced from progesterone by reactions that involve members of the P450 family.

The principal biologically important products of adrenal cortical steroid synthesis are the glucocorticoid cortisol, and the mineralocorticoid aldosterone. The principal steroid synthesized in the ovary is estradiol (although progesterone is an important ovarian hormone and some testosterone is synthesized there as well). Testosterone is the principal hormone synthesized in the testicle.

Fig. 43.7. Synthesis of the catecholamines. BH_4 and BH_2 = tetra- and dihydrobiopterin; PLP = pyridoxal phosphate.

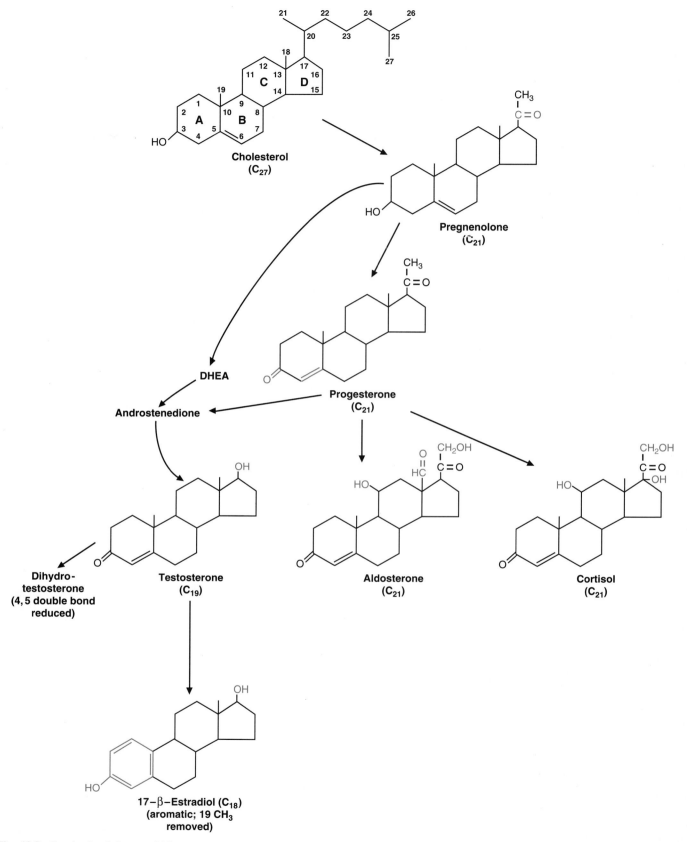

Fig. 43.8. Synthesis of the steroid hormones. The rings of the precursor, cholesterol, are lettered. Dihydrotestosterone is produced from testosterone by reduction of the carbon-carbon double bond in ring A. Structural changes between the precursor and final hormone are noted in blue. DHEA = dehydroepiandrosterone.

SYNTHESIS OF CORTISOL

The adrenocortical biosynthetic pathway which leads to cortisol synthesis occurs in the middle layer of the adrenal cortex known as the zona fasciculata. Free cholesterol is transported by an intracellular carrier protein to the inner mitochondrial membrane of cells (Fig. 43.9), where the side chain is cleaved to form pregnenolone. Pregnenolone returns to the cytosol where it forms progesterone.

In the membranes of the endoplasmic reticulum, a 17,20-lyase catalyzes the hydroxylation of C17 of progesterone or pregnenolone and can also catalyze the cleavage of the 2-carbon side chain of these compounds at C17. These two separate functions of the same enzyme allow further steroid synthesis to proceed along two separate pathways: the 17-hydroxylated steroids which retain their side chains are precursors of cortisol, whereas those from which the side chain was cleaved (C19 steroids) are precursors of androgens (male sex hormones) and estrogens (female sex hormones).

In the pathway of cortisol synthesis, the 17-hydroxylation of progesterone yields 17-OH-progesterone which, along with progesterone, is transported to the smooth endoplasmic reticulum where the membrane-bound $P450_{C21}$ enzyme catalyzes hydroxylation of C21 of 17-OH-progesterone to form 11-deoxycortisol (and of progesterone to form deoxycorticosterone (DOC), a precursor of the mineralocorticoid, aldosterone).

 Cytochrome $P450_{11}$, another enzyme located in the mitochondrial membrane, catalyzes β-hydroxylation at C11. Hydroxylations at C17 and C21 are catalyzed by two enzymes located in the membranes of the endoplasmic reticulum ($P450_{C17}$ for 17α-hydroxylation and $P450_{C21}$ for 21-hydroxylation).

Vera Leizd consulted her gynecologist, who confirmed that her problems were the result of an excess production of androgens (virilization) and ordered blood and urine studies to determine whether Vera's adrenal cortices or her ovaries were causing her virilizing syndrome.

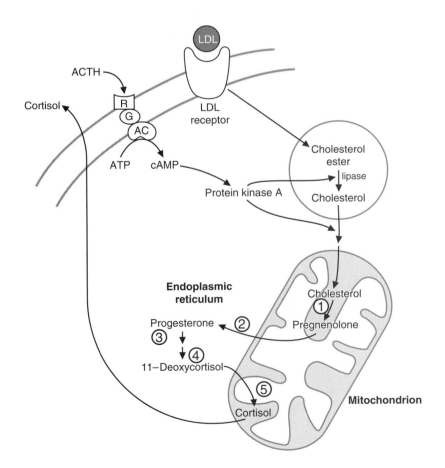

Fig. 43.9. Cellular route for cortisol synthesis. Cholesterol is synthesized from acetyl CoA or derived from low density lipoprotein (LDL), which is endocytosed and digested by lysosomal enzymes. Cholesterol is stored in cells of the adrenal cortex as cholesterol esters. ACTH signals the cell to convert cholesterol to cortisol. **1** = cholesterol desmolase (involved in side chain cleavage); **2** = 3β-hydroxysteroid dehydrogenase; **3** = 17α-hydroxylase; **4** = 21-hydroxylase; **5** = 11β-hydroxylase.

Although aldosterone is the major mineralocorticoid in humans, excessive production of a weaker mineralocorticoid, DOC, which occurs in patients with a deficiency of the 11-hydroxylase (the $P450_{C11}$ enzyme), may lead to clinical signs and symptoms of mineralocorticoid excess even though aldosterone secretion is suppressed in these patients.

Hyperplasia or tumors of the adrenal cortex that produce excess aldosterone result in a condition known as primary aldosteronism, which is characterized by enhanced sodium and water retention, resulting in hypertension.

Biologically, the most potent circulating androgen is testosterone. About 50% of the testosterone in the blood in a normal woman is produced equally in the ovaries and in the adrenal cortices. The remaining half is derived from ovarian and adrenal androstenedione, which, after secretion into the blood, is converted to testosterone in adipose tissue, muscle, liver, and skin. The adrenal cortex, on the other hand, is the major source of the relatively weak androgen dehydroepiandrosterone (DHEA). The serum concentration of its stable metabolite, DHEAS, is used as a measure of adrenal androgen production in hyperandrogenic patients with excessive growth of secondary sexual hair, e.g., facial hair as well as that in the axillae, the suprapubic area, and the chest.

Adrenal

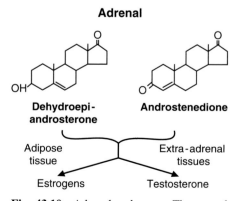

Fig. 43.10. Adrenal androgens. These weak androgens are converted to testosterone or estrogens in other tissues.

The final step in cortisol synthesis requires transport of 11-deoxycortisol back to the inner membrane of the mitochondria, where $P450_{C11}$ (adrenodoxin and adrenodoxin reductase) receives electrons from electron transport protein intermediates. The enzyme then transfers these reducing equivalents by way of oxygen to 11-deoxycortisol for hydroxylation at C11 to form cortisol. The rate of biosynthesis of cortisol and other adrenal steroids is dependent on stimulation of the adrenal cortical cells by adrenocorticotropic hormone (ACTH).

SYNTHESIS OF ALDOSTERONE

The synthesis of the potent mineralocorticoid aldosterone in the zona glomerulosa of the adrenal cortex also begins with the conversion of cholesterol to progesterone. Progesterone is then hydroxylated at C21, a reaction catalyzed by $P450_{C21}$, to yield deoxycorticosterone (DOC). The $P450_{C11}$ enzyme system catalyzes the reactions that convert DOC to corticosterone. The terminal steps in aldosterone synthesis, catalyzed by the P450 aldosterone system, involve the oxidation of corticosterone to 18-hydroxycorticosterone, which is oxidized to aldosterone.

The primary stimulus for aldosterone production is the octapeptide angiotensin II, although alterations in serum Na^+ and K^+ levels may directly influence aldosterone synthesis as well (see Chapter 46). ACTH has a permissive action in aldosterone production. It maintains cells so that they can respond to their primary stimulus, angiotensin II.

SYNTHESIS OF THE ADRENAL ANDROGENS

Adrenal androgen biosynthesis proceeds from cleavage of the 2-carbon side chain of 17-hydroxypregnenolone at C17 to form the 19-carbon adrenal androgen dehydroepiandrosterone (DHEA) and its sulfate derivative (DHEAS) in the zona reticulosum of the adrenal cortex. These compounds, which are weak androgens, represent a significant percentage of the total steroid production by the normal adrenal cortex

Androstenedione, another weak adrenal androgen, is produced when the 2-carbon side chain is cleaved from 17α-hydroxyprogesterone by $P450_{C17}$. This androgen is converted to testosterone primarily in extraadrenal tissues. Although the adrenal cortex makes very little estrogen, the weak adrenal androgens may be converted to estrogens in the peripheral tissues, particularly in adipose tissue (see Fig. 43.10).

SYNTHESIS OF TESTOSTERONE

Luteinizing hormone (LH) from the anterior pituitary stimulates the synthesis of testosterone and other androgens by the human testicle. In many ways the pathways leading to androgen synthesis in the testicle are similar to those described for the adrenal cortex. In the human testicle, the predominant pathway leading to testosterone synthesis is through pregnenolone to 17-hydroxypregnenolone to DHEA (the Δ^5 pathway), and then from DHEA to androstenedione, and from androstenedione to testosterone. As for all steroids, the rate-limiting step in testosterone production is the conversion of cholesterol to pregnenolone. LH controls the rate of side-chain cleavage from cholesterol at carbon 21 to form pregnenolone, and thus regulates the rate of testosterone synthesis. In its target cells, the double bond in ring A of testosterone is reduced, forming the active hormone dihydrotestosterone (DHT) (see Fig. 43.8).

SYNTHESIS OF ESTROGENS AND PROGESTERONE

Ovarian production of estrogens, progestins (compounds related to progesterone), and androgens requires the activity of the cytochrome P450 family of oxidative enzymes used for the synthesis of other steroid hormones. Ovarian estrogens are C18 steroids with a phenolic hydroxyl group at C3 and either a hydroxyl group (estradiol) or a ketone group (estrone) at C17. Although the major steroid-producing compartments of the ovary (the granulosa cell, the thecal cell, the stromal cell, and the cells of the corpus luteum) have all of the enzyme systems required for the synthesis of multiple steroids, the granulosa cells secrete primarily estrogens, the thecal and stromal cells secrete primarily androgens, and the cells of the corpus luteum secrete primarily progesterone.

The ovarian granulosa cell, in response to stimulation by follicle-stimulating hormone (FSH) from the anterior pituitary and through the catalytic activity of P450 aromatase, converts testosterone to estradiol, the predominant and most potent of the ovarian estrogens (see Fig. 43.8). Similarly, androstenedione is converted to estrone in the ovary, although the major site of estrone production from androstenedione occurs in extraovarian tissues, principally skeletal muscle and adipose tissue.

GENERAL MECHANISMS OF HORMONE ACTION

Each hormone has one or more specific physiological actions mediated by target tissues which have the ability to recognize the presence of a particular hormone (often in nano- or picomolar concentrations) in the circulation and to specifically bind and respond to that molecule and not to a multitude of other hormones present in the blood. The specificity of this hormone-target tissue interaction is determined by the presence of cellular receptors located either on the plasma membrane of cells (for peptide hormones and epinephrine) or in the cytosol and nucleus (for steroid and thyroid hormones, active vitamin D_3, and retinoic acid). For hormonal activity to occur, this hormone-receptor binding must be transduced into a postreceptor chemical signal within the cell. This signal causes the specific physiological response to that hormone in the target tissue, such as enzyme activation or new protein synthesis for cellular growth or differentiation.

Mechanism of Action of Hormones That Bind to Cell Surface Receptors

Many of the physicochemical properties of the hormone-cell surface receptor interaction are known. This interaction is swift and reversible, allowing rapid onset and termination of hormone action. Different types of target cells contain different numbers of receptors for a specific hormone, varying from 100 or less to more than a million receptors per cell. Yet for cells of a given tissue, the receptor number is finite. In most target cells, the greater the receptor density on the target cell membrane, the greater the physiological response to the hormone.

Receptor affinity for the ligand (the compound that binds to the receptor) must be high because most hormones circulate in the blood in picomolar to nanomolar concentrations. Receptor specificity depends on the ability of the receptor protein to distinguish the ligand from all other circulating hormones as it approaches the cell surface. Receptors bind the ligand with an affinity which parallels the strength of its biological response.

CELL SURFACE RECEPTOR PROTEINS

The structures of plasma membrane receptor proteins are quite variable. This structural diversity is related to the fact that the hormones capable of interacting with plasma membrane receptors are also structurally diverse. Catecholamines, for example, are small molecules, whereas the glycoprotein hormones such as thyroid-stimulating hormone (TSH) and the gonadotropins, luteinizing hormone (LH) and follicle-stim-

Precursors of a hormone such as proinsulin usually have less affinity for the receptor than the mature hormone and, as a consequence, proportionally less biological potency.

Competitive antagonism of hormone action occurs when a compound competes with the hormone for binding to the hormone receptor but has little or no capacity to activate postreceptor events. Tamoxifen is a drug that competes with estrogen for binding to the estrogen receptor, but has little estrogen activity. It is used in the treatment of advanced estrogen-sensitive breast cancer.

Q 43.1: The results of the blood tests on Vera Leizd revealed that her level of testosterone was normal but that her serum dehydroepiandrosterone sulfate (DHEAS) level was significantly elevated. Which tissue was the most likely source of the androgens that caused Vera's hirsutism (a male pattern of secondary sexual hair growth)?

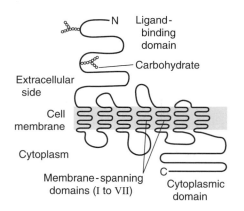

Fig. 43.11. A typical cell membrane hormone receptor. The extracellular domain binds the ligand. In addition, there are seven hydrophobic membrane-spanning domains (I to VII) and an intracellular (cytoplasmic) domain.

ulating hormone (FSH), are structurally complex.

In general, membrane receptor proteins can be divided into three functionally distinct domains, as shown in Figure 43.11. The ligand binding domain, which is often heavily glycosylated, exists on the extracellular side of the cell membrane and, as its name implies, is responsible for binding the circulating hormone. The transmembrane domain consists of seven separate hydrophobic α-helical clusters of amino acid residues that span the membrane and anchor the receptor to the cell. The configuration of the transmembrane helix may form a "pocket" for the bound ligand. The cytoplasmic domain is a chain of amino acids of varying lengths extending from membrane-spanning domain VII. The cytoplasmic domain of some receptors has a catalytic function, such as tyrosine kinase activity.

INTRACELLULAR EFFECTS OF LIGAND BINDING TO CELL SURFACE RECEPTORS

Ligand binding to the receptor initiates a biochemical cascade which ultimately activates an intracellular effector system. Receptors are classified based on which one of a variety of intracellular effector systems or second messengers is induced by the initial hormone receptor binding signal (Fig. 43.12). The major classes of membrane receptor-effector pathways involve cAMP, inositol 1,4,5-trisphosphate (IP_3), diacylglycerol (DAG), or ions, particularly Ca^{2+}, that act as second messengers within the cytosol (Figs. 43.13–43.15). For many receptors, these cytosolic effector systems or second messengers are generated only if intramembrane transducer proteins (known as G proteins because they bind guanosine triphosphate (GTP)) are first activated (see Chapter 24).

A second class of membrane receptors has only one transmembrane domain and with rare exceptions does not require the intervention of separate intramembrane G proteins or enzymes to transduce the physiological action of the ligand (see Fig. 43.12). These receptors contain the effector system as an intrinsic part of their structure. For example, receptors for insulin and for other growth factors, such as insulin-like growth factor I (IGF-I), platelet-derived growth factor (PDGF), and epidermal growth factor (EGF), contain an enzymatic activity within an intracellular domain that phosphorylates tyrosine residues (a tyrosine kinase activity). When the hormone is bound, the tyrosine kinase is stimulated to autophosphorylate tyrosine residues on the receptor, which then phosphorylates other proteins within the cell. A cascade of proteins is activated, and each kinase in the cascade phosphorylates the next protein in the sequence (Fig. 43.16). Many of these proteins are the products of protooncogenes (see Chapter 17).

REGULATION OF CELL SURFACE RECEPTORS

The number of receptors on a cell is controlled by a process known as down-regulation (Fig. 43.17). After the hormone binds to the receptor, the hormone-receptor complex is taken into the cell by the process of endocytosis. The endocytic vesicles fuse with lysosomes, and lysosomal enzymes degrade the peptide hormones. The receptors may also be degraded, or they may be recycled to the cell surface. This internalization of receptors decreases the number that are available on the cell surface to bind hormones. Hence, the receptors are down-regulated.

MECHANISM OF ACTION OF HORMONES THAT ACT ON RECEPTORS WITHIN THE CELL

Steroid hormones (glucocorticoids, mineralocorticoids, estrogens, and androgens), the activated form of vitamin D (calcitriol), thyroid hormone, and retinoic acid (a

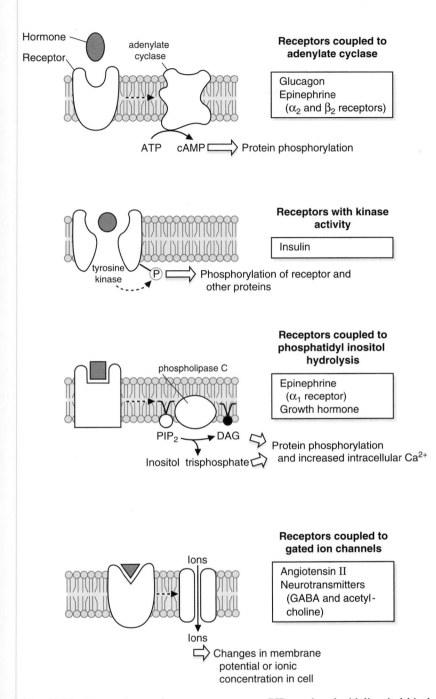

Fig. 43.12. Types of second messenger systems. PIP_2 = phosphatidylinositol bisphosphate; DAG = diacylglycerol; GABA = γ-aminobutyric acid.

A 43.1: **Vera Leizd's** hirsutism was most likely the result of a problem in her adrenal cortex that caused excessive production of DHEA.

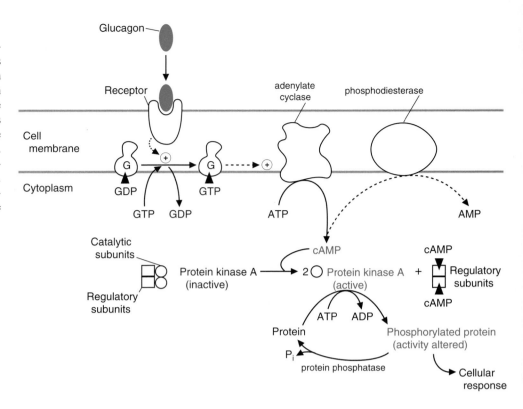

Fig. 43.13. Signal transduction involving cAMP. Hormones bind to receptors and activate G proteins, causing them to release GDP and bind GTP. When GTP is bound, G proteins activate adenylate cyclase, which produces cAMP. cAMP activates protein kinase A by removing regulatory subunits. Protein kinase A phosphorylates proteins, producing the cellular response. G = G proteins; ○ = free catalytic subunits; □ = regulatory subunits; ⊕ = stimulates.

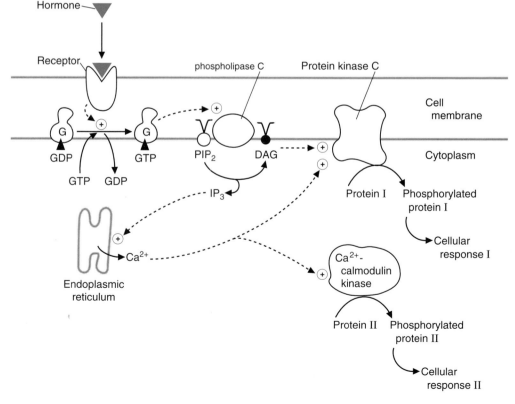

Fig. 43.14. Signal transduction involving Ca^{2+} and the phosphatidylinositol bisphosphate (PIP_2) system. Binding of a hormone to its receptor activates G proteins that stimulate phospholipase C. Phospholipase C cleaves phosphatidylinositol bisphosphate (PIP_2) to DAG and inositol 1,4,5-trisphosphate (IP_3). DAG activates protein kinase C. IP_3 stimulates the release of Ca^{2+} from the endoplasmic reticulum. Ca^{2+} activates protein kinase C and binds to other kinases, activating them. The kinases phosphorylate proteins, which produce the cellular responses. G = G proteins; ⊕ = stimulates.

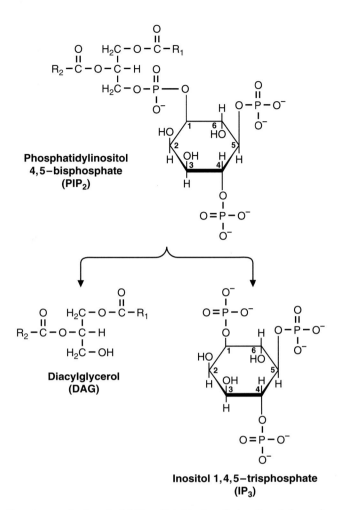

Fig. 43.15. Structures of phosphatidylinositol bisphosphate, diacylglycerol, and inositol trisphosphate.

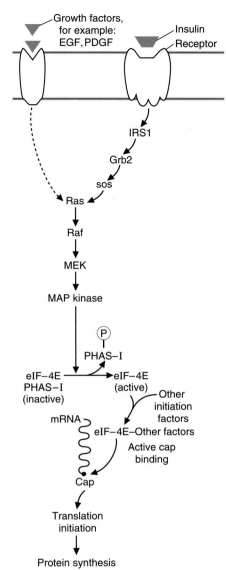

Fig. 43.16. Example of a cascade activated by growth factors. Binding of insulin or growth factors to their cell surface receptors stimulates a cascade. The proteins in the cascade are indicated by three-letter abbreviations. PHAS-I is a protein that binds to eucaryotic initiation factor (eIF)-4E and inhibits the initiation step of protein synthesis. MAP kinase phosphorylates PHAS-I, which then dissociates from eIF-4E. eIF-4E is now active and translation can be initiated. MAP = mitogen-activated protein; IRS = insulin receptor substrate. Based on Travis J. Science 1994;266:542.

form of vitamin A) bind to intracellular receptors and through similar mechanisms have similar ultimate effects, i.e., activation of a specific portion of the genome, inducing RNA and protein synthesis. Because the process is so similar for each of the hormones of this class, a generic model of their mechanism of action will be presented using a steroid hormone as the signal ligand (Fig. 43.18).

Transport of Steroid Hormones in the Blood

Within the blood, steroid hormones are mainly bound to "carrier" or "transport" proteins. Because the steroid hormones are relatively water insoluble, a transport protein is required to deliver the hormone to the target cell. For adrenal corticosteroids, the transporter is corticosteroid-binding globulin (CBG), also known as transcortin.

Binding of Hormones to Intracellular Receptors

The process of steroid hormone action begins with simple diffusion of the unbound hormone through the plasma membrane of the cell, although an active process of cellular uptake of the hormone may occur in some cases. After diffusing into the cell,

 It is generally believed that for most target cells, only the "free" or "unbound" portion of the total amount of circulating hormone can enter cells and have biological effects.

Because steroid hormones circulate in low concentration in the blood (10^{-10} to 10^{-8} M), steroid receptors possess a high binding affinity. For instance, the binding constant for glucocorticoids is about 10^9 M^{-1}.

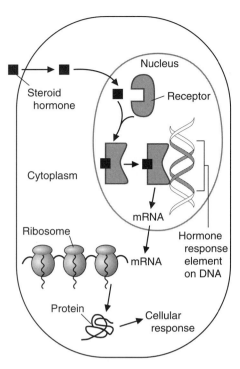

Fig. 43.18. Mechanism of action of hormones that bind to intracellular receptors. These hormones bind to receptors in the nucleus and activate genes. In some cases, receptors are also present in the cytoplasm. The cytoplasmic receptors bind hormone and translocate to the nucleus, where the hormone-receptor complex activates genes.

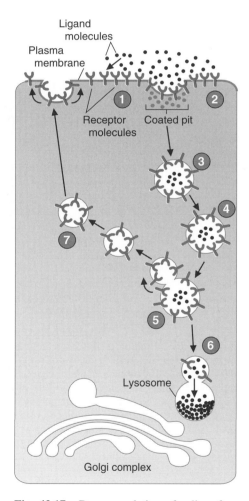

Fig. 43.17. Down-regulation of cell surface receptors. The ligand binds to its receptor and is taken into the cell by endocytosis (**1–5**). Lysosomal enzymes digest the ligand (**6**). The receptor may either be digested (**6**) or recycled to the cell surface (**7**). This process decreases the number of receptors on the cell surface.

the steroid binds to receptor proteins which contain specific binding domains for the hormone. These receptors are found in the nucleus of the cell. For some hormones, they are also present in the cytosol. The receptors for glucocorticoids and probably for mineralocorticoids (aldosterone) are located in the cytosol, whereas receptors for androgens, estrogens, thyroid hormone, activated vitamin D, and retinoic acid appear to reside within the nucleus.

Some of the properties of steroid receptors are well established. The binding of ligand to the receptor is saturable, suggesting that the number of receptors per cell is limited and finite. In addition, these receptors display a high degree of specificity for their respective ligands; however, their capacity for recognition and ability to distinguish between similar steroid structures is not absolute. Only tissues that respond to steroid hormones appear to contain receptors for these ligands. Finally, the extent of the biological response to the hormone is, in general, related to the degree of receptor occupancy.

The steroid hormone binds to an inactive and nontransformed receptor with an unoccupied ligand binding site. The inactive receptor may be complexed with several heat shock proteins (proteins formed in cells undergoing some form of stress) of varying size which cover the DNA binding domain of the inactive unbound receptor molecule.

Binding of the Receptor-Hormone Complex to DNA

When binding of the ligand occurs, the heat shock proteins dissociate from the receptor, thereby exposing the receptor's DNA binding domain. The activated, transformed receptor now binds to DNA. (If the receptor was originally located in the cytosol, it must first translocate to the nucleus.) The activated receptor searches the DNA for a specific high affinity acceptor site (the steroid-receptor complex response element (SRE)).

The DNA sequences that define specific acceptor sites for the binding of the activated steroid hormone-receptor complexes are known for all of the steroid hormones. When binding at these sites occurs, transactivation processes stimulate RNA polymerase activity and, subsequently, transcription occurs (see Chapters 13 and 15). For inhibitory ligands, this process may lead to repression of transcription instead of stimulation.

The newly formed messenger RNAs (mRNAs) bind to the ribosomes in the cytosol, where they are translated, producing specific proteins. These proteins, in turn, will alter target cell function according to the command inherent in the steroid hormone-receptor interaction.

This general model for the actions of glucocorticoids, mineralocorticoids, and the sex steroids also applies to the action of retinoic acid, thyroid hormone, and activated vitamin D.

A major dissimilarity between the general model of steroid hormone action described above and that of vitamin D, thyroid hormone, and retinoic acid is that receptors for the latter hormones do not associate with heat shock proteins. Yet, until these receptors bind their ligands (hormones), they remain inactive. This fact suggests that, when these receptors bind their ligands, a conformational change other than disassociation of heat shock proteins occurs in the receptor protein, which increases the accessibility of its DNA binding domain to its specific hormone response element on DNA.

Steroid-Thyroid Hormone Receptor Superfamily

The receptors for the steroid hormones, thyroid hormone, the active form of vitamin D, and retinoic acid all have three major domains (Fig. 43.19). The ligand binding domain is located near the C-terminus of the receptor. This portion of the protein has 30–60% homology in amino acid sequence with the binding domain of other receptors in this steroid-thyroid receptor superfamily. The DNA binding domain is located near the center of the protein where a 60–95% homology exists with other receptors in this superfamily. This domain contains two finger-like projections from the molecule, each of which has a globular shape and is complexed with zinc. These zinc fingers are the portion of the receptor which interacts with chromatin by fitting into the major groove of the double helix of DNA (see Chapter 8). The third domain is near the N-terminus of the protein. It binds to other proteins that are complexed with their DNA binding sequences in the regulatory region of the gene. Interaction of these DNA-bound proteins with each other causes activation of transcription (see Chapter 15). Because the amino acid sequences in this third domain of the receptor (the transcriptional transactivation segment) are highly variable, this domain is also called the "variable region" of the receptor.

The receptors in the cytosol or nucleus of the cell can be down-regulated if exposure to an increased concentration of ligand is sustained beyond some critical time frame. Unlike membrane receptors, which are down-regulated through a process of endocytosis of the receptor in areas of coated pits in the membrane, the intracellular receptors are probably down-regulated by means of repression of synthesis due to decreased generation of mRNA for the receptor protein. Degradative processes within the cell reduce the amount of the protein.

CLINICAL COMMENTS. The orally administered radioactive iodine used to treat **Ahot Goyta's** hyperthyroidism was deposited in thyroglobulin which is stored in the lumen of the thyroid follicle. From that strategic location with-

Q **43.2:** What characteristics of retinoic acid, thyroid hormone, and the active form of vitamin D suggest that they should behave like steroid hormones rather than like polypeptide hormones?

in the thyroid gland, the β-particle emissions should damage important hormone-synthesizing organelles within the cytosol of Ahot's thyroid acinar cells without permanently damaging the nuclei, which are, of course, necessary for future cell regeneration. Unfortunately, in Ahot's case, the radiation penetration was deep enough to permanently damage enough of his thyroid cell nuclei to cause lifelong hypothyroidism. He was started on a daily replacement dose of synthetic thyroid hormone with the intention of measuring indices of his thyroid function in approximately 3 months to determine if the dose initially selected would maintain his thyroid parameters in the normal range.

Vera Leizd was born with a normal female genotype and phenotype, had normal female sexual development, spontaneous onset of puberty, and regular, although somewhat scanty, menses until the age of 20. At that point, she developed secondary amenorrhea (cessation of menses) and evidence of male hormone excess with early virilization (masculinization).

The differential diagnosis included an ovarian versus an adrenocortical source of the excess androgenic steroids. A screening test to determine whether the adrenal cortex or the ovary is the source of excess male hormone involves the measurement of the concentration of DHEAS in the patient's plasma, since the adrenal cortex makes most of the DHEA, and the ovary makes little or none. Vera's plasma DHEAS level was moderately elevated, identifying her adrenal cortices as the likely source of her virilizing syndrome.

If the excess production of androgens is not the result of an adrenal tumor, but the result of a defect in the pathway for cortisol production, the simple treatment is to administer glucocorticoids by mouth (for rationale, see Biochemical Comments). Vera's adrenal androgen levels in the blood returned to normal after several months of therapy with prednisone (a synthetic glucocorticoid). As a result, her menses

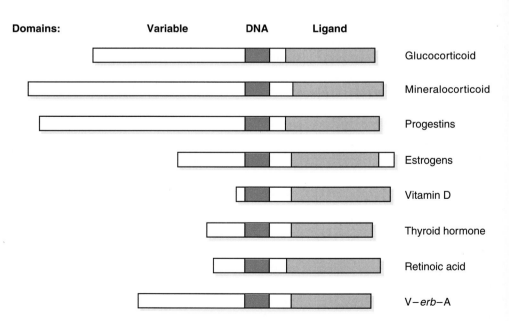

Fig. 43.19. Steroid-thyroid hormone receptor superfamily. These receptors are proteins with three domains: (1) a domain that binds the ligand (listed on the right); (2) a domain that binds to DNA; and (3) a transactivation domain that is of variable length and binds to other proteins associated with the promoter region of the gene. The DNA binding domains have substantial homology (i.e., similar amino acid sequences).

resumed and her virilizing features slowly resolved.

Because Vera's symptoms began in adult life, her genetically determined adrenal hyperplasia is referred to as a "nonclassic" form of the disorder. A more severe enzyme deficiency leads to the "classic" disease, which is associated with excessive fetal adrenal androgen production in utero and, therefore, manifests itself at birth, often with ambiguous external genitalia and virilizing features in the female neonate.

BIOCHEMICAL COMMENTS. Congenital adrenal hyperplasia refers to a group of disorders in adrenal steroidogenesis caused by a genetically determined deficiency in one of the major enzyme systems for the synthesis of cortisol. Because cortisol is the major negative-feedback inhibitor of the secretion of corticotropin (ACTH) by the anterior pituitary, an enzyme deficiency leading to a reduction in cortisol levels results in oversecretion of ACTH. ACTH then acts to increase the synthesis of cortisol as well as that of adrenal androgens and mineralocorticoids. Each specific enzymatic deficiency leads to a unique abnormal profile of adrenal steroids in the blood and, hence, to a distinguishable and definable clinical syndrome.

The most common enzymatic defects include a deficiency of 21-hydroxylase, 11β-hydroxylase, 3β-hydroxysteroid dehydrogenase, 17α-hydroxylase, and cholesterol desmolase (see Fig. 43.9). Through appropriate studies of her urine and plasma, **Vera Leizd** was discovered to have a nonclassic, mild form of 21-hydroxylase deficiency. A partial deficiency in this enzyme will cause precursors of cortisol to accumulate. These compounds will be diverted to the pathway that produces adrenal androgens, particularly dehydroepiandrosterone (DHEA). The androgens caused the virilizing features that prompted Vera to consult her physician.

Prednisone, a synthetic glucocorticoid, feeds back on the anterior pituitary to inhibit ACTH secretion. Thus, oral treatment with prednisone reduces ACTH levels to normal and removes the ACTH-induced overproduction of adrenal androgens. However, when ACTH secretion returns to normal, endogenous cortisol synthesis falls below normal. The administered prednisone brings the net glucocorticoid activity in the blood back to physiological levels.

Suggested Readings

Baxter JD. General concepts of endocrinology. In: Greenspan FS, Baxter JD, eds. Basic and clinical endocrinology. Norwalk, CT: Appleton & Lange, 1994:1–63.

Lin T, Kong X, Haystead TAJ, et al. PHAS-I as a link between mitogen-activated protein kinase and translation initiation. Science 1994;266:653–656.

Strader CD, Fong TM, Tota MR, Underwood D, Dixon RAF. Structure and function of G protein-coupled receptors. Annu Rev Biochem 1995;63:101–132.

Tsai M, O'Malley BW. Molecular mechanisms of action of steroid/thyroid receptor superfamily members. Annu Rev Biochem 1995;63:451–486.

White MF, Kahn CR. The insulin signaling system. J Biol Chem 1994;269:1–4.

PROBLEM

A 25-year-old woman presents with a history of rapidly developing and severe virilization (masculinization). Her serum DHEAS level was 164 μg/dL (normal = 80–340 μg/dL), her serum testosterone level was 374 ng/dL (normal = 30–70 ng/dL), and her 24-hour urinary 17-ketosteroid (17-KS) excretion rate was 14 mg/24 hours (normal = 5–15 mg). A tumor is demonstrated on an abdominal computed tomography (CT) scan. On the basis of these findings, and without a more specific report on the abdom-

A 43.2: These ligands are similar in molecular structure to the steroid hormones. Active vitamin D has a ring system that is very similar to the sterol ring (see Fig. 46.9). Retinoic acid contains a six-membered ring that resembles the A ring of the steroid nucleus, and it contains a side chain composed of 2 isoprene units (see Fig. 47.4). Thyroid hormone has two phenolic rings that are coupled (see Fig. 43.5).

inal CT findings, would an underlying neoplasm causing this syndrome more likely be found in the adrenal gland or in the ovary of this patient?

ANSWER

Virilizing tumors of both the adrenal cortex and of the ovary have the enzymatic capacity to secrete both 17-KS (such as DHEA, DHEAS, and androstenedione) and testosterone. In general, however, virilizing adrenal tumors tend to produce a preponderance of 17-KS (which must be present in large amounts to cause virilization), whereas virilizing ovarian tumors tend to secrete predominantly testosterone. In addition, testosterone is not significantly metabolized to 17-KS. From these considerations, the clinical and laboratory picture presented is more suggestive of an ovarian neoplasm as a cause of the masculinizing changes experienced by this patient. On further review, the CT scan demonstrated normal-appearing adrenal glands but a 2.4-cm mass was seen on the patient's left ovary.

44 Actions of Hypothalamic and Pituitary Hormones

The cell bodies of neurons in the hypothalamus, the region of the brain directly above the pituitary gland, produce peptide and polypeptide hormones (Fig. 44.1). Some of the hypothalamic hormones are stored in the posterior pituitary gland (the neurohypophysis), from which they are released into the blood. Other hypothalamic hormones are released into the hypothalamico-hypophyseal portal vessels and delivered to the anterior pituitary gland (the adenohypophysis), where they have a stimulatory or inhibitory effect on secretion of anterior pituitary hormones (Fig. 44.2).

 Millicent Keeway, a 28-year-old attorney, noted a gradual decrease in the volume of her menstrual flow until, after 7 months of this change, she developed amenorrhea (absence of menses). In the last 2 months she noted breast distension and tenderness. When she noted a small amount of a white milky fluid coming from both breasts while bathing, she consulted her family physician. As a first step in establishing a diagnosis, her physician ordered a fasting serum prolactin level which was reported as 246 ng/mL (normal = 0–25 ng/mL).

 Sam Atotrope, a 42-year-old jeweler, noted increasingly severe headaches behind his eyes sometimes associated with a "flash of light" in his visual fields. At times his vision seemed blurred, making it difficult to perform some of the intricate work required of a jeweler. He consulted his ophthalmologist who was impressed with the striking change in Sam's facial features that had occurred since he last saw the patient 5 years earlier. The normal skin creases in Sam's face had grown much deeper, his nose and lips appeared more bulbous, and his jaw seemed more prominent. The doctor also noted that Sam's hands appeared bulky and his voice had deepened. An eye examination revealed that Sam's optic nerves appeared slightly atrophied and there was a loss of the upper outer quadrants of his visual fields.

HYPOTHALAMIC HORMONES STORED IN THE POSTERIOR PITUITARY

Vasopressin (VP), also known as antidiuretic hormone (ADH), and oxytocin (OT) are peptides synthesized in cells of the hypothalamus. These hormones travel through the axons of the nerves that produce them to the nerve endings in the posterior pituitary, where they are stored. They are released into the blood in response to the appropriate stimuli.

Oxytocin and vasopressin are each encoded by a gene that also encodes a neurophysin, a polypeptide that acts as a specific transport protein. After translation, these hormones are cleaved from their neurophysins, yet remain noncovalently bound to these transport proteins as they travel down the axons of the neurons, which end in the posterior pituitary.

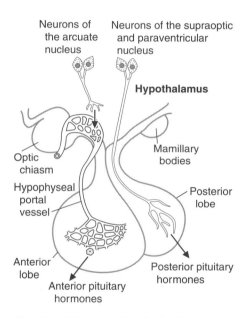

Fig. 44.1. The anatomic relationship between the hypothalamus and anterior and posterior pituitary. Neurons in the hypothalamus secrete hormones that enter the hypophyseal portal vessel. These hormones stimulate (or inhibit) the secretion of hormones from the anterior pituitary that enter the general circulation. Other neurons in the hypothalamus secrete hormones that travel through axons to the posterior pituitary, where they are stored and secreted into the circulation in response to the appropriate stimuli.

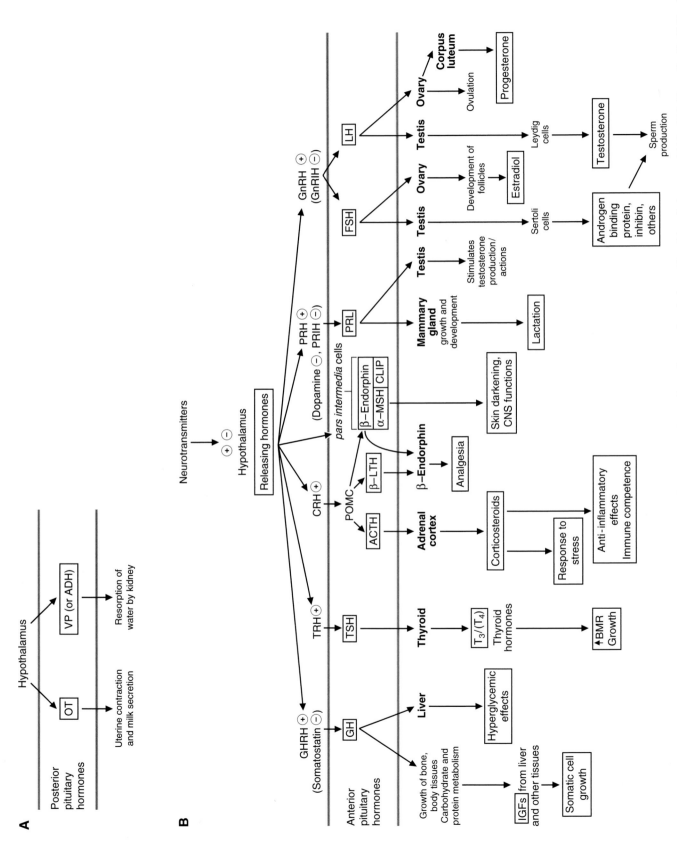

Fig. 44.2. Overview of hormones of the hypothalamus, pituitary, and other endocrine glands. **A.** Hypothalamic hormones stored and released by the posterior pituitary. **B.** Hypothalamic hormones that stimulate (⊕) or inhibit (⊖) the release of hormones from the anterior pituitary. For abbreviations, see Table 43.1. From Devlin T. Textbook of chemistry, 3rd ed. New York: John Wiley, 1992:853.

Vasopressin (Antidiuretic Hormone)

Vasopressin is a peptide containing nine amino acids (Fig. 44.3). It is produced in the supraoptic and paraventricular nuclei of the hypothalamus. Because it contains an arginine residue at position 8, in contrast to some mammalian vasopressins that contain a lysine residue at that position, it is commonly called arginine vasopressin (AVP).

ACTIONS OF VASOPRESSIN

The name vasopressin refers to the ability of the hormone to cause vasoconstriction in most vascular beds of the body. This action is mediated by vasopressin 1 (V_1) receptors in vascular smooth muscle cells. Contraction of these cells is stimulated by activation of phospholipase C, which hydrolyzes phosphatidylinositol 4,5-bisphosphate, forming diacylglycerol (DAG) and inositol 1,4,5-trisphosphate (IP_3). IP_3 stimulates the release of Ca^{2+} from the endoplasmic reticulum. Thus, Ca^{2+} plays a role in eliciting the cellular effects of the hormone (see Chapter 43).

Another major action of vasopressin is to promote water reabsorption through the luminal membrane of the epithelial cells of the cortical and medullary segments of the kidney collecting ducts. This action of vasopressin is reflected in its alternate name, antidiuretic hormone. Binding of vasopressin to vasopressin 2 (V_2) receptors on renal tubular cells activates the adenylate cyclase system, resulting in accumulation of intracellular cAMP. cAMP activates protein kinase A, which phosphorylates proteins, changing the structure of the cytoskeleton of the cell. Channel-containing vesicles within the cytoplasm then fuse with the luminal membrane. These channels, which are formed by the protein aquaporin, are incorporated into the membrane, where they act as conductors that allow increased permeability of these tubular cells to luminal water (see Chapter 46).

STIMULUS FOR RELEASE OF VASOPRESSIN

Changes in osmolality (solute concentration) of the plasma, sensed by osmoreceptors in the hypothalamus, and changes in the pressure within the heart and other parts of

Diabetes insipidus is a condition caused by inadequate secretion or action of antidiuretic hormone. Individuals with this condition produce large volumes of dilute urine.

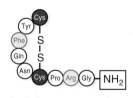

Arginine vasopressin

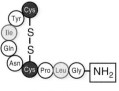

Oxytocin

Fig. 44.3. Structure of arginine vasopressin and oxytocin. These hormones differ in only two amino acid residues (in blue). In each hormone, the N-terminal cysteine forms a disulfide with the internal cysteine residue and the carboxyl group of the C-terminal glycine forms an amide.

the vascular system, sensed by baroreceptors in the atrium and carotid sinus, are the primary stimuli for the release of vasopressin (see Chapter 46).

Oxytocin

Oxytocin, like vasopressin, is a nonapeptide (i.e., it contains nine amino acids). It is synthesized in the supraoptic and paraventricular nuclei of the hypothalamus within neurons that are distinct from those that produce vasopressin. The structures of oxytocin and vasopressin are very similar (see Fig. 44.3).

ACTIONS OF OXYTOCIN

The major actions of oxytocin involve the female reproductive system. The hormone stimulates both the frequency and amplitude of contraction of uterine smooth muscle. This effect is dependent on the presence of estrogen, a hormone that increases in concentration as pregnancy advances. This increase in estrogen may explain the eight- to ninefold increase in uterine responsiveness to oxytocin between the 20th and 39th weeks of pregnancy, which enhances the initiation of labor. Oxytocin also plays a major role during lactation. It causes contraction of the myoepithelial cells of the mammary gland, resulting in the discharge of milk from the alveolar ducts into the sinuses proximal to the nipple. The second messenger system that mediates these actions of oxytocin is incompletely understood.

STIMULUS FOR RELEASE OF OXYTOCIN

Suckling of an infant (i.e., stimulation of the nipples) results in neural impulses that cause the release of oxytocin from the hypothalamus. This stimulus also causes the release of prolactin from the anterior pituitary. Prolactin induces the synthesis of milk proteins (see Fig. 44.10).

HYPOTHALAMIC HORMONES THAT INFLUENCE ANTERIOR PITUITARY FUNCTION

The hypothalamus acts as a key mediator between the higher centers of the central nervous system and the pituitary gland through the synthesis and secretion of peptides which either facilitate the release of hormones from the adenohypophysis (hypothalamic releasing hormones) or inhibit their secretion (hypothalamic release-inhibiting hormones) (Table 44.1). These release and release-inhibiting hormones are delivered to the anterior pituitary cells via the hypothalamico-hypophyseal portal vessels (see Fig. 44.1). Synthesis and secretion of most of the hormones produced by the anterior pituitary are regulated by stimulatory (releasing) hormones. Synthesis and secretion of growth hormone, prolactin, and the gonadotropins (LH and FSH) are also regulated by inhibitory (release-inhibiting) hormones.

The adenohypophyseotropic hormones include growth hormone-releasing hormone (GHRH), growth hormone release-inhibiting hormone (GHRIH) also called somatostatin (SS), prolactin-releasing hormone (PRH), prolactin release-inhibiting hormone (PRIH), dopamine (DA), thyrotropin-releasing hormone (TRH), corticotropin-releasing hormone (CRH), and gonadotropin-releasing hormone (GnRH)

Prolactin-Releasing Hormone and Prolactin Release-Inhibiting Hormone

The secretion of prolactin from the galactotrophs of the anterior pituitary is under bipolar regulation, i.e., the hypothalamus produces hormones that cause prolactin

Mil Keeway has amenorrhea. Chronically elevated levels of prolactin in the blood cause diminished or absent menstrual flow by suppressing the release of the anterior pituitary gonadotropins, LH and FSH, as well as by reducing the stimulatory effects of LH and FSH on ovarian function. The release of GnRH may also be inhibited.

Table 44.1. Hypothalamic Hormones That Influence Anterior Pituitary Function[a]

Hypothalamic Hormone	Anterior Pituitary Hormone	Target Gland Hormone	Process Affected by the Target Gland Hormone
CRH	ACTH and other hormones from the POMC gene	Adrenal Cortisol	Response to stress
TRH	TSH	Thyroid T_3, T_4	Energy production (fuel metabolism)
GnRH	LH, FSH	Gonads Estradiol Progesterone Testosterone	Reproduction Menstrual cycle Pregnancy Production of sperm
GnRIH	⊖ LH, FSH		
GHRH (somatocrinin)	GH	Various cells IGF (somatomedin)	Cell growth
GHRIH (somatotostatin)	⊖ GH		
PRH (?)	PRL		Lactation (mammary gland)
PRIH (dopamine)	⊖ PRL		Lactation inhibited

[a]The hypothalamic hormones in column 1 stimulate the release of the corresponding anterior pituitary hormones in column 2 unless inhibition is indicated by ⊖. The anterior pituitary hormones act on on the target glands in column 3 (or in column 4, in the case of PRL), which release hormones that have the effect listed in column 4. Question marks (?) indicate hormones that have not been fully established.

The most common cause of hyperprolactinemia is the use of drugs that interfere with the synthesis or action of dopamine, a naturally occurring prolactin-inhibiting factor, within the hypothalamus. These agents include neuroleptics (the phenothiazines), antidepressants, opiates, certain antihypertensive drugs, and high doses of estrogen.

After taking a careful history, **Mil Keeway's** physician concluded that the use of such drugs was not the cause of her hyperprolactinemia.

The serum increase in TSH levels in response to intravenously administered TRH occurs within 20–30 minutes after the injection and returns to basal levels within 2–3 hours.

release as well as hormones that inhibit prolactin release. The identity of the major physiological prolactin-releasing hormone has not been established, although a large number of substances with diverse structural characteristics have been shown to cause prolactin release in vivo. These include TRH, vasoactive intestinal peptide (VIP), serotonin, oxytocin, as well as β-endorphin, bradykinin, and acetylcholine. Although other prolactin release-inhibiting factors have been identified, current evidence supports dopamine as the most physiologically important inhibitor.

Dopamine is a catecholamine (Fig. 44.4). When released into the hypothalamicohypophyseal portal venous system from the hypothalamus, dopamine inhibits prolactin secretion from the lactotrophs (prolactin-secreting cells) of the anterior pituitary. The interaction of dopamine with high affinity, specific dopamine receptors lowers intracellular cAMP levels, causing a decrease in prolactin gene transcription and subsequently a reduction in prolactin synthesis and secretion.

Thyrotropin-Releasing Hormone

TRH is a tripeptide, pyroglutamyl-histidyl-prolinamide (Fig. 44.5). It is protected at its N-terminus by cyclization of glutamate to pyroglutamate. TRH is widely distributed in the hypothalamus but is especially concentrated in the paraventricular nucleus. Although TRH appears to regulate the secretion of several other anterior pituitary hormones under a variety of physiological and pathological settings, its major action involves the regulation of thyroid-stimulating hormone (TSH) secretion from the thyrotrophs (anterior pituitary cells which secrete TSH). This action is mediated by specific, high affinity receptors for TRH on the plasma membrane of these cells. Because TRH also plays an important role in the posttranslational processing of the oligosaccharide moieties of TSH, it also has an important influence on the biological activity of TSH.

Corticotropin-Releasing Hormone

The structure of CRH, a 41 amino acid peptide produced primarily in the paraventricular nucleus, was elucidated in 1981 and is shown in Figure 44.6.

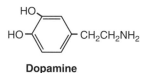

Dopamine

Fig. 44.4. Dopamine. This compound belongs to the class of catecholamines, which also includes epinephrine and norepinephrine. It is produced from tyrosine (see Fig. 43.7).

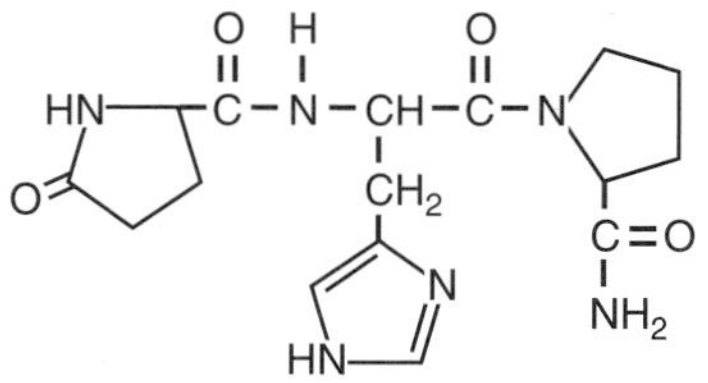

Pyro-glutamyl-histidyl-prolinamide (TRH)

Fig. 44.5. Structure of thyrotropin-releasing hormone (TRH). TRH is a tripeptide with a pyroglutamate at the N terminus and an amide at the C-terminus.

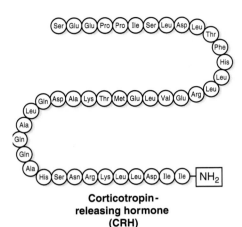

**Corticotropin-
releasing hormone
(CRH)**

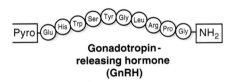

**Gonadotropin-
releasing hormone
(GnRH)**

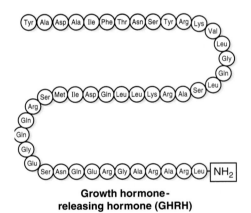

**Growth hormone-
releasing hormone (GHRH)**

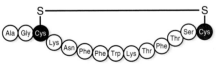

**Growth hormone release-
inhibiting hormone
(GHRIH) (Somatostatin)**

Fig. 44.6. Structures of corticotropin releasing hormone (CRH), gonadotropin releasing hormone (GnRH), growth hormone releasing hormone (GHRH), and growth hormone release-inhibiting hormone (GHRIH, also called somatostatin). These hormones are peptides that differ in sequence and length. GnRH has a pyroglutamate at its N-terminus, and CRH, GnRH, and GHRH have an amide at the C-terminus (see Fig. 44.5).

CRH travels to the corticotrophs (the anterior pituitary cells which secrete ACTH) via the hypothalamico-hypophyseal portal vessels. The peptide binds with a single class of specific CRH receptors on the plasma membrane of these cells. This first messenger signal is probably coupled to adenylate cyclase and causes an increase in intracellular cAMP with a subsequent influx of Ca^{2+} into the cytosol of the corticotrophs. An increase in proopiomelanocortin (POMC) synthesis and in adrenocorticotropic hormone (ACTH) secretion follows (see Fig. 44.9). Evidence suggests that ACTH is then co-secreted with POMC cleavage products, peptides whose biological actions remain poorly understood.

Gonadotropin-Releasing Hormone

GnRH is composed of a single chain of amino acids protected, like TRH, at its N-terminus by cyclization of glutamate to pyroglutamate. It is also amidated at the C-terminus (see Fig. 44.6).

GnRH is secreted episodically, the pulse frequency of secretion varying during different phases of the menstrual cycle in females. This pulsatile release of GnRH is required for optimal luteinizing hormone (LH) and follicle-stimulating hormone (FSH) secretion from the gonadotrophs (the anterior pituitary cells which secrete LH and FSH). Pulsatile release of these gonadotropins is required for a normal gonadal response.

GnRH exerts its actions via specific receptors on the plasma membrane of the gonadotrophs. These receptors are coupled to the hydrolysis of phosphoinositides with the production of inositol trisphosphate and diacylglycerol and the subsequent enrichment of cytosolic Ca^{2+} in the gonadotrophs from both intracellular stores and via calcium channels in the plasma membranes.

Growth Hormone-Releasing Hormone

The structure of GHRH was identified in 1982 (see Fig. 44.6). It exists as both a 40 and a 44 amino acid peptide encoded on chromosome 20 and produced in cells of the arcuate nucleus. Its C-terminal leucine residue is amidated. Full biological activity of this releasing hormone resides in the first 29 amino acids of the N-terminal portion of the molecule. GHRH interacts with specific receptors on the plasma membranes of the somatotrophs (the cells of the anterior pituitary that synthesize and release growth hormone). The intracellular signaling mechanisms that result in growth hormone (GH) synthesis and release appear to be multiple, since cAMP and calcium-calmodulin both stimulate GH release.

Growth Hormone Release-Inhibiting Hormone

GHRIH, also called somatostatin, inhibits the release of GH from the anterior pituitary. It blocks the release of GH ordinarily induced by a variety of physiological GH secretogogues such as exercise, arginine, hypoglycemia, and GHRH. Somatostatin was initially discovered in the hypothalamus. Subsequently, it was found in extrahypothalamic brain centers and in the gastrointestinal tract, particularly in the stomach, intestine, the D cells of the pancreas, and the nerve fibers of the intestine. It has also been found in the peripheral nerves, placenta, adrenal medulla, and the tissues of the retina.

Somatostatin contains 14 amino acid residues with a cyclic structure joined by an intramolecular disulfide bond between 2 cysteine residues (see Fig. 44.6). A family of somatostatin-related peptides exists in addition to the original tetradecapeptide (known as S-14). An active form of the peptide called S-28 contains an N-terminal

14 amino acid extension. Although S-28 may serve as a precursor of S-14, it appears to have distinct biological as well as immunological activity in its own right. The larger molecule, for example, suppresses GH release far longer than does S-14.

Like other peptide hormones, both S-14 and S-28 bind to receptors in the plasma membrane of target cells. At least two classes of somatostatin receptors exist. Binding to either class leads to activation of one or more membrane-bound G proteins, which then reduce levels of intracellular cAMP and the cytosolic free Ca^{2+} concentration in somatostatin-responsive cells.

HORMONES OF THE ANTERIOR PITUITARY

Growth Hormone

Human growth hormone is a polypeptide composed of a single chain of 191 amino acids having two intramolecular disulfide bonds (Fig. 44.7). It is secreted by the somatotroph cells of the anterior pituitary. GH is structurally related to human chorionic somatomammotropin (hCS) from the placenta, a polypeptide that stimulates growth of the developing fetus. Yet the hCS peptide has only 0.1% of the growth-inducing potency of GH. Prolactin is also a member of the GH family, having 199 amino acids (but only 16% homology with GH) and an additional disulfide bond.

The physiological secretion of GH is determined by a balance between GHRH (also called somatocrinin) and GHRIH (also called somatostatin), acting upon the somatotrophs of the anterior pituitary. In addition, insulin-like growth factor I (IGF-

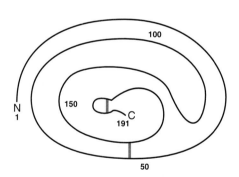

Human growth hormone

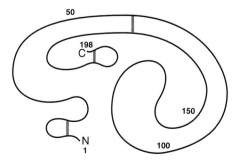

Ovine prolactin

Fig. 44.7. Structures of growth hormone and prolactin. ▌ = disulfide bridges. From Murray RK, et al. Harper's biochemistry, 23rd ed. Stamford, CT: Appleton & Lange, 1993:502.

After 100 µg of ovine CRH is given intravenously as a bolus to elevate the secretory capacity of the pituitary corticotropic cells, plasma ACTH levels rise rapidly, reaching a peak concentration in about 10 minutes.

A persistent nonpulsatile release of GnRH suppresses the pituitary-gonadal axis and hence the production of testosterone. This observation has been used to advantage in patients with metastatic prostate cancer whose tumor growth is enhanced by androgenic steroids. Therefore, the chronic use of exogenous GnRH agonists, designed to maintain pharmacological levels of this releasing hormone in the blood, may slow the growth of the malignancy by reducing testosterone production by the testicles.

The ophthalmologist ordered a morning fasting serum GH level on **Sam Atotrope**, which was elevated at 56 ng/mL (normal = 0–5 ng/mL)

In addition to its effects on normal GH secretion, somatostatin also suppresses the pathological increase in GH which occurs in acromegaly (caused by a GH-secreting pituitary tumor), diabetes mellitus, and carcinoid tumors (tumors that secrete serotonin). Somatostatin also suppresses the basal secretion of TSH, TRH, insulin, and glucagon. The hormone also has a suppressive effect on a wide variety of nonendocrine secretions.

The major limitation in the clinical use of native somatostatin is its short half-life of less than 3 minutes in the circulation. Analogues of native somatostatin, however, have been developed which are resistant to degradation and, therefore, have a longer half-life. One such analogue is octreotide, an octapeptide variant of somatostatin with a half-life of about 110 minutes.

Q **44.1:** Three months after therapy with oral thyroid hormone (thyroxine (T_4)) was started, **Ahot Goyta's** TSH levels were 23 ng/mL (normal = 0.1–5 ng/mL). Was his dose of thyroxine adequate?

Sam Atotrope was given an oral dose of 100 g of glucose syrup. This dose would suppress serum GH levels to less than 2 ng/mL in normal subjects, but not in patients with acromegaly who have an autonomously secreting pituitary tumor making GH. Because Sam's serum GH level was 43 ng/mL after the oral glucose load, a diagnosis of acromegaly was made. The patient was referred to an endocrinologist for further evaluation.

GH not only stimulates IGF-I gene expression in the liver but in a number of extrahepatic tissues as well. In acromegalics, rising levels of IGF-I cause a gradual generalized increase in skeletal, muscular, and visceral growth. As a consequence, there is a diffuse increase in the bulk of all tissues (enlargement = "megaly") especially in the "acral" (most peripheral) tissues of the body, such as the face, the hands, and the feet, hence the term "acromegaly."

Sam Atotrope's coarse facial features and bulky hands are typical of patients with acromegaly.

A 44.1: An elevated TSH level indicates that thyroid hormone levels in the blood are not high enough to suppress TSH secretion by the anterior pituitary. Therefore, **Ahot Goyta's** dose of thyroid hormone is not adequate and should be increased to a level that further suppresses his serum TSH level, bringing it into the normal range.

I; also called somatomedin C), produced primarily in the liver in response to the action of GH on hepatocytes, feeds back negatively on the somatotrophs to limit GH secretion. Other physiological factors (e.g., exercise, sleep, hypoglycemia) and many pathological factors control its release.

The actions of GH can be classified as those which occur as a consequence of the hormone's direct effect on target cells and those which occur indirectly through the ability of GH to generate other factors, particularly IGF-I (see Chapter 47).

The direct actions of GH are exerted primarily in hepatocytes. GH administration is followed by an early increase in the synthesis of 8 to 10 proteins among which are IGF-I, α_2-macroglobulin, and the serine protease inhibitors Spi 2.1 and Spi 2.3. Expression of the gene for ornithine decarboxylase, an enzyme active in polyamine synthesis (and, therefore, in the regulation of cell proliferation), is also significantly increased by GH.

Muscle and adipocyte cell membranes contain GH receptors which mediate direct, rapid metabolic effects on glucose and amino acid transport as well as on lipolysis (see Chapter 45). GH also has growth-promoting effects. GH receptors are present on a variety of tissues where GH increases IGF-I gene expression. The subsequent rise in IGF-I levels contributes to cell multiplication and differentiation by autocrine and/or paracrine mechanisms. These, in turn, lead to skeletal, muscular, and visceral growth. These actions are accompanied by a direct anabolic influence of GH on protein metabolism with a diversion of amino acids from oxidation to protein synthesis and a shift to a positive nitrogen balance.

Thyroid-Stimulating Hormone

TSH belongs to a family of pituitary and placental glycoproteins that includes FSH, LH, and human chorionic gonadotropin (hCG) (Fig. 44.8). Each contains a common α-subunit and a structurally distinct β-subunit. The β-subunit determines the specific biological activity of the dimer.

TSH is synthesized in the thyrotropic cells of the anterior pituitary. Its secretion is primarily regulated by a balance between the stimulatory action of hypothalamic TRH and the inhibitory (negative feedback) influence of thyroid hormone at levels above a critical threshold in the blood bathing the pituitary thyrotrophs.

TSH secretion occurs in a circadian pattern, a surge beginning late in the afternoon and peaking before the onset of sleep. In addition, TSH is secreted in a pulsatile fashion with intervals of 2–6 hours between peaks.

TSH stimulates all phases of thyroid hormone synthesis by the thyroid gland including iodide trapping from the plasma, organification of iodide, coupling of mono- and diiodotyrosine, endocytosis of thyroglobulin, and proteolysis of thyroglobulin to release triiodothyronine (T_3) and T_4 (see Fig. 43.6). In addition, the vascularity of the thyroid gland increases as TSH stimulates hypertrophy and hyperplasia of the thyroid acinar cells.

The predominant mechanism of action of TSH is mediated by binding of TSH to its specific receptor on the plasma membrane of the thyroid acinar cell, leading to an increase in the concentration of cytosolic cAMP. Recent evidence indicates, however, that TSH also increases the cellular levels of inositol trisphosphate and diacylglycerol, causing a rise in cytosolic Ca^{2+} within the thyroid cell.

Gonadotropins

The anterior pituitary gland produces glycoproteins which control the maturation of the male and female gametes and the production of gonadal sex steroids, facilitating normal sexual function and maturation (see Chapter 47). These glycoprotein hormones belong to a family of endocrine substances known as the gonadotropins, which include the pituitary hormones FSH and LH, and the placental hormone chorionic gonadotropin (hCG or choriogonadotropin). Each of these hormones contains a common α-subunit and a unique β-subunit (see Fig. 44.8). hCG maintains the corpus luteum during the early stages of pregnancy (see Chapter 47).

Follicle-Stimulating Hormone

In females, FSH stimulates the maturation of the follicle (see Chapter 47). The hormone acts on the FSH receptors on the granulosa cells of the ovary to increase the conversion of androgenic steroids to estrogens (primarily estradiol) as well as to induce cell proliferation. As estradiol and FSH levels rise, the granulosa cells become increasingly sensitive to the actions of FSH. Certain follicles are more sensitive than others to these stimulatory effects and develop more rapidly. Even as FSH levels decline, these dominant follicles continue to mature in the second half of the follicular phase of the menstrual cycle.

Follicles less sensitive to estradiol and FSH undergo apoptosis or "programmed cell death." When the dominant follicle reaches the later stages of maturation, FSH promotes the formation of the antrum (the fluid-filled central cavity of the developing follicle). FSH also promotes the induction of the granulosa cell LH receptors in preparation for the midcycle surge of LH which stimulates ovulation and differentiation of the granulosa and thecal cells of the follicle into a corpus luteum.

In immature males, FSH contributes to the initiation of spermatogenesis. FSH binds to receptors on the cell membrane of Sertoli cells and stimulates the synthesis of proteins that promote the maturation of the most immature form of the testicular germ cells known as spermatogonia. In sexually mature males, FSH also binds to Sertoli cells, but sperm development can be maintained in the absence of FSH.

Luteinizing Hormone

In females, the major action of LH involves the induction of ovulation and luteinization of the mature Graafian follicle. In addition, LH stimulates steroidogenesis by the interstitial (thecal) cells of the ovary. Androgens produced by these thecal cells serve as precursors for estradiol synthesis by the granulosa cells of the follicle (see Chapter 47).

In males, LH induces androgen production by the Leydig cells of the testis. These androgens help initiate and maintain spermatogenesis as well as induce the development of male secondary sexual characteristics.

Adrenocorticotropin and Proopiomelanocortin

ACTH is a peptide hormone composed of 39 amino acid residues. The hormone is synthesized in the corticotrophic cells of the anterior pituitary gland. Its secretion is stimulated primarily by CRH from the hypothalamus and inhibited by levels of cortisol above a critical threshold in the blood bathing the anterior pituitary gland.

ACTH is produced in the corticotrophic cells by cleavage of proopiomelanocortin (POMC), a macromolecule with a molecular weight of 28,500 (Fig. 44.9). POMC consists of 265 amino acids including a signal peptide of 26 amino acids. The factors that regulate POMC synthesis are similar to those regulating the production of ACTH.

The processing of this large precursor molecule to form ACTH, β-lipotropin (β-LPH), and other degradation products of POMC, including both α- and β-MSH, is shown in Figure 44.9. In the anterior pituitary, the major endproducts are the N-terminal peptide, the joining peptide, ACTH, and β-LPH. β-LPH is further processed to β-endorphin.

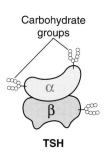

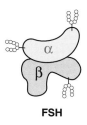

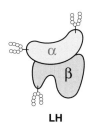

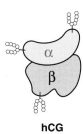

Fig. 44.8. Structures of TSH, FSH, LH, and hCG. The α-subunits are the same and are experimentally interchangeable. The β-subunits differ and confer biological specificity. These hormones are glycoproteins.

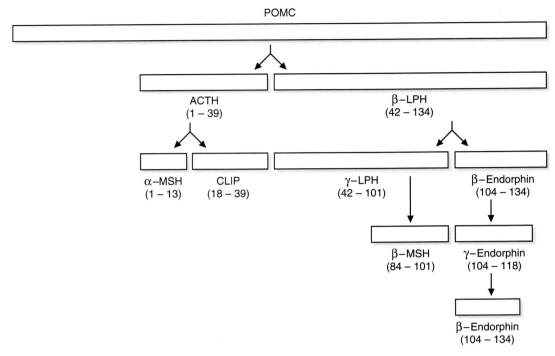

Fig. 44.9. Processing of proopiomelanocortin (POMC). The protein POMC is produced by the anterior pituitary in response to corticotropin releasing hormone (CRH). The N-terminal region is removed, and the remainder is cleaved to form adrenocorticotropic hormone (ACTH) (residues 1–39) and β-lipotropin (β-LPH) (residues 42–134). Additional cleavages produce the melanocyte stimulating hormones (α- and β-MSH), endorphins, corticotropin-like intermediate lobe peptide (CLIP), and γ-lipotropin (γ-LPH). These additional cleavages may not all occur in the human (see text).

 β-Melanocyte-stimulating hormone (β-MSH) is not produced in the human pituitary. Process-ing of ACTH to form α-MSH and corticotropin-like intermediate lobe poly-peptide (CLIP) occurs to a minor extent in the rat but not in the human pituitary. The latter processing, however, does occur quite extensively in the intermediate lobe of the pituitary of some species, but this lobe is vestigial in adult humans.

The first 13 amino acid residues of human ACTH are identical to those of α-MSH of some mammals, and excessive levels of ACTH in the blood are associated with hyperpigmentation of the skin in humans (i.e., with dermal melanocyte stimulation). Therefore, it is likely that normal production of the skin pigment melanin is stimulated by ACTH in humans.

The precise physiological actions of all of the degradation products of POMC in various tissues remain to be determined. The proposed actions of β-endorphin include a role as an endogenous opiate, which modulates pain perception. It may also regulate the secretion of other pituitary hormones as well as the neural control of breathing. In addition, β-endorphin has been proposed to influence feeding and sexual behavior as well as the learning process. Less is known about the physiological actions of β-LPH. It has weak lipolytic activity and some opiate-like actions.

The major biological action of ACTH is to stimulate synthesis and secretion of adrenocortical steroids. The secretion of the major glucocorticoid cortisol is stimulated by ACTH. Signaling occurs through the activation of adenylate cyclase, which produces cAMP. Steroidogenesis is regulated primarily at the step involving the oxidative cleavage of the side chain of cholesterol, a reaction that forms pregnenolone. ACTH also enhances the production of adrenal androgens, and has a permissive effect on aldosterone production (i.e., it is required for optimal synthesis of this mineralocorticoid in response to other stimuli).

Prolactin

STRUCTURE OF PROLACTIN

Human prolactin is composed of 199 amino acid residues having three internal disulfide bridges (see Fig. 44.7). Numerous isoforms of the hormone exist, each with differing biological potency. This structural diversity results both from posttranscriptional and posttranslational modifications. Some isoforms are glycosylated, some phosphorylated, and others deamidated, while others are partially cleaved.

SYNTHESIS AND SECRETION OF PROLACTIN

Prolactin is synthesized in the lactotrophs of the anterior pituitary. Prolactin, like all anterior pituitary hormones, is secreted episodically with a distinctive 24-hour pattern of release, showing a nocturnal peak related to sleep.

The control of prolactin secretion is bipolar, with PRH acting as a stimulator and PRIHs, such as dopamine, acting as inhibitors. TRH, VIP, and possibly serotonin also act as prolactin-releasing factors (PRFs).

ACTIONS OF PROLACTIN

The actions of prolactin in milk production occur as a consequence of the binding of prolactin to receptors on the plasma membrane of the secretory cells of the mammary gland. Prolactin is also capable of binding to receptors in the liver, kidneys, adrenals, testicles, ovaries, uterus, and other tissues. This broad spectrum of prolactin-sensitive tissues may explain the wide array of biological activities of the hormone. The predominant mechanism of postreceptor signaling that mediates these actions, however, remains to be determined.

The actions of prolactin in the breast are essential to the initiation and maintenance of lactation. Prolactin specifically induces the synthesis of the milk proteins (both the major protein of human milk, α-lactalbumin, and casein), an action enhanced by the 20-fold increase in the number of prolactin receptors in breast tissue which occurs at parturition (delivery of an infant). Extensive turnover of phospholipids occurs in the breast during lactation, reflecting the fact that a major component of breast milk is triacylglycerol. Prolactin, in conjunction with insulin and cortisol, increases the rate of fatty acid synthesis, maintains the level of activity of lipoprotein lipase, and enhances phospholipid synthesis in the breast. Although prolactin was originally thought to have a mitogenic effect on breast epithelial cells, increasing their number, it now appears that the latter action is caused by GH, not prolactin.

In the male, physiological levels of prolactin increase and maintain the concentration of LH receptors on the Leydig cell membrane in the testis, thereby helping to sustain normal testosterone production. The hormone also influences normal sperm motility and enhances fertility.

Minor actions of prolactin in the human include a decrease in renal water, sodium, and potassium excretion without renal hemodynamic changes occurring within the kidney, suggesting a direct osmoregulatory effect.

Finally, an immunoregulatory action of prolactin has been proposed. Hypophysectomized animals display a reduction in immune competence which is restored with daily treatment with either GH or prolactin. Evidence suggests that prolactin stimulates both humoral and cell-mediated immunity and that lymphocytes are an important target cell for this action.

STIMULUS FOR RELEASE OF PROLACTIN

Release of prolactin is stimulated by suckling of an infant, the same stimulus that promotes oxytocin release. As oxytocin causes contraction of myoepithelial cells in the mammary gland, forcing milk to be ejected through the nipple, prolactin stimulates the production of milk. Thus, the stimulus for the release of milk from the mammary gland also serves to replenish the milk supply (Fig. 44.10).

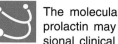 The molecular heterogeneity of prolactin may explain the occasional clinical syndrome of sustained hyperprolactinemia as measured by radioimmunoassay in a patient with few, if any, specific signs or symptoms of excess prolactin secretion. In this case, the antibodies used for the radioimmunoassay bind not only to prolactin but also to isoforms that have little biological activity.

A magnetic resonance imaging (MRI) scan of **Mil Keeway's** pituitary gland was performed. This scan demonstrated a mass in the pituitary approximately 7 mm in diameter. Because none of the nonneoplastic ("functional") causes of an elevation in serum prolactin (such as the prolonged use of high dose estrogen therapy, severe hypothyroidism, or chronic renal insufficiency) was present; a diagnosis of a prolactin-secreting pituitary tumor was made. An endocrinologist was consulted for advice with regard to further diagnostic steps and appropriate therapy.

In the female, ovulation may be inhibited by high blood levels of prolactin via impairment of follicular development and indirectly by reduction of ovarian estrogen synthesis. High levels of prolactin also decrease the amplitude and frequency of LH pulses possibly at the level of the hypothalamic GnRH pulse generator.

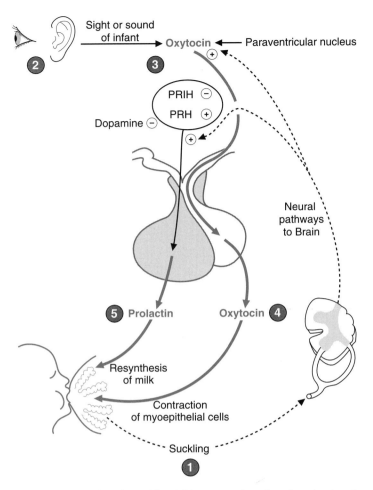

Fig. 44.10. Regulation of lactation. **1.** Suckling initiates nerve impulses that stimulate the production of oxytocin (OT) in the hypothalamus and its release from the posterior pituitary. **2** and **3.** The sight or sound of the infant also cause OT release. In addition, suckling stimulates the release of prolactin releasing hormone (PRH) from the hypothalamus, which stimulates the release of prolactin (PRL) from the anterior pituitary. **4.** OT causes myoepithelial cells of the mammary gland to contract, forcing milk from the gland. **5.** PRL stimulates the resynthesis of milk.

CLINICAL COMMENTS. Hyperprolactinemia, as found in **Mil Keeway**, is present in approximately 25% of women presenting with secondary amenorrhea (the cessation of menstrual periods), in 10% of those with oligomenorrhea (diminished menstrual flow and/or regularity), and in 3% with unexplained infertility. The use of drugs that interfere with the synthesis of dopamine is the most common cause of an elevated serum prolactin level. In a patient who is not using such drugs, the cause is most likely a benign secretory tumor of the galactotroph cells in the anterior pituitary gland. Although these tumors are generally small, they may progress in secretory capacity and size over many years. Nevertheless, a substantial number of these patients will show either no change or even a decrease in serum prolactin levels over time. Those with more aggressive tumors may be treated with stereotactic radiotherapy, surgical resection, or the chronic use of the drug bromocriptine. In those patients with longstanding and moderately severe tumor-related hyperprolactinemia, the cure rate with radiotherapy and/or surgical resection may be less than 50%. Although bromocriptine often normalizes the serum prolactin level with long term administration, serum prolactin levels almost always rise into the abnormal range soon after the drug is discontinued.

An MRI scan of **Sam Atotrope's** brain revealed a macroadenoma (a tumor greater than 10 mm in diameter) in the pituitary gland, with superior extension that compressed the optic nerve as it crossed above the sella turcica, causing his visual problems. The skeletal and visceral changes noted by the ophthalmologist are characteristic of acromegalic patients with chronically elevated serum levels of GH and IGF-I.

Therapeutic alternatives for acromegaly caused by a GH-secreting tumor of the anterior pituitary gland are similar to those for a prolactinoma. These alternatives include lifelong medical therapy with the somatostatin analogue octreotide. Other therapeutic options include stereotactic radiotherapy, or surgical resection of the neoplasm. If the excessive secretion of GH is controlled successfully, some of the visceral changes of acromegaly may slowly subside to varying degrees. The skeletal changes, on the other hand, cannot be reversed.

BIOCHEMICAL COMMENTS. To establish the diagnosis of a secretory tumor of an endocrine gland, one must first demonstrate that basal serum levels of the hormone in question are regularly elevated. More importantly, one must show that the hypersecretion of the hormone (and, hence, its elevated level in the peripheral blood) cannot be adequately inhibited by "maneuvers" which are known to suppress secretion from a normally functioning gland (i.e., one must demonstrate that the hypersecretion is "autonomous").

To ensure that both the basal and the postsuppression levels of the specific hormone to be tested will reflect the true secretory rate of the suspected endocrine tumor, all of the known factors that can stimulate the synthesis of the hormone must be eliminated. For GH, for example, the secretogogues (stimulants to secretion) include nutritional factors; the patient's level of activity, consciousness, and stress; and certain drugs. GH secretion is stimulated by a high protein meal or by a low level of fatty acids or of glucose in the blood. Vigorous exercise, stage III–IV sleep, psychological and physical stress, and levodopa, clonidine, and estrogens also increase GH release.

The suppression test used to demonstrate the autonomous hypersecretion of GH involves giving the patient an oral glucose load and, subsequently, measuring GH levels. A sudden rise in blood glucose suppresses serum GH to 2 ng/mL or less in normal subjects, but not in patients with active acromegaly.

If one attempts to demonstrate autonomous hypersecretion of GH in a patient suspected of having acromegaly, therefore, before drawing the blood for both the basal (pre-glucose load) serum GH level and the post-glucose load serum GH level, one must be certain that the patient has not eaten for 6–8 hours, has not done vigorous exercise for at least 4 hours, remains fully awake during the entire testing period (in a nonstressed state to the extent possible), and has not taken any drugs known to increase GH secretion for at least 1 week.

Under these carefully controlled circumstances, if both the basal and postsuppression serum levels of the suspect hormone are elevated, one can conclude that autonomous hypersecretion is probably present. At this point, localization procedures (such as an MRI of the pituitary gland in an acromegalic suspect) are performed to further confirm the diagnosis.

Suggested Readings

DeGroot LJ. Endocrinology. Philadelphia: WB Saunders, 1995:151–406.

Goodman HM. Basic medical endocrinology. New York: Raven Press, 1994:28–45.

PROBLEMS

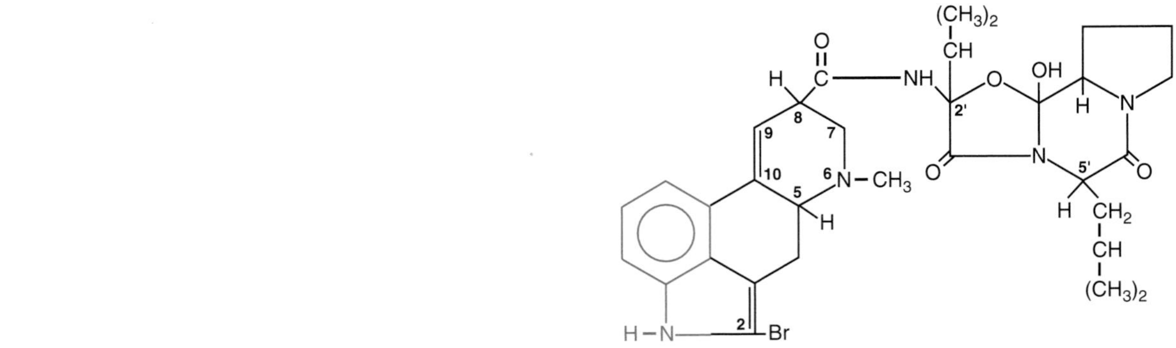

Bromocriptine

1. The structure of the drug bromocriptine is shown above. Based on its structure, suggest a mechanism for its action.

2. A woman was scheduled for a growth hormone suppression test. If each of the following occurred the morning of the test, which would be most likely to cause a decrease in growth hormone levels?

   A. She ate 4 large doughnuts for breakfast.

   B. She was on estrogen replacement therapy and took her tablets after breakfast.

   C. While unlocking her car, she was chased by the neighbor's vicious dog.

   D. She fell asleep at the start of the test and slept soundly until it was completed 1.5 hours later.

ANSWERS

1. Bromocriptine is a structural analogue of dopamine (see Fig. 44.4). Bromocriptine mimics the action of this natural inhibitor of prolactin secretion.

2. The answer is **A.** High blood glucose levels cause a decrease in growth hormone levels in the blood. This fact serves as the basis for the glucose suppression test for growth hormone. B, C, and D all would cause growth hormone levels to increase.

45 Actions of Hormones That Regulate Fuel Metabolism

Many hormones affect fuel metabolism, including those that regulate appetite as well as those that influence absorption, transport, and oxidation of foodstuffs. The major hormones that influence nutrient metabolism are listed in Table 45.1.

Insulin is the major anabolic hormone. It promotes the storage of nutrients as glycogen in liver and muscle, and as triacylglycerols in adipose tissue. It also stimulates the synthesis of proteins in tissues such as muscle. At the same time, insulin acts to inhibit fuel mobilization.

Glucagon is the major counterregulatory hormone. The term "counterregulatory" means that its actions are generally opposed to those of insulin (contrainsular). The major action of glucagon is to mobilize fuel reserves by stimulating glycogenolysis and gluconeogenesis. These actions ensure that glucose will be available to glucose-dependent tissues between meals.

Epinephrine, norepinephrine, cortisol, somatostatin, and growth hormone also have contrainsular activity. Thyroid hormone must also be classified as an insulin counterregulatory hormone because it increases the rate of fuel consumption and also increases the sensitivity of the target cells to other insulin counterregulatory hormones.

Insulin and the counterregulatory hormones exert two types of metabolic regulation (see Chapter 24). The first type of control occurs within minutes to hours of the hormone-receptor interaction and usually results from changes in the catalytic activity or kinetics of key preexisting enzymes, caused by phosphorylation or dephosphorylation of these enzymes. The second type of control involves regulation of the synthesis of key enzymes by mechanisms that stimulate or inhibit transcription and translation of mRNA. These processes are slow and require hours to days.

Table 45.1. Major Hormones That Regulate Fuel Metabolism

Anabolic hormone
       Insulin
Counterregulatory hormones[a]
       Glucagon
       Epinephrine
       Norepinephrine
       Cortisol
       Somatostatin
       Growth hormone
       Thyroid hormone

[a]Hormones with actions that are generally opposed to those of insulin.

Ron Templeton, now a third-year medical student, was assigned to do a history and physical examination on a newly admitted 47-year-old patient named **Corti Solemia**. Mr. Solemia had consulted his physician for increasing weakness and fatigue and was found to have a severely elevated serum glucose level. While examining the patient, Ron noted marked redness of the patient's facial skin as well as reddish-purple stripes (striae) in the skin of the patient's lower abdomen and thighs. The patient's body fat was unusually distributed in that it appeared to be excessively deposited in his cheeks, upper back, and abdomen, while his distal arms and legs appeared to be almost devoid of fat. The patient's skin appeared thinned and large bruises were present over many areas of his body, for which Mr. Solemia had no explanation. The neurological examination revealed severe muscle weakness, especially in the proximal arms and legs, where the muscles seemed atrophied.

While **Sam Atotrope** was trying to decide which of the major alternatives for the treatment of his growth hormone (GH)-secreting pituitary tumor to choose, he noted progressive fatigue and the onset of increasing urinary frequency associated with a marked increase in thirst. In addition, he had lost 4 lb over the course of the last 6 weeks in spite of a good appetite. His physician suspected that Mr. Atotrope had developed diabetes mellitus, perhaps related to the chronic hypersecretion of GH. This suspicion was confirmed when Sam's serum glucose level, drawn prior to breakfast, was reported to be 236 mg/dL.

PHYSIOLOGICAL EFFECTS OF INSULIN

The effects of insulin on fuel metabolism and substrate flux were considered in many of the earlier chapters of this book, particularly in Chapter 24. Insulin stimulates the storage of glycogen in liver and muscle, and the synthesis of fatty acids and triacylglycerols and their storage in adipose tissue. In addition, insulin stimulates the synthesis in various tissues of over 50 proteins, some of which contribute to the growth of the organism. In fact, it is difficult to separate the effects of insulin on cell growth from those of insulin-like growth factors I and II (IGF-I and IGF-II) (see Chapter 47).

Finally, insulin has paracrine actions within the pancreatic islet cells. When insulin is released from the B cells, it suppresses glucagon release from the A cells.

PHYSIOLOGICAL EFFECTS OF GLUCAGON

Glucagon is one of several counterregulatory (contrainsular) hormones. It is synthesized as part of a large precursor protein, proglucagon. Proglucagon is produced in the A cells of the islets of Langerhans in the pancreas and in the L cells of the intestine. It contains a number of peptides linked in tandem: glicentin-related peptide, glucagon, glucagon-related peptide 1 (GLP-1), and glucagon-related peptide-2 (GLP-2). Proteolytic cleavage of proglucagon releases various combinations of its constituent peptides. Glucagon is cleaved from proglucagon in the pancreas and constitutes 30–40% of the immunoreactive glucagon in the blood. The remaining immunoreactivity is due to other cleavage products of proglucagon released from the pancreas and the intestine. Pancreatic glucagon has a plasma half-life of 3–6 minutes and is removed mainly by the liver and kidney.

Glucagon promotes glycogenolysis, gluconeogenesis, and ketogenesis by stimulating the generation of cAMP in target cells. The liver is the major target organ for glucagon, in part because the concentrations of this hormone bathing the liver cells in the portal blood are higher than in the peripheral circulation. Portal vein levels of glucagon may reach concentrations as high as 500 pg/mL.

Finally, glucagon stimulates insulin release from the B cells of the pancreas. Whether this is a paracrine effect or endocrine effect has not been established. The pattern of blood flow in the pancreatic islet cells is believed to bathe the B cells first and then the A cells. Therefore, the B cells may influence A-cell function via an endocrine mechanism, whereas the influence of A-cell hormone on B-cell function is more likely to be paracrine.

PHYSIOLOGICAL EFFECTS OF OTHER COUNTERREGULATORY HORMONES

Somatostatin

BIOCHEMISTRY

Preprosomatostatin, a 116 amino acid peptide, is encoded on the long arm of chromosome 3. Somatostatin (S-14), a cyclic peptide with a molecular weight of 1,600, is produced from the 14 amino acids at the C-terminus of this precursor molecule. S-14 was first isolated from the hypothalamus and named for its ability to inhibit the release of GH (somatotropin) from the anterior pituitary. It also inhibits the release of insulin. In addition to the hypothalamus, somatostatin is also secreted from the D cells (δ cells) of the pancreatic islets and is found in many areas of the central nervous system, and in gastric and duodenal mucosal cells as well as in the circulation. S-14 predominates in the central nervous system (CNS) and in the D cells of the pancreas. In the gut, however, prosomatostatin (S-28), which has 14 additional amino acids from the C-terminal of the precursor, makes up 70–75% of the immunoreactivity (the amount of hormone that reacts with antibodies to S-14). The prohormone S-28 is 7–10 times more potent in inhibiting the release of GH and that of insulin than is S-14.

SECRETION OF SOMATOSTATIN

The secretogogues for somatostatin are similar to those that cause secretion of insulin. The metabolites that increase somatostatin release include glucose, arginine, and leucine. The hormones that stimulate somatostatin secretion include glucagon, vasoactive intestinal polypeptide (VIP), and cholecystokinin (CCK). Insulin, on the other hand, does not influence somatostatin secretion.

Tolbutamide, a sulfonylurea drug which increases insulin secretion, also increases the secretion of pancreatic somatostatin.

PHYSIOLOGICAL EFFECTS OF SOMATOSTATIN

Somatostatin binds to its plasma membrane receptors on target cells. These "activated" receptors interact with inhibitory G proteins of adenylate cyclase. As a result, the production of cAMP is inhibited and protein kinase A is not activated. This inhibitory effect suppresses secretion of GH and thyroid-stimulating hormone (TSH) from the anterior pituitary gland as well as the secretion of insulin and glucagon from the pancreatic islets. In addition to these effects on hormones that regulate fuel metabolism, somatostatin also reduces nutrient absorption from the gut by prolonging gastric emptying time, by decreasing stomach acid and gastrin secretion, by diminishing pancreatic exocrine secretions (i.e., digestive enzymes, bicarbonate, and water), and by decreasing splanchnic blood flow. Thus, somatostatin exerts a broad, albeit indirect, influence on the utilization of fuels.

Catecholamines (Epinephrine, Norepinephrine, Dopamine)

The catecholamines are secretory products of the sympathoadrenal system which are required for the body to adapt to a great variety of acute and chronic stresses. Epinephrine (80–85% of stored catecholamines) is synthesized primarily in the cells of the adrenal medulla, whereas norepinephrine (15–20% of stored catecholamines) is synthesized and stored not only in the adrenal medulla but also in various areas of the CNS and in the nerve endings of the adrenergic nervous system. Dopamine acts primarily as a neurotransmitter and has little effect on fuel metabolism.

SYNTHESIS OF THE CATECHOLAMINES

Tyrosine is the precursor of the catecholamines (see Chapter 41, Fig. 41.40).

SECRETION OF THE CATECHOLAMINES

Secretion of epinephrine and norepinephrine from the adrenal medulla is stimulated by a variety of stresses, including pain, hemorrhage, exercise, hypoglycemia, and hypoxia. Release is mediated by stress-induced transmission of nerve impulses emanating from adrenergic nuclei in the hypothalamus. These impulses stimulate the release of acetylcholine from preganglionic neurons that innervate the adrenomedullary cells. This neurotransmitter depolarizes the plasma membranes of these cells, allowing the rapid entry of extracellular calcium (Ca^{2+}) into the cytosol. Ca^{2+} stimulates the synthesis and release of epinephrine and norepinephrine from the chromaffin granules into the extracellular space by exocytosis.

PHYSIOLOGICAL EFFECTS OF EPINEPHRINE AND NOREPINEPHRINE

The catecholamines act through two major types of receptors on the plasma membrane of target cells, the α-adrenergic and the β-adrenergic receptors (see Chapter 24 and Table 24.4).

The actions of epinephrine and norepinephrine in the liver, the adipocyte, the skeletal muscle cell, and the A and B cells of the pancreas directly influence fuel metabolism (Fig. 45.1). These catecholamines are counterregulatory hormones which have metabolic effects directed toward mobilization of fuels from their storage sites for oxidation by cells in order to meet the increased energy requirements of acute and chronic stress. They simultaneously suppress insulin secretion, which ensures that fuel fluxes will continue in the direction of fuel utilization rather than storage as long as the stressful stimulus persists.

In addition, the effects of catecholamines on the heart and blood vessels serve to increase cardiac output and systemic blood pressure, hemodynamic changes that facilitate the delivery of these fuels to metabolically active tissues.

METABOLISM AND INACTIVATION OF CATECHOLAMINES

Catecholamines have a relatively low affinity for both α- and β-receptors. After binding, the catecholamine disassociates from its receptor quickly, causing the duration of the biological response to be brief. The free hormone is degraded in several ways. Catecholamines secreted by the terminus of the adrenergic neurons may be taken up again by these same nerve endings. After reuptake, the catecholamine may be reutilized (re-secreted) or it may be deaminated by monoamine oxidase (MAO) to form dihydroxymandelic acid (see Fig. 41.24). Following deamination, this inactive metabolite is either released from the cytosol of the adrenergic nerve cell as such or it is methylated by catechol O-methyltransferase (COMT) to form 3-methoxy-4-hydroxymandelic acid within the nerve terminus and then released.

Other tissues (primarily liver and kidney) may take up the circulating catecholamines. In these tissues, COMT and MAO, acting in concert, form 3-methoxy-4-hydroxymandelic acid (also called vanillylmandelic acid or VMA).

In patients suspected of having a neoplasm of the adrenal medulla (a pheochromocytoma) which is secreting excessive quantities of epinephrine and/or norepinephrine, either the catecholamines themselves (epinephrine, norepinephrine, and dopamine) or their metabolites (the metanephrines and VMA) may be measured in a 24-hour urine collection, or the level of catecholamines in the blood may be measured. A patient who has consistently elevated levels in the blood and/or urine should be considered to have a pheochromocytoma, particularly if the patient has signs and symptoms of catecholamine excess, such as excessive sweating, palpitations, tremulousness, and hypertension.

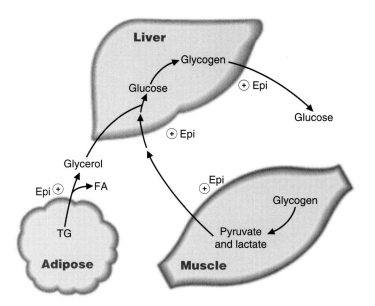

Fig. 45.1. Effects of epinephrine on fuel metabolism. Epinephrine (Epi) stimulates glycogen breakdown in muscle and liver, gluconeogenesis in liver, and lipolysis in adipose tissue.

Glucocorticoids, such as cortisol, were named for their ability to raise blood glucose levels. These steroids are among the "counterregulatory" hormones that protect the body from insulin-induced hypoglycemia.

Free catecholamines may also be inactivated through a process of conjugation. The hydroxyl group on the phenol ring may be conjugated with sulfate or glucuronide primarily in the liver and the gut.

Glucocorticoids

BIOCHEMISTRY

Cortisol (hydrocortisone) is the major physiological glucocorticoid (GC) in humans, although corticosterone also has some glucocorticoid activity. The biosynthesis of steroid hormones and their basic mechanism of action is described in Chapter 43.

SECRETION OF GLUCOCORTICOIDS

The synthesis and secretion of cortisol is controlled by a cascade of neural and endocrine signals linked in tandem in the cerebrocortical-hypothalamic-pituitary-adrenocortical axis. Cerebrocortical signals to the midbrain are initiated in the cerebral cortex by "stressful" signals such as pain, hypoglycemia, hemorrhage, and exercise (Fig. 45.2). These nonspecific "stresses" elicit the production of monoamines in the cell bodies of neurons of the midbrain. Those which stimulate the synthesis and release of corticotropin-releasing hormone (CRH) are acetylcholine and serotonin. These neurotransmitters then induce the production of CRH by neurons originating in the paraventricular nucleus. These neurons discharge CRH into the hypothalamico-hypophyseal portal blood. CRH is delivered through these portal vessels to specific receptors on the cell membrane of the adrenocorticotropic hormone (ACTH)-secreting cells of the anterior pituitary gland (corticotrophs). This hormone-receptor interaction causes ACTH to be released into the general circulation to eventually interact with specific receptors for ACTH on the plasma membranes of cells in the zona fasciculata and zona reticulosum of the adrenal cortex. The major trophic influence of ACTH on cortisol synthesis is at the level of the conversion of cholesterol to pregnenolone, from which the adrenal steroid hormones are derived.

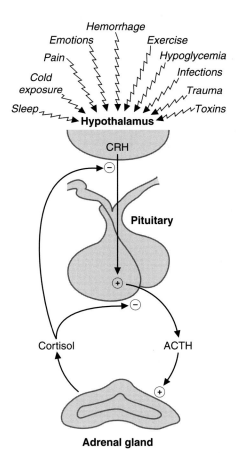

Fig. 45.2. Regulation of cortisol secretion. Various factors act on the hypothalamus to stimulate the release of CRH. CRH stimulates the release of ACTH from the anterior pituitary, which stimulates the release of cortisol from the adrenal cortex. Cortisol inhibits the release of CRH and ACTH.

When Ron was writing his list of differential diagnoses to explain the clinical presentation of **Corti Solemia**, he suddenly thought of a relatively rare endocrine disorder which could explain all of the presenting signs and symptoms. He made a provisional diagnosis of excessive secretion of cortisol caused either by an excess secretion of ACTH (Cushing's disease) or by an increase of cortisol production by an adrenocortical tumor (Cushing's syndrome).

Ron suggested that resting, fasting plasma cortisol and ACTH levels be measured at 8:00 the next morning. These studies showed that Mr. Solemia's morning plasma ACTH and cortisol levels were both significantly above the reference range. Therefore, Ron concluded that Mr. Solemia probably had a tumor that was producing ACTH autonomously (i.e., not subject to normal feedback inhibition by cortisol). The high plasma levels of ACTH were stimulating the adrenal cortex to produce excessive amounts of cortisol. Additional laboratory and imaging studies revealed that the hypercortisolemia was caused by a benign ACTH-secreting adenoma of the anterior pituitary gland (Cushing's disease).

 Ron was now able to explain the mechanism for most of **Corti Solemia's** signs and symptoms. For example, Ron knew the metabolic explanation for the patient's hyperglycemia. Some of Mr. Solemia's muscle wasting and weakness were caused by the catabolic effect of hypercortisolemia on protein stores, such as those in skeletal muscle, to provide amino acids as precursors for gluconeogenesis. This catabolic action also resulted in the degradation of elastin, a major supportive protein of the skin, as well as an increased fragility of the walls of the capillaries of the cutaneous tissues. These changes resulted in the easy bruisability and the torn subcutaneous tissues of the lower abdomen, which resulted in red striae or stripes. The plethora (redness) of Mr. Solemia's facial skin was also caused in part by the thinning of the skin as well as by a cortisol-induced increase in the bone marrow production of red blood cells, which enhanced the "redness" of the subcutaneous tissues.

Cortisol is secreted from the adrenal cortex in response to ACTH. The concentration of free (unbound) cortisol which bathes the CRH-producing cells of the hypothalamus and the ACTH-producing cells of the anterior pituitary acts as a negative feedback signal which has a regulatory influence on the release of CRH and ACTH (see Fig. 45.2). High cortisol levels in the blood suppress CRH and ACTH secretion and low cortisol levels stimulate secretion. In severe stress, however, the negative feedback signal on ACTH secretion exerted by high cortisol levels in the blood is overridden by the stress-induced activity of the higher portions of the axis (see Fig. 45.2).

The effects of glucocorticoids on fuel metabolism in liver, skeletal muscle, and adipose tissue are outlined in Figure 45.3. Their effects on other tissues are diverse and in many instances, essential for life. Some of the nonmetabolic actions of GCs are listed in Table 45.2.

EFFECTS OF GLUCOCORTICOIDS

Glucocorticoids have diverse actions that affect most tissues of the body. At first glance, some of these effects may appear to be contradictory, but taken together they promote survival in times of stress.

In many tissues, GCs inhibit DNA, RNA, and protein synthesis and stimulate the degradation of these macromolecules. In response to chronic stress, GCs act to make fuels available, so that when the acute alarm sounds and epinephrine is released, the organism can fight or flee. When GCs are elevated, glucose uptake by the cells of many tissues is inhibited, lipolysis occurs in adipose tissue, and proteolysis occurs in skin, lymphoid cells, and muscle. The fatty acids which are released are oxidized by the liver for energy, and the glycerol and amino acids serve in the liver as substrates for the production of glucose, which is converted to glycogen and stored. The alarm

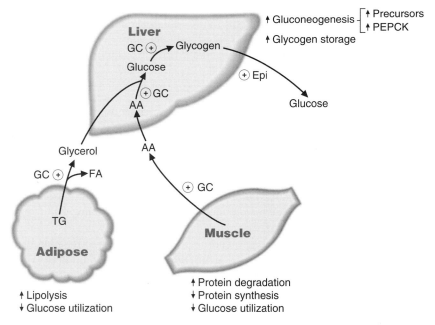

Fig. 45.3. Effects of glucocorticoids (GC) on fuel metabolism. Glucocorticoids stimulate lipolysis in adipose tissue and the release of amino acids from muscle protein. In liver, glucocorticoids stimulate gluconeogenesis and the synthesis of glycogen. The breakdown of liver glycogen is stimulated by epinephrine.

Table 45.2. Some Nonmetabolic Physiological Actions of Glucocorticoids

On electrolyte and water balance:
Increase sodium and water retention (1/3000 the potency of aldosterone)
Increase renal glomerular filtration rate to maintain water excretion rate
Suppress ADH release from posterior pituitary (?)

On cardiovascular system:
Indirect effect of glucocorticoid actions on sodium and water metabolism (above)
Maintain volume of microcirculation to tissues (cardiac output)
Maintain normal vasomotor response to vasoconstricting agents

On skeletal muscle:
Maintain muscle function by providing normal microcirculation to muscle
Influence muscle mass via enhancing protein catabolism and suppressing protein synthesis

On central nervous system:
Indirect
Maintain normal cerebral microcirculation
Direct
Influence mood, behavior
Influence sensitivity of special senses to stimuli
Suppress CRH, ACTH, and ADH secretion

On formed elements in blood:
Increase red blood cell mass and granulocyte proliferation
Decrease lymphocyte, monocyte, and basophil proliferation

Antiinflammatory actions:
Inhibit early inflammatory process (i.e., edema, fibrin deposition, capillary dilatation, leukocyte migration, and phagocytic action)
Inhibit late inflammatory process (proliferation of capillaries and fibroblasts, deposition of collagen, and, later, scar formation)

Immune suppressant actions (of questionable significance at physiological levels):
Prevent manifestations of humoral and cellular immunity
Interfere with production of cytokines needed for immune competence via cell-to-cell communication

Q 45.1: If **Corti Solemia's** problem had been caused by a neoplasm of the adrenal cortex, what would his levels of blood ACTH and cortisol have been?

The "central" deposition of fat in patients, such as **Corti Solemia,** with Cushing's disease or syndrome is not readily explained because GCs actually cause lipolysis in adipose tissue. The increased appetite caused by an excess of GC and the lipogenic effects of the hyperinsulinemia that accompanies the GC-induced chronic increase in blood glucose levels have been suggested as possible causes. Why the fat is deposited centrally under these circumstances, however, is not understood. This central deposition leads to the development of a large fat pad at the center of the upper back ("buffalo hump"), to accumulation of fat in the cheeks and jowls ("moon facies"), and to a marked increase in abdominal fat. Simultaneously, there is a loss of adipose tissue below the elbows and knees, exaggerating the appearance of "central obesity" in Cushing's disease or syndrome.

signal of epinephrine stimulates liver glycogen breakdown, making glucose available as fuel to combat the acute stress.

The mechanism by which GCs exert these effects involves binding of the steroid to intracellular receptors, interaction of the steroid-receptor complex with GC response elements on DNA, transcription of genes, and synthesis of specific proteins (see Chapter 43). In some cases, the specific proteins responsible for the GC effect are known (e.g., the induction of phosphoenolpyruvate carboxykinase that stimulates gluconeogenesis). In other cases, the proteins responsible for the GC effect have not yet been identified.

Growth Hormone

BIOCHEMISTRY

Growth hormone is a polypeptide which, as its name implies, stimulates growth. Many of its effects are mediated by insulin-like growth factors (IGFs) that are produced by cells in response to the binding of GH to its cell membrane receptors. However, GH also has direct effects on fuel metabolism.

GH is synthesized primarily in the lateral areas of the anterior pituitary and is the most abundant trophic hormone in the gland, being present in concentrations of 5–15 mg/g of tissue compared to microgram per gram quantities for the other anterior pituitary hormones. GH is a water-soluble protein with a plasma half-life of 20–50 minutes.

A 45.1: If **Corti Solemia's** problem had resulted from primary hypersecretion of cortisol by a neoplasm of the adrenal cortex, his blood cortisol levels would have been elevated. The cortisol would have acted on the CRH-producing cells of the hypothalamus and the ACTH-secreting cells of the anterior pituitary by a negative feedback mechanism to decrease ACTH levels in the blood.

Because his cortisol and ACTH levels were both high, Mr. Solemia's tumor was most likely in the pituitary gland or possibly in extrapituitary tissue that was secreting ACTH "ectopically." (Ectopic means that the tumor is producing and secreting a substance that is not made by the normal tissue from which the tumor developed.) Mr. Solemia's tumor was in the anterior pituitary.

CONTROL OF SECRETION OF GROWTH HORMONE

Although the regulation of GH secretion is complex, the major influence is hormonal (Fig. 45.4). Release is stimulated by growth hormone-releasing hormone (GHRH), while secretion is suppressed by growth hormone release-inhibiting hormone (somatostatin). Whereas the synthesis of GHRH is confined to the hypothalamus, somatostatin is produced in various nuclei of the brain as well as in the D (δ) cells of the pancreatic islets and in intestinal mucosal cells.

GH release is modulated by plasma levels of all of the metabolic fuels including proteins, fats, and carbohydrates. A rising level of glucose in the blood normally suppresses GH release, whereas hypoglycemia increases GH secretion in normal subjects. Amino acids, such as arginine, stimulate release of GH when their concentrations rise in the blood. Rising levels of fatty acids may blunt the GH response to arginine or a rapidly dropping blood glucose level. However, prolonged fasting, in which fatty acids are mobilized in an effort to spare protein, is associated with a rise in GH secretion. Some of the physiological, pharmacological, and pathological influences on GH secretion are given in Table 45.3.

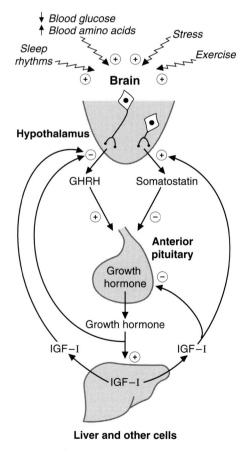

Fig. 45.4. Control of growth hormone secretion. Various factors stimulate the release of GHRH from the hypothalamus. The hypothalamus also releases somatostatin in response to other stimuli. GHRH stimulates and somatostatin inhibits the release of growth hormone from the anterior pituitary. Growth hormone causes the release of IGF-I from liver and other tissues. IGF-I inhibits GHRH release and stimulates somatostatin release.

Table 45.3.   Some Factors Affecting Growth Hormone Secretion

	Stimulate	Supress
Physiological	Low blood glucose after meals High blood amino acids after meals Exercise Sleep Stress	High blood glucose after meals High blood fatty acids
Pharmacological	GHRH Estrogens α-Adrenergic agonists β-Adrenergic antagonists Dopamine agonists Serotonin precursors K+ infusion	Somatostatin Progesterone α-Adrenergic antagonists β-Adrenergic agonists Dopamine antagonists Growth hormone and IGF-I
Pathological	Starvation Anorexia nervosa Ectopic GHRH production Acromegaly Chronic renal failure Hypoglycemia	Obesity Hypothyroidism Hyperthyroidism

These modulators of GH secretion provide the basis for clinical suppression and stimulation tests in patients suspected of having excessive or deficient GH secretion.

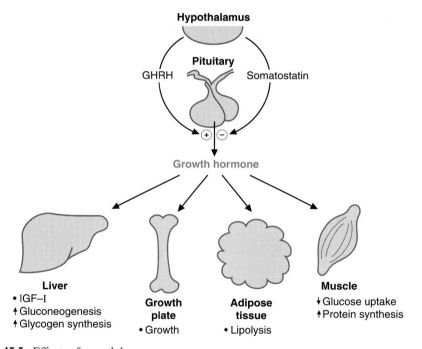

Fig. 45.5. Effects of growth hormone.

EFFECTS OF GROWTH HORMONE ON ENERGY METABOLISM

GH affects the uptake and oxidation of fuels in adipose tissue, muscle, and liver, and indirectly influences energy metabolism through its actions on the islet cells of the pancreas. In summary, GH increases the availability of fatty acids, which are oxidized for energy. This and other effects of GH spare glucose and protein, i.e., GH indirectly decreases the oxidation of glucose and amino acids (Fig. 45.5).

EFFECTS OF GROWTH HORMONE ON ADIPOSE TISSUE

Growth hormone increases the sensitivity of the adipocyte to the lipolytic action of the catecholamines, and decreases its sensitivity to the lipogenic action of insulin.

As a result of the metabolic effects of GH, the clinical course of acromegaly may be complicated by impaired glucose tolerance or even overt diabetes mellitus as occurred with **Sam Atotrope.**

45.2: A patient presents with the following clinical and laboratory profile: the serum free and total T_3 and T_4 and the serum TSH levels are elevated but the patient has symptoms of mild hypothyroidism, including a diffuse, palpable goiter. What single abnormality in the pituitary-thyroid-thyroid hormone target cell axis would explain all of these findings?

These actions lead to the release of free fatty acids and glycerol into the blood to be metabolized by the liver. GH also decreases esterification of fatty acids, thereby reducing triacylglycerol synthesis within the fat cell. Recent evidence suggests that GH may impair glucose uptake by both fat and muscle cells by a postreceptor inhibition of insulin action.

EFFECTS OF GROWTH HORMONE ON MUSCLE

The lipolytic effects of GH increase free fatty acid levels in the blood bathing muscle. These fatty acids are preferentially utilized as fuel, indirectly suppressing glucose uptake by muscle cells. Through the effects on glucose uptake, the rate of glycolysis is proportionately reduced.

GH increases the transport of amino acids into muscle cells, providing substrate for protein synthesis. Through a separate mechanism, GH increases the synthesis of DNA and RNA. The positive effect on nitrogen balance is reinforced by the protein-sparing effect of GH-induced lipolysis that makes fatty acids available to muscle as an alternative fuel source.

EFFECTS OF GROWTH HORMONE ON THE LIVER

When plasma insulin levels are low, as in the fasting state, GH enhances fatty acid oxidation to acetyl CoA. This effect in concert with the increased flow of fatty acids from adipose tissue enhances ketogenesis. The increased amount of glycerol reaching the liver as a consequence of enhanced lipolysis acts as a substrate for gluconeogenesis.

Hepatic glycogen synthesis is also stimulated by GH in part because of the increased gluconeogenesis in the liver. Finally, glucose metabolism is suppressed by GH at several steps in the glycolytic pathway.

A major effect of GH on liver is to stimulate production and release of IGFs. Their action in promoting growth is described in Chapter 47.

Thyroid Hormone

BIOCHEMISTRY

The biochemical reactions involved in the synthesis of triiodothyronine (T_3) and tetraiodothyronine (T_4) from tyrosine as well as their chemical structures and basic mechanism of action are described in Chapter 43.

The plasma half-life of T_4 is approximately 7 days and that of T_3 is 1–1.5 days. These relatively long plasma half-lives result from binding of T_3 and T_4 to several transport proteins in the blood. Of these transport proteins, thyroid binding globulin (TBG) has the highest affinity for these hormones and carries about 70% of bound T_3 and T_4. Only 0.03% of total T_4 and 0.3% of total T_3 in the blood are in the unbound state. This free fraction of hormone has biological activity since it is the only form which is capable of diffusing across target cell membranes to interact with intracellular receptors. The transport proteins, therefore, serve as a large reservoir of hormone which can release additional free hormone as the metabolic need arises.

The thyroid hormones are degraded in liver, kidney, muscle, and other tissues by deiodination, which produces compounds with no biological activity.

SECRETION OF THYROID HORMONE

The large protein thyroglobulin, which contains T_3 and T_4 in peptide linkage, is stored extracellularly in the colloid which fills the central space of each thyroid follicle (see Chapter 43). Each of the biochemical reactions which leads to the release

 Normally, the thyroid gland secretes 80–100 μg of T_4 and approximately 5 μg of T_3 per day. The additional 22–25 μg of T_3 "produced" daily is the result of the deiodination of the 5′-carbon of T_4 in peripheral tissues. T_3 is believed to be the predominant biologically active form of thyroid hormone in the body.

 Approximately 35% of T_4 is deiodinated at the 5′ position to form T_3, and 45% is deiodinated at the 5 position to form the inactive "reverse" T_3. Further deiodination and/or oxidative deamination leads to formation of compounds that have no biological activity.

and eventual secretion of T_3 and T_4, like those which lead to their formation in thyroglobulins, is TSH-dependent. Rising levels of serum TSH stimulate the endocytosis of thyroglobulin into the thyroid acinar cell. Lysosomal enzymes then cleave T_3 and T_4 from thyroglobulin. T_3 and T_4 are secreted into the bloodstream in response to rising levels of TSH.

As the free T_3 level in the blood bathing the thyrotrophs of the anterior pituitary gland rises, the feedback loop is closed. Secretion of TSH is inhibited until the free T_3 levels in the systemic circulation fall just below a critical level, which once again signals the release of TSH. This feedback mechanism ensures an uninterrupted supply of biologically active free T_3 in the blood (Fig. 45.6). High levels of T_3 also inhibit the release of TRH from the hypothalamus.

PHYSIOLOGICAL EFFECTS OF THYROID HORMONE

Only those physiological actions of thyroid hormone that influence fuel metabolism will be considered here. It is important to stress the term "physiological" since the effects of supraphysiological concentrations of thyroid hormone on fuel metabolism may not be simple extensions of their physiological effects. In general, the following comments apply to the effects of thyroid hormone on energy metabolism in individuals with normal thyroid hormone levels in the blood.

Effects of Thyroid Hormone on the Liver

Several of the actions of thyroid hormone affect carbohydrate and lipid metabolism in the liver. Thyroid hormone increases glycolysis and cholesterol synthesis and increases the conversion of cholesterol to bile salts. Through its action of increasing the sensitivity of the hepatocyte to the gluconeogenic and glycogenolytic actions of epinephrine, T_3 indirectly increases hepatic glucose production (permissive or facilitatory action). Because of its ability to sensitize the adipocyte to the lipolytic action of epinephrine, T_3 increases the flow of fatty acids to the liver and thereby indirectly increases hepatic triacylglycerol synthesis. The concurrent increase in the flow of glycerol to the liver (as a result of increased lipolysis) further enhances hepatic gluconeogenesis.

Effects of Thyroid Hormone on the Adipocyte

T_3 has an amplifying or facilitatory effect on the lipolytic action of epinephrine on the fat cell. Yet thyroid hormone has a bipolar effect on lipid storage, since it increases the availability of glucose to the fat cell, which serves as a precursor for fatty acid and glycerol 3-phosphate synthesis. The major determinant of the rate of lipogenesis, however, is not T_3, but rather the amount of glucose and insulin available to the adipocyte for triacylglycerol synthesis.

Effects of Thyroid Hormone on Muscle

In physiological concentrations, T_3 increases glucose uptake by muscle cells. It also stimulates protein synthesis, and, therefore, growth of muscle, through its stimulatory actions on gene expression.

In physiological concentrations, thyroid hormone sensitizes the muscle cell to the glycogenolytic actions of epinephrine. Glycolysis in muscle is increased by this action of T_3.

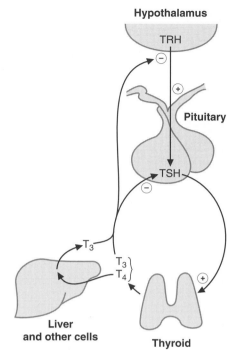

Fig. 45.6. Feedback regulation of thyroid hormone levels. TRH from the hypothalamus stimulates the release of TSH from the anterior pituitary, which stimulates the release of T_3 and T_4 from the thyroid. T_4 is converted to T_3 in the liver and other cells. T_3 and T_4 inhibit the release of TSH from the anterior pituitary and of TRH from the hypothalamus.

A 45.2: A generalized (i.e., involving all of the target cells for thyroid hormone in the body), but incomplete resistance of cells to the actions of thyroid hormone could explain the profile of the patient. In Refetoff's disorder, a mutation in the portion of the gene that encodes the ligand binding domain of the β-subunit of the thyroid hormone receptor protein causes a relative resistance to thyroid hormone action within the thyrotrophs of the anterior pituitary gland. Therefore, the gland releases more TSH than normal into the blood. The elevated level of TSH causes an enlargement of the thyroid gland (goiter) as well as an increase in the serum levels of both T_3 and T_4. The increase in the secretion of thyroid hormone may or may not be adequate to fully compensate for the relative resistance of the peripheral tissues to thyroid hormone. If not, the patient may manifest the signs and symptoms of hypothyroidism.

When present in excess, T$_3$ has severe catabolic effects which increase the flow of amino acids from muscle into the blood and eventually to the liver.

 In hypothyroid patients, insulin release may be suboptimal, although glucose intolerance on this basis alone is uncommon.

In hyperthyroidism, the degradation and the clearance of insulin are increased. These effects, plus the increased demand for insulin caused by the changes in glucose metabolism, may lead to varying degrees of glucose intolerance in these patients (a condition called metathyroid diabetes mellitus). The patient with uncomplicated hyperthyroidism, however, rarely develops significant diabetes mellitus.

Effects of Thyroid Hormone on the Pancreas

Thyroid hormone increases the sensitivity of the B cells of the pancreas to those stimuli which normally promote insulin release and is required for optimal insulin secretion.

CALORIGENIC EFFECTS OF THYROID HORMONE

The oxidation of fuels converts about 25% of the potential energy present in the foods ingested by humans to ATP. This relative inefficiency of the human "engine" leads to the production of heat as a consequence of fuel utilization. This inefficiency, in part, allows homeothermic animals to maintain a constant body temperature in spite of rapidly changing environmental conditions. The acute response to cold exposure is shivering, which is probably secondary to increased activity of the sympathetic nervous system in response to this "stressful" stimulus.

Thyroid hormone participates in this acute response by sensitizing the sympathetic nervous system to the stimulatory effect of cold exposure. The ability of T$_3$ to increase heat production is related to its effects on the pathways of fuel oxidation, which both generate ATP and release energy as heat. The effects of T$_3$ on the sympathetic nervous system increase the release of norepinephrine. Norepinephrine stimulates the uncoupling protein thermogenin in brown adipose tissue (BAT), resulting in increased heat production from the uncoupling of oxidative phosphorylation (see Chapter 20).

Norepinephrine also increases the permeability of BAT and skeletal muscle to sodium. Because an increase of intracellular Na$^+$ is potentially toxic to cells, Na$^+$,K$^+$-ATPase is stimulated to transport Na$^+$ out of the cell in exchange for K$^+$. The increased hydrolysis of ATP by Na$^+$,K$^+$-ATPase stimulates the oxidation of fuels and the regeneration of more ATP and heat from oxidative phosphorylation. Over a longer time course, thyroid hormone also increases the level of Na$^+$,K$^+$-ATPase and many of the enzymes of fuel oxidation. Since even at normal room temperature ATP utilization by Na$^+$,K$^+$-ATPase accounts for 20% or more of our BMR, changes in its activity can cause relatively large increases in heat production.

Thyroid hormone may also increase heat production by stimulating ATP utilization in futile cycles (in which reversible ATP-consuming conversions of substrate to product and back to substrate utilize fuels and, therefore, produce heat).

CLINICAL COMMENTS. One of the functions of cortisol is to prepare the body to deal with periods of stress. In response to cortisol, the body re-sorts its fuel stores, so that they can rapidly be made available for the "fight or flight" response to the alarm signal sounded by epinephrine. Cortisol causes gluconeogenic substrates to move from peripheral tissues to the liver, where they are converted to glucose and stored as glycogen. The release of epinephrine stimulates the breakdown of glycogen, increasing the supply of glucose to the blood. Thus fuel becomes available for muscle to fight or flee.

Cushing's disease, the cause of **Corti Solemia's** current problems, results from prolonged hypersecretion of ACTH from a benign pituitary tumor. ACTH stimulates the adrenal cortex to produce cortisol, and blood levels of this steroid hormone rise.

Causes of Cushing's syndrome, on the other hand, include a primary tumor of the adrenal cortex secreting excessive amounts of cortisol directly into the bloodstream. This disorder can also result from the release of ACTH from secretory nonendocrine neoplasms ("ectopic" ACTH syndrome). Cushing's syndrome is often caused by excessive doses of synthetic GCs used to treat a variety of disorders because of their potent antiinflammatory effects (iatrogenic Cushing's syndrome).

The diabetogenic potential of chronically elevated GH levels in the blood is manifest by the significant incidence of diabetes mellitus (25%) and impaired glucose tolerance (33%) in patients with acromegaly, such as **Sam Atotrope**. Yet, under normal circumstances, physiological concentrations of GH (as well as cortisol and thyroid hormone) have a facilitatory or permissive effect on the quantity of insulin released in response to hyperglycemia and other insulin secretogogues. This "proinsular" effect is probably intended to act as a "brake" to dampen any potentially excessive "contrainsular" effects that increments in GH and the other counterregulatory hormones exert.

BIOCHEMICAL COMMENTS. Most hormones are present in body fluids in picomolar to nanomolar amounts, requiring highly sensitive assays to determine their concentration in the blood or urine. Radioimmunoassays (RIAs), developed in the 1960s, use an antibody, generated in animals, against a specific antigen (the hormone to be measured). Determining the concentration of the hormone in the sample involves incubating the plasma or urine sample with the antibody and then quantitating the level of antigen-antibody complex formed during the incubation by one of several techniques.

The classic RIA utilizes very high affinity antibodies, which have been fixed (immobilized) on the inner surface of a test tube, a Teflon bead, or a magnetized particle. A standard curve is prepared, using a set amount of the antibody and various known concentrations of the unlabeled hormone to be measured. In addition to a known concentration of the unlabeled hormone, each tube contains the same small, carefully measured amount of radiolabeled hormone. The labeled hormone and the unlabeled hormone compete for binding to the antibody. The higher the amount of unlabeled hormone in the sample, the less radiolabeled hormone is bound. A standard curve is plotted (Fig. 45.7). The unknown sample from the patient's blood or urine, containing the unlabeled hormone to be measured, is incubated with the immobilized antibody in the presence of the same small, carefully measured amount of radiolabeled hormone. The amount of radiolabeled hormone bound to the antibody is determined, and the standard curve is used to quantitate the amount of unlabeled hormone in the patient sample.

The same principle is used in immunoradiometric assays (IRMAs), but with this technique the antibody, rather than the antigen to be measured, is radiolabeled.

The sensitivity of RIAs can be enhanced using a "sandwich technique." This method utilizes two different monoclonal antibodies (antibodies generated by a single clone of plasma cells rather than multiple clones), each of which recognizes a different specific portion of the hormone's structure. The first antibody, attached to a solid support matrix such as a plastic culture dish, binds the hormone to be assayed. Following exposure of the patient sample to this first antibody, the excess plasma is washed away, and the second antibody (which is radiolabeled) is then incubated with the first antibody-hormone complex. The amount of binding of the second (labeled) antibody to the first complex is proportional to the concentration of the hormone in the sample.

The sandwich technique can be improved even further if the second antibody is attached to an enzyme, such as alkaline phosphatase. The enzyme rapidly converts an added colorless substrate into a colored product, or a nonfluorescent substrate into a highly fluorescent product. These changes can be quantitated if the degree of change in color or fluorescence is proportional to the amount of hormone present in the patient sample. Less than a nanogram (10^{-9} g) of a protein can be measured by such an enzyme-linked immunosorbent assay (ELISA).

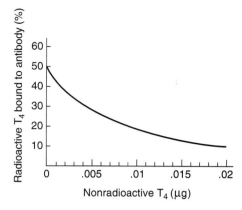

Fig. 45.7. Standard curve for a radioimmunoassay. A constant amount of radioactive T_4 is added to a series of tubes, each of which contains a different amount of nonradioactive T_4. The amount of radioactive hormone that binds to an antibody specific for the hormone is measured and plotted against the nonradioactive hormone concentration. When more nonradioactive T_4 is present in the tube, less radioactive T_4 binds to the antibody.

Suggested Reading

Goodman HM. Hormonal regulation of fuel metabolism. In: Basic medical endocrinology. New York: Raven Press, 1994:203–224.

PROBLEMS

1. A patient consults her physician because of nervousness combined with rapid weight loss in spite of a voracious appetite. She is sweating, her hands are shaking, and she complains of palpitations. The physician can feel a goiter and, suspecting a problem in thyroid function, orders a total serum T_4. The standard curve for the radioimmunoassay is shown in Figure 45.7.

For the patient's sample, 12% of the radioactive T_4 was bound to the antibody. Was the patient's serum T_4 level within the normal range (4–10 µg/dL)?

RIA was also used to measure the patient's TSH level. Based on the patient's T_4 level, would you expect the patient's TSH level to be high or low? (Assume that her pituitary function is normal.) How should the patient be treated?

2. As a third year medical student, you examine your first patient. You find that he is 52 years old, has a round face, acne, and a large hump of fat on the back of his neck. He complains that he is too weak to mow his lawn. His fasting blood glucose level was 170 mg/dL (reference range = 80–100 mg/dL). Plasma cortisol levels were 62 µg/mL (reference range = 3–31 µg/mL). Plasma ACTH levels were 0 pg/mL (reference range = 0–100 pg/mL).

Based on the information given above, if the patient's problem is due to a single cause, the most likely diagnosis is

    A. non-insulin-dependent diabetes mellitus

    B. insulin-dependent diabetes mellitus

    C. a secretory tumor of the anterior pituitary

    D. a secretory tumor of the posterior pituitary

    E. a secretory tumor of the adrenal cortex

ANSWERS

1. If the patient's antibody-bound radioactive T_4 is 12%, according to the standard curve, her serum T_4 level is about 18 µg/dL. Therefore, she is hyperthyroid. Her TSH should be lower than normal, and she requires treatment with oral antithyroid drugs or radioactive iodine, or subtotal resection of her thyroid gland.

2. The answer is **E**. Uncomplicated non-insulin-dependent and insulin-dependent diabetes mellitus can be eliminated as possible diagnoses because they are not associated with elevated plasma cortisol levels and low plasma ACTH levels. In this patient, hyperglycemia resulted from the diabetogenic effects of chronic hypercortisolemia. An ACTH-secreting tumor of the anterior pituitary gland would cause hypercortisolemia which, in turn, could adversely affect glucose tolerance, but, in this case, the plasma ACTH levels would have been high, rather than 0 pg/mL. The posterior pituitary gland secretes oxytocin and vasopressin, neither of which influences blood glucose, cortisol, or ACTH levels.

The correct answer is that a tumor of the adrenal cortex is secreting excessive amounts of cortisol into the blood, which adversely affects glucose tolerance, suppresses pituitary secretion of ACTH, and, through chronic hypercortisolemia, causes the physical changes described in this patient.

46 Actions of Hormones That Affect Sodium and Calcium Levels

Ingested water and solutes are distributed into three body compartments: the intravascular, the interstitial, and the intracellular spaces.

SODIUM AND WATER BALANCE

Acute changes in the amount of water or solutes such as sodium in the body compartments are potentially life-threatening. Survival depends upon our ability to compensate for these sudden changes by activating homeostatic mechanisms designed to return the water and solute concentrations to normal as quickly as possible. The major hormones that contribute to the regulatory processes which control sodium and water balance, (antidiuretic hormone (ADH), atrial natriuretic peptide (ANP), angiotensins II and III, and aldosterone) will be presented in this chapter, with emphasis on their biochemical and molecular characteristics (Table 46.1).

Sodium salts are the principal osmotically active solutes of the extracellular fluid (ECF). Sodium and its anions account for 95% of the osmotic pressure of the plasma and interstitial fluid.

Deviations of the ECF sodium concentration from normal stimulate mechanisms that return sodium and water levels to normal. An increase in ECF sodium concentration is not only a potent stimulus to thirst and, hence, to water intake but to ADH secretion as well. ADH causes renal retention of water. Increased sodium concentrations also lead to decreased resorption of sodium by the kidney, the result of decreased aldosterone production via the renin-angiotensin system. These reactions to sodium overload are designed to normalize an excess of total body sodium through a dilutional process. A decrease in ECF sodium has the opposite effect. A normal total body sodium content is necessary if normal ECF and intravascular volume are to be maintained.

 In a 70-kg person, about 42 liters of water are present in the body (total body water (TBW)). Roughly two-thirds of TBW resides in the intracellular space (28 liters). The remaining 14 liters of TBW are extracellular and are partitioned into the intravascular compartment (in blood vessels) which contains 3.5 liters of fluid (8–9% of TBW) and the interstitial compartment (the fluid surrounding cells) which contains 10–11 liters of fluid (25% of TBW).

 Osmotic pressure is generated by the flow of water through a semipermeable membrane from an aqueous compartment containing solute at a lower concentration to one containing solute at a higher concentration.

Table 46.1. Hormones That Regulate Sodium and Water Balance

Hormone	Major Actions Related to Fluid and Electrolyte Balance	Tissue(s) Affected
ADH	↑ H_2O resorption	Kidney
Aldosterone	↑ Na^+ resorption	Kidney, salivary and sweat glands, distal colon
	↑ K^+ excretion	
ANP	↑ Na^+ excretion	Kidney
	↑ Urine volume	
	↓ Renin	
	↓ Angiotensin II	Adrenal glomerulosa
	↓ Aldosterone production	
Angiotensin II	↑ Aldosterone production	Adrenal glomerulosa
	↑ Vasoconstriction	Peripheral resistance vessels
Angiotensin III	↑ Aldosterone production	Adrenal glomerulosa

The vasoconstrictor action of angiotensin II and of ADH and the vasodilatory actions of ANP allow the size or capacity of the vascular bed to be altered so that it can accommodate increases (through vasodilation) and decreases (through vasoconstriction) in intravascular volume. Maintenance of a normal vascular volume ensures that the tissues will be adequately perfused with oxygen-rich and nutrient-rich arterial blood, but not to the extent that overexpansion of plasma volume occurs. Overexpansion could lead to an increase in blood pressure and eventually to congestion of the heart and lungs.

CALCIUM METABOLISM

In spite of a widely fluctuating dietary intake of calcium from day to day, the calcium concentration in the intracellular and extracellular fluids is remarkably constant. Of the ionic components of the ECF, only sodium is more tightly regulated than calcium. However, within the cell, the concentration of calcium is more strictly controlled than that of sodium. For example, whereas the concentration of sodium in the ECF is 16–20 times greater than that in the cytosol of cells, the concentration of calcium is 10,000–12,000 times greater outside the cell than in the cell. A common denominator of cell death, regardless of the nature of the insult (e.g., hypoxia, trauma, intoxication) is an increase of intracellular calcium above a critical concentration.

The critical intracellular calcium concentration as well as the calcium concentration in the ECF is controlled by the integrated activity of two polypeptide hormones, parathyroid hormone (PTH) and calcitonin (CT), and by the activated form of vitamin D_3 (1,25-dihydroxycholecalciferol; 1,25-$(OH)_2D_3$), a sterol hormone (Table 46.2). A feedback loop exists between the concentration of "free" (elemental, non-protein-bound) Ca^{2+} in the blood and the synthesis and secretion of these calcitropic hormones.

The calcium ion (Ca^{2+}) has important physiological effects in almost every tissue of the body. Calcium influences the permeability of membranes to water and other ions, it couples neural excitation stimuli with muscular contraction at the neuromuscular junction, it is an important component of the blood coagulation cascade, it serves as a stable component of crystals within the skeleton, providing structural support, and it participates in the coupling of hormonal signals with their intracellular effects.

Table 46.2. Actions of Hormones That Regulate Calcium Balance

Tissue	Parathyroid Hormone (PTH)	Calcitonin (CT)	Active Vitamin D (1,25-$(OH)_2D_3$)
Bone	↑ Ca^{2+} resorption ↑ PO_4^{2-} resorption	↓ Ca^{2+} resorption ↓ PO_4^{2-} resorption	Promotes mobilization of Ca^{2+} from bone by increasing the number of osteoclasts
Kidney	↑ Ca^{2+} resorption ↓ PO_4^{2-} resorption ↓ HCO_3^- resorption ↑ conversion of 25-$(OH)D_3$ to 1,25-$(OH)_2D_3$	↓ Ca^{2+} resorption ↓ PO_4^{2-} resorption	↑ Ca^{2+} resorption
Intestine			↑ Ca^{2+} absorption ↑ PO_4^{2-} absorption

Rena Lischemia, a 72-year-old retired librarian, was in good health when she noted the onset of severe pulsatile headaches accompanied by blurring of vision. During a particularly severe episode associated with dizziness, she came to her physician's office where Erna Nemdy, now a third-year medical student, was taking a private office clerkship. When Erna took Mrs. Lischemia's blood pressure, which had always been normal, she found it to be extremely elevated, with an average reading of 215/124 mm Hg. Erna also heard a systolic-diastolic bruit (a sound, heard with a stethoscope, which is caused by turbulence of the blood as it flows through a narrowed segment of a major artery) to the left of the patient's umbilicus. Erna related her findings to the physician, and told him that she suspected that the sudden increase in blood pressure was caused by a relatively recent significant reduction in blood flow to Rena's left kidney, possibly caused by rapid growth of an atherosclerotic plaque within the lumen of her left main renal artery. The doctor agreed and ordered appropriate functional and anatomic imaging studies of the kidneys, which confirmed Erna's suspicions.

Teresa Livermore recovered fully from her bout of hepatitis and, through a balanced diet, managed to regain 14 lb. One evening, however, as she attempted to rise from a soft chair, she experienced an excruciating pain in the high lumbar spine area which radiated laterally to both the right and left flank. Because of the unrelenting severity of the pain, she was rushed to the hospital emergency room. The physician on duty ordered an x-ray of the lumbosacral spine. The film revealed a severe compression fracture of the second lumbar vertebra. In addition, severe osteopenia (a generic term indicative of a loss of mineralized bone) was noted throughout Teresa's spine and pelvis. She was admitted to the hospital and placed at bed rest. Parenteral analgesics were given and, in addition, she received daily subcutaneous injections of salmon calcitonin (CT). Over the next 3 days, the pain gradually improved and she was discharged on a therapeutic regimen designed to promote mineralization of her depleted skeleton.

HORMONES INVOLVED IN REGULATING SODIUM AND WATER BALANCE

Normal cellular function requires that cell volume and osmolality (solute concentration per liter of intracellular fluid) be maintained within very narrow limits. These parameters are, in part, established by factors which determine the gradient of solute concentration (e.g., for Na^+) across the plasma membrane of the cell. Such factors include the passive diffusion of water and some solutes across cell membranes and the active transport of ions by energy-requiring pumps located within the cell membrane. The constancy of cell volume and osmolality is also determined to some extent by the osmolality of the ECF, which is partly determined by ADH acting on the distal tubules of the kidneys to regulate the excretion of solute-free water into the urine.

If maintenance of a normal ECF solute concentration (osmolality) were dependent on this single endocrine mechanism alone for its regulation, however, the volume of blood in the vascular compartment (the plasma volume) would fluctuate widely throughout the day because of the episodic nature of our daily intake of water and solutes. As a result of these dietary fluctuations, the relative constancy of our blood volume must be guarded and, therefore, under the control of multiple regulatory processes. The factors which accomplish this constancy, other than ADH, are also primarily endocrine in nature. They include the renin-angiotensin-aldosterone system (RAAS) and ANP. These regulatory hormones have their major action in determining

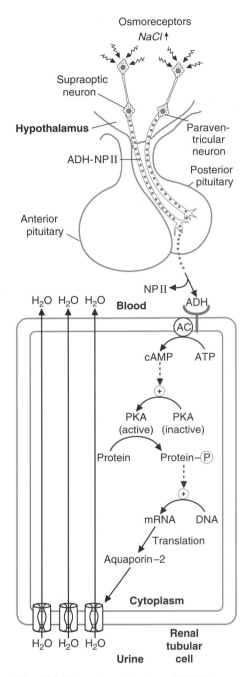

Fig. 46.1. Secretion and action of ADH is produced by neurons in the hypothalamus and stored bound to its neurophysin (NPII) in the posterior pituitary. ADH is synthesized and released in response to increased sodium concentration and decreased plasma volume. ADH binds to cell surface receptors, stimulating the activation of protein kinase A (PKA). PKA phosphorylates proteins that stimulate synthesis of aquaporin, a protein that forms channels in the renal tubular membrane. Water, resorbed through these channels from the urine, enters the blood.

blood volume through their effect on renal handling of sodium and water, which determines the amount of sodium and water in the extracellular space.

Antidiuretic Hormone

ADH, also called arginine vasopressin (AVP), is a peptide that contains 9 amino acids with a disulfide bridge (see Fig. 44.3). It is synthesized as a prohormone in hypothalamic neurons whose cell bodies originate in the supraoptic and paraventricular nuclei. The gene for ADH also encodes neurophysin II, a carrier protein that transports ADH down the axons of neurons which terminate in the posterior pituitary where ADH is stored.

The release of ADH from its storage vesicles in the neurohypophysis (posterior pituitary, pars nervosa), is regulated primarily by the plasma osmolality (osmotically active solute concentration in millimoles/kg of plasma water) (Fig. 46.1). The average "set point" for normal plasma osmolality is 282 mmol/kg with normal limits of 1.8% on either side of this mean. If plasma osmolality rises above a critical osmotic threshold of 287 mmol/kg, ADH release increases rapidly. This release is a consequence of the activity of osmoreceptors located on the cell membrane of the supraoptic and paraventricular neurons of the hypothalamus and probably in cells of the carotid arterial system as well. These osmostats are capable of detecting increments as small as 3–5% above the "set point" in plasma osmolality, particularly if the rate of increase is rapid (>2%/hour).

Hemodynamic factors also have a significant regulatory influence on ADH release. A fall in mean arterial blood pressure and/or "effective" plasma volume as small as 10% can be detected by pressure-sensitive receptors (baroreceptors) located in cells of the left atrium of the heart and to a lesser extent in the carotid sinus. Through a multisynaptic afferent pathway, neural impulses generated by decreased "stretch" on these baroreceptors impact on neurons in the supraoptic and paraventricular nuclei of the hypothalamus, causing ADH release.

The major biological effect of ADH is to increase the resorption of free water from the urine in the lumen of the distal portion of the kidney tubules into the tubular cells (see Fig. 46.1). ADH binds to its specific V_2 receptors on the nonluminal (basolateral) membrane of these cells, causing activation of adenylate cyclase, which forms cAMP. cAMP activates protein kinase A, which phosphorylates proteins that stimulate expression of the gene for aquaporin-2, a member of a family of similar proteins that form water channels. Aquaporin-2 migrates to the luminal membrane of the tubular cell, where it inserts, forming pores or channels through which tubular water diffuses freely into the tubular cell. Water then passes through channels in the plasma membrane into the interstitial space. Eventually the water moves back into the blood.

Renin-Angiotensin-Aldosterone System (RAAS)

The RAAS is a major determinant of the constancy of ECF volume and osmolality as well as the luminal diameter of the vasculature and the level of tissue perfusion (Fig. 46.2). This enzyme (renin)-peptide hormone (angiotensin II)-steroid hormone (aldosterone) cascade accomplishes this important function through its specific capacity to detect and reverse even subtle expansion or contraction of the sodium and water compartments of the body.

The physiology of the complex homeostatic function of the RAAS can be briefly summarized using acute volume contraction as the stimulus for its activation. If a patient vomits frequently for several hours or more and cannot retain replacement liquids by mouth, the ECF volume acutely contracts. As a result, the perfusion pressure

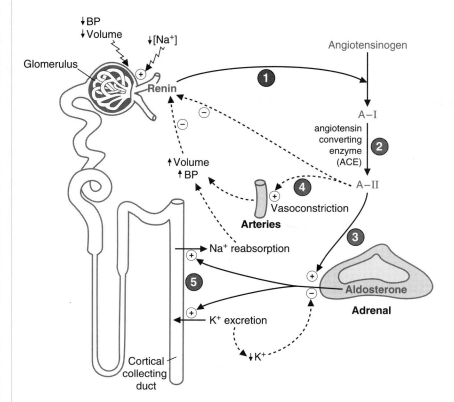

The most common clinical disorder caused by dysfunction of the hypothalamic-posterior pituitary axis in humans is caused by a deficiency of vasopressin (ADH) secretion. This deficiency leads to a condition known as diabetes insipidus, in which large volumes of a dilute urine are excreted, causing a concentration of body fluids unless exogenous ADH is administered.

Less commonly, inappropriate and excessive amounts of ADH may be secreted as a result of a variety of pathological processes (e.g., a central nervous system (CNS) infection that stimulates ADH release). This syndrome of inappropriate ADH secretion (SIADH) leads to marked renal water retention and dilution of body fluids.

Fig. 46.2. Renin-angiotensin-aldosterone system (RAAS). Decreases in blood pressure, blood volume, or sodium concentration in the blood bathing the juxtaglomerular (JG) cells of the kidney stimulate the release of renin from the JG cells. **1.** Renin catalyzes the conversion of angiotensinogen to angiotensin I (AI). **2.** AI is converted to AII by angiotensin-converting enzyme (ACE). AII (**3**) stimulates the release of aldosterone from the adrenal cortex, and (**4**) causes vasoconstriction of peripheral arteries. **5.** Aldosterone stimulates Na^+ resorption and K^+ excretion by renal tubular cells. Dashed lines indicate feedback regulation of the RAAS system.

to the afferent arterioles that lie proximal to each kidney glomerular capillary tuft falls. The juxtaglomerular cells located in the wall of these arterioles sense decreased elastic "stretch" on the vessel wall and, as a result, secrete the enzyme renin into the glomerular capillary blood. The polypeptide angiotensinogen (renin substrate) is produced and secreted by the liver. Renin cleaves a decapeptide, angiotensin I (AI), from angiotensinogen within the kidney. Angiotensin I, which has no intrinsic biological action, acts as a substrate for angiotensin-converting enzyme (ACE), which cleaves two additional amino acids from AI, primarily in the lungs, to form the octapeptide, angiotensin II (AII).

AII has several actions which contribute to correction of the contracted ECF volume. One action of AII is to increase aldosterone synthesis and secretion by the adrenal glomerulosa cells. AII can be converted to angiotensin III (AIII), a heptapeptide which has a similar ability to stimulate adrenal aldosterone release and, like AII, inhibits renin secretion. Aldosterone, a potent mineralocorticoid produced by the adrenal cortex, causes sodium and water reabsorption by the distal portion of the kidney tubule (as well as the distal colon and sweat and salivary glands), acting to correct the contracted ECF volume. Second, AII causes a direct increase in renal tubular Na^+ and water reabsorption. Third, AII (but not AIII) has a potent direct vasoconstrictor action on the resistance vessels of the body, allowing the vascular bed to contract to accommodate the vomiting-induced constricted vascular volume. As a result, blood pressure and tissue perfusion are maintained. AII also activates the adrenergic (sympathetic) nervous system, causing release of norepinephrine, which also causes vasoconstriction and further compensates for any vomiting-induced tendencies to hypotension and hypoperfusion. Finally, AII secreted in the CNS stimulates thirst, which, once the vomiting subsides, causes the patient to drink and thus to replete the ECF volume.

Had the insult to the body been ECF volume overexpansion (e.g., excessive blood transfusions) rather than contraction, the activity of the RAAS would have been suppressed because the resulting expansion of ECF volume would have caused an "excessive stretch" signal in the renin-producing juxtaglomerular cells of the kidney, and renin secretion would have been decreased. As a consequence, AII and aldosterone levels in the blood would also be decreased, leading to vasodilation and increased sodium and water excretion into the urine (as well as stool, sweat, and saliva), all of which would help to normalize the overexpanded ECF volume.

RENIN

Renin is a protease that is highly specific for angiotensinogen (renin substrate). A preproenzyme form (called "prorenin") is believed to be the biological precursor of mature renin. Angiotensinogen is an α_2-globulin secreted by the liver. Its 14 N-terminal amino acid residues contain the amino acid sequence of AI.

ANGIOTENSIN-CONVERTING ENZYME

Angiotensin-converting enzyme (ACE) is a peptidase with a molecular weight of 50,000 that removes the C-terminal dipeptide of AI to form AII. ACE is present in great excess on the endothelial lining cells of pulmonary capillaries and is, therefore, not rate-limiting in the generation of AII.

ANGIOTENSINS

Angiotensin II is an octapeptide with multiple biological actions. AII binds to plasma membrane receptors of cells in the glomerulosa layer of the adrenal cortex, vascular smooth muscle cells, and other target tissues. The activated receptor stimulates G proteins that activate phospholipase C, which cleaves phosphatidylinositol bisphosphate (PIP_2), forming inositol trisphosphate (IP_3) and diacylglycerol (DAG). IP_3 activates ligand-gated Ca^{2+} channels, releasing Ca^{2+} from the endoplasmic reticulum into the cytosol. Both DAG and Ca^{2+} activate protein kinase C, which then phosphorylates target cell proteins, leading to the specific AII-stimulated biological response (e.g., aldosterone secretion, vasoconstriction).

ALDOSTERONE

Aldosterone is the most potent mineralocorticoid in the human body. This steroid hormone diffuses from the blood into the cytosol of target cells and interacts with its specific receptor, probably located both in the cytosol and the nucleus. The hormone-receptor complex binds to a specific response element in DNA, activating certain genes. Specific proteins are produced that change the flux of Na^+, K^+, Mg^{2+}, and water across target cell membranes.

The precise mechanisms by which these aldosterone-induced proteins mediate these changes is not completely established, but three possible mechanisms have been presented (Fig. 46.3). The first, called the "permease theory," suggests that the

The plasma ACE concentration is decreased in patients with a variety of disorders involving lung parenchyma, such as emphysema and cystic fibrosis, and increased in granulomatous disease involving the lungs, such as sarcoidosis.

ACE inhibitors are drugs used in the treatment of certain types of hypertension. They act by inhibiting angiotensin-converting enzyme.

Hypertension or high blood pressure can occur if the amount of blood pumped out of the heart per minute (the cardiac output) is increased and/or the luminal diameter of the muscular resistance vessels in the peripheral circulation is decreased secondary to vasoconstriction (causing a rise in total peripheral resistance, or TPR). The atherosclerotic plaque in **Rena Lischemia's** left main renal artery significantly reduced the perfusion pressure of the blood reaching her left kidney, activating her RAAS, which caused a rise in both cardiac output and TPR.

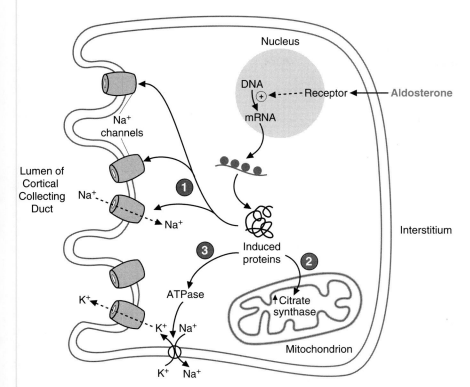

Fig. 46.3. Proposed action of aldosterone. Aldosterone stimulates the synthesis of proteins in kidney tubular cells. These proteins may be (**1**) components of Na⁺ channels that increase the resorption of Na⁺ from the urine; (**2**) enzymes of the TCA cycle that increase the capacity for ATP production; and (**3**) Na⁺,K⁺-ATPases that increase the rate at which Na⁺ and K⁺ are exchanged between the intracellular compartment and the blood. The net result is that more Na⁺ is resorbed from the urine and more K⁺ is excreted.

Rena Lischemia's cardiac output rose because the increased secretion of aldosterone (which occurred as a consequence of the activation of her RAAS) caused marked renal sodium and water retention. Sodium and water retention increased her plasma volume and, therefore, increased the volume of blood pumped from her heart each minute (increased cardiac output).

Before modern isotopic, duplex color Doppler and magnetic resonance angiographic renal blood flow determinations became available, the functional diagnosis of renal artery stenosis was made by demonstrating a higher level of plasma renin activity in the blood of the renal vein on the side of the stenotic renal artery compared to the level in the venous blood draining the normal kidney.

activity (or, less likely, the number) of Na⁺-conducting channels in the luminal membrane of distal renal tubular cells is increased, causing an increase in the passive movement of Na⁺ from the urine into the tubular cell. The second hypothesis, the "energy theory," suggests that aldosterone induces synthesis of enzymes (e.g., citrate synthase) which increase the capacity of the TCA cycle to deliver electrons to the mitochondrial electron transport chain and thus the capacity to generate ATP to provide increased energy for active ion transport. The third hypothesis suggests that new proteins synthesized in the target cell through the action of aldosterone either activate Na⁺,K⁺-ATPase pumps already in existence in the basolateral membrane of the distal tubular cell or cause the synthesis of new pumps.

The balance of current evidence suggests that the primary action of aldosterone is to increase the activity of Na⁺-conducting channels in the luminal membrane and that ATP generation and increased activity of the Na⁺,K⁺-ATPase pumps are secondary effects. The resolution of this question awaits additional experimental evidence.

ATRIAL NATRIURETIC PEPTIDE

Atrial natriuretic peptide (ANP) is a 28 amino acid peptide (also called atriopeptin I) with a single cysteine-cysteine disulfide bridge (Fig. 46.4). It is synthesized and stored as a 126 amino acid preprohormone by cardiocytes in the right (and perhaps the left) atrium and secreted as an inactive dimer which is converted to the active

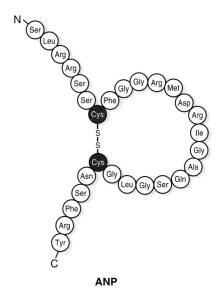

ANP

Fig. 46.4. Structure of atrial natriuretic peptide (ANP). N is the N-terminus, and C is the C-terminus of the peptide.

Q 46.1: A 23-year-old man had a nonsecretory tumor removed from the superior portion of his anterior pituitary gland via a transsphenoidal sinus surgical approach. The neurosurgeon had to put rather severe downward tension on the pituitary stalk in order to expose the tumor. Although all anterior pituitary hormone function was normal postoperatively, the patient developed severe polyuria (large urine volume). What hormone deficiency was responsible for the polyuria?

monomer in the plasma. Enzymatic processing to remove amino acids from both the C- and N-terminal ends yields a 20 amino acid peptide, atriopeptin II, which may be the species with greatest biological potency.

Several factors regulate the secretion of ANP, but increased blood volume and central venous pressure are the major secretagogues. Other stimuli include high blood pressure, increased serum osmolality, increased heart rate, and increased levels of catecholamines in the blood. Glucocorticoids also increase ANP synthesis through a regulating action on the ANP gene.

As its name implies, the kidney is the primary target for ANP but it also acts on peripheral resistance arteries. In the kidney, ANP increases the tone of the efferent (exiting) while decreasing that of the afferent (entering) glomerular arterioles, leading to an increase in glomerular filtration pressure. In addition, ANP raises the glomerular filtration rate without significantly increasing renal blood flow. These actions produce increased sodium excretion (natriuresis) in a large volume of relatively dilute urine. Sodium excretion is further enhanced through the suppressive action of ANP on renin secretion from the juxtaglomerular cells of the kidney. Suppression of the RAAS causes increased sodium excretion and peripheral vasodilation. Sodium excretion is further increased through a direct action of ANP in the proximal renal tubule as well as an indirect inhibitory action on adrenal aldosterone synthesis and release.

Finally, ANP inhibits the secretion of ADH from cells in the posterior pituitary. The sum of these actions of ANP are designed to reverse any pathological processes causing expansion of the sodium and water compartments in the body (Fig. 46.5). The signals which activate ANP are opposite to those which stimulate AII formation.

The mechanism of action of ANP is unique in several ways. No intermediary G proteins are activated by ligand-receptor binding. Instead, the plasma membrane receptor is a protein with intrinsic guanylate cyclase activity. Its ligand binding domain is located in the extracellular space, and it has only one membrane-spanning domain.

The intracellular domain of the ANP receptor is heavily phosphorylated in the inactive unbound state. Following ANP binding to the receptor, guanylate cyclase is activated and catalyses the formation of cyclic GMP (cGMP) from GTP. In the cells

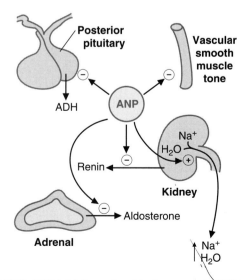

Fig. 46.5. Actions of ANP. ANP inhibits renin, aldosterone, and ADH (AVP) production and secretion. ANP also relaxes vascular smooth muscles. The net result is that more Na^+ and water are excreted by the kidneys and blood pressure is reduced.

of the adrenal glomerulosa, cGMP inhibits aldosterone synthesis directly as well as indirectly (the latter through a suppressive effect on cAMP formation). In addition, cGMP inhibits the secretion of preformed aldosterone into the extravascular space.

In target cells of the kidney and blood vessels, activation of cGMP leads to phosphorylation of proteins, which, through mechanisms yet to be determined, produces the biological action of ANP in these tissues.

HORMONES THAT INFLUENCE CALCIUM METABOLISM

Three overlapping regulatory systems or loops are tightly integrated by changes in the level of unbound calcium, of parathyroid hormone (PTH), and of calcitonin (CT) in the blood. Each system operates through a calcitropic hormone-sensitive target tissue (bone, intestine, kidney). In the process, the activation of vitamin D is either stimulated or suppressed depending upon the circulating level of phosphorus, PTH, and perhaps CT. The primary physiological actions of these three major calcium-regulating hormones are given in Table 46.2.

The integrated activities of the three target organs of the calcium-active hormones and the four controlling factors (plasma free Ca^{2+}, PTH, CT, and 1,25-$(OH)_2D_3$) can best be described using a model in which the free Ca^{2+} level in the blood acutely falls below normal. This hypocalcemic stimulus causes an increase in PTH secretion from the chief cells of the parathyroid glands and a decrease in the release of CT from the parafollicular cells of the thyroid. These hormonal changes cause increased resorption of Ca^{2+} from bone, a reduction in the renal excretion of calcium, and an increase in the absorption of Ca^{2+} from the gut. PTH stimulates renal generation of 1,25-$(OH)_2D_3$ from 25-$(OH)D_3$, which increases production of a Ca^{2+}-transporting protein in the cells of the small bowel that facilitates the entry of Ca^{2+} into the blood.

Through these three mechanisms, the previously subnormal free Ca^{2+} in the blood rises to a level slightly above the set point for the upper normal range. As a consequence, PTH secretion is suppressed and CT release is stimulated, changes that decrease bone resorption, increase Ca^{2+} excretion into the urine, and reduce intestinal absorption of dietary Ca^{2+}. These homeostatic forces operate until the previously elevated concentration of free Ca^{2+} in the blood falls to just below physiological levels, bringing the model full cycle. All of the reactions in this cascade occur in less than a second and serve to maintain the free Ca^{2+} levels in the blood within a narrow range of normal without major fluctuations in spite of a wide variability in dietary calcium intake.

Transport processes play a role in regulating the concentration of free Ca^{2+} in the cytosol and in the subcellular organelles. Small changes (in the micromolar range) in intracellular free Ca^{2+} concentration help to mediate the action of hormones in their target tissues. Cytosolic Ca^{2+} concentrations are maintained at submicromolar levels despite the millimolar Ca^{2+} concentration of the extracellular fluid. The continuous Ca^{2+} "leak" or influx of Ca^{2+} which occurs down this strong electrochemical gradient into the cell interior requires that intracellular Ca^{2+} be constantly pumped from the cytosol to the exterior of the cell. It also moves from the cytosol into subcellular organelles. To this end, membranes contain Ca^{2+} transport mechanisms such as the Ca^{2+}-ATPase transporter and the Ca^{2+}-Na^+ antiport for plasma membranes, a Ca^{2+}-Na^+ antiport for mitochondrial membranes, and a Ca^{2+}-ATPase for the membranes of both the endoplasmic and sarcoplasmic reticula. These interactions are summarized in Figure 46.6.

The "modulator protein" depicted in Figure 46.6 is represented by one of several proteins which bind with Ca^{2+} to carry out a variety of cellular functions. For example, calmodulin (CM) is a small protein with a molecular weight of about 16,700

When a physician orders a "calcium level" in the blood, unless otherwise specified, the number reported by the laboratory represents the "total" calcium present. This "total" calcium is distributed in three major fractions: the protein-bound, the free (elemental, unbound, or ionized), and the complexed fractions. The protein-bound fraction makes up 40–48% of the total serum Ca^{2+}. Seventy-five to 85% of bound Ca^{2+} is linked to albumin and 15–25% to globulin. Unbound or free Ca^{2+} makes up 45–50% of total Ca^{2+}. Finally, approximately 8% of total Ca^{2+} is complexed in the plasma mainly with bicarbonate, citrate, lactate, or sulfate.

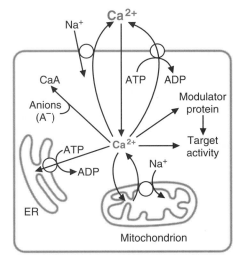

Fig. 46.6. Calcium transport processes. See text for description.

46.1: Trauma to the pituitary stalk led to a temporary inability of the hypothalamic-posterior pituitary axis to produce and release ADH. As a result, excessive volumes of water were lost into the urine.

In the case of this patient, the polyuria lasted 5 days, during which urinary losses were replaced with intravenous fluids. Then urine excretion returned to normal as his ability to secrete ADH returned spontaneously.

which can complex 4 Ca^{2+} ions, thereby undergoing a conformational change which allows the Ca^{2+}-calmodulin complex to bind strongly to a variety of target proteins (see Chapter 9). If cytosolic Ca^{2+} increases for any reason, CM complexes the incoming Ca^{2+} and the complex binds to the Ca^{2+}-ATPase pump on the plasma membrane, increasing transport of Ca^{2+} from the cytosol to the ECF, thereby returning cytosolic Ca^{2+} levels to normal. The Ca^{2+}-CM may also bind to enzymes, thereby activating the enzymes and influencing the metabolism of a variety of substrates. Ca^{2+}-CM may have other functions, such as inhibition of microtubular assembly.

Another family of regulatory or modulator proteins, the troponin-tropomyosin proteins (T-TM), is physically positioned in the interface of the contractile proteins, actin and myosin, preventing their physical contact and hence their shortening. If muscle cytosolic Ca^{2+} increases, T-TM binds Ca^{2+}, altering its configuration in a way that allows actin-myosin coupling and muscle contraction.

Parathyroid Hormone

PTH is a polypeptide with 84 amino acids and a molecular weight of 9,500. It is synthesized in the parathyroid chief cells as a preprohormone that is cleaved to form mature PTH, which is stored in secretory vesicles for later discharge into the blood (see Fig. 43.4). These stores of intact PTH may be degraded within the gland to a variety of fragments, a process which may be regulated in part by the concentration of free Ca^{2+} ions in the plasma. (Degradation is increased by high and suppressed by low free Ca^{2+} levels.) These fragments are secreted from the gland along with mature PTH. Fragments that contain the 34 amino acids from the N-terminus of PTH have full biological activity.

Radioimmunoassays are available to measure several species of PTH, including the whole molecule (biologically active), an N-terminal fragment (biologically active), and a mid-molecule fragment and a C-terminal fragment (both of which are biologically inactive). The inactive C-terminal fragment has a much longer half-life than the active fragments. Therefore, measurement of its concentration in the blood is used to assess the secretion rate of the parathyroid glands.

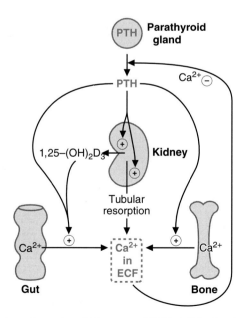

Fig. 46.7. Regulation of parathyroid hormone (PTH). PTH stimulates ($\oplus$) the resorption of calcium from bone and from the urine. It also stimulates the hydroxylation of 25-hydroxycholecalciferol in the kidney to form 1,25-dihydroxycholecalciferol (1,25-(OH)$_2$D$_3$), which increases Ca^{2+} absorption by the intestine. Increased concentrations of Ca^{2+} in the extracellular fluid (ECF) inhibit PTH secretion ($\ominus$).

As shown in Figure 46.7, intact PTH and its fragments are secreted into the blood in response to subnormal levels of free Ca^{2+} in the circulation. These hormones cause the concentration of free serum Ca^{2+} to increase to a level just above the normal range (above a critical set point). The latter acts as a "negative feedback" signal to the chief cells of the parathyroid gland, inhibiting further release of PTH and its fragments until the free Ca^{2+} level in the blood again falls below a specific threshold or set point.

After secretion into the blood, intact PTH is inactivated by proteolysis. Enzymes in the liver and kidneys form additional fragments of the 84 amino acid molecule.

The biological actions of PTH and its active N-terminal fragments (see Table 46.2) in the kidney, the skeleton, and indirectly in the gut are mediated by binding of PTH (or its active fragments) to receptors on the plasma membrane of these target tissues. This binding leads to activation of adenylate cyclase and a series of phosphorylations which result in the cellular response to PTH (e.g., Ca^{2+} reabsorption in the proximal tubule of the kidney, stimulation of osteoclastic activity in bone). cAMP may not be the only or even the predominant second messenger for PTH. Inositol trisphosphate, DAG, and cytosolic Ca^{2+} itself may also mediate some or all of the biological actions of PTH.

Parathyroid Hormone-Related Protein

Parathyroid hormone-related protein (PTHrP) in humans exists as several peptides containing 139–173 amino acid residues. Eight of the first amino acid residues of the N-terminus of PTHrP are identical to those of PTH, but no significant homology exists in the remainder of these molecules. These structural characteristics explain why the biochemical features of nonmetastatic hypercalcemia associated with certain cancers which produce PTHrP ectopically simulate those of primary hyperparathyroidism. The dissimilarities of the remainder of the molecule explain why most antisera against PTH do not detect PTHrP activity in plasma or tumors of patients with the humoral hypercalcemia of malignancy.

PTH and PTHrP compete for plasma membrane receptor binding in traditional target cells for PTH. PTHrP, like PTH, activates adenylate cyclase in bone and kidney. Both hormones bind specifically to receptors on skeletal osteoblastic cells to promote bone resorption and to receptors on kidney tubular cells to promote excretion of phosphate and to reduce calcium excretion.

Like PTH, PTHrP causes relaxation of vascular smooth muscle as well as that in the stomach, uterus, and urinary bladder. Acting via a paracrine mechanism, PTHrP, therefore, may modulate tissue perfusion as well as gastric, uterine, and urinary bladder tone.

Calcitonin

Calcitonin is a linear polypeptide with a molecular weight of 3,700. It is produced in the parafollicular or C cells of the thyroid gland. Calcitonin has 32 amino acids with a disulfide bridge between residues 1 and 7 on its N-terminus. Almost all of the 32 amino acids (but not the disulfide bridge) are required for full biological activity. A high molecular weight precursor protein is synthesized which contains CT plus two other peptides, katacalin (carboxy-adjacent peptide, or CT carboxy protein) which can lower serum calcium, and CT gene-related peptide (CGRP) found in the nervous system (see Fig. 15.20). The biological significance of these peptides in humans is not clear.

The regulation of CT secretion depends upon changes in free Ca^{2+} levels in the blood; levels above a high set point stimulate and levels below a lower set point inhibit release.

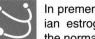 In premenopausal women, ovarian estrogens help to maintain the normal mineral density of the skeleton, in part, by blunting the osteolytic (bone resorbing) action of a variety of cytokines produced locally in bone. As gonadal estrogen production wanes in the perimenopausal female, this protective action diminishes. As a result, a rapid increase in bone turnover accompanied by an annual loss of 1–2% of the total calcified skeleton occurs. This loss can, in part, be reversed through the use of estrogen replacement therapy, which was used to treat **Teresa Livermore's** osteoporosis.

PTHrP was discovered as a consequence of research into the mechanisms by which cancers cause hypercalcemia. It is secreted by many tumors, and its actions on bone and kidney are similar to those of native PTH and result in hypercalcemia. Subsequently, mRNA for PTHrP was demonstrated in normal tissues such as epithelial cells (e.g., skin, lung, gut, kidney), endocrine cells (e.g., parathyroid, thyroid, gonad, pancreas, adrenal), muscle (e.g., myocardium, skeletal muscle, smooth muscle), as well as brain, bone, and liver.

Parenteral CT has limited efficacy as chronic therapy for osteoporosis, but its apparent analgesic effect at the site of an acute fracture prompted its temporary use in **Teresa Livermore.**

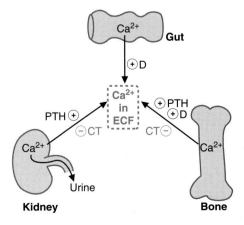

Fig. 46.8. Actions of calcitonin. Calcitonin inhibits the release of Ca^{2+} from bone and stimulates its excretion in the urine.

Ergosterol is the provitamin of vitamin D_2 which differs from 7-dehydrocholesterol and vitamin D_3, respectively, only by having a double bond between C22 and C23 and a methyl group at C24. Vitamin D_2 is the constituent in many commercial vitamin preparations and in irradiated milk and bread. The antirachitic potencies of D_2 and D_3 in humans are equal, but both must be converted to 25-(OH)-cholecalciferol and eventually to the active form calcitriol (1,25-$(OH)_2D_3$) for biological activity.

The nonpharmacological approach to postmenopausal osteoporosis includes dietary calcium and vitamin D supplementation as well as exercises that encourage bone remodeling and renewal. This approach, in addition to pharmacological therapy, was used to treat **Teresa Livermore.**

Rickets is a disorder of young children caused by a deficiency of vitamin D. Low levels of calcium and phosphorus in the blood are associated with skeletal deformities in these patients.

The actions of CT are depicted in Figure 46.8. The hormone acts on osteoclastic cells in bone (bone-resorbing cells) to suppress their osteolytic activity. As a consequence, the egress of calcium and phosphorus from bone is reduced, causing a fall in serum Ca^{2+} and phosphorus levels. Calcitonin may also cause phosphorus to move into liver and other cells, suggesting that this hormone has an important role in the regulation of phosphorus metabolism independent of calcium homeostasis. The physiological importance of its renal action (and intestinal action, if any) remains to be determined.

Vitamin D

The calciferols, including several forms of vitamin D, are a family of steroids that affect calcium homeostasis (Fig. 46.9). Cholecalciferol (vitamin D_3) requires ultraviolet light for its production from 7-dehydrocholesterol in animals and from ergosterol in plants. This irradiation cleaves the carbon-carbon bond at C9–C10 to open the B ring to form cholecalciferol, an inactive precursor of 1,25-$(OH)_2$-cholecalciferol (calcitriol). Calcitriol is the most potent biologically active form of vitamin D (see Fig. 46.9).

The formation of calcitriol begins in the liver and ends in the kidney, where the pathway is regulated. In this activation process, carbon 25 of D_2 or D_3 is hydroxylated in the microsomes of the liver to form 25-hydroxycholecalciferol (calcidiol). Calcidiol circulates to the kidney bound to vitamin D binding globulin (transcalciferin). In the proximal convoluted tubule of the kidney, a mixed function oxidase, which requires molecular O_2 and NADPH as cofactors, hydroxylates carbon 1 on the A ring to form calcitriol. This step is tightly regulated and is the rate-limiting step in the production of the active hormone. Factors that increase this hydroxylation step include a declining level of serum and renal tubular phosphate and calcium (the latter probably mediated by PTH). Calcitonin may inhibit this activation reaction.

1,25-$(OH)_2D_3$ (calcitriol) is about 100 times more potent than 25-$(OH)D_3$ in its actions, yet 25-$(OH)D_3$ is present in the blood in a concentration that may be 100 times greater, which suggests it may play some role in calcium and phosphorus homeostasis.

The biologically active forms of vitamin D are sterol hormones and, like other steroids, diffuse passively through the plasma membrane. In the intestine, bone, and kidney, the sterol then moves into the nucleus and binds to specific vitamin D_3 receptors. This complex activates genes that encode proteins mediating the action of active vitamin D_3. In the intestinal mucosal cell, for example, transcription of genes encoding calcium-transporting proteins is activated. These proteins are capable of carrying Ca^{2+} (and phosphorus) absorbed from the gut lumen across the cell, making it available for eventual passage into the circulation. The physiological actions of active vitamin D_3 on the gut, bone, and kidney are summarized in Table 46.2.

CLINICAL COMMENTS. A balloon angioplasty of the obstructing atherosclerotic lesion within the lumen of the left main renal artery was successfully performed on **Rena Lischemia.** Compression of the atherosclerotic plaque against the side walls of the vessel permitted increased blood flow to her left kidney. As a result, less renin was secreted, which led to a decrease in AII and aldosterone and, consequently, a decrease in blood pressure. Within several days, her blood pressure returned to the normal range.

Osteoporosis, the most common form of osteopenia or bone loss, affects the majority of postmenopausal women, such as **Teresa Livermore**, to varying degrees. When the bone mineral content falls below a critical level, the supportive function of the skeleton is diminished and fractures occur at brittle sites in the skeleton. The ver-

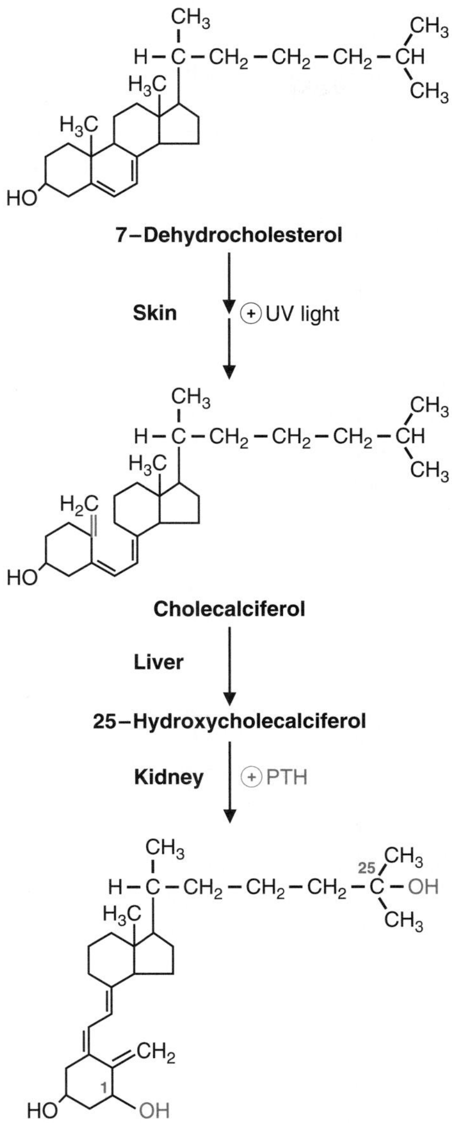

Fig. 46.9. Synthesis of active vitamin D. ($1,25$-di$(OH)_2D_3$) is produced from 7-dehydrocholesterol, a precursor of cholesterol. In the skin, ultraviolet (UV) light produces cholecalciferol, which is hydroxylated at the 25-position in the liver and the 1-position in the kidney to form the active hormone.

tebral bodies of the thoracic and lumbar spine and of the bones of the hip are two of the most common sites of fractures in severely affected patients. These fractures often lead to significant morbidity and mortality, resulting in an estimated 10 billion dollars in health care expenditure annually.

The presence and course of this disorder can be determined by serial measurements of bone mineral density using such techniques as dual energy x-ray absorptiometry (DEXA) of the lumbosacral spine and/or a hip joint. Teresa's bone density in both her lower spine and in the bones of her left hip was only 65% that of age-matched controls.

The mainstay of the pharmacological approach to postmenopausal osteoporosis is lifelong estrogen replacement therapy (ERT), provided that no absolute contraindications to its use, such as a personal or close family history of breast cancer, are present. In a postmenopausal woman who still has a uterus, a progestational agent such as medroxyprogesterone acetate must be added to ERT to prevent the 4–8-fold increase in endometrial (uterine lining) cancer that would otherwise occur with chronic unopposed estrogen use. A class of drugs known as the bisphosphonates may also speed the process of bone replacement.

BIOCHEMICAL COMMENTS. Changes in the concentration of the free (ionized) calcium level in the cytosol ($[Ca^{2+}]_I$) mediate many cellular processes, such as secretion, contraction, and gene transcription. Normally, the $[Ca^{2+}]_I$ in the resting nonstimulated cell is approximately 100 nanomolar (nM, or 1×10^{-7} M), which is 10,000–12,000-fold less than the concentration of Ca^{2+} in the ECF. This tightly controlled low cytosolic Ca^{2+} concentration is maintained through the activity of a number of cellular pumps (see Fig. 46.6). The plasma membrane of the cell is highly impermeable to Ca^{2+}. Any movement of extracellular Ca^{2+} into the cell must occur primarily via the ion channels in the plasma membrane of the cell which can be opened or activated by specific signals. In addition, the plasma membrane contains two energy-dependent mechanisms that regulate $[Ca^{2+}]_I$ by pumping Ca^{2+} from the cell into the ECF. These are the Ca^{2+},Mg^{2+}-ATPase pump and the Na^+-Ca^{2+} exchanger. The intensity of the activity of the latter is determined by the magnitude of the Na^{2+} gradient established by the plasma membrane Na^+,K^+-ATPase.

The low $[Ca^{2+}]_I$ of the resting, unstimulated cell is also maintained by several intracellular organelles (primarily the endoplasmic reticulum and the mitochondria), which can sequester Ca^{2+} from the cytosol. Ca^{2+} is taken up by the endoplasmic reticulum via the operation of a membrane-linked Ca^{2+},Mg^{2+}-ATPase, distinct from that in the plasma membrane. The mechanism for mitochondrial sequestration of Ca^{2+} is related to the proton gradient across the membranes of these organelles. The electrical potential difference drives Ca^{2+} into mitochondria via a uniport. The efflux of Ca^{2+} from the mitochondrion to the cytosol involves either a Ca^{2+}-Na^+ antiport or a Na^+ and ATP independent mechanism, depending on the cell type.

When the first messenger-second messenger cascade is activated by binding of a hormone to its plasma membrane receptor, the Ca^{2+} concentration inside the cell ($[Ca^{2+}]_I$) rapidly increases above the ambient, unstimulated level either through entry via the plasma membrane Ca^{2+} channels (primarily the voltage-sensitive channels) and/or through release from the endoplasmic reticulum. This elevation in $[Ca^{2+}]_I$ activates cellular responses (e.g., secretion, contraction, gene transcription), which are specific for the first messenger signal that initiated activation of the cellular cascade.

Unlike the rapidly changing concentration of Ca^{2+} in the intracellular compartments, Ca^{2+} must be maintained at near constant levels in the extracellular fluid. In part, this constancy is determined through the activity of recently described calcium ion-sensing receptors on the plasma membrane of such cells as the chief cells of the parathyroid gland, the C cells of the thyroid gland, and the tubular cells of the kidney. Accordingly, in response to hypercalcemia, parathyroid chief cells secrete less PTH (a classic negative endocrine feedback loop), the C cells of the thyroid gland increase their secretion of CT, and the renal tubular cells increase the secretion of Ca^{2+} into the tubular urine. As a consequence of these responses, the ECF Ca^{2+}_I concentration returns to normal. The opposite responses would occur if the ECF Ca^{2+} concentration were initially suppressed.

The physiological importance of the normal function of these calcium ion-sensing receptors is clear from studies demonstrating that point mutations in the genes for these receptors is associated with clinical disorders such as familial hypocalciuric hypercalcemia and familial isolated hypoparathyroidism.

Suggested Readings

Brown EM, Pollak M, Seidman CE, et al. Calcium-ion-sensing cell-surface receptors. N Engl J Med 1995;333:234–240.

Goodman HM. Basic medical endocrinology. New York: Raven Press, 1994:152–202.

Greenspan FS, Baxter JD. Basic and clinical endocrinology. Norwalk, CT: Appleton & Lange, 1994:227–306, 347–369.

Kanno K, Sasaki S, Hirata Y, et al. Urinary excretion of aquaporin-2 in patients with diabetes insipidus. N Engl J Med 1995;332:1540–1545.

Martin TJ, Moseley JM. Parathyroid hormone-related protein. In: DeGroot LJ, ed. Endocrinology. Philadelphia: WB Saunders, 1995:967–977.

PROBLEMS

1. A 46-year-old man was discovered to have a recent increase in his blood pressure associated with a spontaneous drop in his serum potassium level (hypokalemia). His plasma renin activity was low and his plasma aldosterone level was elevated. An MRI of his adrenal glands revealed a 1.8-cm nodule on the left adrenal gland. Which one of the following statements regarding this patient is **false**?

   A. His plasma angiotensin II (AII) level would be expected to be low.

   B. His plasma volume would be increased.

   C. His urine potassium concentration would be inappropriately high in relation to the serum potassium level.

   D. Treatment of his high blood pressure with a drug that inhibits the conversion of angiotensin I (AI) to AII (e.g., an ACE inhibitor) would be appropriate therapy from a pathophysiological point of view.

   E. The low serum potassium level should be accompanied by a metabolic alkalosis.

2. A 48-year-old man complains of fatigue, muscle aches, constipation, and a recent episode of renal colic (flank pain caused by a kidney stone passing down a ureter). Appropriate studies determined that he has primary hyperparathyroidism caused by a benign hypersecretory tumor of his left inferior parathyroid gland. Which one of the following laboratory or imaging findings is **not** consistent with this diagnosis?

   A. His serum free (unbound) Ca^{2+} level is increased.

   B. Mild osteopenia (loss of bone mineral) is noted on a bone densitometry study.

   C. His serum parathyroid hormone level is elevated.

   D. His **total** (free plus bound) serum Ca^{2+} level is persistently normal.

   E. His serum phosphate level is low.

ANSWERS

1. **A, B, C, and E are true.** In a patient who has primary aldosteronism (an aldosterone-producing adenoma of one adrenal cortex), the plasma volume is expanded because of the excess secretion of aldosterone. High aldosterone levels cause sup-

pression of renin secretion which, in turn, reduces AI and AII synthesis. Therefore, the plasma AII level would be low. The increased mineralocorticoid activity of excess aldosterone on the distal portions of the renal tubules enhances sodium reabsorption from the tubular luminal urine with a proportional increase in the excretion of potassium (and hydrogen) into the urine. Thus the patient has a hypokalemia (and a metabolic alkalosis) and an inappropriate excretion of potassium into the urine.

D is false. Because both AI and AII levels in the blood are already low in primary aldosteronism, a drug that lowers blood pressure by inhibiting the conversion of AI to AII would not be appropriate therapy in this patient.

2. **A, B, C, and E are consistent with the diagnosis.** The secretory parathyroid tumor leads to an elevation of parathyroid hormone (PTH) in the blood. This, in turn, causes an increase in both the total and the free Ca^{2+} levels in the blood through the hormone's actions on the gut, the skeleton and the kidney. The osteolytic (bone resorbing) action of excess PTH on the skeleton leads to a decrease in bone density. The serum phosphate level tends to fall in these patients primarily as a result of the phosphate-excreting action of PTH on the renal tubule.

D is not consistent with the diagnosis. Hypersecretion of PTH would cause an increase in both the free and the total Ca^{2+} levels in the blood.

47 Actions of Hormones That Affect Growth, Differentiation, and Reproduction

Many hormones are involved in growth and differentiation of cells in the human organism. However, growth hormone is the major hormone that regulates growth, in part by stimulating the synthesis and secretion of insulin-like growth factors (somatomedins). Hormones involved in differentiation of cells include retinoic acid, which is derived from dietary vitamin A.

Reproduction is regulated mainly by testosterone in males and the estrogens and progestins in females. Luteinizing hormone (LH) and follicle-stimulating hormone (FSH) from the anterior pituitary regulate the production of these sex steroids.

 Yetta Bloom, a 4-year-old girl, was brought to her pediatrician by her mother, who felt that her daughter's growth was slow although her cognitive and motor development appeared to be normal. The physician plotted Yetta's linear growth velocity and body weight against her age on a standard nomogram and found that Yetta's growth plots fell into the 60th percentile from birth until about 18 months of age, when they fell dramatically to the 5th percentile and remained at that level.

Yetta's mother could not identify any events that could have precipitated growth retardation except for an automobile accident in which Yetta was thrown head-first into the car's dashboard, fracturing her left cheek bone and her nose when she was about 18 months old. The pediatrician suspected that Yetta's pituitary area was injured in that crash, causing a deficiency of growth hormone (GH) secretion.

 Yuri Nader, a 66-year-old architect, had an increasing urgency to urinate on arising from sleep and every 4 or 5 hours thereafter. His urinary stream was growing less forceful, he had occasional difficulty initiating urination, and he "dribbled" urine after he thought he had completely emptied his bladder. He was now reluctant to take a long automobile trip without first determining where he could find a restroom along the way.

His physician suspected that Yuri's symptoms were the result of a rather rapidly progressing benign hyperplasia of his prostate gland. A digital rectal examination revealed a moderate to severe diffuse anodular enlargement of both lobes of the prostate.

 As part of their medical school training, Erna Nemdy and Ron Templeton were required to follow a patient throughout her pregnancy and to participate in the delivery. Their patient was **Jessica Tayshun**, a 20-year-old nul-

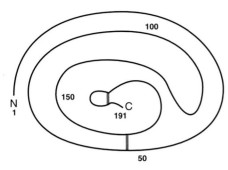

Human growth hormone

Fig. 47.1. Structure of growth hormone. From Murray RK, et al. Harper's biochemistry, 23rd ed. Stamford, CT: Appleton & Lange, 1993:502.

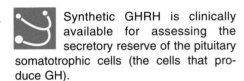 Synthetic GHRH is clinically available for assessing the secretory reserve of the pituitary somatotrophic cells (the cells that produce GH).

Excessive secretion of growth hormone (GH) is usually the result of the overproduction of GH by a benign tumor of the anterior pituitary gland. If the hypersecretion begins before the growth centers (epiphyses) located near the ends of the long bones have closed, gigantism occurs. Individuals with gigantism can reach 8 feet or more in height. If hypersecretion begins after the bone growth centers have closed, the result is acromegaly, the problem for which **Sam Atotrope** was treated. The characteristics of acromegaly are thickness of the skin, coarseness of the facial features, organomegaly, and a general increase in skeletal and muscle mass. Diabetes mellitus may also be caused by excess GH. If the pituitary tumor grows superiorly and encroaches on the optic nerves, visual loss can result. If further expansion of the tumor occurs, dysfunction of other cranial nerves, severe headaches, and symptoms of increased intracranial pressure may develop.

lipara (first pregnancy), who thought she was about 3 weeks pregnant at the time of her first visit.

The patient had a long list of questions she wanted answered. Her first urgent concern was related to the potentially harmful effect of a derivative of vitamin A she had taken for the treatment of acne 3 years earlier. Ms. Tayshun, a biology major at a local university, also wanted to know what tests are performed to confirm that conception has actually occurred and if a series of these tests could be used to determine if her pregnancy was proceeding normally, what hormones could be given to maintain pregnancy if she should show signs of aborting early, what hormonal changes would occur in her body as her gestation progressed, what hormonal signals initiated labor, and, finally, would she be "knocked out" just before the baby was born. Erna and Ron both realized that Ms. Tayshun was going to be a major challenge for them over the next 8 months.

GROWTH HORMONE

Growth hormone, produced in the anterior pituitary, is the major hormone that regulates growth in the human. Insulin and thyroid hormone also have growth-promoting effects and are necessary for optimal growth to occur. During adolescence, androgens and estrogens accelerate growth, stimulating the adolescent "growth spurt."

Structure of Growth Hormone

Human growth hormone (GH, also called somatotropin) is a member of a family of hormones, which, in addition to GH, includes prolactin (PRL) and human chorionic somatomammotropin (hCS; human placental lactogen). Although each has potential growth-promoting and lactogenic activity, only GH has a significant influence on growth (see Chapter 44).

Growth hormone is a 191 amino acid polypeptide (molecular weight about 22,000) which has two disulfide bridges (Fig. 47.1). (See Fig. 44.7 for a comparison of GH and PRL structure.)

Both GH and hCS are encoded as prehormones on chromosome 17, while prolactin is encoded on chromosome 6. Pregrowth hormone has a molecular weight of 28,000 and, although secreted, is without biological activity.

Regulation of Secretion of Growth Hormone

The synthesis and secretion of GH is regulated by GHRH and somatostatin. Growth hormone-releasing hormone (GHRH) is a 44 amino acid peptide with its biological activity residing in the first 27 residues at the N-terminus (see Fig. 44.6). GHRH is produced in the hypothalamus and acts on the anterior pituitary to promote the release of GH.

Somatostatin (growth hormone release-inhibiting hormone) is a tetradecapeptide which inhibits GH synthesis and secretion. It also suppresses the synthesis and release of such hormones as thyroid-stimulating hormone (TSH), gastrin, secretin, vasoactive intestinal polypeptide (VIP), as well as insulin and glucagon. Somatostatin is produced by a number of cells in the body (see Chapter 44).

Effects of Growth Hormone

Prior to 1957, GH was believed to directly increase growth of both skeletal and soft tissues. When GH was discovered to increase growth of tissues in vivo but to be inactive in vitro, the existence of a GH-induced "mediator" of growth was suggested. Eventually, two such compounds were identified. Because they mediated growth of somatic tissues, they were designated "somatomedins."

The dual effector hypothesis for cellular growth suggests that GH may promote the growth of cells both by a direct and an indirect action. Through its proposed direct effect, GH causes cells to differentiate, and through its indirect effect, i.e., by stimulating somatomedin synthesis, GH causes growth of these precursor cells (Fig. 47.2).

Insulin-Like Growth Factors

The two somatomedins in humans share structural homologies with proinsulin and both have substantial insulin-like growth activity, hence the designations, insulin-like growth factor I (human IGF-I, or somatomedin-C) and insulin-like growth factor II (human IGF-II, or somatomedin A). IGF-I is a single-chain basic peptide having 70 amino acids, and IGF-II is slightly acidic with 67 amino acids. These two peptides are identical to insulin in half of their residues. In addition, they contain a structural domain that is homologous to the C-peptide of proinsulin.

A broad spectrum of normal cells respond to high doses of insulin by increasing thymidine uptake and initiating cell propagation. In most instances, IGF-I causes the same response as insulin in these cells but at significantly smaller, more physiological concentrations. Thus, the IGFs are more potent than insulin in their growth-promoting actions.

One form of dwarfism is caused by a deficiency in GH production. The deficiency may be due to a variety of mechanisms, including autoimmune (antibody)-mediated damage to the somatotrophs, head trauma, or irradiation damage to the normal pituitary cells which occurs in the course of radiation therapy to a tumor in the vicinity of the pituitary gland. These GH-deficient individuals have early onset of growth failure, and their adult height is often less than 4 feet. If they are able to secrete gonadotropins, they undergo puberty, although it may be somewhat delayed. Except for a juvenile appearance and small stature, they are otherwise normal and can reproduce.

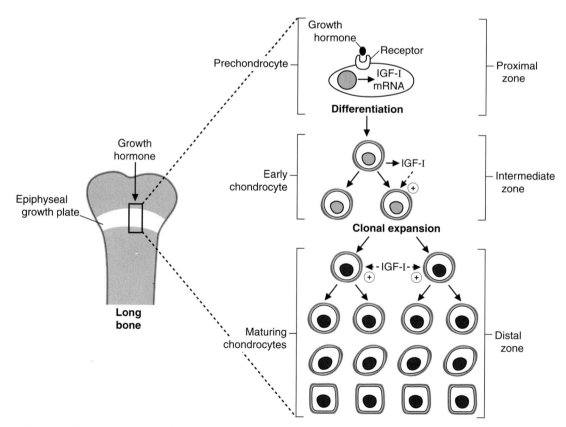

Fig. 47.2. Dual effects of growth hormone. Growth hormone directly acts on cells to cause differentiation and the release of IGFs, which stimulate cell division. The effects of GH and IGFs are illustrated. From Wilson JW, Foster DW. Williams textbook of endocrinology, 8th ed. Philadelphia: WB Saunders, 1992:235.

Q 47.1: Laron dwarfs differ from pituitary dwarfs in that they have high levels of GH. Like pituitary dwarfs, their insulin-like growth factor levels are low. What could be the molecular basis for their growth failure?

Because serum concentrations of GH fall to nearly undetectable levels between the two to five secretory bursts which regularly occur each day in normal children, the doctor performed two pharmacological stimulation tests on **Yetta Bloom** designed to determine Yetta's pituitary reserve capacity for the release of GH. The first test was an insulin tolerance test. An injection of insulin causes hypoglycemia, which normally increases GH secretion. The second test was an arginine infusion test. Arginine directly stimulates the release of GH. Both tests failed to cause the expected rise in the serum GH level to 7 ng/mL or more. These results were interpreted as showing at least a partial GH deficiency. After further studies confirmed the diagnosis, treatment was initiated with a series of injections using GH produced by recombinant DNA techniques.

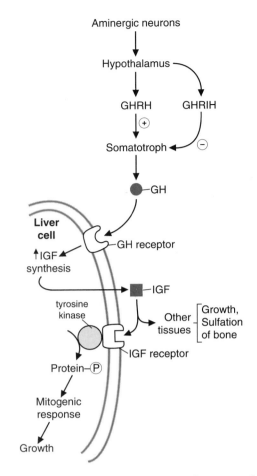

Fig. 47.3. Production and action of IGFs. The hypothalamus produces growth hormone-releasing hormone (GHRH) which stimulates somatotrophs in the anterior pituitary to release growth hormone (GH). Growth hormone release-inhibiting hormone (GHRIH, also called somatostatin) inhibits GH release. GH binds to cell surface receptors and stimulates IGF production and release by liver and other tissues. IGF binds to cell surface receptors and stimulates the phosphorylation of proteins that cause mitosis and growth.

Vitamin A and its derivatives are known as retinoids because of the importance of this vitamin to the retina.

Evidence suggests that the IGFs exert their effects through either an endocrine or a paracrine/autocrine mechanism. IGF-I appears to stimulate cell propagation and growth by binding to specific IGF-I receptors on the plasma membrane of target cells, rather than binding to GH receptors (Fig. 47.3).

Like insulin, the intracellular portion of the plasma membrane receptor for IGF-I (but not IGF-II) has intrinsic tyrosine kinase activity. The fact that the receptors for insulin and a number of other growth factors have intrinsic tyrosine kinase activity indicates that tyrosine phosphorylation initiates the process of cellular replication and growth. Subsequently, a chain of kinases is activated, which include a number of proto-oncogene products (see Fig. 43.16).

Most cells of the body have mRNA for IGF, but the liver has the greatest concentration of these messengers, followed by kidney and heart. The synthesis of IGF-I is regulated, for the most part, by GH, whereas hepatic production of IGF-II is independent of GH levels in the blood.

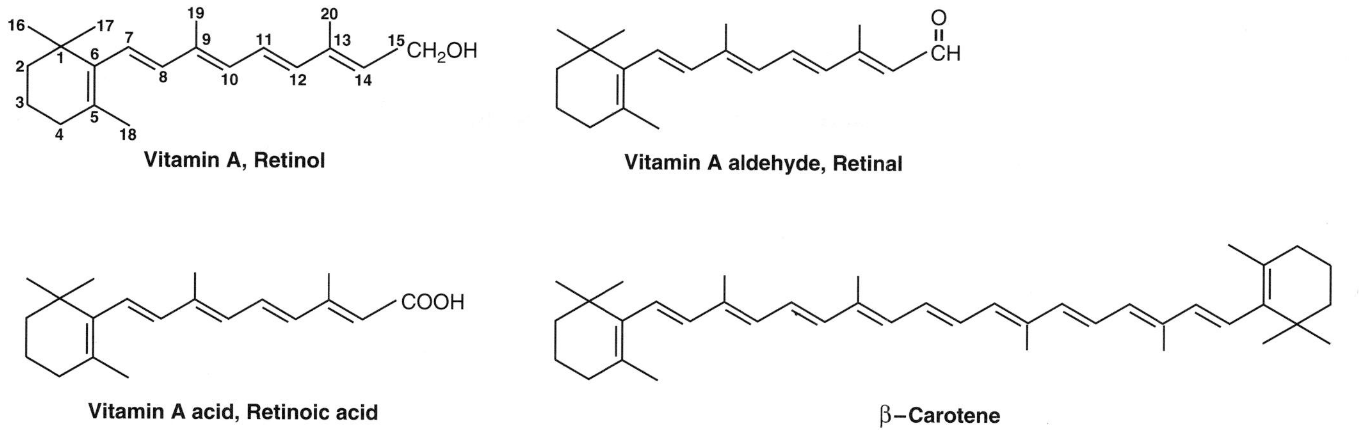

Vitamin A, Retinol

Vitamin A aldehyde, Retinal

Vitamin A acid, Retinoic acid

β—Carotene

Fig. 47.4. Structures of β-carotene, retinol, retinal, and retinoic acid. β-Carotene is the major carotenoid synthesized in plants that are the main source of vitamin A in the diet. β-Carotene is cleaved to form 2 molecules of retinol. Dietary sources of retinol and retinal include liver, egg yolks, milk fat, and fish oils.

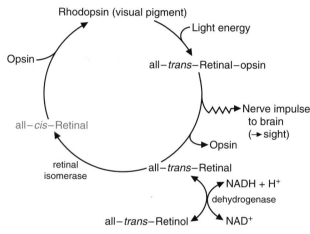

Excessive intake of vitamin A can result in toxic symptoms, including redness of the skin and desquamation.

Polar bear liver contains toxic amounts of vitamin A, and some Arctic explorers who ate this liver lost the soles of their feet as a consequence of vitamin A toxicity.

Fig. 47.5. Role of retinal in the visual cycle. All-*cis*-retinal binds to the protein opsin to form rhodopsin. Light converts all-*cis*-retinal to all-*trans*-retinal. This reaction stimulates nerves to transmit impulses to the brain that result in visual images. Opsin is released, and all-*trans*-retinal is reconverted to all-*cis*-retinal.

VITAMIN A

Retinoic acid, derived from vitamin A, functions like a steroid hormone. It promotes normal growth and differentiation of epithelial tissue, optimal bone growth, and embryonic development. Other forms of vitamin A are required for normal vision and may enhance the competence of the immune system as well as protect against certain malignancies.

Vitamin A is required in the diet. It is obtained from animal fat, fish oils, and certain plants. The major plant form of the vitamin, β-carotene, is cleaved to 2 molecules of vitamin A, mainly by intestinal cells (Fig. 47.4).

In the body, vitamin A exists in three oxidation states: an alcohol, an aldehyde, and an acid (see Fig. 47.4). It is absorbed and transported as the alcohol form, retinol, and stored as retinyl esters mainly in the stellate cells of the liver. Retinol is oxidized to the aldehyde form, retinal by a reversible reaction requiring NAD^+. Retinal forms the light-sensing component of the visual cycle (Fig. 47.5). Retinal is oxidized to retinoic acid by an irreversible reaction.

A 47.1: Laron dwarfs have structural or functional abnormalities in GH receptors. When IGF-I is administered to a Laron dwarf, typical growth stimulation is observed.

Erna and Ron had done their homework and were ready for **Jess Tayshun** when she returned for her second prenatal visit. They first discussed the potential for fetal abnormalities related to her use of a derivative of vitamin A for the treatment of acne 3 years earlier. Erna explained that 13-*cis*-retinoic acid, the form of retinoic acid in the drug she had taken, should be cleared from her body by now and should not have teratogenic effects on her developing baby.

Yuri Nader has benign prostatic hyperplasia (BPH), a common cause of symptoms of urinary bladder muscle irritability (e.g., urgency, frequency, nocturia) and eventually of varying degrees of obstruction of the flow of urine from the bladder through the prostatic portion of the distal urethra (e.g., hesitancy, weak urinary stream, urinary retention).

Although the precise etiology is not completely understood, testosterone, the major androgen produced by the testes, is certainly involved in the pathogenesis of BPH. Testosterone secreted by the Leydig cells of the testes crosses the plasma membrane of the stromal cells of the prostate gland. An enzyme located in the nuclear membrane of these cells, 5α-reductase, reduces testosterone to DHT, a potent androgen which induces the transcription of mRNAs for growth-promoting cytokines such as transforming growth factor β and basic fibroblast growth factor. These cytokines not only cause growth of the stromal cells by an autocrine effect but also cause growth of the epithelial cells of the prostate by a paracrine effect. The increasing estrogen/androgen ratio common in the aging male may enhance this growth process through the putative action of estrogen in increasing the number of DHT receptors in the nuclei of the stromal cells of the prostate.

Retinoic acid behaves like a steroid hormone. It associates with receptors in the nucleus of its target cells, and the receptor-retinoic acid complex binds to response elements in DNA, stimulating the transcription of genes. The receptors for retinoic acid belong to the steroid-thyroid receptor superfamily (see Fig. 43.19). The proteins produced from genes activated by retinoic acid are responsible for the effects of vitamin A on growth, differentiation, reproduction, and embryonic development.

SEX STEROIDS

Androgenic Steroids

The male sex hormones, or androgens, are responsible for normal male sexual development, including masculinization of the internal and external genital tracts, the development of male secondary sexual characteristics (such as beard growth), fertility, and the anabolic character of somatic tissues (such as the male type skeletal shape and size and heavier muscle bulk). Over 95% of circulating testosterone, the principal androgen in the blood, is synthesized in the testis in men and in the ovary in women. The remainder is produced in the adrenal cortex of both sexes.

BIOCHEMICAL PROPERTIES OF THE ANDROGENS

Testosterone serves as a precursor for the formation of two other sex steroids. About 4% of circulating testosterone is converted to dihydrotestosterone (DHT), which serves as the intracellular mediator of most of testosterone's androgenic actions. A smaller proportion (about 0.2%) of circulating testosterone is converted to estrogens in various tissues containing the aromatase enzyme. These estrogens have either androgen-like or antiandrogen effects. These molecular interconversions ultimately determine the full spectrum of physiological actions of the androgenic steroids.

Approximately 2% of the total testosterone in the blood is in an unbound or free, easily diffusible state. This free hormone is the most biologically active form of the total hormone in the circulation because of its ability to move passively into the cytosol of target cells. A fraction of the total testosterone is loosely bound to sex hormone binding globulin and makes up a readily accessible pool for the diffusible free fraction.

PHYSIOLOGICAL ACTIONS OF THE ANDROGENS

The physiological actions of the androgens differ at different stages of life. In the embryo, androgens induce virilization of the male urogenital tract in which the Wolffian ducts differentiate into the epididymis, vas deferens, and the seminal vesicles. In the neonate, a surge of androgen secretion occurs which may influence masculine organizational and developmental functions in the brain. In the prepubertal male, minimal androgen release from the testis and adrenal cortex chronically suppresses pituitary gonadotropin release until the onset of puberty, at which time the gonadotrophs of the anterior pituitary become increasingly less sensitive to feedback inhibition by circulating androgens. This loss of sensitivity allows a cyclic release of LH and FSH. LH stimulates testosterone production by the testicular Leydig cells, and FSH stimulates maturation of the spermatogonia. Virilization and fertility follow.

The growth-promoting actions of rising androgen levels in the prepubertal male lead to a spurt in height and to growth of skeletal muscle and bone mass. These anabolic actions of male hormone are mediated by the same androgen receptors that mediate the actions of male hormone in other target tissues. As a result of these effects, the skin thickens and sebaceous gland secretion increases.

Secondary sexual characteristics develop including growth of the larynx, the appearance of pubic, axillary, facial, and extremity hair, and growth of the penis. Androgens may also contribute to the more aggressive behavior of the pubertal male. In the late teens or early twenties, genetically predisposed males may develop initial evidence of male pattern baldness.

REGULATION OF TESTOSTERONE PRODUCTION AND SPERMATOGENESIS

Androgens are required for spermatogenesis and the maturation of sperm as they pass through the epididymis and the vas deferens. Androgens also control the growth and function of the seminal vesicles and of the prostate gland.

Gonadotropin-releasing hormone (GnRH), secreted episodically during the day from the hypothalamus, stimulates the anterior pituitary to release luteinizing hormone (LH) and follicle-stimulating hormone (FSH). LH acts on the Leydig cells in the testes, stimulating the production and secretion of testosterone. This hormone enters the Sertoli cells of the testes and is reduced to DHT. FSH and DHT act to stimulate synthesis of proteins in the Sertoli cells that promote spermatogenesis in the spermatogonia. Sertoli cells also produce inhibin, a protein that feeds back and inhibits FSH release. Testosterone has a negative feedback effect on LH secretion (Fig. 47.6).

In immature males, FSH contributes to the initiation of spermatogenesis. The hormone binds to receptors on the plasma membrane of Sertoli cells, which are attached to the basement membrane of the seminiferous tubules of the testes. These cells not only provide physical support for the contiguous germ cells through the rigidity of their cytoskeleton but also respond to FSH stimulation with the production of proteins that promote the maturation of spermatogonia within the tubules.

In the sexually mature male, FSH also binds to specific receptors on Sertoli cell membranes, but once spermatogenesis is underway, testosterone can maintain sperm development in the absence of FSH.

Estrogens

STRUCTURE OF ESTROGENS

Estrogenic activity is shared by many steroidal compounds (e.g., estradiol, mestranol, quinestrol) and by certain nonsteroidal compounds (e.g., synthetic diethylstilbestrol and the naturally occurring plant estrogens known as the phytoestrogens). The most potent naturally occurring steroidal estrogen in humans is 17β-estradiol, followed by estrone, and, finally estriol. Their structures are shown in Figure 47.7. Each is an 18-carbon steroid with a phenolic A ring (an aromatic ring with a hydroxyl group at carbon 3). This configuration gives these steroids selective, high affinity binding to estrogen receptors. These compounds also have a β-hydroxy group or ketone at position 17 of the D ring, which further contributes to their binding capacity.

REGULATION OF SECRETION OF ESTROGENS

Estrogen production occurs mainly in the granulosa cells of the ovary (Fig. 47.8). Secretion of estrogen increases in response to release of FSH from the anterior pituitary gland. In the arcuate nucleus of the hypothalamus and in the gonadotrophs of the anterior pituitary gland, a rising level of serum estradiol suppresses GnRH release and FSH release through a negative feedback effect. These follicular cells also produce inhibin, which has a negative feedback effect on FSH release.

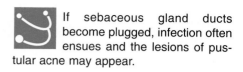 If sebaceous gland ducts become plugged, infection often ensues and the lesions of pustular acne may appear.

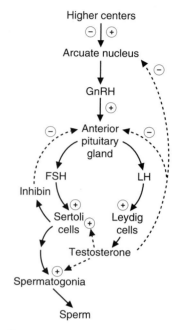

Fig. 47.6. Actions of LH and FSH on spermatogenesis. Gonadotropin-releasing hormone (GnRH) stimulates the hypothalamus to release both FSH and LH. FSH stimulates Sertoli cells in the testes to produce proteins involved in sperm production. Sertoli cells also produce inhibin, which feeds back on the anterior pituitary to inhibit FSH release. LH stimulates Leydig cells in the testes to produce testosterone, which, in turn, stimulates Sertoli cells and also spermatogonia, promoting sperm production.

 The nonsteroidal estrogens, such as the synthetic estrogen diethylstilbestrol, often contain a phenolic ring which simulates the A ring of the steroidal estrogens and probably imparts estrogenic activity to these compounds.

Diethylstilbestrol

ACTIONS OF ESTROGENS

Like other sterol hormones, estrogens act by regulating the transcription of a limited number of steroid-responsive genes. Estrogens are believed to induce the synthesis of 50 to 100 different proteins, which are responsible for the physiological actions of the estrogenic hormones. They affect a wide variety of tissues.

Estrogens induce cellular proliferation (growth) in labial, vaginal, uterine, Fallopian tubal, and breast tissue. Estrogens also induce differentiation of the mammary glands, increasing ductal growth, stromal cell development, and accretion of adipose tissue within the breast. Through unknown mechanisms, estrogens contribute to the development of feminine body contours and to the size and shape of the female skeleton (e.g., influencing growth characteristics at the epiphyseal plate of the long bones) and eventually contribute to fusion of the epiphyseal plates with cessation of linear growth.

Estrogens play a role in the appearance and growth of secondary sexual hair and to the increase in pigmentation of the skin of the vaginal labia majora as well as that of the areola and nipples of the breasts after puberty.

Estrogens regulate the transcription of progestin receptor genes, making more receptor available for enhancement of target cell response to the release of progestins during the menstrual cycle. In uterine endometrial cells, estrogens, along with progestins, prepare and maintain the uterine endometrium for implantation of the fertilized egg. Estrogens sensitize the uterine muscle or myometrium to the contractile action of oxytocin at parturition (working in concert with prostaglandin $F_{2\alpha}$).

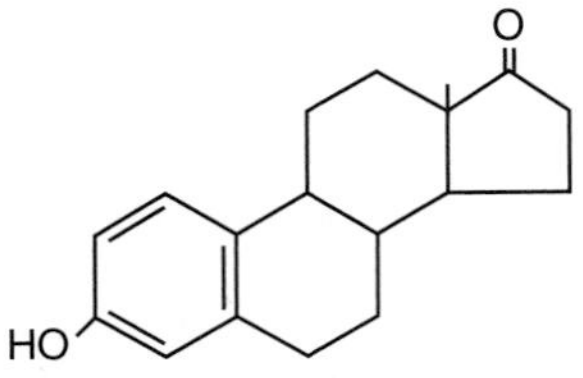

Estrone

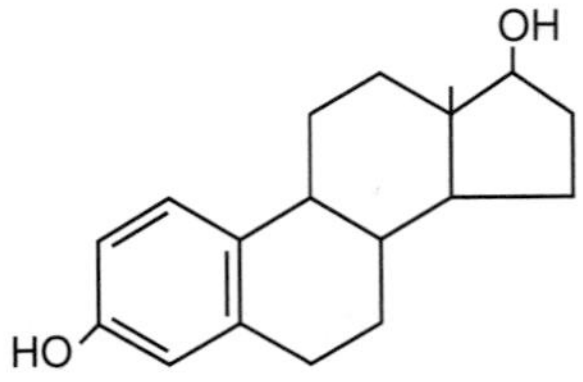

Estradiol

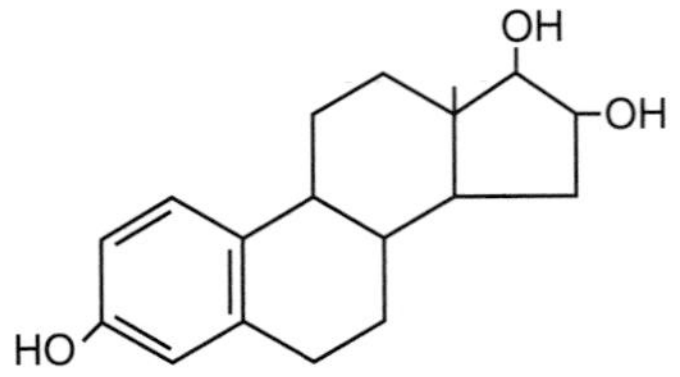

Estriol

Fig. 47.7. Structures of the major human estrogens.

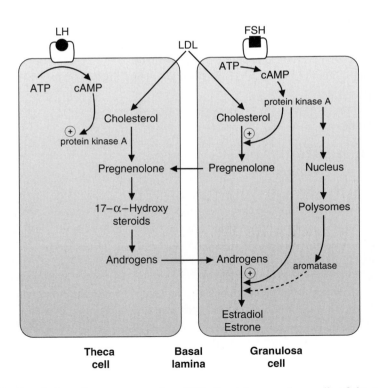

Fig. 47.8. Regulation of estrogen secretion. FSH stimulates granulosa cells of the ovary to produce pregnenolone, which is converted to androgens in theca cells under the influence of LH. These androgens are converted to estrogens in granulosa cells. Production of the aromatase enzyme that converts androgens to estrogens is stimulated by FSH. From Goodman MH. Basic medical endocrinology, 2nd ed. Philadelphia: JB Lippincott, 1994:281.

Estrogens also affect neurochemical and receptor protein synthesis in the central nervous system, perhaps contributing to the psychological and emotional alterations which occur premenstrually in some women.

Other metabolic effects of estrogens include the maintenance of the normal structure of the skin and blood vessels in women. Estrogens may promote the generation of nitric oxide within vascular smooth muscle, helping to maintain normal blood flow in a variety of vascular beds.

Estrogens reduce the motility of the gut and stimulate hepatic synthesis of binding or transport proteins such as thyroid binding globulin (TBG) and sex hormone binding globulin (SHBG). Estrogens may enhance the coagulability of the blood, raising the levels of coagulation factors II, VII, IX, and X in the blood while decreasing levels of antithrombin III.

Finally, estrogens also influence lipid metabolism, increasing serum high density lipoprotein (HDL) and triacylglycerol levels and lowering total and low density lipoprotein (LDL) levels.

Progestational Steroids

SOURCE OF PROGESTINS

The progestational steroids or progestins are produced in the ovary, the testis, the adrenal cortex, and, during pregnancy, the placenta. 17α-Hydroxyprogesterone was the first progestin to be isolated from the adrenal cortex (in 1940). Although inactive, its esters have the biological effects characteristic of the progestins.

In the female, progesterone (a progestin) is secreted by the ovary primarily from the corpus luteum during the luteal phase (second half) of the menstrual cycle. Its synthesis and secretion from the corpus luteum are stimulated by LH via the adenylate cyclase-cAMP effector system.

ACTIONS OF PROGESTINS

The actions of the progestins are primarily directed toward normal reproductive function. Unlike the estrogen receptor, which requires a phenolic A ring for binding, the progesterone receptor favors a Δ^4-3-one A-ring configuration. In the luteal phase of the menstrual cycle, progestins (along with estrogens) promote the development of a secretory endometrium in preparation for the implantation of the fertilized egg. The progestins also control the movement of the egg within the lumen of the Fallopian tube and, during labor, regulate uterine contractions indirectly by inhibiting oxytocin release from the posterior pituitary gland. These steroids act as a differentiation factor for mammary gland secretory cell development.

The progestins are responsible for the increase in basal body temperature of 1.0–1.5°F that begins shortly after the time of ovulation and persists throughout the luteal phase of the menstrual cycle.

Natural progestins can also compete with mineralocorticoid hormones, such as aldosterone, for mineralocorticoid receptors on the distal portions of the renal tubules. This competitive inhibitory effect leads to a modest loss of sodium and water into the urine. Progestins also enhance the ventilatory response to a rising level of CO_2 in the blood causing a decrease in arterial and alveolar pCO_2 during the latter half of the menstrual cycle and during pregnancy. Finally, progesterone may have hypnotic effects in the brain, an action which could contribute to the emotional and physical changes sometimes seen during the immediate premenstrual interval (the "premenstrual syndrome" or PMS).

By antagonizing the osteolytic action of skeletal cytokines on bone, estrogens decrease the rate of bone resorption in premenopausal women and in postmenopausal women, like **Teresa Livermore**, receiving estrogen replacement therapy.

The increase in blood coagulation factors promoted by estrogens predisposes some women taking oral contraceptives to venous thromboses (clots), particularly in the veins of the lower extremities.

Synthetic progestational agents, such as norethindrone acetate, are active when given orally. They are used, along with estrogens, for oral contraception in women of reproductive age. In postmenopausal women who still have a uterus, estrogen replacement therapy is combined with the progestin medroxyprogesterone acetate, a synthetic derivative of 17α-hydroxyprogesterone.

An increase in body temperature taken immediately upon awakening (the basal body temperature) can be used to estimate the time of ovulation.

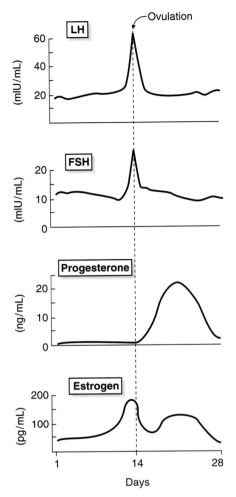

Fig. 47.9. Hormone levels during the menstrual cycle. The cycle begins on day 1, ovulation occurs on day 14, and menstruation starts on day 28.

HORMONAL REGULATION OF THE MENSTRUAL CYCLE

During the first part of the menstrual cycle (the follicular phase), FSH, secreted by the anterior pituitary, stimulates estradiol production by the granulosa cells of the ovary (Fig. 47.9). FSH and estradiol cause proliferation of these cells, and estradiol production increases. These hormones also stimulate production of LH receptors. Estradiol acts on the uterine endometrium, causing it to thicken and vascularize in preparation for implantation of a fertilized egg.

The peak of estradiol near the midpoint of the menstrual cycle (about 14 days) triggers a surge of LH from the anterior pituitary. LH stimulates ovulation (i.e., the release of the ripe egg from the follicle). The remaining cells in the postovulatory follicle form the corpus luteum, which begins to secrete both progesterone and estradiol.

During the second or luteal phase of the menstrual cycle, progesterone, along with estradiol, causes the endometrium to continue to thicken. Increased vascularization also occurs, and the endometrial cells differentiate and become secretory.

Approximately 1 week after its formation, the corpus luteum begins to regress and to produce less estradiol and progesterone. By day 28 of the cycle, the levels of ovarian steroids are inadequate to support the thickened endometrium, and it is sloughed into the uterine cavity and excreted. This discharge of blood through the vagina is known as menstruation. It lasts from 3 to 5 days and produces a maximum of about 50 mL of fluid.

The low levels of estradiol and progesterone at the end of a menstrual cycle relieve the feedback inhibition of GnRH secretion by the hypothalamus. GnRH levels rise and stimulate FSH and LH secretion by the anterior pituitary, and a new cycle begins.

HORMONAL CHANGES DURING PREGNANCY

If the egg is fertilized, an event that occurs shortly after ovulation, the corpus luteum is maintained by human chorionic gonadotropin (hCG), produced initially by the trophoblast cells of the developing embryo (Fig. 47.10). This hormone is similar to LH in its actions.

As the placenta develops, it begins to secrete hCG and progesterone, and is the source of progesterone after the corpus luteum ceases to function (see Fig. 47.10). Estrogens (estradiol, estrone, and estriol) are produced by the placenta from androgens secreted both by the maternal and fetal adrenals (Fig. 47.11).

Near term (about 40 weeks after fertilization), parturition occurs. Uterine contractions stimulated by oxytocin force the fetus from the uterus through the vaginal canal.

At **Jess Tayshun's** second visit, Ron told Jess that her serum human chorionic gonadotropin (hCG) level drawn at the time of the previous visit, was reported as 70 mIU/mL, a level consistent with a 3-week gestation. (hCG is not detectable in the nonpregnant, healthy female.) Ron also explained that the concentration of hCG in the maternal blood normally doubles every 36 to 48 hours early in pregnancy and that serial measurements, therefore, can be used as a sensitive index of placental differentiation if the health of the placenta should come into question.

CLINICAL COMMENTS. Failure to grow because of a deficiency in GH secretion can be a very subtle form of growth retardation because the child may be normal in all other aspects of development. "Primary" GH-related growth failure can result from a congenital partial or complete deficiency in the capacity of the somatotrophs of the anterior pituitary to secrete GH, from production of a bioinactive form of GH, or from a resistance of peripheral tissues to the actions of a bioactive GH. In **Yetta Bloom's** case, the deficiency of GH secretion was not primary but instead was "secondary" to the earlier head trauma which partially compromised the ability of her pituitary somatotrophic cells to secrete GH.

The prostate gland participates in normal reproductive function by producing secretions which promote sperm motility as well as protect the sperm from damage as they traverse the distal urethra. These secretions also contribute to the eventual lysis of those sperm which did not participate in fertilizing the ovum following sexual intercourse.

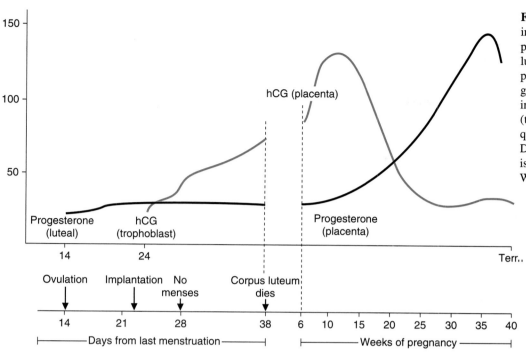

Fig. 47.10. Hormone levels during pregnancy. Progesterone is produced initially by the corpus luteum and subsequently by the placenta. Human chorionic gonadotropin (hCG) is produced initially by cells of the embryo (trophoblast cells) and subsequently by the placenta. From Devlin T. Textbook of biochemistry, 3rd ed. New York: John Wiley, 1992:880.

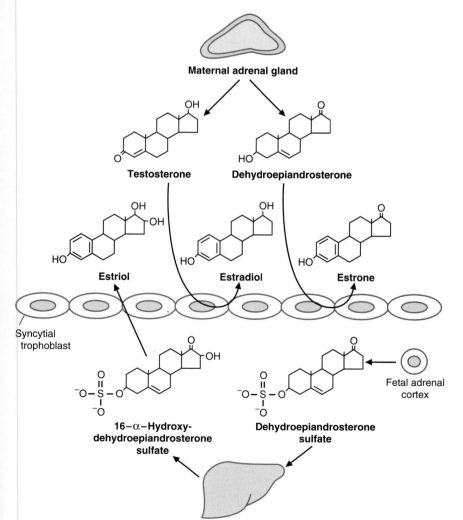

The placenta provides nutritional and hormonal communication between the mother and the fetus. It secretes hormones into the maternal blood which can be measured to determine whether the pregnancy is proceeding normally.

Erna explained to **Jess Tayshun** that the corpus luteum secretes progesterone for the first 6 or 7 weeks after conception. Then the placenta produces progesterone. This hormone enhances implantation of the fertilized ovum and suppresses uterine muscle contractility. Progesterone may be used, therefore, to prevent an early threatened abortion, caused by a deficiency of progesterone production.

Ron told Jess that a mother's total serum cortisol level approximately triples by term, her thyroid hormone levels do not change, and her insulin levels increase while her glucagon levels remain unchanged (see Biochemical Comments).

Fig. 47.11. Production of estrogens during pregnancy. Estrogens are produced by the placenta from androgens synthesized in the maternal adrenal and the fetal adrenal and liver. From Goodman MH. Basic medical endocrinology, 2nd ed. Philadelphia: JB Lippincott, 1994:307.

Erna addressed the issue of the hormonal signals which initiate labor, telling **Jess Tayshun** that the key inciting hormonal signal had not yet been fully determined. Suggested signals include an increase in the estrogen/progesterone ratio in the maternal blood near term and the placental production of certain prostaglandins and catecholamines.

As to the control of pain during labor and delivery, Erna and Ron told Ms. Tayshun that this important issue would be the focus of a series of classes on childbirth that she would be invited to attend closer to the time of delivery.

Excessive growth of the prostate gland (benign prostatic hyperplasia) causes obstruction of the flow of urine from the distal urethra. These symptoms may be slowed, and to some degree reversed, by chronic use of a 5α-reductase inhibitor, finasteride. This drug was used to treat **Yuri Nader**. It inhibits the conversion of testosterone to dihydrotestosterone (DHT). Because testosterone levels may rise with the use of finasteride and since a normal libido is dependent upon testosterone and not DHT, men treated with this drug do not generally experience sexual dysfunction.

During the 39th week of **Jess Tayshun's** pregnancy, Erna and Ron were notified by the patient's obstetrician that Jess had been admitted to the delivery suite of the hospital in early labor. Erna and Ron went immediately to the hospital's obstetrical unit. The patient was very relieved to have them with her during her labor and delivery.

In part because of her excellent prenatal care and Erna and Ron's detailed explanations and concern throughout her pregnancy, Ms. Tayshun went through labor relatively easily. Ten hours after her first contractions, Erna and Ron assisted in the delivery of a healthy 7 pound, 2 ounce baby girl, **Erna R. Tayshun.**

BIOCHEMICAL COMMENTS. The levels of many hormones change during pregnancy. Total cortisol levels in the blood triple, in part because of an estrogen-induced increase in the synthesis of cortisol-binding globulin (transcortin). Free cortisol levels also increase slightly, but whether this increase occurs because of an increase in pituitary ACTH release or some other secretagogue is unknown. The thyroid gland becomes palpably enlarged, possibly secondary to a poorly characterized TSH-like glycoprotein produced in the placenta. A second factor causing thyroid enlargement is a slight increase in the secretion of pituitary TSH related to a relative iodide deficiency. This deficiency is caused by the increased renal clearance of iodide that occurs even in a normal pregnancy. In spite of these changes, free thyroid hormone levels in the blood remain normal throughout pregnancy.

During the second trimester, insulin secretion from the pancreatic B cells increases, leading to a hyperinsulinemic state. This increase is, in part, the result of a relative degree of resistance to the metabolic actions of insulin in maternal tissues. This change in maternal insulin sensitivity serves to reserve glucose for fetal needs, while maternal energy requirements are increasingly met through the peripheral metabolism of fatty acids.

Pancreatic glucagon production, on the other hand, remains sensitive to the usual stimuli and is normally suppressed when maternal serum glucose levels rise. Because the major biological role of insulin and glucagon is the intracellular transport of nutrients, the changing insulin/glucagon ratio of pregnancy provides both the mother and her fetus with appropriate nutrient fluxes after the mother has eaten and during fasting.

Suggested Readings

Goodman HM. Basic medical endocrinology. New York: Raven Press, 1994:225–318.

Greenspan FS, Baxter JD. Basic and clinical endocrinology. Norwalk, CT: Appleton & Lange, 1994:128–159, 391–550.

Means AL, Gudas LJ. The roles of retinoids in vertebrate development. Annu Rev Biochem 1995;64:201–233.

Russell DW, Wilson JD. Steroid 5α-reductase: two genes/two enzymes. Annu Rev Biochem 1995;63:25–61.

PROBLEMS

1. A sexually active 21-year-old college student consulted her doctor about the use of oral contraceptive (OC) drugs. After describing the efficacy and safety of these agents, the physician wrote a prescription for a commonly used birth control pill. Which of the following statements related to the use of OCs are true and which are false?

    A. Estrogen therapy induces the liver to increase the production of the carrier proteins for thyroid hormone and for cortisol and could, therefore, increase the total T_4 and cortisol levels in the blood.

    B. The administration of the combination of estrogen and progesterone in OCs for the first 25 days of each month will induce a monthly menstrual period after the 25th day (when the OCs are not taken).

    C. The principle which underlies the use of OCs for birth control is to cause a constant rather than cyclic release of the gonadotropins, LH and FSH, thereby suppressing ovulation.

    D. The amount of estrogen in OCs is higher than that used as estrogen replacement therapy for postmenopausal women.

    E. OC use is sometimes associated with fluid retention.

2. A 24-year-old woman was found to have a large nonsecretory tumor of the pituitary gland that invaded the surrounding tissue, causing progressive visual loss. In order to adequately debulk the mass, the neurosurgeon could not avoid causing an irreversible loss of all anterior pituitary hormones. With regard to the general therapy and the lifelong hormonal replacement that will be required postoperatively, which of the following statements are true and which are false?

    A. TSH and ACTH should be given orally.

    B. Water intake should be restricted to compensate for low vasopressin levels.

    C. Thyroxine tablets should be prescribed and taken regularly by the patient.

    D. Cortisol should be administered daily except during periods of increased stress.

    E. Estrogen and progesterone are the only hormones needed by women to ensure fertility.

ANSWERS

1. **A is true.** Estrogens induce the liver to produce the carrier proteins that bind thyroid hormone and cortisol in the blood and, thereby, raise the concentration of **total** (free plus protein bound) hormone in the blood. The concentration of the biologically active (free) fraction of the hormone remains within normal limits, however, so estrogen therapy is not associated with hyperthyroidism or hypercortisolism.

    B is true. The cyclic use of the estrogen-progesterone combination causes a "build-up" of the endometrium (uterine lining) on the days that the OC pills are taken. When the OC pill is discontinued each month, the endometrial lining is sloughed, resulting in a monthly drug-induced menstrual period.

    C is false, and D is true. The pharmacological principle by which OCs inhibit ovulation relates to the negative feedback action of the increased serum estrogen levels on the production of gonadotropin releasing hormone and of the gonadotropins by the hypothalamic-pituitary axis. To accomplish this, the estrogen content in OCs must be greater than that used in estrogen replacement therapy in postmenopausal women.

E is true. The natural progestins are usually natriuretic (cause sodium and water excretion), but the synthetic progestins often found in OCs may cause sodium and water retention. In addition, the estrogenic component of OCs may also cause sodium and water retention and contribute to edema.

2. **A is false.** To treat her inability to produce TSH (and, hence, thyroid hormone) and ACTH (and, hence, cortisol) one would not use TSH or ACTH replacement since these hormones have relatively short half-lives and would, therefore, have to be given very frequently. In addition, these peptide hormones must be given parenterally (by injection) since, when given orally, they are cleaved and thereby inactivated by digestive enzymes in the gut.

B is false. The low vasopressin (ADH) levels in the blood would result in the loss of large amounts of free water through the kidneys. Until ADH is administered, water intake must, therefore, be increased to avoid severe volume depletion.

C is true. A TSH deficiency is treated through the administration of thyroid hormone. Tetraiodothyronine (T_4, thyroxine) and triiodothyronine (T_3) are not degraded by digestive enzymes and, therefore, are effective when given orally. The patient must be cautioned to take thyroid hormone replacement every day for the rest of her life.

D is false. Although the loss of the ability to produce ACTH can be treated through the oral administration of cortisol, the amount of cortisol should be increased during stress. The importance of increasing the daily dosage of this steroid during times of increased physical or psychological stress cannot be overemphasized since the normal stress-related increase in ACTH secretion can no longer occur in this patient because of the irreparable surgical damage done to the corticotropic cells of her anterior pituitary gland.

E is false. This patient cannot be made fertile through estrogen and progesterone replacement therapy. The cyclic administration of the gonadotropins LH and FSH in a pattern that simulates the patient's normal cycle would be required to successfully stimulate ovulation.

Patient Index

Note: Page numbers followed by "t" denote tables; those followed by "f" denote figures. The number behind the patient's name indicates the page where the patient first appears.

A

Appleman, Thomas, 3
  abdominal fat to hip ratio in, 387
  antibiotic selection for, 207, 209
  aspirin use in, 555
  basal metabolic rate of, 8, 9
  calorie consumption by, 6, 7
  carbohydrate diet in, 25
  cholesterol level in, 21, 25
  coronary heart disease risks in, 527, 527t
  daily energy expenditure of, 10, 11
  dental caries in, 342, 346, 349, 352–353
  erythromycin for, 162, 164, 200, 209
  ethanol consumption in
    caloric content of, 284, 285, 286, 298
  glucose intolerance in, 25
  high density lipoprotein levels in, 538
  hyperglycemia in, 534
  hyperlipidemia in, 25
  lipid levels in, 534
  low density lipoprotein levels in
    therapy for, 542
  noninsulin-dependent diabetes mellitus in, 25
  obesity in, 25
  protein glycation in, 534
  Streptococcus pneumoniae infection in, 150, 164, 200
  triacylglycerol level in, 25
  weight gain in, 10, 13, 276
  weight reduction in, 18, 21, 25–26
Atotrope, Sam
  acromegaly in, 696
  ACTH-secreting pituitary adenoma in, 709
  diabetes mellitus in, 704, 711
  growth hormone levels in, 714–715
  growth hormone suppression test in, 695
  hypercortisolemia in, 709
  pituitary macroadenoma in, 701
  visual disturbance in, 689

B

Beatty, Dianne, 37
  blood glucose monitoring in, 52, 64
  diabetic ketoacidosis in, 35, 40, 43, 52, 370, 558, 565
    insulin therapy for, 567
  fatigue in, 388
  glucagon levels in, 563
  glucose administration for, 474
  glucose production in, 563
  glycogen stores in, 417
  hypertriglyceridemia in, 561
  hyperventilation in, 40
  insulin deficiency in, 141, 561
  insulin excess in, 471, 474
  insulin levels in, 380, 563
  insulin release in
    eating and, 477
  insulin therapy for, 143
  insulin-dependent diabetes mellitus in, 35, 37, 40, 387
    genetic defect in, 378
  ketone bodies in, 35, 43, 44, 49
  Kussmaul breathing in, 40
  laboratory values in, 35, 43
  lipolysis in, 564
  macrovascular complications in, 483
  metabolic acidosis in, 43
  nitroprusside reaction test in, 49
  peripheral neuropathy in, 447
  postprandial blood glucose levels in, 129
  urinary tract infection in, 168, 179
    norfloxacin for, 169
Bewser, Doug, 243
  HIV testing in, 243
Bloom, Yetta, 736
  growth failure in, 733
  growth hormone deficiency in, 742
  growth hormone levels in, 736
Bodie, Jim, 408
  androgen use by, 420
  blood glucose levels in
    exercise and, 408
  exogenous insulin administration in, 418, 420
  hypoglycemia in, 408, 418, 420
  seizure in, 408

Bolic, Katta, 648
  acute phase response in, 648, 662
  catabolism in, 648
  negative nitrogen balance in, 648, 662
  ruptured viscus in, 648
  septicemia in, 648
Burne, Lofata, 358
  dicarboxylic acid excretion by, 366
  medium chain acyl CoA dehydrogenase deficiency in, 358, 363, 370–371

C

Carbo, Getta, 408
  blood glucose levels in, 408
  hypoglycemia in, 419–420
  liver glycogen stores in, 417
Colamin, Katie, 625
  catecholamine levels in, 640, 643–644
  pheochromocytoma in, 625
    treatment of, 644

D

Dopaman, Les
  Parkinson's disease in, 327–328
    dopaminergic neurons in
      oxidative damage to, 332, 335
      oxygen free radical formation in, 332
    treatment of, 337–338
D'Souder, Sellie
  cartilage synthesis/degradation imbalance in, 462, 466–467
  joint pain in, 458, 462
  systemic lupus erythematosus in, 182, 190, 196, 462, 466–467

F

Felya, Rena, 624
  metabolic acidosis in, 648, 654, 656
  poststreptococcal glomerulonephritis in, 624, 642–643, 662
    glomerular filtration rate in, 625
  rapid progressive glomerulonephritis in, 647–648, 663
Fibrosa, Sissy, 239
  cystic fibrosa in, 239–240
    gene mutation in, 254, 256

Subject Index

Note: Page numbers followed by "t" denote tables; those followed by "f" denote figures.

Hybridization
of DNA, 156, 157f
Hydride ion
in oxidation-reduction reactions, 48
Hydrochloric acid
gastric secretion of
H$_2$ blockers for, 555
Hydrogen, 43
in oxidation-reduction reactions, 48
in water, 45
Hydrogen bonds
amino acid residues and, 85, 85f
in α-helix, 82, 82f
in hydroxy-containing amino acids, 71, 71f
nitrogen in, 64, 64f
in β-sheets, 83, 83f
types of, 38, 38f
between water molecules, 38, 38f
Hydrogen ion
concentration of
kidneys/lungs and, 40, 40f
oxygen-hemoglobin binding and, 92f
pH and, 38, 38f
water concentration of, 41
water dissociation and, 38, 38f
Hydrogen peroxidase, 332
Hydrogen peroxide, 330, 330t
formation of, 329, 329f
in peroxisomes, 138, 138f
removal of, 335f, 336–337
Hydrogenases
NAD$^+$-dependent
in catalytic reactions, 112, 112f
Hydrolases
catalysis by, 101t
Hydronium ion, 38
Hydroperoxyeicosatetraenoic acid, 552, 553f
Hydroxide ion
water dissociation and, 38, 38f
L-β-Hydroxyacyl CoA
formation of
fatty acid β-oxidation and, 361, 362f
3-Hydroxybutyrate, 48, 50f
β-Hydroxybutyrate, 48, 50f
acetoacetate from, 49, 50, 369, 369f
from acetyl CoA, 29, 29f
functional groups in, 44
β-Hydroxybutyric acid, 44
25-Hydroxycholecalciferol
hydroxylation of
parathyroid hormone in, 726f
synthesis of, 728
Hydroxyl free radical, 330
Hydroxyl group, 53, 54
Hydroxyl radical, 330t
formation of, 329, 329f
generation of, 330, 330f

7α-Hydroxylase
catalysis by, 538, 538f
21-Hydroxylase
deficiency of
in congenital adrenal hyperplasia, 687
Hydroxymethylglutaryl CoA
carbon structure of, 586
formation of, 525
in ketone body synthesis, 366–367, 367f
mevalonate from, 530, 530f
Hydroxymethylglutaryl CoA reductase
in cholesterol synthesis, 525, 530, 530f
Hydroxymethylglutaryl CoA reductase
inhibitors, 531, 535, 542
Hydroxyurea
hemoglobin F and, 91
Hyperammonemia
neurologic effects of, 661
Hyperbilirubinemia, 644
Hypercalcemia
in multiple myeloma, 96
Hypercatabolic states
amino acid metabolism in, 661f, 661–662
insulin resistance in, 664
nitrogen balance in, 661
Hypercholesterolemia
familial, 521
low density lipoprotein receptor defect
in, 534
type IIA, 528
familial type IIA, 540–541
LDL receptor defects in, 541, 542, 543f
treatment for, 541
Hypercortisolemia
in Cushing's disease, 708
hyperglycemia in, 716
Hyperglycemia, 25
ATP deficits in, 388
complications of, 375
in Cushing's disease, 708
glucagon levels in, 563
glucocorticoids and, 433, 435
glucose production in, 563
glycation in, 534
glycogen storage inability in, 417
hypercortisolemia in, 716
insulin deficiency and, 273
insulin resistance in, 563
lens glucose levels in, 448
terminology in, 52
vascular changes from, 482–483
weight balance and, 374
Hyperlipidemia
familial combined, 514, 521
lipoprotein lipase deficiency in, 514, 515
Hypermethioninemia, 611

Hyperparathyroidism
parathyroid tumor and, 731
Hyperphenylalaninemia
dihydropteridine reductase deficiency in,
606
incidence of, 608
Hyperprolactinemia
bromocriptine for, 700–701
drug usage and, 693
radioimmunoassay of, 699
tumor-related, 700
Hypertension
chloride/sodium intake and, 15
Hyperthyroidism
ATP utilization in, 279
basal metabolic rate and, 8
heat production in, 319
insulin metabolism in, 714
oxidative metabolism in, 279
presentation of, 276
radioactive iodine for, 685–686
radioimmunoassay of, 716
Hypertriglyceridemia
in diabetes mellitus, 561
lipoprotein lipase deficiency and, 560, 561
Hyperuricemia
uric acid production/excretion and, 643
Hyperventilation
anxiety and, 40
metabolic acidosis and, 40
Hypochlorous acid, 330, 330t
Hypoglycemia
adrenergic response to, 376, 381
alcohol ingestion and, 434–435
aldolase B defects and, 448
blood-brain barrier glucose transport and,
403
fasting, 374, 376
liver glycogen phosphorylase deficiency
and, 413
glucagon secretion in, 381
in glycogen storage diseases, 413
glycogenolysis and, 390
hypoglycin and, 371
hypoketotic
in medium chain acyl CoA
dehydrogenase deficiency, 371
insulin administration and, 420
insulin excess and, 420, 474
glucocorticoids and, 707
neuroglycopenic, 374, 435, 474
phosphoglucomutase inhibition and, 452,
455
seizure in, 420, 423
stress of, 381
symptoms of, 388f
terminology in, 52

dietary protein and, 381, 381f
fasting and, 28
glucagon in, 705
glucose blood levels and, 376, 377f, 379, 416
glucose phosphorylation and, 379
in pregnancy, 744
regulators of, 380, 380t
signal transduction by, 385, 386f
structure of, 95, 96f
synthesis of, 378–379, 379f
therapeutic, 143
glucose blood levels and, 88, 89
in very low density lipoprotein synthesis, 475, 475f
Insulin counterregulatory hormones, 377–378, 378f
Insulin receptor, 387
Insulin resistance, 387
in hypercatabolic states, 664
in noninsulin-dependent diabetes mellitus, 477
Insulin substrate receptor, 385, 386f
Insulin tolerance test
growth hormone secretion and, 736
Insulin/glucagon ratio
in liver glycogen regulation, 412
in liver glycogen synthesis, 413
in metabolism regulation, 557
phosphofructokinase-2/fructose 2,6-bisphosphatase and, 425, 425f
Insulin-like growth factors
action of, 735–736, 736f
in growth hormone regulation, 709
synthesis of, 736, 736f
Insulinoma
C-peptide levels in, 379
hereditary, 565
insulin hypersecretion from, 377, 378
weight gain in, 562
Insulin-sensitive hormone response element, 387
Interferon-α, 232
Interferon(s), 229
in eukaryotic initiation factor 2 phosphorylation, 235
Interleukin-1
amino acid mediation by
in sepsis, 663, 664f
Interleukin(s)
recombinant DNA production of, 252
Intestinal cells
in protein digestion, 575
Intestines
amino acid metabolism in, 657–658, 658f
dietary protein and, 660, 660f
amino acid transport and, 576, 577f

brush-border membrane of
glucoamylase complex in, 396–397
glycosidases of, 395–398, 396f–398f, 398t
lactase in, 397f, 397–398, 398t
sucrase-isomaltase complex in, 396, 397f
trehalase in, 398, 398f
epithelial cells of
absorption by, 22, 23
facilitative transport in, 399–400, 401f, 402
villi of
absorptive cells of, 396f
Intracellular fluid
calcium concentration in, 730
Intracellular space
water content of, 717
Intrinsic factor
deficiency of, 618
in vitamin B_{12} absorption, 618, 619f
Introns, 224
in mRNA, 189, 189f
in rRNA, 191
in tRNA, 193f, 193–194
Iodide
deficiency of
in pregnancy, 744
in thyroid cell, 674
in thyroid hormone synthesis, 673, 674f
Iodine
deficiencies of, 17t
sources of, 17t
131Iodine
for hyperthyroidism, 685–686
therapeutic action of, 674
Ion channels
gated
receptor binding to, 383f
Ions
transport of
through inner mitochondrial membrane, 320, 322, 322f
Iron
absorption of, 627, 629f
phytate and, 628
deficiency of, 17t, 236
anemia from, 15, 215, 630, 631
in heme synthesis, 206
levels of
transferrin receptor synthesis and, 234f, 234–235
loss of, 628
metabolism of, 627, 629f
requirements for, 627
sources of, 17t, 627–628
storage of, 628

hemochromatosis and, 630
in iron deficiency anemia, 633
Ischemia-reperfusion injury, 328
antioxidants for, 338
xanthine oxidase in, 336
Islets of Langerhans
B cells of, 379, 380f
insulin release in, 378, 379, 393–394
insulin synthesis in, 378, 379, 393–394
A cells of, 379, 380f
glucagon release in, 373–374, 378, 380–381
glucagon synthesis in, 373–374, 380, 380f
Isocitrate
from citrate, 293
in tricarboxylic acid cycle, 293f
Isocitrate dehydrogenase
allosteric regulation of, 302, 304f, 305
carbon dioxide release from, 294, 295
formation of, 294
oxidative decarboxylation of, 294, 294f
regulatory activity of, 121
in tricarboxylic acid cycle regulation, 303f
Isoelectric point, 74, 75f
for glycine, 76–77
for histidine, 76–77
Isoenzymes, 99, 123–124
in tissue injury diagnosis, 124, 124f
tissue-specific, 354
Isoforms
glucose transport proteins, 399–400, 401f, 402t
Isoleucine, 70, 70f
acetyl CoA from, 605, 606f
dietary requirements for, 13, 13t
propionyl CoA from, 605, 606f
side chains of, 69f
Isomaltase
in sucrase-isomaltase complex, 396, 397f
Isomerases
catalysis by, 101t
Isopentenyl pyrophosphate, 530, 530f
Isoprene units
in plants, 529
as precursor, 51

J

Jamaican vomiting sickness, 371
Jaundice, 446
alcoholism and, 583
bile duct obstruction and, 498, 643
bilirubin levels in, 449
in hepatitis, 644, 645
causes of, 623, 644
extrahepatic obstructive, 624
neonatal, 631

positive charges on, 45, 45f
reactivity of, 46f, 46–47, 47f
single bonds in, 43, 43f
solubility of, 45–46
Molybdenum
deficiencies of, 17t
sources of, 17t
Monoacylglycerols
formation of, 60
from triacylglycerols, 21, 23
Monoamine oxidase
in oxidative deamination, 639, 641f
Monoamine oxidase inhibitors
free radical reduction by, 338
for parkinsonism, 338
Monoiodotyrosine, 674
Monooxygenase, 332, 333, 333f
Monophosphate, 51
Monosaccharides, 4
carbohydrate digestion and, 21
digestion and, 22
generation of, 393, 394
glycosidic bonds of, 55–56, 56f
mutarotation of, 53–54, 54f
phosphorylated, 54f, 55
ring structure of, 53–54, 54f
structure of, 5f, 51, 52f–56f, 52–56
sulfated, 55, 55f
transport of, 393, 394, 395f, 402
types of, 52, 52f
D-Monosaccharides
structure of, 52f, 52–53, 53f
L-Monosaccharides
structure of, 52f, 52–53, 53f
Monosodium urate crystals
deposition of, 137
Monoxygenase
NADPH use by, 334, 335
Mucin
salivary
in starch digestion, 394
structure of, 463, 463f
Mucopolysaccharidosis
defective enzymes in, 466, 466t
lysosomal enzyme deficiency and, 138
lysosomal enzyme deficiency in, 469
Mucosal cells
amino acid requirements of, 657–658, 658f
Multiple myeloma, 96–97
Muscle
amino acid release from
during fasting, 649–650, 650f, 651f
ATP concentration in, 319
ATP generation in
aerobic vs. anaerobic glycolysis for, 349
branched chain amino acid oxidation in, 655–656, 656f

contraction of
ATP hydrolysis in, 29, 279, 280f, 480, 480f
eicosanoids in, 545
fatty acid oxidation in, 27, 29, 370
fasting and, 27
fuel usage of
via blood, 482, 482f
glucose oxidation in, 24, 24f, 26f
glucose transport to
insulin in, 402, 402f, 405–406
glutamine synthesis in, 655
glycogen stores in, 3, 6, 7, 7f, 21, 481
degradation of, 418
in diabetes mellitus, 417
function of, 407f, 409, 412
glycogen loading and, 486
regulation of, 412, 413t, 418–419, 419f
use of, 480
glycogen synthesis in, 407, 418, 476, 476f
glycogenolysis in. (see also
Glycogenolysis)
in exercise, 418, 480f, 480–481, 481f
regulation of, 418–419, 419f
growth hormone effects on, 712
heme and, 89
lactate production in
ATP demands and, 349
lipoprotein lipase in, 497
oxidative capacity of
exercise and, 306
protein concentration in, 649
protein degradation in, 654–655
protein stores in, 3, 6, 7f
fasting and, 27
protein synthesis in, 650, 654
slow twitch fibers in, 481–482
sodium permeability of
norepinephrine and, 714
starvation and, 31, 31t
thyroid hormone effects on, 713
wasting of
hypercortisolemia and, 708
water content of, 7
weakness in
glucocorticoids and, 427
Muscle cells
ATP hydrolysis in
energy from, 278, 279
glucose 6-phosphate:glucose in, 281
Mushroom poisoning, 181, 188, 196, 197, 198
Mutagens
DNA damage by, 173
Mutarotation, 54, 54f
Mutations, 147
antibiotic resistance and, 213

in cancer, 267, 268, 268f
carcinogens and, 174
chemicals and, 264, 265f
detection of
by allele-specific oligonucleotide probes, 249
hypervariable regions and, 250, 250f, 252
by polymerase chain reaction, 249–250
frameshift, 204, 204f
mitochondrial dysfunction from, 324
molecular damage and, 167
nonsense
in thalassemia, 204, 205
point, 203, 203t
missense, 203, 203t
in myoclonic epileptic ragged red fiber disease, 326
nonsense, 203, 203t
in OXPHOS diseases, 324, 325f
in restriction enzyme recognition site, 249
silent, 203, 203t
radiation and, 264, 265f
replication errors and, 167
in Tay-Sachs disease, 214
in thalassemia, 232, 236, 237t
in translation, 203t, 203–204
Myocardial infarction, 80, 85
ATP generation in, 278, 351
creatine kinase isoenzymes in, 124, 124f
creatine kinase levels in, 124, 125, 323
creatine phosphokinase levels in, 85, 625
presentation of, 276
prevention of
aspirin in, 552
tissue plasminogen activator in, 322–323
Myoclonic epileptic ragged red fiber disease, 326
Myoglobin
oxygen binding to, 90, 91f
oxygen saturation of, 89, 90f
structure of, 89, 90f
vs. hemoglobin, 90, 91f
Myosin ATPase, 279, 280f
ATP hydrolysis and, 305
Myosin filaments
movement of
high energy phosphate bonds in, 285f

N

NAD. (see under Nicotinamide-adenine dinucleotide)
NAD+ dehydrogenase
in catalytic reactions, 112, 112f
NADH. (see under Nicotinamide-adenine dinucleotide)